NURSE'S REFERENCE LIBRARY®

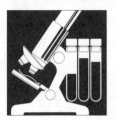

Diagnostics

Second Edition

Nursing91 Books™
Springhouse Corporation
Springhouse, Pennsylvania

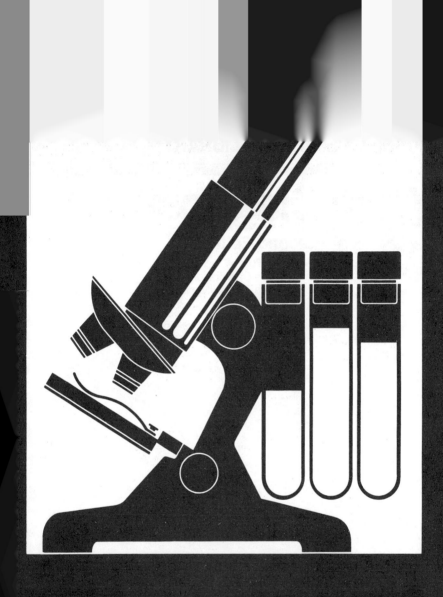

NURSE'S REFERENCE LIBRARY®

Diagnostics
Second Edition

Nursing91 Books™
Springhouse Corporation
Springhouse, Pennsylvania

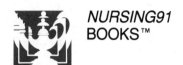

NURSING91
BOOKS™

Springhouse Corporation Book Division

CHAIRMAN
Eugene W. Jackson

PRESIDENT
Daniel L. Cheney

VICE-PRESIDENT AND DIRECTOR
Timothy B. King

VICE-PRESIDENT, BOOK OPERATIONS
Thomas A. Temple

VICE-PRESIDENT, PRODUCTION AND PURCHASING
Bacil Guiley

PROGRAM DIRECTOR, REFERENCE BOOKS
Stanley E. Loeb

First edition published 1981; second edition, 1986
© 1989 by Springhouse Corporation, 1111 Bethlehem Pike, Springhouse, Pa. 19477

Library of Congress Cataloging in Publication Data
Main entry under title:

Diagnostics.

    (Nurse's reference library)
    "Nursing86 books."
    Includes bibliographies and index.
    1. Diagnosis.   2. Nursing.   I. Springhouse Corporation.   II. Series.   [DNLM: 1.
Diagnosis—nurses' instruction.   WB 141 D53663]
RT48.D5   1986   616.07′5   85-12626
ISBN 0-87434-007-1

NURSE'S REFERENCE LIBRARY®

Staff for this edition

EDITORIAL DIRECTOR
Helen Klusek Hamilton

EXECUTIVE EDITOR
Matthew Cahill

CLINICAL DIRECTOR
Minnie Bowen Rose, RN, BSN, MEd

ART DIRECTOR
Sonja E. Douglas

Editorial Manager: Jill Lasker

Clinical Editor: Joanne Patzek DaCunha, RN

Contributing Clinical Editors: Margaret L. Belcher, RN, BSN; Mary Gyetvan, RN, BSEd; Judith A. McCann, RN, BSN; Sandra L. Nettina, RN, BSN; Susan Weiner, RN, BSN; Nina P. Welsh, RN

Drug Information Manager: Larry Neil Gever, PharmD

Associate Editors: Kevin J. Law, Elizabeth L. Mauro

Assistant Editor: Loralee Choman Moclock

Contributing Editors: Andrea Barrett, Barbara Hodgson, Roberta Kangilaski, Nancy Priff

Copy Supervisor: David R. Moreau

Copy Editors: Traci A. Deraco, Diane M. Labus, Jo Lennon, Doris Weinstock

Production Coordinator: Kathleen P. Luczak

Designers: Carol Cameron-Sears, Jacalyn Bove Facciolo, Christopher Laird, Matie Anne Patterson

Art Production: Robert Perry (manager), Don Knauss, Sandra Sanders, Joan Walsh, Bob Wieder

Typography: David C. Kosten (manager), Amanda C. Erb, Ethel Halle, Diane Paluba, Nancy Wirs

Production: Wilbur D. Davidson, Deborah C. Meiris (managers); T.A. Landis

Assistant: Maree E. DeRosa

Staff for the preceding edition

Editorial Director: Helen Klusek Hamilton

Clinical Director: Minnie Bowen Rose, RN, BSN, MEd

Editorial Managers: Matthew Cahill, Martin DiCarlantonio, Thomas J. Leibrandt

Clinical Editors: Regina Daley Ford, RN, BSN, MA; Susan M. Glover, RN, BSN

Clinical Consultants: Anita Chinnici, RN, MSN; Helen D'Angelo, RN, MSN; Barbara Egoville, RN, MSN; Judith E. Meissner, RN, MSN; Helene Nawrocki, RN; Paula Okun, RN, MSN

Clinical Pharmacy Editor: Larry N. Gever, PharmD

Senior Editors: Peter Johnson, Jerome Rubin

Assistant Editors: Nancy Holmes, William Kelly, Patricia Minard, Brenda Moyer

Graphics Coordinator: Lisa Z. Cohen

Copy Editor: Barbara Hodgson

Designer: Kathaleen Motak Singel

Art Production Manager: Wilbur D. Davidson

Illustrators: Jacquelyn Diotte, Darcy Feralio, Jean Gardner, Robert Jackson, Marsha Jessup, Thomas Lewis, Cynthia Mason, Sandi Pierantozzi, Jim Story, Barry Wimberly, Bud Yingling

Typography Manager: David C. Kosten

Production Manager: Robert L. Dean

Contents

SECTION I: BLOOD TESTS

1 Hematology

2 Hemostasis

3 Blood Gases and Electrolytes

4 Enzymes

5 Hormones

SECTION II: URINE TESTS

SECTION III: HISTOLOGIC AND MICROBIOLOGIC TESTS

SECTION IV: ORGAN TESTS

SECTION V: BODY SYSTEM TESTS

23 Respiratory System

24 Skeletal System

25 Reproductive System

26 Nervous System

27 Gastrointestinal System

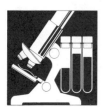

Advisory Board

At the time of publication, the advisors, clinical consultants, and contributors held the following positions.

xiii

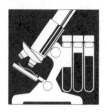

Clinical Consultants

Doris G. Bartuska, MD, FACP, Professor of Medicine; Director, Division of Endocrinology and Metabolism, Medical College of Pennsylvania, Philadelphia

George J. Brodmerkel, Jr., MD, Head, Division of Gastroenterology, Allegheny General Hospital, Pittsburgh

A. Bruce Campbell, MD, PhD, Hematologist/Oncologist, Scripps Memorial Hospital, La Jolla, Calif.

Ricardo L. Camponovo, MD, Consultant in Anatomic and Clinical Pathology, Scottsdale (Ariz.) Community Hospital

James Robert Cronmiller, BS, MA, Medical Technologist, The Genesee Hospital, Rochester, N.Y.

Leonard V. Crowley, MD, Clinical Assistant Professor, Department of Laboratory Medicine and Pathology and Department of Family Practice and Community Health, University of Minnesota Medical School, Minneapolis; Pathologist, St. Mary's Hospital, Minneapolis

Elise C. Deutsch, MD, Instructor, Department of Otolaryngology and Head and Neck Surgery, University of Illinois, Chicago

William M. Dougherty, BS, Manager, Technical and Customer Services, Worldwide Geometric Data, Wayne, Pa.

Paul R. Finley, MD, Professor, Department of Pathology, University of Arizona Medical Center, Tucson

Ruth Ann Fitzpatrick, MD, Director, Division of Endocrinology, Crozer-Chester Medical Center, Chester, Pa.; Clinical Assistant Professor of Medicine, Hahnemann Medical College, Philadelphia

Sandra K. Crabtree Goodnough, RN, MSN, Pulmonary Clinical Nurse Specialist, Hermann Hospital, Houston

Margaret J. Griffiths, MSN, PhD, Professor, Thomas Jefferson University School of Nursing, Philadelphia

John J. Hagarty, MD, Surgical Pathologist; Emeritus Director of Laboratories and Attending Pathologist, Holy Redeemer Hospital, Meadowbrook, Pa.

Clare Hastings, RN, BSN, Head Nurse, Ambulatory Care, Clinical Center, National Institutes of Health, Bethesda, Md.

Mary Frances Keen, RN, DNSc, Associate Professor, University of Miami School of Nursing, Coral Gables, Fla.

Rose M. Kenny, MD, Associate Pathologist, Doylestown (Pa.) Hospital

Paul M. Kirschenfeld, MD, Pulmonary Fellow, Hahnemann University, Philadelphia; Private Practice in Pulmonary Disease, Absecon, N.J.

Marc S. Lapayowker, MD, Chairman, Department of Radiology, Abington (Pa.) Memorial Hospital

Peter G. Lavine, MD, Director, Coronary Care Unit, Crozer-Chester Medical Center, Chester, Pa.

Thomas E. Mackell, MD, FAAOS, Orthopedic Surgeon, Doylestown (Pa.) Hospital

Kenneth J. Mamot, RN, BS, Infection Control Consultant, The Genesee Hospital, Rochester, N.Y.

Molly J. Moran, RN, MS, Hematology Clinical Nurse Specialist, The Ohio State University Hospitals, Columbus

John E. Nestler, MD, Fellow in Endocrinology, University of Pennsylvania, Philadelphia

John F. O'Brien, PhD, Consultant, Department of Laboratory Medicine, Mayo Clinic, Rochester, Minn.

Gary M. Oderda, PharmD, MPH, Director, Maryland Poison Control Center; Associate Professor, University of Maryland School of Pharmacy, Baltimore

Paula Stephens Okun, RN, MSN, Instructor, Gwynedd-Mercy College, Gwynedd Valley, Pa.

John J. O'Shea, Jr., MD, Chief Medical Staff Fellow, Clinical Immunology Section, Laboratory of Clinical Investigation, National Institute of Allergy and Infectious Disease, Bethesda, Md.

Janice Hiscar Overdorff, RN, BSN, Administrative Nurse III, University of Illinois, Chicago

Gizell Maria Rossetti, MD, Instructor, Department of Neurology, Medical College of Pennsylvania, Philadelphia

Grannum R. Sant, MD, Assistant Professor of Urology, Tufts University School of Medicine, Boston

Harrison J. Shull, Jr., MD, FACP, Assistant Professor of Medicine, Vanderbilt University, Nashville, Tenn.

Barbara L. Solomon, RN, MS, Clinical Nurse Specialist, Endocrinology, National Institutes of Health, Bethesda, Md.

June L. Stark, RN, BSN, CCRN, Critical Care Instructor; Renal Nurse Consultant, New England Medical Center, Boston

Richard W. Tureck, MD, Assistant Professor of Obstetrics and Gynecology, University of Pennsylvania School of Medicine, Philadelphia

Cheryl A. Walker, RN, MN, CFNP, C-ANP, MBA, Assistant Professor, School of Nursing, University of Colorado Health Science Center, Denver

Joseph B. Warren, RN, BSN, Neurosurgical Nurse Consultant, Kinetic Concepts, Inc., San Antonio, Tex.

Harvey F. Watts, MD, Director, Pathology Department, Bryn Mawr (Pa.) Hospital

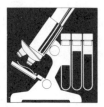# Contributors

Lolita M. Adrien, RN, MS, ET, Clinical Nurse Specialist, Surgery/Enterostoma Clinic, Stanford (Calif.) University Medical Center

Bonnie L. Anderson, MD, Resident, Bowman Gray School of Medicine, North Carolina Baptist Hospital, Winston-Salem

Barbara A. Ankenbrand, RN, BS, MA, Assistant Professor of Nursing, Mt. Mercy College, Cedar Rapids, Iowa

Wendy L. Baker, RN, BSN, MS, Staff, Critical Care Medicine Unit, University of Michigan Hospitals, Ann Arbor

Carol K. Barker, RN, MSN, MEd, Associate Professor, Bergen Community College, Paramus, N.J.

Patricia L. Baum, RN, BSN, Research and Clinical Consultant, Peripheral Vascular Nursing, University of Massachusetts Medical Center, Worcester

Deborah M. Berkowitz, RN, MSN, FNP, Nurse Practitioner, Columbia University Health Service, New York

Donna R. Blackburn, RN, RVT, Assistant Director, Blood Flow Laboratory, Northwestern Memorial Hospital, Chicago

Debra C. Broadwell, RN, PhD, ET, Associate Professor of Nursing, Emory University, Atlanta

Frank Lowell Brown, CUT, Chief Urology Technician, Department of Surgery, Division of Urology, Maricopa Medical Center, Phoenix, Ariz.

Judith Byrne, BS, MT(ASCP), Affiliate Member, American Society of Clinical Pathologists

Donald C. Cannon, MD, PhD, Resident in Internal Medicine, University of Kansas School of Medicine, Wichita

Deborah L. Dalrymple, RN, MSN, Assistant Professor of Nursing, Montgomery County Community College, Blue Bell, Pa.; Staff, Doylestown (Pa.) Hospital

William M. Dougherty, BS, Manager, Technical and Customer Services, Worldwide Geometric Data, Wayne, Pa.

Patricia A. Dowen, BA, COT, OT, Ophthalmic Technician, Franklin Eye Consultants, Southfield, Mich.

Barbara Boyd Egoville, RN, MSN, Former Instructor, Critical Care Nursing, Lankenau Hospital School of Nursing, Philadelphia

Jane Farrell, RN, BS, Orthopedic Nursing Specialist, Bellin Memorial Hospital, Green Bay, Wis.

John J. Fenton, PhD, DABcc, FNACB, Director of Chemistry, Crozer-Chester Medical Center, Chester, Pa.; Associate Professor of Clinical Chemistry, West Chester University of Pennsylvania

Sr. Rebecca Fidler, MT(ASCP), PhD, Chairperson, Health Sciences, Salem (W.Va.) College

Margaret C. Fisher, MD, Assistant Professor of Pediatrics, Temple University School of Medicine, Philadelphia; Epidemiologist, St. Christopher's Hospital for Children, Philadelphia

Regina Daley Ford, RN, BSN, MA, Developmental Editor, Springhouse Corporation, Springhouse, Pa.

Cynthia G. Fowler, PhD, Audiologist and Assistant Clinical Instructor, Veterans Administration Medical Center/University of California, Irvine

Katherine L. Fulton, RN, Clinical Supervisor, Gastrointestinal Unit, The Genesee Hospital, Rochester, N.Y.

Shirley Given, HT(ASCP), Supervisor of Histology, Crozer-Chester Medical Center, Chester, Pa.

Mary Chapman Gyetvan, RN, BSEd, Clinical Consultant, Nurse's Reference Library, Springhouse Corporation, Springhouse, Pa.

Thad C. Hagen, MD, Chief, Medical Service; Veterans Administration Medical Center, Milwaukee; Professor and Co-chairman, Department of Medicine, Medical College of Wisconsin, Milwaukee

Patrice M. Harman, RN, Staff Builders Registry, Ventura, Calif.

Annette L. Harmon, RN, MSN, CEN, Assistant Director of Nursing, Newton-Wellesley Hospital, Newton–Lower Falls, Mass.

Lenora R. Haston, RN, MSN, Former Clinical Editor, Nurse's Reference Library, Springhouse Corporation, Springhouse, Pa.

Kathy A. Hausman, RN, MS, CNRN, Neuroscience Consultant and Program Planner, Resource Applications, Baltimore

Tobie Virginia Hittle, RN, BSN, CCRN, Head Nurse, Intensive Care Unit, The Genesee Hospital, Rochester, N.Y.

Sr. Eileen Marie Hollen, RN, BSN, CCRN, Special Care Unit Supervisor, Nazareth Hospital, Philadelphia

Richard Edward Honigman, MD, FAAP, Pediatrician, Levittown, N.Y.

Susan A. Kayes, BS, SM(ASCP), Supervisor, Microbiology Department, Southwestern Vermont Medical Center, Bennington

Sr. Mary Brian Kelber, RN, SM, DNS, Associate Professor, School of Nursing, University of San Francisco

Dana Kathryn Kelly, RN, BSN, Teaching Assistant, Psychomotor Skills Laboratory, Rush University School of Nursing, Chicago

Catherine E. Kirby, RN, MSN, Nurse Consultant, Nursing Technomics of National Technomics, Inc., West Chester, Pa.

William E. Kline, MS, MT(ASCP), SBB, Director, Technical Services, St. Paul (Minn.) Red Cross

Clarke Lambe, MD, Clinical Assistant III, Department of Pathology, University of Arizona, Tucson

Laurel Kareus Lambe, MS, RD, Nutrition Consultant, Tucson, Ariz.

Dennis E. Leavelle, MD, Associate Professor and Consultant, Mayo Medical Laboratories, Department of Laboratory Medicine, Mayo Clinic, Rochester, Minn.

Cheryl Longinotti, PhD, Audiologist, Veterans Administration Westside Medical Center, Chicago

Marylou K. McHugh, RN, MSN, Academic Counselor, Department of Nursing, LaSalle University, Philadelphia

Joan C. McManus, RN, MA, Assistant Professor of Nursing, Bergen Community College, Paramus, N.J.

Claire B. Mailhot, RN, MS, Director of Operating Room Services and Assistant Director of Nursing, Stanford (Calif.) University Hospital

Elizabeth Anne Mallon, MS, MT(ASCP), Transplant Coordinator, Thomas Jefferson University Hospital, Philadelphia

Nancy L. Mauldin, RN, Nurse-Technician, St. Mary's Hospital, Galveston, Tex.

Malinda S. Mitchell, RN, MS, Associate Director of Nursing, Stanford (Calif.) University Hospital

Marilee Warner Mohr, RN, MSN, Assistant Director of Nursing, Mercy Catholic Medical Center, Misericordia Division, Philadelphia

S. Breanndan Moore, MD, DCH, FCAP, Staff Physician in Blood Bank and Transfusion Service, Mayo Clinic, Rochester, Minn.

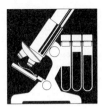

Foreword

More than ever before, your professional responsibility for patient care is likely to involve laboratory tests and other diagnostic procedures. Such involvement may include multiple aspects of preparing for the test, assisting during its course, and monitoring its effects. For example, you are often responsible for ensuring that patients are correctly prepared for testing; for ensuring that tests are correctly ordered; for assisting the examiner during the actual procedure; for supporting and reassuring the patient during difficult or painful procedures; for quickly transmitting properly prepared specimens to the laboratory in appropriate containers; for assisting with the monitoring of test results; for monitoring complications during and after the test; and finally, for providing appropriate post-test care.

To meet these responsibilities effectively, you need much more than a superficial familiarity with any given test. You must have a ready source of fundamental information about the test itself: why it is useful, how it is performed, how it is likely to affect the patient, and what the test results indicate. DIAGNOSTICS, another volume of the Nurse's Reference Library, provides this information in a comprehensive and readily accessible form.

This book is organized into five major sections that include virtually all available diagnostic tests, ranging from routine procedures, such as CBC and urinalysis, to the most complex tests, such as the latest variants of computed tomography and magnetic resonance imaging. Section I (chapters 1 through 11) presents tests that are performed on a blood sample. Section II (chapters 12 through 17) presents tests that require a urine specimen. Section III (chapters 18 and 19) presents tests concerning histology, microbiology, and parisitology. Section IV (chapters 20 to 22) presents tests on body organs—the thyroid gland, the eye, and the ear. Section V (chapters 23 to 29) presents tests that evaluate structure and function of the body systems. The final section (chapters 30 and 31) presents special tests, including skin tests, tests for determining therapeutic and toxic blood levels, and miscellaneous tests.

Each chapter begins with an *Introduction* that summarizes general information about the tests that follow, describing the relevant groups of tests, telling why they are useful, summarizing test methods, and providing supplementary information, such as anatomy and physiology.

Each individual test entry that follows includes significant information about the test; specific indications for the test; and relevant physiology that supports understanding of the test, its clinical importance, and other pertinent facts. The entry continues with *Purpose*—a brief summary of common indications for the test—followed by *Patient preparation,* which summarizes the necessary physical and psychological preparation for the test, including dietary and drug restrictions. The next section, *Equipment,* lists the equipment you may use while performing the test or must have ready before the test. *Procedure* describes in detail the test procedure and, when appropriate, describes the nurse's role. Next, *Values* or *Findings* summarizes normal results of each test and is graphically highlighted for easy reference. (Some numerical values listed in this section may vary by laboratory and by method and are provided as a general guide.) *Implications of results* summarizes abnormal results and their clinical significance. *Post-test care* describes nursing actions needed to help the patient resume pretest activity or diet, or to deal with adverse effects of the test. Finally, *Interfering factors* summarizes elements of preparation or procedure that can invalidate the test or make its interpretation difficult or unreliable.

Throughout the volume, a special graphic device, the *Nursing Alert,* calls your attention to conditions that involve potential hazard to the patient and how to deal with them. When appropriate, each entry also includes helpful information on patient teaching, anatomic illustrations, and graphs and charts that isolate and emphasize useful supplementary information. A special introductory section on *Collection Techniques* summarizes recommended procedures and offers practical guidelines for obtaining and handling blood and urine samples—the two most common laboratory specimens.

DIAGNOSTICS provides a clear, concise, and comprehensive presentation of information concerning current diagnostic tests. I highly recommend this volume not only to nurses, but to all medical professionals who deal with diagnostic testing in any way. A thorough knowledge of its contents will promote your understanding of diagnostic procedures and enhance your effectiveness as a member of the health-care team.

DENNIS E. LEAVELLE, MD
Mayo Medical Laboratories
Department of Laboratory Medicine
Mayo Clinic
Rochester, Minnesota

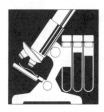

Overview:
New Diagnostic Challenges

Traditionally, doctors and laboratory technicians have dominated the field of diagnostic testing. Nurses have been limited to a peripheral, strictly supportive role. Many of us have been allowed merely to carry out the patient's physical preparations for a test and perhaps gather necessary equipment. Occasionally, we'd be asked to assist with a diagnostic procedure; the extent of the doctor's communication on these memorable occasions was usually "Hold this for me, please."

Changing responsibilities
Today the scene is changing. The recent dramatic proliferation in the number and complexity of diagnostic tests has vastly enlarged their potential benefits and applications, and consequently, has required wider sharing of clinical responsibility. We now find the sanctums of diagnostics—the hematology and the microbiology laboratories, the radiology and the ultrasound departments—opening to us. More nurses than ever before are not only assisting with sophisticated diagnostic tests, but are ordering tests for patients and performing many procedures formerly restricted to other members of the health-care team.

These changes reflect the upheaval in diagnostic medicine during the past 15 years. Computed tomography, introduced in 1972 and now refined to a remarkable degree, represents a quantum leap in modern medicine's diagnostic capabilities. Cardiac catheterization laboratories have become commonplace; nuclear medicine has made it possible to study the structures and functions of the heart with astonishing precision. New technology has multiplied the uses of di-

agnostic testing and, inevitably, has enlarged nursing responsibility in the diagnostic process. To meet this responsibility, we need to *know* more about diagnostic testing than in the past.

I could cite several examples of nurses performing procedures formerly restricted to others: in Maryland, a recent state requirement that every female hospital patient be offered the opportunity to have a Pap test has extended routine performance of this test to staff nurses. In some hospitals, nurse clinicians perform bone marrow examinations and colposcopic examinations. ICU nurses routinely perform radial artery punctures; obstetrical department nurses do fetal monitoring; and neurology department nurses monitor intracranial pressure using transducers. The list of new responsibilities is expanding rapidly.

Patient preparation critical
Even when nurses do not perform or assist with some diagnostic tests, they are generally responsible for preparing patients for tests performed in other areas and for caring for these patients after the tests are complete. Knowing how to prepare patients for testing is an important benefit derived from a thorough working knowledge of diagnostic processes. Such preparation must be physical, intellectual, and emotional. We are accustomed to providing physical preparation for diagnostic tests and can do so readily. But many of us are less confident about intellectual and emotional preparation. These less tangible aspects of preparation are no less important and may be critical. Patients facing a diagnostic test they don't fully understand need a clear, nonthreatening explanation of its pur-

pose. Better understanding promotes better cooperation and, in turn, produces better, more reliable test results.

Teaching guidelines

You can help such patients by observing the following teaching guidelines:

□ Explain the purpose of the test and the procedure in words the patient can understand. A clear explanation can dispel needless anxiety, confusion, and embarrassment.

□ If your hospital provides an informational pamphlet about the test to be performed, make sure the patient has received a copy in time to read it before preparation for the test begins. Tell him everything that common sense and discretion dictate. How much you should tell him about the test varies, of course, with his capacity to understand—based on age, education, familiarity with medical terms and procedures, and on conditions that could interfere with intellectual function, such as stress, drugs, or trauma.

□ On the morning of the test—or sooner—inform the patient who will perform the test (tell him their names, if you know them) and where it will be performed.

□ Refer to the test by its full name. Don't overwhelm the patient by using abbreviations and medical jargon. Terms like PBI and EKG are useful shortcuts for communicating with your peers, but they're likely to intimidate the average patient and discourage discussion.

□ Keep in mind that the patient has a legal right to know the test's benefits and dangers *before* he signs a consent form.

□ Tell the patient it's appropriate for him to ask the doctor for the test results. Some patients are timid about asking.

□ Make sure your understanding of the test is adequate before you attempt explaining it to the patient. To provide useful explanations, we must be familiar with the various purposes of diagnostic tests. For example, when a child with poststreptococcal glomerulonephritis is scheduled for serial blood urea nitrogen and creatinine tests, you should be able to explain to his parents that these tests are necessary to monitor their child's response to treatment by measuring improvement in kidney function.

Sensory instruction

Sensory instruction means telling the patient what he will see, hear, smell, taste, and feel during a test. The rapid-fire clacking sound of an X-ray machine exposing a series of consecutive radiographs, the characteristic burning sensation that follows infusion of contrast material, the formidable appearance of a CT scanner—you should tell a patient to expect these things before a test.

Wise and clinically experienced nurses have instinctively included sensory instruction in test preparation. But only recently have we known how valuable such instruction can be. Psychologists and behaviorists report that emotional distress during a threatening situation depends on how closely expectations match the actual experience. The closer the match between expectation and actual perception, the less severe the distress. Evidence shows that pretest instruction minimizes the patient's anxiety and helps him withstand even rigorously uncomfortable procedures.

Responsibility for interpretation

Results of diagnostic tests have little meaning unless we know normal values. We are expected to recognize abnormal values in laboratory reports and to understand their clinical significance. Fortunately, some laboratory forms include this information, specifying the upper and lower limits of the normal range. But even when they don't, it's a nursing responsibility to know what test results mean. You should recognize, for example, that a serum sodium level of 153 mEq is high, that it necessitates your notifying the patient's doctor, and that you should obtain orders to replace the I.V. infusion of 5% dextrose in 0.9% normal saline solution with one containing less or no sodium. Failure to do so can precipitate congestive heart failure in certain patients. After cardiac enzyme determinations to identify myocardial damage, you should recognize elevated enzyme levels and know what they imply for continuing assessment of chest pain, skin and color changes, and arrhythmias. To know the nursing implications of bleeding, venous congestion, weakness, and hypoxia, your understanding of normal blood values must go beyond the routine hemoglobin, hematocrit, and WBC; it must include understanding of abnormal values for reticular cell count, platelet count, and so forth.

In many institutions, particularly in small community hospitals or institutions without constant medical supervision, you are commonly expected to read chest X-ray films. To do so effectively, you must recognize terminology for X-ray interpretation (anterior, posterior, oblique, lateral, and so forth). You must be familiar with the location of lung outlines, heart border, trachea, and mediastinum. You must know how to recognize the signs of congestion, pneumothorax, and effusion.

Long-term implications
In chronic care settings, such as nursing homes, diagnostic tests also figure prominently in patient care, with the emphasis on long-term implications. In these settings, special tests monitor physical and chemical changes and assess drug reactions during prolonged treatment. Nurses who care for cardiac patients receiving Coumadin or dipyridamole need to know how to monitor their effects on coagulation. To do this requires familiarity with normal and abnormal values of prothrombin or partial thromboplastin times. When caring for patients who receive prolonged treatment with phenothiazines, we must know how to monitor and recognize adverse effects on the bone marrow and on liver function.

Diagnostic tests maintain health
Preventive health care is of increasing importance for applying our knowledge of diagnostic testing. For some time we have performed routine examinations of "well patients" to help them maintain good health and to screen for common diseases like hypertension and diabetes mellitus. Today we must be able to screen seemingly healthy persons for many more diseases, such as glaucoma (through tonometry) and carcinoma (through the Pap test). And we must expect to perform these tests in just about any setting—clinics, offices, schools and hospitals.

To meet this growing diagnostic responsibility, we need reliable testing and interpretation skills, and the ability to educate the public about the importance of screening programs. For example, we must be able to persuade the 50-year-old man with no sign of heart disease that he will benefit from taking a stress test every 3 years.

New day
Clearly, rigorous application of the many aspects of diagnostic medicine is indispensable to effective health care, and nurses are obliged to participate in it fully. We must accept the challenge of diagnostic testing as still another tool to help us care for our patients more knowledgeably, more efficiently, and more compassionately. There is much to know, but there is much worth knowing. Its greatest value, as always, is in helping us carry out our unique commitment as patient advocates.

FRANCES J. STORLIE, RN, PhD, ANP

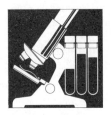

Collection Techniques: Blood and Urine Samples

Blood

The type of blood sample that's required—whole blood, plasma, or serum—depends on the nature of the test. *Whole blood*—containing all blood elements—is the sample of choice for blood gas analysis, determination of hemoglobin derivatives, and measurement of RBC constituents. In addition, most routine hematologic studies, such as complete blood count, erythrocyte sedimentation rate, reticulocyte and platelet counts, and the osmotic fragility test, require whole blood samples.

Plasma is the liquid part of whole blood, which contains all the blood proteins; *serum*, the liquid that remains after whole blood clots. Plasma and serum samples, which contain most of the physiologically and clinically significant substances found in blood, are used for most biochemical, immunologic, and coagulation studies. They also provide useful electrolyte evaluation, enzyme analysis, glucose concentration, protein determination, and bilirubin level.

Venous, arterial, and capillary blood

Venous blood returns to the heart through the veins. It carries a high concentration of carbon dioxide from the cells back to the lungs, for exhalation. Since venous blood represents physiologic conditions throughout the body and is relatively easy to obtain, it's used for most laboratory procedures.

Arterial blood, replenished with oxygen from the lungs, leaves the heart through the arteries, to distribute nutrients throughout the capillary network. Although an arterial puncture increases the risks of hematoma and arterial spasm, arterial blood samples are necessary for pH, PaO_2, and $PaCO_2$ determinations, and oxygen saturation studies.

Capillary, or peripheral, blood does the real work of the circulatory system—exchanging fluids, nutrients, and wastes between blood and tissues. Capillary blood samples are most useful for studies such as hemoglobin and hematocrit determinations; blood smears; microtechniques for clinical chemistry; and platelet, RBC, and WBC counts requiring only small amounts of blood.

Quantities and containers

Sample quantities needed for diagnostic studies depend on the laboratory, available equipment, and the type of test. Some laboratories, for example, use automated analyzer systems that require a serum sample of 100 µl or less; others use manual systems that require a larger amount. The desired sample quantity determines the collection procedure, and the type and size of the container. A single venipuncture with a conventional glass or disposable plastic syringe can provide 15 ml of blood—sufficient for many hematologic, immunologic, chemical, and coagulation tests, but hardly enough for a series of tests.

To avoid multiple venipunctures when tests require a large blood sample, use an evacuated tube system (Vacutainer, Corvac) with interchangeable glass tubes, optional draw capacities, and a selection

COMMON ARTERIAL AND VENOUS PUNCTURE SITES

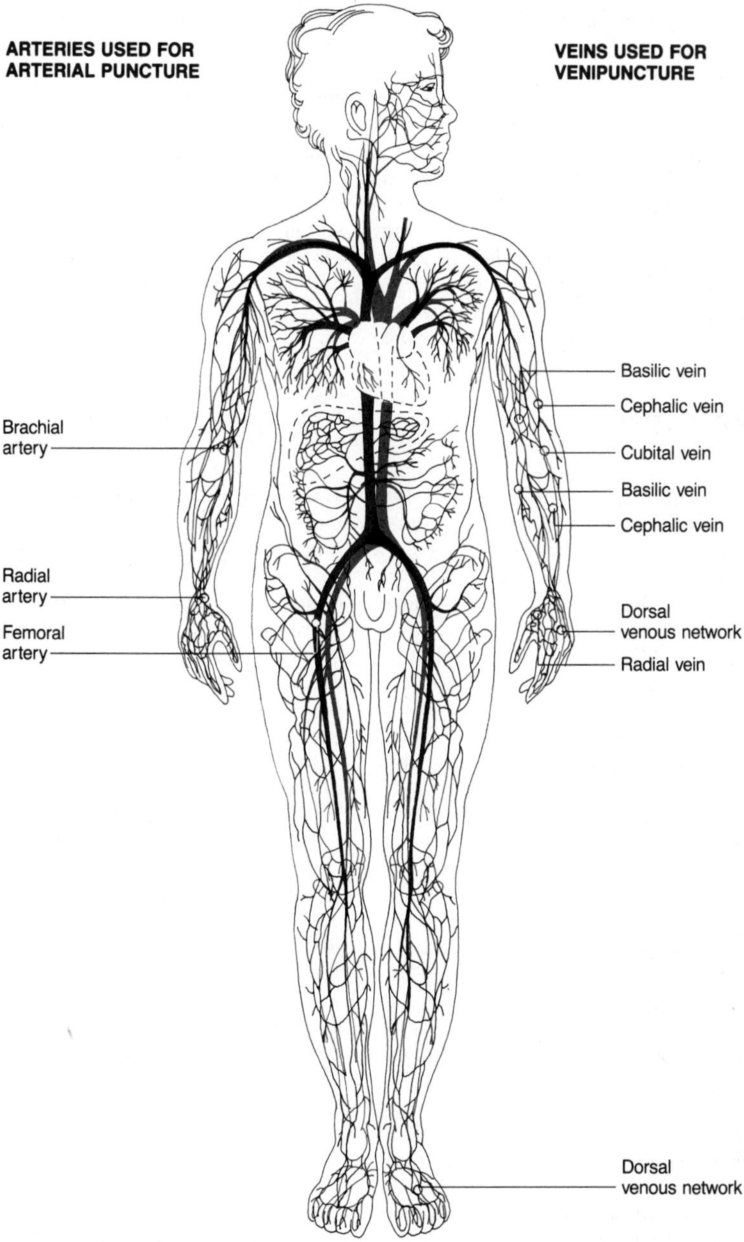

**ARTERIES USED FOR
ARTERIAL PUNCTURE**

**VEINS USED FOR
VENIPUNCTURE**

Basilic vein

Cephalic vein

Cubital vein

Basilic vein

Cephalic vein

Brachial
artery

Radial
artery

Femoral
artery

Dorsal
venous network

Radial vein

Dorsal
venous network

of additives. Evacuated tubes are commercially prepared with or without additives (indicated by their color-coded stoppers), and with enough vacuum to draw a predetermined blood volume (2 to 20 ml per tube). (For a guide to the uses of color-coded stoppers, see pages 1068 and 1069.)

Microanalysis of minute amounts of capillary blood collected with micropipettes or glass capillary tubes allows numerous hematologic and routine laboratory studies on infants, children, and patients with severe burns or poor veins. Micropipettes are color-coded by sample capacity and hold 30 to 50 μl of whole blood; glass capillary tubes hold 80 to 130 μl of serum or plasma.

Equipment

Venipuncture: tourniquet/70% alcohol or povidone-iodine solution/sterile syringes or evacuated tubes/sterile needle—20G or 21G for forearm; 25G for wrist, hand, or ankle, or for children/color-coded tubes containing appropriate additives/labels for identification/2″ x 2″ gauze pads/small adhesive bandage.

Arterial blood: 10-ml Luer-Lok glass syringe/1-ml ampul heparin/20G, 1½″ short bevel needle/23G, 1″ short bevel needle/rubber stopper or cork/antiseptic swabs/70% alcohol or povidone-iodine solution/2″ x 2″ gauze pads/tape or adhesive bandage/iced specimen container/labels (for syringe and specimen bag) for patient's name and room number (if applicable), doctor's name, date, collection time, and details of oxygen therapy.

Capillary blood: sterile, disposable blood lancet/2″ x 2″ gauze pads/70% alcohol or povidone-iodine solution/glass slides, heparinized capillary tubes, or pipettes/appropriate solutions.

Venous sample

The nature of the test and the patient's age and condition determine the appropriate blood sample, collection site, and technique. Most tests require a venous sample. Although a relatively simple procedure, venipuncture must be performed carefully to avoid hemolysis or hemo-

concentration of the sample, to prevent hematoma formation, and to prevent damage to the patient's veins.

Label all test tubes clearly with the patient's name and room number, doctor's name, date, and collection time.

Select a venipuncture site. The most common site is the antecubital fossa area; other sites include the wrist and the dorsum of the hand or foot. When drawing the sample at bedside, instruct the patient to lie on his back, with his head slightly elevated and his arms resting at his sides. When drawing blood from an ambulatory patient, tell him to sit in a chair, with his arm supported securely on an armrest or table.

When using an evacuated tube, attach the needle to the holder before applying the tourniquet. Apply a soft rubber tourniquet above the puncture site to prevent venous blood return and to increase venous pressure, thus making the veins more prominent and increasing the volume of blood at the puncture site. Make sure the tourniquet is snug but not tight enough to constrict arteries. Using a tourniquet for a patient with large, distended, and highly visible veins increases the risk of hematoma. If the patient's veins appear distinct, you may not need to apply a tourniquet.

Instruct the patient to make a fist several times to further enlarge the veins. Select a vein by palpation and inspection.

If you can't feel a vein distinctly, *don't* attempt venipuncture. Working in a circular motion from the center outward, clean the puncture site with alcohol or povidone-iodine solution, and dry it with a gauze pad. If you must touch the cleansed puncture site again to relocate the vein, palpate with an antiseptically clean finger, and wipe the area again with an alcohol swab.

Draw the skin tautly over the vein by pressing just below the puncture site with your thumb, to keep the vein from moving.

Hold the syringe or tube with the needle bevel up and the shaft parallel to the path of the vein at a 15° angle to the

HOW TO COLLECT A VENOUS SAMPLE

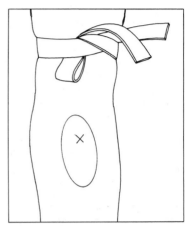

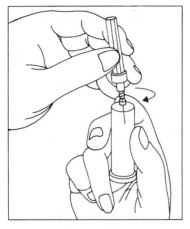

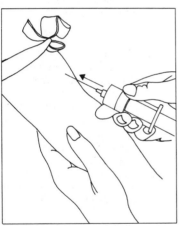

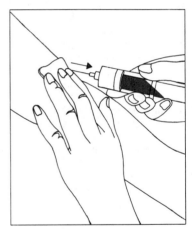

- Select a venipuncture site, usually the antecubital fossa.

- Using a circular motion, cleanse the area first with povidone-iodine solution and then alcohol.

- Screw the Vacutainer needle into the sleeve (top left).

- Apply a soft rubber tourniquet above the venipuncture site (top right).

- Remove the needle cover. With the bevel facing up, insert the needle into the patient's vein at a 15° angle (bottom left). When a drop of blood appears just inside the needle holder, gently push the Vacutainer tube into the needle sleeve, so the blood enters the tube. Try to keep the needle still to prevent it from perforating the patient's vein.

- When the tube is filled, remove the tourniquet, and pull the Vacutainer tube off the needle end. Withdraw the needle, using a dry sponge to apply direct pressure to the puncture site (bottom right). After 2 or 3 minutes, remove the sponge, and cover the site with an adhesive bandage.

arm. Enter the vein with a single direct puncture of the skin and vein wall. If you use a syringe, venous blood will appear in the hub. Withdraw the blood slowly, gently pulling on the syringe to create steady suction until you obtain the desired amount. For an evacuated tube, when a drop of blood appears just inside the needle holder, grasp the needle holder securely and push down on the collection tube until the needle punctures the rubber stopper; blood flows into the tube automatically. When the tube is filled, remove it, and if drawing multiple samples, repeat the procedure with additional tubes.

To prevent stasis, release the tourniquet as soon as you establish adequate blood flow. If the flow is sluggish, you may want to leave the tourniquet in place longer. However, always remove the tourniquet before withdrawing the needle.

After drawing the sample, ask the patient to open his fist as soon as you collect the desired amount. Release the tourniquet. Place a gauze pad over the puncture site, then withdraw the needle slowly and gently. Apply gentle pressure to the puncture site. If the patient is alert and cooperative, tell him to hold the gauze in place for several minutes until the bleeding stops, to prevent hematoma. If the patient is not alert or cooperative, hold the pad in place, or apply a small adhesive bandage.

After collection with a syringe, remove the needle and carefully empty the sample into the appropriate test tube, without delay. To prevent foaming and possible hemolysis, *don't* eject the blood through the needle or force it out of the syringe.

Place the appropriate color-coded stoppers on the tubes. Gently invert a tube containing anticoagulant several times to mix the sample thoroughly. Examine the sample for clots or clumps; if none appears, send the sample to the laboratory. *Don't* shake the tube.

Before leaving the patient, check his condition. If a hematoma develops at the puncture site, apply warm soaks. If the patient has lingering discomfort or undue bleeding, instruct him to lie down. Watch for anxiety or signs of shock, such as hypotension and tachycardia.

Make sure the specimen is sent to the laboratory immediately.

Arterial sample

Arterial blood is rarely required for routine studies. Since arterial puncture carries risks, samples are generally collected by a doctor or a specially trained nurse.

Before drawing an arterial blood sample, administer a local anesthetic at the puncture site, if necessary.

To heparinize the syringe, first attach a 20G needle to the syringe; then, break open the ampul of heparin and draw 1 ml into the syringe. While rotating the barrel, pull the plunger back past the 7-

---

SAFEGUARDS FOR VENIPUNCTURE

- Make sure the patient is adequately supported, in case of syncope.
- When using a syringe to draw a sample, avoid injecting air into a vein by checking that the plunger is fully depressed before injection.
- If possible, avoid drawing blood from an arm or leg used for I.V. infusion of blood, dextrose, or electrolyte solutions, since this dilutes the blood sample. If you must collect blood near an I.V. site, choose a location below it.
- For easier identification of veins in patients with tortuous or sclerosed veins, or with veins damaged by repeated venipuncture, antibiotic therapy, or chemotherapy, apply warm, wet compresses

15 minutes before attempting venipuncture.
- If you aren't successful after two attempts, ask another nurse to perform the venipuncture.
- When you can't find a vein quickly, release the tourniquet temporarily, to avoid tissue necrosis and circulation problems.
- Be sure to insert the needle at the correct angle to reduce the risk of puncturing the opposite wall of the vein and causing a hematoma.
- Always release the tourniquet before withdrawing the needle, to prevent a hematoma. When drawing multiple samples, release the tourniquet within 1 minute after beginning to draw blood to prevent a hemoconcentration sample.

THE ALLEN'S TEST: HOW TO PERFORM IT

Before inserting an arterial line in one of your patient's radial arteries, assess the blood supply to your patient's hand. If the radial artery is blocked by a blood clot—a frequent complication of arterial lines—the ulnar artery alone must supply blood to the hand. The Allen's test is a simple, reliable procedure that quickly assesses arterial function.

Just follow these steps:

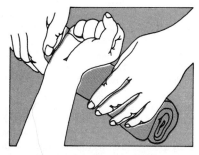

1 First, have the patient rest his arm on the bedside table. Support his wrist with a rolled towel. Ask him to clench his fist.

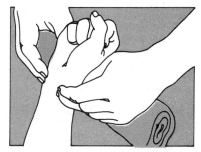

2 Now, use your index and middle fingers to exert pressure over both the radial and the ulnar arteries.

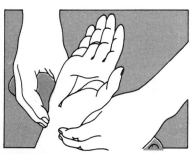

3 Without removing your fingers, ask the patient to unclench his fist. You'll notice his palm is blanched because you've impaired the normal blood flow with your fingers.
Nursing tip: Suppose your patient's unconscious or unable to clench his fist for some other reason. You can encourage his palm to blanch by occluding both arteries, elevating his hand, and massaging his palm.

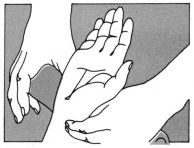

4 Release the pressure on the ulnar artery, and ask the patient to open his hand. If the ulnar artery's functioning well, his palm will turn pink in about 5 seconds, even though the radial artery's still occluded. But if blood return is slow and his fingers begin to contract, blood supply from the ulnar artery may not be adequate. In that case, try the Allen's test on his other wrist; you may get better results. *Note:* Slow blood return doesn't always indicate arterial occlusion. It may indicate poor cardiac output or poor capillary refill, resulting from shock.

ml mark. Hold the syringe in an upright position, and slowly force the heparin toward the hub of the syringe, as you continue to rotate the barrel. Leave enough heparin—about 0.1 ml—to fill the syringe tip.

Heparinize the needle by removing the first needle and replacing it with a 23G needle. Continue to hold the syringe upright, but tilt it slightly. Then push the plunger all the way up to eject the remaining heparin.

Perform Allen's test (see page xxix) to assess circulation in the radial artery. Choose either the radial or brachial artery, whichever has the better circulation. *Don't* choose a site where the patient has had a vascular graft or has an atrioventricular fistula in situ.

Next, using a circular motion, clean the puncture site with a swab soaked in povidone-iodine solution. Then wipe the site with a swab soaked in alcohol to remove the povidone-iodine solution, which is sticky and may hinder palpation. Palpate the artery with the forefinger and middle finger of one hand, while holding the syringe over the puncture site with the other hand.

With the needle bevel up, puncture the skin at a 45° angle for the radial artery and at a 60° angle for the brachial artery. For a femoral arterial puncture, the needle is inserted at a 90° angle.

Advance the needle, but don't pull the plunger back. When you've punctured the artery, blood will pulsate into the syringe. Allow it to fill 5 to 10 ml. If the syringe doesn't fill immediately, you may have pushed the needle through the artery. Pull the needle back slightly, but don't pull the plunger back. If the syringe still doesn't fill, withdraw the needle and start over with a fresh heparinized needle. Never make more than two attempts to draw blood from one site.

After drawing the sample, remove the needle and apply firm pressure to the puncture site with a gauze pad for at least 5 minutes, to prevent hematoma (a significant risk after arterial puncture). If the patient is receiving an anticoagulant or has a bleeding disorder, apply pressure for at least 15 minutes. *Don't* ask the patient to apply pressure to the site. The patient may not apply the continuous, firm pressure that's needed.

Rotate the syringe to mix the heparin with the sample. If air bubbles appear, try to remove them by holding the syringe upright and tapping it lightly with your finger. If the bubbles don't disappear, hold the syringe upright and pierce a 2″ x 2″ gauze pad or alcohol swab with the needle (slowly forcing some of the blood out of the syringe eliminates the bubbles, and the gauze pad catches the ejected blood). After removing air bubbles, plunge the needle into a rubber stopper to seal it from the air, and trans-

AUTOMATIC TEST SERIES: SMA 12/60 AND SMAC

Many laboratories now use automated electronic systems, such as the sequential multiple analyzer (SMA) 12/60 and the sequential multiple analyzer with computer (SMAC), chemistry, blood banking, and serologic and bacteriologic procedures. These systems perform blood studies rapidly, economically, and comprehensively. They can detect unsuspected abnormalities and indicate the need for additional tests.

• The SMA 12/60 can make 12 determinations on 60 serum specimens in 1 hour: glucose, cholesterol, albumin, and total protein levels (nutritional status); bilirubin levels (liver function); BUN and uric acid levels (kidney function); SGOT and LDH enzyme levels (tissue injury); alkaline phosphatase (bone tissue injury); and calcium and phosphate levels (parathyroid function).

• The SMAC can perform 20 to 40 biochemical determinations on 120 serum specimens in 1 hour. It can analyze selected blood components, singly or in combination, as well as provide an entire test profile on each specimen. This system also automatically reports special cardiac, renal, hepatic, lipid, bone, enzyme, and electrolyte profiles. With SMAC, tests performed on a 450-μl sample include cholesterol, triglycerides, glucose, BUN, calcium, phosphorus, sodium, potassium, chloride, CO_2, total protein, total bilirubin, albumin, creatinine, GGT, SGOT, SGPT, LDH, uric acid, acid and alkaline phosphatase, and iron.

fer the sample to the iced specimen container.

Note on the laboratory slip the patient's temperature, hemoglobin count, and the type and amount of oxygen he's receiving. Send the sample to the laboratory immediately.

After releasing pressure on the puncture site, tape a bandage firmly over it. (Don't tape the entire wrist, as this may restrict circulation.)

 After arterial puncture, observe carefully for signs of circulatory impairment distal to the puncture site, such as swelling, discoloration, pain, numbness, or tingling in the bandaged extremity.

Before drawing an arterial blood sample for blood gas studies, carefully check the patient's oxygen therapy. If ABG levels are being measured to monitor response to withdrawal of oxygen, but the patient continues to receive it, results will be misleading. For the same reason, don't draw an arterial sample immediately after suctioning or after placement on a ventilator. Wait at least 15 minutes to allow circulating blood levels to accurately reflect response to mechanical ventilation.

Capillary sample

Collection of a capillary blood sample requires skin puncture of the fingertip or earlobe of adults, or puncture of the great toe or the heel of newborns.

To facilitate collection of a capillary sample, first dilate the vessels by applying warm, moist compresses to the area for about 10 minutes. Select the puncture site, wipe it with gauze and alcohol, and dry it thoroughly with another gauze pad so the blood will well up. Avoid cold, cyanotic, or swollen sites, to ensure an adequate blood sample.

To draw a sample from the fingertip, use a lancet smaller than 2 mm, and make the puncture perpendicular to the lines of the patient's fingerprints.

After drawing the sample, wipe away the first drop of blood to reduce the chance of sample dilution with tissue fluid. For the same reason, avoid squeezing the puncture site. After collecting the sample, briefly apply pressure to the puncture site to prevent painful extravasation of blood into the subcutaneous tissues. Ask the adult patient to hold a sterile gauze pad over the puncture site until bleeding has stopped. Then apply a small adhesive bandage.

Interfering factors

Food or medications can interfere with test methods, so be sure to check the patient's diet and medication history before tests, and to schedule them after an overnight fast of 12 to 14 hours. Although the concentration of most blood constituents doesn't change significantly after a meal, fasting is customary, because blood collected shortly after eating often appears cloudy (turbid) from a temporary increase in triglyceride levels that can interfere with many chemical reactions. Transient, food-related lipemia usually disappears 4 to 6 hours after a meal, making such short fasts acceptable before blood collection.

Baseline studies often depend on the patient's diet. For example, valid glucose tolerance test results require an adequate daily carbohydrate intake (250 mg) for 3 days before testing. Similarly, recent protein and fat consumption influences uric acid, urea, and lipid levels.

Numerous drugs and their metabolites affect test results by pharmacologic or chemical interference. Pharmacologic interference results from temporary or permanent drug-induced physiologic change in a blood component. For example, long-term administration of such drugs as erythromycin can damage the liver and alter the results of liver function studies. Chemical interference results from a drug's physical characteristic that alters the test reaction. For example, high dosages of ascorbic acid may raise blood glucose levels. To identify such interference with test results, all unexpected changes in blood values require a meticulous review of the patient's drug and dietary history and of his clinical status.

JUDITH BYRNE, BS, MT(ASCP)

Urine

The type of urine specimen required—random, second-voided, clean-catch midstream, first morning, fasting, or timed—depends on the patient's condition and age, and the purpose of the test. Random, second-voided, and clean-catch midstream specimens can be collected at any time; first morning, fasting, or timed specimens require collection at specific times.

To collect a *random* specimen (for such routine tests as urinalysis), the patient simply collects one voiding in a specimen container. Although this method provides quick laboratory results, the information it provides is less reliable than that from a controlled specimen.

To collect a *second-voided* specimen, the patient voids, discards the urine, and then 30 minutes later voids again into a specimen container.

To collect a *clean-catch* specimen, the patient voids first into either a bedpan or toilet, and collects a sample in midstream. Originally used mainly to test for bacteriuria and pyuria, this specimen is now replacing the random specimen because it's aseptic.

First morning and *fasting* specimens must be collected when the patient awakes. Since the *first morning* specimen is the most concentrated of the day, it's the specimen of choice for nitrate, protein, and urinary sediment analyses. For this specimen, the patient voids and discards the urine just before going to bed, then collects the first voiding of the morning. For the *fasting* specimen, which is used for glucose testing, the patient maintains an overnight fast and collects a *first morning* specimen.

The *timed* specimen determines the urinary concentration of such substances as hormones, proteins, creatinine, and electrolytes over a specified period—usually 2, 12, or 24 hours. The 24-hour collection, the most common timed specimen, provides a measure of average excretion for substances eliminated in variable amounts during the day, such

as hormones. Timed specimens may also be collected after administration of a challenge dose of a chemical, to measure physiologic efficiency—for example, ingestion of glucose to test for incipient diabetes mellitus or hypoglycemia. This type of specimen is also preferred for quantitative analysis of urobilinogen, xylose, amylase, phenolsulfonphthalein dye excretion, or an Addis count.

Equipment

Random, second-voided, first morning, or fasting collection: clean, dry bedpan or urinal (for nonambulatory patients)/specimen container/specimen labels/laboratory request slip.

Clean-catch midstream collection: commercially prepared kit containing necessary equipment and directions to patient in several languages (English, Spanish, French) or antiseptic solution (green soap or povidone-iodine solution)/water/cotton balls/sterile gloves/specimen labels/laboratory request slip.

Timed collection (24-hour specimen): clean, dry gallon containers or commercial urine collection containers/preservative, as ordered/labels for collection container/display signs.

Pediatric urine collection: plastic disposable collection bags/specimen containers/laboratory request slip/cotton swabs/soap and water/diapers.

Random and second-voided collections

For random collection, tell the ambulatory patient to urinate directly into a clean, dry specimen container. Tell the nonambulatory patient to void into a clean bedpan or urinal, to minimize bacterial or chemical contamination; then transfer about 30 ml of urine to the specimen container, and secure the cap.

For second-voided collection, instruct the patient to void and discard the urine. Then, offer him at least one glass of water, to stimulate urine production. Collect urine 30 minutes later, using the random collection technique.

Label the container with the patient's name and room number (if applicable), doctor's name, date, and collection time. Send the specimen and a completed request slip to the laboratory immediately. On the chart, record the procedure and the time the specimen was sent.

First morning and fasting collections

Unless the patient is an infant or is catheterized or unable to urinate, the following collection techniques are used for first morning and fasting specimens.

For fasting specimen collection, instruct the patient to restrict food and fluids after midnight before the test. For both collection procedures, instruct the patient to void and discard the urine before retiring for the night; then collect the first voiding of the next day in a clean, dry specimen container. (If the patient must void during the night, note it on the specimen label—for example, "Urine specimen, 2:15 a.m. to 8:00 a.m.")

Label the container with the patient's name and room number (if applicable),

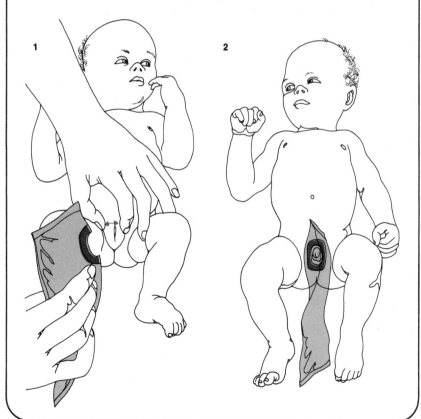

APPLYING A PEDIATRIC URINE COLLECTOR

To attach a plastic urine collector to an infant girl (1), stretch the perineum to smooth the skin around the vagina. Working upward from the perineum, press the bag's adhesive ring inside the labia. To attach the catheter to an infant boy (2), make sure the adhesive seal attaches firmly to the skin and does not pucker.

HOW TO OBTAIN A CLEAN-CATCH
MIDSTREAM SPECIMEN

Dear Patient:
Your doctor has requested a urine specimen. To minimize its contamination by organisms outside the urinary tract, you must obtain what's called a clean-catch midstream specimen. To collect this specimen, follow the instructions below:

Procedure for males

1 Before attempting to collect this specimen, make sure your bladder is moderately full. This minimizes the risk of contamination by prostatic fluid.

2 Retract your foreskin, and clean the tip of your penis (urethral meatus and glans) with an antiseptic-moistened swab, wiping in a circular motion away from the urinary opening. Discard this swab, and use another swab to remove excess antiseptic.

3 Begin voiding into a toilet or urinal, and without interrupting the flow, catch about 1 oz (30 ml) of urine in a sterile specimen container. (To prevent contamination of the specimen, don't touch the inner surface of the container or lid.)

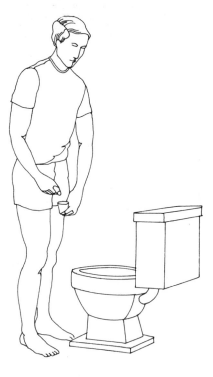

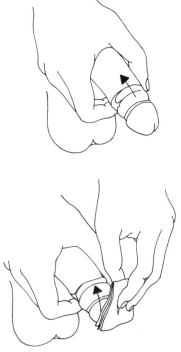

4 Replace the lid of the specimen container. If you're not going to deliver the specimen to a laboratory immediately, refrigerate the specimen.

Procedure for females

1 If you're menstruating, inform the doctor. He may want to postpone this test until after your menstrual period ends. However, if he wants to perform the test immediately, you can prevent contamination of the urine specimen with vaginal discharge or menstrual flow by inserting a tampon.

2 Kneel or squat over a bedpan or straddle the toilet bowl, to facilitate separating the folds of skin (labia) that cover the vagina and urinary opening.

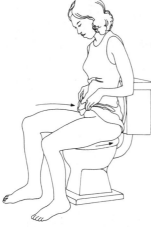

3 Expose the urinary opening (urethral meatus) by separating the labia with your thumb and forefinger. Keep the labial folds separated during the collection.

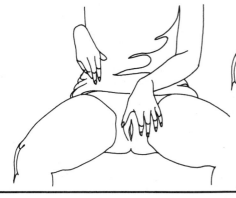

4 Clean the area around the urinary opening with three antiseptic-moistened swabs: one for each side of the urethral meatus and the third for the meatus itself. Wipe with a front-to-back motion. Remove excess antiseptic with another swab.

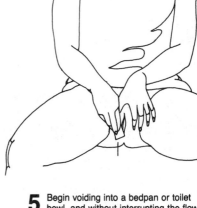

5 Begin voiding into a bedpan or toilet bowl, and without interrupting the flow, catch about 1 oz (30 ml) of urine in a sterile specimen container. (To prevent contamination of the specimen, don't touch the inner surface of the container or lid.)

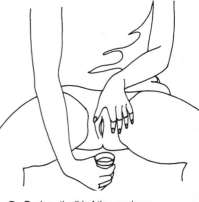

6 Replace the lid of the specimen container. If you're not going to deliver the specimen to a laboratory immediately, refrigerate the specimen.

INSERTING A STRAIGHT CATHETER

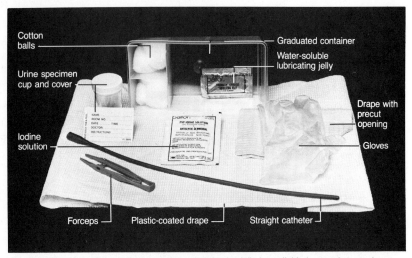

Cotton balls
Graduated container
Water-soluble lubricating jelly
Urine specimen cup and cover
Drape with precut opening
Iodine solution
Gloves
Forceps
Plastic-coated drape
Straight catheter

1 Assemble the equipment displayed above. Lubricating jelly is available in a packet, as shown, or in a prefilled syringe. In addition to the equipment shown above, to wash your patient, you'll need examining gloves, two bedsaver pads, a washcloth, a basin, a towel, mild soap, and warm water. Make sure you have strong, direct lighting. Explain the procedure and reassure your patient. Wash your hands. (For instructional purposes, this patient is shown undraped, but normally the patient is draped, to ensure comfort and privacy.)

---

doctor's name, date, and collection time. Send the specimen and a completed request slip to the laboratory immediately. On the chart, record the procedure and the time the specimen was sent.

Clean-catch midstream collection

This aseptic technique for obtaining a clean-catch midstream urine specimen has recently become the acceptable procedure for collecting a random urine specimen. It's especially valuable for collecting urine specimens in women, since it provides a specimen that's virtually free of bacterial contamination.

Instruct the patient how to obtain a clean-catch midstream specimen (see patient teaching aid on pages xxxiv and xxxv). After obtaining the specimen, send it to the laboratory immediately or refrigerate it to prevent proliferation of any bacteria that is present. On the chart,

record the procedure and the time the specimen was sent.

Timed collection

All timed specimens—2-, 12-, and 24-hour—are collected in virtually the same way. This procedure is applicable for uncatheterized adults and continent children.

Explain the procedure to the patient, and instruct him to collect all urine during the test period, to notify you after each voiding, and to avoid contaminating the specimen with toilet tissue or stool. Also, provide him with written instructions for home collection. Explain any necessary dietary, drug, or activity restrictions.

Obtain the proper preservative from the laboratory. Write down the test requirements on the nursing-care Kardex.

Label a gallon jug or commercial urine collection container with the patient's

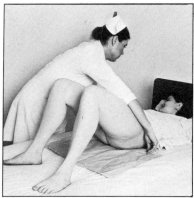

2 Position a female patient flat on her back, with her knees bent and her legs abducted. Put a bedsaver pad under her buttocks, and place her feet about 24" (61 cm) apart. Direct the light toward the perineal area.

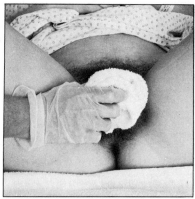

3 Put on the clean examining gloves. Using a washcloth, wash the perineum with soap and water; pat dry with a towel. Replace the wet bedsaver pad with a dry one, and remove the gloves.

Place the sterile catheter kit between the patient's legs. Open the kit, using aseptic technique. If the catheter is packaged separately, open the package and drop the catheter into the open kit.

name and room number (if applicable); doctor's name; date and time the collection begins and ends; a warning "Do Not Discard"; and instructions to keep the container refrigerated. Prominently display signs indicating that a 24-hour urine collection is in progress: one at the head of the patient's bed, a second over the toilet bowl in his bathroom, and a third over the utility room bedpan hopper.

Tell the patient to void and discard the urine; then begin 24-hour collection with the next voiding. After placing the first voiding in the container, add the preservative. Add each voiding to the container immediately. If any urine is lost, restart the test, but remember the test should end at a time the laboratory is open. Just before the end of the collection period, instruct the patient to void, and add the urine to the gallon jug.

Send the labeled container to the laboratory immediately after the collection period. On the chart, record the time urine collection ended and when the specimen was sent to the laboratory.

Special timed collections

Some tests require specimen collection at specified times—for example, the glucose tolerance test requires collection of urine at ½ hour, 1 hour, 2 hours, 3 hours, and occasionally, 4 and 5 hours after a test meal. To ensure that the patient can void at the specified times, provide water at least every hour. Other tests, including urea clearance, require only 2-hour collection periods. For these tests, give the patient at least 20 oz (600 ml) of water 30 minutes before the test, and instruct him to drink at least one full glass each hour during the test.

Pediatric urine collection

Pediatric urine collection is used to obtain a random, second-voided, first

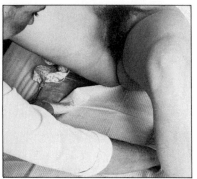

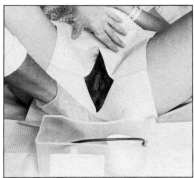

4 Continuing to use aseptic technique, put on sterile gloves, and pick up the sterile plastic-coated drape. Ask the patient to raise her pelvis by pushing down with her feet. Slide the drape under her buttocks, taking care not to touch her buttocks with your gloved hands.

Now, instruct her to lower her pelvis onto the drape.

5 Position the precut drape so that the opening is over the perineal area.

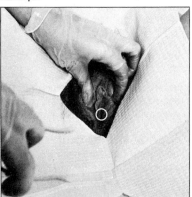

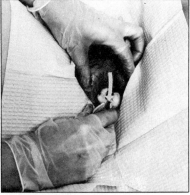

6 To clean the perineal area, use your nondominant hand to spread apart the patient's labia. Separate the labia with the thumb and index finger of the same hand to expose the urethral meatus.

Be extremely careful not to confuse the urethral opening with the vaginal opening. Look for the meatus between the clitoris and vagina. If you can't see it, it may be hidden in the anterior part of the vagina. If you can't find it there, slightly exert downward pressure when you clean between the labia (see step 7). This should open the meatus briefly.

Important: The hand used to spread apart the labia is now contaminated. Don't use it to insert the catheter.

7 With your uncontaminated hand, use the forceps to pick up a saturated cotton ball. By doing this, you keep the hand sterile for catheter insertion. With a downward stroke, clean the right labium minora, as shown.

To preserve the sterile field, discard the cotton ball into a wastebasket. Use another saturated cotton ball to clean the left labium minora. Discard this cotton ball, too. Repeat the procedure again, stroking down the middle between the labia minora.

Now, pick up the last cotton ball in the forceps, making one last stroke between the labia.

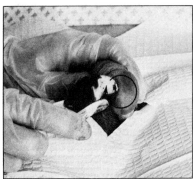

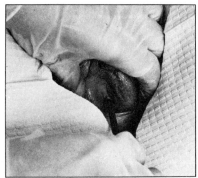

7a If the patient is a male, take his penis in your contaminated hand.

With your uncontaminated hand, use the forceps to pick up a saturated cotton ball. Clean around the meatus, using a circular motion. Then, with another cotton ball, clean in a spiral motion to the corona of the glans penis.

8 Now, with your uncontaminated hand, grasp the catheter as you would a pencil. This gives you greater control. Making sure the catheter doesn't touch the un-prepped areas of the perineum, gently insert it 2″ to 3″ (5 to 7.6 cm) into the meatus. Angle the catheter slightly upward as you advance it. *Note:* Never force the catheter.

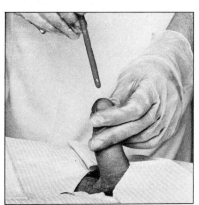

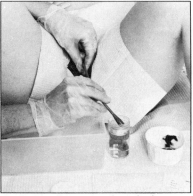

8a To prepare a male patient for catheter insertion, hold his penis at a 90° angle to his thighs. Grasp the catheter with your uncontaminated hand, and gently insert the catheter into the meatus. Advance the catheter 7″ to 10″ (17.8 to 25.4 cm) along the anterior wall of the urethra. A few inches into the urethra (at the external sphincter, which is just below the prostate), you'll encounter resistance from most patients. If your patient shows discomfort, reassure him.

Important: Never forcibly insert a catheter. If you encounter an obstruction, call the doctor. The doctor will introduce the catheter, using a guide.

9 As the catheter enters the patient's bladder, urine begins to drain. Release the labia. Using your sterile hand, place the free end of the catheter in the specimen container. Make sure you grasp the catheter high enough to prevent contamination of the specimen. Let the container fill to the three-quarters mark.

When the specimen container is filled, allow the remainder of urine to drain into a graduated container.

morning, fasting, or timed specimen from infants.

Position the patient on his back, with his hips externally rotated and abducted, and knees flexed. Clean the perineal area with cotton swabs, soap, and water. Rinse the area with warm water; dry it thoroughly.

For *boys,* apply the collection device over the penis and scrotum, and closely press the flaps of the collection bag against the perineum to ensure a tight fit.

For *girls,* tape the pediatric collection device to the perineum, starting at the point between the anus and the vagina and working anteriorly.

Place a diaper over the collection bag to discourage the child from tampering with it. Elevate the head of the bed to facilitate drainage.

Remove the bag immediately after collection is complete to prevent skin excoriation. Transfer the urine to a clean, dry specimen container. Label the container with the patient's name and room number (if applicable), doctor's name, date, and collection time. Send the specimen and the completed request slip to the laboratory immediately, and note the collection time on the chart.

Catheter collection

Although catheter collection increases the risk of bacterial infection in the lower genitourinary tract, it may be necessary to obtain a random, second-voided, first morning, fasting, or timed specimen in a patient who can't void voluntarily.

Have ready the following equipment: Sterile catheterization set (sterile gloves, sterile catheter [for adults, #16F; for children, #8F])/sterile forceps/soap, water, towelette/sterile water-soluble lubricant/sterile cotton balls/antiseptic solution/sterile drapes/sterile specimen container/labels for specimen container.

Tell the patient that you will collect a urine sample by inserting a small tube into the bladder through the urethra and that, although this procedure may cause some discomfort, it takes only a few minutes.

Male catheterization: Wash the perineal area with soap and water. Place a sterile drape under the patient's buttocks and around the penis, making sure not to contaminate the drape. Put on sterile gloves. Place sterile cleaning solution on the cotton balls. Arrange all sterile articles within easy reach on a sterile wrapper. Open the sterile specimen container, and lubricate the sterile catheter.

Grasp the shaft of the penis in one hand and elevate it about 90°, to the upright position; hold it in this position until the procedure is completed.

Retract the foreskin and, with the forceps, grasp an antiseptic-moistened cotton ball. Clean the urethral meatus, wiping with a circular motion away from the urethral opening, toward the glans. Repeat twice, each time with a clean cotton ball. *Gently* insert the lubricated catheter until urine flows. Allow a few milliliters to drain into the basin, then collect 10 to 60 ml in a sterile plastic container, depending on test requirements. After gently removing the catheter, clean and dry the periurethral area.

Send the specimen and the completed request slip to the laboratory within 10 minutes, or refrigerate the specimen. On the chart, record the procedure and the time the specimen is sent.

Female catheterization: After washing the perineal area with soap and water, place the patient in supine position, with knees flexed and feet on the bed. Place a sterile drape under the patient's buttocks and around the perineal area, making sure not to contaminate the drape. Put on sterile gloves, and place sterile cleaning solution on the cotton balls. Lubricate the sterile catheter. Arrange all sterile articles within easy reach on a sterile wrapper, and open the sterile specimen container. Separate and keep the labia majora open with one hand. With the forceps, grasp an antiseptic-moistened cotton ball. Make two vertical swipes on the labia minora. (Use a new cotton ball for *each* swipe, cleaning from the urethral meatus toward the anus.)

Position the sterile tray with the lubricated catheter on the sterile field between the patient's legs. *Gently* insert the catheter into the urethra until urine flows. Allow a few milliliters of urine to flow into a basin, then collect 10 to 60 ml in a sterile plastic container, depending on the test requirements. Gently remove the catheter; clean and dry the urethral area.

Send the specimen and a completed request slip to the laboratory within 10 minutes after collection, or refrigerate the specimen. On the chart, record the procedure and the time the specimen was sent.

Collection from an indwelling catheter

You can minimize the risk of bacterial contamination by aspirating a urine specimen from a Foley catheter made of self-sealing rubber or from a collection tube with a special sampling port. However, *don't* aspirate a Silastic, silicone, or plastic catheter. This technique can provide a random, second-voided, first morning, fasting, or timed specimen.

Have ready the following equipment: Sterile syringe (10 to 20 ml)/sterile needle (21G to 25G)/alcohol sponge/sterile specimen container/specimen labels/laboratory request slip.

About 30 minutes before collecting the specimen, clamp the collection tube. (This procedure is contraindicated for patients who've just undergone genitourinary surgery.) If the collection tube has a sampling port, wipe the sampling port with an alcohol sponge, insert the needle at a 90° angle, and aspirate the urine into the syringe. If it doesn't have a port, but if the catheter is made of rubber, you can obtain the specimen from the catheter. To do this, wipe the catheter with alcohol just above the connection of the collection tube to the catheter. Insert the needle at a 45° angle into the rubber catheter, and withdraw the urine specimen. Never insert the needle into the shaft of the catheter since this may puncture the lumen leading to the balloon.

Be sure to unclamp the tube after collecting the specimen. Failure to do so can cause bladder distension and may predispose the patient to a bladder infection. If you can't draw any urine, lift the tube a little, but make sure urine doesn't return to the bladder. Aspirate urine, and transfer the specimen to a sterile container.

Interfering factors

A common interfering factor in urine collection, especially in timed collections, is the patient's failure to follow the correct collection procedure. Improper specimens may result from *overcollection,* by failing to discard the last voiding before the test period; *undercollection,* by failing to include all urine voided during the test; *contamination,* by including toilet tissue or stool in the specimen; or, for procedures requiring collection at specified times or for the second-voided collection, the patient's *inability to urinate on demand.* In urine specimens collected from females, vaginal drainage—such as menses, which elevates RBCs—can alter the results of a urinalysis.

Improper collection or handling of the specimen can also produce unreliable results. For instance, failure to thoroughly clean the urethral meatus and glans before collection can contaminate a clean-catch midstream specimen. Similarly, failure to send a urine specimen to the laboratory immediately allows bacterial proliferation and thus invalidates the colony count on bacterial culture.

Obviously, foods and drugs can also affect test results by changing the composition of the urine. For example, ingestion of sugar increases urine glucose. Drugs can cause chemical or pharmacologic interference with the laboratory analysis. For example, aspirin causes false-positive results with Clinitest, and corticosteroids tend to elevate glucose levels.

ELAINE GILLIGAN WHELAN, RN, BS, MA

1 Hematology

LEARNING OBJECTIVES

After completing this chapter, the reader will be able to:
- describe the formation, components, and functions of red blood cells (RBCs).
- describe the types and functions of white blood cells (WBCs).
- explain how hypoxia stimulates erythropoiesis.
- list drugs that decrease the WBC count.
- list five disorders that affect serum iron and total iron-binding capacity.
- identify the causes of abnormal blood cell production.
- discuss the significance of the complete blood count and differential.
- state the purpose of each test discussed in the chapter.
- prepare the patient physically and psychologically for each test.
- describe the procedure for performing each test.
- specify appropriate precautions for accurate administration of each test.
- implement appropriate post-test care.
- state the normal values for each test.
- discuss the implications of abnormal test results.
- list factors that may interfere with accurate test results.

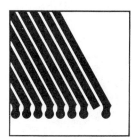

Hematology

Introduction

Blood is a continuously circulating tissue that performs many vital functions as it flows through the body. Most important is its ability to transport oxygen (bound to hemoglobin in RBCs) from the lungs to the body tissues and to return carbon dioxide from the tissues to the lungs. Blood also produces and delivers antibodies formed by plasma cells and lymphocytes; contains leukocytes that consume pathogens by phagocytosis; and provides complement, a group of immunologically significant protein substances.

Other functions performed by blood include maintenance of hemostasis with platelets and with coagulation factors, which repair tissue injuries and prevent bleeding; regulation of body temperature and of acid-base and fluid balances; movement of nutrients and regulatory hormones to body tissues; and disposal of metabolic wastes through the kidneys, lungs, and skin.

Blood is three times as viscous as water, tastes slightly salty, and has an alkaline pH of 7.35 to 7.45. Oxygenated arterial blood is bright red; oxygen-poor venous blood is dark red.

Blood has two major components; plasma, the clear, straw-colored liquid portion; and the formed elements, erythrocytes (red blood cells), leukocytes (white blood cells), and thrombocytes (platelets).

Red cells

Also known as erythrocytes and red corpuscles, red blood cells (RBCs) appear in the embryonic yolk sac during the first weeks of development. During the second trimester, the fetal liver produces most red cells, with the spleen and the lymph nodes acting as backup suppliers. Starting just before birth and continuing through adulthood, the marrow of membranous bones (sternum, ribs, vertebrae, and pelvis) becomes the primary source of red cells; the marrow of long bones (humerus, femur, tibia) acts as a secondary source. Red cell production declines with advancing age.

Current theory states that hemocytoblasts are the progenitors of red cells. Hemocytoblasts repeatedly change shape and function until they become mature red cells. Most circulating red cells are biconcave, range in color from pale pink at the center to deep pink at the periphery, and are disk-shaped. Abnormal red cells may vary in size (anisocytosis) or in color (anisochromia), or may assume permanent changes in shape (poikilocytosis). In *anisocytosis*, cell diameter ranges from about 6 microns (microcytic) to 9 microns (macrocytic), with slight, moderate, or marked gradations. In *anisochromia*, RBC color ranges from insufficient (hypochromic) to excessive (hyperchromic). In *poikilocytosis*, bizarre shapes—teardrop, dumbbell, or

BLOOD CELL DISORDERS

RED CELL DISORDERS

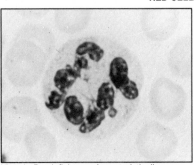

Vitamin B₁₂ deficiency: characteristically marked by a macrocytic neutrophil cell with increased lobulation, interspersed with macrocytic erythrocytes

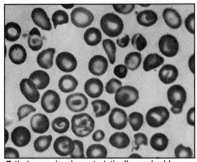

B-thalassemia: characteristically marked by erythrocytes which vary in size and shape and include target cells (dark centers encircled by pale rings)

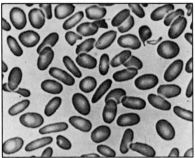

Hereditary ovalocytosis: characteristically marked by oval erythrocytes with pale centers

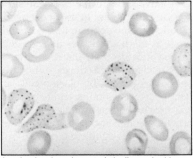

Lead poisoning: characteristically marked by basophilic stippling of red blood cells

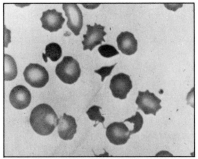

Thrombotic thrombocytopenic purpura: characteristically marked by helmet, thorn, burr and fragmented erythrocytes and diffusely basophilic cells

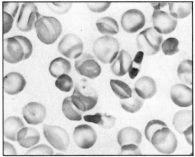

Hemoglobin S-C disease: characteristically marked by "SC" red cells (dense staining finger-like protrusions in center), many target cells (dark centers encircled by pale rings) and several folded and irregular spherical cells

WHITE CELL DISORDERS

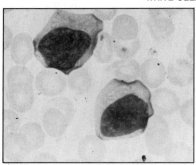

Infectious mononucleosis: characteristically marked by large, reactive lymphocytes interspersed with normal erythrocytes

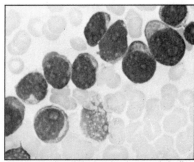

Acute granulocytic leukemia: characteristically marked by myeloblasts showing early chromatin pattern and nucleoli

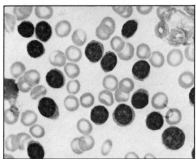

Chronic lymphocytic leukemia: characteristically marked by increased numbers of mature lymphocytes and thrombocytopenia, shown in the photograph by two disintegrated cells (smudges)

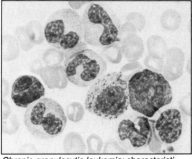

Chronic granulocytic leukemia: characteristically marked by leukocytosis shown in the photograph by the presence of a progranulocyte, a neutrophilic myelocyte, a neutrophilic metamyelocyte, neutrophilic bands, and basophils

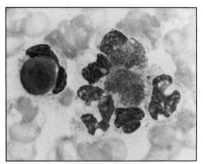

Lupus erythematosus: characteristically marked by LE rosette and LE cell

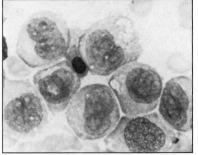

Acute monocytic leukemia: characteristically marked by monoblasts, promonocytes, prominent nucleoli, nuclear folding, abundant blue cytoplasm, vacuoles, and pseudopods

pear—generally reflect abnormal cell formation and development in the bone marrow.

The number of red cells in an adult varies according to sex, age, and geographic location. Men usually have higher counts than women, and the elderly have fewer red cells than young adults. Persons living at high altitudes generally have more red cells than those living at sea level—a compensatory adaptation to the thinner air.

Red cell function

A primary function of red cells is to maintain a high concentration of circulatory hemoglobin. Hemoglobin—the main component of the red cell—is a conjugated protein that enables red cells to carry oxygen from the lungs to the tissues, and to carry carbon dioxide from the tissues back to the lungs, for excretion. Red cells also transport large quantities of carbon dioxide through the activity of carbonic anhydrase, a red cell enzyme. By accelerating the reaction between carbon dioxide and water, this enzyme promotes absorption into the blood of large quantities of carbon dioxide. Thus, red cells help maintain the body's acid-base balance.

Mature red cells circulate in the blood for about 120 days. As they age, these cells become fragile, finally rupture and decompose, and then are removed by the spleen and the liver.

Hemoglobin

Hemoglobin (Hgb), which constitutes about 90% of the mature red cell's dry weight, is composed of 4% heme—an iron and porphyrin complex that colors it—and 96% globin—a simple water-soluble protein. Hemoglobin synthesis depends on the metabolisms of heme, globin, and iron.

The body contains about 4 g of iron; more than half this amount is in the hemoglobin of red cells. Absorption is strictly limited by the iron storage capacity of the liver, spleen, and bone marrow. In a normal iron ingestion cycle, iron is absorbed from food in the upper intestine, primarily the duodenum. For transport, iron combines with a glycoprotein, transferrin. Some iron is transported to the bone marrow for hemoglobin synthesis; some goes to needy tissues, such as muscle, for myoglobin synthesis; and unused iron is converted to ferritin and is stored in the liver, spleen, bone marrow, and reticuloendothelial system. The iron in the hemoglobin of aging red cells is recycled by the spleen, either for inclusion in new red cells or for storage in the liver. Normally, less than 1 mg of iron is lost daily through the skin, feces, and urine.

Three major types of hemoglobin are found in normal blood: Hgb A, Hgb A_2, and Hgb F. Hgb A accounts for more than 95% of adult hemoglobin, with Hgb A_2 comprising 2% to 3%. Although traces of Hgb F appear in adult blood, this type of hemoglobin appears predominately in the fetus and neonate, thereafter decreasing to 2% to 3% of the infant's blood at age 6 months.

Hemoglobin variants

Because one molecule of hemoglobin is composed of four heme groups, it can carry four molecules of oxygen. It also consists of two pairs of polypeptide chains, called *globins*. Variations occur, however, creating abnormal hemoglobins. Since the heme portion of all hemoglobin is identical, variations are possible only in the polypeptide segments, resulting from substitutions in any of the amino acid chains. Such substitutions may result in hemoglobin with an unstable structure (unstable hemoglobin). An identical substitution in both polypeptide pairs produces a *homozygous* variation; a substitution in one pair or nonidentical changes in both pairs result in *heterozygous* variation. Overall, genetic and acquired variations account for more than 200 abnormal hemoglobins.

Except for the normal Hgb F and Hgb A, and the abnormal Hgb S (present in sickle cell anemia), hemoglobins are identified by sequential letters of the alphabet. When hemoglobins show elec-

ABNORMAL HEMOGLOBIN VARIANTS

CLASSIFICATION	ABNORMAL HEMOGLOBIN	CLINICAL EFFECTS
Homozygous (double complement of genes)	S	Sickle cell anemia
	C	Three variants, two of which cause sickling
	D, E	Mild hemolytic anemia
	M	Methemoglobinemia and cyanosis
Heterozygous (bearing a single gene)	Chesapeake, Hiroshima, Capetown, Bethesda	Increased oxygen affinity and polycythemia
	Kansas, Seattle, Bristol, Yoshizuka	Decreased oxygen affinity, cyanosis, and anemia
	Torino, Ann Arbor, Hasharon	Congenital Heinz body hemolytic anemia
	H, Bart's	Thalassemias

trophoretic migration, their names reflect their places of discovery—for example, Hgb D Punjab. In addition, the Greek letters alpha and beta identify a known abnormal polypeptide chain.

Abnormal red cell production

Erythropoietin, a glycoprotein of low molecular weight originating in the kidneys, stimulates production, maturation, and release of red cells from bone marrow and other blood-forming tissues. Low oxygen levels in the kidneys and in other tissues (hypoxia) cause secretion of this glycoprotein, which accelerates red cell production. Hypoxia can result from severe anemia, heart failure, pulmonary disease, or living at high altitudes.

Anemias, characterized by abnormally low hemoglobin concentration, red cell count, and hematocrit, may reflect acute or chronic blood loss, excessive hemolysis, or deficient blood production. Anemias are classified by their causes or by the typical structural changes they produce in the blood. Red cells are classified by size as normocytic (normal), microcytic (small), or macrocytic (large), and by hemoglobin content as normochromic (normal color) or hypochromic (pale).

These classifications, considered together, can describe anemia accurately. If the size, shape, hemoglobin content and concentration, and mean corpuscular volume of RBCs are normal but RBC production is depressed, the patient has *normocytic normochromic anemia.* Such anemia results from debilitating disorders, such as cancer and chronic infection. If RBCs have normal color but are abnormally large, the patient has *macrocytic normochromic anemia,* commonly associated with vitamin B_{12} or folic acid deficiency. If RBCs are small and pale from hemoglobin deficiency, the patient has *microcytic hypochromic anemia,* which most often results from iron deficiency.

Hemolytic anemia, with red cell destruction, may result from a congenital defect (such as sickle cell anemia or thalassemia) or as an acquired response to certain drugs (such as methyldopa); to certain disorders (Hodgkin's disease, lupus erythematosus, or lymphomas); or to antigens (transfusion reaction).

Similarly, reduced erythropoiesis may result from various disease states and deficiencies. For example, chronic bone marrow hypoplasia and varying degrees of pancytopenia (aplastic anemia) can result from prolonged X-ray therapy. Impairment or destruction of bone marrow by cancer, thymic tumor, or chloramphenicol creates deficiency of hemocytoblasts, causing anemia. Deficient erythropoiesis also results from deficiency of iron, folic acid, or vitamin B_{12}. A major cause of deficient erythropoiesis, particularly in renal failure, is impaired secretion of erythropoietin, the hormone that stimulates bone marrow

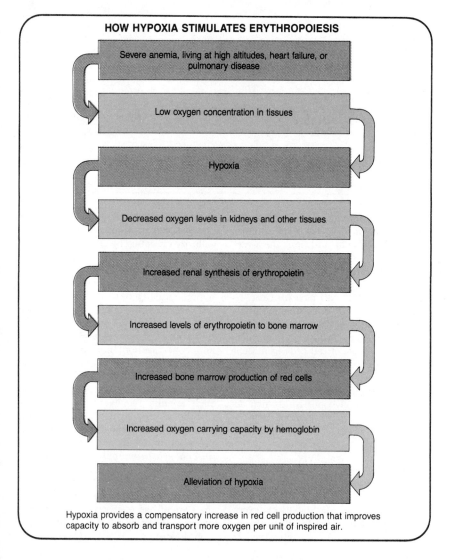

HOW HYPOXIA STIMULATES ERYTHROPOIESIS

Severe anemia, living at high altitudes, heart failure, or pulmonary disease

Low oxygen concentration in tissues

Hypoxia

Decreased oxygen levels in kidneys and other tissues

Increased renal synthesis of erythropoietin

Increased levels of erythropoietin to bone marrow

Increased bone marrow production of red cells

Increased oxygen carrying capacity by hemoglobin

Alleviation of hypoxia

Hypoxia provides a compensatory increase in red cell production that improves capacity to absorb and transport more oxygen per unit of inspired air.

production. The renal mechanism in erythropoietin production is still unclear, but erythropoietin levels drop markedly when the kidneys are removed.

Polycythemias

The body reacts to hypoxia by a compensatory increase in red cell production. Severe and chronic hypoxia, such as results from congenital heart disease and pulmonary disease, can lead to overcompensation and overproduction of red cells, a condition called polycythemia.

Polycythemias may be relative, absolute, or primary, and either reactive or secondary. In *relative polycythemia* (also called spurious polycythemia), hematocrit is elevated and circulating plasma volume is decreased, but total red cell mass is normal. Relative polycythemia develops after dehydration from vomiting, diarrhea, or heatstroke, and in massive fluid loss following extensive burns. In *absolute* or *primary polycythemia* (polycythemia vera), the red cell count may rise to 8 million as the circulating mass of red cells increases, and hematocrit rises to 70% to 80%. *Secondary* or *reactive polycythemia* develops in persons who live at altitudes higher than 14,000 feet; to compensate for less atmospheric oxygen, the blood needs a greater number of RBCs to meet the body's oxygen requirements. Secondary polycythemia results from abnormal conditions, including certain hemoglobinopathies, cardiopulmonary disease, and certain renal cysts and tumors.

Five types of white cells

White blood cells (leukocytes, WBCs) are known as neutrophils, eosinophils, basophils, monocytes, and lymphocytes. The names of the first three cell types reflect their affinity for certain dyes and stains. For example, *neutrophils* accept both acidic and basic stains. White cells that develop an orange-red cytoplasm when stained with the coal tar dye eosin are called *eosinophils* (eosin-loving cells). *Basophils* are so called because their cytoplasm readily accepts a basic dye. These three cell types are collectively known as *granulocytes,* because they have irregularly shaped nuclei and granules dispersed in their cytoplasm.

Monocytes and *lymphocytes* are mononuclear cells. Monocytes are phagocytic and develop into macrophages. Most lymphocytes are formed in lymphoid tissue, but a few lymphocytes, as well as neutrophils, basophils, eosinophils, and monocytes, are formed only in bone marrow.

The special function of white cells, particularly neutrophils, is to protect the body against infection. WBCs respond to inflammation by chemotaxis, a process of chemical attraction or repulsion. Inflamed tissue causes positive chemotaxis, a biochemical alarm that draws white cells to the infected area. White cells move about by amoeboid motion or diapedesis. In amoeboid motion, one end of the cell alternately protrudes and pulls the remainder of the cell along with it. In diapedesis, the cell squeezes itself through pores or interstitial spaces in the capillary endothelium. Once at the infection site, white cells engulf and digest any foreign matter by a process called phagocytosis.

Granulocytes

Produced in the bone marrow and stored there until the body needs them, granulocytes normally circulate for about 12 hours, but during severe stress, they survive only 2 or 3 hours. Several abnormal cellular inclusions can appear in granulocytes:

☐ *Toxic granulations:* Patients with severe bacterial infection or fever associated with extensive tissue damage may have neutrophils with deeply staining granules. These granules may be abnormally activated neutrophilic granules rather than inclusion bodies or phagocytized material.

☐ *Döhle's inclusion bodies:* Patients with severe burns, bacterial infection, malignant disease, or extensive cytolysis may have neutrophils with large, round, blue cytoplasmic masses. These bodies reflect a too-rapid proliferation of neutrophils but may also occur in normal pregnancy.

PHAGOCYTOSIS—
ENGULFMENT AND DESTRUCTION OF FOREIGN PARTICLES

1 — Opsonizing antibodies
— Bacterium
— Opsonized bacteria
— Pseudopod
2 — Phagosome
4
— Release of digestive debris
3 — Phagolysosome

In response to infection, chemotaxis directs macrophages to the site of inflammation. At the infection site, phagocytosis—engulfment and destruction of the bacteria or other foreign particles—occurs.

First, bacteria attach to the cell surface, initiating opsonization (figure 1), antibody coating of the bacteria that enables phagocytosis. Then, macrophages surround the bacteria by forming pseudopods—footlike extensions (figure 2). Phagosomes digest the foreign particle and merge with lysosomes, becoming phagolysosomes (figure 3), which release enzymes that help iodine, bromide, and chloride bind to the cell wall to destroy the bacteria. Finally, macrophages release digestive debris (figure 4), so they can continue to fight infection.

□ *Azurophil granules:* Small, smoothly rounded granules that contain diverse lysosomal enzymes, azurophil granules appear in lymphocytes, monocytes, and immature granulocytes. After such cells mature and specific granulation develops, a few azurophil granules persist in the cells but reflect no pathology.

□ *Auer bodies (Auer rods):* Composed of slender, rodlike masses of pink or purple cytoplasmic material, Auer bodies indicate abnormal cellular development of granulocytes or monocytes. Since these bodies never appear in lymphocytes, their presence makes possible the classification of very immature, undifferentiated leukemic cells as belonging to the myelomonocytic series.

□ *Hypersegmentation and macropolycytes:* Abnormal metabolism of folic acid and vitamin B_{12} may induce production of abnormally large granulocytes and erythrocytes. Hypersegmented neutrophils may have seven or eight lobes in their nuclei, instead of the normal three to five.

Neutrophils

More than half the white cells in the peripheral circulation are neutrophils. Since they quickly phagocytize significant quantities of microorganisms, neutrophils are the body's first line of defense against infection. Each mature neutrophil can inactivate 5 to 20 bacteria.

A small number of slightly immature neutrophils, known as *band cells,* normally appears in peripheral blood. In a differential count, the presence of many band cells and their precursors is known as a shift to the left and indicates infection. A shift to the right describes the presence of mature, hypersegmented neutrophils that have more nuclear segments than normal; this commonly occurs with pernicious anemia and hepatic disease. Increased band cells and a low total WBC count reflect bone marrow depression (as in typhoid fever), known as a degenerative shift. A regenerative shift implies stimulation of the bone marrow (as in pneumonia and appendicitis), and may be noted by increased band cells, metamyelocytes, and myelocytes, together with a high WBC count.

Eosinophils

Although eosinophils are phagocytic, they proliferate in response to allergic conditions rather than to bacterial infection. In allergic reactions, eosinophils pour into the blood and collect at the site of tissue inflammation. Eosinophils detoxify foreign protein matter and ingest antigen-antibody complexes before they can damage the body. The most common causes of eosinophilia are allergic disorders and parasitic infections.

Basophils

Basophils contain large amounts of histamine. Although their function isn't fully understood, they're thought to help the body resist systemic allergic reactions and anaphylactoid states by being transported by the blood to tissues, where they become mast cells. They proliferate during inflammation, releasing histamine as well as bradykinin and serotonin.

Monocytes to macrophages

The body's second line of defense, monocytes arrive at infection sites in smaller numbers than do neutrophils. Bone marrow releases immature monocytes into the circulation. Within a few hours, they enter the tissue, where they perform their phagocytic function. As a monocyte matures into a macrophage, it enlarges; its lysosome and hydrolytic enzymes increase, enhancing its bactericidal activity. These macrophages ingest debris, and depending on the amount ingested, they may eventually become so engorged that they die. Immature monocytes that become fixed in the tissue are called *tissue macrophages,* or *histiocytes;* they become part of the reticuloendothelial system and establish themselves in the lymph nodes, alveoli of the lungs, the spleen, the bone marrow, and the hepatic sinuses (in the latter, they are known as *Kupffer cells*).

Lymphocytes

Important in both humoral and cell-mediated immunity, lymphocytes are produced in the lymph glands, spleen, thymus, tonsils, and lymphoid tissue of the gut. Together with neutrophils, lymphocytes comprise the majority of white cells. In cellular immunity, sensitized T-(thymus-derived) lymphocytes attach to and destroy specific foreign antigens. Humoral immunity refers to the production of circulating antibodies by B-(bone marrow–derived) lymphocytes that attack invading microorganisms.

Abnormal immune reactions to viral infections may cause characteristic changes in the appearance of mature lymphocytes, which are then called *reactive* or *atypical lymphocytes.* These cells may appear in infectious mononucleosis, hepatitis, viral pneumonia, and allergic conditions.

Plasma cells

Usually found in the lymphoid tissue but rarely in the peripheral circulation, plasma cells produce antibodies to help fight disease. Contact with a specific antigen causes certain lymphocytes to become plasma cells and stimulates their immune activity. Plasma cells may appear in the circulation during severe infection, to reinforce immunity when sufficient antibodies are not available. The presence of such cells in the blood may indicate multiple myeloma, plasma cell leukemia, scarlet fever, measles, or chickenpox.

Reticuloendothelial system

The reticuloendothelial system (RES) is made up of tissue histiocytes, macrophages, and lymphatic tissue. Reticuloendothelial cells are much less mobile than circulating white cells, but like them, RES cells remove foreign matter and endogenous debris from the blood, lymph, and interstitial spaces of the body. For example, when hemoglobin enters the blood from ruptured red cells, reticuloendothelial cells digest it.

Abnormal white cell production

Malignant mutation of the blood-forming tissues can cause unrestrained white cell production, better known as *leukemia.* This condition is marked by a sharp rise in the number of abnormal white cells, first in the tissues of origin and then throughout the body.

Leukemias are classified according to the type of white cell proliferation: lymphocytic, granulocytic, or monocytic. The more immature the blood cell—that is, the more primitive its development— the more severe the disease; the older the cell, the more chronic the disease. For example, abnormal, excessive granulocyte production results in *chronic granulocytic leukemia.* Abnormally high levels of immature lymphocytes and their precursors (lymphoblasts) predominate in *acute lymphoblastic leukemia.*

In *agranulocytosis,* bone marrow stops producing granulocytes, leaving the body virtually defenseless against infection. Acute agranulocytosis, which is fatal if untreated, may result from infection; the effect of certain antibodies; or certain drugs (such as clindamycin, sulfonamides, melphalan, and other chemotherapeutic agents, and barbiturates).

Blood platelets

Derived from megakaryocytes in bone marrow and also known as thrombocytes, platelets protect vascular surfaces and help the blood clot to stop bleeding. Abnormal platelet function (thrombasthenia) and decreased platelet counts (thrombocytopenia) can interfere with hemostasis. (The significance of platelets is discussed in chapter 2, HEMOSTASIS.)

Complete blood count (CBC)

This often requested test gives a fairly complete picture of all the blood's formed elements. The CBC generally is composed of two sections: direct measurement of cellular components, including hemoglobin and erythrocyte indices, and differentiation of white blood cells, with an assessment of WBC, RBC, and platelet morphology. The following tests are usually included: hemoglobin concentration, hematocrit, red and white counts, differential white cell count, and stained red cell examination. Besides pointing the way toward further definitive studies, CBC data have proven extremely valuable in themselves.

CBC data can detect anemias, determine their severity, and compare the status of specific blood elements. Thus, the CBC is especially useful for evaluating conditions in which hematocrit does not parallel the red cell count. Normally, as the red cell count rises, so does hematocrit. However, in patients with microcytic or macrocytic anemia, this natural correlation does not hold true. For example, the patient with iron deficiency anemia has undersized red cells that cause his hematocrit to decrease, even though his red cell count may be reported as nearly normal. Conversely, the patient with pernicious anemia has many oversized red cells that cause his hematocrit to be higher than his red cell count.

White cell differential

Although the white cell count alone can detect infection, a white cell differential adds a detailed evaluation of white cell distribution and morphology that can help identify specific infections. Thus, while a WBC count merely confirms moderate infection, a white cell differential can aid in positively identifying the infection. A differential also detects abnormal white cells, revealing neutrophil shifts.

The stained red cell examination often accompanies the white cell differential as part of the CBC. After the differential, the same stained slide is evaluated for RBC distribution and morphology, including changes in cell contents, color, size, and shape, providing additional information for detecting leukemia, anemia, and thalassemia. Variations in size and shape are reported as occasional, slight, moderate, marked, or very marked; structural variations are reported as the number of immature or nucleated RBCs/100 WBCs, noting cell inclusions.

WILLIAM M. DOUGHERTY, BS
MARYLOU K. MCHUGH, RN, MSN

RED CELL TESTS

Red Blood Cell Count

[Erythrocyte count]

This test reports the number of red blood cells (RBCs) found in a microliter (cubic millimeter) of whole blood, and is included in the complete blood count. Traditionally counted by hand with a hemacytometer, RBCs are now commonly counted with electronic devices such as the Coulter counter, which provide faster, more accurate results. The RBC count itself provides no qualitative information regarding the size, shape, or concentration of hemoglobin within the corpuscles but may be used to calculate two erythrocyte indices: mean corpuscular volume (MCV) and mean corpuscular hemoglobin (MCH).

Purpose

□ To supply figures for computing the erythrocyte indices, which reveal RBC size and hemoglobin content
□ To support other hematologic tests in diagnosis of anemia and polycythemia.

Patient preparation

Explain to the patient that this test evaluates the number of RBCs to detect suspected blood disorders. Inform him that he needn't restrict food or fluids. Tell him this test requires a blood sample; who will perform the venipuncture and when; and that he may experience transient discomfort from the needle puncture and the pressure of the tourniquet. If the patient is an infant or child, explain to the parents (and to the child if he is old enough to understand) that a small amount of blood will be drawn from his finger or earlobe. Reassure the patient that collecting the sample takes less than 3 minutes.

Procedure

For adults and older children, draw venous blood into a 7-ml *lavender-top* tube. For younger children, collect capillary blood in a pipette or Microtainer.

Precautions

□ Completely fill the collection tube, and invert it gently several times to mix the sample and the anticoagulant.
□ Handle the sample gently to prevent hemolysis.

Values

Normal RBC values vary, depending on age, sex, sample, and geographic location. In adult males, red cell counts range from 4.5 to 6.2 million/μl of venous blood; in adult females, 4.2 to 5.4 million/μl of venous blood; in children, 4.6 to 4.8 million/μl of venous blood. In full-term infants, values range from 4.4 to 5.8 million/μl of capillary blood at birth; fall to 3 to 3.8 million/μl at age 2 months; and increase slowly thereafter. Values are generally higher in persons living at high altitudes.

Implications of results

An elevated RBC count may indicate primary or secondary polycythemia, or dehydration; a depressed count may indicate anemia, fluid overload, or recent hemorrhage. Further tests, such as stained cell examination, hematocrit, hemoglobin, red cell indices, and white cell studies, are needed to confirm diagnosis.

Post-test care

If a hematoma develops at the venipuncture site, apply warm soaks.

Interfering factors

The following factors may interfere with accurate determination of test results:
☐ failure to use the proper anticoagulant in the collection tube and to adequately mix the sample and anticoagulant
☐ hemolysis due to rough handling of the sample
☐ hemoconcentration due to prolonged tourniquet constriction
☐ hemodilution caused by drawing the sample from the same arm that is being used for I.V. infusion of fluids
☐ high white cell count, which falsely elevates red cell count in semiautomated and automated counters
☐ diseases that cause RBCs to agglutinate or form rouleaux, which falsely decreases red cell count.

WILLIAM M. DOUGHERTY, BS

Hematocrit

Hematocrit (Hct), a common, reliable test, may be done by itself or as part of a complete blood count. It measures the percentage by volume of packed RBCs in a whole blood sample; for example, an Hct of 40% means that a 100-ml sample contains 40 ml of packed RBCs. This packing is achieved by centrifugation of anticoagulated whole blood in a capillary tube, so that red cells are tightly packed without hemolysis.

Most commonly, Hct is measured electronically, producing results 3% lower than when Hct is measured manually. (Manual measurement traps plasma in the column of packed RBCs.) Test results may be used to calculate two erythrocyte indices: mean corpuscular volume (MCV) and mean corpuscular hemoglobin concentration (MCHC).

Purpose
☐ To aid diagnosis of abnormal states of hydration, polycythemia, and anemia
☐ To aid in calculating red cell indices.

Patient preparation

Explain to the patient that this test detects anemia and other abnormal conditions of the blood. Inform him he needn't restrict food or fluids before the test. Tell him the test requires a blood sample; who will perform the venipuncture and when; and that he may experience transient discomfort from the needle puncture and the pressure of the tourniquet. If the patient is an infant or child, explain to the parents (and to the child if he's old enough to understand) that a small amount of blood will be drawn from his finger or earlobe. Reassure the patient that collecting the sample will take less than 3 minutes.

Procedure

Perform a finger stick, using a heparinized capillary tube with a red band on the anticoagulant end.

Precautions

Fill the capillary tube from the red-banded end to about two-thirds capacity, and seal this end with clay. Send the sample to the laboratory immediately. Or, if you perform the test, place the tube in the centrifuge, with the red end pointing outward.

Values

Hematocrit values vary, depending on the

patient's sex and age, type of sample, and the laboratory performing the test. See the accompanying chart for normal values within age groups.

Implications of results

Low Hct may indicate anemia or hemodilution; high Hct suggests polycythemia or hemoconcentration due to blood loss.

Post-test care

If a hematoma develops at the veni-

puncture site, apply warm soaks.

Interfering factors

□ Failure to use the proper anticoagulant in the collection tube and to fill it appropriately may interfere with accurate determination of test results.

□ Hemolysis due to rough handling of the sample may affect test results.

□ Tourniquet constriction for longer than 1 minute causes hemoconcentration and typically raises Hct by 2.5% to 5%.

□ Taking the blood sample from the

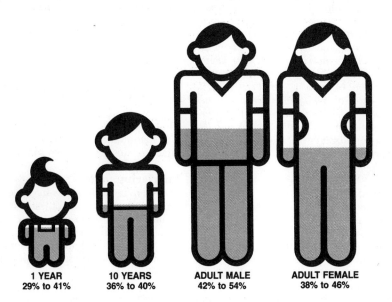

NORMAL HEMATOCRIT VARIES ACCORDING TO AGE

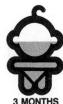

NEWBORN
55% to 68%

1 WEEK
47% to 65%

1 MONTH
37% to 49%

3 MONTHS
30% to 36%

1 YEAR
29% to 41%

10 YEARS
36% to 40%

ADULT MALE
42% to 54%

ADULT FEMALE
38% to 46%

same arm that is being used for I.V. infusion of fluids causes hemodilution.

☐ Failure to adequately mix the sample and anticoagulant may hinder accurate determination of test results.

☐ Excessive centrifugation of the sample results in hemolysis.

WILLIAM M. DOUGHERTY, BS

Red Cell Indices

[Erythrocyte indices]

Using the results of the RBC count, hematocrit, and total hemoglobin tests, the red cell indices provide important information about the size, hemoglobin concentration, and hemoglobin weight of an average red cell. The indices include mean corpuscular volume (MCV), mean corpuscular hemoglobin (MCH), and mean corpuscular hemoglobin concentration (MCHC).

MCV, the ratio of hematocrit (packed cell volume) to the RBC count, expresses the average size of the erythrocytes and indicates whether they are undersized (microcytic), oversized (macrocytic), or normal (normocytic). MCH, the hemoglobin-RBC ratio, gives the weight of hemoglobin in an average red cell. MCHC, the ratio of hemoglobin weight to hematocrit, defines the concentration of hemoglobin in 100 ml of packed red cells. It helps distinguish normally colored (normochromic) red cells from paler (hypochromic) red cells.

Purpose
☐ To aid diagnosis and classification of anemias.

Patient preparation
Explain to the patient that this test helps determine if he has anemia. Tell him the test requires a blood sample; who will perform the venipuncture and when; and that he may experience transient discomfort from the needle puncture and tour-

niquet pressure. However, collecting the sample takes less than 3 minutes.

Procedure
Perform a venipuncture, and collect the sample in a 7 ml *lavender-top* tube.

Precautions
☐ Completely fill the collection tube, and invert it gently several times to adequately mix the sample and anticoagulant.

☐ Handle the sample gently to prevent hemolysis.

Values
The range of normal red cell indices is as follows:
☐ MCV: 84 to 99 μ^3/red cell
☐ MCH: 26 to 32 pg/red cell
☐ MCHC: 30% to 36%.

Implications of results
The red cell indices aid in classification of anemias. Low MCV and MCHC indicate microcytic, hypochromic anemias caused by iron deficiency anemia, pyridoxine-responsive anemia, and thalassemia. A high MCV suggests macrocytic anemias caused by megaloblastic anemias, due to folic acid or vitamin B_{12} deficiency, inherited disorders of DNA synthesis, and reticulocytosis. Because MCV reflects average volume of many cells, a value within normal range can encompass RBCs of varying size, from microcytic to macrocytic.

Post-test care
If a hematoma develops at the venipuncture site, apply warm soaks.

Interfering factors
The following factors may interfere with accurate determination of test results:
☐ failure to use the proper anticoagulant in the collection tube, and to adequately mix the sample and anticoagulant
☐ hemolysis due to rough handling of the sample
☐ hemoconcentration due to prolonged tourniquet constriction
☐ high white cell count, which falsely elevates red cell count in semiautomated

COMPARATIVE RED CELL INDICES IN ANEMIAS

	NORMAL VALUES (Normocytic, normochromic)	IRON DEFICIENCY ANEMIA (Microcytic, hypochromic)	PERNICIOUS ANEMIA (Macrocytic, normochromic)
MCV	84 to 99μ³	60 to 80μ³	95 to 150μ³
MCH	26 to 32 pg	5 to 25 pg	33 to 53 pg
MCHC	30% to 36%	20% to 30%	33% to 38%

and automated counters, invalidates MCV and MCH results
□ falsely elevated hemoglobin values invalidate MCH and MCHC results
□ diseases that cause RBCs to agglutinate or form rouleaux falsely decrease red cell count and invalidate test results.

WILLIAM M. DOUGHERTY, BS

Erythrocyte Sedimentation Rate

The erythrocyte sedimentation rate (ESR) measures the time required for erythrocytes in a whole blood sample to settle to the bottom of a vertical tube. As the red cells descend in the tube, they displace an equal volume of plasma upward, which retards the downward progress of other settling blood elements. Factors affecting ESR include red cell volume, surface area, density, aggregation, and surface charge. Plasma proteins (notably fibrinogen and globulin) en- *courage aggregation, increasing ESR.*

The ESR is a sensitive but nonspecific test that is frequently the earliest indicator of disease when other chemical or physical signs are normal. It often rises significantly in widespread inflammatory disorders due to infection or autoimmune mechanisms; such elevations may be prolonged in localized inflammation and malignancy.

Purpose
□ To monitor inflammatory or malignant disease
□ To aid detection and diagnosis of occult disease, such as tuberculosis, tissue necrosis, or connective tissue disease.

Patient preparation
Explain to the patient that this test evaluates the condition of RBCs. Inform him that he needn't restrict food or fluids. Tell him the test requires a blood sample; who will perform the venipuncture and when; and that he may experience transient discomfort from the needle puncture and the pressure of the tourniquet. Collecting the sample takes less than 3 minutes.

Procedure
Perform a venipuncture, and collect the sample in a 7-ml *lavender-top*, 4.5-ml *black-top*, or 4.5-ml *blue-top* tube. (Check with the laboratory to determine its preference.)

Precautions
☐ Completely fill the collection tube, and invert it gently several times to adequately mix the sample and the anticoagulant.

☐ Since prolonged standing decreases the ESR, after examining the sample for clots or clumps, send it to the laboratory immediately (it must be tested within 2 hours).

☐ Handle the sample gently to prevent hemolysis.

Values
Normal sedimentation rates range from 0 to 20 mm/hour; rates gradually increase with age.

Implications of results
The ESR rises in pregnancy, acute or chronic inflammation, tuberculosis, paraproteinemias (especially multiple myeloma and Waldenström's macroglobulinemia), rheumatic fever, rheumatoid arthritis, and some malignancies. Anemia

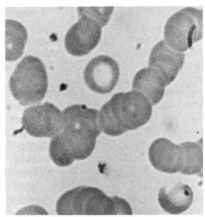

As erythrocytes settle to the bottom of a vertical tube, they may line up in a rouleau formation, resembling a pile of coins. This formation usually indicates paraproteinemia, plasma cell myeloma, or macroglobulinemia.

also tends to raise ESR, since less upward displacement of plasma occurs to retard the relatively few sedimenting RBCs. Polycythemia, sickle cell anemia, hyperviscosity, or low plasma protein level tends to depress ESR.

Post-test care
If a hematoma develops at the venipuncture site, apply warm soaks.

Interfering factors
☐ Failure to use the proper anticoagulant in the collection tube, to adequately mix the sample and anticoagulant, and to send the sample to the laboratory immediately may interfere with accurate determination of test results.

☐ Hemolysis due to rough handling or excessive mixing of the sample may affect the sedimentation.

☐ Prolonged tourniquet constriction may cause hemoconcentration.

WILLIAM M. DOUGHERTY, BS

Reticulocyte Count

Reticulocytes are nonnucleated, immature RBCs that remain in the peripheral blood for 24 to 48 hours, while maturing. They are generally larger than mature RBCs, and contain ribosomes, the centriole, particles of Golgi vesicles, and mitochondria that produce hemoglobin. Because reticulocytes retain remnants of normoblasts (their precursors) that absorb supravital stains, such as new methylene blue or brilliant cresyl blue, they sometimes can be distinguished from other blood cells in a peripheral blood smear.

In this test, reticulocytes in a whole blood sample are counted and expressed as a percentage of the total red cell count. The reticulocyte count is useful in the evaluation of anemia and is an index of effective erythropoiesis and bone marrow response to anemia. Because the manual method for reticulocyte counting is imprecise, values may be reported as being below normal, normal, or above normal.

Purpose
□ To aid in distinguishing between hypo- and hyperproliferative anemias
□ To help assess blood loss, bone marrow response to anemia, and therapy for anemia.

Patient preparation
Tell the patient this test helps detect anemia, or monitors its treatment. Inform him that he needn't restrict food or fluids. Tell him the test requires a blood sample; who will perform the venipuncture and when; and that he may experience transient discomfort from the needle puncture and the pressure of the tourniquet. If the patient is an infant or child, explain to the parents (and to the child if he's old enough to understand) that a small amount of blood will be drawn from his finger or earlobe. Collecting the sample will take less than 3 minutes.

Withhold ACTH, antimalarials, antipyretics, azathioprine, chloramphenicol, dactinomycin, furazolidone (from infants), levodopa, methotrexate, phenacetin, and sulfonamides, as ordered. If such medications must be continued, note this on the laboratory slip.

Procedure
Perform a venipuncture, and collect the sample in a 7 ml *lavender-top* tube.

Precautions
□ Completely fill the collection tube and invert it gently several times to mix the sample and the anticoagulant.
□ Handle the sample gently to prevent hemolysis.

Values
Reticulocytes comprise 0.5% to 2% of the total RBC count. In infants, the percentage is normally higher, ranging from 3.2% at birth to 0.7% at age 12 weeks.

Implications of results
A low reticulocyte count indicates hypo-

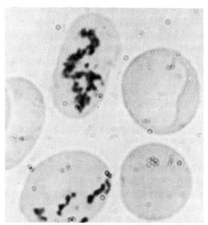

In the bright-field microscopy (x 2,500) photograph above, reticulocytes—immature, nonnucleated RBCs—are identifiable by their characteristic granular network. Methylene blue staining makes these reticulocytes visible.

proliferative bone marrow (hypoplastic anemia) or ineffective erythropoiesis (pernicious anemia). A high reticulocyte count indicates a bone marrow response to anemia caused by hemolysis or blood loss. The reticulocyte count may also rise after effective therapy for iron deficiency anemia or pernicious anemia.

Post-test care
□ If a hematoma develops at the venipuncture site, ease discomfort by applying warm soaks.
□ As ordered, resume administration of any medications that were withheld before the test.
□ When following a patient with an abnormal reticulocyte count, look for trends in repeated tests or very gross changes in the numerical value.

Interfering factors
□ False-negative test results can be caused by azathioprine, chloramphenicol, dactinomycin, and methotrexate. False-positive results can be caused by ACTH, antimalarials, antipyretics, furazolidone (in infants), and levodopa. Sulfonamides can cause false-negative or false-positive results.
□ Failure to use the proper anticoagu-

lant in the collection tube, or to adequately mix the sample and anticoagulant may interfere with accurate determination of the reticulocyte count.

☐ Prolonged tourniquet constriction may influence accurate determination of test results.

☐ Hemolysis due to rough handling of the sample may affect test results.

WILLIAM M. DOUGHERTY, BS

Osmotic Fragility

Osmotic fragility measures red cell resistance to hemolysis when exposed to a series of increasingly dilute saline solutions. The test is based on osmosis—movement of water across a membrane from a less concentrated solution to a more concentrated one, in a natural tendency to correct the imbalance.

Red cells suspended in an isotonic saline solution—one with the same salt concentration (osmotic pressure) as normal plasma (0.85 g/dl)—keep their shape. If red cells are added to a hypotonic (less concentrated) solution, they take up water until they burst; if placed in a hypertonic solution, they shrink.

The degree of hypotonicity needed to produce hemolysis varies inversely with the red cells' osmotic fragility; the closer saline tonicity is to normal physiologic values when hemolysis occurs, the more fragile the cells. In some cases, red cells do not hemolyze immediately, and their

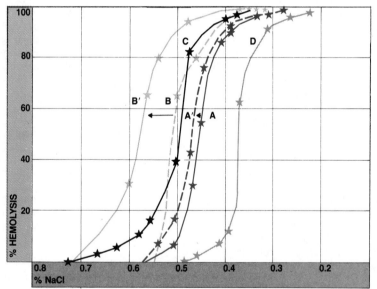

PATTERNS OF HEMOLYTIC RESPONSE TO VARYING SALINE HYPOTONICITY

These curves show what happens when red cells are subjected to increasingly dilute (hypotonic) saline solution concentrations. Normal red cells behave as in curve A, and incubation for 24 hours (to improve test sensitivity) produces only a slight increase in their osmotic fragility (curve A'). But in hereditary spherocytosis, the cells burst easily (curve B), and even more easily upon incubation (curve B'). Acquired hemolytic anemia produces a line like curve C. Lowered osmotic fragility and, hence, increased resistance to hemolysis occur in thalassemia (curve D).

Adapted with permission from Maxwell M. Wintrobe, et al, *Clinical Hematology,* 7th ed. (Philadelphia: Lea & Febiger, 1974).

CONCENTRATION AND FLUID FLOW

ISOTONIC	HYPERTONIC	HYPOTONIC
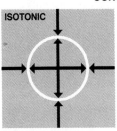	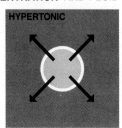	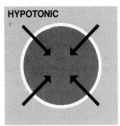

An isotonic fluid has a concentration of dissolved particles, or tonicity, equal to that of intracellular fluid. When isotonic fluids, such as 5% dextrose in water or 0.9% sodium chloride, enter the circulation, they cause no net movement of water across the semi-permeable cell membrane. And because the osmotic pressure is the same inside and outside the cells, they neither swell or shrink.

A hypertonic fluid has a concentration greater than that of intracellular fluid. When a hypertonic solution, such as 50% dextrose or 3% sodium chloride, is rapidly infused into the body, water rushes out of the cells to the area of greater concentration, and the cells shrivel. Dehydration can also make extracellular fluid hypertonic, leading to the same kind of cellular shrinking.

A hypotonic fluid has a concentration less that that of intracellular fluid. When a hypotonic solution, such as 2.5% dextrose or 0.45% sodium chloride, surrounds a cell, water diffuses into the intracellular fluid, causing the cell to swell. Inappropriate use of intravenous fluids or severe electrolyte loss makes body fluids hypotonic.

---

incubation in solution for 24 hours improves test sensitivity.

This test offers quantitative confirmation of red cell morphology and should supplement the stained cell examination.

Purpose
☐ To aid diagnosis of hereditary spherocytosis
☐ To confirm morphologic red cell abnormalities.

Patient preparation
Explain to the patient that this test helps identify the cause of anemia. Inform him that he needn't restrict food or fluids. Tell the patient the test requires a blood sample; who will perform the venipuncture and when; and that he may experience transient discomfort from the needle puncture and the pressure of the tourniquet. Reassure him that collecting the sample takes less than 3 minutes.

Procedure
Perform a venipuncture, and collect the sample in a 7 ml *green-top* (heparinized)

tube, or secure a special heparinized tube for collecting defibrinated blood.

Precautions
☐ Since this is not a routine test, notify the laboratory before drawing the sample, so the staff can be prepared for it.
☐ Completely fill the tube, and invert it gently several times to mix the sample and anticoagulant adequately.
☐ Handle the sample gently to prevent hemolysis.

Values
Osmotic fragility values (percent of RBCs hemolyzed) that have been obtained photometrically are plotted against decreasing saline tonicities to produce an S-shaped curve with a slope characteristic of the disorder (see chart).

Implications of results
Low osmotic fragility (increased resistance to hemolysis) is characteristic of thalassemia, iron deficiency anemia, sickle cell anemia, and other red cell disorders in which codocytes (target

cells) and leptocytes are found. Low osmotic fragility also occurs after splenectomy.

High osmotic fragility (increased tendency to hemolysis) is characteristic in patients with hereditary spherocytosis, in spherocytosis associated with autoimmune hemolytic anemia, severe burns, chemical poisoning, and in hemolytic disease of the newborn (erythroblastosis fetalis).

Post-test care
If a hematoma develops at the venipuncture site, apply warm soaks.

Interfering factors
The following factors may affect the accurate determination of test results:
□ failure to use the proper anticoagulant in the collection tube, to fill the tube completely, or to mix the sample and anticoagulant adequately
□ hemolysis due to rough handling of the sample
□ presence of hemolytic organisms in the sample
□ severe anemia, or other condition in which fewer red cells are available for testing.

WILLIAM M. DOUGHERTY, BS

HEMOGLOBIN TESTS
Total Hemoglobin

This test measures the grams of hemoglobin (Hgb) found in a deciliter (100 ml) of whole blood. Hgb concentration correlates closely with the RBC count, and is affected by the Hgb-RBC ratio (mean corpuscular hemoglobin [MCH]) and free plasma Hgb. In the laboratory, Hgb is chemically converted to pigmented compounds and is measured by spectrophotometric or colorimetric technique.

The test is usually performed as part of a complete blood count.

Purpose
□ To measure the severity of anemia or polycythemia and monitor response to therapy
□ To supply figures for calculating MCH and mean corpuscular hemoglobin concentration.

Patient preparation
Explain to the patient that this test helps determine if he has anemia or polycythemia, or assesses his response to treatment. Inform him that he needn't restrict food or fluids. Tell him the test requires a blood sample; who will perform the venipuncture and when; and that he may experience some discomfort from the needle puncture and the pressure of the tourniquet. If the patient is an infant or a young child, explain to the parents (and to the child if he's old enough to understand) that a small amount of blood will be drawn from his finger or earlobe. However, collecting the sample takes less than 3 minutes.

Procedure
For adults and older children, perform a venipuncture, and collect the sample in a 7 ml *lavender-top* tube. For younger children and infants, collect capillary blood in a pipette.

Precautions
□ Completely fill the collection tube, and invert it gently several times to adequately mix the sample and the anticoagulant.
□ Handle the sample gently to prevent hemolysis.

Values
Hgb concentration varies, depending on the patient's age and sex, and on the type of blood sample drawn. Except for infants, values for age groups listed in the accompanying chart are based on venous blood samples.

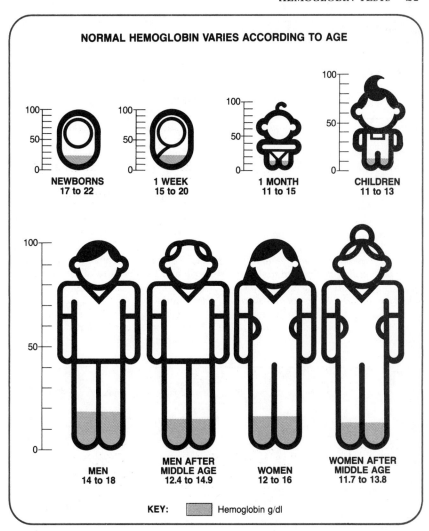

NORMAL HEMOGLOBIN VARIES ACCORDING TO AGE

NEWBORNS
17 to 22

1 WEEK
15 to 20

1 MONTH
11 to 15

CHILDREN
11 to 13

MEN
14 to 18

MEN AFTER
MIDDLE AGE
12.4 to 14.9

WOMEN
12 to 16

WOMEN AFTER
MIDDLE AGE
11.7 to 13.8

KEY: Hemoglobin g/dl

Implications of results

Low Hgb concentration may indicate anemia, recent hemorrhage, or fluid retention, causing hemodilution; elevated Hgb suggests hemoconcentration from polycythemia or dehydration.

Post-test care

If a hematoma develops at the venipuncture site, apply warm soaks.

Interfering factors

☐ Failure to use the proper anticoagulant in the collection tube, or to adequately mix the sample and anticoagulant may interfere with accurate determination of test results.

☐ Hemolysis due to rough handling of the sample may adversely affect the test results.

☐ Prolonged tourniquet constriction may cause hemoconcentration.

☐ Very high white cell counts, lipemia, or red cells that are resistant to lysis will falsely elevate Hgb values.

WILLIAM M. DOUGHERTY, BS

Hemoglobin Electrophoresis

Hemoglobin (Hgb) electrophoresis is probably the most useful laboratory method for separating and measuring normal and certain abnormal hemoglobins. Electrophoresis apparatus consists of an anode (+) and a cathode (−), separated by cellulose acetate, on which hemoglobin molecules migrate when an electrical current is passed through the medium. Different groups migrate toward the anode at different speeds, creating a series of distinctively pigmented bands in the medium that are then compared with a normal sample.

In practice, the laboratory may change the medium (from cellulose acetate to starch gel), or its pH (from 6.2 to 8.6), to clearly separate hemoglobins and to expand the range of this test beyond those hemoglobins routinely checked: hemoglobins A, A_2, S, and C.

Purpose
☐ To measure the amount of Hgb A and to detect abnormal hemoglobins
☐ To aid diagnosis of thalassemias.

Patient preparation
Explain to the patient that this test evaluates the type and distribution of hemoglobins in the blood. Inform him that he needn't restrict food or fluids. Tell him that the test requires a blood sample; who will perform the venipuncture and when; and that he may experience transient discomfort from the needle puncture and the pressure of the tourniquet. Collecting the sample takes less than 3 minutes.

Check the patient's history for recent blood transfusion (within the past 4 months).

VARIATIONS OF HEMOGLOBIN TYPE AND DISTRIBUTION

HEMOGLOBIN	PERCENTAGE OF TOTAL HEMOGLOBIN	CLINICAL IMPLICATIONS
Hgb A_2	4% to 5.8%	β-thalassemia minor
	Under 2%	Hgb H disease
Hgb F	2% to 5%	β-thalassemia minor
	10% to 90%	β-thalassemia major
	5% to 15%	β-δ-thalassemia minor
	5% to 35%	Heterozygous hereditary persistence of fetal hemoglobin (HPFH)
	100%	Homozygous HPFH
	15%	Homozygous Hgb S
Homozygous Hgb S	70% to 98%	Sickle cell disease
Homozygous Hgb C	90% to 98%	Hgb C disease
Heterozygous Hgb C	24% to 44%	Hemoglobin C trait

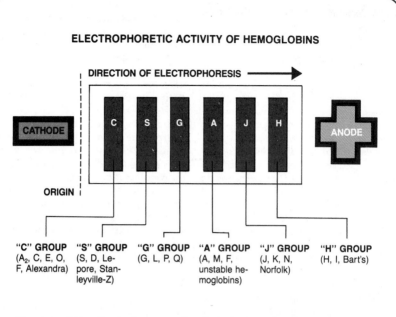

ELECTROPHORETIC ACTIVITY OF HEMOGLOBINS

DIRECTION OF ELECTROPHORESIS ⟶

CATHODE

C S G A J H

ANODE

ORIGIN

"C" GROUP	"S" GROUP	"G" GROUP	"A" GROUP	"J" GROUP	"H" GROUP
(A₂, C, E, O, F, Alexandra)	(S, D, Lepore, Stanleyville-Z)	(G, L, P, Q)	(A, M, F, unstable hemoglobins)	(J, K, N, Norfolk)	(H, I, Bart's)

Since hemoglobin molecules have a negative charge, in electrophoresis, hemoglobin molecules move toward the anode at a rate equal to the strength of their electrical charge. The electrophoretic patterns above show the relative activity of the known hemoglobin groups. Group C is the slowest and has the weakest negative charge; group H is the fastest, with the strongest negative charge.

Procedure

Perform a venipuncture, and collect the sample in a 7 ml *lavender-top* tube.

Precautions

Completely fill the collection tube, and invert it gently several times to mix the sample and anticoagulant adequately. Don't shake the tube vigorously, since hemolysis may result.

Values

In adults, Hgb A accounts for over 95% of all hemoglobins; A₂, 2% to 3%; and F, less than 1%. In neonates, Hgb F normally accounts for half the total. Hemoglobins S and C are normally absent.

Implications of results

Hemoglobin electrophoresis allows identification of various types of hemoglobin, many of which clinically may imply a hemolytic disease. The accompanying chart shows some possible results and their associated conditions.

Post-test care

If a hematoma develops at the venipuncture site, apply warm soaks.

Interfering factors

☐ If the patient has received a blood transfusion within the past 4 months, this may invalidate test results.

☐ Failure to use the proper anticoagulant in the collection tube, to fill the tube completely, or to mix the sample and the anticoagulant adequately may interfere with the accurate determination of test results.

☐ Hemolysis due to rough handling of the sample may hinder accurate determination of test results.

WILLIAM M. DOUGHERTY, BS

Sickle Cell Test
[Hemoglobin S test]

Sickle cells are severely deformed erythrocytes. The sickling phenomenon results from a hemoglobinopathy—most commonly, the polymerization of hemoglobin (Hgb) S, in the presence of low pH, low oxygen tension, elevated osmolarity, and elevated temperature, to form elongated structures (tactoids) that deform red cells. Reversing these conditions depolymerizes Hgb S and allows the red cells to resume their normal shape. However, repeated sickling leads to permanent red cell deformity. Hgb S is found almost exclusively in Blacks; and 0.2% of the Blacks born in the United States have sickle cell anemia.

Persons with sickle cell disease (who are homozygous Hgb S) usually show abundant spontaneously sickled red cells on a peripheral blood smear. Persons with sickle cell trait (who are heterozygous Hgb S) or those who are doubly heterozygous may have normal red cells that can be easily changed to sickled forms by lowering oxygen tension. This tendency to sickling can be identified by sealing a drop of blood between a glass slide and coverslip, and adding a reducing agent, such as sodium metabisulfite. The red cells can then be observed under a microscope and compared to a central slide containing blood and saline solution. The prevalence and rapidity of the sickling that follows are governed by the concentration of Hgb S.

Although this test is useful as a rapid screening procedure, it may produce false-positive and false-negative results; consequently, a Hgb electrophoresis should be performed if the presence of Hgb S is strongly suspected.

Purpose
□ To identify sickle cell disease and sickle cell trait.

Patient preparation
Explain to the patient that this test helps detect sickle cell disease. Inform him

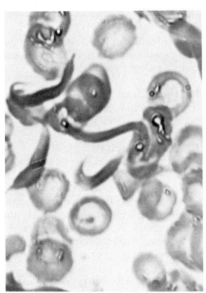

This photograph shows sickle cells—severely deformed, rigid erythrocytes in venous circulation—which may slow blood flow.

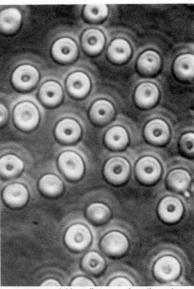

In contrast to sickle cells, normal erythrocytes are circular, flat, and bilaterally indented disks (often called biconcave disks).

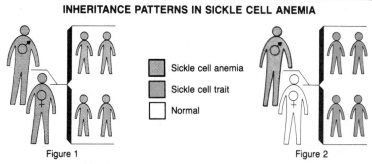

INHERITANCE PATTERNS IN SICKLE CELL ANEMIA

Sickle cell anemia

Sickle cell trait

Normal

Figure 1   Figure 2

The most serious risk occurs when both parents have sickle cell anemia (figure 1); childbearing—if possible at all—is dangerous for the mother, and all offspring will have sickle cell anemia. When one parent has sickle cell anemia and one is normal (figure 2), all offspring will be carriers of sickle cell anemia.

that he needn't restrict food or fluids. Tell him the test requires a blood sample; who will perform the venipuncture and when; and that he may experience transient discomfort from the needle puncture and the pressure of the tourniquet. Reassure him that collecting the sample takes less than 3 minutes.

Check patient history for blood transfusion within the past 3 months.

Procedure

Perform a venipuncture, and collect the sample in a 7 ml *lavender-top* tube.

Precautions

Completely fill the collection tube, and invert it gently several times to adequately mix the sample and the anticoagulant. Don't shake the tube vigorously, since hemolysis may result.

Values

Results of this test are reported as positive or negative. A normal, or negative, test suggests the absence of Hgb S.

Implications of results

A positive test may indicate the presence of sickle cells, but a Hgb electrophoresis is needed to distinguish between homozygous and heterozygous forms. Rarely, other abnormal Hgbs cause sickling of erythrocytes in the absence of Hgb S.

Post-test care

If a hematoma develops at the venipuncture site, apply warm soaks.

Interfering factors

☐ Hgb concentration under 10%, ele-

FETAL SICKLE CELL TEST

When both parents of a developing fetus are suspected carriers of sickle cell trait, a reliable test is now available that can detect whether the fetus has the sickle cell trait or the disease. This test, developed in 1979 at the University of California at San Francisco, was the first diagnostic tool resulting from recombinant DNA research. Many major medical centers throughout the United States currently perform the test. In addition, any doctor can request the fetal sickle cell test if he suspects that both parents are carriers. He need only mail the appropriate samples to the nearest location.

The test requires a venous blood sample from both parents and an amniotic fluid sample. Diagnosis is based on analysis of the genes and the DNA in the fetal cells, and on the DNA in parental leukocytes. About 1 week is required to complete the test, which can generally be performed between the 14th and 18th weeks of pregnancy. This provides a sufficient opportunity for the couple to seek genetic counseling.

vated Hgb F levels in infants under age 6 months, and blood transfusion within the past 3 months may produce false-negative test results.
□ Failure to use the proper anticoagulant in the collection tube, to completely fill the tube, or to adequately mix the sample and the anticoagulant may interfere with accurate determination of test results.
□ Hemolysis due to rough handling of the sample may affect test results.

WILLIAM M. DOUGHERTY, BS

Unstable Hemoglobins

Unstable hemoglobins are rare, congenital red cell defects caused by amino acid substitutions in the normally stable structure of hemoglobin. These abnormal replacements produce a molecule that spontaneously denatures into clumps and aggregations called Heinz bodies, which separate from the red cell cytoplasm and accumulate at the cell membrane. Although Heinz bodies are usually efficiently removed by the spleen or liver,
they may cause mild to severe hemolysis.

Unstable hemoglobins are best detected by precipitation tests (heat stability or isopropanol solubility) performed in the laboratory. Although a hemoglobin electrophoresis and the Heinz body test can demonstrate certain unstable hemoglobins, these tests don't always confirm the presence of such hemoglobins. Globin chain analysis identifies them more reliably, but this procedure is time-consuming and technically complex and, therefore, is not performed routinely.

Purpose
□ To detect unstable hemoglobins.

Patient preparation
Explain to the patient that this test detects abnormal hemoglobin in the blood. Inform him that he needn't restrict food or fluids. Tell him the test requires a blood sample; who will perform the venipuncture and when; and that he may experience transient discomfort from the needle puncture and the pressure of the tourniquet. Reassure him that collecting the sample takes less than 3 minutes.

As ordered, withhold antimalarials, furazolidone (from infants), nitrofurantoin, phenacetin, procarbazine, and sulfonamides before the test, since these drugs may induce hemolysis. If these medications must be continued, note this on the laboratory slip.

Procedure
Perform a venipuncture, and collect the sample in a 7 ml *lavender-top* tube.

Precautions
Completely fill the collection tube, and invert it gently several times to mix the sample and the anticoagulant adequately. Don't shake the tube vigorously, since hemolysis may result.

Values
When no unstable hemoglobins appear in the sample, the heat stability test is reported as negative; the isopropanol solubility test, as stable.

Implications of results

A positive heat stability or unstable solubility test, especially with hemolysis, strongly suggests the presence of unstable hemoglobins.

Post-test care

☐ If a hematoma develops at the venipuncture site, apply warm soaks.
☐ As ordered, resume administration of medications withheld before the test.

Interfering factors

☐ Antimalarials, furazolidone (in infants), nitrofurantoin, phenacetin, procarbazine, and sulfonamides can induce Heinz body formation and result in a positive or unstable test.
☐ High levels of Hgb F may cause a false-positive isopropanol test.
☐ Failure to use the proper anticoagulant in the collection tube, to fill the tube completely, or to mix the sample and the anticoagulant adequately may interfere with accurate determination of test results.
☐ Hemolysis due to rough handling of the sample, or hemoconcentration due to prolonged tourniquet constriction may influence test results.

WILLIAM M. DOUGHERTY, BS

Heinz Bodies

Heinz bodies are particles of denatured hemoglobin that have precipitated out of the cytoplasm of RBCs, and that have collected in small masses and attached to the cell membranes. They form as a result of drug injury to red cells, the presence of unstable hemoglobins, unbalanced globin chain synthesis due to thalassemia, or a red cell enzyme deficiency (such as glucose 6-phosphate dehydrogenase deficiency). Although Heinz bodies are rapidly removed from red cells in the spleen, they are a major factor in causing hemolytic anemias.

Using a whole blood sample, Heinz

CLINICAL SIGNS OF UNSTABLE HEMOGLOBINS

More than 60 varieties of unstable hemoglobins exist, each named after the city in which it was discovered. Their effects vary according to their number, severity of instability, the condition of the spleen, and the oxygen-binding abilities of the unstable hemoglobin. Common indications of unstable hemoglobins include pallor, jaundice, splenomegaly, and with severely unstable hemoglobins, cyanosis, pigmenturia, and hemoglobinuria. Thalassemia often causes similar clinical effects, but the molecular bases of the two diseases differ greatly.

---

bodies can be detected by phase microscopy or with supravital stains, such as crystal violet, brilliant cresyl blue, or new methylene blue. However, when Heinz bodies do not form spontaneously, various oxidant drugs are added to the whole blood sample to induce their formation.

Purpose

☐ To help detect causes of hemolytic anemia.

Patient preparation

Explain to the patient that this test helps determine the cause of anemia. Inform him that he needn't restrict food or fluids before the test. Tell him this test requires a blood sample; who will perform the venipuncture and when; and that he may experience transient discomfort from the needle puncture and the pressure of the tourniquet. Reassure him that collecting the blood sample takes less than 3 minutes.

Review the patient's drug history for medications that may interfere with accurate determination of test results. Withhold antimalarials, furazolidone, nitrofurantoin, phenacetin, procarbazine, and sulfonamides, as ordered. If these medications must be continued, note this on the laboratory slip.

Procedure

Perform a venipuncture, and collect the sample in a 7 ml *lavender-top* tube.

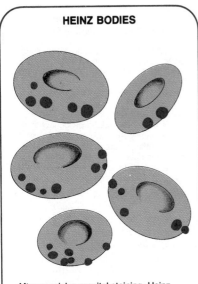

HEINZ BODIES

After special supravital staining, Heinz bodies (particles of denatured hemoglobin generally attached to the cell membrane) appear as small, purple inclusions at cell margins. Heinz bodies are present in certain hemolytic anemias.

Precautions
Completely fill the sample collection tube, and invert it gently several times to adequately mix the sample and the anticoagulant.

Values
Absence of Heinz bodies is the normal (negative) test result.

Implications of results
The presence of Heinz bodies—a positive test result—may indicate an inherited red cell enzyme deficiency, the presence of unstable hemoglobins, thalassemia, or drug-induced red cell injury. Heinz bodies may also be present after splenectomy.

Post-test care
☐ If a hematoma develops at the venipuncture site, ease discomfort by applying warm soaks.
☐ As ordered, resume administration of medications withheld before the test.

Interfering factors
☐ Antimalarials, furazolidone (in infants), nitrofurantoin, phenacetin, procarbazine, and sulfonamides can cause false-positive results.
☐ Failure to use the appropriate anticoagulant in the collection tube, to fill the collection tube completely, to adequately mix the sample and the anticoagulant, or to send the sample immediately to the laboratory may interfere with the accurate determination of test results.

WILLIAM M. DOUGHERTY, BS

Serum Iron and Total Iron-binding Capacity

Iron is essential to the formation and function of hemoglobin, as well as many other heme and nonheme compounds. After iron is absorbed by the intestine, it's distributed to various body compartments for synthesis, storage, and transport. Since iron appears in the plasma, bound to a glycoprotein called transferrin, it is easily sampled and measured. The sample is treated with buffer and color reagents.

Serum iron assay measures the amount of iron bound to transferrin; total iron-binding capacity (TIBC) measures the amount of iron that would appear in plasma if all the transferrin were saturated with iron. The percentage of saturation is obtained by dividing the serum iron result by the TIBC, which reveals the actual amount of saturated transferrin. Normally, transferrin is about 30% saturated.

Serum iron and TIBC are of greater diagnostic usefulness when performed with the serum ferritin assay, but together these tests may not accurately reflect the state of other iron compartments, such as myoglobin iron and

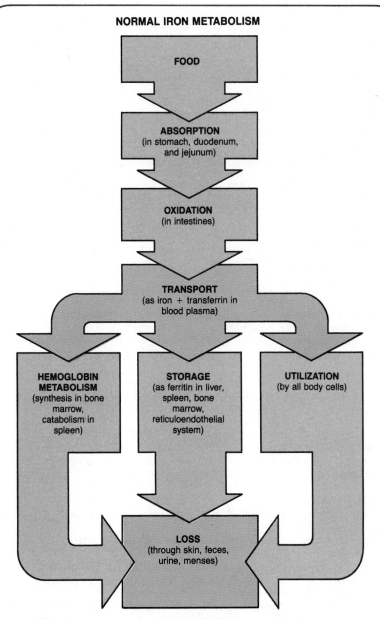

NORMAL IRON METABOLISM

FOOD

ABSORPTION
(in stomach, duodenum,
and jejunum)

OXIDATION
(in intestines)

TRANSPORT
(as iron + transferrin in
blood plasma)

HEMOGLOBIN
METABOLISM
(synthesis in bone
marrow,
catabolism in
spleen)

STORAGE
(as ferritin in liver,
spleen, bone
marrow,
reticuloendothelial
system)

UTILIZATION
(by all body cells)

LOSS
(through skin, feces,
urine, menses)

Ingested iron, absorbed and oxidated in the bowel, bonds with transport protein transferrin for circulation to bone marrow for hemoglobin synthesis, and to all iron-hungry body cells. In the spleen, hemoglobin breakdown recycles iron back to the bone marrow or into storage. The body conserves iron, losing small amounts through skin, feces, urine, and menses. Storage areas in the liver, spleen, bone marrow, and reticuloendothelial system hold iron as ferritin until the body needs it; the liver alone stores about 60%. Normal iron metabolism is essential for red cell function.

SIDEROCYTE STAIN

Siderocytes are red blood cells (RBCs) containing particles of nonhemoglobin iron known as siderocytic granules. In newborn infants, siderocytic granules are normally present in normoblasts and reticulocytes during hemoglobin synthesis. However, the spleen removes most of these granules from normal RBCs, and they disappear rapidly with age. In adults, an elevated siderocyte level usually indicates abnormal erythropoiesis, as in congenital spherocytic anemia, chronic hemolytic anemias such as the thalassemias, pernicious anemia, hemochromatosis, toxicities such as lead poisoning, infection, or severe burns. Elevated levels may also follow splenectomy, since the spleen normally removes siderocytic granules.

The siderocyte stain test measures the number of circulating siderocytes. Venous blood is drawn into a 7-ml *lavender-top* tube or, for infants and children, collected in a Microtainer or a pipette and smeared directly on a 3″ by 1″ glass slide. When the blood smear is stained, siderocytic granules appear as purple-blue specks clustered around the periphery of mature erythrocytes. Cells containing these granules are counted as a percentage of total RBCs. The results aid differential diagnosis of the anemias and hemochromatosis, and help detect toxicities.

Normally, newborn infants have a slightly elevated siderocyte level that reaches the normal adult value of 0.5% of total RBCs in 7 to 10 days. In patients with pernicious anemia, the siderocyte level is 8% to 14%; in chronic hemolytic anemia, 20% to 100%; in lead poisoning, 10% to 30%; and in hemochromatosis, 3% to 7%. A high siderocyte level mandates additional testing—including bone marrow examination—to determine the cause of abnormal erythropoiesis.

---

the labile iron pool. Bone marrow or liver biopsy, and iron absorption or excretion studies may yield more information.

Purpose
☐ To estimate total iron storage
☐ To aid diagnosis of hemochromatosis
☐ To help distinguish between iron deficiency anemia and anemia of chronic disease
☐ To provide data for evaluating nutritional status.

Patient preparation
Explain to the patient that this test evaluates his body's capacity to store iron. Inform him that he needn't restrict food or fluids before the test. Tell him that the test requires a blood sample and who will perform the venipuncture and when. Explain to him that he may experience transient discomfort from the needle puncture and the pressure of the tourniquet. And reassure him that collecting the blood sample takes less than 3 minutes.

Review the patient's drug history for medications that may interfere with accurate determination of test results. Withhold chloramphenicol, ACTH, iron supplements, and oral contraceptives, as ordered. If such medications must be continued, note this on the laboratory slip.

Procedure
Perform a venipuncture, and collect the sample in a 7 ml *red-top* tube.

Precautions
Handle the sample gently to prevent hemolysis, and send it to the laboratory immediately.

Values
Normal serum iron and TIBC values are as follows:

Serum iron (mcg/dl)	TIBC (mcg/dl)	Saturation (%)
Men: 70 to 150	300 to 400	20 to 50
Women: 80 to 150	300 to 450	20 to 50

Implications of results
In iron deficiency, serum iron levels drop and TIBC increases to decrease the saturation. In cases of chronic inflammation (such as in rheumatoid arthritis), serum iron may be low in the presence of adequate body stores, but TIBC may be unchanged or may drop to preserve

normal saturation. Iron overload may not alter serum levels until relatively late, but in general, serum iron increases and TIBC remains the same to increase the saturation.

Post-test care
□ If a hematoma develops at the venipuncture site, ease discomfort by applying warm soaks.
□ As ordered, resume administration of medications withheld before the test.

Interfering factors
□ Chloramphenicol and oral contraceptives can cause false-positive test results; ACTH can produce false-negative results. Iron supplements can cause false-positive serum iron values but false-negative TIBC.
□ Hemolysis due to rough handling of the sample, or failure to send the sample to the laboratory immediately may interfere with accurate determination of test results.

WILLIAM M. DOUGHERTY, BS

Serum Ferritin

Ferritin, a major iron-storage protein found in reticuloendothelial cells, normally appears in small quantities in serum. In healthy adults, serum ferritin levels are directly related to the amount of available iron stored in the body and can be measured accurately by radioimmunoassay. Unlike many other blood studies, the serum ferritin test isn't affected by moderate hemolysis of the sample or by any known drugs.

Purpose
□ To screen for iron deficiency and iron overload
□ To measure iron storage
□ To distinguish between iron deficiency (a condition of low iron storage) and chronic inflammation (a condition of normal storage).

Patient preparation
Explain to the patient that the test assesses the available iron stored in the body. Inform him that he needn't restrict food, fluids, or medications before the test. Tell him the test requires a blood sample; who will perform the venipuncture and when; and that he may experience transient discomfort from the needle puncture and the pressure of the tourniquet. Reassure the patient that collecting the blood sample generally takes less than 3 minutes. Review the patient's history for recent transfusion.

Procedure
Perform a venipuncture, and collect the sample in a 10 ml *red-top* tube.

Values
Normal serum ferritin values vary with age. According to the Mayo Medical Laboratories, serum ferritin levels range as follows:
- *men:* 20 to 300 ng/ml
- *women:* 20 to 120 ng/ml
- *6 months to 15 years:* 7 to 140 ng/ml
- *2 to 5 months:* 50 to 200 ng/ml
- *1 month:* 200 to 600 ng/ml
- *neonates:* 25 to 200 ng/ml.

Implications of results
High serum ferritin levels may indicate acute or chronic hepatic disease, iron overload, leukemia, acute or chronic infection or inflammation, Hodgkin's disease, or chronic hemolytic anemias; in these disorders, iron stores in the bone marrow may be normal or significantly increased. Serum ferritin levels are characteristically normal or slightly elevated in those patients who have chronic renal disease. Low serum ferritin levels indicate chronic iron deficiency.

Post-test care
If a hematoma develops at the venipuncture site, apply warm soaks.

Interfering factors
Recent transfusion may cause elevated serum ferritin levels.

WILLIAM M. DOUGHERTY, BS

WHITE CELL TESTS

White Blood Cell Count

[Leukocyte count]

Part of the complete blood count, the white blood cell (WBC) count reports the number of white cells found in a microliter (cubic millimeter) of whole blood by using a hemacytometer or an electronic device, such as the Coulter counter.

On any given day, WBC counts may vary by as much as 2,000. Such variation can be the result of strenuous exercise, stress, or digestion. The WBC count may rise or fall significantly in certain diseases, but is diagnostically useful only when interpreted in light of the white cell differential and of the patient's current clinical status.

Purpose
□ To determine infection or inflammation
□ To determine the need for further tests, such as the WBC differential or bone marrow biopsy
□ To monitor response to chemotherapy or radiation therapy.

Patient preparation
Explain to the patient that the test helps detect an infection or inflammation. Inform him that he needn't restrict food or fluids but should avoid strenuous exercise for 24 hours before the test. Also tell him that he should avoid ingesting a heavy meal before the test. Explain to him that the test requires a blood sample; who will perform the venipuncture and when; and that he may experience some transient discomfort from the needle puncture and the pressure of the tourniquet. Reassure him, however, that collecting the blood sample takes less than 3 minutes.

If the patient is being treated for an infection, advise him that this test will be repeated to monitor his progress. Review his drug history for medications that may interfere with accurate determination of test results. Note use of such medications on the laboratory slip.

Procedure
Perform a venipuncture, and collect the sample in a 7 ml *lavender-top* tube.

Precautions
Completely fill the sample collection tube, and invert it gently several times to adequately mix the sample and the anticoagulant.

Values
The WBC count ranges from 4,100 to 10,900/μl.

Implications of results
An elevated WBC count (leukocytosis) usually signals infection, such as an abscess, meningitis, appendicitis, or tonsillitis. A high count may also result from leukemia and tissue necrosis due to burns, myocardial infarction, or gangrene.

A low WBC count (leukopenia) indicates bone marrow depression that may result from viral infections or from toxic reactions, such as those following treatment with antineoplastics, ingestion of mercury or other heavy metals, or exposure to benzene or arsenicals. Leukopenia characteristically accompanies influenza, typhoid fever, measles, infectious hepatitis, mononucleosis, and rubella.

Post-test care
□ If a hematoma develops at the venipuncture site, ease discomfort by applying warm soaks.
□ As ordered, advise the patient that he may resume normal activity that he discontinued before the test.

LEUKOCYTE ALKALINE PHOSPHATASE STAIN

Levels of leukocyte alkaline phosphatase (LAP), an enzyme found in neutrophils, may be altered by infection, stress, chronic inflammatory diseases, Hodgkin's disease, and hematologic disorders. Most of these conditions elevate LAP levels; only a few, notably chronic myelogenous leukemia (CML), depress them. Thus, this test is most often used to differentiate CML from other disorders that produce an elevated white blood cell count.

To perform this test, a blood sample is obtained by venipuncture or finger stick. The venous blood sample is collected in a 7-ml *green-top* tube and transported immediately to the laboratory, where a blood smear is prepared; the peripheral blood sample is smeared on a 3″ x 1″ glass slide and fixed in cold formalin-methanol. The blood smear is then stained to show the amount of LAP present in the cytoplasm of the neutrophils. One hundred neutrophils are counted and assessed; each is assigned a score of 0 to 4, according to the degree of LAP staining. Normally, values for LAP fall in the range of 40 to 100, depending upon the laboratory's standards.

Depressed LAP values typically indicate CML; however, low values may also occur in paroxysmal nocturnal hemoglobinuria, aplastic anemia, and infectious mononucleosis. Elevated values may indicate Hodgkin's disease, polycythemia vera, or a neutrophilic leukemoid reaction— a response to conditions such as infection, chronic inflammation, or pregnancy.

After a diagnosis of CML, the LAP stain may also be used to help detect onset of the blastic phase of the disease, when LAP levels typically rise. However, LAP levels also increase toward normal in response to therapy; because of this, test results must be correlated with the patient's condition.

CLARKE LAMBE, MD

□ Patients with severe leukopenia may have little or no resistance to infection and, therefore, require reverse isolation.

Interfering factors

□ Hemolysis caused by rough handling of the sample may interfere with accurate determination of test results.

□ Exercise, stress, or digestion raises the WBC count, thus yielding inaccurate results.

□ Some drugs, including most antineoplastic agents; anti-infectives, such as metronidazole and flucytosine; anticonvulsants, such as phenytoin derivatives; thyroid hormone antagonists; and nonsteroidal anti-inflammatories, such as indomethacin, lower the WBC count, altering results.

MARYLOU K. MCHUGH, RN, MSN

White Blood Cell Differential

Because the white blood cell (WBC) differential evaluates the distribution and morphology of white cells, it provides more specific information about a patient's immune system than the WBC count. In this test, the laboratory classifies 100 or more white cells in a stained film of peripheral blood according to two major types of leukocytes—granulocytes (neutrophils, eosinophils, and basophils), and nongranulocytes (lymphocytes and monocytes)—and determines the percentage of each type. The differential count is the relative number of each type of white cell in the blood. By multiplying the percentage value of each type by the total WBC count, the investigator obtains the absolute number of each type of white cell. Although little is known about the function of eosinophils in the blood, abnormally high levels of these cells are associated with various allergic diseases and reactions to parasites. In such cases, an eosinophil count is sometimes ordered as a follow-up to the white cell differential. This test is also appropriate if the differential white blood cell count shows a depressed eosinophil level.

Purpose

□ To evaluate the body's capacity to resist and overcome infection

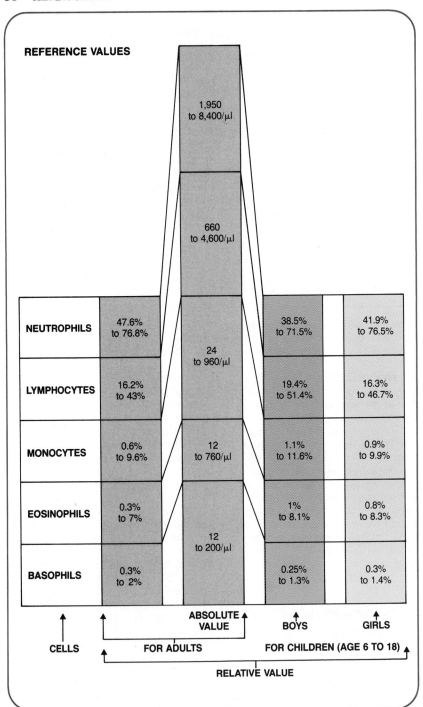

REFERENCE VALUES

| CELLS | FOR ADULTS | | FOR CHILDREN (AGE 6 TO 18) | |
	RELATIVE VALUE	ABSOLUTE VALUE	BOYS	GIRLS
NEUTROPHILS	47.6% to 76.8%	1,950 to 8,400/µl	38.5% to 71.5%	41.9% to 76.5%
LYMPHOCYTES	16.2% to 43%	660 to 4,600/µl	19.4% to 51.4%	16.3% to 46.7%
MONOCYTES	0.6% to 9.6%	24 to 960/µl	1.1% to 11.6%	0.9% to 9.9%
EOSINOPHILS	0.3% to 7%	12 to 760/µl	1% to 8.1%	0.8% to 8.3%
BASOPHILS	0.3% to 2%	12 to 200/µl	0.25% to 1.3%	0.3% to 1.4%

□ To detect and identify various types of leukemia

□ To determine the stage and severity of an infection

□ To detect allergic reactions and parasitic infections, and assess their severity (eosinophil count).

Patient preparation

Explain to the patient that the test evaluates the immune system. Inform him that he needn't restrict food or fluids but should refrain from strenuous exercise for 24 hours before the test. Tell him the test requires a blood sample; who will perform the venipuncture and when; and that he may experience transient discomfort from the needle puncture and the pressure of the tourniquet. Reassure him that collecting the sample takes less than 3 minutes.

Review the patient's history for use of medications that may interfere with test results.

Procedure

Perform a venipuncture, and collect the sample in a 7 ml *lavender-top* tube.

Precautions

Completely fill the collection tube, and invert it gently several times to mix the sample and the anticoagulant adequately. Handle the tube gently to prevent hemolysis.

INTERPRETING THE DIFFERENTIAL

To make an accurate diagnosis, the examiner must consider both relative and absolute values of the differential. Considered alone, relative results may point to one disease, while masking the true pathology that would be revealed by considering the results of the white cell count. For example, consider a patient whose WBC count is 6,000/μl, and whose differential shows 30% neutrophils and 70% lymphocytes. His relative lymphocyte count would seem to be quite high (lymphocytosis); but when this figure is multiplied by his white cell count—6,000 × 70% = 4,200 lymphocytes/μl—it is well within the normal range.

This patient's neutrophil count, however, is low (30%) and when this is multiplied by the white cell count—6,000 × 30% = 1,800 neutrophils/μl—the result is a low absolute number.

This low result indicates decreased neutrophil production, which may mean depressed bone marrow.

Values

Normal values for the five types of WBCs that are classified in the differential—neutrophils, eosinophils, basophils, lymphocytes, and monocytes—are given for adults and children in the accompanying tables. For an accurate diagnosis, differential test results must always be interpreted in relation to the total WBC count.

DRUGS THAT INFLUENCE THE EOSINOPHIL COUNT

MAY INCREASE OR DECREASE EOSINOPHIL COUNT:	DECREASE EOSINOPHIL COUNT:	INCREASE EOSINOPHIL COUNT BY PROVOKING AN ALLERGIC REACTION:	
methysergide	indomethacin	anticonvulsants	novobiocin
desipramine	procainamide	capreomycin	para-aminosalicylic acid
		cephalosporins	paromomycin
		D-penicillamine	penicillins
		gold compounds	phenothiazines
		isoniazid	rifampin
		nalidixic acid	streptomycin
			sulfonamides
			tetracyclines

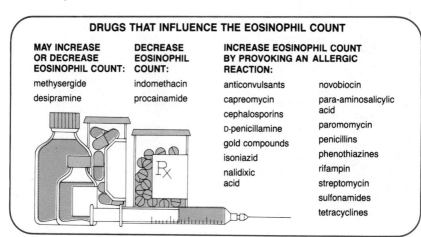

INFLUENCE OF DISEASE ON BLOOD CELL COUNT

CELL TYPE	HOW AFFECTED

Neutrophils

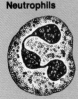

Increased by:
- Infections: osteomyelitis, otitis media, salpingitis, septicemia, gonorrhea, endocarditis, smallpox, chickenpox, herpes, Rocky Mountain spotted fever
- Ischemic necrosis due to myocardial infarction, burns, carcinoma
- Metabolic disorders: diabetic acidosis, eclampsia, uremia, thyrotoxicosis
- Stress response due to acute hemorrhage, surgery, excessive exercise, emotional distress, third trimester of pregnancy, childbirth
- Inflammatory disease: rheumatic fever, rheumatoid arthritis, acute gout, vasculitis and myositis

Decreased by:
- Bone marrow depression due to radiation or cytotoxic drugs
- Infections: typhoid, tularemia, brucellosis, hepatitis, influenza, measles, mumps, rubella, infectious mononucleosis
- Hypersplenism: hepatic disease and storage diseases
- Collagen vascular disease, such as systemic lupus erythematosus
- Deficiency of folic acid or vitamin B_{12}

Eosinophils

Increased by:
- Allergic disorders: asthma, hay fever, food or drug sensitivity, serum sickness, angioneurotic edema
- Parasitic infections: trichinosis, hookworm, roundworm, amebiasis
- Skin diseases: eczema, pemphigus, psoriasis, dermatitis herpes
- Neoplastic diseases: chronic myelocytic leukemia, Hodgkin's disease, metastases and necrosis of solid tumors
- Miscellaneous: collagen vascular disease, adrenocortical hypofunction, ulcerative colitis, polyarteritis nodosa, postsplenectomy, pernicious anemia, scarlet fever, excessive exercise

Decreased by:
- Stress response due to trauma, shock, burns, surgery, mental distress
- Cushing's syndrome

Basophils

Increased by:
- Chronic myelocytic leukemia, polycythemia vera, some chronic hemolytic anemias, Hodgkin's disease, systemic mastocytosis, myxedema, ulcerative colitis, chronic hypersensitivity states, and nephrosis

Decreased by:
- Hyperthyroidism, ovulation, pregnancy, stress

Lymphocytes

Increased by:
- Infections: pertussis, brucellosis, syphilis, tuberculosis, hepatitis, infectious mononucleosis, mumps, German measles, cytomegalovirus
- Other: thyrotoxicosis, hypoadrenalism, ulcerative colitis, immune diseases, lymphocytic leukemia

Decreased by:
- Severe debilitating illness, such as CHF, renal failure, advanced TB
- Defective lymphatic circulation, high levels of adrenal corticosteroids, immunodeficiency due to immunosuppressives

Monocytes

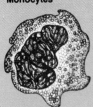

Increased by:
- Infections: subacute bacterial endocarditis, tuberculosis, hepatitis, malaria, Rocky Mountain spotted fever
- Collagen vascular disease: systemic lupus erythematosus, rheumatoid arthritis, polyarteritis nodosa
- Carcinomas
- Monocytic leukemia
- Lymphomas

Implications of results
Evidence for a wide range of disease states and other conditions is revealed by abnormal differential patterns, as shown in the chart.

Post-test care
If a hematoma develops at the venipuncture site, apply warm soaks.

Interfering factors
□ Hemolysis caused by rough handling of the sample may affect test results.
□ Failure to use the proper anticoagulant, to completely fill the collection tube, or to mix the sample and anticoagulant adequately may influence accurate determination of test results.

MARYLOU K. MCHUGH, RN, MSN

Selected References

Brown, Barbara A. *Hematology: Principles and Procedures,* 3rd ed. Philadelphia: Lea & Febiger, 1980.

Byrne, C. Judith, et al. *Laboratory Tests: Implications for Nurses and Allied Health Professionals.* Reading, Mass.: Addison-Wesley Publishing Co., 1981.

Diseases, 2nd ed. Nurse's Reference Library. Springhouse, Pa.: Springhouse Corp., 1986.

Fischbach, Frances. *A Manual of Laboratory Diagnostic Tests,* 2nd ed. Philadelphia: J.B. Lippincott Co., 1984.

French, Ruth M. *Guide to Diagnostic Procedures,* 5th ed. New York: McGraw-Hill Book Co., 1980.

Guyton, Arthur C. *Textbook of Medical Physiology,* 6th ed. Philadelphia: W.B. Saunders Co., 1981.

Henry, John Bernard, ed. *Todd-Sanford-Davidsohn Clinical Diagnosis and Management by Laboratory Methods,* 17th ed., Philadelphia: W.B. Saunders Co., 1984.

Lamb, Jane O. *Laboratory Tests for Clinical Nursing.* Bowie, Md.: Robert J. Brady Co., 1984.

Nursing85 Drug Handbook. Springhouse, Pa.: Springhouse Corp., 1985.

Petersdorf, Robert G., and Adams, Raymond D., eds. *Harrison's Principles of Internal Medicine,* 10th ed. New York: McGraw-Hill Book Co., 1983.

Platt, William R. *Color Atlas and Textbook of Hematology,* 2nd ed. Philadelphia: J.B. Lippincott Co., 1979.

Price, Sylvia, and Wilson, Lorraine. *Pathophysiology: Clinical Concepts of Disease Processes,* 2nd ed. New York: McGraw-Hill Book Co., 1982.

Ravel, Richard A. *Clinical Laboratory Medicine,* 4th ed. Chicago: Year Book Medical Pubs., 1984.

Selkurt, Ewald E. *Basic Physiology for the Health Sciences,* 2nd ed. Boston: Little, Brown & Co., 1981.

Tilkian, Sarko M., et al. *Clinical Implications of Laboratory Tests,* 3rd ed. St. Louis: C.V. Mosby Co., 1983.

Wallach, Jacques B. *Interpretation of Diagnostic Tests: A Handbook Synopsis of Laboratory Medicine,* 3rd ed. Boston: Little, Brown & Co., 1978.

Widmann, Frances K. *Clinical Interpretation of Laboratory Tests,* 9th ed. Philadelphia: F.A. Davis Co., 1983.

Williams, William J., et al. *Hematology,* 2nd ed. New York: McGraw-Hill Book Co., 1977.

Wintrobe, Maxwell M., et al. *Clinical Hematology,* 8th ed. Philadelphia: Lea & Febiger, 1981.

2 Hemostasis

LEARNING OBJECTIVES

After completing this chapter, the reader will be able to:
- describe how hemostasis protects the body against excessive blood loss.
- discuss common coagulation defects, platelet disorders, and vascular defects.
- name the deficient factor in eight hereditary coagulation disorders.
- describe the sequence of physiologic events in blood coagulation.
- state the purpose of each test discussed in the chapter.
- prepare the patient physically and psychologically for each test.
- describe the procedure for performing each test.
- specify appropriate precautions for accurate administration of each test.
- implement appropriate post-test care.
- state the normal values for each test.
- discuss the implications of abnormal test results.
- list factors that may interfere with accurate test results.

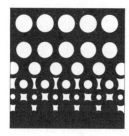

Hemostasis

Introduction

Hemostasis is the process whereby the circulatory system protects itself from excessive blood loss. In this process, vascular injury activates a complex chain of events—vasoconstriction, platelet aggregation, and coagulation—leading to clotting that stops the bleeding without hindering blood flow through the injured vessel.

Vasoconstriction: Primary response

Within seconds of vascular injury, neural reflexes and local smooth-muscle spasms cause the walls of the damaged vessel to contract, aided by secretion of serotonin, epinephrine, and lipoproteins. Constriction lasts about 10 minutes in a small vessel, and up to 30 minutes in a larger one. The extent of tissue damage determines the extent of vasospasm; for example, a blood vessel that suffers a clean cut bleeds more than one that is crushed. However, vasoconstriction slows blood flow only briefly in small vessels and is insufficient to prevent blood loss from large ones. Permanent repair requires a hemostatic plug formed of platelet aggregates, and a fibrin clot.

Aggregation of platelets

Circulating platelets converge on the wound site, first touching and then adhering to the collagen fibers of the torn vessel lining (endothelium). This contact of platelets with collagen stimulates the platelets to secrete adenosine diphosphate (ADP), which causes them to break down and become adhesive, sticking together in clumps. Additional ADP activates greater numbers of platelets, which also collect at the site. This aggregation loosely plugs the wound to prevent further blood loss.

Coagulation (clotting)

When platelet aggregation is underway, blood loses its fluidity and forms a gelatinous clot. More than a score of agents in blood and in tissues influence this process. Some promote coagulation (procoagulants) and others inhibit it (anticoagulants). When vascular injury causes bleeding, procoagulants gather at the injury site and stimulate formation of a stable fibrin clot.

Clotting begins within 60 seconds of injury and proceeds through the interaction of two parallel pathways—the extrinsic and the intrinsic clotting systems. The *extrinsic* system is activated when tissue thromboplastin is released at the injury site. At the same time, procoagulants already in the blood are activated, in the *intrinsic* system, to produce plasma thromboplastin and several other factors. Both systems then interact to build a meshwork of fibrin strands that traps blood cells, more platelets, and plasma, to form a clot.

Three crucial steps

Normal clotting proceeds in three stages:
1. Trauma to blood vessels or tissues triggers thromboplastin activity through intrinsic and extrinsic pathways.
2. Thromboplastin activity converts prothrombin to thrombin.
3. Thrombin converts fibrinogen in the surrounding plasma to a fibrin plug.

Formation of thromboplastin

When blood contacts injured tissue, the tissue frees Factor III (tissue thromboplastin), which is an ill-defined, clot-promoting substance. Factor III alone is ineffective and requires additional plasma factors to complete its activity. Factor III interacts with Factor VII (proconvertin) in the presence of calcium ions. Factor IV (calcium ions [Ca^{++}]) and tissue phospholipids form a complex that initiates the reactions of the extrinsic system. This complex then activates Factor X (Stuart-Prower factor), at the end of the extrinsic pathway.

In intrinsic clotting, plasma thromboplastin results from progressive activation of several procoagulants. When stimulated by surface contact or vascular injury, Factor XII (Hageman factor) activates Factor XI (plasma thromboplastin antecedent), which, in the presence of calcium, initiates activity of Factor IX (Christmas factor). The activated form of this plasma protein, in the presence of platelet phospholipids, converts Factor VIII (antihemophilic factor) to its active state and forms a complex that activates Factor X.

Almost simultaneously, Factor X—stimulated by both extrinsic and intrinsic pathways—reacts with Factor V (proaccelerin), in the presence of Ca^{++} and platelet phospholipids, to form a prothrombin-converting complex. Within 15 seconds of its formation, this protein begins to split Factor II (prothrombin) to form thrombin.

Conversion of prothrombin to thrombin

Prothrombin is converted to thrombin by Factor X with the aid of Factor V (which accelerates this conversion), in the presence of Ca^{++} and platelets. Prothrombin splits into two parts: one is inert and the other is thrombin. Thrombin is a potent enzyme that converts fibrinogen to fibrin, helps stabilize the final clot, and starts clot breakdown (fibrinolysis) after healing.

Conversion of fibrinogen to fibrin

After thrombin is formed in adequate amounts, it hydrolyzes fibrinogen (Factor I), splitting two low–molecular-weight peptides from each fibrinogen molecule. The remaining peptides are fibrin monomers, which automatically combine end to end and side by side to form fibrin threads that eventually build a weak, soluble polymer meshwork.

To strengthen this weak fibrin clot, thrombin activates another plasma enzyme called Factor XIII (fibrin stabilizing factor). In the presence of Ca^{++}, this enzyme strengthens the fibrin polymer by forming covalent bonds and causing cross-linkage of peptide bonds. This stabilizing action results in a firm, insoluble clot.

Coagulation defects and bleeding disorders

Coagulation defects due to *Factor I* (fibrinogen) deficiency may be hereditary or acquired. Hereditary errors are classified as quantitative (afibrinogenemia or hypofibrinogenemia) or qualitative (dysfibrinogenemia). Afibrinogenemia causes severe bleeding that may be life-threatening. This disorder, thought to be transmitted as an autosomal recessive trait, first occurs in the newborn as umbilical bleeding. Acquired hypofibrinogenemia can result from conditions such as disseminated intravascular coagulation (DIC), hyperfibrinolysis, and hepatic disease.

Factor II deficiency, or hypoprothrombinemia, can also be hereditary or acquired. The former, transmitted as an autosomal recessive trait, is rare. The acquired form can result from vitamin K deficiency, warfarin therapy, and hepatic disease. Acquired prothrombin

BLOOD COAGULATION FACTORS

FACTOR	SYNONYM	PROFILE	SITE OF SYNTHESIS
I	Fibrinogen	Precursor of fibrin	Liver
II	Prothrombin	Precursor of thrombin	Liver
III	Tissue thromboplastin	Activator of prothrombin	All tissues
IV	Ca++	Essential for prothrombin activation and formation of fibrin	From diet
V	Proaccelerin	Accelerates conversion of prothrombin to thrombin	Liver
VII	Serum prothrombin (proconvertin)	Accelerates conversion of prothrombin to thrombin	Liver
VIII	Antihemophilic factor (AHF, hemophilic factor A)	Associated with factors IX, XII, and XI; aids in formation of plasma thromboplastin and conversion of prothrombin to thrombin	Reticuloendothelial system
IX	Christmas factor (hemophilic factor B, plasma thromboplastin component [PTC])	Activated by Factor XI; essential to formation of plasma thromboplastin; associated with factors XII, XI, and VIII	Liver
X	Stuart-Prower factor	Triggers prothrombin conversion; requires vitamin K	Liver
XI	Plasma thromboplastin antecedent (PTA)	Activated by Factor XII; associated with factors XII, IX, and VIII in formation of plasma thromboplastin	Unknown
XII	Hageman factor	First factor activated in the intrinsic pathway; activates Factor XI in formation of plasma thromboplastin	Unknown
XIII	Fibrin stabilizing factor (FSF)	Produces stronger urea-insoluble fibrin clot	Unknown

deficiency is frequently associated with deficiencies of Factor VII, Factor IX, and Factor X.

Factor VII deficiency can also be inherited as an autosomal recessive trait. Although the clinical effects of this hereditary defect may vary, it commonly causes overt symptoms of abnormal coagulation, such as epistaxis, easy bruising, and bleeding from the gums. An acquired form of Factor VII deficiency can result from vitamin K deficiency, warfarin therapy, and hepatic disease.

A defect of *Factor VIII* causes two congenital disorders: hemophilia A (classic hemophilia) and von Willebrand's disease. Hemophilia A, a sex-linked recessive disorder transmitted by females that occurs almost exclusively in males, is marked by severe bleeding (hemarthroses, and muscular and gastrointestinal bleeding). Von Willebrand's disease, which causes a milder coagulation dysfunction than hemophilia A, is characterized by abnormal platelet function and a mild-to-moderate deficiency of

COMMON COAGULATION SCREENING TESTS

TEST	WHAT ABNORMAL FINDINGS USUALLY MEAN
Bleeding Time	Prolonged bleeding time: thrombocytopenia, disseminated intravascular coagulation, or von Willebrand's disease. Abnormal bleeding time, with normal platelet count: platelet function disorder.
Capillary Fragility	Excessive number of petechiae in 2" (5-cm) circle of skin: capillary wall weakness or platelet disorder.
Activated Partial Thromboplastin Time (APTT)	Prolonged APTT: presence of anticoagulant, fibrin split products, fibrinolysins, or antibodies to specific clotting factors; or deficiency of clotting factor other than Factor VII or Factor XIII.
Prothrombin Time (PT)	Prolonged PT: deficiency of fibrinogen (Factor I), prothrombin (Factor II), or factors V, VII, or X; hepatic disease; vitamin K deficiency; or ongoing anticoagulant therapy.
Plasma Thrombin Time	Prolonged thrombin time: hepatic disease, disseminated intravascular coagulation, effective heparin therapy, hypo- or dysfibrinogenemia.
Fibrin Split Products (FSP)	Elevated FSP: pulmonary embolus, myocardial infarction, deep venous thrombosis, disseminated intravascular coagulation, or primary fibrinolysis syndrome.

Factor VIII, and is transmitted to both sexes as an autosomal dominant trait. Symptoms of this disorder include epistaxis, ecchymoses, and oozing after tooth extraction. Both DIC and fibrinolysis may induce acquired Factor VIII deficiency.

Congenital deficiency of *Factor IX* can cause hemophilia B (Christmas disease), a severe bleeding disorder transmitted as a sex-linked recessive trait from mothers to sons. Because Factor IX is formed in the liver and depends on the presence of sufficient vitamin K, an acquired deficiency of this factor can result from lack of vitamin K or from warfarin therapy and hepatic disease.

A *Factor X* deficiency, inherited as an autosomal recessive trait (rare), is generally associated with depressed levels of vitamin K, hepatic disease, and anticoagulant therapy.

Congenital deficiency of *Factor XI*, transmitted as an autosomal recessive trait, does not usually produce symptoms. A transient form of this defect is sometimes detectable in newborns. Congenital *Factor XII* deficiency, also transmitted as an autosomal recessive trait, is similarly unlikely to cause symptoms. An acquired form of this deficiency sometimes develops in nephrosis, vitamin K deficiency, anticoagulant therapy, and hepatic disease.

Platelet disorders

Platelets, oval or rod-shaped cytoplasmic fragments about 2 to 4 microns in diameter, are derived from bone marrow megakaryocytes. Platelet disorders stemming from abnormalities of number (thrombocytopenia and thrombocytosis) or function (thrombasthenia and thrombocytopathia) impair vascular integrity and the coagulation mechanism. However, serious coagulopathy is likely only when large numbers of platelets are dysfunctional or deficient.

In *thrombocytopenia*, the most common platelet deficiency, the number of platelets is abnormally low (less than 150,000/mm³); nevertheless, overt bleeding doesn't generally develop until the count drops below 50,000/mm³. Throm-

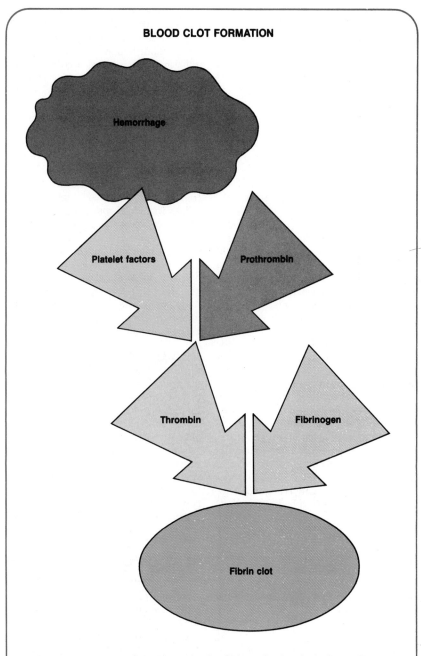

BLOOD CLOT FORMATION

- Hemorrhage
- Platelet factors
- Prothrombin
- Thrombin
- Fibrinogen
- Fibrin clot

When injury occurs, platelets gather at the site of injury, releasing platelet factors. These factors combine with the protein prothrombin to form thrombin. Then, thrombin—also a protein—combines with fibrinogen to form fibrin, the essential part of the clot.

CALCIUM IONS AND CLOTTING

Calcium ions are needed for nearly all re-actions in the clotting process. Decreased plasma calcium levels may result from hypoparathyroidism, vitamin D deficiency, magnesium deficiency, or chronic laxative ingestion, or after a massive transfusion of citrated blood. However, coagulopathy seldom results from hypocalcemia, since clotting can occur with less calcium than is required for other physiologic functions. Calcium levels low enough to cause defective coagulation are incompatible with life.

---

bocytopenia may result from decreased bone marrow production of platelets related to aplastic anemia, leukemia, and vitamin B_{12} or folic acid deficiency; from accelerated destruction of platelets by the spleen; from exaggerated destruction of platelets caused by antiplatelet or drug-induced antibodies; and from severe blood loss.

Antiplatelet antibodies stimulate the reticuloendothelial system to sequester circulating platelets. Proliferation of antibodies may result from treatment with medications such as quinidine, quinine, and thiazide derivatives. Sulfonamides and phenylbutazone may exert a direct toxic effect on platelets, through an unknown mechanism. Drug toxicity is likely to induce bleeding from capillaries rather than from larger vessels. This tendency causes small hemorrhages that appear on the skin as purple discolorations (purpura).

In *thrombocytosis*, which is usually secondary to other disorders, the platelet count is abnormally high (more than 400,000/mm³), and is associated with inflammatory response, iron deficiency, or splenectomy. Abnormally elevated platelet counts also appear in myeloproliferative disorders, such as polycythemia vera, myelofibrosis, and chronic granulocytic leukemia. Thrombocytosis does not generally cause symptoms but may occasionally lead to bleeding or thrombosis.

Qualitative platelet disorders may be congenital or acquired. Congenital disorders include *thrombasthenia*, a rare autosomal recessive trait; *storage-pool disease*, typified by decreased ADP levels in blood platelets; and *Bernard-Soulier (giant platelet) syndrome*, marked by abnormally large platelets that fail to aggregate with the reagent ristocetin. Acquired defects may result from aspirin ingestion, uremia, dysproteinemias, and chronic hepatic disease.

Vascular defects

Bleeding due to vascular defects results from abnormal vascular permeability (as in vitamin C deficiency) or fragility (as in purpura senilis). Blood vessels can also rupture and bleed after certain abrupt movements, because blood vessels are lightly anchored to surrounding tissue. In allergic purpura, increased vascular permeability and tissue hemorrhage result from an inflammatory capillary reaction.

ELIZABETH ANNE MALLON, BS, MT (ASCP)

PLATELET ACTIVITY TESTS

Bleeding Time

This test measures the duration of bleeding after a standardized skin incision. Bleeding time depends on the elasticity of the blood vessel wall and on the number and functional capacity of platelets.

Although this test is usually performed on patients with personal or family histories of bleeding disorders, it is also useful for preoperative screening, along with a platelet count. Bleeding time may be measured by one of four methods: Duke, Ivy, template, or modified template. The template methods are the most frequently used and the most accurate, since they standardize the incision size, making test results reproducible.

Usually, the test isn't recommended for a patient whose platelet count is less than 75,000/mm³. However, some patients with altered platelet morphology may have normal bleeding times despite low platelet counts.

Purpose
□ To assess overall hemostatic function (platelet response to injury and functional capacity of vasoconstriction)
□ To detect congenital and acquired platelet function disorders.

Patient preparation
Explain to the patient that this test measures the time required to form a clot and stop bleeding. Tell him who will perform the test and when. Inform him he needn't restrict food or fluids before the test. Reassure him that, although he may feel some discomfort from the incisions, the antiseptic, and the tightness of the blood pressure cuff, the test takes only 10 to 20 minutes to perform. Advise the patient that the incisions will leave two small, hairline scars that should be barely visible when healed.

Check patient history for recent ingestion of drugs that prolong bleeding time. If the patient has taken such drugs, check with the laboratory for special instructions. If the test is being used to identify a suspected bleeding disorder, it should be postponed and the drugs discontinued, as ordered; if it's being used preoperatively, to assess hemostatic function, it should proceed as scheduled.

Equipment
Blood pressure cuff/disposable lancet/template with 9 mm slits (template method) or 5 mm slits (modified template method)/spring-loaded blade (modified template method)/70% alcohol or povidone-iodine solution/filter paper/small pressure bandage/stopwatch.

Procedure
□ *Template and modified template methods:* Wrap the pressure cuff around the upper arm and inflate the cuff to 40 mmHg. Select an area on the forearm that is free of superficial veins, and cleanse it with antiseptic. Allow the skin to dry *completely* before making the incision. Apply the appropriate template lengthwise to the forearm. For the template method, use the lancet to make two incisions, 1 mm deep and 9 mm long. For the modified template method, use the spring-loaded blade to make two incisions, 1 mm deep and 5 mm long. Start the stopwatch. Taking care not to touch the cuts, gently blot the drops of blood with filter paper every 30 seconds, until the bleeding stops in both cuts. Average the bleeding time of the two cuts, and record the result.

□ *Ivy method:* After applying the pressure cuff and preparing the test site, make three small punctures with a disposable lancet. Start the stopwatch immediately. Taking care not to touch the punctures, blot each site with filter paper every 30 seconds, until the bleeding stops. Average the bleeding time of the three punctures, and record the result.

□ *Duke method:* Drape the patient's shoulder with a towel. Clean the earlobe, and let the skin air-dry. Then, make a puncture wound 2 to 4 mm deep on the earlobe, with a disposable lancet. Start the stopwatch. Being careful not to touch the ear, blot the site with filter paper every 30 seconds, until bleeding stops. Record bleeding time.

Precautions
If the bleeding doesn't diminish after 15 minutes, discontinue the test by applying compression to the incision site.

Values
The normal range of bleeding time is from 2 to 8 minutes in the template method; from 2 to 10 minutes in the modified template method; from 1 to 7 minutes in the Ivy method; and from 1 to 3 minutes in the Duke method.

Implications of results
Prolonged bleeding time may indicate the presence of many disorders associ-

ated with thrombocytopenia, such as Hodgkin's disease, acute leukemia, disseminated intravascular coagulation, hemolytic disease of the newborn, Schönlein-Henoch purpura, severe hepatic disease (cirrhosis, for example), or severe deficiency of factors I, II, V, VII, VIII, IX, and XI. Prolonged bleeding time in a person with a normal platelet count suggests a platelet function disorder (thrombasthenia, thrombocytopathia) and requires further investigation with clot retraction, prothrombin consumption, and platelet aggregation tests.

Post-test care
□ In a patient with a bleeding tendency (hemophilia, for example), maintain a pressure bandage over the incision for 24 to 48 hours to prevent further bleeding. Keep the edges of the cuts aligned to minimize scarring. Otherwise, a piece of gauze held in place by an adhesive bandage is sufficient. Check the test area frequently.
□ As ordered, resume administration of medications discontinued before the test.

Interfering factors
Sulfonamides, thiazides, antineoplastics, anticoagulants, nonsteroidal antiinflammatory drugs, aspirin and aspirin compounds, and some nonnarcotic analgesics may prolong bleeding times.
ELIZABETH ANNE MALLON, BS, MT(ASCP)

Platelet Count

Platelets, or thrombocytes, are the smallest formed elements in the blood. They are vital to the formation of the hemostatic plug in vascular injury and promote coagulation by supplying phospholipids to the intrinsic thromboplastin pathway. Platelet count is one of the most important screening tests of platelet function. Accurate counts are vital for monitoring chemotherapy, radiation therapy, or severe thrombocytosis and

thrombocytopenia. A platelet count that falls below 50,000 can cause spontaneous bleeding; when it drops below 5,000, fatal CNS bleeding or massive gastrointestinal hemorrhage is possible.

Properly prepared and stained peripheral blood films provide a reliable estimate of platelet number if the sample shows at least one platelet for every 10 to 20 RBCs visible in an oil-immersion field. A more accurate visual method involves use of a hemacytometer counting chamber and a phase microscope. The most accurate measurement, however, employs the voltage pulse or electro-optical counting system. Nevertheless, results from such automated systems should always be checked against a visual estimate from a stained blood film.

Purpose
□ To evaluate platelet production
□ To assess effects of chemotherapy or radiation therapy on platelet production
□ To aid diagnosis of thrombocytopenia and thrombocytosis
□ To confirm visual estimate of platelet number and morphology from a stained blood film.

Patient preparation
Explain to the patient that this test helps determine if his blood clots normally. Inform him that he needn't restrict food or fluids before the test. Tell him the test requires a blood sample; who will perform the venipuncture and when; and that he may experience transient discomfort from the needle puncture and the pressure of the tourniquet. Reassure him that collecting the sample takes less than 3 minutes.

Check patient history for use of medications that may affect test results. Notify the laboratory if such drugs have been used.

Procedure
Perform a venipuncture, and collect the sample in a 7 ml *lavender-top* tube.

Precautions
□ To prevent hemolysis, handle the sam-

ple gently and avoid excessive probing at the venipuncture site.

☐ Completely fill the collection tube, and invert it gently several times to mix the sample and the anticoagulant adequately.

Values

Normal platelet counts range from 130,000 to 370,000/mm³.

Implications of results

A decreased platelet count (thrombocytopenia) can result from aplastic or hypoplastic bone marrow; infiltrative bone marrow disease, such as carcinoma, leukemia, or disseminated infection; megakaryocytic hypoplasia; ineffective thrombopoiesis due to folic acid or vitamin B_{12} deficiency; pooling of platelets in an enlarged spleen; increased platelet destruction due to drugs or immune disorders; disseminated intravascular coagulation; Bernard-Soulier syndrome; or mechanical injury to platelets.

An increased platelet count (thrombocytosis), can result from hemorrhage; infectious disorders; malignancies; iron deficiency anemia; recent surgery, pregnancy, or splenectomy; and inflammatory disorders, such as collagen vascular disease. In such cases, the platelet count returns to normal after the patient recovers from the primary disorder. However, the count remains elevated in primary thrombocytosis, myelofibrosis with myeloid metaplasia, polycythemia vera, and chronic myelogenous leukemia. When the platelet count is abnormal, diagnosis usually requires further studies, such as a complete blood count, bone marrow biopsy, direct antiglobulin test (direct Coombs' test), and serum protein electrophoresis.

Post-test care

If a hematoma develops at the venipuncture site, apply warm soaks.

Interfering factors

☐ Failure to use the proper anticoagulant or to mix the sample and antico-

agulant promptly and adequately may interfere with the accurate determination of test results.

☐ Hemolysis due to rough handling of the sample or to excessive probing at the venipuncture site may alter test results.

☐ Medications that may decrease platelet count include acetazolamide, acetohexamide, antimony, antineoplastics, brompheniramine maleate, carbamazepine, chloramphenicol, ethacrynic acid, furosemide, gold salts, hydroxychloroquine, indomethacin, isoniazid, mephenytoin, mefenamic acid, methazolamide, methimazole, methyldopa, oral diazoxide, oxyphenbutazone, penicillamine, penicillin, phenylbutazone, phenytoin, pyrimethamine, quinidine sulfate, quinine, salicylates, streptomycin, sulfonamides, thiazide and thiazide-like diuretics, and tricyclic antidepressants. Heparin causes transient, reversible thrombocytopenia.

☐ Platelet counts normally increase at high altitudes, with persistent cold temperature, and during strenuous exercise and excitement; the count decreases just before menstruation.

ELIZABETH ANNE MALLON, BS, MT(ASCP)

Capillary Fragility
[Tourniquet test, Rumpel-Leede capillary fragility test]

A nonspecific method for evaluating bleeding tendencies, the capillary fragility test (positive-pressure test) measures capillaries' ability to remain intact under increased intracapillary pressure. In this test, a laboratory technician or other specially trained person places a blood pressure cuff around the patient's upper arm and raises the pressure to a point midway between the systolic and diastolic blood pressures but no higher than 100 mmHg. At this pressure, blood can enter the arm and hand but can't easily return to circu-

lation. Pressure is maintained for 5 minutes. This temporary increase in pressure may cause rhexis bleeding of the capillaries and formation of petechiae on the arm, wrist, or hand. The number of petechiae within a given circular space is recorded as the test result.

Purpose
□ To assess the fragility of capillary walls
□ To identify platelet deficiency (thrombocytopenia).

Patient preparation
Explain to the patient that this test helps identify abnormal bleeding tendencies. Inform him that he needn't restrict food or fluids. Tell him who will perform the procedure and when, and that he may feel discomfort from the pressure of the blood pressure cuff.

Procedure
If you perform this test, select and mark a 2″ (5-cm) space on the patient's forearm. Select a site that's free of petechiae; otherwise, record the number of petechiae present on the site before starting the test. The patient's skin temperature and the room temperature should be normal to ensure accurate results.

Fasten the cuff around the arm, and raise the pressure to a point midway between the systolic and diastolic blood pressures. Maintain this pressure for 5 minutes; then release the cuff. Count the number of petechiae that appear in the 2″ (5-cm) space. Record test results.

Precautions
□ Don't repeat this test on the same arm within 1 week.
□ This test is contraindicated in patients with disseminated intravascular coagulation (DIC) or other bleeding disorders, and in those with significant petechiae.

Values
A few petechiae may normally be present before the test. Less than 10 petechiae on the forearm 5 minutes after the test is considered normal, or negative; more than 10 petechiae is considered a positive result. The following scale may also be used to report test results:

Number of petechiae	Score
0 to 10	1+
10 to 20	2+
20 to 50	3+
50	4+

Implications of results
A positive finding (more than 10 petechiae present, or a score of 2+ to 4+) indicates weakness of the capillary walls (vascular purpura) or a platelet defect, and occurs in conditions such as thrombocytopenia, thrombasthenia, purpura senilis, scurvy, DIC, von Willebrand's

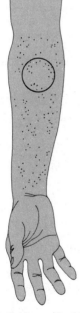

POSITIVE CAPILLARY FRAGILITY TEST

Hemorrhagic disorders, such as thrombocytopenia, produce a strong showing of petechiae below the site of application of the blood pressure cuff. Both size (greater than 1 mm) and number of petechiae indicate abnormality.

disease, vitamin K deficiency, dysproteinemia, polycythemia vera, and in severe deficiencies of Factor VII, fibrinogen, or prothrombin. Conditions unrelated to bleeding defects, such as scarlet fever, measles, influenza, chronic renal disease, hypertension, and diabetes with coexistent vascular disease, may also increase capillary fragility. An abnormal number of petechiae sometimes appears before onset of menstruation and at other times in some healthy persons, especially in women over age 40.

Post-test care
Encourage the patient to open and close his hand a few times to hasten return of blood to the forearm.

Interfering factors
☐ Decreased estrogen levels in postmenopausal women may increase capillary fragility.
☐ Glucocorticoids may increase capillary resistance, even in a patient with thrombocytopenia.
☐ A high number of pretest petechiae may be caused by allergy to certain foods or drugs.
☐ Repeating the test on the same arm within 1 week may lead to an error in counting the number of petechiae.
ELIZABETH ANNE MALLON, BS, MT(ASCP)

Platelet Aggregation

After vascular injury, platelets gather at the injury site and clump together to form an aggregate—a plug—that helps maintain hemostasis and promotes healing. The platelet aggregation test, an in vitro procedure, measures the rate at which the platelets in a sample of citrated platelet-rich plasma form a clump after the addition of an aggregating reagent (adenosine diphosphate, epinephrine, thrombin, collagen, or ristocetin). Since evenly suspended platelets aggregate and fall to the bottom of the tube,

the greater the aggregation, the less turbid the sample. A spectrophotometer measures changes in turbidity and prints a graphic record of the results. This test is a major diagnostic tool for detecting von Willebrand's disease; persons with this disorder lack the ristocetin cofactor that enables platelets to aggregate in the presence of ristocetin.

Purpose
☐ To assess platelet aggregation
☐ To detect congenital and acquired platelet bleeding disorders.

Patient preparation
Explain to the patient that this test helps determine if his blood clots properly. Instruct him to fast or to maintain a nonfat diet for 8 hours before the test, since lipemia can affect test findings. Tell him the test requires a blood sample; who will perform the venipuncture and when; and that he may experience some transient discomfort from the needle puncture and the pressure of the tourniquet. Reassure him that collecting the sample takes less than 3 minutes.

Withhold aspirin and aspirin compounds for 14 days, and phenylbutazone, sulfinpyrazone, phenothiazines, antihistamines, anti-inflammatory drugs, and tricyclic antidepressants for 48 hours, as ordered. If these medications must be continued, note this on the laboratory slip. Since the list of medications known to alter the results of this test is long and continually growing, the patient should be as free of drugs as possible before the test.

Procedure
Perform a venipuncture, and collect the sample in a 7 ml *blue-top* siliconized tube.

Precautions
☐ If a coagulation defect is suspected, avoid excessive probing at the venipuncture site; don't leave the tourniquet on too long (it causes bruising); and apply pressure to the venipuncture site for 5 minutes, or until the bleeding stops.

PLATELET AGGREGATION CURVES

NORMAL

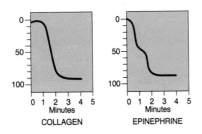

| COLLAGEN | EPINEPHRINE | ADP | RISTOCETIN |

STORAGE POOL DISEASE

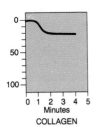
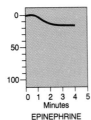
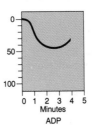
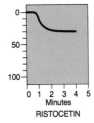

| COLLAGEN | EPINEPHRINE | ADP | RISTOCETIN |

VON WILLEBRAND'S DISEASE   ## BERNARD-SOULIER SYNDROME

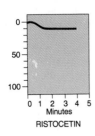
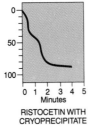
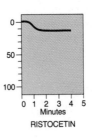
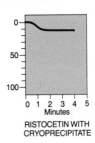

| RISTOCETIN | RISTOCETIN WITH CRYOPRECIPITATE | RISTOCETIN | RISTOCETIN WITH CRYOPRECIPITATE |

A spectrophotometer measures the degree of platelet aggregation, from 0% to 100%, over a 5-minute period and plots the rate curve on a graph. Normal platelet aggregation occurs in 3 to 5 minutes. But in a patient suspected of having a platelet aggregation defect, the rate is greatly reduced. The addition of reagents, such as adenosine diphosphate (ADP), epinephrine, or collagen, helps distinguish various disorders. For instance, in samples treated with ristocetin, there is almost no difference between the poor reactions obtained in von Willebrand's disease and in Bernard-Soulier syndrome; but the addition of cryoprecipitate causes a dramatic improvement only in the former, because cryoprecipitate contains the portion of Factor VIII molecule that is lacking in patients with von Willebrand's disease.

Courtesy of the Clinical Hemostasis Laboratory, Cardeza Foundation for Hematologic Research, Thomas Jefferson University, Philadelphia.

☐ Completely fill the collection tube, and invert it gently several times to mix the sample and the anticoagulant adequately.

☐ Handle the sample gently to prevent hemolysis, and keep it between 71.6° F. (22° C.) and 98.6° F. (37° C.) to prevent aggregation.

☐ If the patient has taken aspirin within the past 14 days and the test can't be postponed, notify the laboratory. The technician will then use arachidonic acid as the reagent, to verify the presence of aspirin in the plasma. If test results are abnormal for such a sample, the use of aspirin must be discontinued and the test repeated in 2 weeks.

Values

Normal aggregation occurs in 3 to 5 minutes, but findings are temperature-dependent and vary with the laboratory. Aggregation curves obtained by using different reagents help to distinguish various qualitative platelet defects, as shown in the accompanying chart.

Implications of results

Abnormal findings may indicate von Willebrand's disease, Bernard-Soulier syndrome, storage pool disease, Glanzmann's thrombasthenia, or polycythemia vera.

Post-test care

☐ If a hematoma develops at the venipuncture site, apply warm soaks.

☐ As ordered, resume diet and administration of medications withheld before the test.

Interfering factors

☐ Hemolysis caused by rough handling of the sample or by trauma at the venipuncture site may interfere with accurate determination of test results.

☐ Failure to use the proper anticoagulant or to mix the sample and anticoagulant adequately may alter test results.

☐ Failure to observe restrictions of diet and medications may hinder accurate determination of test results. Platelet aggregation is inhibited by aspirin and aspirin compounds, phenylbutazone, sulfinpyrazone, phenothiazines, antihistamines, anti-inflammatory drugs, and tricyclic antidepressants.

ELIZABETH ANNE MALLON, BS, MT(ASCP)

Platelet Survival

The platelet survival test measures the rate at which platelets are destroyed and renewed in the peripheral circulation. Platelets labeled with radioactive chromium-51 (^{51}Cr) are injected into the bloodstream. For 8 to 10 days, labeled platelets remaining in circulation are counted in serial samples of peripheral blood and are plotted to obtain a platelet survival curve. Findings are easily reproducible and closely express the life span of circulating platelets. This test provides important information for diagnosis of idiopathic thrombocytopenic purpura, a disorder marked by shortened platelet life span.

Purpose

☐ To aid diagnosis of idiopathic thrombocytopenic purpura

☐ To assess platelet survival and life span.

Patient preparation

Explain to the patient that this test provides information about platelets that allows asessment of the clotting mechanism. Advise him that he needn't restrict food or fluids. Tell him the test requires a series of blood samples. A laboratory technologist will perform three or four venipunctures on the first day of the test and one venipuncture daily for the next 8 to 10 days. Reassure the patient that while he may experience some discomfort from the needle puncture and the pressure of the tourniquet, collecting each sample takes less than 3 minutes.

Check history for repeated pregnancies or transfusions, and report such information to the laboratory.

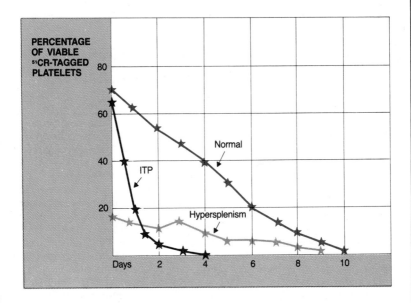

PLATELET SURVIVAL PATTERNS

Labeling blood platelets with radioactive chromium can monitor their active life span in the bloodstream. A normal survival curve is nearly linear. In idiopathic thrombocytopenic purpura (ITP), platelets are thought to be attacked by antigen-antibody complexes and destroyed by the liver or spleen. An overactive spleen (hypersplenism) pulls platelets out of circulation, temporarily retaining up to 90% of them.

Reproduced with permission from A.D. Ginsburg and R.H. Aster, "Platelet Function: Its Clinical Significance," in H.F. Dowling, et al, eds., *Disease-A-Month.* Copyright © 1970, Year Book Medical Publishers, Inc., Chicago.

Procedure

Three or four venipunctures are performed on the first day, and the samples collected in 7 ml *lavender-top* tubes. The first venipuncture is performed to obtain platelets for tagging with ^{51}Cr isotope (donor platelets from a blood bag may be used instead). The ^{51}Cr-tagged platelets are injected into the bloodstream. Then, two samples are drawn: one at 30 minutes and another at 2 hours after the platelet injection.

A venipuncture is performed daily for the next 8 to 10 days, and the blood samples are collected in 7 ml *lavender-top* tubes.

Precautions

If the patient has a suspected coagulation defect, avoid excessive probing during venipuncture; don't leave the tourniquet on too long (it will cause bruising); and be sure to apply pressure to the venipuncture site for 5 minutes, or until the bleeding stops.

Values

Normally, half the radiolabeled platelets disappear from circulation in 84 to 116 hours. The remaining radioactivity normally disappears in 8 to 10 days, which is thought to be the normal platelet life span.

Implications of results

Diminished platelet survival time—which may be as brief as 1 to 4 hours—occurs in idiopathic thrombocytopenic purpura, systemic lupus erythematosus, consumptive coagulopathy, and in some cases of Hodgkin's disease and lymphosarcoma.

Post-test care

If a hematoma develops at the venipuncture site, ease discomfort by applying warm soaks.

Interfering factors

Presence of antiplatelet antibodies after multiple transfusions, platelet transfusion, or repeated pregnancies may interfere with accurate determination of test results by shortening platelet survival time.

ELIZABETH ANNE MALLON, BS, MT(ASCP)

COAGULATION TESTS

Whole Blood Clotting Time and Clot Retraction Time

[Lee-White coagulation time, coagulation time, venous clotting time]

Whole blood clotting time measures the interval required for fresh whole blood to clot in vitro at 98.6° F. (37° C.) and grossly evaluates the intrinsic clotting mechanism. Developed in 1939, clotting time is nonspecific for any coagulation factor, time-consuming, difficult to standardize, subject to technical error, and is unreliable as a screening test. Other tests, such as the activated partial thromboplastin time (APTT), are more useful. Using the same whole blood sample, the clot retraction study measures the time needed for the platelet and fibrinogen network to contract into a firm clot. Successful retraction is based on the number and activity of platelets, fibrinogen and other intrinsic factor levels, and hematocrit.

Purpose

☐ To assess the intrinsic system of blood coagulation

☐ To monitor effectiveness of heparin therapy (but less reliable than the APTT).

Patient preparation

Explain to the patient that this test helps determine if his blood clots normally. Inform him he needn't restrict food or fluids before the test. Tell him the test requires a blood sample; who will perform the venipuncture and when (a laboratory technologist usually performs this test); and that he may experience discomfort from the needle puncture and the pressure of the tourniquet. Collecting the sample takes less than 3 minutes.

Check the patient's history for medications that may affect test results. Notify the laboratory, when appropriate.

Procedure

Perform a venipuncture, using a two-syringe technique. Draw 3 ml of blood with a plastic syringe; disconnect the syringe from the needle and discard it (to minimize contamination of the sample with tissue thromboplastin). Attach a new syringe, and start a stopwatch as soon as blood enters the new syringe. Apply pressure to the puncture site after withdrawing the needle, and instruct the patient to continue this pressure until the bleeding stops.

Remove the needle from the syringe, and immediately transfer 1-ml portions of the sample into three 12 x 75 mm plain glass tubes set in a water bath at 98.6° F. (37° C.). Take the last tube filled and tilt it gently every 30 seconds until a clot forms; next, do the same with the second tube filled, and finally, with the first.

CLOT RETRACTION

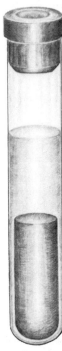

The illustration above shows normal clotting after 4 hours. As the clot firms, it retracts from the sides and top of the tube, occupying about half the original blood volume.

Stop the watch when clotting has occurred in all three tubes, and record the time elapsed as the whole blood clotting time.

Observe the three samples at hourly intervals for signs of clot retraction. Record retraction as complete when the clot has separated from the sides and bottom of the tube.

Precautions

□ If a coagulation defect is suspected, avoid excessive probing during venipuncture; don't leave the tourniquet on too long (it will cause bruising); and apply pressure to the venipuncture site for 5 minutes, or until the bleeding stops.
□ Since the inside surface of the collec-

tion tube affects clot retraction, use only plain glass tubes.
□ Handle the sample gently to prevent hemolysis.

Values

Normal whole blood clotting time ranges from 5 to 15 minutes. After 1 hour, the clot becomes firm and retracted from the sides of the tube, occupying about half the original blood volume (most of the serum has been expressed from the clot). Record the retraction as normal, doubtful, or defective; approximately 50% retraction is normal.

Implications of results

Prolonged clotting time indicates a severe deficiency of coagulation factors (except Factor VII and Factor XIII) or the presence of anticoagulants. Abnormal clotting time necessitates further tests, including prothrombin time, APTT, and specific factor assays.

Slow or incomplete clot retraction may indicate thrombocytopenia; thrombasthenia also produces reduced retraction and a characteristically soft clot. Abnormal retraction also occurs in hyperfibrinogenemia and anemia. The clot may appear soft and ill-defined in a patient with secondary fibrinolysis or DIC.

Post-test care

If a hematoma develops at the venipuncture site, apply warm soaks.

Interfering factors

□ Failure to record the sample collection time, to maintain the sample at 98.6° F. (37° C.), or to fill the collection tubes to the proper level may interfere with accurate determination of test results.
□ Hemolysis due to poor venipuncture technique or rough handling of the sample may affect test results.
□ Contamination of the sample with tissue thromboplastin may interfere with accurate determination of test results.
□ Use of a plastic or silicone-coated collection tube, instead of glass, prolongs clotting time.
□ Depressed fibrinogen levels (less than

100 mg/dl) prolong clotting time.
□ Anticoagulants increase clotting time.
ELIZABETH ANNE MALLON, BS, MT(ASCP)

Activated Partial Thromboplastin Time

The activated partial thromboplastin time (APTT) test evaluates all the clotting factors of the intrinsic pathway—except Factor VII and Factor XIII—by measuring the time required for formation of a fibrin clot after the addition of calcium and phospholipid emulsion to a plasma sample. The APTT relies on an activator, such as kaolin, to shorten clotting time. The partial thromboplastin time (PTT) test, which is similar but less sensitive and less frequently performed, relies on contact with the glass surface of a test tube to activate the sample. Since most congenital coagulation deficiencies occur in the intrinsic pathway, APTT is valuable in preoperative screening for bleeding tendencies. It's also the test of choice for monitoring heparin therapy.

Purpose
□ To screen for deficiencies of the clotting factors in the intrinsic pathways (except Factor VII and Factor XIII)
□ To monitor heparin therapy.

Patient preparation
Explain to the patient that this test helps determine if his blood clots normally. Advise him that he needn't restrict food or fluids. Tell him the test requires a blood sample; who will perform the venipuncture and when; and that he may experience discomfort from the needle puncture and the pressure of the tourniquet. Reassure him that collecting the sample takes less than 3 minutes.

When appropriate, tell the patient receiving heparin therapy that this test may be repeated at regular intervals to assess response to treatment.

Procedure
Perform a venipuncture, and collect the sample in a 7 ml *blue-top* tube.

Precautions
□ To prevent hemolysis, avoid excessive probing at the venipuncture site and handle the sample gently.
□ Completely fill the collection tube, invert it gently several times, and send it to the laboratory or place it on ice.

Values
Normally, a fibrin clot forms 25 to 36 seconds after addition of reagent.

Implications of results
Prolonged times may indicate a deficiency of certain plasma clotting factors; the presence of heparin; or the presence of fibrin split products, fibrinolysins, or circulating anticoagulants that are antibodies to specific clotting factors.

HEPARIN NEUTRALIZATION ASSAY

This complex, quantitative test is sometimes used to monitor heparin therapy. It can also help determine if prolonged thrombin time results from effective heparin therapy or from the presence of circulating anticoagulants, such as fibrin split products. To perform this test, a specimen is divided into small plasma samples. Thrombin time is determined on one sample; the other samples are added to various dilutions of protamine sulfate. After a brief incubation, equal amounts of thrombin are added to each solution and thrombin time is measured. Because protamine sulfate neutralizes heparin, reduced thrombin time in the protamine-treated samples indicates the presence of heparin.

A fibrometer is used to select the sample with the thrombin time closest to standard. Then, a chart or formula is used to convert the sample's protamine concentration to units of heparin/ml, providing an accurate measurement of heparin blood levels. If none of the samples shows a reduced thrombin time, no heparin is present, indicating that the prolonged thrombin time is due to other anticoagulants, such as fibrin split products.

WILLIAM E. KLINE, MS, MT(ASCP), SBB

Post-test care
If a hematoma develops at the venipuncture site, apply warm soaks.

Interfering factors
□ Failure to use the proper anticoagulant, to fill the collection tube completely, or to mix the sample and the anticoagulant adequately may interfere with accurate determination of test results.
□ Hemolysis due to rough handling of the sample or to excessive probing at the venipuncture site may alter test results.
□ Failure to send the sample to the laboratory immediately or to place it on ice may cause spurious test results.

ELIZABETH ANNE MALLON, BS, MT (ASCP)

Prothrombin Time
[Pro time]

This test measures the time required for a fibrin clot to form in a citrated plasma sample after addition of calcium ions and tissue thromboplastin (Factor III), and compares this time with the fibrin clotting time in a control sample of plasma. Since the test reaction bypasses the intrinsic coagulation pathway (plasma thromboplastin formation in Stage I) and doesn't involve platelets, the prothrombin time (PT) indirectly measures prothrombin, and is an excellent screening procedure for overall evaluation of extrinsic coagulation factors V, VII, and X, and of prothrombin and fibrinogen. Prothrombin time is the test of choice for monitoring oral anticoagulant therapy.

Although test results are frequently reported as "percent of normal activity," compared with a curve of the clotting rate of normal diluted plasma, this method is inaccurate, because dilution of the sample affects the coagulation mechanism. The most reliably accurate method reports both the patient's and the control clotting times in seconds.

Purpose
□ To evaluate the extrinsic coagulation system
□ To monitor response to oral anticoagulant therapy.

Patient preparation
Explain to the patient that this test helps determine if his blood clots normally. Advise him that he needn't restrict food or fluids. Tell him the test requires a blood sample; who will perform the venipuncture and when; and that he may experience discomfort from the needle puncture and the pressure of the tourniquet. Collecting the sample takes less than 3 minutes.

Check patient history for use of medications that may interfere with accurate determination of test results.

When appropriate, explain to the patient that this test monitors the effects of medications (oral anticoagulants). Tell him the test will be performed daily when therapy begins, and will be repeated at longer intervals when medication levels stabilize.

Procedure
Perform a venipuncture, and collect the sample in a 7 ml *blue-top* tube.

Precautions
□ To prevent hemolysis, avoid excessive probing during venipuncture and handle the sample gently.
□ Completely fill the collection tube, and invert it gently several times to mix the sample and the anticoagulant adequately. If the tube isn't filled to the correct volume, an excess of citrate appears in the sample.
□ Send the sample to the laboratory promptly. If transport is delayed more than 4 hours, and the sample is kept at room temperature, Factor V may deteriorate, prolonging the PT; however, if the sample is refrigerated, Factor VII may be activated, shortening the PT.

Values
Normally, PT values range from 9.6 to 11.8 seconds in males, and from 9.5 to

11.3 seconds in females. However, values vary, depending on the source of tissue thromboplastin and the type of sensing devices used to measure clot formation. In a patient receiving oral anticoagulants, PT is usually maintained between one and a half and two times the normal control.

Implications of results

Prolonged PT may indicate deficiencies in fibrinogen, prothrombin, or factor V, VII, or X (specific assays can pinpoint such deficiencies); vitamin K deficiency; and hepatic disease. Or, it may result from ongoing oral anticoagulant therapy. Prolonged PT that exceeds two and a half times the control value is commonly associated with abnormal bleeding.

Post-test care

If a hematoma develops at the venipuncture site, apply warm soaks.

Interfering factors

□ Hemolysis caused by excessive probing during venipuncture or by rough handling of the sample may interfere with the accurate determination of test results.

□ Failure to mix the sample and anticoagulant adequately or to send the sample to the laboratory promptly may alter test results.

□ Fibrin or fibrin split products in the sample, or plasma fibrinogen levels less than 100 mg/dl can prolong PT.

□ Falsely prolonged results may occur if the collection tube is not filled to capacity with blood; then the amount of anticoagulant is excessive for the blood sample.

□ Prolonged PT can also result from the use of ACTH, alcohol (large quantities), anabolic steroids, cholestyramine resin, heparin I.V. (within 5 hours of sample collection), indomethacin, mefenamic acid, para-aminosalicylic acid, methimazole, oxyphenbutazone, phenylbutazone, phenytoin, propylthiouracil, quinidine, quinine, thyroid hormones, and vitamin A.

□ Shortened PT can result from the use of antihistamines, chloral hydrate, corticosteroids, digitalis, diuretics, glutethimide, griseofulvin, progestin-estrogen combinations, pyrazinamide, vitamin K, and xanthines (caffeine, theophylline).

□ Prolonged or shortened PT results can follow ingestion of antibiotics, barbiturates, hydroxyzine, sulfonamides, salicylates (more than 1 g/day prolongs PT), mineral oil, or clofibrate.

ELIZABETH ANNE MALLON, BS, MT(ASCP)

Prothrombin Consumption Time

In normal coagulation, the thromboplastin formed in the intrinsic coagulation pathway converts most plasma prothrombin into thrombin, leaving little or no prothrombin in normal serum. Consequently, the presence of prothrombin in serum indicates deficiency of platelets or of the clotting factors that generate thromboplastin. Such deficiencies allow only a small amount of prothrombin to be converted to thrombin, shortening the prothrombin consumption time (PCT).

Using a serum sample, this test measures the rate and the amount of prothrombin activation in the clotting process.

Purpose

□ To detect deficiencies of platelets or clotting factors essential to thromboplastin formation (factors VIII, IX, XI, and XII).

Patient preparation

Explain to the patient that this test helps determine if his blood clots normally. Advise him that he needn't restrict food or fluids. Tell him the test requires a blood sample; who will perform the venipuncture and when; and that he may experience discomfort from the needle puncture and the pressure of the tourniquet. Collecting the sample takes less than 3 minutes.

Check patient history for ingestion of anticoagulants, such as coumarin, and note such drugs on the laboratory slip.

Procedure

Perform a venipuncture, and collect the sample in a 7 ml *red-top* tube.

Precautions

Handle the sample gently to prevent hemolysis, and send it to the laboratory immediately, or place it on ice.

Values

Prothrombin consumption is normally complete after 20 seconds.

Implications of results

Excess prothrombin in the serum indicates shortened consumption time, usually caused by deficiency in some or all the Stage I clotting factors (factors VIII, IX, XI, and XII), or platelet abnormalities. A shortened interval also suggests that one or more of these clotting factors is at 10% or less of its normal concentration. Prolonged prothrombin consumption time may result from hemolysis or from contamination of the sample with tissue thromboplastin.

Patients with abnormal results require factor assays, platelet studies, and further tests of thromboplastin function (activated partial thromboplastin time, for example) to confirm diagnosis.

Post-test care

If a hematoma develops at the venipuncture site, ease discomfort by applying warm soaks.

Interfering factors

□ Traumatic venipuncture, hemolysis caused by rough handling of the sample, or failure to send the sample to the laboratory immediately or to place it on ice may interfere with accurate determination of test results.

□ Anticoagulant therapy may alter test results.

ELIZABETH ANNE MALLON, BS, MT(ASCP)

One-stage Assay: Extrinsic Coagulation System

[Factor II assay, Factor V assay, Factor VII assay, Factor X assay]

When prothrombin time (PT) and activated partial thromboplastin time (APTT) are abnormal (prolonged), a one-stage assay helps detect deficiency of Factor II, Factor V, or Factor X. If PT is abnormal but APTT is normal, Factor VII may be deficient.

In this test, samples of the patient's plasma are added to normal plasma controls, each deficient in a single factor. The activity of each factor in the patient's plasma is compared with normal activity plotted on a predetermined standard curve for each factor. Observing which factor corrects the coagulation deficiency can identify disorders of factors II, V, VII, and X.

Purpose

□ To identify a specific factor deficiency in persons with prolonged PT or APTT
□ To study patients with congenital or acquired coagulation defects
□ To monitor the effects of anticoagulant therapy.

Patient preparation

Explain to the patient that this test assesses the function of the blood coagulation mechanism. Inform him that he needn't restrict food or fluids. Tell him the test requires a blood sample; who will perform the venipuncture and when; and that he may experience discomfort from the needle puncture and the pressure of the tourniquet. Reassure him that collecting the sample takes less than 3 minutes.

When appropriate, tell the patient a series of tests will be needed to monitor the effects of anticoagulant therapy.

THE MISSING LINK: FACTOR XIII ASSAY

When the patient shows poor wound healing and other symptoms of a bleeding disorder, despite normal results of coagulation screening tests, a Factor XIII assay is recommended. In this test, a plasma sample is incubated with either chloracetic acid or a urea solution, after normal clotting takes place. The clot is observed for 24 hours. If the clot dissolves, a severe Factor XIII deficiency exists.

Factor XIII is responsible for stabilizing the fibrin clot, the final step in the clotting process. If the clot is unstable, it breaks loose, resulting in scarring and poor wound healing. Deficiency of this factor is usually transmitted as an autosomal recessive trait but may result from hepatic disease or from tumors. Clinical effects of Factor XIII deficiency include umbilical bleeding in neonates; recurrent ecchy-

moses, hematomas, and poor wound healing; prolonged bleeding after trauma; hemarthrosis; spontaneous abortion (rarely); and intraovarial bleeding (more common in Factor XIII deficiency than in other bleeding disorders). Bleeding after trauma may begin immediately or may be delayed as long as 12 to 36 hours. Treatment with infusions of plasma or cryoprecipitate has improved the prognosis; some patients may even live normal lives.

Before appropriate treatment for Factor XIII deficiency can begin, diagnostic evaluation must rule out other bleeding disorders. Dysfibrinogenemia, hyperfibrinogenemia, and disseminated intravascular coagulation also cause rapid clot dissolution in this assay, but unlike Factor XIII deficiency, they also cause an abnormal fibrinogen level and thrombin time.

Procedure

Perform a venipuncture, and collect the sample in a 7 ml *blue-top* tube.

Precautions

□ If the patient has a suspected coagulation defect, avoid excessive probing during venipuncture; don't leave the tourniquet on too long (it will cause bruising); and apply pressure to the puncture site for 5 minutes, or until the bleeding stops.

□ Completely fill the collection tube, and invert it gently several times to mix the sample and the anticoagulant adequately.

□ Handle the sample gently to prevent hemolysis, and send it to the laboratory immediately, or place it on ice.

Values

Factor V activity ranges from 50% to 150% of the control; Factor VII, from 65% to 135%; and Factor X, from 45% to 155%. The Factor II assay is performed differently, and its values range from 225 to 290 u/ml. (One unit of Factor II [prothrombin] equals one unit of thrombin that clots 1 ml of standard fibrinogen in 15 seconds.)

Implications of results

Deficiency of Factor II, Factor VII, or Factor X may indicate hepatic disease, vitamin K deficiency, or for Factor X, disseminated intravascular coagulation (DIC). Factor V deficiency suggests severe hepatic disease, DIC, or fibrinolysis. Deficiencies of all four factors may be congenital, although congenital Factor II deficiency is rare. Absence of Factor II is lethal; hypoprothrombinemia is rare.

Post-test care

If a hematoma develops at the venipuncture site, apply warm soaks.

Interfering factors

□ Hemolysis caused by rough handling of the sample may interfere with accurate determination of test results.

□ Failure to mix the sample and anticoagulant adequately, or to send the sample to the laboratory immediately or to place it on ice may alter test results.

□ Oral anticoagulant therapy may increase bleeding time by inhibiting vitamin K–dependent synthesis and activation of clotting factors II, VII, and X, which are formed in the liver.

ELIZABETH ANNE MALLON, BS, MT(ASCP)

One-stage Assay: Intrinsic Coagulation System

[Factor VIII assay, Factor IX assay, Factor XI assay, Factor XII assay]

When prothrombin time (PT) is normal but activated partial thromboplastin time (APTT) is abnormal, a one-stage assay helps identify a deficiency in the intrinsic coagulation system—Factor VIII, Factor IX, Factor XI, or Factor XII.

In this test, samples of the patient's plasma are added to normal plasma controls, each lacking a single factor. The activity of each factor in the patient's plasma is compared with normal activity plotted on a predetermined standard curve for each factor. Observing which factor corrects the coagulation deficiency

can identify disorders of factors VIII, IX, XI, and XII.

Purpose
□ To identify a specific factor deficiency
□ To study patients with congenital or acquired coagulation defects.

Patient preparation
Explain to the patient that this test assesses the function of the blood coagulation mechanism. Inform him he needn't restrict food or fluids. Tell him the test requires a blood sample; who will perform the venipuncture and when; and that he may experience discomfort from the needle puncture and the pressure of the tourniquet. Collecting the sample takes less than 3 minutes.

Withhold oral anticoagulants before the test, as ordered. If such medications must be continued, note this on the laboratory slip.

Procedure
Perform a venipuncture, and collect the sample in a 7 ml *blue-top* tube.

Precautions
□ If a coagulation defect is suspected, avoid excessive probing during venipuncture, don't leave the tourniquet on too long (it will cause bruising), and apply pressure to the puncture site for 5 minutes, or until the bleeding stops.
□ Completely fill the collection tube, and invert it gently several times to mix the sample and the anticoagulant adequately.
□ Handle the sample gently to prevent hemolysis, and send it to the laboratory immediately, or place it on ice.

Values
Factor VIII activity values range from 55% to 145% of the control; Factor IX, from 60% to 140%; Factor XI, from 65% to 135%; and Factor XII, from 50% to 150%.

Implications of results
Factor VIII deficiency may indicate hemophilia A, von Willebrand's disease,

HEREDITARY COAGULATION DEFECTS

DEFICIENT FACTOR	COAGULATION DISORDER
II	Hypoprothrombinemia
V	Parahemophilia
VII	Factor VII deficiency
VIII	Hemophilia A (classic hemophilia), von Willebrand's disease (vascular hemophilia)
IX	Hemophilia B (Christmas disease)
X	Stuart factor deficiency
XI	Plasma thromboplastin antecedent deficiency (PTA deficiency)
XII	Hageman trait

or Factor VIII inhibitor. An acquired deficiency of Factor VIII may result from disseminated intravascular coagulation or fibrinolysis. Factor VIII antigen and ristocetin cofactor tests distinguish between hemophilia A (and its carrier state) and von Willebrand's disease.

Factor IX deficiency may suggest hemophilia B, or it may be acquired as a result of hepatic disease, Factor IX inhibitor, vitamin K deficiency, or coumarin therapy. (Factors VIII and IX inhibitors occur after transfusions in patients deficient in either factor, and are antibodies specific to each factor.)

Factor XI deficiency may appear transiently in neonates. Factor XII deficiency may be inherited or acquired (as in nephrosis) and, like Factor XI deficiency, may appear transiently in neonates.

Post-test care

□ If a hematoma develops at the venipuncture site, apply warm soaks.

□ A patient with a bleeding disorder may require a pressure bandage to stop bleeding at the venipuncture site.

□ As ordered, resume administration of medications discontinued before the test.

Interfering factors

□ Hemolysis caused by rough handling of the sample may interfere with accurate determination of test results.

□ Failure to mix the sample and the anticoagulant adequately, or to send the sample to the laboratory immediately or to place it on ice may alter test results.

□ Oral anticoagulants decrease Factor IX levels; pregnancy elevates Factor VIII.

ELIZABETH ANNE MALLON, BS, MT(ASCP)

Plasma Thrombin Time

[Thrombin clotting time]

The thrombin time test measures how quickly a clot forms when a standard

---

FACTOR VIII–RELATED ANTIGEN TEST

Bleeding time tests and patient history can usually distinguish between classic hemophilia and von Willebrand's disease. But when bleeding time tests prove inconclusive and the patient has no family history of bleeding, the Factor VIII–related antigen test can provide helpful diagnostic information. In this test, a sample of the patient's plasma is compared with a control sample after both are placed in an agarose gel impregnated with Factor VIII antibody. Electrophoresis is performed; then the gel is examined for rocket-shaped immunoprecipitates indicative of Factor VIII antigen response.

Persons with hemophilia and carriers of hemophilia demonstrate normal activity: 45% to 185% of the control sample. Patients with von Willebrand's disease, however, show absent or deficient levels of Faction VIII antigen.

---

amount of bovine thrombin is added to a platelet-poor plasma sample from the patient and to a normal plasma control sample. After thrombin is added, the clotting time for each sample is compared and recorded. Since thrombin rapidly converts fibrinogen to a fibrin clot, this test allows a quick but imprecise estimation of plasma fibrinogen levels, which are a function of clotting time.

Purpose

□ To detect fibrinogen deficiency or defect

□ To aid diagnosis of DIC and hepatic disease

□ To monitor the effectiveness of treatment with heparin, streptokinase, or urokinase.

Patient preparation

Explain to the patient that this test helps determine if his blood clots normally. Inform him he needn't restrict food or fluids. Tell him the test requires a blood sample; who will perform the venipuncture and when; and that he may experience discomfort from the needle puncture and the pressure of the tourniquet. Collecting the sample takes less than 3 minutes.

Procedure
Perform a venipuncture, and collect the sample in a 7 ml *blue-top* tube.

Precautions
☐ To prevent hemolysis, avoid excessive probing during venipuncture and rough handling of the sample.
☐ Fill the collection tube, invert it gently several times, and send it to the laboratory immediately or place it on ice.

Values
Normal thrombin times range from 10 to 15 seconds. Test results are usually reported with a normal control value.

Implications of results
A thrombin time greater than 1.3 times the control may indicate effective heparin therapy, hepatic disease, DIC, hypofibrinogenemia, or dysfibrinogenemia.

Patients with prolonged thrombin times require quantitation of fibrinogen levels; in suspected DIC, the test for fibrin split products is also necessary.

Post-test care
If a hematoma develops at the venipuncture site, apply warm soaks.

ANTITHROMBIN III TEST

This test helps detect the cause of impaired coagulation, especially hypercoagulation. Antithrombin III (AT III) inactivates thrombin and inhibits coagulation. Normally, a balance between AT III and thrombin creates hemostasis, whereas AT III deficiency increases coagulation.

Using a fresh, citrated blood sample, this test measures the ability of AT III to inhibit thrombin's enzymatic cleavage of *p*-nitroaniline (*p*-NA) from a small polypeptide chain. Cleavage of colored *p*-NA is measured spectrophotometrically and compared to control samples. Normal values exceed 50% of control. Decreased AT III levels can indicate DIC or thromboembolic, hypercoagulation, or hepatic disorders. Slightly decreased levels can result from use of oral contraceptives. Elevated levels can result from kidney transplant and use of oral anticoagulants or anabolic steroids.

WILLIAM E. KLINE, MS, MT(ASCP), SBB

Interfering factors
☐ Hemolysis caused by excessive probing during venipuncture or rough handling of the sample may alter test results.
☐ Failure to use the proper anticoagulant in the collection tube, to mix the sample and the anticoagulant adequately, to send the sample to the laboratory immediately, or to place it on ice may interfere with the accurate determination of test results.
☐ Administration of heparin may prolong clotting time.

ELIZABETH ANNE MALLON, BS, MT(ASCP)

Plasma Fibrinogen

Fibrinogen (Factor I), a plasma protein originating in the liver, isn't normally present in serum; it's converted to fibrin by thrombin during clotting. Since fibrin is a necessary part of a blood clot, fibrinogen deficiency can produce mild-to-severe bleeding disorders. When fibrinogen levels drop below 100 mg/dl, accurate interpretation of all coagulation tests having a fibrin clot as an end point becomes most difficult.

In this test, thrombin is added to a citrated plasma sample. The resulting clot is rinsed to rid it of soluble proteins and is dissolved in biuret reagent. The amount of protein in the clot is then assayed photometrically, allowing quantitation of fibrinogen. Several other tests, involving immunologic or heat-precipitation techniques, are also in use.

Purpose
☐ To aid the diagnosis of suspected bleeding disorders.

Patient preparation
Explain to the patient that this test helps determine if his blood clots normally. Inform him that he needn't restrict food or fluids before the test. Tell him a blood sample is required; who will perform the venipuncture and when; and that he may

experience transient discomfort from the needle puncture and the pressure of the tourniquet. Reassure him that collecting the sample usually will take less than 3 minutes. Check patient history for use of heparin and oral contraceptives. Note such drugs on the laboratory slip.

Procedure

Perform a venipuncture, and collect the sample in a 7 ml *blue-top* tube.

Precautions

☐ This test is contraindicated in patients with active bleeding and acute infection or illness, and in those who have received blood transfusions within 4 weeks.

☐ If the patient is receiving heparin therapy, notify the laboratory; such therapy requires use of a different reagent.

☐ Completely fill the collection tube, invert it gently several times, and send it immediately or place it on ice.

☐ To prevent hemolysis, avoid excessive probing during venipuncture and rough handling of the sample.

Values

Fibrinogen levels normally range from 195 to 365 mg/dl.

Implications of results

Depressed fibrinogen levels may indicate congenital afibrinogenemia; hypofibrinogenemia or dysfibrinogenemia; disseminated intravascular coagulation; fibrinolysis; severe hepatic disease; cancer of the prostate, pancreas, or lung; or bone marrow lesions. Low levels may also follow obstetric complications or trauma. Elevated levels may indicate cancer of the stomach, breast, or kidney; or inflammatory disorders, such as membranoproliferative glomerulonephritis or pneumonia.

Prolonged activated partial thromboplastin time, coagulation time, prothrombin time, or thrombin time also points to fibrinogen deficiency.

Post-test care

If a hematoma develops at the venipuncture site, apply warm soaks.

Interfering factors

☐ Fibrinogen levels may also be elevated during pregnancy (third trimester) and in postoperative patients.

☐ Hemolysis caused by traumatic venipuncture or rough handling of the sample may affect test results.

☐ Failure to fill the collection tube completely, to mix the sample and anticoagulant adequately, to send the sample to the laboratory promptly, or to place it on ice may interfere with accurate determination of test results.

ELIZABETH ANNE MALLON, BS, MT(ASCP)

Fibrin Split Products
[Fibrinogen degradation products (FDP)]

After a fibrin clot forms in response to vascular injury, the fibrinolytic system acts to prevent excessive clotting by converting plasminogen into the fibrin-dissolving enzyme plasmin. Plasmin breaks down fibrin and fibrinogen into fragments, or split products, labeled X, Y, D, and E, in order of decreasing molecular weight. These products may combine with fibrin monomers to prevent polymerization; that is, the fragments retain some anticoagulant activity. An excess of such products in circulation leads to abnormally active fibrinolysis and to coagulation disorders, such as disseminated intravascular coagulation (DIC).

Fibrin split products (FSP) are detected by an immunoprecipitation reaction, in which the serum left in a blood sample after clotting is mixed on a slide with latex particles that carry D and E split products. These products adhere in clumps if fibrin or fibrinogen degradation products are present in serum.

Purpose

☐ To detect FSP in the circulation
☐ To help diagnose DIC and distinguish

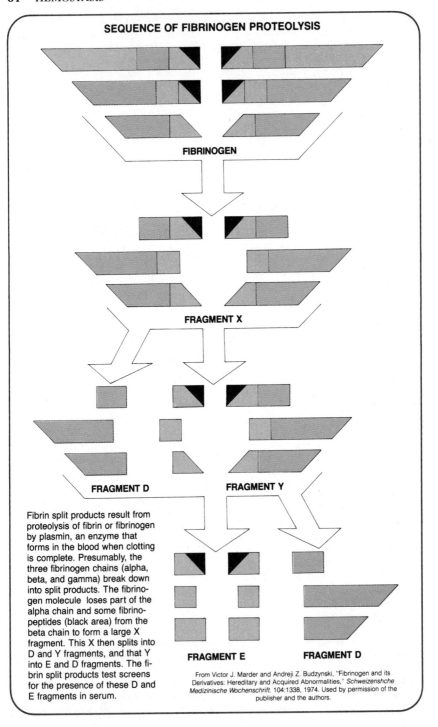

SEQUENCE OF FIBRINOGEN PROTEOLYSIS

FIBRINOGEN

FRAGMENT X

FRAGMENT D

FRAGMENT Y

FRAGMENT E

FRAGMENT D

Fibrin split products result from proteolysis of fibrin or fibrinogen by plasmin, an enzyme that forms in the blood when clotting is complete. Presumably, the three fibrinogen chains (alpha, beta, and gamma) break down into split products. The fibrinogen molecule loses part of the alpha chain and some fibrinopeptides (black area) from the beta chain to form a large X fragment. This X then splits into D and Y fragments, and that Y into E and D fragments. The fibrin split products test screens for the presence of these D and E fragments in serum.

From Victor J. Marder and Andreji Z. Budzynski, "Fibrinogen and its Derivatives: Hereditary and Acquired Abnormalities," *Schweizerishche Medizinische Wochenschrift.* 104:1338, 1974. Used by permission of the publisher and the authors.

CAUSES OF DISSEMINATED INTRAVASCULAR COAGULATION

Obstetric:	Amniotic fluid embolism, eclampsia, retained dead fetus, retained placenta, abruptio placentae, and toxemia
Neoplastic:	Sarcoma, metastatic carcinoma, acute leukemia, prostatic cancer, and giant hemangioma
Infectious:	Acute bacteremia, septicemia, rickettsemia, and infection from virus, fungi, or protozoa
Necrotic:	Trauma, destruction of brain tissue, extensive burns, heatstroke, rejection of transplant, and hepatic necrosis
Cardiovascular:	Fat embolism, acute venous thrombosis, cardiopulmonary bypass surgery, hypovolemic shock, cardiac arrest, and hypotension
Other:	Snakebite, cirrhosis, transfusion of incompatible blood, purpura, and glomerulonephritis

it from other coagulation disorders
□ To determine the degree of fibrinolysis during coagulation.

Patient preparation
Explain to the patient that this test helps determine if his blood clots normally. Inform him that he needn't restrict food or fluids. Tell him the test requires a blood sample; who will perform the venipuncture and when; and that he may experience transient discomfort from the needle puncture and the pressure of the tourniquet. Reassure him that collecting the sample takes less than 3 minutes.

Check patient history for use of medications that may interfere with accurate determination of test results.

Procedure
Perform a venipuncture, and draw 2 ml of blood into a plastic syringe. Transfer the sample to the tube provided by the laboratory, which contains a soybean tryspin inhibitor and bovine thrombin.

Precautions

□ Draw the sample before administering heparin, which may cause false-positive test results.
□ Gently invert the collection tube several times to mix the contents adequately; don't shake the tube vigorously or hemolysis may result. The blood clots within 2 seconds and must then be immediately sent to the laboratory, to be incubated at 98.6° F. (37° C.) for 30 minutes before testing proceeds.

Values
In a screening assay, serum contains less than 10 mcg/ml of FSP. A quantitative assay shows normal levels of less than 3 mcg/ml.

Implications of results
FSP levels rise in primary fibrinolytic states, due to increased levels of circulating profibrinolysin; in secondary states, due to DIC and subsequent fibrinolysis; and in alcoholic cirrhosis, postcesarean birth, preeclampsia, abruptio placentae, congenital heart disease, sunstroke, burns, intrauterine death, pulmonary embolus, deep-vein thrombosis (transient increase), and myocardial infarction (after 1 or 2 days). FSP levels usually exceed 100 mcg/ml in active renal disease or renal transplant rejection.

Post-test care
If a hematoma develops at the venipuncture site, apply warm soaks.

Interfering factors

□ Pretest administration of heparin causes false-positive results.

□ Fibrinolytic drugs, such as urokinase, and large doses of barbiturates increase FSP levels.

□ Failure to fill the collection tube completely, to mix the sample and anticoagulant adequately, or to send the sample to the laboratory immediately may interfere with the accurate determination of test results.

□ Hemolysis caused by rough handling of the sample may alter test results.

ELIZABETH ANNE MALLON, BS, MT(ASCP)

Plasma Plasminogen

Plasminogen, the precursor molecule of plasmin, is measured to assess fibrinolysis. During fibrinolysis, plasmin dissolves fibrin clots to prevent excessive coagulation and resultant impairment of blood flow. However, because plasmin doesn't circulate in active form, it can't be measured directly; its circulating precursor, plasminogen, can be measured and provides an estimate of fibrinolysis.

This test assesses plasminogen levels by adding streptokinase, a plasminogen activator, to a plasma sample. Streptokinase converts plasminogen to active plasmin; the plasmin then converts substrate a-casein to tyrosine, a colored substance that's measured spectrophotometrically. The amount of color that develops represents the amount of functional plasminogen in the sample.

Purpose

□ To assess fibrinolysis

□ To detect congenital and acquired fibrinolytic disorders.

Patient preparation

Explain to the patient that this test evaluates blood clotting. Inform him that he needn't restrict food or fluids. Tell him the test requires a blood sample; who will perform the venipuncture and when; and that he may experience minor discomfort from the needle puncture and the pressure of the tourniquet. Reassure him that collecting the sample takes less than 3 minutes. Check patient history for use of streptokinase or other drugs that may cause inaccurate test results. If these drugs must be continued, note this on the laboratory slip.

Procedure

Perform a venipuncture and collect the sample in a 7-ml *blue-top* tube.

Precautions

□ Collect the sample as quickly as possible to prevent stasis, which can slow blood flow, causing coagulation and plasminogen activation.

□ To prevent hemolysis, avoid excessive probing during venipuncture and rough handling of the specimen.

□ Immediately after collection, invert the tube gently several times; send the sample to the laboratory. If testing must be delayed, plasma must be separated and frozen at −94°F. (−70°C.).

Values

Normal plasminogen levels are 65% or greater (expressed as a percentage of normal), or 2.7 to 4.5 μ/ml (expressed as activity units).

Implications of results

Diminished plasminogen levels can result from DIC, tumors, preeclampsia, and eclampsia, which accelerate plasminogen conversion to plasmin and increase fibrinolysis. Some liver diseases prevent formation of sufficient plasminogen, decreasing fibrinolysis.

Post-test care

□ If a hematoma develops at the venipuncture site, apply warm soaks.

□ Resume medications, as ordered.

Interfering factors

□ Failure to use the proper tube, to mix the sample and citrate adequately, to send the sample immediately, or to have it

separated and frozen may alter results.
□ Hemolysis caused by excessive probing during venipuncture or by rough handling of the sample may alter results.
□ Prolonged tourniquet use before venipuncture may cause stasis, falsely decreasing plasminogen levels.
□ Oral contraceptives may slightly increase plasminogen levels. Thrombolytic drugs, such as streptokinase or urokinase, may decrease levels also.

WILLIAM E. KLINE, MS, MT(ASCP), SBB

Euglobulin Lysis Time

This test measures the interval between clot formation and dissolution in the euglobulin fraction of plasma. In the laboratory, a blood sample is acidified and mixed with calcium to form a clot. The time required for this clot to lyse is recorded.

Purpose
□ To assess systemic fibrinolysis
□ To help detect abnormal fibrinolytic states.

Patient preparation
Explain to the patient that this test evaluates the blood clotting mechanism. Tell him the test requires a blood sample; who will perform the venipuncture and when; and that, although he may have some discomfort from the needle puncture and the tourniquet pressure, collection takes less than 3 minutes.

Procedure
Perform a venipuncture. Collect a 4.5 ml sample in a *blue-top* tube or in a chilled tube with 0.5 ml sodium oxalate.

Precautions
□ When drawing the sample, be careful not to rub the area over the vein too vigorously, to pump the fist excessively, or to leave the tourniquet in place too long. Avoid excessive probing during venipuncture; handle the sample gently.
□ If a blue-top tube is used, mix the sample and anticoagulant thoroughly. If a chilled tube containing 0.5 ml sodium oxalate is used, mix the sample and preservative adequately, pack the sample in ice, and send it to the laboratory immediately.

Values
Normal lysis time is at least 2 hours.

Implications of results
Clot lysis within 1 hour indicates increased plasminogen activator activity. In pathologic fibrinolysis, lysis time may be as brief as 5 to 10 minutes.

Post-test care
If a hematoma develops at the venipuncture site, apply warm soaks.

Interfering factors
□ Prolonged tourniquet constriction, vigorous vein preparation, or excessive pumping of the fist shortens lysis time.
□ Hemolysis due to excessive probing during venipuncture or to rough handling of the sample may alter test results.
□ Failure to follow appropriate precautions for the type of collection tube used may hinder accurate results.
□ Depressed fibrinogen levels (less than 100 mg/dl) can shorten lysis time.

ELIZABETH ANNE MALLON, BS, MT(ASCP)

Selected References

Beck, William S., ed. *Hematology,* 3rd ed. Cambridge, Mass.: MIT Press, 1981.
Lamb, Jane O. *Laboratory Tests for Clinical Nursing.* Bowie, Md.: Robert J. Brady Co., 1984.

Nursing85 Drug Handbook. Springhouse, Pa.: Springhouse Corp., 1985.
Wintrobe, Maxwell M., et al. *Clinical Hematology,* 8th ed. Philadelphia: Lea & Febiger, 1981.

3 Blood Gases and Electrolytes

LEARNING OBJECTIVES

After completing this chapter, the reader will be able to:
- identify the three major fluid compartments.
- state the ABG results commonly associated with respiratory acidosis and alkalosis and with metabolic acidosis and alkalosis.
- identify the functions of the major serum electrolytes.
- list and define 11 key terms for understanding blood gases and electrolytes.
- explain the physiology of calcium absorption.
- state the causes, signs, and symptoms of hypovolemia and hypervolemia.
- explain how the sodium pump works.
- state the purpose of each test discussed in the chapter.
- prepare the patient physically and psychologically for each test.
- describe the procedure for performing each test.
- specify appropriate precautions for safe administration of each test.
- recognize signs of abnormal serum levels of the major electrolytes and respond appropriately.
- implement appropriate post-test care.
- state the normal values for each test.
- discuss the implications of abnormal test results.
- list factors that may interfere with accurate test results.

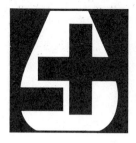

Blood Gases and Electrolytes

Introduction

Laboratory analysis of blood gases and electrolytes helps evaluate the respiratory and metabolic states of the body. Arterial blood gas measurements provide important diagnostic information concerning the adequacy of gas exchange in the lungs, the integrity of the ventilatory control system, and the blood pH and acid-base balance. Measuring serum concentrations of electrolytes also supplies valuable data about the body's acid-base balance and fluid balance.

Metabolic processes continually form acids, which must be eliminated to maintain acid-base balance. To maintain this balance, the lungs and kidneys control excretion of electrolytes to keep pH within an acceptable range. Blood gas studies measure the lungs' capacity to regulate carbon dioxide concentration in the blood; serum electrolyte assays determine the kidneys' capacity to retain or excrete metabolic acids and bases. Because these functions are so closely interwoven, accurate assessment of homeostasis requires simultaneous interpretation of blood gas and electrolyte studies.

Arterial blood gases

Blood gas studies are usually performed on arterial blood, which contains oxygen (O_2) and carbon dioxide (CO_2). Arterial blood gases (ABGs) are measurements of the partial pressure (PaO_2 and $PaCO_2$)

that each gas exerts in the blood. As the concentration of the gas rises, so does its partial pressure. To understand the clinical significance of ABG values, one must first understand the phenomenon of gas exchange in the lungs.

Environmental oxygen, about 21% of inspired air, travels through the airways into the lungs; the waste product, carbon dioxide, travels from the lungs to the surrounding air. Consequently, the alveoli in the lungs contain a mixture of inspired oxygen moving through the capillaries and into circulation, and carbon dioxide (waste product of metabolism) moving through the capillaries for exhalation.

Oxygen taken up in the lungs is transported to the tissues through the circulatory system. Only a small amount of inspired oxygen can dissolve in arterial blood; how much dissolves depends on the partial pressure of the oxygen. The remainder combines chemically with hemoglobin. *Oxygen content* (O_2CT) measures the amount of oxygen combined with hemoglobin; this value is used infrequently. *Oxygen saturation* (O_2 Sat) is the ratio of the amount of oxygen in the blood that is combined with hemoglobin, to the total amount of oxygen that the hemoglobin could carry; this value is used most often.

Carbon dioxide is produced by cellular metabolism and is released into the

IMPORTANT DEFINITIONS FOR UNDERSTANDING BLOOD GASES AND ELECTROLYTES

Partial pressure	A measure of the force that a gas exerts on the fluid in which it is dissolved
Pao_2	Partial pressure of oxygen in arterial blood
$Paco_2$	Partial pressure of carbon dioxide in arterial blood
pH	A measure of acid-base balance or the concentration of free hydrogen ions in the blood
O_2CT	Oxygen content, or the volume of oxygen combined with hemoglobin in arterial blood
O_2 Sat	Oxygen saturation, a measure of the percentage of oxygen combined with hemoglobin to the total amount of oxygen with which hemoglobin could combine
Electrolytes	Substances that dissociate into ions when fused or in solution, and thus conduct electricity
Cations	Positively charged ions
Anions	Negatively charged ions
Acidosis	Metabolic or respiratory changes that result in a loss of base or accumulation of acid
Alkalosis	Metabolic or respiratory changes that result in a loss of acid or accumulation of base

bloodstream. Because carbon dioxide is more soluble than oxygen, it dissolves in the blood, the majority forming bicarbonate (HCO_3^-), and lesser amounts constituting carbonic acid (H_2CO_3) and carbamino compounds (bound to hemoglobin).

Acid-base balance

Enzymes that control vital cellular functions perform most efficiently when the body's pH ranges between 7.35 and 7.45. Therefore, the carbonic acid/bicarbonate buffer system helps maintain body pH at this desirable level. The system may be represented by these equations:

$$CO_2 + H_2O \leftrightarrow H_2CO_3$$
carbon dioxide + water ↔ carbonic acid

In turn, carbonic acid can undergo the following change:

$$H_2CO_3 \leftrightarrow H^+ + HCO_3^-$$
carbonic acid ↔ hydrogen ion + bicarbonate

Bicarbonate and carbonic acid normally exist in a 20:1 ratio. Any change in this ratio causes a blood pH that is abnormally acidic or alkaline.

The lungs control carbonic acid levels by converting carbonic acid to carbon dioxide and water, for excretion. By changing the rate and depth of respiration, the lungs can adjust the amount of carbon dioxide lost, to maintain the normal ratio. This compensatory mechanism is rapidly effective. For example, in metabolic acidosis, the lungs increase their rate and depth in order to "blow off" excess carbon dioxide (carbonic acid).

When the lungs are functioning inadequately, they can actually produce an acid-base imbalance. For example, they cause *respiratory acidosis* by hypoventilation and retaining too much carbon dioxide (carbonic acid excess); they cause *respiratory alkalosis* by hyperventilation and exhaling too much carbon dioxide (carbonic acid deficit).

The kidneys—primary regulators of bicarbonate—excrete, reabsorb, or regenerate the amount of bicarbonate needed to maintain the normal carbonic acid/bicarbonate ratio. This can be a source of effective compensation for an imbalance that results from pulmonary dysfunction. However, this compensatory response is notably slower than pulmonary compensation and may take hours or even days.

The kidneys have another important role to play: Since the acids resulting from metabolic processes—with the exception of carbonic acid—cannot be converted to gases for exhalation by the lungs, they must be excreted by the kidneys. Thus, renal dysfunction can cause metabolic acid-base imbalance. Summarized briefly, metabolic acidosis results when the body loses too much base (bicarbonate) or retains excessive acid; metabolic alkalosis results when the body retains too much base (bicarbonate) or loses too much acid.

Clinical significance of ABGs

Abnormal variations in ABGs may result from respiratory or metabolic causes. Compensatory mechanisms, such as those in the lungs and kidneys, automatically attempt to correct an imbalance. But compensation is not correction, and compensatory mechanisms are limited.

Although valuable in assessing overall respiratory and metabolic status, ABG measurements are not diagnostically specific. For example, taken alone, ABG values do not distinguish between pulmonary and cardiac disorders. These values are most useful when considered with other factors, such as cardiac out-

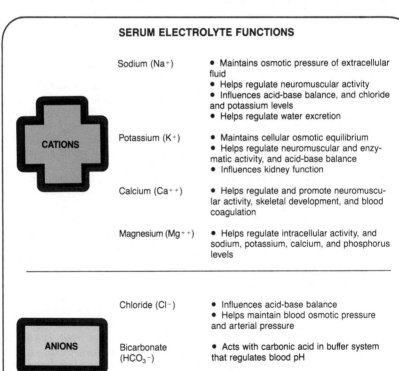

SERUM ELECTROLYTE FUNCTIONS

CATIONS

Sodium (Na+)
- Maintains osmotic pressure of extracellular fluid
- Helps regulate neuromuscular activity
- Influences acid-base balance, and chloride and potassium levels
- Helps regulate water excretion

Potassium (K+)
- Maintains cellular osmotic equilibrium
- Helps regulate neuromuscular and enzymatic activity, and acid-base balance
- Influences kidney function

Calcium (Ca++)
- Helps regulate and promote neuromuscular activity, skeletal development, and blood coagulation

Magnesium (Mg++)
- Helps regulate intracellular activity, and sodium, potassium, calcium, and phosphorus levels

ANIONS

Chloride (Cl−)
- Influences acid-base balance
- Helps maintain blood osmotic pressure and arterial pressure

Bicarbonate (HCO_3^-)
- Acts with carbonic acid in buffer system that regulates blood pH

Phosphate (HPO_4^{--})
- Helps regulate calcium levels, energy metabolism, and acid-base balance

BODY FLUIDS

Fluids, mainly water, account for 60% of an adult's total body weight. Body fluids contain substances that dissociate in solutions and conduct a weak electric current (electrolytes), and those that don't break down into smaller substances. Electrolytes with a positive charge are called cations; those carrying a negative charge are anions. A cation-anion balance results in electric neutrality.

Two main compartments house the body's fluids. Within its 100 trillion cells, the intracellular compartment accounts for 40% of the total body weight (approximately 25 liters of fluid). In the spaces between the cells, the extracellular compartment comprises 15% of the total body weight (approximately 15 liters of interstitial fluid). Intravascular fluid, or plasma, accounts for the final 5%. A change in the amount or composition of these compartments can be fatal.

Electrolytes play a crucial role in the body's water distribution, osmolality, acid-base balance, and neuromuscular irritability. As shown, potassium (K^+) is the principal cation, and phosphate (HPO_4^{--}) the dominant anion in the intracellular compartment. Like plasma, the interstitial fluid contains high concentrations of sodium (Na^+) and chloride (Cl^-). Together, fluids and electrolytes nourish and maintain the body.

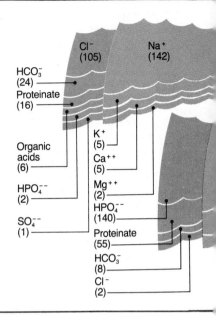

Cl^- (105)
Na^+ (142)
HCO_3^- (24)
Proteinate (16)
K^+ (5)
Organic acids (6)
Ca^{++} (5)
Mg^{++} (2)
HPO_4^{--} (2)
HPO_4^{--} (140)
SO_4^{--} (1)
Proteinate (55)
HCO_3^- (8)
Cl^- (2)

put, regional blood flow, and tissue oxygen consumption.

The significance of ABG studies is also limited by the fact that these studies don't necessarily detect disease. For example, the lungs may continue to function properly, with unchanged ABG values, despite the presence of pulmonary disease. Therefore, other diagnostic screening tests, such as spirometry or chest X-ray, must be performed. When dealing with ABG values, make sure you check the accepted values for your hospital. Normal range may vary, according to the laboratory method.

Serum electrolytes

Electrolytes are substances that dissociate into ions when dissolved in the blood. Electrolytes that carry a positive charge are called cations; those that carry a negative charge are called anions. Sodium, calcium, chloride, and bicarbonate are the major extracellular electrolytes. Sodium is the most abundant extracellular cation; chloride, the most abundant anion. Potassium, magnesium, and phosphate are the major intracellular electrolytes. Potassium is the most abundant intracellular cation; phosphate, the most abundant anion.

Serum concentrations of electrolytes influence movement of fluid within and between body compartments. Such movement depends on osmolality—the concentration of electrolytes in the respective fluid compartments. Total electrolyte concentration (usually expressed in milliequivalents [mEq] per liter of serum) plus other dissolved substances, such as glucose, determine the osmolality of a given compartment. During osmosis, water flows from a compartment of lower osmolality to one of higher osmolality, until the osmotic pressure in the two compartments is equal.

Electrolytes and homeostasis

The body can function properly only if the kidneys and lungs (with the aid of endocrine hormones) maintain electrolyte balance between intracellular and extracellular compartments. The hypothalamus and the pituitary control osmolality by regulating antidiuretic hormone, which promotes water reab-

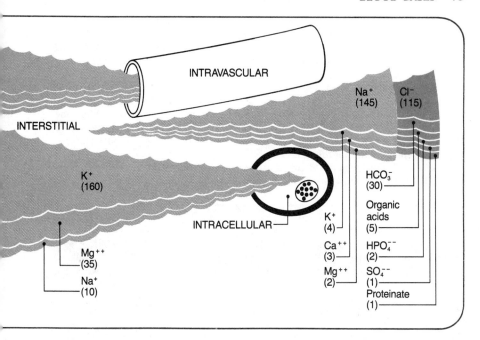

sorption by the kidneys. The kidneys govern fluid and electrolytes through filtration, reabsorption, and excretion.

Electrolytes also help maintain acid-base balance. The kidneys may exchange potassium or sodium for hydrogen, and absorb or excrete bicarbonate or chloride ions to maintain a proper pH. Serum electrolyte concentrations affect all metabolic activity in some way. Also, electrolyte concentration differences between intracellular fluid and extracellular fluid regulate neuromuscular function. Consequently, serum electrolyte studies are essential to routine medical evaluation in all hospitalized patients. Abnormal electrolyte values may reflect fluid or acid-base imbalance, or kidney, neuromuscular, endocrine, or skeletal dysfunction.

LYNDA PALMER, RN, BHS
ANNETTE L. HARMON, RN, MSN

BLOOD GASES

Arterial Blood Gas Analysis

Arterial blood gas (ABG) analysis evaluates gas exchange in the lungs by measuring the partial pressures of oxygen (PaO_2) and carbon dioxide ($PaCO_2$), and the pH of an arterial sample. PaO_2 indicates how much oxygen the lungs are delivering to the blood. $PaCO_2$ indicates how efficiently the lungs eliminate carbon dioxide. The pH indicates the acid-base level of the blood, or the hydrogen ion (H^+) concentration. Acidity indicates H^+ excess; alkalinity, H^+ deficit. Oxygen content (O_2CT), oxygen saturation (O_2 Sat), and bicarbonate (HCO_3^-) values also aid diagnosis. A blood sample for ABG analysis may be drawn by percutaneous arterial puncture or from an arterial line.

Purpose

□ To evaluate the efficiency of pulmonary gas exchange
□ To assess integrity of the ventilatory control system
□ To determine the acid-base level of the blood
□ To monitor respiratory therapy.

Patient preparation

Explain to the patient that this test evaluates how well the lungs are delivering oxygen to blood and eliminating carbon dioxide. Inform him he needn't restrict food or fluids. Tell him the test requires a blood sample; who will perform the arterial puncture and when; and which site—radial, brachial, or femoral artery—has been selected for the puncture. Instruct the patient to breathe normally during the test, and warn him that he may experience a brief cramping or throbbing pain at the puncture site.

Procedure

Perform an arterial puncture.

ACID-BASE DISORDERS

DISORDERS AND ABG FINDINGS	POSSIBLE CAUSES	SIGNS AND SYMPTOMS
Respiratory acidosis (excess CO_2 retention) pH < 7.35 HCO_3^- > 26 mEq/liter (if compensating) $Paco_2$ > 45 mmHg	• CNS depression from drugs, injury, or disease • Asphyxia • Hypoventilation due to pulmonary, cardiac, musculoskeletal, or neuromuscular disease	• Diaphoresis, headache, tachycardia, confusion, restlessness, apprehension
Respiratory alkalosis (excess CO_2 excretion) pH > 7.42 HCO_3^- < 22 mEq/liter (if compensating) $Paco_2$ < 35 mmHg	• Hyperventilation due to anxiety, pain, or improper ventilator settings • Respiratory stimulation by drugs, disease, hypoxia, fever, or high room temperature • Gram-negative bacteremia	• Rapid, deep respirations; paresthesias; lightheadedness; twitching; anxiety; fear
Metabolic acidosis (HCO_3^- loss, acid retention) pH < 7.35 HCO_3^- < 22 mEq/liter $Paco_2$ < 35 mmHg (if compensating)	• HCO_3^- depletion due to renal disease, diarrhea, or small bowel fistulas • Excessive production of organic acids due to hepatic disease; endocrine disorders, including diabetes mellitus; hypoxia; shock; or drug intoxication • Inadequate excretion of acids due to renal disease	• Rapid, deep breathing; fruity breath; fatigue; headache; lethargy; drowsiness; nausea; vomiting; coma (if severe)
Metabolic alkalosis (HCO_3^- retention, acid loss) pH > 7.42 HCO_3^- > 26 mEq/liter $Paco_2$ > 45 mmHg (if compensating)	• Loss of hydrochloric acid from prolonged vomiting, gastric suctioning • Loss of potassium due to increased renal excretion (as in diuretic therapy), steroid overdose • Excessive alkali ingestion	• Slow, shallow breathing; hypertonic muscles; restlessness; twitching; confusion; irritability; apathy; tetany; convulsions; coma (if severe)

Precautions
□ If the patient has recently had an intermittent positive-pressure breathing treatment, wait at least 20 minutes before drawing arterial blood, because such treatment alters blood gas values.
□ If the patient is receiving oxygen therapy, find out whether the order for ABG measurements specifies that these be obtained on room air or on oxygen therapy. If the order indicates room air, discontinue oxygen therapy for 15 to 20 minutes before drawing the sample.

Before sending the sample to the laboratory, include the following information on the requisition slip:
□ Indicate whether the patient was breathing room air or receiving oxygen therapy when the sample was drawn. If he was receiving oxygen therapy, give the flow rate.
□ If the patient's on a ventilator, note the FIO_2 and tidal volume.
□ Record the patient's rectal temperature and respiratory rate.

Values
Normal ABG values fall within the following ranges:

PaO_2	75 to 100 mmHg
$PaCO_2$	35 to 45 mmHg
pH	7.35 to 7.42
O_2CT	15% to 23%
O_2 Sat	94% to 100%
HCO_3^-	22 to 26 mEq/liter

Implications of results
Low PaO_2, O_2CT, and O_2 Sat levels, in combination with a high $PaCO_2$ value, may be due to conditions that impair respiratory function, such as respiratory muscle weakness or paralysis (as in Guillain-Barré syndrome or myasthenia gravis), respiratory center inhibition (from head injury, brain tumor, or drug abuse, for example), and airway obstruction (possibly from mucous plugs or a tumor). Similarly, low readings may result from bronchiole obstruction caused by asthma or emphysema, from an abnormal ventilation-perfusion ratio due to partially blocked alveoli or pulmonary capillaries, or from alveoli that are damaged or filled with fluid because of disease, hemorrhage, or near-drowning.

When inspired air contains insufficient oxygen, PaO_2, O_2CT, and O_2 Sat also decrease, but $PaCO_2$ may be normal. Such findings are common in pneumothorax, impaired diffusion between alveoli and blood (due to interstitial fibrosis, for example), or in an arteriovenous shunt that permits blood to bypass the lungs.

Low O_2CT—with normal PaO_2, O_2 Sat, and possibly, $PaCO_2$ values—may result from severe anemia, decreased blood volume, and reduced hemoglobin oxygen-carrying capacity.

In addition to clarifying blood oxygen disorders, ABGs can give considerable information about acid-base disorders, as shown in the accompanying chart.

Post-test care
□ After applying pressure to the puncture site, tape a gauze pad firmly over it. (If the puncture site is on the arm, don't tape the entire circumference; this may restrict circulation.)

□ Monitor vital signs, and observe for signs of circulatory impairment, such as swelling, discoloration, pain, numbness, or tingling in the bandaged arm or leg. Watch for bleeding from the puncture site.

Interfering factors
□ Exposing the sample to air affects PaO_2 and $PaCO_2$ levels, and interferes with accurate determination of results.
□ Failure to heparinize the syringe, to place the sample correctly in an iced bag, or to send the sample to the laboratory immediately adversely affects the test results.
□ Venous blood in the sample may lower PaO_2 and elevate $PaCO_2$.
□ Bicarbonate, ethacrynic acid, hydrocortisone, metolazone, prednisone, and thiazides may elevate $PaCO_2$ levels. Acetazolamide, methicillin, nitrofurantoin, and tetracycline may decrease $PaCO_2$ levels.

LYNDA PALMER, RN, BHS

Total Carbon Dioxide Content

Carbon dioxide (CO_2) is present in small amounts in the air, and in the body as an end product of food metabolism. When the pressure of CO_2 in the red cells exceeds 40 mmHg, CO_2 spills out of the cells and dissolves in plasma. There it may combine with water (H_2O) to form carbonic acid (H_2CO_3), which, in turn, can dissociate into hydrogen (H^+) and bicarbonate ions (HCO_3^-).

This test measures the total concentration of all such forms of CO_2 in serum, plasma, or whole blood samples. Since about 90% of CO_2 in serum is in the form of bicarbonate, this test closely assesses bicarbonate levels. Total CO_2 content reflects the adequacy of gas exchange in the lungs and the efficiency of the carbonic acid-bicarbonate buffer system, which maintains acid-base balance and normal pH. Consequently, this test is commonly ordered for patients with respiratory insufficiency and is usually included in any assessment of electrolyte balance. For maximum clinical significance, test results must be considered with both pH and arterial blood gas values.

Purpose
☐ To help evaluate acid-base balance.

Patient preparation
Explain to the patient that this test measures the amount of CO_2 in the blood. Inform him that he needn't restrict food or fluids. Tell him this test requires a blood sample; who will perform the venipuncture and when; and that he may feel some transient discomfort from the needle puncture and the pressure of the tourniquet. Reassure him that collecting the sample usually takes only a few minutes. Check the patient's history for use of medications that may influence CO_2 blood levels.

Procedure
Perform a venipuncture. Since CO_2 content is usually measured along with electrolytes, a 10 to 15 ml *red-top* tube may be used. When this test is performed alone, a *green-top* (heparinized) tube is appropriate.

Precautions
Completely fill the tube, to prevent diffusion of CO_2 into the vacuum.

Values
Normally, total CO_2 levels range from 22 to 34 mEq/liter.

Implications of results
High CO_2 levels may occur in metabolic alkalosis (due to excessive ingestion or retention of base bicarbonate), respiratory acidosis (from hypoventilation, for example, as in emphysema or pneumonia), primary aldosteronism, and Cushing's syndrome. CO_2 levels may also rise above normal after excessive loss of acids, as in severe vomiting and continuous gastric drainage.

Decreased CO_2 levels are common in metabolic acidosis (as in diabetic acidosis, or renal tubular acidosis resulting from renal failure). Decreased total CO_2 levels in metabolic acidosis also result from loss of bicarbonate (as in severe diarrhea or intestinal drainage). Levels may fall below normal in respiratory alkalosis (from hyperventilation, for example, after trauma).

Post-test care
If a hematoma develops at the venipuncture site, apply warm soaks.

Interfering factors
☐ CO_2 levels rise with administration of excessive ACTH, cortisone, or thiazide diuretics, or with excessive ingestion of alkalis or licorice.
☐ CO_2 levels decrease with administration of salicylates, paraldehyde, methicillin, dimercaprol, ammonium chloride, acetazolamide, and accidental ingestion of ethylene glycol or methyl alcohol.

PATRICE M. HARMAN, RN

ELECTROLYTES

Serum Calcium

This test measures serum levels of calcium, a predominantly extracellular cation that helps regulate and promote neuromuscular and enzyme activity, skeletal development, and blood coagulation. The body absorbs calcium from the gastrointestinal tract, provided sufficient vitamin D is present, and excretes it in the urine and feces. Over 98% of the body's calcium is found in the bones and teeth. However, calcium can shift in and out of these structures. For example, when calcium concentrations in the blood fall below normal, calcium ions can move out of the bones and teeth to help restore blood levels.

Parathyroid hormone, vitamin D, and to a lesser extent, calcitonin and adrenal steroids control calcium blood levels. Calcium and phosphorus are closely related, usually reacting together to form insoluble calcium phosphate. To prevent formation of a precipitate in the blood, calcium levels vary inversely with phosphorus; as serum calcium levels rise, phosphorus levels should decrease through renal excretion. Since the body excretes calcium daily, regular ingestion of calcium in food (at least 1 g/day) is necessary for normal calcium balance.

Purpose
☐ To aid diagnosis of neuromuscular, skeletal, and endocrine disorders; arrhythmias; blood-clotting deficiencies; and acid-base imbalance.

Patient preparation
Explain to the patient that this test determines blood calcium level. Inform him he needn't restrict food or fluids. Tell him the test requires a blood sample; who will perform the venipuncture and when; and that he may feel some discomfort from the needle puncture and

the pressure of the tourniquet. Reassure him that collecting the sample takes less than 3 minutes.

Procedure
Perform a venipuncture, and collect the sample in a 10 to 15 ml *red-top* tube.

Precautions
None.

Values
Normally, serum calcium levels range from 8.9 to 10.1 mg/dl (atomic absorption), or from 4.5 to 5.5 mEq/liter. In children, serum calcium levels are higher than in adults. Calcium levels can rise as high as 12 mg/dl or 6 mEq/liter during phases of rapid bone growth.

Implications of results
Abnormally high serum calcium levels (hypercalcemia) may occur in hyperparathyroidism and parathyroid tumors (due to oversecretion of parathyroid hormone), Paget's disease of the bone, multiple myeloma, metastatic carcinoma, multiple fractures, or prolonged immobilization. Elevated serum calcium levels may also result from inadequate excretion of calcium, as in adrenal insufficiency and renal disease; from excessive calcium ingestion; or from overuse of antacids such as calcium carbonate.

 Observe the patient with hypercalcemia for deep bone pain, flank pain due to renal calculi, and muscle hypotonicity. Hypercalcemic crisis begins with nausea, vomiting, and dehydration, leading to stupor and coma, and can end in cardiac arrest.

Low calcium levels (hypocalcemia) may result from hypoparathyroidism, total parathyroidectomy, or malabsorption. Decreased serum levels of calcium may follow calcium loss in Cushing's syndrome, renal failure, acute pancreatitis, and peritonitis.

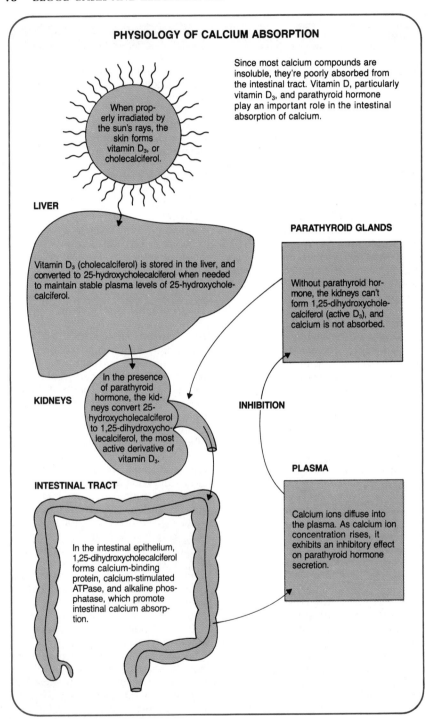

PHYSIOLOGY OF CALCIUM ABSORPTION

Since most calcium compounds are insoluble, they're poorly absorbed from the intestinal tract. Vitamin D, particularly vitamin D_3, and parathyroid hormone play an important role in the intestinal absorption of calcium.

When properly irradiated by the sun's rays, the skin forms vitamin D_3, or cholecalciferol.

LIVER

Vitamin D_3 (cholecalciferol) is stored in the liver, and converted to 25-hydroxycholecalciferol when needed to maintain stable plasma levels of 25-hydroxycholecalciferol.

PARATHYROID GLANDS

Without parathyroid hormone, the kidneys can't form 1,25-dihydroxycholecalciferol (active D_3), and calcium is not absorbed.

KIDNEYS

In the presence of parathyroid hormone, the kidneys convert 25-hydroxycholecalciferol to 1,25-dihydroxycholecalciferol, the most active derivative of vitamin D_3.

INHIBITION

INTESTINAL TRACT

PLASMA

Calcium ions diffuse into the plasma. As calcium ion concentration rises, it exhibits an inhibitory effect on parathyroid hormone secretion.

In the intestinal epithelium, 1,25-dihydroxycholecalciferol forms calcium-binding protein, calcium-stimulated ATPase, and alkaline phosphatase, which promote intestinal calcium absorption.

In a patient with hypocalcemia, be alert for circumoral and peripheral numbness and tingling, muscle twitching, Chvostek's sign (facial muscle spasm), tetany, muscle cramping, Trousseau's sign (carpopedal spasm), seizure activity, and arrhythmias.

Post-test care

If a hematoma develops at the venipuncture site, ease discomfort by applying warm soaks.

Interfering factors

☐ Excessive ingestion of vitamin D or its derivatives (dihydrotachysterol, calcitriol), and the use of androgens, calciferol-activated calcium salts, progestins-estrogens, and thiazides can elevate serum calcium levels.

☐ Chronic use of laxatives, excessive transfusions of citrated blood, and administration of acetazolamide, corticosteroids, and mithramycin can suppress calcium levels.

ANNETTE L. HARMON, RN, MSN

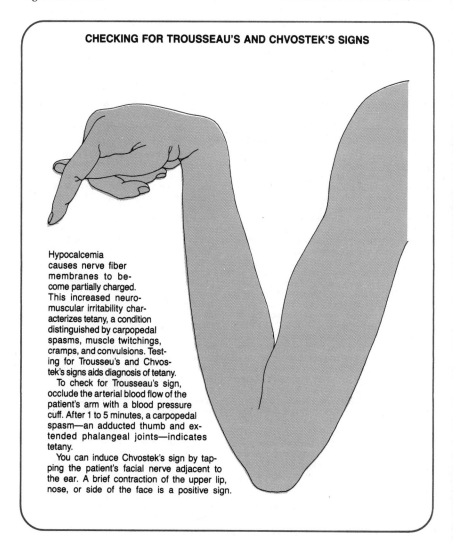

CHECKING FOR TROUSSEAU'S AND CHVOSTEK'S SIGNS

Hypocalcemia causes nerve fiber membranes to become partially charged. This increased neuromuscular irritability characterizes tetany, a condition distinguished by carpopedal spasms, muscle twitchings, cramps, and convulsions. Testing for Trousseu's and Chvostek's signs aids diagnosis of tetany.

To check for Trousseau's sign, occlude the arterial blood flow of the patient's arm with a blood pressure cuff. After 1 to 5 minutes, a carpopedal spasm—an adducted thumb and extended phalangeal joints—indicates tetany.

You can induce Chvostek's sign by tapping the patient's facial nerve adjacent to the ear. A brief contraction of the upper lip, nose, or side of the face is a positive sign.

Serum Chloride

This test, a quantitative analysis, measures serum levels of chloride, the major extracellular fluid anion. Interacting with sodium, chloride helps maintain the osmotic pressure of blood and therefore helps regulate blood volume and arterial pressure. Chloride levels also affect acid-base balance. Serum concentrations of this electrolyte are regulated by aldosterone secondarily to regulation of sodium. Chloride is absorbed from the intestines and is excreted primarily by the kidneys.

Purpose
□ To detect acid-base imbalance (acidosis and alkalosis) and to aid evaluation of fluid status and extracellular cation-anion balance.

Patient preparation
Explain to the patient that the test evaluates the chloride content of blood. Tell him this test requires a blood sample; who will perform the venipuncture and when; and that he may feel some transient discomfort from the needle puncture and pressure of the tourniquet. Reassure the patient that collecting the sample usually takes only a few minutes.

Check the patient's medication history for recent therapy with drugs that may influence chloride levels.

Procedure
Perform venipuncture, and collect the sample in a 10 to 15 ml *red-top* tube.

BALANCING pH LEVELS

To measure the acidity or alkalinity of a solution, chemists use a pH scale of 1 to 15 that measures hydrogen ion concentrations. As hydrogen ions and acidity increase, pH falls below 7.0, which is neutral. Conversely, pH and alkalinity increase when hydrogen ions decrease. Acid-base balance, or homeostasis of hydrogen ions, is mandatory if the body's enzyme systems are to work properly.

The slightest change in ionic hydrogen concentration alters the rate of cellular chemical reactions and, if sufficiently severe, can be fatal. To maintain a normal blood pH—generally between 7.35 and 7.45—the body relies on the following three mechanisms:
- *Buffers,* chemically composed of two substances, prevent radical pH changes by replacing strong acids added to a solution (such as blood) with weaker ones. For example, strong acids capable of yielding many hydrogen ions are replaced by weaker ones that yield fewer hydrogen ions. Because of the principal buffer coupling of bicarbonate and carbonic acid—normally in a ratio of 20:1—the plasma acid-base level rarely fluctuates. Increased bicarbonate, however, indicates alkalosis, while a decrease in bicarbonate points to acidosis. Increased carbonic acid indicates acidosis, while a decrease indicates alkalosis.
- *Respiration* is important in maintaining blood pH. The lungs convert carbonic acid to carbon dioxide and water. With every expiration, carbon dioxide and water leave the body, decreasing the carbonic acid content of the blood. Consequently fewer hydrogen ions are formed, and blood pH increases. When the blood's hydrogen ion or carbonic acid content increases, neurons in the respiratory center stimulate respiration. Hyperventilation eliminates carbon dioxide and hence carbonic acid from the body, reduces hydrogen ion formation, and increases pH. Conversely, increased blood pH from alkalosis—decreased hydrogen ion concentration—causes hypoventilation, which restores blood pH to its normal level by retaining carbon dioxide and thus increasing hydrogen ion formation.
- *Urinary excretion* is the third factor in acid-base balance. Since the kidneys excrete varying amounts of acids and bases, they control urine pH, which, in turn, affects blood pH. For example, when blood pH is decreased, the distal and collecting tubules remove excessive hydrogen ions—carbonic acid forms in the tubular cells and dissociates into hydrogen and bicarbonate—and displace them in urine, thereby eliminating hydrogen from the body. In exchange, basic ions in the urine—most often sodium—diffuse into the tubular cells, where they combine with bicarbonate. This sodium bicarbonate is then reabsorbed in the blood, resulting in decreased urine pH and, more importantly, increased blood pH.

Precautions

Handle the sample gently to prevent hemolysis.

Values

Normally, serum chloride levels range from 100 to 108 mEq/liter.

Implications of results

Chloride levels relate inversely to those of bicarbonate and thus reflect acid-base balance. Excessive loss of gastric juices or of other secretions containing chloride may cause hypochloremic metabolic alkalosis; excessive chloride retention or ingestion may lead to hyperchloremic metabolic acidosis.

Elevated serum chloride levels (hyperchloremia) may result from severe dehydration, complete renal shutdown, head injury (producing neurogenic hyperventilation), and primary aldosteronism.

Low chloride levels (hypochloremia) are usually associated with low sodium and potassium levels. Possible underlying causes include prolonged vomiting, gastric suctioning, intestinal fistula, chronic renal failure, and Addison's disease. Congestive heart failure, or edema resulting in excess extracellular fluid can cause dilutional hypochloremia.

 Observe a patient with hypochloremia for hypertonicity of muscles, tetany, and depressed respirations. In a patient with hyperchloremia, be alert for signs of developing stupor, rapid deep breathing, and weakness that may lead to coma.

Post-test care

If a hematoma develops at the venipuncture site, ease discomfort by applying warm soaks.

Interfering factors

□ Elevated serum chloride levels may result from administration of ammonium chloride, cholestyramine, boric acid, oxyphenbutazone, phenylbutazone, or excessive I.V. infusion of sodium chloride.

□ Serum chloride levels are decreased by thiazides, furosemide, ethacrynic acid, bicarbonates, or prolonged I.V. infusion of 5% dextrose in water.

□ Hemolysis due to rough handling of the sample may interfere with accurate determination of test results.

ANNETTE L. HARMON, RN, MSN

Serum Magnesium

This test, a quantitative analysis, measures serum levels of magnesium, the most abundant intracellular cation after potassium. Vital to neuromuscular function, this often overlooked electrolyte helps regulate intracellular metabolism, activates many essential enzymes, and affects the metabolism of nucleic acids and proteins. Magnesium also helps transport sodium and potassium across cell membranes and, through its effect on the secretion of parathyroid hormone, influences intracellular calcium levels. Most magnesium is found in bone and in intracellular fluid; a small amount is found in extracellular fluid. Magnesium is absorbed by the small intestine and is excreted in the urine and feces.

Purpose

□ To evaluate electrolyte status
□ To assess neuromuscular or renal function.

Patient preparation

Explain to the patient that this test determines the magnesium content of the blood. Instruct him not to use magnesium salts (such as milk of magnesia or Epsom salt) for at least 3 days before the test, but he needn't restrict food or fluids. Tell him the test requires a blood sample; who will perform the venipuncture and when; and that he may feel some discomfort from the needle puncture and pressure of the tourniquet. Reassure him that collecting the sample takes only a few minutes.

Procedure

Perform a venipuncture, and collect the sample in a 10 to 15 ml *red-top* tube.

Precautions

Handle the sample gently to prevent hemolysis. (*Note:* This is especially important with this test, since 75% of the blood's magnesium is present in RBCs.)

Values

Normally, serum magnesium levels range from 1.7 to 2.1 mg/dl (atomic absorption) or from 1.5 to 2.5 mEq/liter.

Implications of results

Elevated serum magnesium levels (hypermagnesemia) most commonly occur in renal failure, when the kidneys excrete inadequate amounts of magnesium. Adrenal insufficiency (Addison's disease) can also elevate serum magnesium.

In suspected or confirmed hypermagnesemia, observe the patient for lethargy; flushing; diaphoresis; decreased blood pressure; slow, weak pulse; diminished deep tendon reflexes; muscle weakness; and slow, shallow respirations.

Suppressed serum magnesium levels (hypomagnesemia) most commonly result from chronic alcoholism. Other causes include malabsorption syndrome, diarrhea, faulty absorption following bowel resection, prolonged bowel or gastric aspiration, acute pancreatitis, primary aldosteronism, severe burns, hypercalcemic conditions (including hyperparathyroidism), and certain diuretic therapy.

In hypomagnesemia, watch for leg and foot cramps, hyperactive deep tendon reflexes, cardiac arrhythmias, muscle weakness, seizures, twitching, tetany, and tremors.

Post-test care

If a hematoma develops at the venipuncture site, ease discomfort by applying warm soaks.

Interfering factors

☐ Excessive use of antacids or cathartics, or excessive infusion of magnesium sulfate raises magnesium levels.

☐ Prolonged I.V. infusions without magnesium suppress magnesium levels. Excessive use of diuretics, including thiazides and ethacrynic acid, decreases levels by increasing magnesium excretion in the urine.

☐ I.V. administration of calcium gluconate may falsely decrease serum magnesium levels if measured by the Titan yellow method.

☐ Hemolysis due to rough handling of the sample causes falsely elevated serum magnesium levels.

ANNETTE L. HARMON, RN, MSN

Serum Phosphates

This test measures serum levels of phosphates, the dominant cellular anions. Phosphates help store and utilize body energy, and help regulate calcium levels, carbohydrate and lipid metabolism, and acid-base balance. Phosphates are essential to bone formation; about 85% of the body's phosphates are found in bone. The intestine absorbs a considerable amount of phosphates from dietary sources, but adequate levels of vitamin D are necessary for their absorption. The kidneys excrete phosphates and serve as a regulatory mechanism. Since calcium and phosphate interact in a reciprocal relationship, urinary excretion of phosphates increases or decreases in inverse proportion to serum calcium levels. Abnormal concentrations of phosphates result more often from improper excretion than from abnormal ingestion or absorption from dietary sources.

Purpose

☐ To aid diagnosis of renal disorders and acid-base imbalance

☐ To detect endocrine, skeletal, and calcium disorders.

Patient preparation

Explain to the patient that this test determines the blood levels of phosphate. Inform him he needn't restrict food or fluids. Tell him this test requires a blood sample; who will perform the venipuncture and when; and that, although he may feel some discomfort from the needle puncture and the pressure of the tourniquet, collecting the sample takes only a few minutes. Check the patient's medication history for recent therapy with drugs that alter phosphate levels.

Procedure

Perform a venipuncture, and collect the sample in a 10 to 15 ml *red-top* tube.

Precautions

Handle the sample gently to prevent hemolysis.

Values

Normally, serum phosphate levels range from 2.5 to 4.5 mg/dl (atomic absorption), or from 1.8 to 2.6 mEq/liter. Children have higher serum phosphate levels than adults. Phosphate levels can rise as high as 7 mg/dl or 4.1 mEq/liter during periods of increased bone growth.

Implications of results

Since serum phosphate values alone are of limited use diagnostically (only a few rare conditions directly affect phosphate metabolism), they should be interpreted in light of serum calcium results.

Depressed phosphate levels (hypophosphatemia) may result from malnutrition, malabsorption syndromes, hyperparathyroidism, renal tubular acidosis, or treatment of diabetic acidosis. In children, hypophosphatemia can suppress normal growth.

Elevated levels (hyperphosphatemia) may result from skeletal disease, healing fractures, hypoparathyroidism, acromegaly, diabetic acidosis, high intestinal obstruction, and renal failure. Hyperphosphatemia is rarely clinically significant; however, if prolonged, it can alter bone metabolism by causing abnormal calcium phosphate deposits.

Post-test care

If a hematoma develops at the venipuncture site, apply warm soaks.

Interfering factors

□ Excessive vitamin D intake, and drug therapy with anabolic steroids and androgens may elevate serum phosphorus levels.

□ Improper handling of the sample, resulting in hemolysis, falsely increases serum phosphate levels.

□ Suppressed phosphate levels may result from excessive phosphate excretion due to prolonged vomiting and diarrhea, vitamin D deficiency (which interferes with phosphate absorption), extended I.V. infusion of 5% dextrose in water, ingestion of phosphate-binding antacids, and drug therapy with acetazolamide, insulin, and epinephrine.

ANNETTE L. HARMON, RN, MSN

Serum Potassium

This test, a quantitative analysis, measures serum levels of potassium, the major intracellular cation. Small amounts of potassium may also be found in extracellular fluid. Vital to homeostasis, potassium maintains cellular osmotic equilibrium and helps regulate muscle activity (it's essential in maintaining electrical conduction within the cardiac and skeletal muscles). Potassium also helps regulate enzyme activity and acid-base balance, and influences kidney function. Potassium levels are affected by variations in the secretion of adrenal steroid hormones, and by fluctuations in pH, serum glucose levels, and serum sodium levels. A reciprocal relationship appears to exist between potassium and sodium; a substantial intake of one element causes a corresponding decrease in the other. Although it readily conserves sodium, the body has no efficient method for conserving potassium. Even in potassium depletion, the kidneys con-

---

TREATING POTASSIUM IMBALANCE

HYPOKALEMIA
Most patients with potassium deficiency can be treated with oral potassium chloride replacements and increased dietary intake. In severe cases, replace potassium I.V. no faster than 20 mEq/hour and at a concentration of no more than 80 mEq/liter of I.V. fluid. Mix the potassium well in the I.V. solution, since it can settle near the neck of the bottle or plastic bag. Failure to mix the solution adequately or to infuse it properly can cause a burning sensation at the I.V. site or can even cause fatal hyperkalemia. Monitor EKG, urinary output, and serum potassium levels frequently during infusion. Never administer I.V. potassium replacement to a patient with inadequate urine flow, since diminished excretion can rapidly lead to hyperkalemia.

HYPERKALEMIA
Dangerously high potassium levels may be reduced with sodium polystyrene sulfonate—a potassium-removing resin—administered orally, rectally, or through a nasogastric tube. A patient with hyperkalemia may also be treated with an I.V. infusion of sodium bicarbonate or of glucose and insulin, which lowers blood potassium by causing potassium to move into cells. A calcium I.V. infusion provides fast but transient relief from the cardiotoxic effects of hyperkalemia; however, it does not directly lower serum potassium. In a patient with renal failure, dialysis may help remove excess potassium, but this corrects the imbalance much more slowly.

---

tinue to excrete potassium; therefore, potassium deficiency can develop rapidly and is quite common.

Since the kidneys daily excrete nearly all the ingested potassium, a dietary intake of at least 40 mEq/day is essential. (A normal diet usually includes 60 to 100 mEq potassium.)

Purpose
☐ To evaluate clinical signs of potassium excess (hyperkalemia) or potassium depletion (hypokalemia)
☐ To monitor renal function, acid-base balance, and glucose metabolism
☐ To evaluate neuromuscular and endocrine disorders
☐ To detect the origin of arrhythmias.

Patient preparation
Explain to the patient that this test determines the potassium content of blood. Inform him he needn't restrict food or fluids. Tell him the test requires a blood sample; who will perform the venipuncture and when; and that he may feel some transient discomfort from the needle puncture and the pressure of the tourniquet. Reassure the patient that collecting the sample usually takes only a few minutes.

Check the patient's medication history for use of diuretics or other drugs that may influence test results. If these medications must be continued, note this on the laboratory slip.

Procedure
Perform a venipuncture, and collect the sample in a 10 to 15 ml *red-top* tube.

Precautions
☐ Draw the sample immediately after applying the tourniquet, since a delay may elevate the potassium level by allowing leakage of intracellular potassium into the serum.
☐ Handle the sample gently to avoid hemolysis.

Values
Normally, serum potassium levels range from 3.8 to 5.5 mEq/liter.

Implications of test results
Abnormally high serum potassium levels (hyperkalemia) are common in patients with burns, crushing injuries, diabetic ketoacidosis, and myocardial infarction—conditions in which excessive cellular potassium enters the blood. Hyperkalemia may also indicate reduced sodium excretion, possibly due to renal failure (preventing normal sodium/potassium exchange) or Addison's disease (due to the absence of aldosterone, with consequent potassium buildup and sodium depletion).

DIETARY SOURCES OF POTASSIUM

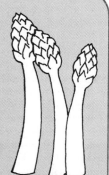

MEATS	SERVING SIZE	mEq
Beef	4 oz (112 g)	11.2
Chicken	4 oz (112 g)	12.0
Scallops	5 large	30.0
Veal	4 oz (112 g)	15.2

VEGETABLES

Artichokes	1 large bud	7.7
Asparagus, fresh, frozen, cooked	½ cup	5.5
raw	6 spears	7.7
Beans, dried, cooked	½ cup	10.0
Beans, lima	½ cup	9.5
Broccoli, cooked	½ cup	7.0
Carrots cooked	½ cup	5.7
raw	1 large	8.8
Mushrooms, raw	4 large	10.6
Potato, baked	1 small	15.4
Spinach, fresh, cooked	½ cup	8.5
Squash, winter, baked	½ cup	12.0
Tomato, raw	1 medium	10.4

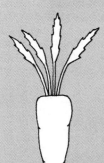

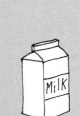

FRUITS

Apricots, dried	4 halves	5.0
fresh	3 small	8.0
Banana	1 medium	12.8
Cantaloupe	½ small	13.0
Figs, dried	7 small	17.5
Peach, fresh	1 medium	6.2
Pear, fresh	1 medium	6.2

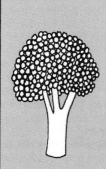

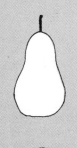

BEVERAGES

Apricot nectar	1 cup (240 ml)	9.0
Grapefruit juice	1 cup (240 ml)	8.2
Orange juice	1 cup (240 ml)	11.4
Pineapple juice	1 cup (240 ml)	9.0
Prune juice	1 cup (240 ml)	14.4
Tomato juice	1 cup (240 ml)	11.6
Milk, whole, skim	1 cup (240 ml)	8.8

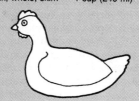

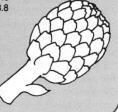

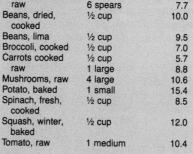

Observe a patient with hyperkalemia for weakness, malaise, nausea, diarrhea, colicky pain, muscle irritability progressing to flaccid paralysis, oliguria, and bradycardia. EKG reveals a prolonged P-R interval; wide QRS; tall, tented T wave; and S-T depression.

Below-normal potassium values often result from aldosteronism or Cushing's syndrome (marked by hypersecretion of adrenal steroid hormones), loss of body fluids (as in long-term diuretic therapy), or excessive licorice ingestion (due to the aldosterone-like effect of glycyrrhizic acid). Although serum values and clinical symptoms can indicate a potassium imbalance, an EKG provides the definitive diagnosis.

 Observe a patient with hypokalemia for decreased reflexes; rapid, weak, irregular pulse; mental confusion; hypotension; anorexia; muscle weakness; and paresthesia. EKG shows a flattened T wave, S-T depression, and U wave elevation. In severe cases, ventricular fibrillation, respiratory paralysis, and cardiac arrest can develop.

Post-test care
If a hematoma develops at the venipuncture site, apply warm soaks.

Interfering factors
☐ Excessive or rapid potassium infusion, spironolactone or penicillin G potassium therapy, or renal toxicity from administration of amphotericin B, methicillin, or tetracycline elevates serum potassium levels.
☐ Insulin and glucose administration, diuretic therapy (especially with thiazides, but not with triamterine, amiloride, or spironolactone), or I.V. infusions without potassium suppress serum potassium levels.
☐ Excessive hemolysis of the sample or delay in drawing blood following the application of a tourniquet elevates potassium levels.

ANNETTE L. HARMON, RN, MSN

Serum Sodium

This test measures serum levels of sodium, the major extracellular cation. Sodium affects body water distribution, maintains osmotic pressure of extracellular fluid, and helps promote neuromuscular function; it also helps maintain acid-base balance and influences chloride and potassium levels. Sodium is absorbed by the intestines and is excreted primarily by the kidneys; a small amount is lost through the skin.

Since extracellular sodium concentration helps the kidneys to regulate body water (decreased sodium levels promote water excretion and increased levels promote retention), serum levels of sodium are evaluated in relation to the amount of water in the body. For example, a sodium deficit (hyponatremia) refers to a decreased level of sodium in relation to the body's water level. The body normally regulates this sodium-water balance through aldosterone, which inhibits sodium excretion and promotes its resorption (with water) by the renal tubules, to maintain balance. Low sodium levels stimulate aldosterone secretion; elevated sodium levels depress aldosterone secretion.

Purpose
☐ To evaluate fluid-electrolyte and acid-base balance, and related neuromuscular, renal, and adrenal functions.

Patient preparation
Explain to the patient that this test determines the sodium content of blood. Inform him that he needn't restrict food or fluids. Tell him this test requires a blood sample; who will perform the venipuncture and when; and that, while he may feel some discomfort from the needle puncture and pressure of the tourniquet, collecting the sample takes only a few minutes.

Check the patient's medication history

for use of diuretics and other drugs that influence sodium levels. If these medications must be continued, note this on the laboratory slip.

Procedure
Perform a venipuncture, and collect the sample in a 10 to 15 ml *red-top* tube.

Precautions
Handle the sample gently to prevent hemolysis.

Values
Normally, serum sodium levels range from 135 to 145 mEq/liter.

Implications of results
Sodium imbalance can result from a loss or gain of sodium, or from a change in water volume. Remember, *serum sodium results must be interpreted in light of the patient's state of hydration.*

Elevated serum sodium levels (hypernatremia) may be due to inadequate water intake, water loss in excess of sodium (as in diabetes insipidus, impaired renal function, prolonged hyperventilation, and occasionally, severe vomiting or diarrhea), and sodium retention (as in aldosteronism). Hypernatremia can also result from excessive sodium intake.

 In a patient with hypernatremia and associated loss of water, observe for signs of thirst, restlessness, dry and sticky mucous membranes, flushed skin, oliguria, and diminished reflexes. However, if increased total body sodium causes water retention, observe for hypertension, dyspnea, and edema.

Abnormally low serum sodium levels (hyponatremia) may result from inadequate sodium intake or excessive sodium loss due to profuse sweating, gastrointestinal suctioning, diuretic therapy, diarrhea, vomiting, adrenal insufficiency, burns, or chronic renal insufficiency with acidosis. Urine sodium determinations are frequently more sensitive to early changes in sodium balance and should always be evaluated simultaneously with serum sodium findings.

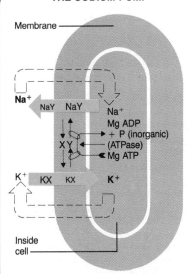

THE SODIUM PUMP

According to the laws of diffusion, a substance spreads from an area of higher concentration to one of lower concentration. Thus, when stimuli, such as heat, cold, electricity, or mechanical damage, cause the cellular membrane to become very permeable, sodium ions—normally most abundant outside the cells—diffuse inward, and potassium ions—normally most abundant inside the cells—diffuse outward. To combat this ionic diffusion and maintain normal sodium and potassium concentrations, an active sodium transportation mechanism is constantly at work.

Since sodium and potassium can't easily penetrate the cellular membrane, they're forced to combine with a single lipoprotein carrier. (This carrier is called Y in combination with sodium and X following a chemical transformation allying it with potassium.) In the cellular membrane, sodium from inside the cells combines with carrier Y to form large quantities of NaY, which move toward the cell's outer surface. Because of energy provided by adenosine triphosphate (ATP) and adenosine triphosphatase (ATPase), the sodium is released outside the cells, and the Y is chemically transformed to X. X joins potassium, forming KX. As the KX within the membrane moves inward, ATP and ATPase provide the energy needed to split K from X. K enters the cells, X is reconverted to Y, and the cycle continues indefinitely. This system, known as the sodium pump, helps prevent cellular swelling, stimulate glandular secretions, and transmit neuromuscular impulses.

WATER IMBALANCES

HYPERVOLEMIA
(Water and electrolyte retention resulting in increased extracellular fluid volume)

CAUSES	SIGNS AND SYMPTOMS	LABORATORY FINDINGS
• Increased water intake	• Increased... —blood pressure	• Decreased... —red cell count
• Decreased water output due to renal disease	—pulse rate	—hemoglobin concentration
• Congestive heart failure	—body weight	—packed cell volume
• Excessive ingestion or infusion of sodium chloride	—respiratory rate	—serum sodium concentration (dilutional decrease)
• Long-term administration of adrenocortical hormones	• Bounding peripheral pulses	—urine specific gravity
• Excessive infusion of isotonic solutions	• Moist pulmonary rales	
	• Moist mucous membranes	
	• Moist respiratory secretions	
	• Edema	
	• Weakness	
	• Convulsions and coma due to swelling of brain cells	

HYPOVOLEMIA
(Decreased extracellular fluid volume due to loss of water and electrolytes)

CAUSES	SIGNS AND SYMPTOMS	LABORATORY FINDINGS
• Decreased water intake	• Increased... —pulse rate	• Increased... —red cell count
• Fluid loss due to diarrhea, fever, vomiting	—respiratory rate	—hemoglobin concentration
• Systemic infection	• Decreased...	—packed cell volume
• Impaired renal concentrating ability	—blood pressure	—serum sodium concentration
• Fistulous drainage	—body weight	—urine specific gravity
• Severe burns	• Weak and thready peripheral pulses	
• Hidden fluid in body cavities	• Thick, slurred speech	
	• Thirst	
	• Oliguria (diminished urine output compared with fluid intake)	
	• Anuria	
	• Dry skin	

In a patient with hyponatremia, watch for apprehension, lassitude, headache, decreased skin turgor, abdominal cramps, and tremors that may progress to convulsions.

Post-test care
If a hematoma develops at the venipuncture site, apply warm soaks.

Interfering factors
☐ Most diuretics suppress serum sodium levels by promoting sodium excretion; lithium, chlorpropamide, and vasopressin suppress levels by inhibiting water excretion.
☐ Corticosteroids elevate serum sodium levels by promoting sodium retention. Antihypertensives, such as methyldopa, hydralazine, and reserpine, may cause sodium and water retention.
☐ Hemolysis due to rough handling of the sample may interfere with accurate determination of test results.

ANNETTE L. HARMON, RN, MSN

Anion Gap

The anion gap reflects serum anion-cation balance and helps distinguish types of metabolic acidosis without expensive, time-consuming measurement of all serum electrolytes. This test uses serum levels of routinely measured electrolytes—sodium (Na^+), chloride (Cl^-), and bicarbonate (HCO_3^-)—for a quick calculation based on a simple physical principle: Total concentrations of cations and anions are normally equal, thereby maintaining electrical neutrality in serum. Since sodium accounts for more than 90% of circulating cations, whereas chloride and bicarbonate together account for 85% of the counterbalancing anions, the "gap" between measured cation and anion levels represents those anions not routinely measured (sulfate, phosphates, organic acids

such as ketone bodies and lactic acid, and proteins).

An increased anion gap indicates an increase in one or more of these unmeasured anions, which may occur with acidoses characterized by excessive organic or inorganic acids, such as lactic acidosis or ketoacidosis.

A normal anion gap occurs in hyperchloremic acidoses, renal tubular acidosis, and severe bicarbonate-wasting conditions, such as biliary or pancreatic fistulas and poorly functioning ileal loops.

Purpose
☐ To distinguish types of metabolic acidosis
☐ To monitor renal function and I.V. hyperalimentation.

Patient preparation
Explain to the patient that this test helps determine the cause of acidosis. Inform him that he needn't restrict food or fluids before the test. Tell the patient that the test requires a blood sample; who will perform the venipuncture and when; and that he may feel transient discomfort from the needle puncture and the pressure of the tourniquet. Reassure him that collecting the sample takes only a few minutes.

Check the patient's history for recent use of drugs (such as diuretics, corticosteroids, and antihypertensives) that may influence sodium, chloride, or bicarbonate blood levels. If these drugs must be continued, be sure to note this on the laboratory slip.

Procedure
Perform a venipuncture, and collect the sample in a 10- to 15-ml *red-top* tube.

Precautions
Handle the sample gently to prevent hemolysis, which can interfere with accurate determination of test results.

Values
Normally, the anion gap ranges from 8 to 14 mEq/liter.

Implications of results

A normal anion gap doesn't rule out metabolic acidosis. When acidosis results from loss of bicarbonate in the urine or other body fluids, renal reabsorption of sodium promotes retention of chloride, and the anion gap remains unchanged. Thus, metabolic acidosis resulting from excessive chloride levels is known as a *normal anion gap acidosis.*

   When acidosis results from accumulation of metabolic acids—as occurs in lactic acidosis, for example—the anion gap increases (above 14 mEq/liter) with the increase in unmeasured anions. Metabolic acidosis caused by such accumulation is known as a *high anion gap acidosis.* (See *How Anion Gap Results Distinguish Causes of Metabolic Acidosis* on this page for the possible causes of both normal and high anion gap acidoses.)

   Because the anion gap only determines total anion-cation balance, it doesn't necessarily reflect abnormal values for individual electrolytes. Further investigation and diagnostic tests are usually necessary to determine the specific cause of metabolic acidosis.

   A decreased anion gap (below 8 mEq/liter) is rare. However, it may occur with hypermagnesemia and with paraproteinemic states, such as multiple myeloma and Waldenström's macroglobulinemia.

Post-test care
□ If a hematoma develops at the venipuncture site, ease discomfort by applying warm soaks.
□ As ordered, instruct the patient to resume use of any drugs discontinued before the test.

Interfering factors
□ Diuretics, lithium, chlorpropamide, and vasopressin suppress serum sodium, possibly decreasing the anion gap; corticosteroids and antihypertensives elevate serum sodium and may increase the anion gap.
□ Salicylates, paraldehyde, methicillin, dimercaprol, ammonium chloride, acetazolamide, ethylene glycol, and methyl alcohol decrease serum bicarbonate, possibly increasing the anion gap; ACTH, cortisone, mercurial or chlorthiazide diuretics, and excessive ingestion of alkalis or licorice elevate serum bicarbonate and may decrease the anion gap.
□ Ammonium chloride, cholestyramine, boric acid, oxyphenbutazone, phenylbutazone, and excessive I.V. infusion of sodium chloride may elevate serum chloride and possibly decrease the anion gap.
□ Thiazides, furosemide, ethacrynic acid, bicarbonates, or prolonged I.V. infusion of 5% dextrose in water can lower serum chloride and may increase the anion gap.
□ Iodine absorption from wounds packed with povidone-iodine, or excessive use of magnesium-containing antacids (especially by patients with renal failure) may cause a spuriously low anion gap.
□ Hemolysis due to rough handling of the sample may interfere with accurate determination of test results.

ANNETTE L. HARMON, RN, MSN

Selected References

Bauer, John D., and Ackerman, Philip G. *Clinical Laboratory Methods,* 9th ed. St. Louis: C.V. Mosby Co., 1982.

Berkow, Robert, ed. *The Merck Manual of Diagnosis and Therapy,* 14th ed. Rahway, N.J.: Merck, Sharp and Dohme Research Laboratories, 1982.

Brunner, Lillian S., and Suddarth, Doris S. *Textbook of Medical-Surgical Nursing,* 5th ed. Philadelphia: J.B. Lippincott Co., 1984.

Byrne, C. Judith, et al. *Laboratory Tests: Implications for Nurses and Allied Health Professionals.* Reading, Mass.: Addison-Wesley Publishing Co., 1981.

Diseases, 2nd ed. Nurse's Reference Library. Springhouse, Pa.: Springhouse Corp., 1986.

Drugs, 2nd ed., Nurse's Reference Library. Springhouse, Pa.: Springhouse Corp., 1984.

Fischbach, Frances. *A Manual of Laboratory Diagnostic Tests,* 2nd ed. Philadelphia: J.B. Lippincott Co., 1984.

French, Ruth M. *Guide to Diagnostic Procedures,* 5th ed. New York: McGraw-Hill Book Co., 1980.

Griffiths, Mary. *Introduction to Human Physiology,* 2nd ed. New York: Macmillan Publishing Co., 1981.

Guyton, Arthur C. *Textbook of Medical Physiology,* 6th ed. Philadelphia: W.B. Saunders Co., 1981.

Hansten, Philip D. *Drug Interactions,* 5th ed. Philadelphia: Lea & Febiger, 1984.

Harvey, A. McGehee, ed. *The Principles and Practice of Medicine,* 21st ed. East Norwalk, Conn.: Appleton-Century-Crofts, 1984.

Henry, John Bernard, ed. *Todd-Sanford-Davidsohn Clinical Diagnosis and Management by Laboratory Methods,* vol. 1, 17th ed. Philadelphia: W.B. Saunders Co., 1984.

Immune Disorders, Nurse's Clinical Library. Springhouse, Pa.: Springhouse Corp., 1985.

Lamb, Jane O. *Laboratory Tests for Clinical Nursing.* Bowie, Md.: Robert J. Brady Co., 1984.

Leavelle, Dennis E., ed. *Mayo Medical Laboratories Test Catalog.* Rochester, Minn.: Mayo Medical Laboratories, 1984.

Luckmann, Joan, and Sorensen, Karen C. *Medical-Surgical Nursing: A Psychophysiologic Approach,* 2nd ed. Philadelphia: W.B. Saunders Co., 1980.

Maxwell, Morton H., and Kleeman, Charles R. *Clinical Disorders of Fluid and Electrolyte Metabolism,* 3rd ed. New York: McGraw-Hill Book Co., 1983.

McFarland, Mary Brambilla, and Grant, Marcia Moeller. *Nursing Implications of Laboratory Tests.* New York: John Wiley & Sons, 1982.

Monitoring Fluid and Electrolytes Precisely, 2nd ed. New Nursing Skillbook series. Springhouse, Pa.: Springhouse Corp., 1983.

Nursing85 Drug Handbook, Springhouse, Pa.: Springhouse Corp., 1985.

Petersdorf, Robert G., and Adams, Raymond D., eds. *Harrison's Principles of Internal Medicine,* 10th ed. New York: McGraw-Hill Book Co., 1983.

Price, Sylvia Anderson, and Wilson, Lorraine McCarthy. *Pathophysiology: Clinical Concepts of Disease Processes,* 2nd ed. New York: McGraw-Hill Book Co., 1982.

Ravel, Richard A. *Clinical Laboratory Medicine,* 4th ed. Chicago: Year Book Medical Pubs., 1984.

Rose, Burton David. *Clinical Physiology of Acid Base and Electrolyte Disorders.* New York: McGraw-Hill Book Co., 1977.

Sumner, Sara M. "Refining Your Technique for Drawing Arterial Blood Gases," *Nursing80* 10:65-69, April 1980.

Tietz, Norbert W., ed. *Fundamentals of Clinical Chemistry,* 2nd ed. Philadelphia: W.B. Saunders Co., 1976.

Tilkian, Sarko M., et al. *Clinical Implications of Laboratory Tests,* 3rd ed. St. Louis: C.V. Mosby Co., 1983.

Wade, Jacqueline F. *Comprehensive Respiratory Nursing Care: Physiology and Technique,* 3rd ed. St. Louis: C.V. Mosby Co., 1982.

Wallach, Jacques B. *Interpretation of Diagnostic Tests: A Handbook Synopsis of Laboratory Medicine,* 3rd ed. Boston: Little, Brown & Co., 1978.

Wegener, Lee T., ed. *Mayo Medical Laboratories Interpretive Handbook,* Rochester, Minn.: Mayo Medical Laboratories, 1984.

Widmann, Frances K. *Clinical Interpretation of Laboratory Tests,* 9th ed. Philadelphia: F.A. Davis Co., 1983.

Wyngaarden, James, and Smith, Lloyd. *Cecil Textbook of Medicine,* 16th ed. Philadelphia: W.B. Saunders Co., 1982.

4 Enzymes

LEARNING OBJECTIVES

After completing this chapter, the reader will be able to:
- define the terms *enzyme* and *isoenzyme*.
- identify the major enzymes and isoenzymes of the heart and liver.
- explain how enzymes function.
- describe the changes in serum enzyme and isoenzyme levels after a myocardial infarction.
- list drugs that may elevate serum amylase levels.
- explain the renin-angiotensin feedback system.
- state the purpose of each test discussed in the chapter.
- prepare the patient physically and psychologically for each test.
- describe the procedure for performing each test.
- specify appropriate precautions for accurate administration of each test.
- recognize signs of adverse reaction and respond appropriately.
- implement appropriate post-test care.
- state the normal values for each test.
- discuss the implications of abnormal test results.
- list factors that may interfere with accurate test results.

Enzymes

Introduction

Enzymes are reusable proteins that catalyze the thousands of chemical reactions needed to keep a single cell alive and functioning. They accelerate and control reaction rates without being destroyed themselves in the process.

Different kinds of cells produce different enzymes; and most tissues contain many different enzymes. When tissue cells are damaged by disease or some other defect, they release enzymes specific to that area into the bloodstream, where they can be readily detected. For example, leakage from dying cells is the source of elevated serum enzymes in myocardial infarction, infectious hepatitis, and other disease states. Although serum levels of any one enzyme may not identify its tissue of origin, comparing serum levels of several enzymes may give important diagnostic information, since individual enzymes are present in different tissues in different ratios. Such analysis may reveal the extent of pathology and monitor progress of healing.

Sensitivity and specificity define usefulness

Because certain diseases that produce similar symptoms cause distinctively different enzyme abnormalities, enzyme tests can be used to separate them. Their diagnostic value depends on their sensitivity and specificity. Sensitivity indicates how reliably the test gives a positive result when a particular disease is present; specificity indicates how often the test is "normal" when the disease is absent. Thus, enzyme tests with low sensitivity produce negative readings when the disease is present; tests with low specificity show positive readings when the disease is absent.

Some enzymes—creatine phosphokinase (CPK) and lactic dehydrogenase (LDH), for instance—occur in multiple forms—isoenzymes—that differ in molecular details while retaining their basic identity. Certain organs or tissues contain greater or lesser amounts of one isoenzyme than another; therefore, testing for isoenzymes sometimes provides better sensitivity or specificity than measuring an entire enzyme group. CPK is present in heart muscle, skeletal muscle, and brain tissue. CPK isoenzymes are combinations of the subunits M (muscle) and B (brain). For example, CPK-BB is found primarily in brain and nerve tissue, CPK-MB in heart muscle, and CPK-MM in skeletal muscle. Therefore, if an acute myocardial infarction (MI) is suspected, elevated CPK-MB levels reliably indicate cardiac damage, since this isoenzyme isn't prevalent in other tissues.

LDH has five isoenzymes that are formed from different combinations of two subunits—M (muscle) and H (heart). The patterns of LDH_1 and LDH_2 levels are monitored—along with other serum enzyme levels—to trace the progress of MI. LDH_3 levels are elevated primarily in patients with pulmonary infarction, while LDH_4 and LDH_5 elevations are characteristic of skeletal muscle and hepatic disorders.

Isoenzymes may be separated and assayed by several laboratory methods including electrophoresis, column chromatography, heat stability, substrate alterations, and use of inhibitors. These techniques take advantage of some physical or chemical property of the isoenzyme molecule.

Enzyme test batteries

Some enzymes and isoenzymes are routinely tested in groups to aid identification of disorders such as myocardial infarction, and hepatic and pancreatic diseases. Nevertheless, because some enzymes are present in many organs and disease states, positive test results are meaningful only in light of the patient's overall clinical status.

Cardiac enzymes and isoenzymes

CPK-MB levels rise 4 to 8 hours after onset of infarction, peak after 24 hours, and may remain elevated for as long as 72 hours. LDH_1 and LDH_2 levels usually rise within 24 hours after an episode, tapering off 72 to 96 hours later. Some laboratories also measure hydroxybutyric dehydrogenase (HBD) in suspected acute MI when electrophoresis equipment is not available or when the total LDH is not diagnostic. Serum HBD levels rise 8 to 10 hours after infarction, peak in 48 to 96 hours, and return to normal in 16 to 18 days.

Serum glutamic-oxaloacetic transaminase (SGOT) also rises during acute MI, increasing 6 to 10 hours after the infarction and peaking in 24 to 48 hours. The SGOT level may increase to 4 to 10 times normal but returns to normal in 4 to 6 days. In some patients, SGOT rises as a result of severe angina or arrhythmia and does not indicate MI. Thus, correct interpretation of enzyme analyses always requires careful correlation with the patient's clinical status.

Since the diagnostic value of some enzyme tests depends on the sequence of analysis, each sample must be labeled with the time of collection, the date, and the patient's name and room number. For example, in acute MI, the first set of tests is ordered immediately to obtain a baseline. Subsequent sets of tests are ordered serially, perhaps at 6, 12, and 24 hours after the episode and daily thereafter, to monitor enzyme elevations and peaks. Writing "Rule out MI" on the requisition slip will help, but it's also essential to specify the time the sample was drawn. Specifying "4 hours post-suspected time of MI" helps place test results in their chronologic order.

Liver enzymes and isoenzymes

The liver is the site of many biochemical reactions that are controlled by numerous enzymes. Many of these reactions occur at diagnostically significant levels in the serum in a spectrum of hepatobiliary disorders ranging from minute

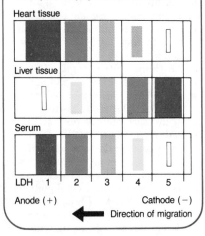

ELECTROPHORESIS SEPARATES LDH ISOENZYMES

Lactic dehydrogenase (LDH) occurs in five different forms, or isoenzymes, which differ in certain molecular details, such as the rate of electrophoretic migration, while retaining their basic identity. Each organ or tissue contains more or less of one LDH isoenzyme than of another, as shown below by the varying densities of color.

Heart tissue

Liver tissue

Serum

LDH 1 2 3 4 5

Anode (+) Cathode (−)

Direction of migration

changes within hepatic cells (hepatitis) to extrahepatic disorders, such as biliary obstruction.

Although neither SGOT nor *serum glutamic-pyruvic transaminase* (SGPT) is confined to the liver, both reliably identify hepatic disease. In severe necrosis (as in viral hepatitis), SGOT levels may rise as high as 100 times the normal range, because of massive tissue destruction. SGPT levels may rise even higher and remain elevated longer than SGOT. These enzyme changes become detectable early in the disease and persist longer than changes in other liver function studies.

Gamma glutamyl transferase is a sensitive indicator of early hepatocellular damage, obstruction, or alcohol-induced hepatic disease, and is usually measured with other enzymes to confirm hepatic disease. Elevated levels rise in patterns similar to those of serum alkaline phosphatase.

The enzyme *alkaline phosphatase* can be separated into five isoenzymes, each of which is found in different tissues. Alkaline phosphatase isoenzyme type 1 is specific to hepatic disorders. Serum levels rise dramatically in biliary cirrhosis, and in bile duct obstruction that impedes phosphatase excretion. When alkaline phosphatase is elevated, measuring another phosphatase enzyme— *5'-nucleotidase* (5'NT), which is formed mostly in the liver—can determine whether alkaline phosphatase levels are liver- or bone-related. Usually, both 5'NT and alkaline phosphatase are elevated in hepatic disease, while only alkaline phosphatase rises in skeletal disease.

Two isoenzymes of LDH—LDH_4 and LDH_5—occur predominantly in the liver. Their serum levels are commonly elevated even before jaundice appears and return to normal while clinical symptoms are still evident.

Another enzyme, *ornithine carba-*

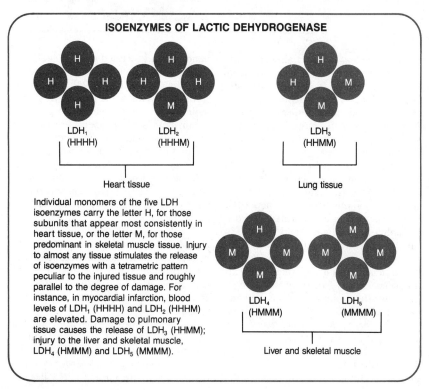

ISOENZYMES OF LACTIC DEHYDROGENASE

LDH₁ (HHHH) — LDH₂ (HHHM)

Heart tissue

LDH₃ (HHMM)

Lung tissue

LDH₄ (HMMM) — LDH₅ (MMMM)

Liver and skeletal muscle

Individual monomers of the five LDH isoenzymes carry the letter H, for those subunits that appear most consistently in heart tissue, or the letter M, for those predominant in skeletal muscle tissue. Injury to almost any tissue stimulates the release of isoenzymes with a tetrametric pattern peculiar to the injured tissue and roughly parallel to the degree of damage. For instance, in myocardial infarction, blood levels of LDH₁ (HHHH) and LDH₂ (HHHM) are elevated. Damage to pulmonary tissue causes the release of LDH₃ (HHMM); injury to the liver and skeletal muscle, LDH₄ (HMMM) and LDH₅ (MMMM).

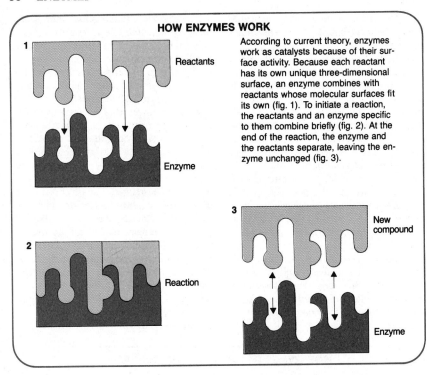

HOW ENZYMES WORK

According to current theory, enzymes work as catalysts because of their surface activity. Because each reactant has its own unique three-dimensional surface, an enzyme combines with reactants whose molecular surfaces fit its own (fig. 1). To initiate a reaction, the reactants and an enzyme specific to them combine briefly (fig. 2). At the end of the reaction, the enzyme and the reactants separate, leaving the enzyme unchanged (fig. 3).

moyltransferase, is found almost exclusively in the liver. Marked elevations of this enzyme occur in hepatic necrosis, such as in acute viral hepatitis, while lesser elevations may be present in cirrhosis, or obstructive jaundice. This test is notably specific for and sensitive to hepatocellular injury.

Leucine aminopeptidase (LAP) levels are elevated in most hepatic diseases, such as obstructive jaundice, cirrhosis, carcinoma of the liver, and hepatitis. LAP levels tend to rise parallel to those of alkaline phosphatase, and this test is sometimes used to separate hepatic disease from skeletal disease when alkaline phosphatase levels are elevated from an unknown cause. *Isocitrate dehydrogenase,* another enzyme, is greatly increased in patients with viral hepatitis. The test offers no advantages over SGPT and is used mainly in research.

Pancreatic enzymes

Amylase and *lipase* are produced by the pancreas and secreted into the small intestine, where they break down starches and fats, respectively. Both appear in serum following acute pancreatitis, and their concentrations tend to be parallel. Serum amylase levels rise rapidly in acute pancreatitis, reaching twice normal values just 4 hours after onset of symptoms; however, levels also drop quickly, returning to normal 48 to 72 hours later. Serum lipase levels rise similarly, but lipase concentrations persist for as long as 14 days.

Prostatic and other enzymes

Acid phosphatase is found mainly in the adult prostate gland. Elevated levels of this enzyme usually indicate prostatic cancer that has penetrated the prostatic capsule.

Special enzyme tests that aren't part of specific organ test profiles include *plasma renin activity, cholinesterase, glucose-6-phosphate dehydrogenase* (G-6-PD), *pyruvate kinase* (PK), *hexos-*

aminidase A and B, uroporphyrinogen 1 synthase, galactose-1-phosphate uridyl transferase, and angiotensin converting enzyme. Plasma renin testing helps identify primary aldosteronism. Pseudocholinesterase may aid diagnosis of hepatobiliary diseases and pesticide poisonings. G-6-PD, PK, uroporphyri-nogen 1 synthase, and galactose-1-phosphate uridyl transferase assays detect inherited enzyme deficiencies. Hexosaminidase A and B testing diagnoses Tay-Sachs disease. The angiotensin converting enzyme test is mainly used to detect sarcoidosis.

SR. MARY BRIAN KELBER, RN, DNS

CARDIAC ENZYMES

Creatine Phosphokinase

[Creatine kinase (CK)]

Creatine phosphokinase (CPK) is an enzyme that catalyzes the creatine-creatinine metabolic pathway in muscle cells and brain tissue. Because of its intimate role in energy production, CPK reflects normal tissue catabolism; an increase above normal serum levels indicates trauma to cells with high CPK content. CPK may be separated into three isoenzymes with distinct molecular structures: CPK-BB (CPK$_1$), CPK-MB (CPK$_2$), and CPK-MM (CPK$_3$). CPK-BB is found primarily in brain tissue; CPK-MB, in cardiac muscle (a small amount also appears in skeletal muscle); and CPK-MM, in skeletal muscle.

An assay of total serum CPK was once widely used to detect acute myocardial infarction (MI), but elevated serum CPK levels caused by skeletal muscle damage reduce the test's specificity for this disorder. Fractionation and measurement of CPK isoenzymes is rapidly replacing use of total CPK to accurately localize the site of increased tissue destruction.

Purpose

☐ To detect and diagnose acute MI and reinfarction (CPK-MB primarily used)
☐ To evaluate possible causes of chest pain and to monitor the severity of myocardial ischemia after cardiac surgery, cardiac catheterization, or cardioversion (CPK-MB primarily used)
☐ To detect skeletal muscle disorders that are not neurogenic in origin, such as Duchenne muscular dystrophy (total CPK primarily used), and early dermatomyositis.

Patient preparation

Explain to the patient that this test helps assess myocardial and skeletal muscle function, and that multiple blood samples are required to detect fluctuations in serum levels. Inform him that he need not restrict food or most fluids before the test. If the patient is being evaluated for skeletal muscle disorders, advise him to avoid exercising for 24 hours before the test. Tell him who will perform the venipuncture and when. Reassure him that although he may experience discomfort from the needle puncture or the pressure of the tourniquet, collecting the sample takes less than 3 minutes.

Withhold alcohol, aminocaproic acid, and lithium, as ordered, before the test. If these substances must be continued, note this on the laboratory slip.

Procedure

Perform a venipuncture, and collect the sample in a 7 ml *red-top* tube.

Precautions

☐ Draw the sample before or within 1 hour of giving I.M. injections, as muscle trauma raises total CPK levels.
☐ Obtain the sample on schedule. Note, on the laboratory slip, the time the sample was drawn and the hours elapsed since onset of chest pain.

☐ Handle the collection tube gently to prevent hemolysis, and send the sample to the laboratory immediately (CPK activity diminishes significantly after 2 hours at room temperature).

Values

Total CPK values determined by ultraviolet or kinetic measurement range from 23 to 99 u/liter for men, and from 15 to 57 u/liter for women. CPK levels may be significantly higher in very muscular people. Infants up to age 1 have levels two to four times higher than adult levels, possibly reflecting birth trauma and striated muscle development. Normal ranges for isoenzyme levels are as follows: CPK-BB, undetectable; CPK-MB, undetectable to 7 IU/liter; CPK-MM, 5 to 70 IU/liter.

Implications of results

CPK-MM constitutes over 99% of total CPK normally present in serum. Detectable CPK-BB isoenzyme may indicate brain tissue injury, certain widespread malignant tumors, severe shock, or renal failure. However, such elevations don't confirm a specific diagnosis.

CPK-MB isoenzyme greater than 5% of total CPK (or more than 10 IU/liter) indicates MI, especially if the LDH_1/LDH_2

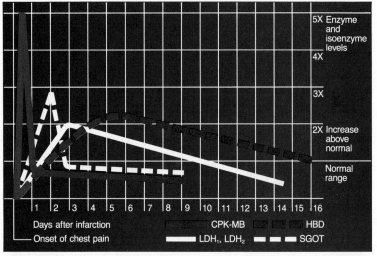

SERUM ENZYME AND ISOENZYME LEVELS AFTER MYOCARDIAL INFARCTION

Since they're released by damaged tissue, serum enzymes and isoenzymes—catalytic proteins that vary in concentration in specific organs—can help identify the compromised organ and assess the extent of damage. The following serum enzyme and isoenzyme determinations are most significant in myocardial infarction:

Isoenzymes:
- Creatine phosphokinase-MB (CPK-MB): in the heart muscle, and a small amount in skeletal muscle
- Lactic dehydrogenase 1 and 2 (LDH_1, LDH_2): in the heart, brain, kidneys, liver, skeletal muscles, and RBCs.

Enzymes:
- Hydroxybutyric dehydrogenase (HBD): an indirect measurement of LDH_1 and LDH_2
- Serum glutamic-oxaloacetic transaminase (SGOT): heart muscle and liver, and less extensively in skeletal muscles, kidneys, pancreas, and RBCs.

isoenzyme ratio is greater than 1 (flipped LDH). In acute MI and following cardiac surgery, CPK-MB begins to rise in 2 to 4 hours, peaks in 12 to 24 hours, and usually returns to normal in 24 to 48 hours; persistent elevations or increasing levels indicate ongoing myocardial damage. Total CPK follows roughly the same pattern but rises slightly later. CPK-MB levels don't rise in congestive heart failure or during angina pectoris not accompanied by myocardial cell necrosis (not all investigators agree on this, however). Serious skeletal muscle injury that occurs in certain muscular dystrophies, polymyositis, and severe myoglobinuria may produce mild CPK-MB elevation, since a small amount of this isoenzyme is present in some skeletal muscles.

Rising CPK-MM values follow skeletal muscle damage from trauma, such as surgery and I.M. injections, or from diseases, such as dermatomyositis and muscular dystrophy (values may be 50 to 100 times normal). A moderate rise in CPK-MM levels develops in patients with hypothyroidism; sharp elevations occur with muscular activity caused by agitation, such as an acute psychotic episode.

Total CPK levels may be elevated in patients with severe hypokalemia, carbon monoxide poisoning, malignant hyperthermia, postconvulsions, alcoholic cardiomyopathy, and occasionally, in those who have suffered pulmonary or cerebral infarctions.

Post-test care
☐ If a hematoma develops at the venipuncture site, apply warm soaks to help ease discomfort.
☐ Resume administering medications that were discontinued before the test, as ordered.

Interfering factors
☐ Hemolysis due to rough handling of the sample may affect CPK levels.
☐ Failure to send the sample to the laboratory immediately or to refrigerate the serum if testing will be delayed for more than 2 hours may hinder accurate determination of CPK levels.
☐ Failure to draw the samples at the scheduled time, missing peak levels, may interfere with accurate determination of test results.
☐ Halothane and succinylcholine, alcohol, lithium, and large doses of aminocaproic acid reportedly cause elevated CPK levels. Intramuscular injections, cardioversion, invasive diagnostic procedures, surgery, trauma, recent vigorous exercise or muscle massage, and severe coughing also increase total CPK values.

SR. MARY BRIAN KELBER, RN, DNS

Lactic Dehydrogenase

Lactic dehydrogenase (LDH) is an enzyme that catalyzes the reversible conversion of muscle lactic acid into pyruvic acid. This essential final step in the Embden-Meyerhof glycolytic pathway provides the metabolic bridge to the Krebs cycle (citric acid or tricarboxylic acid cycle), ultimately producing cellular energy. Because LDH is present in almost all body tissues, cellular damage causes an elevation of total serum LDH, thus limiting the diagnostic usefulness of LDH. However, five tissue-specific isoenzymes can be identified and measured, using heat inactivation or electrophoresis: two of these isoenzymes, LDH_1 and LDH_2, appear primarily in the heart, RBCs, and kidneys; LDH_3, primarily in the lungs; and LDH_4 and LDH_5, in the liver and the skeletal muscles.

The specificity of LDH isoenzymes and their distribution pattern is useful in diagnosing hepatic, pulmonary, and erythrocytic damage. But its widest clinical application (with other cardiac enzyme tests) is in diagnosing acute myocardial infarction (MI). LDH isoenzyme assay is also useful when creatine phosphokinase (CPK) hasn't been measured within 24 hours of an acute MI. The myocardial LDH level rises later than CPK (12 to 48 hours after infarction begins), peaks in 2 to 5 days, and drops to normal in 7 to 10 days, if tissue necrosis doesn't persist.

DIAGNOSTIC LDH ISOENZYME VARIATIONS IN DISEASE

DISEASE	LDH 1	LDH 2	LDH 3	LDH 4	LDH 5
Cardiovascular					
Myocardial infarction	▨	▨			
Myocardial infarction with hepatic congestion	▨	▨			▨
Rheumatic carditis	▨				
Myocarditis	▨				
Congestive heart failure (decompensated)					▨
Shock	▨	▨	▨	▨	▨
Angina pectoris	■				
Pulmonary					
Pulmonary embolism		▨	▨		
Pulmonary infarction			▨		
Hematologic					
Pernicious anemia	▨	▨			
Hemolytic anemia	▨	▨			
Sickle cell anemia	▨	▨			
Hepatobiliary					
Hepatitis					▨
Active cirrhosis					▨
Hepatic congestion					▨

■ Normal   ▨ Diagnostic   ☐ Not diagnostic

Adapted with permission from information from Helena Laboratories, 1513 Lindberg Dr., Beaumont, Tex.

Purpose
☐ To aid differential diagnosis of MI, pulmonary infarction, anemias, and hepatic disease
☐ To support CPK isoenzyme test results in diagnosing MI, or to provide diagnosis when CPK-MB samples are drawn too late to display elevation
☐ To monitor patient response to some forms of chemotherapy.

Patient preparation
Explain to the patient that this test is used primarily to detect tissue alterations. Inform him he needn't restrict food or fluids before the test. Tell him the test requires a blood sample; who will perform the venipuncture and when; and that he may experience transient discomfort from the needle puncture and the pressure of the tourniquet. Reassure him that collecting the sample takes less than 3 minutes. Tell the patient suspected of having an MI that the test will be repeated on the next two mornings to monitor progressive changes.

Procedure
Perform a venipuncture, and collect the sample in a 7 ml *red-top* tube.

Precautions
☐ Draw the samples on schedule to avoid missing peak levels, and mark the collection time on the laboratory slip.
☐ Handle the sample gently to prevent artifact blood sample hemolysis, since RBCs contain LDH_1.
☐ Send the sample to the laboratory immediately or, if transport is delayed, keep the sample at room temperature. Changes in temperature reportedly inactivate LDH_5, thus altering isoenzyme patterns.

Values
Total LDH levels normally range from 48 to 115 IU/liter. Normal distribution is as follows:

LDH_1	18.1% to 29% of total
LDH_2	29.4% to 37.5% of total
LDH_3	18.8% to 26% of total
LDH_4	9.2% to 16.5% of total
LDH_5	5.3% to 13.4% of total

Implications of results

Since many common diseases cause elevations in total LDH levels, isoenzyme electrophoresis is usually necessary for diagnosis. In some disorders, total LDH may be within normal limits, but abnormal proportions of each enzyme indicate specific organ tissue damage. For instance, in acute MI, the concentration of LDH_1 is greater than LDH_2 within 12 to 48 hours after onset of symptoms. This reversal of normal isoenzyme patterns is typical of myocardial damage and is referred to as flipped LDH.

Post-test care

If a hematoma develops at the venipuncture site, apply warm soaks.

Interfering factors

□ Hemolysis due to rough handling of the sample may affect accurate determination of LDH levels.

□ For diagnosis of acute MI, failure to draw the sample on schedule may interfere with test results.

□ Failure to send the sample to the laboratory immediately may influence determination of LDH isoenzyme patterns.

□ Recent surgery or pregnancy can cause elevated LDH levels. Prosthetic heart valves may also increase LDH levels, from chronic hemolysis.

SR. MARY BRIAN KELBER, RN, DNS

Hydroxybutyric Dehydrogenase

[Alpha-hydroxybutyric dehydrogenase]

Hydroxybutyric dehydrogenase (HBD) is actually total lactic dehydrogenase (LDH) that is tested using a hydroxybutyric acid substrate instead of lactic or pyruvic acid. With this substrate, the electrophoretically fast-moving LDH_1 and LDH_2 (cardiac) isoenzymes exhibit
more activity than the slow-moving LDH_5 (liver) fraction, so that HBD activity roughly parallels LDH_1 and LDH_2 activity. Measurement of serum HBD is sometimes used as a substitute for LDH isoenzyme fractionation because this analysis is easier to perform and less expensive than LDH electrophoresis.

Although HBD concentration predominately reflects LDH_1 and LDH_2 activity, it may also show LDH_5 activity, if enough of this isoenzyme is present (as it is in some forms of hepatic disease). Therefore, this test isn't consistently reliable in distinguishing between myocardial and hepatic cellular damage, and is less popular than it used to be.

Purpose

□ To aid diagnosis of myocardial infarction (MI) when LDH isoenzyme assay is unavailable

□ To monitor cardiac isoenzyme activity after LDH_1 is proven to be elevated

□ To detect MI after other enzyme levels drop to normal (HBD remains elevated longer)

□ To aid in differentiating between cardiac and hepatic cellular damage when total LDH is elevated (LDH/HBD ratio is commonly used).

Patient preparation

Explain to the patient that this test evaluates the function of the heart or liver. Inform him he need not restrict food or fluids before the test. Tell him the test requires a blood sample; who will perform the venipuncture and when; and that he may experience transient discomfort from the needle puncture and the pressure of the tourniquet. Collecting the sample takes less than 3 minutes. Tell the patient suspected of having an MI that the test will be repeated on subsequent mornings to monitor his progress.

Procedure

Perform a venipuncture, and collect the sample in a 7 ml *red-top* tube.

Precautions

□ For patients with MI, draw blood at

SGOT ELEVATIONS IN MYOCARDIAL INFARCTION AND HEPATIC DISEASE

In acute myocardial infarction (MI), SGOT levels rise 6 to 10 hours after onset of chest pain, peak in 24 to 48 hours, and if the infarct doesn't extend or another MI doesn't occur, drop to normal in 4 or 5 days. The degree of elevation is roughly proportional to the number of damaged cells, and to the interval between the beginning of the infarction and the time the sample is drawn. Values 15 to 20 times normal indicate extensive myocardial damage and a guarded prognosis. Variable increases occur in congestive heart failure and shock, due to hypoxia and hepatic congestion.

In hepatic disease, SGOT levels usually rise within 4 to 8 hours of onset of acute disease, peak in 24 to 48 hours, and drop to normal in 4 to 8 days or longer, depending on the disease. Subsequent elevations generally indicate a relapse. Serum levels commonly rise before symptoms (such as jaundice) appear.

the same time each morning.

□ Handle the collection tube gently to prevent hemolysis, since RBCs contain LDH_1. Because HBD activity is unstable at room temperature, send the sample to the laboratory immediately or refrigerate it at 32° to 39.2° F. (0° to 4° C.).

Values

Serum HBD values range from 114 to 290 u/ml. Ratio of serum LDH to HBD normally varies from 1.2 to 1.6:1.

Implications of results

In MI, HBD levels peak 72 hours after onset of chest pains and remain elevated for 2 weeks. The LDH/HBD ratio is decreased due to greater activity of LDH_1 and LDH_2, as reflected in HBD levels; total LDH rises less markedly. HBD levels are also raised by artifact blood sample hemolysis, hemolytic or megaloblastic anemia, muscular dystrophy, and moderate-to-severe acute hepatocellular damage. Acute hepatitis increases the LDH/HBD ratio, since HBD levels are less sensitive to hepatocellular damage than LDH levels, which increase moderately.

Post-test care

If a hematoma develops at the venipuncture site, apply warm soaks.

Interfering factors

□ Failure to draw the sample on schedule, missing peak levels, may interfere with accurate determination of values.

□ If the sample is not sent to the laboratory promptly or is not refrigerated, test results may be affected.

□ Extensive surgery, or cardioversion can elevate HBD levels.

SR. MARY BRIAN KELBER, RN, DNS

Serum Glutamic-Oxaloacetic Transaminase

[Aspartate aminotransferase, aspartate transaminase]

Serum glutamic-oxaloacetic transaminase (SGOT) is one of two enzymes that catalyze the conversion of the nitrogenous portion of an amino acid to an amino acid residue. It is essential to energy production in the Krebs cycle (tricarboxylic acid or citric acid cycle). SGOT is found in the cytoplasm and mitochondria of many cells, primarily in the liver, heart, skeletal muscles, kidneys, pancreas, and to a lesser extent, in RBCs. It is released into serum in proportion to cellular damage.

Although a high correlation exists between myocardial infarction (MI) and elevated SGOT, this test is sometimes considered superfluous for diagnosing MI because of its relatively low organ specificity; it doesn't enable differentiation between acute MI and the effects of hepatic congestion due to heart failure.

Purpose

□ To detect recent MI (together with creatine phosphokinase and lactic dehydrogenase)

☐ To aid detection and differential diagnosis of acute hepatic disease

☐ To monitor patient progress and prognosis in cardiac and hepatic diseases.

Patient preparation

Explain to the patient that this test helps assess heart and liver function. Inform him that he needn't restrict food or fluids. Tell him the test usually requires three venipunctures: one at admission and one each day for the next 2 days. Reassure him that although he may experience transient discomfort from the needle puncture and the pressure of the tourniquet, collecting each sample takes less than 3 minutes.

Withhold morphine, codeine, meperidine, chlorpropamide, methyldopa, phenazopyridine, and antitubercular drugs (isoniazid, para-aminosalicylates and pyrazinamide), as ordered. If any of these medications must be continued, note this on the laboratory slip.

Procedure

Perform a venipuncture, and collect the sample in a 7 ml *red-top* tube.

Precautions

☐ To avoid missing peak SGOT levels, draw serum samples at the same time each day.

☐ Handle the collection tube gently to prevent hemolysis, and send the sample to the laboratory immediately.

Values

SGOT levels range from 8 to 20 u/liter. Normal values for infants are as high as four times those of adults.

Implications of results

SGOT levels fluctuate in response to the extent of cellular necrosis and therefore may be transiently and minimally elevated early in the disease process, and extremely elevated during the most acute phase. Depending on when during the course of the disease the initial sample was drawn, SGOT levels can rise—indicating increasing disease severity and tissue damage—or fall—indicating disease resolution and tissue repair. Thus, the relative change in SGOT values serves as a reliable monitoring mechanism.

Maximum elevations are associated with certain diseases and conditions. For example, very high elevations (more than 20 times normal) may indicate acute viral hepatitis, severe skeletal muscle trauma, extensive surgery, drug-induced hepatic injury, and severe passive liver congestion.

High levels (ranging from 10 to 20 times normal) may indicate severe myocardial infarction, severe infectious mononucleosis, and alcoholic cirrhosis. High levels also occur during the prodromal or resolving stages of conditions that cause maximal elevations.

Moderate-to-high levels (ranging from 5 to 10 times normal) may indicate Duchenne muscular dystrophy, dermatomyositis, and chronic hepatitis. Moderate-to-high levels also occur during prodromal and resolving stages of diseases that cause high elevations.

Low-to-moderate levels (ranging from 2 to 5 times normal) may indicate hemolytic anemia, metastatic hepatic tumors, acute pancreatitis, pulmonary emboli, delirium tremens, and fatty liver. SGOT levels rise slightly after the first few days of biliary duct obstruction. Also, low-to-moderate elevations occur at some time during any of the preceding conditions or diseases.

Post-test care

☐ If hematoma develops, apply warm soaks.

☐ Resume medications discontinued before the test, as ordered.

Interfering factors

☐ Chlorpropamide, opiates, methyldopa, erythromycin, sulfonamides, pyridoxine, dicumarol, antitubercular agents, large doses of acetaminophen, salicylates, and vitamin A, and many other drugs known to affect the liver cause elevated SGOT levels. Strenuous exercise and muscle trauma caused by intramuscular injections also raise SGOT levels.

☐ Hemolysis due to rough handling of the sample may hinder accurate determination of SGOT levels.

☐ Failure to draw the sample as scheduled, missing peak SGOT levels, may interfere with accurate determination of test results.

SR. MARY BRIAN KELBER, RN, DNS

HEPATIC ENZYMES

Serum Glutamic-Pyruvic Transaminase

[Alanine aminotransferase, alanine transaminase]

Serum glutamic-pyruvic transaminase (SGPT), one of the two enzymes that catalyzes a reversible amino group transfer reaction in the Krebs cycle (citric acid or tricarboxylic acid cycle), is necessary for tissue energy production. Unlike serum glutamic-oxaloacetic transaminase (SGOT), the other aminotransferase, SGPT primarily appears in hepatocellular cytoplasm, with lesser amounts in the kidneys, heart, and skeletal muscles, and is a relatively specific indicator of acute hepatocellular damage. When such damage occurs, SGPT is released from the cytoplasm into the bloodstream, often before jaundice appears, resulting in abnormally high serum levels that may not return to normal for days or weeks. This test measures serum SGPT levels, using the spectrophotometric or the colorimetric method.

Purpose

☐ To help detect and evaluate treatment of acute hepatic disease—especially hepatitis, and cirrhosis without jaundice

☐ To help distinguish between myocardial and hepatic tissue damage (used with SGOT)

☐ To assess hepatotoxicity of some drugs.

Patient preparation

Explain to the patient that this test helps assess liver function. Inform him that he need not restrict food or fluids. Tell him the test requires a blood sample; who will perform the venipuncture and when; and that he may experience transient discomfort from the needle puncture and the pressure of the tourniquet. Reassure him that collecting the sample takes less than 3 minutes.

Withhold hepatotoxic or cholestatic drugs such as methotrexate, chlorpromazine, salicylates, and narcotics. If these medications must be continued, note this on the laboratory slip.

Procedure

Perform a venipuncture, and collect the sample in a 7 ml *red-top* tube.

Precautions

Handle the sample gently to prevent hemolysis. SGPT activity is stable in serum for up to 3 days at room temperature.

Values

Serum SGPT levels in men range from 10 to 32 u/liter; in women, from 9 to 24 u/liter. The normal range for infants is twice that of adults.

Implications of results

Very high SGPT levels (up to 50 times normal) suggest viral or severe drug-induced hepatitis, or other hepatic disease with extensive necrosis. (SGOT levels are also elevated but usually to a lesser degree.) Moderate-to-high levels may indicate infectious mononucleosis, chronic hepatitis, intrahepatic cholestasis or cholecystitis, early or improving acute viral hepatitis, or severe hepatic congestion due to heart failure. Slight-to-moderate elevations of SGPT (usually with higher increases in SGOT levels) may appear in any condition that produces acute hepatocellular injury—such as active cirrhosis, and drug-induced or alcoholic hepatitis. Marginal elevations occasionally occur in acute myocardial infarction, reflecting secondary hepatic congestion or the release of small amounts of SGPT from myocardial tissue.

Post-test care
☐ If a hematoma develops at the venipuncture site, apply warm soaks.
☐ As ordered, resume administration of drugs that were withheld before the test.

Interfering factors
☐ Many medications produce hepatic injury by competitively interfering with cellular metabolism. Falsely elevated SGPT levels can follow use of barbiturates, griseofulvin, isoniazid, nitrofurantoin, methyldopa, phenothiazines, phenytoin, salicylates, tetracycline, chlorpromazine, para-aminosalicylic acid, and other drugs that affect the liver. Narcotic analgesics (morphine, codeine, meperidine) may also falsely elevate SGPT levels by increasing intrabiliary pressure.
☐ Ingestion of lead or exposure to carbon tetrachloride causes direct injury to hepatic cells and sharp elevations of SGPT.
☐ Hemolysis caused by rough handling of the sample may interfere with accurate determination of SGPT levels.

SR. MARY BRIAN KELBER, RN, DNS

Alkaline Phosphatase

This test measures serum levels of alkaline phosphatase, an enzyme that is most active at about pH 9.0. Alkaline phosphatase influences bone calcification and lipid and metabolite transport. Total serum levels reflect the combined activity of several alkaline phosphatase isoenzymes found in the liver, bones, kidneys, intestinal lining, and placenta. Bone and liver alkaline phosphatase are always present in adult serum, with liver alkaline phosphatase most prominent—except during the third trimester of pregnancy (when the placenta originates about half of all alkaline phosphatase). The intestinal variant of this enzyme can be a normal component (in less than 10% of normal patterns; a genetically controlled characteristic found almost exclusively in the sera of blood groups B and O); or it can be an abnormal finding associated with hepatic disease.

The alkaline phosphatase test is particularly sensitive to mild biliary obstruction and is a primary indicator of space-occupying hepatic lesions. However, since both skeletal and hepatic diseases can raise alkaline phosphatase levels, its most specific clinical application is in the diagnosis of metabolic bone disease; additional liver function studies are usually required to identify hepatobiliary disorders.

Purpose
☐ To detect and identify skeletal diseases, primarily characterized by marked osteoblastic activity
☐ To detect focal hepatic lesions causing biliary obstruction, such as tumor or abscess
☐ To supplement information from other liver function studies and gastrointestinal enzyme tests
☐ To assess response to vitamin D in the treatment of deficiency-induced rickets.

Patient preparation
Explain to the patient that this test assesses liver or bone function. Instruct him to fast for 10 to 12 hours before the test, since fat intake stimulates intestinal alkaline phosphatase secretion. Tell him this test requires a blood sample; who will perform the venipuncture and when; and that he may experience discomfort from the needle puncture and the pressure of the tourniquet. Reassure him that collecting the sample usually takes less than 3 minutes.

Procedure
Perform a venipuncture, and collect the sample in a 7 ml red-top tube.

ALKALINE PHOSPHATASE ISOENZYMES

Separation of alkaline phosphatase isoenzymes in the laboratory, using heat inactivation, electrophoresis, or chemical means, is sometimes used in place of serum gamma glutamyl transferase, leucine aminopeptidase, or 5′-nucleotidase to differentiate hepatic and skeletal diseases. Sixteen molecularly distinct isoenzyme fractions have been identified electrophoretically in human serum, stimulating continuing controversy about the origins, proportions, and methods of isoenzyme determination. Although the number and concentration of alkaline phosphatase isoenzymes in total serum levels vary with the laboratory separation method used, the five isoenzymes of greatest clinical significance originate in the liver (includes kidney and bile fractions), bone (may also include bile fraction), intestine, and placenta.

On electrophoresis, the liver isoenzyme usually measures from 20 to 130 u/liter; the bone isoenzyme, from 20 to 120 u/liter; and the intestinal fraction—which occurs almost exclusively in individuals with blood group B or O and is markedly elevated 8 hours after a fatty meal—from undetectable to 18 u/liter. The placental isoenzyme first appears in the second trimester of pregnancy, accounts for roughly half of all alkaline phosphatase during the third trimester, and drops to normal levels the first month postpartum. Another isoenzyme, Regan, resembles the placental isoenzyme and appears in a small percentage of patients with cancer; it may be used as a tumor marker.

Precautions

Handle the collection tube gently to prevent hemolysis, and send the sample to the laboratory immediately, since alkaline phosphatase activity increases at room temperature due to a rise in pH.

Values

The normal range of serum alkaline phosphatase varies with the laboratory method used. Total alkaline phosphatase levels, when measured by chemical inhibition, range from 90 to 239 u/liter for males; for females under age 45, from 76 to 196 u/liter; for women over age 45,

the range widens from 87 to 250 u/liter, for unknown reasons. Since alkaline phosphatase concentrations rise during active bone formation and growth, infants, children, and adolescents normally have levels that may be three times as high as those of adults. Pregnancy also causes a physiologic rise in alkaline phosphatase levels.

When the Bodansky method is used, normal range is from 1.5 to 4 Bodansky units/dl; for the King-Armstrong method, normal adult values range from 4 to 13.5 King-Armstrong units/dl.

Implications of results

Although significant alkaline phosphatase elevations are possible with diseases that affect many organs, they are most likely to indicate skeletal disease, or extra- or intrahepatic biliary obstruction causing cholestasis. Many acute hepatic diseases cause alkaline phosphatase elevations before they result in any change in serum bilirubin levels. Moderate rise in alkaline phosphatase levels may reflect acute biliary obstruction from hepatocellular inflammation in active cirrhosis, mononucleosis, and viral hepatitis. Moderate increases are also seen in osteomalacia and deficiency-induced rickets.

Sharp elevations of alkaline phosphatase levels may result from complete biliary obstruction by malignant or infectious infiltrations or fibrosis. Such markedly high levels are most common in Paget's disease and, occasionally, in biliary obstruction, extensive bone metastases, or hyperparathyroidism. Metastatic bone tumors resulting from pancreatic cancer raise alkaline phosphatase levels without a concomitant rise in serum glutamic-pyruvic transaminase levels.

Isoenzyme fractionation and additional enzyme tests—serum gamma glutamyl transferase, acid phosphatase, 5′-nucleotidase, and leucine aminopeptidase—are sometimes performed when the cause of alkaline phosphatase elevations (skeletal or hepatic disease) is in doubt. Rarely, low levels of serum alkaline phosphatase are associated with hypophosphatasia, and protein or magnesium deficiency.

Post-test care
☐ If a hematoma develops at the venipuncture site, apply warm soaks.
☐ Diet may be resumed.

Interfering factors
☐ Recent ingestion of vitamin D may increase levels of alkaline phosphatase, due to the effect of vitamin D on osteoblastic activity.
☐ Recent infusion of albumin prepared from placental venous blood causes extreme increases in serum alkaline phosphatase levels.
☐ Drugs that influence liver function or cause cholestasis, such as barbiturates, chlorpropamide, oral contraceptives, isoniazid, methyldopa, phenothiazines, phenytoin, and rifampin, can mildly elevate alkaline phosphatase levels; halothane sensitivity may increase levels drastically. Clofibrate decreases alkaline phosphatase levels.
☐ Healing long bone fractures, age (infants, children, adolescents, and women over 45), and pregnancy (third trimester) can produce physiologic elevations of alkaline phosphatase levels.
☐ Hemolysis due to rough handling of the sample or a delay of more than 8 hours in sending the sample to the laboratory may interfere with accurate determination of alkaline phosphatase levels.

SR. MARY BRIAN KELBER, RN, DNS

Gamma Glutamyl Transferase
[Gamma glutamyl transpeptidase]

Gamma glutamyl transferase (GGT) participates in the transfer of amino acids across cellular membranes and, possibly, in glutathione metabolism.

Highest concentrations of GGT exist in the renal tubules, where amino acids are reabsorbed from glomerular filtrate, but the enzyme also appears in the liver, biliary tract epithelium, pancreas, lymphocytes, brain, and testes. At least four isoenzyme forms exist, but fractionation is not clinically useful or practical at present.

This test, which measures serum GGT levels, is a somewhat more sensitive indicator of hepatic necrosis than serum glutamic-oxaloacetic transaminase, and is as sensitive as or more sensitive than alkaline phosphatase, as GGT is not elevated in bone growth or pregnancy. However, the test is nonspecific, providing little data about the type of hepatic disease; increased levels also occur in renal, cardiac, and prostatic disease. Certain medications also elevate serum levels. GGT is particularly sensitive to the effects of alcohol in the liver, and levels may be elevated after moderate alcohol intake and in chronic alcoholism, even without clinical evidence of hepatic injury.

Purpose
☐ To provide information about hepatobiliary diseases, to assess liver function, and to detect alcohol ingestion
☐ To distinguish between skeletal disease and hepatic disease when serum alkaline phosphatase is elevated. (A normal GGT level suggests such elevation stems from skeletal disease.)

Patient preparation
Explain to the patient that this test evaluates liver function. (Depending on the purpose of the test, some laboratories require 12-hour fasting and abstinence from alcohol before the test.) Tell him who will perform the venipuncture and when, and that he may experience discomfort from the needle puncture and the pressure of the tourniquet. Collecting the sample takes less than 3 minutes.

Procedure
Perform a venipuncture, and collect the sample in a 7 ml *red-top* tube.

Precautions

Handle the collection tube gently to prevent hemolysis. GGT activity is stable in serum at room temperature for 5 days.

Values

Serum GGT values vary with the assay method used (colorimetric or kinetic method). In females under age 45, nor-

BILIRUBIN AND ENZYME CHANGES IN HEPTOBILIARY DISEASE

	Viral hepatitis	Infectious mononucleosis	Drug-induced hepatitis	Chronic hepatitis	Alcoholic cirrhosis	Extrahepatic obstruction (pancreatic carcinoma, common duct stones)	Metastatic carcinoma
LDH	slight, moderate; LDH$_5$ marked	slight		normal, marked; LDH$_5$ slight	normal, marked; LDH$_5$ normal		slight, moderate
SGOT (AST) (reflects acute obstructive disease)	marked	slight	marked	normal, slight	normal, slight	normal — rises late	normal
SGPT (ALT) (reflects chronic infective disease)	marked, marked	slight, moderate, marked	marked	normal, slight	normal, slight	moderate — rises late	normal
Alkaline phosphatase	moderate — after 4 to 7 days	slight	slight	normal, slight	normal, slight	marked	marked — with biliary involvement
Bilirubin	normal		slight, marked		normal, moderate	moderate, marked	normal
Direct	moderate		moderate, marked			moderate, marked	
Indirect	moderate		slight, marked			slight, moderate	
GGT	normal — elevated longest	normal, slight	moderate, marked	slight, moderate	moderate, marked	moderate, marked	marked
ICD	marked	moderate	slight	normal	normal, moderate	moderate	slight
LAP	normal	normal, slight	normal	normal	normal, slight	normal, slight, moderate	moderate, marked
5'NT	normal	normal, slight	normal	slight	normal, slight	moderate	moderate, marked
OCT	marked	moderate	moderate	normal	marked	normal	normal

Legend:
○ Normal · ◔ Slight elevation · ◕ Moderate elevation · ● Marked elevation · ▦ Significant in differential diagnosis

mal levels range from 5 to 27 u/liter; in females over age 45, and in males, levels range from 6 to 37 u/liter.

Implications of results

Serum GGT rises in any acute hepatic disease, as enzyme production increases in response to hepatocellular injury. Moderate increases occur in acute pancreatitis, renal disease, prostatic metastases, postoperatively, and in some patients, with epilepsy or brain tumors. Levels also increase due to enzyme induction after alcohol ingestion. The sharpest elevations occur in patients with obstructive jaundice and hepatic metastatic infiltrations. GGT may increase 5 to 10 days after acute myocardial infarction, either as a result of tissue granulation and healing, or as an indication of the effects of cardiac insufficiency on the liver.

Post-test care

If a hematoma develops at the venipuncture site, apply warm soaks.

Interfering factors

□ Clofibrate and oral contraceptives decrease serum GGT levels. Aminoglycosides, barbiturates, and phenytoin produce elevated values.
□ Moderate intake of alcohol causes increased serum GGT levels that may persist for at least 60 hours.
□ Hemolysis due to rough handling of the sample may interfere with accurate determination of serum GGT levels.

SR. MARY BRIAN KELBER, RN, DNS

Isocitrate Dehydrogenase

Isocitrate dehydrogenase (ICD), an enzyme involved in the Krebs cycle (tricarboxylic acid or citric acid cycle), appears primarily in the liver in a stable, electrophoretically fast-moving form, and in the heart in a heat-labile form that quickly loses its activity when released into serum. It's also present in skeletal muscles, platelets, RBCs, and the placenta. This test, which measures total ICD levels in a serum sample, is as sensitive as but more specific for hepatic disease than measurement of serum glutamic-oxaloacetic transaminase (SGOT): ICD levels generally rise in acute hepatocellular damage but remain normal in acute myocardial infarction. However, since ICD offers no advantages over serum glutamic-pyruvic transaminase (SGPT), it's rarely ordered, and no clinical significance has been associated with isoenzyme fractionation.

Purpose

□ To aid diagnosis of acute hepatocellular damage
□ To detect early viral hepatitis and infectious mononucleosis
□ To distinguish between hepatic disease and myocardial infarction when SGOT is elevated.

Patient preparation

Explain to the patient that this test helps assess liver function. Inform him he needn't restrict food or fluids. Tell him this test requires a blood sample; who will perform the venipuncture and when; and that he may experience some discomfort from the needle puncture and the pressure of the tourniquet. Reassure him that collecting the sample takes less than 3 minutes.

Procedure

Perform a venipuncture, and collect the sample in a 7 ml *red-top* tube.

Precautions

Handle the sample gently to prevent hemolysis, and send it to the laboratory immediately. Stability of this enzyme in serum has not been established.

Values

Serum ICD values range from 1.2 to 7 u/liter at 86° F. (30° C.), as measured by continuous monitoring. Neonates may have serum levels four times as high as normal adult values for the first 2 weeks after birth.

Implications of results

Marked serum elevations (10 to 40 times normal) occur as early as the incubation period in acute viral hepatitis and return to normal during the third week of illness, unless the infection becomes chronic. Moderately high levels are found in other conditions that result in liver cell damage, such as hepatic metastases, moderate or severe passive hepatic congestion, active cirrhosis, biliary tract inflammation, neonatal biliary duct atresia, drug-induced hepatic injury, and infectious mononucleosis.

Although the heart contains ICD, myocardial infarction isn't usually associated with high serum levels due to instability of the heart isoenzyme or rapid clearance from serum. The placenta also contains ICD, but normal pregnancy doesn't elevate serum levels. However, in preeclampsia and placental infarction, serum levels do rise.

Post-test care

If a hematoma develops at the venipuncture site, apply warm soaks.

Interfering factors

□ Alcohol, aminosalicylic acid, isoniazid, methotrexate, and phenylbutazone increase ICD levels due to their effect on liver cells.
□ Hemolysis due to rough handling of the sample may interfere with accurate determination of ICD levels.

SR. MARY BRIAN KELBER, RN, DNS

Leucine Aminopeptidase

[Amino acid arylamidase]

Leucine aminopeptidase (LAP) is a proteolytic enzyme found in all body tissues but concentrated in several isoenzyme forms in the liver, pancreas, and small intestine. Its metabolic function in the body is to hydrolyze the peptide bonds of alpha-amino acids involved in cellular energy production. LAP levels tend to parallel those of alkaline phosphatase in hepatic disease and normal pregnancy; but unlike alkaline phosphatase, LAP remains normal in skeletal disease. Despite its relative hepatobiliary specificity, this test—which measures serum LAP levels—isn't commonly performed. In the past, it has been used to diagnose pancreatic cancer but has proven unreliable for this purpose. Recent research suggests that LAP isoenzyme determination may be beneficial in evaluating neonatal jaundice.

Purpose

□ To aid in differentiating hepatic disease from skeletal disease when LAP is elevated from an unknown cause
□ To help distinguish between congenital biliary atresia and neonatal hepatitis.

Patient preparation

Tell the patient (or his parents) that this test helps assess liver function. Advise him whether or not he must restrict food or fluids (this varies with individual laboratory procedure). Tell him this test requires a blood sample; who will perform the venipuncture and when; and that he may experience some discomfort from the needle puncture and the pressure of the tourniquet. Reassure him that collecting the sample takes less than 3 minutes.

Determine if the patient is taking estrogen-progesterone drugs, since they elevate LAP levels.

Procedure

Perform a venipuncture, and collect the sample in a 7 ml *red-top* tube.

Precautions

Handle the sample gently to prevent hemolysis, since LAP is contained in serum.

Values

LAP levels should be less than 50 u/liter

or, in Goldberg-Rutenberg units, 80 to 200 u/ml for males and 75 to 185 u/ml for females.

Implications of results

Since alkaline phosphatase rises in both skeletal and hepatic diseases, and LAP rises only in the latter, normal LAP with elevated alkaline phosphatase indicates skeletal disease. High LAP levels occur with obstructive jaundice resulting from intrahepatic cholestasis (such as liver metastases) and extrahepatic diseases, such as common bile duct calculus or cancer of the head of the pancreas. Slight elevations occur when hepatocellular damage doesn't cause biliary obstruction, and in hepatitis, cirrhosis, and pancreatitis. However, LAP levels may rise before alkaline phosphatase levels in persons without jaundice. In infants with jaundice, high total LAP (more than 500 u/liter) and two zones of electrophoretic activity suggest biliary atresia. Neonatal hepatitis causes milder LAP elevation (less than 500 u/liter), and only a single isoenzyme is detected by fractionation.

Post-test care

If a hematoma develops at the venipuncture site, apply warm soaks.

Interfering factors

☐ Estrogens, progesterone, pregnancy, and oral contraceptives can cause elevated LAP levels.
☐ Hemolysis due to rough handling of the sample may hinder accurate determination of test results.
SR. MARY BRIAN KELBER, RN, DNS

5′-Nucleotidase

The enzyme 5′-nucleotidase (5′NT) is a phosphatase formed almost entirely in the hepatobiliary tract. Unlike alkaline phosphatase, an enzyme that is nonspecific, this enzyme hydrolyzes nucleoside 5′-phosphate groups only. Although serum 5′NT, alkaline phosphatase, and leucine aminopeptidase (LAP) levels rise in hepatic metastases, hepatocarcinoma, and biliary tract obstruction, only 5′NT remains normal in skeletal disease and pregnancy, and so is more specific for hepatic dysfunction than alkaline phosphatase or LAP.

This test, which measures serum 5′NT levels, is technically more difficult than the alkaline phosphatase assay, and has not been widely used as a liver function study, although some authorities consider 5′NT more sensitive than alkaline phosphatase to cholangitis, biliary cirrhosis, and malignant infiltrations of the liver. However, 5′NT is used most often to determine whether alkaline phosphatase elevation originates from skeletal or hepatic disease.

Purpose

☐ To distinguish between hepatobiliary and skeletal disease when the source of elevated alkaline phosphatase levels is uncertain
☐ To help differentiate biliary obstruction from acute hepatocellular damage
☐ To detect hepatic metastasis in the absence of jaundice.

Patient preparation

Explain to the patient that this test evaluates liver function. Inform him he need not restrict food or fluids. Tell him the test requires a blood sample; who will perform the venipuncture and when; and that he may experience discomfort from the needle puncture and the pressure of the tourniquet. Collecting the sample takes less than 3 minutes.

Procedure

Perform a venipuncture, and collect the sample in a 7 ml red-top tube.

Precautions

Handle the sample gently to prevent hemolysis, since RBCs contain this enzyme.

Values

Serum 5′NT values for adults range from

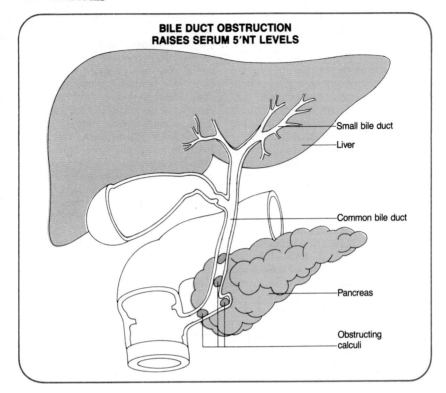

**BILE DUCT OBSTRUCTION
RAISES SERUM 5'NT LEVELS**

Small bile duct

Liver

Common bile duct

Pancreas

Obstructing calculi

2 to 17 u/liter; values for children may be lower.

Implications of results

Highest 5'NT elevations occur in common bile duct obstruction by calculi or tumors in diseases that cause severe intrahepatic cholestasis, such as neoplastic infiltrations of the liver. Slight-to-moderate increases may reflect acute hepatocellular damage or active cirrhosis.

Post-test care

If a hematoma develops at the venipuncture site, apply warm soaks.

Interfering factors

☐ Hemolysis due to rough handling of the sample may interfere with accurate determination of serum levels.
☐ Ingestion of cholestatic drugs, such as phenothiazines, morphine, meperidine, and codeine, elevates 5'NT levels.

SR. MARY BRIAN KELBER, RN, DNS

Ornithine Carbamoyltransferase

Ornithine carbamoyltransferase (OCT), an enzyme involved in urea metabolism in the Krebs cycle (tricarboxylic acid or citric acid cycle), is found almost exclusively in the liver; small amounts are also found in the intestine. This test measures serum OCT levels and is one of the most sensitive indicators of acute hepatocellular dysfunction. Since only trace amounts of OCT occur normally in serum, any increase is clinically significant. Although serum OCT reveals hepatocellular damage with greater sensitivity than tests such as serum glutamic-oxaloacetic transaminase and serum glutamic-pyruvic transaminase, the test isn't commonly performed—de-

spite recent technologic advances that make possible routine laboratory measurement of OCT. Even when an ultra–high-sensitivity analysis is required, gamma glutamyl transferase or bile acid assay is more likely to be ordered.

Purpose
□ To detect minimal hepatocellular damage in such disorders as chronic viral hepatitis or drug-induced hepatic dysfunction
□ To confirm that abnormal values in other serum enzyme tests result from hepatic disease.

Patient preparation
Explain to the patient that this test evaluates liver function. Inform him he need not restrict food or fluids. Tell him the test requires a blood sample; who will perform the venipuncture and when; and that he may experience some discomfort from the needle puncture and the pressure of the tourniquet. Reassure him that collecting the sample takes less than 3 minutes.

Procedure
Perform a venipuncture, and collect the sample in a 7 ml *red-top* tube.

Precautions
Handle the collection tube gently to prevent hemolysis.

Values
Serum OCT levels range from undetectable to 500 Sigma units/ml, by colorimetric measurement.

Implications of results
Rising serum OCT levels almost always reflect hepatocellular necrosis. Marked increases (10 to 200 times normal) occur in acute viral hepatitis; mild or moderate increases, in cholecystitis, cirrhosis, obstructive jaundice, and metastatic carcinoma. Hepatotoxicity resulting from drugs or alcoholism is demonstrated by increased OCT levels. Rarely, elevated OCT levels indicate extensive intestinal infarction and massive release of enzymes from necrotic tissue.

Post-test care
If a hematoma develops at the venipuncture site, apply warm soaks.

Interfering factors
Hemolysis due to rough handling of the sample may interfere with accurate determination of OCT levels.

WILLIAM M. DOUGHERTY, BS

PANCREATIC ENZYMES

Serum Amylase

Alpha-amylase (amylase), synthesized primarily in the pancreas and the salivary glands, is secreted into the gastrointestinal tract. This enzyme helps digest starch and glycogen in the mouth, stomach, and intestine. In cases of suspected acute pancreatic disease, measurement of serum or urine amylase is the most important laboratory test.

More than 20 methods of measuring serum amylase exist, with different ranges of normal values. Unfortunately, test values can't always be converted to a standard measurement. The classic saccharogenic method described here reports serum amylase in Somogyi units/dl.

Purpose
□ To diagnose acute pancreatitis
□ To distinguish between acute pancreatitis and other causes of abdominal pain that require immediate surgery
□ To evaluate possible pancreatic injury caused by abdominal trauma or surgery.

Patient preparation
Explain to the patient that this test helps

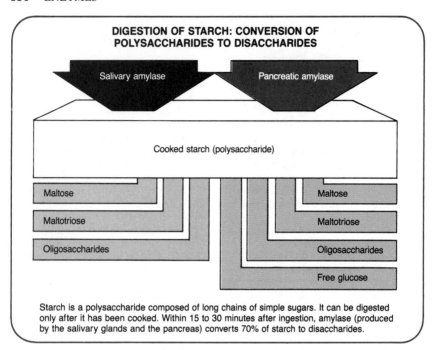

DIGESTION OF STARCH: CONVERSION OF POLYSACCHARIDES TO DISACCHARIDES

Salivary amylase

Pancreatic amylase

Cooked starch (polysaccharide)

Maltose

Maltotriose

Oligosaccharides

Maltose

Maltotriose

Oligosaccharides

Free glucose

Starch is a polysaccharide composed of long chains of simple sugars. It can be digested only after it has been cooked. Within 15 to 30 minutes after ingestion, amylase (produced by the salivary glands and the pancreas) converts 70% of starch to disaccharides.

assess pancreatic function. Inform him that he needn't fast before the test, but must abstain from alcohol, as ordered. Tell him this test requires a blood sample; who will perform the venipuncture and when; and that he may experience transient discomfort from the needle puncture and the pressure of the tourniquet. Reassure him that collecting the sample takes less than 3 minutes. Withhold drugs that may elevate amylase levels, as ordered. If these must be continued, note this on the laboratory slip.

Procedure

Perform a venipuncture, and collect the sample in a 7 ml *red-top* tube.

Precautions

☐ If the patient has severe abdominal pain, draw the sample before diagnostic or therapeutic intervention. For accurate results, it's important to obtain an early sample.

☐ Handle the sample gently to prevent hemolysis.

Values

Serum levels range from 60 to 180 Somogyi units/dl.

Implications of results

Highest amylase levels occur 4 to 12 hours after onset of acute pancreatitis, then drop to normal in 48 to 72 hours. Determination of urine levels should follow normal serum amylase results, to rule out pancreatitis. Moderate serum elevations may accompany obstruction of the common bile duct, the pancreatic duct, or the ampulla of Vater; pancreatic injury from perforated peptic ulcer; pancreatic cancer; and acute salivary gland disease. Impaired renal function may raise serum levels.

Levels may be slightly elevated in a patient who is asymptomatic or who is responding unusually to therapy. An amylase fractionation test helps determine the source of the amylase and aids selection of additional tests.

Depressed levels can occur in chronic pancreatitis, pancreatic cancer, cirrhosis, hepatitis, and toxemia of pregnancy.

Post-test care
☐ If a hematoma develops at the venipuncture site, apply warm soaks.
☐ As ordered, resume administration of drugs discontinued before the test.

Interfering factors
☐ The following conditions may produce false-positive test results:
—ingestion of ethyl alcohol in large amounts; certain drugs, such as aminosalicylic acid, asparaginase, azathioprine, corticosteroids, cyproheptadine, narcotic analgesics, oral contraceptives, rifampin, sulfasalazine, or thiazide and loop diuretics
—recent peripancreatic surgery, perforated ulcer or intestine, or abscess
—spasm of the sphincter of Oddi or, rarely, macroamylasemia
—coughing, sneezing, or talking near an open collection tube (saliva contains amylase).
☐ Hemolysis due to rough handling of the sample may alter test results.

SR. MARY BRIAN KELBER, RN, DNS

Lipase

Lipase is produced in the pancreas and secreted into the duodenum, where it converts triglycerides and other fats into fatty acids and glycerol. Destruction of pancreatic cells, which occurs in acute pancreatitis, releases large amounts of lipase into the blood.

This test measures serum lipase levels by the kinetic turbidimetric technique; it's most useful in diagnosing acute pancreatitis when performed with a serum or urine amylase test.

Purpose
☐ To aid diagnosis of acute pancreatitis.

Patient preparation
Explain to the patient that this test evaluates pancreatic function. Instruct him to fast overnight before the test. Tell him the test requires a blood sample; who

---

MACROAMYLASEMIA: RARE CAUSE OF ELEVATED SERUM AMYLASE

Macroamylasemia doesn't cause any symptoms, but it occasionally causes elevated serum amylase levels. This uncommon, benign condition occurs when macroamylase—a complex of amylase and an immunoglobulin or other protein—is present in a patient's serum.

A typical patient with macroamylasemia has an elevated serum amylase level and a normal or slightly decreased urine amylase level. This characteristic pattern helps differentiate macroamylasemia from conditions such as pancreatitis, in which both serum and urine amylase levels rise. But it doesn't differentiate macroamylasemia from hyperamylasemia due to impaired renal function, which may raise serum levels and lower urine levels. Chromatographic, ultracentrifugation, or precipitation tests are necessary to detect macroamylase in serum and definitively confirm macroamylasemia.

---

will perform the venipuncture and when; and that he may experience transient discomfort from the needle puncture and the pressure of the tourniquet. Collecting the sample takes less than 3 minutes.

Withhold cholinergics, codeine, meperidine, and morphine, as ordered. If such medications must be continued, note this on the laboratory slip.

Procedure
Perform a venipuncture, and collect the sample in a 7 ml *red-top* tube.

Precautions
Handle the collection tube gently to prevent hemolysis.

Values
Serum levels range from 32 to 80 u/liter.

Implications of results
High lipase levels suggest acute pancreatitis or pancreatic duct obstruction. After an attack of acute pancreatitis, levels frequently remain elevated up to 14 days.

Lipase levels may also rise in pancreatic injury not due to acute pancre-

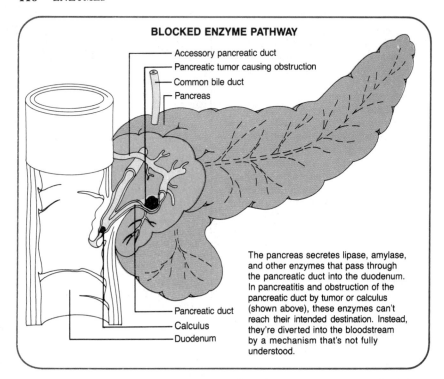

BLOCKED ENZYME PATHWAY

- Accessory pancreatic duct
- Pancreatic tumor causing obstruction
- Common bile duct
- Pancreas

- Pancreatic duct
- Calculus
- Duodenum

The pancreas secretes lipase, amylase, and other enzymes that pass through the pancreatic duct into the duodenum. In pancreatitis and obstruction of the pancreatic duct by tumor or calculus (shown above), these enzymes can't reach their intended destination. Instead, they're diverted into the bloodstream by a mechanism that's not fully understood.

atitis, such as perforated peptic ulcer with chemical pancreatitis due to gastric juices, and in patients with high intestinal obstruction, pancreatic cancer, or renal disease with impaired excretion.

Post-test care
□ If a hematoma develops at the venipuncture site, apply warm soaks.
□ As ordered, resume administration of drugs discontinued before the test.

Interfering factors
□ Cholinergics, codeine, meperidine, and morphine cause spasm of the sphincter of Oddi, producing false-positive results.
□ Hemolysis due to rough handling of the sample may interfere with accurate determination of lipase values.

SR. MARY BRIAN KELBER, SM, RN, DNS

SPECIAL ENZYMES

Acid Phosphatase

Acid phosphatase, a group of phosphatase enzymes most active at a pH of about 5.0, appears primarily in the prostate gland and semen, and to a lesser extent, in the liver, spleen, RBCs, bone marrow, and platelets. Prostatic and erythrocytic enzymes are this group's two major isoenzymes, which can be separated in the laboratory; the prostatic isoenzyme is more specific for prostatic cancer. The more widespread the tumor, the more likely it is to produce high serum acid phosphatase levels. The acid phosphatase assay is usually restricted to adult males to detect prostatic cancer.

This test measures total acid phosphatase and the prostatic fraction in serum by radioimmunoassay or biochemical enzyme assay.

Purpose

☐ To detect prostatic cancer
☐ To monitor response to therapy for prostatic cancer; successful treatment decreases acid phosphatase levels.

Patient preparation

Explain to the patient that this test helps evaluate prostate function. Inform him he needn't restrict food or fluids before the test. Tell him the test requires a blood sample; who will perform the venipuncture and when; and that he may experience discomfort from the needle puncture and the tourniquet. However, sample collection takes less than 3 minutes.

Withhold fluorides, phosphates, and clofibrate, as ordered. If they must be continued, note it on the laboratory slip.

Procedure

Perform a venipuncture, and collect the sample in a 7 ml *red-top* tube.

Precautions

☐ Don't draw the sample within 48 hours of prostate manipulation (rectal exam).
☐ Handle the collection tube gently to prevent hemolysis, and send the sample to the laboratory immediately. Acid phosphatase levels drop by 50% within 1 hour if the sample remains at room temperature without the addition of a preservative or if it's not packed in ice.

Values

Serum values for total acid phosphatase depend on the method and range from: 0 to 1.1 Bodansky units/ml; 1 to 4 King Armstrong units/ml; and 0.13 to 0.63 Bessey-Lowery-Brock (BLB) units/ml.

Implications of results

Generally, high prostatic acid phosphatase levels indicate a tumor that has spread beyond the prostatic capsule. If the tumor has metastasized to bone, high acid phosphatase levels are accompanied by high alkaline phosphatase levels, reflecting increased osteoblastic activity.

Misleading results may occur if alkaline phosphatase levels are high, because acid and alkaline phosphatase enzymes are very similar and differ mainly in their optimum pH ranges. Some alkaline phosphatase may react at a lower pH and thus be detected as acid phosphatase. Acid phosphatase levels rise moderately in prostatic infarction, Paget's disease (some patients), Gaucher's disease, and occasionally, in other conditions, such as multiple myeloma.

Post-test care

☐ If a hematoma develops at the venipuncture site, apply warm soaks.
☐ As ordered, resume administration of medications discontinued before the test.

Interfering factors

☐ Fluorides and phosphates can cause false-negative test results; clofibrate can cause false-positive results.
☐ Prostate massage, catheterization, or rectal examination within 48 hours of the test may interfere with test results.
☐ Hemolysis due to rough handling of the sample, or improper sample storage may interfere with test results.

SR. MARY BRIAN KELBER, RN, DNS

Plasma Renin Activity

Renin secretion is the first stage of the renin-angiotensin-aldosterone cycle that controls the body's sodium-potassium balance, fluid volume, and blood pressure. Renin is released by the juxtaglomerular cells of the kidneys into the renal veins in response to sodium depletion and blood loss. It catalyzes the conversion of angiotensinogen, an alpha$_2$-globulin plasma protein, to angiotensin I, which in turn is converted by hydrolysis into angiotensin II, a vasoconstric-

tor that stimulates aldosterone production in the adrenal cortex. When present in excessive amounts, angiotensin II causes renal hypertension.

The plasma renin activity (PRA) test is a screening procedure for renovascular hypertension but does not unequivocally confirm it. When supplemented by other special tests, the PRA can help establish the cause of hypertension. For instance, sampling blood obtained from both renal veins by renal vein catheterization and analyzing the renal venous renin ratio can identify renovascular disorders. Indexing renin levels against urinary sodium excretion can help identify primary aldosteronism. A sodium-depleted plasma renin test can then confirm this.

Some experts believe that essential hypertension with low, normal, and high renin levels should be treated differently, and the PRA test can categorize the disease for appropriate therapy.

Plasma renin activity is measured by radioimmunoassay of a peripheral or renal blood sample, and results are expressed as the rate of angiotensin I formation per unit of time. Patient preparation is crucial and may take up to 1 month.

Purpose
☐ To screen for renal origin of hypertension
☐ To help plan the best treatment of essential hypertension, a genetic disease often aggravated by excess sodium intake
☐ To help identify hypertension linked to unilateral (sometimes bilateral) renovascular disease by renal vein catheterization
☐ To help identify primary aldosteronism (Conn's syndrome) resulting from aldosterone-secreting adrenal adenoma
☐ To confirm primary aldosteronism (sodium-depleted plasma renin test).

Patient preparation
Explain to the patient that this test helps determine the cause of hypertension. As ordered, tell the patient to discontinue use of diuretics, antihypertensives, vasodilators, oral contraceptives, and licorice for 2 to 4 weeks before the test, and to maintain a normal-sodium diet (3 g/ day) during this period. For the sodium-depleted renin test, tell the patient he'll receive furosemide or, if he has angina or cerebrovascular insufficiency, that he'll receive chlorthiazide and follow a low-sodium diet for 3 days. Inform him that the test requires a blood sample; who will perform the venipuncture and when; and that he may experience some transient discomfort from the needle puncture and the pressure of the tourniquet. Reassure the patient that collecting the blood sample takes less than 3 minutes.

If a recumbent sample is ordered, instruct the patient to remain in bed until the sample is obtained. (Posture influences renin secretion.) If an upright sample is ordered, instruct him to stand or sit upright for 2 hours before the test is performed.

If renal catheterization is ordered, make sure the patient has signed an informed consent form. Tell him the procedure will be done in the X-ray department and that a local anesthetic will be given.

Procedure
Peripheral vein sample: Perform a venipuncture, and collect the sample in a 7 ml *lavender-top* tube.

Renal vein catheterization: A catheter is advanced to the kidneys through the femoral vein, under fluoroscopic control, and samples are obtained from both renal veins and the vena cava.

Precautions
☐ Since renin is very unstable, the sample must be drawn into a chilled syringe and collection tube, placed on ice, and sent to the laboratory immediately.
☐ Completely fill the collection tube, and invert it gently several times to mix the sample and the anticoagulant.

Values
Levels of plasma renin activity and of

PATIENT TEACHING AID

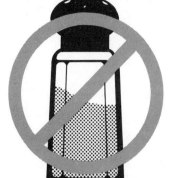

Low-sodium Diet
for Renin Testing

Dear Patient:
Before undergoing renin testing, you must
severely restrict your intake of sodium
for 3 days. This restriction is important to the
accuracy of the test. If you are following
this diet at home, observe these precautions:

• Eat only the foods included in the meal plan provided by the doctor.
• Measure all portions, using standard measuring cups and spoons.
• Use 4 oz (112 g) *unsalted* beefsteak or ground beef for lunch and 4 oz (112 g) *unsalted*
chicken for dinner. (Amount refers to weight before cooking.)
• You may eat the following *unsalted* (fresh or frozen) vegetables: asparagus, green or wax
beans, cabbage, cauliflower, lettuce, and tomatoes.
• Use only the specified amount of coffee.
• If you are thirsty between meals, drink distilled water (no other food or beverage is
allowed).
• Prepare all foods without salt; don't use salt at the table.

Breakfast:
1 egg, poached or boiled, or fried in *unsalted* fat
2 slices *unsalted* toast
1 shredded wheat biscuit or ⅔ cup *unsalted* cooked cereal
4 oz (120 ml) half-and-half or milk
8 oz (240 ml) coffee
Sugar, jam or jelly, and *unsalted* butter, as desired.

Lunch:
4 oz (120 ml) *unsalted* tomato juice
4 oz (112 g) *unsalted* beefsteak or ground beef; may be broiled, or fried in *unsalted* fat
½ cup *unsalted* potato
½ cup *unsalted* green beans or other allowed vegetable
1 serving fruit
8 oz (240 ml) coffee
1 slice *unsalted* bread
Sugar, jam or jelly, and *unsalted* butter, as desired

Dinner:
4 oz (112 g) *unsalted* chicken; may be baked or broiled, or fried in *unsalted* fat
½ cup *unsalted* potato
1 slice *unsalted* bread
Lettuce salad (vinegar and oil dressing)
1 serving fruit
8 oz (240 ml) coffee
Sugar, jam or jelly, and *unsalted* butter, as desired

Reprinted with permission of Mayo Foundation.

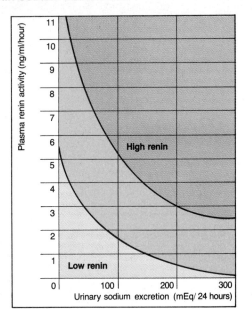

THE RENIN-SODIUM CONNECTION

In the normal kidney, urinary sodium excretion is inversely related to plasma renin activity. The range of normal function with stable levels of salt intake lies within the shaded zone.

Adapted with permission from H.R. Laragh, et al, "Essential Hypertension: Renin and Aldosterone, Heart Attack and Stroke," *New England Journal of Medicine.* 286:441, 1972.

aldosterone decrease with advancing age.

Sodium-depleted, upright, peripheral vein: For ages 20 to 39, the range is from 2.9 to 24 ng/ml/hour; mean, 10.8 ng/ml/hour. For age 40 and over, range is from 2.9 to 10.8 ng/ml/hour; mean, 5.9 ng/ml/hour.

Sodium-replete, upright, peripheral vein: For ages 20 to 39, range is from 0.1 to 4.3 ng/ml/hour; mean, 1.9 ng/ml/hour. For age 40 and over, the range is from 0.1 to 3 ng/ml/hour; mean, 1 ng/ml/hour.

In renal vein catheterization, the renal venous renin ratio (the renin level in the renal vein compared to the level in the inferior vena cava) is less than 1.5 to 1.

Implications of test results

Elevated renin levels may occur in essential hypertension (uncommon), malignant and renovascular hypertension, cirrhosis, hypokalemia, hypovolemia due to hemorrhage, renin-producing renal tumors (Bartter's syndrome), and adrenal hypofunction (Addison's disease). High renin levels may also be found in chronic renal failure with parenchymal disease, end-stage renal disease, and transplantation rejection. Decreased renin levels may indicate hypervolemia due to a high-sodium diet, salt-retaining steroids, primary aldosteronism, Cushing's syndrome, licorice ingestion syndrome, or essential hypertension with low renin levels.

High serum and urine aldosterone levels, with low plasma renin activity, help identify primary aldosteronism: in the sodium-depleted renin test, low plasma renin confirms this and differentiates it from secondary aldosteronism (characterized by increased renin.)

Post-test care

☐ If a hematoma develops at the peripheral venipuncture site, apply warm soaks.
☐ After renal vein catheterization, apply pressure to the catheterization site for 10

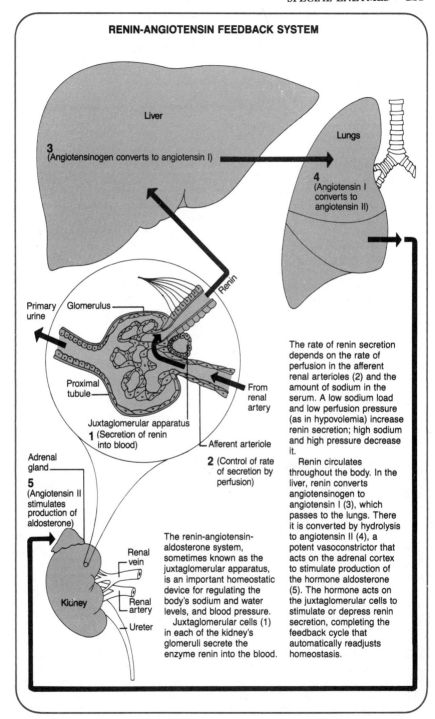

RENIN-ANGIOTENSIN FEEDBACK SYSTEM

Liver

Lungs

3
(Angiotensinogen converts to angiotensin I)

4
(Angiotensin I
converts to
angiotensin II)

Primary urine

Glomerulus

Renin

Proximal tubule

From renal artery

Juxtaglomerular apparatus
1 (Secretion of renin into blood)

Afferent arteriole

2 (Control of rate of secretion by perfusion)

Adrenal gland

5
(Angiotensin II stimulates production of aldosterone)

Renal vein

Kidney

Renal artery

Ureter

The rate of renin secretion depends on the rate of perfusion in the afferent renal arterioles (2) and the amount of sodium in the serum. A low sodium load and low perfusion pressure (as in hypovolemia) increase renin secretion; high sodium and high pressure decrease it.

Renin circulates throughout the body. In the liver, renin converts angiotensinogen to angiotensin I (3), which passes to the lungs. There it is converted by hydrolysis to angiotensin II (4), a potent vasoconstrictor that acts on the adrenal cortex to stimulate production of the hormone aldosterone (5). The hormone acts on the juxtaglomerular cells to stimulate or depress renin secretion, completing the feedback cycle that automatically readjusts homeostasis.

The renin-angiotensin-aldosterone system, sometimes known as the juxtaglomerular apparatus, is an important homeostatic device for regulating the body's sodium and water levels, and blood pressure.
Juxtaglomerular cells (1) in each of the kidney's glomeruli secrete the enzyme renin into the blood.

to 20 minutes to prevent extravasation. Monitor vital signs, and check the catheterization site every half hour for 2 hours, then every hour for 4 hours, to ensure that the bleeding has stopped. Check distal pulse for signs of thrombus formation and arterial occlusion (cyanosis, loss of pulse, coolness of skin).
□ Resume diet and administration of medications, as ordered.

Interfering factors

□ Failure to use the proper anticoagulant in the collection tube, to completely fill it, or to adequately mix the sample and the anticoagulant may influence renin levels. (EDTA helps preserve angiotensin I; heparin does not.)
□ Failure to chill the collection tube and syringe, or failure to chill and send the sample to the laboratory immediately promotes breakdown of renin.
□ Renin levels may be affected by failure to observe diet restrictions and by improper patient positioning during tests.
□ Levels are increased by salt intake, diuretic therapy, oral contraceptives, severe blood loss, antihypertensives, vasodilators, licorice, and pregnancy.
□ Salt-retaining steroid therapy and antidiuretic therapy decrease levels.

SR. MARY BRIAN KELBER, SM, RN, DNS

Cholinesterase

The cholinesterase test measures the amounts of two similar enzymes that hydrolyze acetylcholine: pseudocholinesterase (also known as PCHE or serum cholinesterase) and acetylcholinesterase (or true cholinesterase). Acetylcholinesterase—present in nerve tissue, red cells of the spleen, and the gray matter of the brain—inactivates acetylcholine at nerve junctions and helps transmit impulses across nerve endings to muscle fibers. Pseudocholinesterase—which is produced primarily in the liver and appears in small amounts in the pancreas, in-testine, heart, and white matter of the brain—has no known function; however, its measurement is significant, because certain chemicals that inactivate acetylcholinesterase also affect pseudocholinesterase.

Two groups of anticholinesterase chemicals—organophosphates and muscle relaxants—are important. Organophosphates, which are used by the military as nerve gases and are common ingredients in many insecticides, inactivate acetylcholinesterase directly. Muscle relaxants (such as succinylcholine), which interfere with acetylcholine-mediated transmission across nerve endings, are normally destroyed by pseudocholinesterase.

When poisoning by an organophosphate (such as parathion) is suspected, either cholinesterase may be measured. For technical reasons, pseudocholinesterase is generally tested (although this analysis is less sensitive than the one for acetylcholinesterase).

In "muscle relaxant poisoning", prolonged apnea develops not from the drug itself, but because the patient lacks adequate pseudocholinesterase, which normally inactivates the muscle relaxant. In this case, measurement of pseudocholinesterase is required.

Purpose

□ To evaluate, preoperatively or before electroconvulsive therapy, the patient's potential response to succinylcholine, which is hydrolyzed by cholinesterase
□ To identify atypical forms of pseudocholinesterase to detect those patients who may have reactions to muscle relaxants
□ To assess overexposure to insecticides containing organophosphate compounds
□ To assess liver function and aid diagnosis of liver disease (a rare purpose).

Patient preparation

Explain to the patient that this test assesses muscle function or the extent of exposure to poisoning. Inform him that he needn't fast. Tell him the test requires a blood sample; and who will perform

ACETYLCHOLINESTERASE IN THE TRANSMITTAL OF NERVE IMPULSES

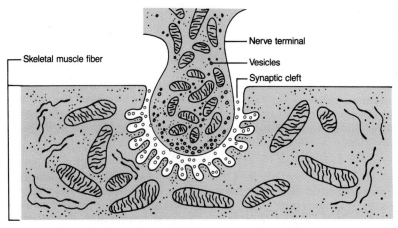

Nerve terminal

Skeletal muscle fiber

Vesicles

Synaptic cleft

Each time a nerve impulse arrives at the neuromuscular junction (between a myelinated nerve fiber and a skeletal muscle fiber), the nerve terminals release about 300 vesicles (bubbles) of acetylcholine into the synaptic clefts. Then acetylcholinesterase (one enzyme component of cholinesterase) inactivates acetylcholine by hydrolyzing it to acetate and choline. This action is necessary to allow the muscle fiber to recover between excitation by acetylcholine. Without acetylcholinesterase, muscle excitation would be continuous.

Adapted with permission from William Bloom and Don W. Fawcett, *Textbook of Histology*, 10th ed. (Philadelphia: W.B. Saunders Co., 1975); originally from J.D. Robertson, in *Journal of Biochemical Psychology*, Vol. 2, 1956.

the venipuncture and when. Reassure him that although he may experience discomfort from the needle puncture and the pressure of the tourniquet, collecting the sample takes less than 3 minutes.

Withhold substances that affect serum cholinesterase levels, as ordered. If such substances must be continued, note this on the laboratory slip.

Procedure

Perform a venipuncture, and collect the sample in a 7 ml *red-top* tube.

Precautions

☐ Handle the collection tube gently to prevent hemolysis.
☐ If the sample can't be sent to the laboratory within 6 hours after being drawn, refrigerate it.

Values

Pseudocholinesterase levels range from 8 to 18 u/ml (when determined by ki-

netic colorimetric technique).

Implications of results

Severely depressed pseudocholinesterase levels suggest a congenital deficiency or organophosphate insecticide poisoning; levels near zero necessitate emergency treatment.

Pseudocholinesterase levels are usually normal in early extrahepatic obstruction, and are variably decreased in hepatocellular damage, such as hepatitis or cirrhosis (especially cirrhosis with ascites and jaundice). Levels also decline in acute infections, chronic malnutrition, anemia, myocardial infarction, obstructive jaundice, and metastasis.

Post-test care

☐ If a hematoma develops at the venipuncture site, apply warm soaks.
☐ As ordered, resume administration of medications that were discontinued before the test.

Interfering factors
☐ Hemolysis due to rough handling of the sample may interfere with accurate determination of test results.
☐ Pregnancy or recent surgery may hinder accurate determination of test results.
☐ Serum cholinesterase levels can be falsely depressed by cyclophosphamide, echothiophate iodide, MAO inhibitors, succinylcholine, neostigmine, quinine, quinidine, chloroquine, caffeine, theophylline, epinephrine, ether, barbiturates, atropine, morphine, codeine, phenothiazines, vitamin K, and folic acid.

SR. MARY BRIAN KELBER, RN, DNS

Glucose-6-Phosphate Dehydrogenase

Glucose-6-phosphate dehydrogenase (G-6-PD), an enzyme found in most body cells, is part of the pentose phosphate pathway (hexose monophosphate shunt) that metabolizes glucose. This test, which measures serum G-6-PD levels, detects deficiency of this enzyme. Such deficiency is a hereditary, sex-linked condition carried on the female X chromosome (with clinical disease found mostly in males) that impairs the stability of the red cell membrane and makes red cells susceptible to destruction by strong oxidizing agents. Red cell enzyme levels normally decrease as cells age, but G-6-PD deficiency accelerates this process, making older red cells more prone to destruction than younger ones. In mild deficiency, young red cells retain enough G-6-PD to ward off destruction; in severe deficiency, all red cells fail to survive.

About 10% of all black males in the United States inherit mild G-6-PD deficiencies; certain peoples of Mediterranean origin inherit severe deficiencies. In some Caucasians, fava beans may produce hemolytic episodes. Although deficiency of G-6-PD provides partial immunity to falciparum malaria, it precipitates an adverse reaction to antimalarials.

Purpose
☐ To detect hemolytic anemia caused by G-6-PD deficiency
☐ To aid differential diagnosis of hemolytic anemia.

Patient preparation
Explain to the patient that this test detects inherited enzyme deficiency that may affect the life span of RBCs. Inform him that he needn't restrict food or fluids. Tell him the test requires a blood sample; who will perform the venipuncture and when; and that he may experience some transient discomfort from the needle puncture and the pressure of the tourniquet. Reassure him that collecting the sample takes less than 3 minutes.

Check patient history, and report recent blood transfusion, or recent ingestion of aspirin, sulfonamides, phenacetin, nitrofurantoin, vitamin K derivatives, antimalarials such as primaquine, or fava beans, since these substances can provoke hemolysis in G-6-PD–deficient persons.

Procedure
Perform a venipuncture, and collect the sample in a 7 ml *lavender-top* tube.

Precautions
☐ Completely fill the collection tube, and invert it gently several times to adequately mix the sample and the anticoagulant.
☐ Handle the sample gently to prevent hemolysis.

Values
Serum values of G-6-PD vary with the method used; for example, with the fluorescent spot–screening test, values are simply reported as normal or abnormal.

Implications of results
The following screening tests can detect but not confirm G-6-PD deficiency: the incubated Heinz body test, dye reduction test of Motulsky, methemoglobin reduc-

tion (Brewer's) test, fluorescence of NADPH test, ascorbate cyanide test, or glutathione stability test.

Post-test care
If a hematoma develops at the venipuncture site, ease discomfort by applying warm soaks.

Interfering factors
☐ Performing the test after a hemolytic episode or a blood transfusion can cause false-negative results.
☐ Failure to use a collection tube containing the proper anticoagulant, or to adequately mix the sample and anticoagulant may hinder accurate determination of test results.
☐ Hemolysis caused by rough handling of the sample may affect test results.
☐ The following substances decrease G-6-PD enzyme activity and precipitate hemolytic episodes: aspirin, sulfonamides, nitrofurantoin, vitamin K derivatives, primaquine, and fava beans.

SR. MARY BRIAN KELBER, SM, RN, DNS

Pyruvate Kinase

The erythrocyte enzyme pyruvate kinase (PK) takes part in the anaerobic metabolism of glucose (Embden-Meyerhof pathway). Abnormally low PK levels, revealed by erythrocyte enzyme assay using a serum sample, are inherited as an autosomal recessive trait and may result in a nonspherocytic red cell membrane defect associated with congenital hemolytic anemia.

Although PK deficiency is uncommon, it is the most prevalent congenital nonspherocytic hemolytic anemia, after glucose-6-phosphate dehydrogenase (G-6-PD) deficiency. PK assay confirms PK deficiency when red cell enzyme deficiency is the suspected cause of anemia.

Purpose
☐ To differentiate PK-deficient hemolytic

anemia from other congenital hemolytic anemias (for example, G-6-PD deficiency), or from acquired hemolytic anemia (when patient history or laboratory tests fail to indicate a genetic red cell defect)
☐ To detect PK deficiency in asymptomatic, heterozygous inheritance.

Patient preparation
Explain to the patient that this test is used to detect inherited enzyme deficiencies. Inform him he need not restrict food or fluids. Tell him this test requires a blood sample; who will perform the venipuncture and when; and that he may experience transient discomfort from the needle puncture and the pressure of the tourniquet. Reassure him that collecting the sample takes less than 3 minutes.

Check patient history for recent blood transfusion, and note such information on the laboratory slip.

Procedure
Perform a venipuncture, and collect the sample in a 7 ml *lavender-top* tube.

Precautions
☐ Completely fill the collection tube, and invert it gently several times to mix the sample and the anticoagulant.
☐ Handle the sample gently to prevent hemolysis.

Values
In a routine assay (ultraviolet), serum PK levels range from 2 to 8.8 u/g of hemoglobin; in the low substrate assay, 0.9 to 3.9 u/g of hemoglobin.

Implications of results
Low serum PK levels confirm diagnosis of PK deficiency, and allow differentiation between the PK-deficient hemolytic anemia and other inherited disorders.

Post-test care
If a hematoma develops at the venipuncture site, apply warm soaks.

Interfering factors
☐ Failure to use a collection tube with

the proper anticoagulant, or to adequately mix the sample and anticoagulant may interfere with accurate determination of test results.

☐ Hemolysis caused by rough handling of the sample may affect test results.

☐ Since PK levels in white cells remain normal in hemolytic anemia, the laboratory removes WBCs from the sample to prevent false results.

☐ Failure to notify the laboratory of recent blood transfusions may interfere with accurate determination of serum PK levels.

SR. MARY BRIAN KELBER, RN, DNS

Serum Hexosaminidase A and B

This fluorometric test measures the hexosaminidase A and B content of serum samples drawn by venipuncture or collected from a neonate's umbilical cord, or of amniotic fluid obtained by amniocentesis. Hexosaminidase deficiency can also be identified by testing cultured skin fibroblasts. However, because this procedure is costly and technically complex, analysis of blood or of amniotic fluid is the prevalent method. A reference center for congenital diseases should be consulted for the best current screening method and the preferred specimen it requires. Hexosaminidase is a group of enzymes necessary for the metabolism of gangliosides—water-soluble glycolipids found primarily in brain tissue. Deficiency of hexosaminidase A (one of the two hexosaminidase isoenzymes) causes Tay-Sachs disease. In this autosomal recessive disorder, G_{M2} ganglioside accumulates in brain tissue, resulting in progressive destruction and demyelination of CNS cells and, usually, death before age 5. In the United States, each year fewer than 100 infants are born with Tay-Sachs disease. However, the disorder strikes persons of Ashkenazic Jewish ancestry about 100 times more often than the general population. According to one authority, in New York City, about 1 in 30 such persons is a heterozygous carrier of this defective gene. If two such carriers have a child, this child, as well as subsequent offspring, has a 25% chance of inheriting Tay-Sachs disease. Sandhoff's disease, which results from total hexosaminidase deficiency (both A and B), is uncommon and not prevalent in any ethnic group.

Purpose

☐ To confirm or rule out Tay-Sachs disease in neonates

☐ To screen for Tay-Sachs carriers

☐ To establish prenatal diagnosis of hexosaminidase A deficiency.

Patient preparation

When testing an adult, explain that this test identifies a carrier state of Tay-Sachs disease. Emphasize the test's importance to an Ashkenazic Jewish couple who plan to have children, and explain that they both must carry the defective gene to transmit Tay-Sachs disease to their offspring. Tell the patient the test requires a blood sample; who will perform the venipuncture and when; and that he may experience transient discomfort from the needle puncture and the pressure of the tourniquet. Collecting the sample takes less than 3 minutes.

When testing a neonate, explain to the parents that this test confirms or rules out Tay-Sachs disease. Tell them blood will be drawn from the neonate's arm, neck, or umbilical cord, and explain that the procedure is safe and quickly performed. Tell them the infant will have a small bandage on the site of venipuncture.

Inform the patient or parents that no pretest restrictions of food or fluid are necessary. If the test is being performed prenatally, advise the patient of preparations for amniocentesis.

Procedure

Perform a venipuncture, collect cord

blood, or assist with amniocentesis, as appropriate. Collect the sample in a 7 ml *red-top* tube.

When testing a neonate, check with the laboratory concerning its preferred method for collecting serum samples from the patient. Obtain the sample from the neonate's arm, neck, or umbilical cord, as appropriate.

Precautions

Handle the collection tube gently to prevent hemolysis.

Values

Total serum levels of hexosaminidase range from 5 to 12.9 u/liter, with hexosaminidase A accounting for 55% to 76% of the total.

Implications of results

Absence of hexosaminidase A indicates Tay-Sachs disease (total hexosaminidase levels can be normal).

Absence of hexosaminidase A and hexosaminidase B (the other isoenzyme) indicates Sandhoff's disease, an uncommon, virulent variant of Tay-Sachs disease that produces more rapid deterioration.

Post-test care

☐ If a hematoma develops at the venipuncture site, ease discomfort by applying warm soaks.

☐ If both partners in a couple are carriers of Tay-Sachs disease, refer them for genetic counseling. Be sure to stress the importance of having amniocentesis performed as early as possible during pregnancy.

If only one partner is a carrier, reassure the couple that there's no risk of their offspring inheriting the disease, since both parents must be carriers in order for transmission of Tay-Sachs disease to occur.

Interfering factors

Hemolysis caused by rough handling of the sample may interfere with accurate determination of test results.

WILLIAM M. DOUGHERTY, BS

Uroporphyrinogen I Synthase

[Uroporphyrinogen I synthetase, porphobilinogen deaminase]

This test measures blood levels of uroporphyrinogen I synthase, an enzyme that converts porphobilinogen to uroporphyrinogen during heme biosynthesis. This enzyme is normally present in erythrocytes, fibroblasts, lymphocytes, liver cells, and amniotic fluid cells. However, a hereditary deficiency can reduce uroporphyrinogen I synthase levels by 50% or more, resulting in acute intermittent porphyria (AIP). An autosomal-dominant disorder of heme biosynthesis, AIP can be latent indefinitely, until certain factors (some sex hormones and drugs, a low-carbohydrate diet, or an infection) precipitate active disease.

An improvement over traditional urine tests that can detect AIP only during an acute episode, the uroporphyrinogen I synthase test can detect AIP even during its latent phase. Thus, it can identify affected individuals before their first acute episode. Because it's specific for AIP, this test can also differentiate AIP from other types of porphyria.

Enzyme activity is determined by fluorometrically measuring the conversion rate of porphobilinogen to uroporphyrinogen. If levels are indeterminate, urine and stool tests for aminolevulinic acid (ALA) and porphobilinogen may be ordered to support the diagnosis, since excretion of these porphyrin precursors increases substantially during an acute episode of AIP and may increase slightly during the latent phase.

Purpose

☐ To aid diagnosis of latent or active AIP.

Patient preparation

Explain to the patient that this test helps

detect a red blood cell disorder. Inform the patient that he will need to fast for 12 to 14 hours before the test, but that he may drink water. Tell him the test requires a blood sample; who will perform the venipuncture and when; and that he may experience slight discomfort from the needle puncture and the pressure of the tourniquet. Reassure him that collecting the sample takes less than 3 minutes.

If the patient's hematocrit is available, record this on the laboratory slip. Check the patient's history for any medications that may decrease enzyme levels, and withhold them as ordered. If they must be continued, note this on the laboratory slip.

Procedure
Perform a venipuncture and collect the sample in a 10-ml *green-top* tube.

Precautions
□ Handle the sample gently to prevent hemolysis.
□ Place the sample on dry ice and send it frozen to the laboratory. (If frozen immediately, the sample will remain stable for up to 1 month.)

Values
Normal values for uroporphyrinogen I synthase are 8.1 to 16.8 nm/sec/L for females and 7.9 to 14.7 nm/sec/L for males.

Implications of results
Decreased levels generally indicate latent or active AIP; symptoms differentiate these phases. Levels below 6.0 nm/sec/L confirm AIP, but levels between 6.0 and 8.0 nm/sec/L are indeterminate. When levels are indeterminate, urine and stool tests for the porphyrin precursors ALA and porphobilinogen may be ordered to support the diagnosis.

Post-test care
□ If a hematoma develops at the venipuncture site, apply warm soaks.
□ As ordered, instruct the patient to resume diet and medications.
□ If the patient has AIP, provide nutri-

tional and genetic counseling. Teach him to avoid low-carbohydrate diets, alcohol, and such drugs as steroid hormones, estrogens, barbiturates, sulfonamides, phenytoin, griseofulvin, chlordiazepoxide, meprobamate, glutethimide, methyprylon, and ergot, which may precipitate an acute episode. Remind him to seek care for all infections promptly, since these may also precipitate an acute episode.

Interfering factors
□ Hemolytic and hepatic diseases may elevate uroporphyrinogen I synthase levels.
□ Hemolysis caused by rough handling of the sample may interfere with accurate interpretation of test results.
□ Failure to freeze the sample will cause false-positive results.
□ Failure to fast before the test may increase enzyme levels.
□ A low-carbohydrate diet, alcohol, infection, and certain drugs, such as those listed above, may decrease enzyme levels.

WENDY L. BAKER, RN, BSN, MS

Galactose-1-Phosphate Uridyl Transferase

This enzyme, with galactokinase and UDP glucose 4-epimerase, converts galactose to glucose during lactose metabolism. Deficiency of these enzymes causes galactosemia, an autosomal-recessive disorder marked by elevated serum galactose and decreased serum glucose. Unless detected and treated soon after birth, galactosemia can impair eye, brain, and liver development, causing irreversible cataracts, mental retardation, and cirrhosis.

A deficiency of galactose-1-phosphate uridyl transferase causes the most common and severe form of galactosemia. Both qualitative and quantitative tests are widely used to detect it. The qualitative method, a simple screening test performed at birth, is required in some hospitals for all neonates. Blood collected on specially treated filter paper is checked for fluorescence after 1- and 2-hour exposures under an ultraviolet light. Normal blood fluoresces; transferase-deficient blood does not. The quantitative test requires a blood sample and measures the amount of a fluorescent substance generated during a coupled enzyme reaction. This is generally ordered as soon as possible after a positive screening test, and may occasionally be ordered for an adult to detect a carrier state.

Prenatal testing of amniotic fluid can also detect transferase deficiency. However, such testing is rarely performed because neonatal screening can detect the deficiency in time to prevent irreversible damage.

Purpose
☐ To screen infants for galactosemia
☐ To detect heterozygous carriers of galactosemia.

Patient preparation
When testing a neonate, explain to the parents that the test screens for galactosemia, a potentially dangerous enzyme deficiency. If a blood sample was not taken from the umbilical cord at birth, tell the parents that a small amount of blood will be drawn from their infant's heel. Explain that the procedure is safe and quickly performed.

When testing an adult, explain that the test identifies a carrier state of galactosemia, a genetic disorder that may be transmitted to his offspring. Tell the patient the test requires a blood sample; who will perform the venipuncture and when; and that he may feel some discomfort from the needle puncture and the tourniquet. Reassure him that collecting the sample takes less than 3 minutes.

Procedure
For a qualitative (screening) test, collect cord blood or blood from a heel stick on special filter paper, saturating all three circles.

For a quantitative test, perform a venipuncture and collect a 4-ml sample in a green-top or lavender-top tube, depending on the laboratory method used.

Indicate the patient's age on the laboratory slip. Check his history for a recent exchange transfusion. Note this on the laboratory slip or postpone the test, as ordered.

Precautions
☐ Handle the collection tube gently to prevent hemolysis.
☐ Send the collection tube to the laboratory on wet ice.

Values
Normally, the qualitative test is negative (fluorescence is strong 1 and 2 hours after the test begins).

The normal range for the quantitative test is 18.5 to 28.5 kU/mol of hemoglobin. Check the normal range for your laboratory if a different method is used.

Implications of results
A positive qualitative test (no fluorescence) may indicate a transferase deficiency. A follow-up quantitative test should be performed as soon as possible.

Quantitative test results less than 5 kU/mol of hemoglobin indicate galactosemia. Levels between 5 and 18.5 kU/mol of hemoglobin may indicate a carrier state.

Post-test care
☐ If a hematoma develops at the venipucture site, ease discomfort by applying warm soaks.
☐ If test results indicate galactosemia, provide nutritional counseling for the parents and a galactose- and lactose-free diet for their infant. A soybean or meat-based formula may be substituted for milk.
☐ If one or both partners in a couple are carriers, stress the importance of having a screening test performed on their infant at birth.

Interfering factors

☐ Failure to use the proper tube or to send the sample on wet ice may cause a false-positive result, because heat inactivates the transferase.

☐ A total exchange transfusion causes a transient false-negative result, because normal transfused blood contains the transferase.

☐ Hemolysis caused by rough handling of the sample may alter test results.

CLARKE LAMBE, MD
LAUREL LAMBE, MS, RD

Angiotensin Converting Enzyme

Angiotensin converting enzyme (ACE) is found in high concentrations in lung capillaries and in lesser concentrations in blood vessels and kidney tissue. Its primary function is to help regulate arterial pressure by converting angiotensin I to angiotensin II, a powerful vasoconstrictor.

This test measures serum levels of ACE. Despite ACE's role in blood pressure regulation, this test is of little use in diagnosing hypertension. Instead, it's primarily used to diagnose sarcoidosis, because of the high correlation between elevated serum ACE levels and this disease. Presumably, elevated serum levels reflect macrophage activity. This test also monitors response to treatment in sarcoidosis and helps confirm diagnosis of Gaucher's disease and leprosy.

Purpose

☐ To aid diagnosis of sarcoidosis, especially pulmonary sarcoidosis
☐ To monitor response to therapy in sarcoidosis
☐ To help confirm Gaucher's disease or leprosy.

Patient preparation

Explain to the patient that this test helps diagnose sarcoidosis, Gaucher's disease, or leprosy, or that it checks his response to treatment for sarcoidosis. Inform the patient that he must fast for 12 hours before the test. Tell him the test requires a blood sample; who will perform the venipuncture and when; and that he may experience slight discomfort from the needle puncture and the pressure of the tourniquet. Reassure him that collecting the blood sample takes less than 3 minutes.

Note the patient's age on the laboratory slip. If the patient is under age 20, notify the doctor; he may want to postpone the test.

Procedure

Perform a venipuncture and collect the sample in a 7-ml *red-top* tube (a green-top tube may be required, depending on the laboratory method used).

Precautions

☐ Avoid using a *lavender-top* tube or contaminating the sample with EDTA, because this can decrease ACE levels, altering test results.

☐ Handle the collection tube gently to prevent hemolysis.

☐ Send the sample to the laboratory immediately, or freeze the sample and place it on dry ice until the test can be performed.

Values

In the colorimetric assay, normal values for serum ACE range from 18 to 67 U/L for patients over age 20. (Patients under age 20 have variable ACE levels and are not usually tested.)

Implications of results

Elevated serum ACE levels may indicate sarcoidosis, Gaucher's disease, or leprosy, but results must be correlated with the patient's clinical condition. In some patients, elevated ACE levels may result from hyperthyroidism, diabetic retinopathy, and liver diseases.

Serum ACE levels decline as the patient responds to steroid or prednisone therapy for sarcoidosis.

Post-test care

☐ If a hematoma develops at the venipuncture site, ease discomfort by applying warm soaks.

Interfering factors

☐ Use of a *lavender-top* collection tube or other EDTA contamination can decrease ACE levels.
☐ Hemolysis due to rough handling of the sample may interfere with accurate determination of ACE levels.
☐ Failure to fast before the test may cause significant lipemia of the sample, which may interfere with accurate test measurement.
☐ Failure to send the sample to the laboratory immediately or to freeze it and place it on dry ice may cause enzyme degradation and yield artificially low ACE levels.

CLARKE LAMBE, MD

Selected References

Byrne, C. Judith, et al. *Laboratory Tests: Implications for Nurses and Allied Health Professionals.* Reading, Mass.: Addison-Wesley Publishing Co., 1981.

Cohen, Judith A., et al. "A Message From the Heart: What Isoenzymes Can Tell You About Your Cardiac Patient," *Nursing82* 12:46-49, April 1982.

Fischbach, Frances. *A Manual of Laboratory Diagnostic Tests,* 2nd ed. Philadelphia: J.B. Lippincott Co., 1984.

Hansten, Philip D. *Drug Interactions,* 4th ed. Philadelphia: Lea & Febiger, 1979.

Henry, John Bernard, ed. *Todd-Sanford-Davidsohn Clinical Diagnosis and Management by Laboratory Methods,* vol. 1, 17th ed. Philadelphia: W.B. Saunders Co., 1984.

Lamb, Jane O. *Laboratory Tests for Clinical Nursing.* Bowie, Md.: Robert J. Brady Co., 1984.

Tilkian, Sarko M., et al. *Clinical Implications of Laboratory Tests,* 3rd ed. St. Louis: C.V. Mosby Co., 1983.

Widmann, Frances K. *Clinical Interpretation of Laboratory Tests,* 9th ed. Philadelphia: F.A. Davis Co., 1983.

Wintrobe, Maxwell M., et al. *Clinical Hematology,* 8th ed. Philadelphia: Lea & Febiger, 1981.

5 Hormones

LEARNING OBJECTIVES

After completing this chapter, the reader will be able to:
- identify the major hormones, their secretion sites, and principal actions.
- explain feedback mechanisms that regulate the secretion of hormones.
- state the purpose of each test discussed in the chapter.
- prepare the patient physically and psychologically for each test.
- describe the procedure for performing each test.
- state the normal values for each test.
- list factors that may interfere with accurate test results.

Hormones

Introduction

Hormones are powerful, complex chemicals, normally produced by the endocrine system and transported through the bloodstream to stimulate or inhibit the metabolic activity of target glands or organs. Some hormones, such as epinephrine, have profound and widespread effects on body tissues; others regulate the production and release of another hormone by the target cell and are referred to as trophic hormones; TSH (thyroid-stimulating hormone) is an example. Hormones continuously interact in complicated feedback systems, both negative and positive, to maintain hormonal homeostasis. Thus, a change in the circulating blood level of any one hormone eventually changes the secretion of others. Consequently, the circulating blood levels of hormones have enormous diagnostic significance, and numerous tests have been devised to detect and evaluate abnormal secretion.

In chemical terms, hormones can be divided into three classes of compounds: polypeptides, amines, and steroids. The polypeptides include hormones such as antidiuretic hormone (ADH) and gastrin; the amines include hormones such as thyroxine and the catecholamines; and the steroids include the gonadal hormones—estrogen and testosterone.

Chemical transmitters

Basically, hormones are chemical transmitters, or messengers. Most hormones attach to specific receptor sites on cell membranes, activating adenyl cyclase, an enzyme responsible for production of cyclic adenosine monophosphate (cAMP) within the cell. Just as the hormone travels through the blood with a chemical message for its target gland, cAMP acts as the third messenger within the cell itself. Prostaglandins have been implicated as the second messenger in the response system. The end result of this delicate and intricate communications network is a change in cellular function—increased protein synthesis, for example, or the release of more metabolic fuel, such as glycogen. Hormones are thus indispensable to the maintenance of homeostasis and to the growth and repair of body tissues.

Sites of secretion

Most hormones are secreted by the ductless glands or organs of the endocrine system: the pituitary, thyroid, parathyroid, and adrenal glands, and the pancreas, gonads (ovaries and testes), and placenta. Most of these glands and organs are controlled—directly or indirectly—by the hypothalamus, the clearinghouse or message coordinator for both the endocrine and the autonomic nervous systems. Some hormones are secreted by nonendocrine organs; gastrin, for example, is secreted by the stomach.

SITES OF HORMONAL SECRETION

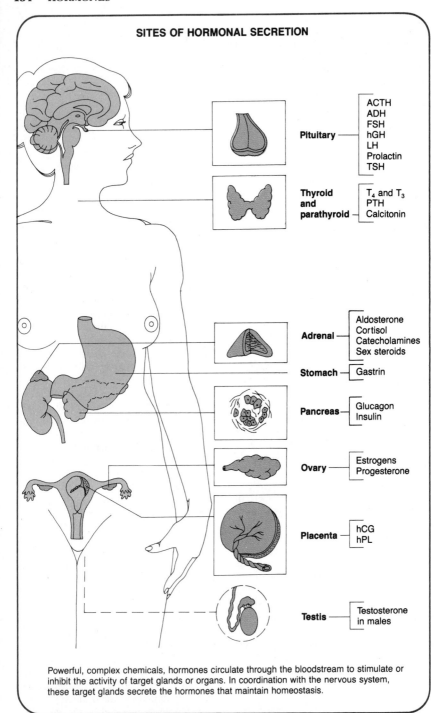

Pituitary	ACTH ADH FSH hGH LH Prolactin TSH
Thyroid and parathyroid	T_4 and T_3 PTH Calcitonin
Adrenal	Aldosterone Cortisol Catecholamines Sex steroids
Stomach	Gastrin
Pancreas	Glucagon Insulin
Ovary	Estrogens Progesterone
Placenta	hCG hPL
Testis	Testosterone in males

Powerful, complex chemicals, hormones circulate through the bloodstream to stimulate or inhibit the activity of target glands or organs. In coordination with the nervous system, these target glands secrete the hormones that maintain homeostasis.

CLINICAL INDICATIONS FOR SERUM HORMONE TESTS

Disease or disorder	Hormones tested
Acromegaly, gigantism	ACTH, hGH, FSH, LH, TSH
Addison's disease	ACTH, cortisol
Aldosteronism	Aldosterone
Congenital adrenal hyperplasia	ACTH, cortisol, androgens, estrogens, hCG, androstenedione
Cushing's syndrome	ACTH, cortisol, androstenedione
Diabetes insipidus	ADH
Diabetes mellitus	Insulin, cortisol, glucagon
Dwarfism	ACTH, hGH, FSH, LH, TSH
Hypogonadism	Estrogens, testosterone, FSH, LH, androstenedione
Hyper- and hypoparathyroidism	PTH
Hypopituitarism	ACTH, hGH, FSH, LH, TSH, T_4, T_3
Hyper- and hypothyroidism	T_4 and T_3, FT_4 and FT_3, TSH
Medullary thyroid carcinoma	Calcitonin
Pituitary tumors	ACTH, hGH, prolactin, FSH, LH
Precocious puberty	FSH, LH, estrogens, androgens, androstenedione
Zollinger-Ellison syndrome	Gastrin

The *pituitary* (or hypophysis) is situated within the sella turcica ("Turkish saddle") of the sphenoid bone, inside the skull. This small but powerful gland dominates and regulates most of the secretory activity of the endocrine system. The pituitary gland is composed of an anterior lobe (adenohypophysis) and a posterior lobe (neurohypophysis). The anterior pituitary is composed of glandular tissue connected to the hypothalamus by a vascular network called the hypothalamic-pituitary portal venous system. The posterior pituitary comprises neural tissue or neuroepithelial cells, and is continuous with the hypothalamus.

The *anterior pituitary* secretes many hormones whose circulating levels in the bloodstream have special diagnostic significance. The basophilic cells of the anterior pituitary secrete four polypeptide hormones that affect other endocrine glands. These include adrenocorticotropic hormone (ACTH), follicle-stimulating hormone (FSH), luteinizing hormone (LH), and thyroid-stimulating hormone (TSH). The acidophilic cells of the anterior pituitary secrete two hormones that affect peripheral tissues directly—prolactin and growth hormone (hGH). Cellular malfunction can cause either hypo- or hypersecretion of these critical hormones, causing serious disorders, from Cushing's syndrome and sterility to gigantism and dwarfism.

The *posterior pituitary* releases stored ADH on neural stimulation by the hypothalamus, where ADH is actually formed. (The posterior pituitary also secretes oxytocin, which stimulates uterine contractions and causes the let-down reflex in lactating women but has no diagnostic significance.)

The *thyroid* gland consists of two lobes, straddling the trachea and connected by an isthmus, that lie just below the cricoid cartilage. About 50% of these glands have a pyramidal lobe; the isthmus may be absent. A primary regulator of body metabolism, the thyroid secretes two vital hormones—thyroxine (T_4) and triiodothyronine (T_3)—to maintain the proper metabolic rate for cellular func-

HYPOTHALAMUS-PITUITARY-TARGET HORMONAL NETWORK

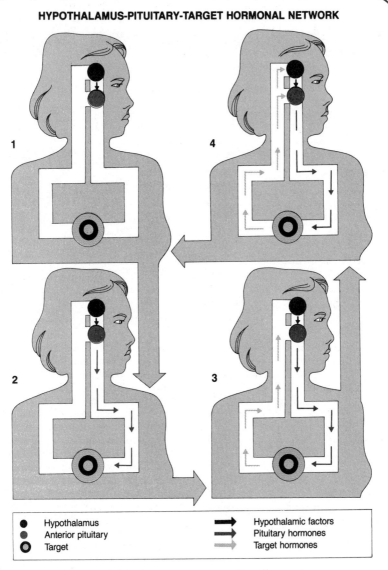

● Hypothalamus	➡ Hypothalamic factors
● Anterior pituitary	➡ Pituitary hormones
◎ Target	➡ Target hormones

1. The hypothalamus secretes releasing and inhibiting hormones (factors), which are carried to the adjoining anterior pituitary gland.

2. The responsive pituitary cells secrete such hormones as ACTH, FSH, hGH, LH, TSH, and prolactin, which travel to receptive target glands or organs.

3. The target gland releases its hormones into the blood. These hormones interact in a complex system of positive and negative feedback, controlled by the hypothalamus and pituitary gland.

4. Thus hormonal homeostasis is achieved through the interaction of hypothalamus, anterior pituitary, and target gland or organ.

tion. Thyroid hormones have a stimulatory effect on calorigenesis (increased oxygen consumption in body tissues), affect the growth and development of the nervous and musculoskeletal systems, and regulate the synthesis, storage, and use of carbohydrates, fats, proteins, vitamins, and body fluids.

Serum T_4 and T_3—probably the most often evaluated hormones—are measured to detect hyper- or hypothyroidism. If confirming tests are needed, free forms of T_4 and T_3 (FT_4 and FT_3)—unbound to thyroxine-binding globulin (TBG)—can be measured. Tests of protein binding, such as the serum T_3 resin uptake or serum TBG electrophoresis, also help assess thyroid function.

The *parathyroids*—four small glands usually located behind the thyroid—release parathyroid hormone (PTH), which maintains calcium and phosphorus homeostasis. PTH, with vitamin D, stimulates the osteocytes to release calcium from the bones in order to raise the serum calcium level. In the opposite direction, calcitonin—a polypeptide hormone secreted by the parafollicular cells of the thyroid gland—and high levels of phosphate stimulate absorption of calcium ions into the bones to lower the calcium level.

The *adrenal glands* secrete mineralocorticoids (aldosterone) to maintain salt and water balance; glucocorticoids (primarily cortisol) to regulate carbohydrate, fat, and protein metabolism; sex steroids (androgenic and estrogenic, such as androstenedione); and catecholamines (mainly epinephrine, norepinephrine, and dopamine) to regulate reaction to stress. The adrenal cortex secretes mineralocorticoids, glucocorticoids, and sex steroids. The adrenal medulla secretes catecholamines as part of the body's fight or flight response.

In the *pancreas,* the islets of Langerhans (beta cells) secrete insulin and the alpha cells secrete glucagon; both hormones have a marked effect on total body metabolism but especially on carbohydrate metabolism. The stomach secretes gastrin, a hormone that plays an indispensable role in facilitating digestion.

The *ovaries* and *testes* secrete the gonadal hormones estrogen and testosterone, respectively, that govern development of secondary sex characteristics and reproductive function. The ovaries also secrete progesterone, which serves mainly to prepare the endometrium for the implantation of the fertilized ovum. During pregnancy, the *placenta* serves as a temporary endocrine organ, secreting the hormones human chorionic gonadotropin (hCG) and human placental lactogen (hPL).

Hormonal "watchdog" mechanisms

Because hormones are so powerful, despite the minute quantities in which they appear in the blood, the body monitors their activities closely to prevent unwanted physiologic effects. Two important "watchdog" mechanisms to control hormonal levels are *neurohumoral regulation* and a closed-loop *feedback system.* In neurohumoral regulation, certain releasing or inhibiting factors produced in the supraoptic hypothalamic nuclei travel to the pituitary, where they regulate secretion of hormones.

The positive loop of the feedback system, which is constantly at work within the endocrine system, encompasses the initial stimulus, such as an elevated blood glucose level, that results in the secretion of the controlling hormone—in this case, insulin. The negative loop goes into action when the desired secretory response or hormonal concentration is achieved. For example, decreased blood glucose levels cause the pancreas to curtail its secretion of insulin.

Hormone assay methods

Radioimmunoassay and competitive protein-binding are two testing methods used by laboratories to measure serum hormone levels. But the assay method is just one consideration that affects reliability of test results. For example, diurnal variations in hormone secretion require careful scheduling of the collection of the sample to coincide with or avoid times of peak secretion. Other important considerations in evaluating serum hormone levels are emotional stress, nutritional status, and medications, all of which may affect the level of the hormone to be tested.

Nursing considerations
□ Assess patients accurately for endocrine disorders, such as hypothyroidism or diabetes.

□ In young patients, watch especially for indications of abnormal growth patterns, such as absent or delayed puberty, irregular bone structure, muscular atrophy, or weight changes.
□ Remember, careful observation, accurate history-taking, and patient teaching are essential to the care of patients scheduled for serum hormone tests.

CAROL K. BARKER, RN, MSN, MEd
RICHARD EDWARD HONIGMAN, MD

PITUITARY HORMONES

Plasma ACTH

[Adrenocorticotropic hormone, corticotropin]

This test measures the plasma levels of adrenocorticotropic hormone (ACTH) by radioimmunoassay. ACTH, a polypeptide hormone released by the basophilic cells of the anterior pituitary, stimulates the adrenal cortex to secrete cortisol and, to a lesser degree, androgens and aldosterone. ACTH also has some melanocyte-stimulating activity and increases the uptake of amino acids by muscle cells, promotes lipolysis by fat cells, stimulates pancreatic beta cells to secrete insulin, and may contribute to the release of growth hormone. ACTH levels vary diurnally, peaking between 6 a.m. and 8 a.m. and ebbing between 6 p.m. and 11 p.m.

Through a negative feedback mechanism, plasma cortisol levels control ACTH secretion—for example, high cortisol levels suppress ACTH secretion. Emotional and physical stress (pain, surgery, insulin-induced hypoglycemia) stimulate secretion and can override the effects of plasma cortisol levels.

The plasma ACTH test may be ordered for patients with signs of adrenal hypofunction (insufficiency) or hyperfunction (Cushing's syndrome). However, ACTH suppression or stimulation testing is usually necessary to confirm diag-

nosis. The instability and unavailability of plasma ACTH greatly limit its diagnostic significance and reliability.

Purpose
□ To facilitate differential diagnosis of primary and secondary adrenal hypofunction
□ To aid differential diagnosis of Cushing's syndrome.

Patient preparation
Explain to the patient that this test helps determine if his hormonal secretion is normal. Advise him that he must fast and limit his physical activity for 10 to 12 hours before the test. Tell him the test requires a blood sample; who will perform the venipuncture and when; and that he may experience some transient discomfort from the needle puncture and the pressure of the tourniquet. Reassure him that collecting the sample takes only a few minutes, although the laboratory requires at least 4 days to complete the analysis.

Check the patient's drug history for the use of any medications that may affect accurate determination of test results, such as corticosteroids, and drugs that affect cortisol levels—estrogens, amphetamines, spironolactone, calcium gluconate, or alcohol (ethanol). Withhold these drugs, as ordered, for 48 hours or longer before the test. If these medications must be continued, note this on the laboratory slip. Arrange with the dietary department to provide a low-carbohydrate diet for 2 days before the test. This requirement may vary, depending on the laboratory.

Procedure
For a patient with suspected adrenal hypofunction, perform the venipuncture for a baseline level between 6 a.m. and 8 a.m. (peak secretion); for a patient with suspected Cushing's syndrome, perform the venipuncture between 6 p.m. and 11 p.m. (low secretion). Collect the sample in a *plastic* tube, since ACTH may adsorb to glass, or in a *green-top* (heparinized) tube. Pack the sample in ice, and send it to the laboratory immediately, where plasma must be rapidly separated from blood cells at 39.2° F. (4° C.). The collection technique may vary, depending on the laboratory.

Precautions
Since proteolytic enzymes in the plasma degrade ACTH, a temperature of 39.2° F. (4° C.) is necessary to retard enzyme activity. Immediate transfer of the sample, packed in ice, to the laboratory is essential for reliable test results.

Values
Reference values are not yet firmly established. The Mayo Clinic sets baseline values at less than 120 pg/ml, but these values may vary, depending on the laboratory.

Implications of results
A higher-than-normal plasma ACTH level may indicate primary adrenal hypofunction (Addison's disease), in which the pituitary gland attempts to compensate for the unresponsiveness of the target organ by releasing excessive ACTH. The underlying cause of adrenocortical hypofunction may be idiopathic atrophy of the adrenal cortex, or partial destruction of the gland by granuloma, neoplasm, amyloidosis, or inflammatory necrosis.

A low-normal plasma ACTH level suggests secondary adrenal hypofunction resulting from pituitary or hypothalamic dysfunction. The primary determinant may be panhypopituitarism, absence of corticotropin-releasing hormone in the hypothalamus, or chronic blunting of ACTH levels by long-term corticosteroid therapy.

In suspected Cushing's syndrome, an elevated plasma ACTH level suggests Cushing's *disease,* in which pituitary dysfunction (due to adenoma) causes continuous hypersecretion of ACTH and, consequently, continuously elevated plasma cortisol levels, without diurnal variations. Moderately elevated ACTH levels suggest pituitary-dependent adrenal hyperplasia, and nonadrenal tumors, such as oat cell carcinoma of the lungs.

A low-normal ACTH level implies adrenal hyperfunction due to adrenocortical tumor or hyperplasia as the source of high cortisol levels; in such hyperfunction, ACTH levels are low-normal (or undetectable) because the high plasma cortisol levels suppress ACTH secretion through negative feedback.

Post-test care
□ If a hematoma develops at the puncture site, ease discomfort by applying warm soaks.
□ Resume diet and administration of medications that were discontinued before the test, as ordered.

Interfering factors
□ Failure to observe restrictions of diet, medications, or physical activity may interfere with accurate determination of the test results. ACTH levels are depressed by corticosteroids, including cortisone and its analogues, and by drugs that increase endogenous cortisol secretion (estrogens, calcium gluconate, amphetamines, spironolactone, and ethanol). Lithium carbonate decreases cortisol levels and may interfere with ACTH secretion. ACTH levels are also affected by the menstrual cycle and pregnancy.
□ Radioactive scan performed within 1 week before the test may influence test results.

CAROL K. BARKER, RN, MSN, MEd

Rapid ACTH Test

[Cosyntropin test]

The rapid ACTH test is gradually replacing the 8-hour ACTH stimulation test as the most effective diagnostic tool for evaluating adrenal hypofunction (insufficiency). Using cosyntropin, a synthetic analogue of the biologically active part of ACTH, the rapid ACTH test provides faster results and causes fewer allergic reactions than the 8-hour test, which uses natural ACTH from animal sources. This test requires prior determination of baseline plasma cortisol levels to evaluate the effect of cosyntropin administration on cortisol secretion. An unequivocally high morning cortisol level rules out adrenal hypofunction and makes further testing unnecessary.

Purpose
□ To aid in identification of primary and secondary adrenal hypofunction.

Patient preparation
Explain to the patient that this test helps determine if his condition is due to a hormonal deficiency. Inform him that he may be required to fast for 10 to 12 hours before the test, and must be relaxed and resting quietly for 30 minutes before the test. Tell him the test, which takes at least 1 hour to perform, requires three venipunctures and an injection.

This test may be given on an outpatient basis. If so, and as ordered, instruct the patient to withhold ACTH and all steroid medications before the test. If the patient is hospitalized, withhold these medications. If they must be continued, note this on the laboratory slip.

Procedure
Draw 5 ml of blood for a baseline value. Collect the sample in a 5 ml *green-top* (heparinized) tube. Label this sample "preinjection," and send it to the labo-
ratory. Inject 250 mcg (0.25 mg) cosyntropin I.V. (preferably) or I.M. (I.V. administration affords more accurate determinations, since ineffective absorption following I.M. administration may cause wide variations in response.) Direct I.V. injection should take 2 minutes.

Draw another 5 ml of blood 30 and 60 minutes following the cosyntropin injection. Collect the samples in 5 ml *green-top* (heparinized) tubes. Label the samples "30 minutes postinjection" and "60 minutes postinjection," then send them to the laboratory. Also include the actual collection times on the laboratory slip.

Precautions
Handle the samples gently to prevent hemolysis. These samples require no special precautions other than avoiding stasis.

Values
Normally, plasma cortisol levels rise 7 or more mcg/dl above the baseline value, to a peak of 18 or more mcg/dl 60 minutes after the cosyntropin injection. Generally, a doubling of the baseline value indicates a normal response.

Implications of results
A normal result excludes adrenal hypofunction (insufficiency). In patients with primary adrenal hypofunction (Addison's disease), cortisol levels remain low. Thus, the rapid ACTH test provides an effective method of screening for adrenal hypofunction. However, if test results show subnormal increases in plasma cortisol levels, prolonged stimulation of the adrenal cortex may be required to differentiate between primary and secondary adrenal hypofunction.

Post-test care
□ If a hematoma develops at the venipuncture sites, apply warm soaks.
□ Observe the patient for signs of an allergic reaction to cosyntropin (rare), such as hives and itching, or tachycardia.
□ As ordered, resume diet and admin-

istration of medications that were discontinued before the test.

Interfering factors

□ Failure to observe restrictions of diet, medications, and physical activity may hinder accurate determination of test results. Drugs that increase plasma cortisol levels—including estrogens (which increase plasma cortisol-binding proteins) and amphetamines—may interfere with test results. Smoking and obesity may also increase plasma cortisol levels. Lithium carbonate decreases plasma cortisol levels.

□ Radioactive scan performed within 1 week before the test may influence test results, since plasma cortisol levels are determined by radioimmunoassay.

□ Hemolysis due to rough handling of the sample may interfere with accurate determination of test results.

CAROL K. BARKER, RN, MSN, MEd

Serum Growth Hormone

[Human growth hormone (hGH), somatotrophic hormone (STH)]

Growth hormone (hGH), a protein secreted by acidophils of the anterior pituitary, is the primary regulator of human growth. Unlike other pituitary hormones, hGH has no easily defined feedback mechanism or single target gland—it affects many body tissues. Like insulin, hGH promotes protein synthesis and stimulates amino acid uptake by cells.

In addition, hGH raises plasma glucose by inhibiting glucose uptake and utilization by cells, and increases free fatty acid concentrations by enhancing lipolysis. Secretion of hGH appears to be regulated by the hypothalamus by means of a growth hormone–releasing factor (GRF) and a growth hormone release–

inhibiting factor (somatostatin). Secretion of hGH is diurnal and varies with such factors as exercise, sleep, stress, and nutritional status. Hypo- or hypersecretion of this hormone may induce pathologic states (such as dwarfism or gigantism). Altered hGH levels are common in patients with pituitary dysfunction.

This test, a quantitative analysis of plasma hGH levels, is usually performed as part of an anterior pituitary stimulation or suppression test. Such testing is crucial, since clinical manifestations of an hGH deficiency can rarely be reversed by therapy.

Purpose

□ To aid differential diagnosis of dwarfism, since retarded growth in children can result from pituitary or thyroid hypofunction

□ To confirm diagnosis of acromegaly and gigantism

□ To aid diagnosis of pituitary or hypothalamic tumors

□ To help evaluate hGH therapy.

Patient preparation

Explain to the patient or his parents (if the patient is a child) that this test measures hormone levels and helps determine the cause of abnormal growth. Instruct him to fast and limit physical activity for 10 to 12 hours before the test. Tell him the test requires a blood sample, and explain who will perform the venipuncture and when. Reassure him that although he may feel some discomfort from the needle puncture, collecting the sample takes less than 3 minutes; however, another sample may have to be drawn the following day for comparison. The laboratory requires at least 2 days for analysis.

Withhold all medications that affect hGH levels, such as pituitary-based steroids, as ordered. If these medications must be continued, note this on the laboratory slip. Make sure the patient is relaxed and recumbent for 30 minutes before the test, since stress and physical activity elevate hGH levels.

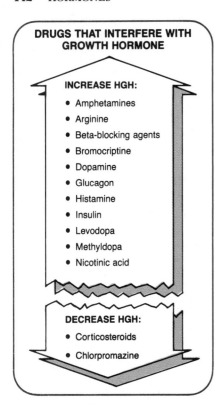

DRUGS THAT INTERFERE WITH GROWTH HORMONE

INCREASE HGH:
- Amphetamines
- Arginine
- Beta-blocking agents
- Bromocriptine
- Dopamine
- Glucagon
- Histamine
- Insulin
- Levodopa
- Methyldopa
- Nicotinic acid

DECREASE HGH:
- Corticosteroids
- Chlorpromazine

Procedure

Between 6 a.m. and 8 a.m. on 2 consecutive days, or as ordered, draw at least 7 ml of venous blood into a 10 ml *red-top* collection tube.

Precautions

Handle the sample gently to prevent hemolysis; send it to the laboratory immediately, since hGH has a half-life of only 20 to 25 minutes.

Values

Normal hGH levels for men range from undetectable to 5 ng/ml; for women, from undetectable to 10 ng/ml. Higher values in women are due to estrogen effects. Children generally have higher hGH levels; nevertheless, they may range from undetectable to 16 ng/ml.

Implications of results

Increased hGH levels may indicate a pi-

tuitary or hypothalamic tumor (frequently an adenoma), which causes gigantism in children and acromegaly in adults and adolescents. Patients with diabetes mellitus sometimes have elevated hGH levels, without acromegaly. Suppression testing is necessary to confirm diagnosis.

Pituitary infarction, metastatic disease, or tumors may reduce hGH levels. Dwarfism may be due to low hGH levels, although only 15% of all cases of growth failure relate to endocrine dysfunction. Confirmation of diagnosis requires stimulation testing with arginine or insulin.

Post-test care

□ If a hematoma develops at the venipuncture site, apply warm soaks.
□ As ordered, resume diet and medications discontinued before the test.

Interfering factors

□ Failure to follow restrictions of diet, medications, or physical activity may alter test results.
□ Arginine, levodopa, insulin (induced hypoglycemia), beta-blockers (propranolol), or estrogens raise hGH secretion.
□ Phenothiazines (chlorpromazine) and corticosteroids reduce hGH secretion.
□ Radioactive scan performed within 1 week before the test may affect results, since plasma hGH levels are determined by radioimmunoassay.
□ Hemolysis due to rough handling of the sample may interfere with accurate determination of test results.

CAROL K. BARKER, RN, MSN, MEd

Growth Hormone Suppression Test
[Glucose loading]

This test evaluates excessive baseline levels of growth hormone (hGH) from the anterior pituitary by measuring the se-

cretory response to a loading dose of glucose. Normally, hGH raises plasma glucose and fatty acid concentrations; in response, insulin secretion increases to counteract these effects. Consequently, a glucose load should suppress hGH secretion. In a patient with excessive hGH levels, failure of suppression indicates anterior pituitary dysfunction and confirms diagnosis of acromegaly and gigantism.

Purpose
☐ To assess elevated baseline hGH levels
☐ To confirm diagnosis of gigantism in children and acromegaly in adults.

Patient preparation
Explain to the patient and to his family (if the patient is a child) that this test helps determine the cause of his abnormal growth. Instruct him to fast and limit physical activity for 10 to 12 hours before the test. Tell him two blood samples will be drawn, and warn that he may experience nausea after drinking the glucose solution and feel some discomfort from the needle punctures. Inform him that the test takes 1 hour, but that the laboratory requires at least another 2 days to complete this analysis.

Before the test, as ordered, withhold all steroids—including estrogens and progestogens—and other pituitary-based hormones. If these or other medications must be continued, note it on the laboratory slip.

Since hGH levels rise after exercise or excitement, make sure the patient is relaxed and recumbent for 30 minutes before the test.

Procedure
Between 6 a.m. and 8 a.m., draw 6 ml of venous blood (basal sample) into a 10 to 15 ml red-top collection tube. Administer 100 g of glucose solution P.O. To prevent nausea, advise the patient to drink the glucose slowly. After 1 or 2 hours, draw another 6 ml of venous blood into a second 10 to 15 ml red-top collection tube. Label the tubes appropriately, and send them to the laboratory.

Precautions
☐ Handle the samples gently to prevent hemolysis.
☐ Send each sample to the laboratory immediately, since hGH has a half-life of only 20 to 25 minutes.

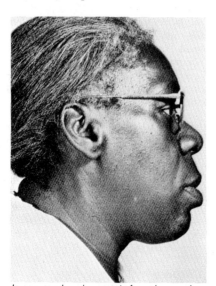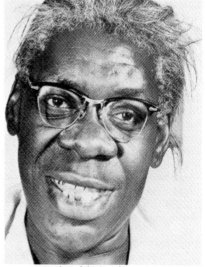

In acromegaly, enlargement of membranous bones causes protrusion of the jaw, forward slanting of the forehead, and enlargement of the nose (to twice normal size).

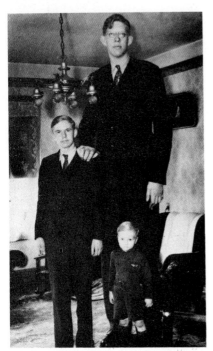

Robert Pershing Wadlow, the tallest person on record, is pictured here at age 14, at which point he was already much taller than his brothers. At his death in 1940 at age 22, he measured 8' 11" (267.5 cm).

Values

Normally, glucose suppresses hGH to levels ranging from undetectable to 3 ng/ml in 30 minutes to 2 hours. In children, rebound stimulation may occur after 2 to 5 hours.

Implications of results

In a patient with active acromegaly, basal levels are elevated (75 ng/ml) and are not suppressed to less than 5 ng/ml during the test. Unchanged or rising hGH levels in response to glucose loading indicate hGH hypersecretion and may confirm suspected acromegaly or gigantism. This response may be verified by repeating the test after a 1 day rest.

Post-test care

☐ If a hematoma develops at the puncture sites, apply warm soaks.
☐ As ordered, resume diet and medi-

cations discontinued before the test.

Interfering factors

☐ Failure to observe restrictions of diet, medications, and physical activity may interfere with accurate determination of test results. Release of hGH may be impaired by corticosteroids and phenothiazines (chlorpromazine), and may be increased by arginine, levodopa, amphetamines, glucagon, niacin, or estrogens.
☐ Radioactive scan performed within 1 week before the test may affect results, since hGH levels are determined by radioimmunoassay.
☐ Hemolysis due to rough handling of the sample may interfere with accurate determination of test results.

CAROL K. BARKER, RN, MSN, MEd

Insulin Tolerance Test

This test measures serum levels of growth hormone (hGH) and adrenocorticotropic hormone (ACTH) after administration of a loading dose of insulin. It's more reliable than direct measurement of hGH and ACTH, because healthy persons often have undetectable fasting levels of these hormones. Insulin-induced hypoglycemia stimulates hGH and ACTH secretion in persons with an intact hypothalamic-pituitary-adrenal axis. Failure of stimulation indicates anterior pituitary or adrenal hypofunction, and helps confirm an hGH or ACTH insufficiency.

Because the insulin tolerance test stimulates an adrenergic response, it's not recommended for patients with cardiovascular or cerebrovascular disorders, epilepsy, or low basal plasma cortisol levels.

Purpose

☐ To aid diagnosis of hGH or ACTH deficiency

□ To identify pituitary dysfunction
□ To aid differential diagnosis of primary and secondary adrenal hypofunction.

Patient preparation
Explain to the patient or to his family that this test evaluates hormonal secretion. Instruct him to fast and to restrict physical activity for 10 to 12 hours before the test. Explain that the test involves I.V. infusion of insulin and the collection of multiple blood samples. Warn him that he may experience an increased heart rate, diaphoresis, hunger, and anxiety after administration of insulin. Reassure him that these symptoms are transient, but that if they become severe the test will be discontinued. Inform him that the test takes about 2 hours and that results are usually available in 2 days.

Since physical activity and excitement increase hGH and ACTH levels, make sure the patient is relaxed and recumbent for 90 minutes before the test.

Procedure
Between 6 a.m. and 8 a.m., collect three 5-ml samples of venous blood for basal levels—one in a *gray-top* tube (for blood glucose) and two in *green-top* tubes (for hGH and ACTH). Then, administer an I.V. bolus of U-100 regular insulin (0.15 U/kg, or as ordered) over a 1- to 2-minute period. Draw additional blood samples 15, 30, 45, 60, 90, and 120 minutes after administration of insulin. Use an indwelling venous catheter to avoid repeated venipunctures. At each interval, collect three samples: one in a *gray-top* and two in *green-top* tubes. Label the tubes appropriately and send them to the laboratory immediately.

Precautions
 □ Have concentrated glucose solution readily available in case of severe hypoglycemic reaction to insulin. To minimize the possibility of such a reaction, use highly purified pork or human insulin.
□ Specify the time of collection on the laboratory slip, and send all samples to the laboratory immediately.
□ Handle the samples gently to prevent hemolysis.

Values
Normally, blood glucose falls to 50% of the fasting level 20 to 30 minutes after insulin administration. This stimulates a 10 to 20 ng/dl increase over baseline values in both hGH and ACTH, with peak levels occurring 60 to 90 minutes after insulin administration.

Implications of results
Failure of stimulation or a blunted response suggests dysfunction of the hypothalamic-pituitary-adrenal axis. An increase in hGH levels below 10 ng/dl above basal suggests hGH deficiency. However, definitive diagnosis of hGH deficiency requires a supplementary stimulation test, such as the arginine test. Additional testing is necessary to determine the site of the abnormality.

An increase in ACTH levels below 10 ng/dl above basal suggests adrenal insufficiency. The metyrapone or ACTH stimulation test then confirms the diagnosis and determines whether insufficiency is primary or secondary.

Post-test care
□ If a hematoma develops at the I.V. or venipuncture site, apply warm soaks.
□ As ordered, instruct the patient to resume diet, activity, and medications.

Interfering factors
□ Failure to follow restrictions of diet, physical activity, and medications can prevent reliable test results.
□ Steroids such as progestogen, estrogen, and pituitary-based drugs elevate hGH levels; glucocorticoids and beta blockers depress hGH levels.
□ Glucocorticoids, estrogens, calcium gluconate, amphetamines, methamphetamines, spironolactone, and ethanol depress ACTH levels.
□ Hemolysis caused by rough handling of the sample may affect test results.

CAROLYN ROBERTSON, RN, MSN

Arginine Test

[Growth hormone stimulation test]

This test measures plasma growth hormone (hGH) levels after I.V. administration of arginine, an amino acid that normally stimulates hGH secretion, and is commonly used to identify pituitary dysfunction in infants and children with growth retardation and to confirm hGH deficiency. This test may be performed concomitantly with an insulin tolerance test or after administration of other hGH stimulants, such as glucagon, vasopressin, and L-dopa.

Purpose

□ To aid diagnosis of pituitary tumors
□ To confirm hGH deficiency in infants and children with low baseline levels.

Patient preparation

Explain to the patient or his parents that this test identifies hGH deficiency. Instruct him to fast and limit physical activity for 10 to 12 hours before the test. Explain that this test requires venous infusion of a drug and collection of several blood samples. The test takes at least 2 hours to perform; results are available in 2 days.

Before the test, as ordered, withhold all steroid medications—including pituitary-based hormones. If these medications must be continued, record this on the laboratory slip. Since hGH levels may rise after exercise or excitement, make sure the patient is relaxed and recumbent for at least 90 minutes before the test.

Procedure

Between 6 a.m. and 8 a.m., draw 6 ml of venous blood (basal sample) into a 10 to 15 ml *red-top* collection tube. Start I.V. infusion of arginine (0.5 g/kg body weight) in normal saline solution, and continue for 30 minutes. Use of an indwelling venous catheter avoids repeated venipunctures and minimizes stress and anxiety. Discontinue I.V. infusion, then draw a total of three 6-ml samples at 30-minute intervals. Collect each sample in a 10 to 15 ml *red-top* collection tube, and label it appropriately.

Precautions

□ Draw each sample at the scheduled time, and specify the collection time on the laboratory slip.
□ Send each sample to the laboratory immediately, since hGH has a half-life of 20 to 25 minutes.
□ Handle the samples gently to prevent hemolysis.

Values

Arginine should raise hGH levels to more than 10 ng/ml in men, 15 ng/ml in women, and 48 ng/ml in children. Such an increase may appear in the first sample drawn 30 minutes after arginine infusion is discontinued, or in the samples drawn 60 and 90 minutes afterward.

Implications of results

Elevated fasting levels, and rises during sleep help to rule out hGH deficiency. Failure of hGH levels to rise after arginine infusion indicates decreased anterior pituitary hGH reserve. In children, this deficiency causes dwarfism; in adults, it can indicate panhypopituitarism. When hGH levels fail to reach 10 ng/ml, retesting is required at the same time of day as the original test.

Post-test care

□ If a hematoma develops at the venipuncture site, apply warm soaks.
□ As ordered, resume diet and medications discontinued before the test.

Interfering factors

□ Failure to observe restrictions of diet, medications, and physical activity may affect test results.
□ Radioactive scan performed within 1 week before the test may affect results.
□ Hemolysis due to rough handling of the sample may affect test results.

CAROL K. BARKER, RN, MSN, MEd

Serum Follicle-stimulating Hormone

This test of gonadal function, performed more often on females than on males, measures plasma follicle-stimulating hormone (FSH) levels by radioimmunoassay and is usually vital to infertility studies. However, its overall diagnostic significance often depends on the results of related hormone tests (for luteinizing hormone, estrogen, or progesterone, for example). A glycoprotein secreted by the anterior pituitary, FSH stimulates gonadal activity in both sexes. In females, FSH spurs development of primary ovarian follicles into graafian follicles for ovulation. Secretion fluctuates rhythmically during the menstrual cycle, peaking at ovulation. In males, continuous secretion of FSH (and testosterone) stimulates and maintains spermatogenesis. Plasma levels fluctuate widely in females, and to obtain a true baseline level, daily testing may be necessary (for 3 to 5 days), or multiple samples can be drawn on the same day.

Purpose
□ To aid in the diagnosis of infertility and disorders of menstruation, such as amenorrhea
□ To aid in the diagnosis of precocious puberty in girls (before age 9) and in boys (before age 10)
□ To aid in the differential diagnosis of hypogonadism.

Patient preparation
Explain to the patient that this test helps determine if her hormonal secretion is normal. Inform her that she needn't fast or limit physical activity before the test. Tell her a blood sample will be drawn and that she may feel some discomfort from the needle puncture. Although collecting the sample takes only a few minutes, advise the patient that the laboratory

requires at least 3 days to complete the analysis.

As ordered, withhold medications, such as estrogens or progestogen, that may interfere with accurate determination of test results for 48 hours before the test. If these medications must be continued, note this on the laboratory slip.

Make sure the patient is relaxed and recumbent for 30 minutes before the test.

Procedure
Perform a venipuncture, preferably between 6 a.m. and 8 a.m., using a 7 ml red-top collection tube, and send the sample to the laboratory immediately.

Precautions
□ Handle the sample gently to prevent hemolysis.
□ If the patient is a female, indicate the phase of her menstrual cycle on the laboratory slip. If she is menopausal, note this on the laboratory slip.

Values
Reference values vary greatly, depending on the patient's age and stage of sexual development, and—for a female—the phase of her menstrual cycle. For menstruating females, approximate values are as follows:
□ follicular phase: 5 to 20 mIU/ml
□ midcycle peak: 15 to 30 mIU/ml
□ luteal phase: 5 to 15 mIU/ml.

Approximate values for adult males are 5 to 20 mIU/ml; for menopausal women, 50 to 100 mIU/ml.

Implications of results
Decreased FSH levels may cause male or female infertility: aspermatogenesis in males and anovulation in females. Low FSH levels may indicate secondary hypogonadotropic states, which can result from anorexia nervosa, panhypopituitarism, or hypothalamic lesions.

High FSH levels in females may indicate ovarian failure associated with Turner's syndrome (primary hypogonadism) or Stein-Leventhal syndrome (polycystic ovary syndrome). Elevated levels may occur in patients with precocious puberty (idiopathic or with CNS lesions) and in postmenopausal women. In males, abnormally high FSH levels may indicate destruction of the testes (from mumps orchitis or X-ray exposure), testicular failure, seminoma, or male climacteric. Congenital absence of the gonads and early-stage acromegaly may cause FSH levels to rise in both sexes.

Post-test care
□ If a hematoma develops at the venipuncture site, apply warm soaks.
□ As ordered, resume medications that were discontinued before the test.

Interfering factors
□ Failure to observe restriction of medications may hinder accurate determination of test results. Ovarian steroid hormones, such as estrogen or progesterone, and related compounds may, through negative feedback, inhibit the flow of releasing hormones from the hypothalamus and pituitary; phenothiazines (such as chlorpromazine) may exert a similar effect.
□ Radioactive scan performed within 1 week before the test may affect results.
□ Hemolysis due to rough handling of the sample may interfere with accurate determination of test results.

CAROL K. BARKER, RN, MSN, MEd

Plasma Luteinizing Hormone

[Interstitial-cell–stimulating hormone (ICSH)]

This test, usually ordered for anovulation and infertility studies and performed most often on females, is a quantitative analysis of plasma luteinizing hormone (LH) levels. For accurate diagnosis, results must be evaluated in light of findings obtained from related hormone tests (follicle-stimulating hormone [FSH], estrogen, and testosterone, for example). LH is a glycoprotein secreted by basophilic cells of the anterior pituitary. In females, cyclic LH secretion (with FSH) causes ovulation and transforms the ovarian follicle into the corpus luteum, which, in turn, secretes progesterone. In males, continuous LH secretion stimulates the interstitial (Leydig) cells of the testes to release testosterone, which stimulates and maintains spermatogenesis (with FSH).

Purpose
□ To detect ovulation
□ To assess male or female infertility
□ To evaluate amenorrhea
□ To monitor therapy designed to induce ovulation.

Patient preparation
Explain to the patient that this test helps determine if her secretion of female hormones is normal.

Since there is no evidence that LH levels are affected by fasting, eating, or exercise, such pretest restrictions may be unnecessary. Tell the patient that this test requires a blood sample; who will perform the venipuncture and when; and that she may feel some discomfort from the needle puncture. Inform her that collecting the sample takes only a few minutes, but the laboratory requires at least 3 days to complete the analysis.

As ordered, withhold drugs, such as steroids (including estrogens or progesterone), that may interfere with plasma LH levels for 48 hours before the test. If these medications must be continued, note this on the laboratory slip.

Procedure
Perform a venipuncture, and collect the sample in a 7 ml *red-top* tube.

Precautions
□ Handle the sample gently to prevent hemolysis.
□ If the patient's a female, indicate the phase of her menstrual cycle on the laboratory slip. If the patient is menopausal, note this on the laboratory slip.

LH SECRETION PEAKS AT OVULATION

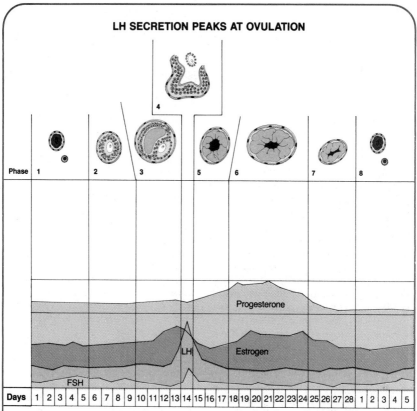

1. Menstrual phase (degeneration of corpus luteum)

2. Early follicular phase (development of follicle)

3. Late follicular phase (development of follicle)

4. Ovulation at midcycle (rupture of follicle)

5. Early luteal phase (development of corpus luteum)

6. Midluteal phase (development of corpus luteum)

7. Late luteal phase (development of corpus luteum)

8. Menstrual phase (degeneration of corpus luteum)

The menstrual cycle is divided into three distinct phases: the menstrual phase (days 1 to 5); the proliferative, or follicular, phase (days 6 to 13); and after ovulation on day 14, the secretory, or luteal, phase (days 15 to 28). The menstrual phase of the normal cycle is characterized by endometrial sloughing, corpus luteum degeneration, and new follicle growth. During this stage, the concentration of both estrogen and progesterone is low, triggering increased follicle-stimulating hormone (FSH) and luteinizing hormone (LH) secretion.

During the follicular phase, the follicle stimulated by FSH reaches full size and increases its secretion of estrogen. Simultaneously with increased estrogen, FSH decreases while LH increases slowly but steadily. During the late follicular phase, LH rises sharply and FSH rises slightly. At about the 14th day, within hours of this abrupt surge in LH, estrogen levels in the plasma drop and ovulation occurs. After ovulation, the concentration of both LH and FSH falls rapidly.

During the final, or luteal, phase, the follicle reorganizes as the corpus luteum secretes progesterone and estrogen. Within 7 or 8 days following ovulation, if fertilization has not occurred, the corpus luteum regresses while progesterone and estrogen levels decrease. The endometrium sloughs, and the menstrual cycle begins again.

Adapted with permission from G.T. Ross. *Recent Progress in Hormone Research.* 26:1, 1970.

Values

Normal values may have a wide range:
- Adult males: 5 to 20 mIU/ml
- Postmenopausal females: 50 to 100 mIU/ml
- Adult females: Values vary, depending on the phase of the patient's menstrual cycle—follicular phase: 5 to 15 mIU/ml; midcycle (ovulation): 30 to 60 mIU/ml; luteal phase: 5 to 15 mIU/ml
- Children: 4 to 20 mIU/ml.

Implications of results

In females, absence of a midcycle peak in LH secretion may indicate anovulation. Decreased or low-normal levels may indicate hypogonadotropism; these findings are commonly associated with amenorrhea. High LH levels may indicate congenital absence of ovaries or ovarian failure associated with Stein-Leventhal syndrome (polycystic ovary syndrome), Turner's syndrome (ovarian dysgenesis), menopause, or early-stage acromegaly. Infertility can result from either primary or secondary gonadal dysfunction.

In males, low values may indicate secondary gonadal dysfunction (of hypothalamic or pituitary origin); high values may indicate testicular failure (primary hypogonadism) or destruction or congenital absence of testes.

Post-test care

- If a hematoma develops at the venipuncture site, apply warm soaks.
- As ordered, resume administration of medications that were discontinued before the test.

Interfering factors

- Failure to observe restrictions of medications may interfere with accurate determination of test results. Steroids (including estrogens, progesterone, and testosterone) may decrease plasma LH levels.
- Radioactive scan performed within 1 week before the test may influence test results, since plasma LH levels are determined by radioimmunoassay.
- Hemolysis due to rough handling of the sample may interfere with accurate determination of test results.

CAROL K. BARKER, RN, MSN, MEd

Prolactin
[Lactogenic hormone, lactogen]

Similar in molecular structure and biologic activity to growth hormone (hGH), prolactin is a polypeptide hormone secreted by the anterior pituitary. It is essential for the development of the mammary glands for lactation during pregnancy, and for stimulating and maintaining lactation postpartum. Prolactin is secreted in males and nonpregnant females, but its function is unknown. Like hGH, prolactin acts directly on tissues, and its levels rise in response to sleep and to physical or emotional stress.

This radioimmunoassay is a quantitative analysis of serum prolactin levels, which normally rise ten- to twentyfold during pregnancy, corresponding to concomitant elevations in human placental lactogen levels. After delivery, prolactin secretion falls to basal levels in mothers who don't breast-feed. However, prolactin secretion increases during breast-feeding, apparently as a result of a stimulus triggered by suckling that curtails the release of prolactin-inhibiting factor (PIF) by the hypothalamus. This, in turn, allows transient elevations of prolactin secretion by the pituitary. This test is considered useful in patients suspected of having pituitary tumors, which are known to secrete prolactin in excessive amounts.

Purpose of the test

- To facilitate diagnosis of pituitary dysfunction, possibly due to pituitary adenoma
- To aid in the diagnosis of hypothalamic dysfunction regardless of cause
- To evaluate secondary amenorrhea and/or galactorrhea.

Patient preparation

Tell the patient that this test helps evaluate hormonal secretion. Advise her that she need not restrict food or fluids, or limit physical activity. But, encourage her to relax for about ½ hour before the test. Tell her who will draw the blood sample and when, and that she may experience some discomfort from the needle puncture. Advise her that collecting the sample takes only a few minutes but the laboratory requires at least 4 days to complete the analysis. As ordered, withhold drugs, such as chlorpromazine and methyldopa, that may influence serum prolactin levels. If they must be contin- ued, note this on the laboratory slip.

Procedure

Perform a venipuncture at least 2 hours after the patient wakes; samples drawn earlier are likely to show sleep-induced peak levels. Collect the sample in a 7 ml *red-top* tube.

Precautions

Handle the sample gently to prevent hemolysis.

Values

Normal values range from undetectable to 23 ng/dl in nonlactating females.

PHYSIOLOGY OF LACTATION

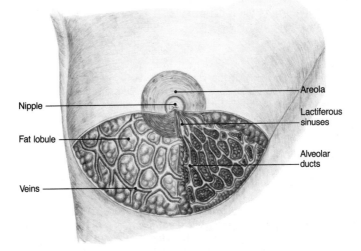

During pregnancy, progesterone and estrogen normally interact to suppress milk secretion while developing the breasts for lactation. Estrogen causes the breasts to grow by increasing their fat content; progesterone causes lobule growth and develops the alveolar cells' secretory capacity.

After childbirth, the mother's anterior pituitary gland secretes prolactin (suppressed during pregnancy), which helps the alveolar epithelium produce and release colostrum. Usually, within 3 days of prolactin release, the breasts secrete large amounts of milk rather than colostrum. The infant's sucking stimulates nerve endings at the nipple, initiating the let-down reflex that allows the expression of milk from the mother's breasts. Sucking also stimulates the release of another pituitary hormone, oxytocin, into the mother's bloodstream. This hormone causes alveolar contraction, which forces milk into the ducts and the lactiferous sinuses beneath the alveolar surface, making milk available to the infant. (It also promotes normal involution of the uterus.) Because the infant's suckling stimulates both milk production and milk expression, the more the infant breast-feeds, the more milk the breast produces.

Implications of results

Abnormally high prolactin levels (100 to 300 ng/ml) suggest autonomous prolactin production by a pituitary adenoma, especially when amenorrhea or galactorrhea is present (Forbes-Albright syndrome). Rarely, hyperprolactinemia may also result from severe endocrine disorders, such as hypothyroidism, acromegaly, and hypothalamic disorders that depress prolactin-inhibiting factor. Idiopathic hyperprolactinemia may be associated with anovulatory infertility.

Decreased prolactin levels in a lactating mother cause failure of lactation and may be associated with postpartum pituitary infarction (Sheehan's syndrome). Abnormally low prolactin levels have also been documented in a few patients with empty-sella syndrome. In patients with empty-sella syndrome, a flattened pituitary gland makes the pituitary fossa look empty.

Post-test care

□ If a hematoma develops at the venipuncture site, apply warm soaks.
□ As ordered, resume administration of medications that were discontinued before the test.

Interfering factors

□ Failure to take into account physiologic variations related to sleep or stress may invalidate test results.
□ Pretest use of ethanol, haloperidol, morphine, methyldopa, estrogens, phenothiazines (such as chlorpromazine), amphetamines, and reserpine—all of which raise prolactin levels—may interfere with accurate determination of test results.
□ Pretest use of apomorphine, ergot alkaloids, and levodopa—which lower prolactin levels—may also affect correct determination of test results.
□ Radioactive scan performed within 1 week before the test, or recent surgery may interfere with test results.
□ Hemolysis due to rough handling of the sample may interfere with accurate determination of test results.

CAROL K. BARKER, RN, MSN, MED

Serum Thyroid-stimulating Hormone
[Thyrotropin]

Thyroid-stimulating hormone (TSH) is a glycoprotein secreted by the anterior pituitary after stimulation by thyrotropin-releasing hormone (TRH) from the hypothalamus. TSH stimulates an increase in the size, number, and secretory activity of thyroid cells; heightens "iodine pump activity" (active transport of iodine across basal cell membrane), often raising the ratio of intracellular to extracellular iodine as much as 350:1; and stimulates the release of triiodothyronine (T_3) and thyroxine (T_4). These hormones exert a generalized effect on total body metabolism and are essential for normal growth and development.

This test measures serum TSH levels by radioimmunoassay. It's a reliable test for primary hypothyroidism and helps determine whether hypothyroidism results from thyroid gland failure, or from pituitary or hypothalamic dysfunction. Normal serum TSH levels rule out primary hypothyroidism because absence of thyroid hormone in the serum stimulates pituitary hypersecretion of TSH through negative feedback. With some laboratory techniques, this test may not distinguish between low-normal and subnormal levels, especially in secondary hypothyroidism.

Purpose

□ To distinguish between primary and secondary hypothyroidism
□ To confirm or rule out primary hypothyroidism
□ To monitor drug therapy in patients with primary hypothyroidism.

Patient preparation

Explain to the patient that this test helps assess thyroid gland function. Tell him the test requires a blood sample; who will perform the venipuncture and when; and that he may feel transient discomfort from the needle puncture. Collecting the sample takes only a few minutes; the laboratory requires at least 2 days to complete the analysis. As ordered, withhold steroids, thyroid hormones, and other drugs that may influence test results. If these medications must be continued, note this on the laboratory slip. Keep the patient relaxed and recumbent for 30 minutes before the test.

Procedure

Between 6 a.m. and 8 a.m., perform a venipuncture. (Some authorities consider diurnal variation insignificant.) Collect the sample in a 5 ml *red-top* tube.

Precautions

Handle the sample gently to prevent hemolysis.

Values

Normal values for adults and children range from undetectable to 15 µIU/ml.

Implications of results

Elevated TSH levels that exceed 20 µIU/ml suggest primary hypothyroidism or, possibly, an endemic goiter (due to dietary iodine deficiency). TSH levels may be slightly elevated in euthyroid patients with thyroid cancer.

Low or undetectable TSH levels may be normal but may occasionally indicate secondary hypothyroidism (with inadequate secretion of TSH or TRH). Low TSH levels may also result from hyperthyroidism (Graves' disease) or thyroiditis; both are marked by hypersecretion of thyroid hormones, which suppresses TSH release. Provocative testing with TRH is necessary to confirm diagnosis.

Post-test care

□ If a hematoma develops at the venipuncture site, apply warm soaks.
□ As ordered, resume administration of drugs discontinued before the test.

Interfering factors

□ Failure to observe restrictions of med-

> ### TRH CHALLENGE TEST
>
> This test, which evaluates thyroid function and is the first direct test of pituitary reserve, is a reliable diagnostic tool in thyrotoxicosis (Graves' disease). The challenge test requires an injection of TRH, normally released by the hypothalamus.
>
> The procedure for this test may vary greatly as to dosage and route of administration. One commonly accepted procedure is the following: After a venipuncture is performed to obtain a baseline TSH reading, synthetic TRH (protirelin) is administered by I.V. bolus in a dosage of 200 to 500 mcg. As many as five samples (5 ml each) are then drawn at 5-, 10-, 15-, 20-, and 60-minute intervals to assess thyroid response. To facilitate blood collection and avoid multiple venipunctures, an indwelling catheter can be used to obtain the required samples.
>
> A sudden spike above the baseline TSH reading indicates a normally functioning pituitary but suggests hypothalamic dysfunction. If the TSH level fails to rise or remains undetectable, pituitary failure is likely. In thyrotoxicosis or thyroiditis, high concentrations of thyroid hormones inhibit TSH secretion. Consequently, TSH levels fail to rise when challenged by TRH.

ications may cause spurious test results. Aspirin, corticosteroids, T_3, and heparin lower TSH levels; lithium carbonate and potassium iodide raise them.
□ Radioactive scan performed within 1 week before the test may influence test results.
□ Hemolysis due to rough handling of the sample may affect test results.

CAROL K. BARKER, RN, MSN, MEd

Neonatal Thyroid-stimulating Hormone

[Neonatal thyrotropin]

This radioimmunoassay confirms congenital hypothyroidism after an initial screening test detects low thyroxine (T_4) levels. Normally, TSH levels surge soon *after birth, triggering a rise in thyroid hormone, which is essential for neurologic development. However, in primary congenital hypothyroidism, the thyroid gland doesn't respond to TSH stimulation, resulting in diminished thyroid hormone levels and elevated TSH levels. Early detection and treatment of congenital hypothyroidism is critical, to prevent mental retardation and cretinism.*

Purpose
☐ To confirm diagnosis of congenital hypothyroidism.

Patient preparation
Explain to the infant's parents that this test helps confirm the diagnosis of congenital hypothyroidism. Emphasize the test's importance in detecting the disorder early, so that prompt therapy can prevent irreversible brain damage.

Equipment
For a filter paper sample: Alcohol or povidone-iodine swabs/sterile lancet/specially marked filter paper/2″ x 2″ sterile gauze pads/adhesive bandage/labels.
For a serum sample: venipuncture equipment.

Procedure
For a filter paper sample: Assemble the necessary equipment and wash your hands thoroughly. Wipe the infant's heel with an alcohol or povidone-iodine swab, then dry it thoroughly with a gauze pad. Perform a heelstick. Squeezing the infant's heel gently, fill the circles on the filter paper with blood. Make sure the blood saturates the paper. Gently apply pressure with a gauze pad to ensure hemostasis at the puncture site. Allow the filter paper to dry, label it appropriately, and send it to the laboratory.
For a serum sample: Perform a venipuncture and collect the sample in a 5-ml *red-top* tube. Label the sample and send it to the laboratory immediately.

Precautions
If a serum sample is taken, handle it carefully to prevent hemolysis.

Values
At age 1 to 2 days, TSH levels are normally 25 to 30 μIU/ml. Thereafter, levels are normally less than 25 μIU/ml.

Implications of results
Neonatal TSH levels must be interpreted in light of T_4 concentrations. Elevated TSH accompanied by decreased T_4 indicates primary congenital hypothyroidism (thyroid gland dysfunction). Depressed TSH and T_4 may be present in secondary congenital hypothyroidism (pituitary or hypothalamic dysfunction). Normal TSH accompanied by depressed T_4 may indicate hypothyroidism due to a congenital defect in thyroxine-binding globulin (TBG), or may indicate transient congenital hypothyroidism due to prematurity or prenatal hypoxia. A complete thyroid workup must be done to confirm the cause of hypothyroidism before treatment can begin.

Post-test care
If a hematoma develops at the venipuncture site, apply warm soaks. Heelsticks require no special care.

Interfering factors
☐ Corticosteroids, T_3, and T_4 lower TSH levels; lithium carbonate, potassium iodide, excessive topical resorcinol, and TSH injection raise TSH levels.
☐ Failure to let a filter paper sample dry completely may alter test results.
☐ Rough handling of a serum sample may cause hemolysis and may interfere with accurate testing.

WENDY BAKER, RN, MS, CCRN

Serum Antidiuretic Hormone
[Vasopressin]

Antidiuretic hormone (ADH) is a polypeptide produced by the hypothalamus and released from storage sites in the

ADH RELEASE AND REGULATION

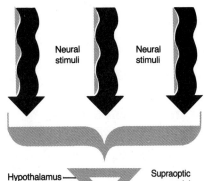

Neural stimuli

Neural stimuli

Hypothalamus

Supraoptic nuclei

Hypothalamico-hypophyseal path

Posterior pituitary

Anterior pituitary

Neural impulses signal the supraoptic nuclei of the hypothalamus to produce ADH. After it is formed, ADH moves along the hypothalamico-hypophyseal tract to the posterior pituitary, where it is stored until needed by the kidneys to maintain fluid balance. In the kidneys, ADH acts on the collecting tubules to retain water.

Homeostasis is maintained by a negative feedback mechanism: ample water or water excess inhibits further ADH secretion by the supraoptic nuclei of the hypothalamus or ADH release from the posterior pituitary. A similar negative feedback mechanism that is vital to hormonal homeostasis prevents oversecretion of other hormones.

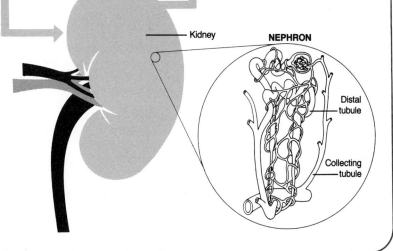

Kidney

NEPHRON

Distal tubule

Collecting tubule

posterior pituitary on neural stimulation. The primary function of ADH is to promote water reabsorption, in response to increased osmolality (water deficiency with high concentration of sodium and other solutes). In response to decreased osmolality (water excess), reduced secretion of ADH allows increased excretion of water to maintain fluid balance. In an interlocking feedback mechanism with aldosterone, ADH helps regulate sodium, potassium, and fluid balance. It also stimulates vascular smooth-muscle contraction, causing an increase in arterial blood pressure.

This relatively rare test, a quantitative analysis of serum ADH level, may identify diabetes insipidus and other causes of severe homeostatic imbalance. It may be ordered as part of dehydration or hypertonic saline infusion testing, which determines the body's response to states of hyperosmolality.

Purpose
□ To aid in the differential diagnosis of pituitary diabetes insipidus, nephrogenic diabetes insipidus (congenital or familial), and syndrome of inappropriate antidiuretic hormone (SIADH).

Patient preparation
Explain to the patient that this test to measure hormonal secretion levels may aid in identifying the cause of his symptoms. Instruct him to fast and limit physical activity for 10 to 12 hours before the test. Tell him a blood sample will be drawn, and reassure him that, although he may feel some discomfort from the needle puncture, collecting the sample takes only a few minutes. The laboratory requires at least 5 days to complete the analysis.

As ordered, withhold conjugated estrogens, morphine, tranquilizers, hypnotics, oxytocin, anesthetics (such as ether), lithium carbonate, vincristine, carbamazepine, cyclophosphamide, and chlorothiazide; these drugs and others may cause SIADH. If these medications must be continued, note this on the laboratory slip.

Make sure the patient is relaxed and recumbent for 30 minutes before the test.

Procedure
Perform a venipuncture, and collect the sample in a *red-top, plastic* collection tube. Immediately send the sample to the laboratory, where serum must be separated from the clot within 10 minutes.

Precautions
The syringe and the collection tube *must* be plastic, since the fragile ADH undergoes degradation when it comes in contact with glass.

Values
Normal ADH values range from 1 to 5 pg/ml.

Implications of results
Absent or below-normal ADH levels indicate pituitary diabetes insipidus, resulting from a neurohypophyseal or hypothalamic tumor, viral infection, metastatic disease, sarcoidosis, tuberculosis, Hand-Schüller-Christian disease, syphilis, neurosurgical procedures, or head trauma.

Normal ADH levels, in the presence of typical clinical features of diabetes insipidus (such as polydipsia, polyuria, and hypotonic urine), may indicate the nephrogenic form of the disease, marked by renal tubular resistance to ADH. Levels may be elevated, however, if the pituitary attempts to compensate for renal resistance.

Elevated ADH levels may also indicate SIADH, possibly as a result of bronchogenic carcinoma, acute porphyria, hypothyroidism, Addison's disease, cirrhosis of the liver, infectious hepatitis, severe hemorrhage, or circulatory shock.

Post-test care
□ If a hematoma develops at the venipuncture site, apply warm soaks.
□ As ordered, resume diet and medications discontinued before the test.

Interfering factors
□ Failure to observe restrictions of diet, medications, or activity may hinder accurate determination of test results. Morphine, anesthetics, estrogens, oxytocin, chlorpropamide, vincristine, carbamazepine, cyclophosphamide, and chlorothiazide elevate ADH levels, as do stress, pain, and positive-pressure ventilation. Alcohol and negative-pressure ventila-

tion inhibit ADH secretion.

☐ Radioactive scan performed within 1 week before the test may influence the results, since serum ADH level is determined by radioimmunoassay.

CAROL K. BARKER, RN, MSN, MEd

THYROID & PARATHYROID HORMONES

Serum Thyroxine

Thyroxine (T₄) is an amine that is secreted by the thyroid gland in response to thyroid-stimulating hormone (TSH) from the pituitary and, indirectly, to thyrotropin-releasing hormone (TRH) from the hypothalamus. The rate of secretion is normally regulated by a complex system of negative and positive feedback involving the thyroid, anterior pituitary, and hypothalamus. The suspected precursor, or prohormone, of triiodothyronine (T₃), T₄ is believed to convert to T₃ by a process known as monodeiodination, during which T₄ loses one of its four iodine atoms. The liver and kidneys—and to a lesser extent certain peripheral tissues—are the sites of this crucial transformation.

Only a fraction of T₄ (about 0.3%) circulates freely in the blood; the rest binds strongly to plasma proteins, primarily thyroxine-binding globulin (TBG). It is

FORMATION OF THYROID HORMONES

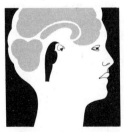

1. Iodine is ingested in seafoods, vegetables, eggs and dairy products, meat, and iodized salt.

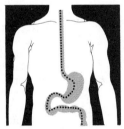

2. After digestion, the iodine contained in these foods is absorbed into the blood from the small bowel.

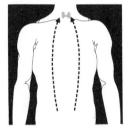

3. Iodine travels through the bloodstream and concentrates within the thyroid gland.

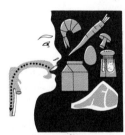

4. Meanwhile, the hypothalamus synthesizes thyrotropin-releasing hormone (TRH), which travels to the pituitary gland.

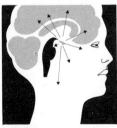

5. Here TRH stimulates the production and release of thyroid-stimulating hormone (TSH).

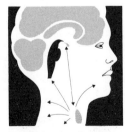

6. TSH then travels to the thyroid gland, where it stimulates synthesis of T₄ and T₃ from iodine, and triggers their release.

DRUGS THAT INTERFERE WITH TESTS FOR THYROXINE (T₄)

Increase T₄:

Clofibrate

Estrogens

Levothyroxine

Methadone

Progestins

Decrease T₄:

Clofibrate

Ethionamide

Free fatty acids

Heparin

Iodides

Liothyronine sodium

Lithium

Methimazole

Methylthiouracil

Phenylbutazone

Phenytoin

Propylthiouracil

Reserpine

Salicylates (high dose)

Steroids

Sulfonamides

Sulfonylureas

this minute fraction that is responsible for the clinical effects of thyroid hormone on body cells and tissues. Because of the tenacity of TBG's binding power, T_4 survives in the plasma for a relatively long time, with a half-life of about 6 days. This radioimmunoassay, one of the most common diagnostic indicators of thyroid function, measures the total circulating T_4 level when TBG is normal. The Murphy-Pattee or T_4(D), a similar test based on competitive protein binding, also provides the same information and may be ordered as an alternate test.

Purpose
□ To evaluate thyroid function
□ To aid diagnosis of hyper- and hypo-thyroidism
□ To monitor response to treatment with antithyroid medication in hyperthyroidism, and to monitor response to thyroid replacement therapy in hypothyroidism. (TSH estimates are needed to confirm hypothyroidism.)

Patient preparation
Explain to the patient that this test helps evaluate thyroid gland function. Inform him that he needn't fast or restrict physical activity before the test. Tell him this test requires a blood sample; who will perform the venipuncture and when; and that he may feel transient discomfort from the needle puncture. Collecting the sample takes only a few minutes.

As ordered, withhold any medications that may interfere with test results. If these medications must be continued, note this on the laboratory slip. (If this test is being performed to monitor thyroid therapy, the patient continues to receive daily thyroid supplements.)

Procedure
Perform a venipuncture, and collect the sample in a 7 ml *red-top* tube. Send the sample to the laboratory immediately so the serum may be separated.

Precautions
Handle the sample gently to prevent hemolysis.

HOW THE THYROID GLAND WORKS

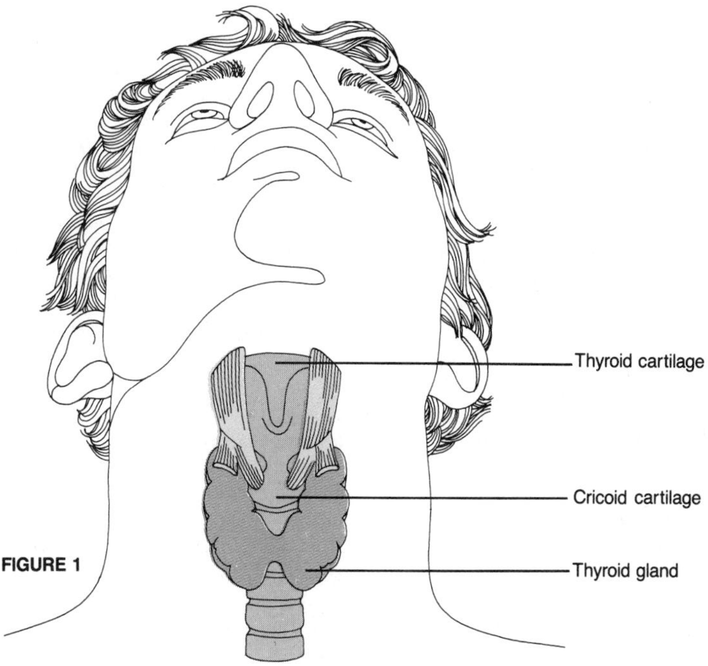

FIGURE 1

Thyroid cartilage

Cricoid cartilage

Thyroid gland

FIGURE 2

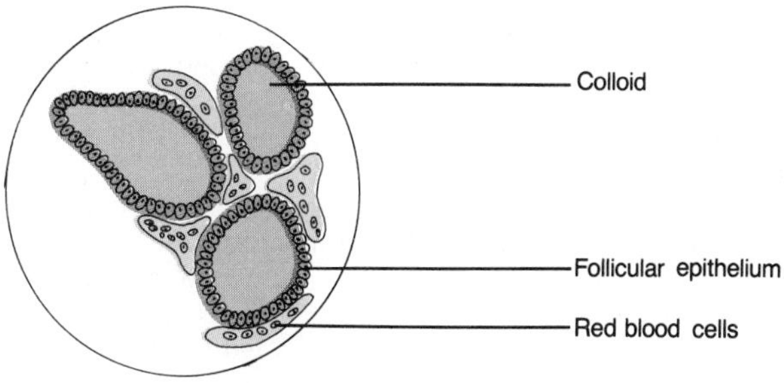

Colloid

Follicular epithelium

Red blood cells

The thyroid gland (figure 1), which straddles the trachea below the cricoid cartilage, is composed of two lateral lobes connected by an isthmus. One of the largest endocrine organs, it secretes two hormones whose primary function is to control growth and metabolism. The closed follicles (microscopic enlargement shown in figure 2) that comprise the thyroid gland contain colloid, a clear protein substance. Thyroglobulin, the main component of colloid, contains the thyroid hormones. Before thyroid hormones can work in the body, the colloid must be reabsorbed by the follicular epithelium (surrounding the follicles) and released into the bloodstream.

Values
Normally, total T_4 levels range from 5 to 13.5 mcg/dl.

Implications of results
Abnormally elevated levels of T_4 are consistent with primary and secondary hyperthyroidism, including excessive T_4 (L-thyroxine) replacement therapy (factitious or iatrogenic hyperthyroidism). Conversely, subnormal levels suggest primary or secondary hypothyroidism, or may be due to T_4 suppression by normal, elevated, or replacement levels of T_3. In doubtful cases of hypothyroidism, TSH levels or TRH test may be indicated.

A normal T_4 level, however, is no guarantee of euthyroidism; for example, normal readings occur in T_3 thyrotoxicosis. In the presence of overt signs of hyperthyroidism, therefore, further testing is necessary.

Post-test care
☐ If a hematoma develops at the venipuncture site, apply warm soaks.
☐ As ordered, resume administration of medications discontinued before the test.

Interfering factors
☐ Hemolysis due to rough handling or stasis of the sample may interfere with accurate determination of test results.
☐ Hereditary factors and some hepatic diseases can decrease or increase TBG concentration; protein-wasting diseases (nephrotic syndrome) and androgens may also reduce TBG. Thus, TBG levels can affect accurate determination of test results.

RICHARD EDWARD HONIGMAN, MD

Serum Triiodothyronine

This highly specific radioimmunoassay measures total (bound and free) serum content of triiodothyronine (T_3) to investigate clinical indications of thyroid dysfunction. T_3, the more potent thyroid hormone, is an amine derived primarily from thyroxine (T_4) through the process of monodeiodination. At least 50% and as much as 90% of T_3 is thought to be derived from T_4 as a result of this pivotal transformation, during which T_4 loses one of its iodine atoms to become T_3. The remaining 10% or more is secreted directly by the thyroid gland. Like T_4 secretion, T_3 secretion occurs in response to thyroid-stimulating hormone (TSH) released by the pituitary and, secondarily, to thyrotropin-releasing hormone from the hypothalamus through a complex negative feedback mechanism.

Although T_3 is present in the bloodstream in minute quantities and is metabolically active for only a short time, its impact on body metabolism dominates that of T_4. Another significant difference between the two major thyroid hormones is that T_3 binds less firmly to thyroxine-binding globulin (TBG). Consequently, T_3 persists in the bloodstream for a short time; half disappears in about 1 day, while half of T_4 disappears in 6 days.

Purpose
☐ To aid diagnosis of T_3 toxicosis
☐ To aid diagnosis of hypo- and hyperthyroidism
☐ To monitor clinical response to thyroid replacement therapy in hypothyroidism.

Patient preparation
Explain to the patient that this test helps to evaluate thyroid gland function and to determine the cause of his symptoms. Tell him this test requires a blood sample; who will perform the venipuncture and when; and that he may experience some transient discomfort from the needle puncture. Collecting the sample takes only a few minutes.

As ordered, withhold medications, such as steroids, propranolol, and cholestyramine, that may influence thyroid function. If such medications must be continued, record this information on the laboratory slip.

Procedure

Draw venous blood into a 7 ml *red-top* tube. Send the sample to the laboratory as soon as possible to avoid stasis and to allow early separation of serum from the clotted blood.

Precautions

Handle the sample gently to prevent hemolysis. If a patient must receive thyroid preparations such as T_3 (liothyronine), note the time of administration of the drug on the laboratory slip. Otherwise, T_3 levels are not reliable.

Values

Serum T_3 levels normally range from 90 to 230 ng/dl. These values may vary with the laboratory performing this test.

Implications of results

Serum T_3 and serum T_4 levels usually rise and fall in tandem. However, in T_3 toxicosis, only T_3 levels rise, while total and free T_4 levels remain normal. T_3 toxicosis occurs in patients with Graves' disease, toxic adenoma, or toxic nodular goiter. T_3 levels also surpass T_4 levels in patients receiving thyroid replacement containing more T_3 than T_4. In iodine-deficient areas, the thyroid may produce larger amounts of the more cellularly active T_3 than of T_4 in an effort to maintain the euthyroid state.

Generally, T_3 levels appear to be a more accurate diagnostic indicator of hyperthyroidism. Although hyperthyroidism increases both T_3 and T_4 levels in about 90% of patients, it causes a disproportionate increase in T_3. In some patients with hypothyroidism, T_3 levels may fall within the normal range and may not be diagnostically significant.

A rise in serum T_3 levels normally occurs during pregnancy. Low T_3 levels may appear in euthyroid patients with systemic illness (especially hepatic or renal disease), during severe acute illness, or following trauma or major surgery; in such patients, however, TSH levels are within normal limits. Low serum T_3 levels are sometimes found in euthyroid patients with malnutrition.

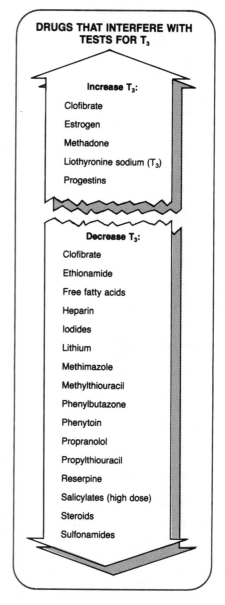

DRUGS THAT INTERFERE WITH TESTS FOR T_3

Increase T_3:

Clofibrate

Estrogen

Methadone

Liothyronine sodium (T_3)

Progestins

Decrease T_3:

Clofibrate

Ethionamide

Free fatty acids

Heparin

Iodides

Lithium

Methimazole

Methylthiouracil

Phenylbutazone

Phenytoin

Propranolol

Propylthiouracil

Reserpine

Salicylates (high dose)

Steroids

Sulfonamides

Post-test care

☐ If a hematoma develops at the venipuncture site, apply warm soaks.
☐ As ordered, resume administration of drugs discontinued before the test.

Interfering factors

These factors influence test results:

ABBREVIATIONS USED IN THYROID FUNCTION TESTS

T$_4$ = thyroxine

FT$_4$ = free thyroxine

T$_4$(D) = T$_4$ measurement by competitive protein-binding displacement radioassay

T$_3$ = triiodothyronine

FT$_3$ = free triiodothyronine

T$_3$ RU = T$_3$ resin uptake

FTI = free thyroxine index; obtained by multiplying T$_4$ (D) times the T$_3$ RU

TBG = thyroxine-binding globulin

TRH = thyrotropin-releasing hormone

TSH = thyroid-stimulating hormone

LATS = long-acting thyroid stimulator

□ markedly increased or decreased TBG levels, regardless of cause
□ failure to take into account medications that affect T$_3$ levels, such as steroids, clofibrate, and propranolol
□ hemolysis due to rough handling of sample.

RICHARD EDWARD HONIGMAN, MD

Serum Thyroxine-binding Globulin

This test measures the serum level of thyroxine-binding globulin (TBG), the predominant protein carrier for circulating thyroxine (T$_4$) and triiodothyronine (T$_3$). Values for TBG levels may be identified by saturating the sample for TBG determination with radioactive thyroxine (T$_4$), then subjecting this to electrophoresis and quantitating the amount of TBG by the amount of T$_4$* bound or by radioimmunoassay.*

Any condition that affects TBG levels and subsequent binding capacity also affects the amount of free T$_4$ (FT$_4$) and free T$_3$ (FT$_3$) in circulation. This can be clinically significant, since only FT$_4$ and FT$_3$ are metabolically active. An underlying TBG abnormality renders tests for total T$_3$ and T$_4$ inaccurate but does not alter tests for FT$_3$ and FT$_4$.

Purpose
□ To evaluate abnormal thyrometabolic states that do not correlate with thyroid hormone (T$_3$ or T$_4$) values (for example, a patient with overt signs of hypothyroidism and a low FT$_4$ level with a high total T$_4$ level due to a marked increase of TBG secondary to oral contraceptives)
□ To identify TBG abnormalities.

Patient preparation
Explain to the patient that this test helps evaluate thyroid function. Tell him the test requires a blood sample; who will perform the test and when; and that he may feel transient discomfort from the needle puncture. Collecting the sample takes only a few minutes.

As ordered, withhold medications that may interfere with accurate determination of test results, such as estrogens, anabolic steroids, phenytoin, salicylates, or thyroid preparations. If these medications must be continued, note this on the laboratory slip. (They may be continued to determine if prescribed drugs are affecting TBG levels.)

Procedure
Draw venous blood into a 10 ml *red-top* tube.

Precautions
Handle the sample gently to prevent hemolysis.

Values
Normal values by electrophoresis range from 10 to 26 mcg T$_4$ (binding capacity)/100 ml to 16 to 24 mcg T$_4$ (binding capacity)/100 ml, depending on the laboratory; by radioimmunoassay, values range from 1.3 to 2 mg/100 ml.

Implications of results

Elevated TBG levels may indicate hypothyroidism and congenital (genetic) excess, some forms of hepatic disease, or acute intermittent porphyria. TBG levels normally rise during pregnancy and are high in neonates. Suppressed levels may indicate hyperthyroidism or congenital deficiency, and can occur in active acromegaly, nephrotic syndrome and malnutrition with hypoproteinemia, acute illness, or surgical stress.

Patients with TBG abnormalities require additional testing, such as the serum FT_3 and serum FT_4 tests, to evaluate thyroid function more precisely.

Post-test care

□ If a hematoma develops at the venipuncture site, apply warm soaks.
□ As ordered, resume administration of medications that were discontinued before the test.

Interfering factors

□ Estrogens (including oral contraceptives) and phenothiazines (perphenazine) elevate TBG levels.
□ Androgens, prednisone, phenytoin, and high doses of salicylates depress TBG levels.
□ Hemolysis due to rough handling of the sample may interfere with accurate determination of test results.

RICHARD EDWARD HONIGMAN, MD

T_3 Resin Uptake

[Resin triiodothyronine uptake, T_3 uptake ratio (T_3UR)]

This test indirectly measures free thyroxine (FT_4) levels by demonstrating the availability of serum protein-binding sites for T_4. A known amount of radioactive triiodothyronine (T_3*), which exceeds the capacity of thyroxine-binding globulin (TBG) to bind to it, and a resin are added to a serum sample. The radioactive hormone combines with unoccupied sites on the TBG; any leftover hormone remains free and available for binding to the resin particles. When the resin is separated from the serum, the amount of radioactivity left on the TBG or bound to resin—measured by radioimmunoassay—is expressed as a percentage of the total amount of the T_3* added initially.

The results of T_3 resin uptake (T_3RU) are frequently combined with a T_4 radioimmunoassay or $T_4(D)$ (competitive protein-binding test) to determine the free thyroxine index, a mathematical calculation that is thought to reflect FT_4 by correcting for TBG abnormalities. The T_3RU is considered a valuable ancillary test for thyroid gland dysfunction.

Purpose

□ To aid diagnosis of hypo- and hyperthyroidism when TBG is normal
□ To aid diagnosis of primary disorders of TBG levels.

Patient preparation

Explain to the patient that this test helps evaluate thyroid function. Tell him the test requires a blood sample; who will perform the venipuncture and when; and that he may experience transient discomfort from the needle puncture. Collecting the sample takes only a few minutes, but the laboratory requires several days to complete the analysis.

As ordered, withhold medications, such as estrogens, androgens, phenytoin, salicylates or thyroid preparations, that may interfere with test results. If these medications must be continued, note this on the laboratory slip.

Procedure

Draw venous blood into a 7 ml *red-top* tube.

Precautions

Handle the collection tube gently to prevent hemolysis.

Values

Normally, 25% to 35% of T_3* binds to the resin.

Implications of results

A high resin uptake percentage in the presence of elevated T_4 levels indicates hyperthyroidism (implying few TBG free binding sites and high FT_4 levels). However, a low resin uptake percentage, together with low T_4 levels, indicates hypothyroidism (implying more TBG free binding sites and low FT_4 levels). Thus, in primary disease of thyroid function, measured T_4 and T_3 RU vary in the same direction; availability of binding sites varies inversely.

Discordant variance in T_4 and T_3 RU suggests abnormality of TBG. For example, a high resin uptake percentage and a low or normal FT_4 suggest decreased TBG levels. Such decreased levels may result from protein loss (as in nephrotic syndrome), decreased production (due to androgen excess, or genetic or idiopathic causes), or competition for T_4 binding sites by certain drugs (salicylates, phenylbutazone, or phenytoin). Conversely, a low resin uptake percentage and a high or normal FT_4 suggest increased TBG levels. Such increased levels may be due to exogenous or endogenous estrogen (pregnancy), or may result from idiopathic causes. Thus, in primary disorders of TBG levels, measured T_4 and free sites change in the same direction.

Post-test care

□ If a hematoma develops at the venipuncture site, apply warm soaks.
□ As ordered, resume administration of medications discontinued before the test.

Interfering factors

□ Therapy with phenylbutazone, phenytoin, high doses of aspirin, anabolic steroids, anticoagulants (heparin), or thyroxine may produce a falsely elevated T_3^* binding percentage.
□ T_3 therapy, oral contraceptives, or estrogen replacement therapy produces a falsely decreased T_3^* binding percentage. (In these cases, FT_4 and FT_3 tests are more valuable in assessing thyroid homeostasis.)
□ Serious illness may influence test results; severe hepatic disease, nephrotic syndrome, or metastatic disease may cause abnormal elevations in T_3^* binding percentage.
□ Hemolysis caused by rough handling of the sample may interfere with accurate determination of test results.

RICHARD EDWARD HONIGMAN, MD

Serum Free Thyroxine and Serum Free Triiodothyronine

These tests, often done simultaneously, measure serum levels of free thyroxine (FT₄) and free triiodothyronine (FT₃), the minute portions of T₄ and T₃ not bound to thyroxine-binding globulin (TBG) and other serum proteins. As the active components of T₄ and T₃, these unbound hormones enter target cells and are responsible for the thyroid's effects on cellular metabolism. Since levels of circulating FT₄ and FT₃ are regulated by a feedback mechanism that compensates for changes in binding protein concentrations by adjusting total hormone levels, measurement of free hormone levels is the best indicator of thyroid function. Disagreement exists as to whether FT₄ or FT₃ is the better indicator; therefore, laboratories commonly measure both. The disadvantages of these tests include a cumbersome and difficult laboratory method, inaccessibility, and cost. This test may be useful in the 5% of patients in whom the standard T₃ or T₄ tests fail to produce diagnostic results.

Purpose

□ To measure the metabolically active form of the thyroid hormones
□ To aid diagnosis of hyper- or hypothyroidism when TBG levels are abnormal.

Patient preparation

Explain to the patient that this special

test helps evaluate thyroid function. Tell him the test requires a blood sample; who will perform the venipuncture and when; and that he may feel transient discomfort from the needle puncture. Collecting the sample takes only a few minutes. The laboratory requires several days to complete the analysis.

Procedure

Draw venous blood into a 7 ml *red-top* tube.

Precautions

Handle the sample gently to prevent hemolysis.

Values

Normal range for FT_4 is from 0.8 to 3.3 ng/dl; for FT_3, from 0.2 to 0.6 ng/dl. Values vary, depending on the laboratory.

Implications of results

Elevated FT_4 and FT_3 levels indicate hyperthyroidism, unless peripheral resistance to thyroid hormone is present. T_3 toxicosis, a distinct form of hyperthyroidism, yields high FT_3 levels, with normal or low FT_4 values. Low FT_4 levels usually indicate hypothyroidism, except in patients receiving replacement therapy with T_3. Patients on thyroid therapy may have varying levels of FT_4 and FT_3, depending on the preparation used and the time of sample collection.

Post-test care

If a hematoma develops at the venipuncture site, apply warm soaks.

Interfering factors

Except for hemolysis due to rough handling of the sample, this test is virtually free of interfering factors. Agents that compete with T_4 and T_3 binding to TBG increase FT_4 fraction; this does not affect in vitro TBG studies due to serum dilution. Depending on the dosage, thyroid therapy may increase FT_4 or FT_3 levels. However, these medications should not be withheld; serial tests may be performed to evaluate thyroid function.

RICHARD EDWARD HONIGMAN, MD

MEASURING FT_4 AND FT_3

FT_4 and FT_3 levels can be determined by adding a known amount of radioactive hormone to the test serum and measuring residual radioactivity—that portion which doesn't bind to TBG. Free fractions of T_4 and T_3 can pass through a dialysis membrane, while the protein-bound fractions cannot. Since radioactive T_4 and T_3 behave the same way, they can be used to measure the amount of T_4 and T_3 that passes through the membrane.

After the known amount of radioactive T_3/T_4 is added to the test serum, and after equilibration with the nonradioactive T_3/T_4 in the patient's serum, the sample is exposed to the dialysis membrane. The free fractions diffuse through, in a process called equilibration dialysis. The percentage of free radioactive hormone is then determined by quantitating the degree of radioactivity and comparing it to the initial radioactive total for T_3 and T_4. This percentage of FT_3 or FT_4, when applied to the total T_4 or T_3 determined by radioimmunoassay, yields an absolute value for FT_3 or FT_4.

Serum Long-acting Thyroid Stimulator

In this test, the McKenzie mouse bioassay method is used to determine whether a patient's serum contains long-acting thyroid stimulator (LATS), an abnormal immunoglobulin (called 75 IgG) that mimics the action of thyroid-stimulating hormone (TSH), although its effects are more prolonged. LATS stimulates the thyroid gland to produce and secrete thyroid hormones in excessive amounts. Thus, through the normal negative feedback mechanism, it inhibits TSH secretion. LATS is often found in a patient with Graves' disease (about 80%), and in a neonate whose mother has Graves' disease, as LATS crosses the placenta.

Some authorities believe that the thyroid gland hyperplasia seen in Graves' disease may be due to LATS or other

---

McKENZIE MOUSE BIOASSAY FOR LATS

In the McKenzie mouse bioassay, samples of the patient's serum are injected into several mice that have received radioactive iodine, so that the T_4 they produce is radioactive. The mice also receive T_3 for several days before the test to suppress endogenous TSH or T_4 production that would interfere with test results. By checking the radioactive counts at 2 hours and at 9 hours after injection, the amount of T_4 released into the mouse serum can be measured. If the patient's serum contains only TSH, radioactive counts in the mouse serum peak within 2 hours. But if long-acting thyroid stimulator (LATS) is also present, high counts persist in the 9-hour sample and exceed the 2-hour reading. A partial measurement of LATS concentration is also obtained during the assay.

□ Note on the laboratory slip if the patient had an ^{131}I radioactive scan within 48 hours before the test.

Values
Normally, LATS does not appear in serum.

Implications of results
LATS in serum indicates Graves' disease, whether or not overt signs of hyperthyroidism are present. About 80% of patients with Graves' disease have detectable LATS in their sera.

Post-test care
If a hematoma develops at the venipuncture site, apply warm soaks.

Interfering factors
□ Radioactive iodine in the serum may affect test results.
□ Hemolysis due to rough handling of the sample may interfere with accurate determination of test results.
                    RICHARD EDWARD HONIGMAN, MD

circulating antibodies. Some consider the clinical significance of this test questionable.

Purpose
□ To confirm diagnosis of Graves' disease. (This test is not done routinely to diagnose thyroid disorders.)

Patient preparation
Explain to the patient (or the infant's parents) that this test helps evaluate thyroid function. Tell him this test requires a blood sample; who will perform the venipuncture and when; and that he may feel transient discomfort from the needle puncture. Reassure him that collecting the sample takes only a few minutes, although the laboratory requires several days to complete the analysis.

Procedure
Draw venous blood into a 5 ml *red-top* tube.

Precautions
□ Handle the sample gently to prevent hemolysis.

Screening Test for Congenital Hypothyroidism

This test measures serum thyroxine (T_4) levels in the neonate to detect congenital hypothyroidism. Characterized by low or absent levels of T_4, congenital hypothyroidism affects roughly 1 in 5,000 neonates, occurring in girls three times more often than in boys. This disorder can result from thyroid dysgenesis or hypoplasia, congenital goiter, or maternal use of thyroid inhibitors during pregnancy. If untreated, it can lead to irreversible brain damage by age 3 months. Because clinical signs are few, in the past, most cases of congenital hypothyroidism went undetected until cretinism became apparent or death followed respiratory distress. Recently,

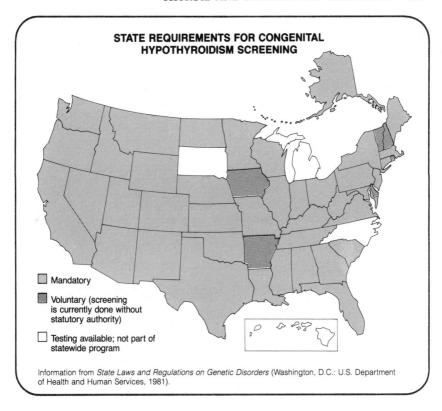

STATE REQUIREMENTS FOR CONGENITAL HYPOTHYROIDISM SCREENING

☐ Mandatory

■ Voluntary (screening is currently done without statutory authority)

☐ Testing available; not part of statewide program

Information from *State Laws and Regulations on Genetic Disorders* (Washington, D.C.: U.S. Department of Health and Human Services, 1981).

however, radioimmunoassays for T_4 and thyroid-stimulating hormone (TSH) have been used effectively to screen neonates for congenital hypothyroidism. This test is now mandatory in some states.

Purpose
☐ To screen neonates for congenital hypothyroidism.

Patient preparation
Explain to the parents that although hypothyroidism is uncommon in infants, this screening test detects the disorder early enough to begin therapy before irreversible brain damage occurs. Tell the parents the test will be performed before the infant is discharged from the hospital and again 4 to 6 weeks later. Emphasize the importance of the screening and the need for following the test protocol.

Since false-positive findings can result from variations in the test procedure or from a congenital thyroxine-binding globulin (TBG) defect, inform the parents that a second test may be necessary before the infant is discharged.

Equipment
Alcohol or povidone-iodine swabs/sterile lancet/specially marked filter paper/ 2″ x 2″ sterile gauze pads/small adhesive bandage strip/labels for infant's and mother's names, doctor's name, room number, and date.

Procedure
After assembling the necessary equipment and washing your hands thoroughly, wipe the infant's heel with an alcohol or povidone-iodine swab. Then dry it thoroughly with a gauze pad.

Perform a heelstick. Squeezing the heel gently, fill the circles on the filter paper with blood. Make sure the blood saturates the paper. Apply gentle pressure with a gauze pad to ensure hemostasis at the puncture site. When the filter paper is dry, label it appropriately and send it to the laboratory.

Precautions
None.

Values
Immediately after birth, neonatal T₄ levels are considerably higher than normal adult levels. By the end of the first week, however, T_4 values decrease markedly:

Age (days)	Normal T_4 level
1 to 5	≤ 4.9 mcg/dl
6 to 8	≤ 4.0 mcg/dl
9 to 11	≤ 3.5 mcg/dl
12 to 120	≤ 3.0 mcg/dl

Implications of results
Low serum T_4 levels in the neonate require TSH testing for clarification of the diagnosis. Decreased T_4 levels accompanied by elevated TSH readings (more than 25 µIU/ml) indicate primary congenital hypothyroidism (thyroid gland dysfunction). If T_4 and TSH levels are depressed, secondary congenital hypothyroidism (resulting from pituitary or hypothalamic dysfunction) should be suspected.

If T_4 levels are subnormal in the presence of normal TSH readings, further testing is required. Serum TBG levels must be analyzed to identify infants with hypothyroidism resulting from congenital defects in TBG. This low T_4-normal TSH pattern also occurs in a transient form of congenital hypothyroidism, which may accompany prematurity, or prenatal hypoxia.

A complete thyroid workup—including serum T_3, TBG, and free T_4 levels—is necessary for unequivocal diagnosis of congenital hypothyroidism before treatment begins.

Post-test care
☐ Heelsticks heal readily and require no special care.
☐ If results of the screening test indicate congenital hypothyroidism, tell the parents additional testing is necessary to determine the cause of the disorder.
☐ If diagnosis is confirmed, inform the parents that replacement therapy can restore normal thyroid gland function. Also tell them that such therapy is lifelong and that dosage will increase until adult requirement is reached.
☐ If the sample is not processed in the hospital laboratory, be sure parents are notified when test results are available.

Interfering factors
The following factors may interfere with accurate determination of test results:
☐ failure to allow the filter paper to dry completely
☐ failure to follow special directions for obtaining the sample.

RICHARD EDWARD HONIGMAN, MD

Plasma Calcitonin
[Thyrocalcitonin]

This radioimmunoassay measures plasma levels of calcitonin, a polypeptide hormone secreted by interstitial or parafollicular cells called specialized C cells of the thyroid gland in response to rising serum calcium levels. The exact role of calcitonin in normal human physiology has not been fully defined. However, calcitonin is known to inhibit bone resorption by osteoclasts and osteocytes, and to increase calcium excretion by the kidneys; thereby, calcitonin acts as an antagonist to parathyroid hormone and lowers serum calcium levels. The usual clinical indication for this test is suspected medullary carcinoma of the thyroid, which causes hypersecretion of calcitonin (without associated hypocalcemia). Equivocal results require provocative testing with I.V. pentagastrin or calcium to rule out disease.

Purpose
☐ To aid diagnosis of thyroid medullary carcinoma or ectopic calcitonin-producing tumors (rare).

Patient preparation

Explain to the patient that this test helps evaluate thyroid function. Instruct him to observe an overnight fast, since eating may interfere with calcium homeostasis and, subsequently, calcitonin levels. Tell him this test requires a blood sample, and advise him who will perform the venipuncture and when. Although he may feel transient discomfort from the needle puncture, collecting the sample takes only a few minutes. The laboratory, however, requires several days to complete the analysis.

Procedure

Draw venous blood into a 10 ml *green-top* (heparinized) tube.

Special precautions

Handle the sample gently to prevent hemolysis, and send it to the laboratory immediately.

Values

Serum calcitonin levels (basal) normally are ≤ 0.155 ng/ml in males; in females, ≤ 0.105 ng/ml.

Values after provocative testing with 4-hour calcium infusion are:
☐ males: 0.265 ng/ml
☐ females: 0.120 ng/ml.

Values after provocative testing with pentagastrin infusion are:
☐ males: 0.210 ng/ml
☐ females: 0.105 ng/ml.

Detection limit of assay is 0.030 ng/ml.

Implications of results

Elevated serum calcitonin levels, in the absence of hypocalcemia, usually indicate medullary carcinoma of the thyroid. Transmitted as an autosomal dominant trait, thyroid medullary carcinoma may occur as part of multiple endocrine neoplasia. Occasionally, increased calcitonin levels may be due to ectopic calcitonin production by oat cell carcinoma of the lung or by breast carcinoma.

Post-test care

If a hematoma develops at the venipuncture site, apply warm soaks.

CALCITONIN STIMULATION TESTING

Stimulation testing is often necessary in patients with medullary thyroid carcinoma when baseline calcitonin levels fail to rise high enough to confirm diagnosis. The most common test is a 4-hour I.V. calcium infusion (15 mg/kg) to provoke calcitonin secretion. Samples are taken just before the infusion and at 3 and 4 hours. After the infusion, calcitonin levels rise rapidly in patients with medullary thyroid carcinoma.

Another test involves I.V. infusion of pentagastrin 0.5 mcg/kg over 5 to 10 seconds. A blood sample is drawn just before the I.V. infusion, and at 90 seconds, 5 minutes, and 10 minutes postinfusion. In patients with medullary thyroid carcinoma, calcitonin levels rise markedly over the baseline reading. This test is now being used in some centers.

Interfering factors

☐ Failure to observe an overnight fast before the test may interfere with accurate determination of test results.
☐ Hemolysis due to rough handling of the sample may interfere with accurate determination of test results.

RICHARD EDWARD HONIGMAN, MD

Serum Parathyroid Hormone

[Parathormone]

Parathyroid hormone (PTH), a polypeptide secreted by the parathyroid glands, regulates plasma concentration of calcium and phosphorus. Normally, PTH release is regulated by a negative feedback mechanism involving serum calcium. Normal or elevated circulating calcium (especially the ionized form) inhibits PTH release; a decrease in calcium ions stimulates PTH release. The overall effect of PTH is to raise plasma levels of calcium while lowering phosphorus levels by stimulating osteoclasts and os-

teocytes to mobilize both calcium and phosphorus from bone; by acting on renal tubular cells to promote calcium reabsorption and phosphorus excretion (phosphaturia); and (with biologic vitamin D [1,25-dihydroxycholecalciferol]) by promoting intestinal absorption of calcium.

Circulating PTH exists in three distinct molecular forms: the intact PTH molecule, which originates in the parathyroids, and two smaller circulating forms—N-terminal fragments and C-terminal fragments—that are cleaved from the intact molecule by the kidneys, liver, and, to a lesser extent for the C-fragment, the parathyroids. Currently, two radioimmunoassays are available to detect intact PTH and the N- and C-terminal fragments. Both tests can be used to confirm diagnosis of hyperpara-

thyroidism and hypoparathyroidism; each test has other specific applications as well. The C-terminal PTH assay is more useful in diagnosing chronic disturbances in PTH metabolism, such as secondary and tertiary hyperparathyroidism; it also better differentiates ectopic from primary hyperparathyroidism. The assay for intact PTH and the N-terminal fragment (both forms are measured concomitantly) more accurately reflects acute changes in PTH metabolism, and thus is useful in monitoring a patient's response to PTH therapy. An inappropriate excess or deficiency of PTH has clinical and diagnostic consequences directly related to the effects of PTH on bone and on the renal tubules, and to its interaction with ionized calcium and biologically active vitamin D. Consequently, measuring

CLINICAL IMPLICATIONS OF ABNORMAL PARATHYROID SECRETION

CONDITIONS	CAUSES	PTH LEVELS	CALCIUM (IONIZED) LEVELS
Primary hyperparathyroidism	• Parathyroid adenoma or carcinoma • Parathyroid hyperplasia	High	High to Normal
Secondary hyperparathyroidism	• Chronic renal disease • Severe vitamin D deficiency • Calcium malabsorption • Pregnancy and lactation	High	Low
Tertiary hyperparathyroidism	• Progressive secondary hyperparathyroidism leading to autonomous hyperparathyroidism	High	High to Normal
Hypoparathyroidism	• Usually, accidental removal of the parathyroid glands during surgery • Occasionally, in association with autoimmune disease	Low	Low
Malignant tumors	• Squamous cell carcinoma of the lung • Renal, pancreatic, or ovarian carcinoma	High to Normal	High

KEY	High ●	Normal ◐	Low ○

serum calcium, phosphorus, and creatine levels with serum PTH is useful in identifying states of pathologic parathyroid function. Suppression or stimulation tests may be of confirming value.

Purpose
□ To aid the differential diagnosis of parathyroid disorders.

Patient preparation
Explain to the patient that this test helps evaluate parathyroid function. Instruct him to observe an overnight fast, because food may affect PTH levels and interfere with the test results. Tell the patient that this test requires a blood sample; who will perform the venipuncture and when; and that although he may experience transient discomfort from the needle puncture, collecting the sample takes only a few minutes. The laboratory requires several days to complete the analysis.

Procedure
Draw 3 ml venous blood into two separate 7 ml *red-top* tubes.

Precautions
Handle the sample gently to prevent hemolysis. Send it to the laboratory immediately so the serum can be separated and frozen for assay.

Values
Normal serum PTH levels vary, depending on the laboratory, and must be interpreted in association with serum calcium levels. Typical values are as follows:
□ Intact PTH: 210 to 310 pg/ml
□ N-terminal fraction: 230 to 630 pg/ml
□ C-terminal fraction: 410 to 1760 pg/ml.

Implications of results
Measured concomitantly with serum calcium levels, abnormally elevated PTH values may indicate primary, secondary, or tertiary hyperparathyroidism. Abnormally low PTH levels may result from hypoparathyroidism and from certain malignant diseases (see chart, opposite page).

Post-test care
□ If a hematoma develops at the venipuncture site, apply warm soaks.
□ As ordered, resume normal diet after the test.

Interfering factors
□ Failure to observe an overnight fast may interfere with the accurate determination of test results.
□ Hemolysis due to rough handling of the sample may interfere with accurate determination of test results.

RICHARD EDWARD HONIGMAN, MD

ADRENAL HORMONES

Serum Aldosterone

This test measures serum aldosterone levels by quantitative analysis and radioimmunoassay. Aldosterone, the principal mineralocorticoid secreted by the zona glomerulosa of the adrenal cortex, regulates ion transport across cell membranes in the renal tubules to promote reabsorption of sodium and chloride in exchange for potassium and hydrogen ions. Consequently, aldosterone helps to maintain blood pressure and blood volume, and to regulate fluid and electrolyte balance.

Aldosterone secretion is controlled primarily by the renin-angiotensin system and by the circulating concentration of potassium. Thus, high serum potassium levels elicit secretion of aldosterone through a potent feedback system; similarly, hyponatremia, hypovolemia, and other disorders that provoke the release of renin stimulate aldosterone secretion.

This test identifies aldosteronism and, when supported by plasma renin levels,

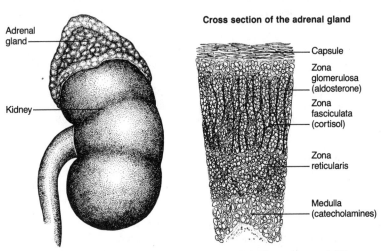

SITES OF ADRENAL HORMONE PRODUCTION

Cross section of the adrenal gland

Adrenal gland

Kidney

Capsule

Zona glomerulosa (aldosterone)

Zona fasciculata (cortisol)

Zona reticularis

Medulla (catecholamines)

The adrenal glands are paired structures located retroperitoneally, one atop each kidney. Each gland consists of the cortex, composed of three layers, and the medulla. The outer layer of the cortex, the zona glomerulosa, produces aldosterone; the first inner layer, the zona fasciculata, produces cortisol; and the medulla stores catecholamines (epinephrine and norepinephrine).

distinguishes between the primary and secondary forms of this disorder. Thus, it's helpful in identifying adrenal adenoma and adrenal hyperplasia, causes of primary aldosteronism. Secondary aldosteronism is commonly associated with salt depletion, potassium excess, congestive heart failure with ascites, or other conditions that characteristically increase activity of the renin-angiotensin system.

Purpose
☐ To aid diagnosis of primary and secondary aldosteronism, adrenal hyperplasia, hypoaldosteronism, and salt-losing syndrome.

Patient preparation
Explain to the patient that this test helps determine if symptoms are due to improper hormonal secretion. Instruct him to maintain a low-carbohydrate, normal-sodium diet (135 mEq or 3 g/day)

for at least 2 weeks or, preferably, for 30 days before the test. Tell him that the test requires a blood sample, and that he may feel some discomfort from the needle puncture. Collecting the sample takes only a few minutes, but the laboratory requires at least 10 days to complete the multistage analysis.

As ordered, withhold all drugs that alter fluid, sodium, and potassium balance—especially diuretics, antihypertensives, steroids, cyclic progestational agents, and estrogens—for at least 2 weeks or, preferably, for 30 days before the test. Also, withhold all renin inhibitors (such as propranolol) for 1 week before the test. If these medications must be continued, note this on the laboratory slip. Licorice produces an aldosterone-like effect and should be avoided for at least 2 weeks before the test.

Procedure
While the patient is still supine after a

night's rest, perform a venipuncture. Collect the sample in a 7 ml *red-top* collection tube, and send it to the laboratory. To evaluate the effect of postural change, draw another sample 4 hours later, after the patient has been up and about, while the patient is standing. Collect the second sample in a 7 ml *red-top* collection tube, and send it to the laboratory.

Precautions
□ Handle the sample gently to prevent hemolysis.
□ Record on the laboratory slip whether the patient was supine or standing during the venipuncture. If the patient is a premenopausal female, specify the phase of her menstrual cycle, since aldosterone levels may fluctuate during the menstrual cycle.

Values
Normally, serum aldosterone levels (in a standing, nonpregnant patient) range from 1 to 21 ng/dl. Specifically, a normal serum aldosterone level for an adult male or female who has been supine for at least 2 hours is 7.4 ± 4.2 ng/dl; for an adult male or female who has been standing for at least 2 hours, 13.2 ± 8.9 ng/dl.

Implications of results
Excessive aldosterone secretion may indicate a primary or secondary disease. Primary aldosteronism (Conn's syndrome) may result from adrenocortical adenoma or carcinoma, or bilateral adrenal hyperplasia. Secondary aldosteronism can result from renovascular hypertension, congestive heart failure, cirrhosis of the liver, nephrotic syndrome, idiopathic cyclic edema, or the third trimester of pregnancy.

Depressed serum aldosterone levels may indicate primary hypoaldosteronism, salt-losing syndrome, toxemia of pregnancy, or Addison's disease.

Post-test care
□ If a hematoma develops at the venipuncture site, apply warm soaks.

□ As ordered, resume diet and medications discontinued before the test.

Interfering factors
□ Hemolysis due to rough handling of the sample may interfere with accurate determination of test results.
□ Failure to observe restrictions of diet, medications, or posture may interfere with accurate determination of test results. Some antihypertensives—methyldopa, for example—promote sodium and water retention, and therefore may reduce aldosterone levels. Diuretics promote sodium excretion and may raise aldosterone levels. Some corticosteroids—fludrocortisone, for example—mimic mineralocorticoid activity and therefore may lower aldosterone levels.
□ Radioactive scan performed within 1 week before the test may influence test results.

CAROL K. BARKER, RN, MSN, MEd

Plasma Cortisol

Cortisol—the principal glucocorticoid secreted by the zona fasciculata of the adrenal cortex, primarily in response to adrenocorticotropic hormone (ACTH) stimulation—helps metabolize nutrients, mediate physiologic stress, and regulate the immune system. Cortisol secretion normally follows a diurnal pattern: levels rise during the early morning hours and peak around 8 a.m., then decline to very low levels in the evening and during the early phase of sleep. Production of this hormone is influenced by physical or emotional stress, which activates ACTH. Thus, intense heat or cold, infection, trauma, exercise, obesity, and debilitating disease influence cortisol secretion.

This radioimmunoassay, a quantitative analysis of plasma cortisol levels, is usually ordered for patients with signs of adrenal dysfunction, but dynamic tests, suppression tests for hyperfunc-

tion, and stimulation tests for hypofunction are generally required for confirmation of diagnoses.

Purpose

□ To aid in the diagnosis of Cushing's disease, Cushing's syndrome, Addison's disease, and secondary adrenal insufficiency.

Patient preparation

Explain to the patient that this test helps determine if his symptoms are due to improper hormonal secretion. Instruct him to maintain a normal salt diet (2 to 3 g/day) for 3 days before the test and to fast and limit physical activity for 10 to 12 hours before the test. Tell him a blood sample is required, who will perform the venipuncture and when, and that he may experience some discomfort from the needle puncture. Give reassurance that collecting the sample takes only a few minutes, although the laboratory requires at least 2 days to complete the analysis.

As ordered, withhold all medications that may interfere with plasma cortisol levels, such as estrogens, androgens, and phenytoin, for 48 hours before the test. If the patient is receiving replacement therapy and is dependent on exogenous steroids for survival, note this on the laboratory slip, as well as any other medications that must be continued.

Make sure the patient is relaxed and recumbent for at least 30 minutes before the test.

Procedure

Between 6 and 8 a.m., perform a venipuncture. Collect the sample in a *green-top* tube, label appropriately, and send to the laboratory immediately. For diurnal variation testing, draw another sample between 4 and 6 p.m. Collect it in a *green-top* tube, label appropriately, and send to the laboratory immediately.

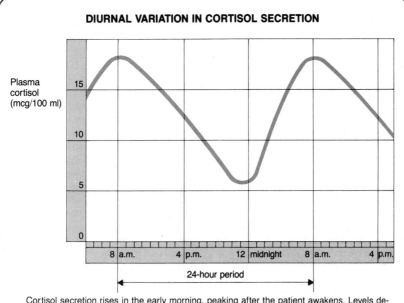

DIURNAL VARIATION IN CORTISOL SECRETION

Plasma cortisol (mcg/100 ml)

15

10

5

0

8 a.m.   4 p.m.   12 midnight   8 a.m.   4 p.m.

24-hour period

Cortisol secretion rises in the early morning, peaking after the patient awakens. Levels decline sharply in the evening and during the early phase of sleep. They rise again during the night and peak by the next morning.

Adapted with permission from Sylvia Price and Lorraine Wilson, *Pathophysiology: Clinical Concepts of Disease Processes* (New York: McGraw-Hill Book Co., 1978).

Precautions

□ Handle the sample gently to prevent hemolysis.

□ Record the collection time on the laboratory slip.

Values

Normally, plasma cortisol levels range from 7 to 28 mcg/dl in the morning, and from 2 to 18 mcg/dl in the afternoon. (The afternoon level is usually half the morning level.)

Implications of results

Increased plasma cortisol levels may indicate adrenocortical hyperfunction in Cushing's disease (a rare disease due to basophilic adenoma of the pituitary gland) or in Cushing's syndrome (glucocorticoid excess from any cause). In most patients with Cushing's syndrome, the adrenal cortex tends to secrete independently of any natural rhythm. Thus, absence of diurnal variation in cortisol secretion is a significant finding in almost all patients with Cushing's syndrome; in these patients, little difference in values, if any, is found between morning samples and those taken in the afternoon. Diurnal variations may also be absent in otherwise healthy persons who are under considerable emotional or physical stress.

Decreased cortisol levels may indicate primary adrenal hypofunction (Addison's disease), most often due to idiopathic glandular atrophy (a presumed autoimmune process). Tuberculosis, fungal invasion, and hemorrhage can cause adrenocortical destruction. Low cortisol levels resulting from secondary adrenal insufficiency may occur in conditions of impaired ACTH secretion, such as hypophysectomy, postpartum pituitary necrosis, craniopharyngioma, or chromophobe adenoma.

Post-test care

□ If a hematoma develops at the venipuncture site, apply warm soaks.

□ As ordered, resume diet and administration of medications that were discontinued before the test.

Interfering factors

□ Failure to observe restrictions of diet, medications, or physical activity may interfere with accurate determination of test results. Plasma cortisol levels are falsely elevated by estrogens (during pregnancy or in oral contraceptives), which increase plasma proteins that bind with cortisol. Obesity, stress, or severe hepatic or renal disease may also increase these levels. Plasma cortisol levels may be decreased by androgens and phenytoin, which decrease cortisol-binding proteins.

□ Radioactive scan performed within 1 week before the test may influence the results.

□ Hemolysis due to rough handling of the sample may interfere with accurate determination of test results.

CAROL K. BARKER, RN, MSN, MEd

Plasma Catecholamines

This test, a quantitative (total or fractionated) analysis of plasma catecholamines, has significant clinical importance in patients with hypertension and signs of adrenal medullary tumor, and in patients with neural tumors that affect endocrine function. Elevated plasma catecholamine levels necessitate supportive confirmation by urinalysis that shows catecholamine degradation products such as vanillylmandelic acid (VMA) and metanephrine.

Major catecholamines include the hormones epinephrine, norepinephrine, and dopamine, which are produced almost exclusively in the brain, sympathetic nerve endings, and adrenal medulla. When secreted into the bloodstream, adrenal medullary catecholamines prepare the body for the fight-or-flight reaction to stress: they increase heart rate and contractility; constrict peripheral and visceral blood vessels, and redistribute circulating blood toward the skeletal and coronary muscles; mobilize carbohydrate and lipid reserves; and sharpen mental alertness. These effects are similar to those produced by direct stimulation of the sympathetic nervous system, although greatly intensified and prolonged.

Since many factors influence catecholamine secretion, diurnal variations are common; for example, plasma levels may fluctuate in response to temperature, stress, postural change, diet, smoking, and many drugs.

Purpose

□ To rule out pheochromocytoma (adrenal medullary or extra-adrenal) in patients with hypertension

□ To help identify neuroblastoma, ganglioneuroblastoma, and ganglioneuroma

□ To distinguish between adrenal medullary tumors and other catecholamine-producing tumors, through fractional analysis. Urinalysis for catecholamine degradation products is recommended to support diagnosis.

□ To aid diagnosis of autonomic nervous system dysfunction, such as idiopathic orthostatic hypotension.

Patient preparation

Explain to the patient that this test helps determine if hypertension or other symptoms are related to improper hormonal secretion. Because the action of catecholamines is so transitory, advise him to strictly follow pretest instructions, for a reliable test result. Instruct him to observe these restrictions before the test: to refrain from using self-prescribed medications (especially cold or hay fever remedies that may contain sympathomimetics) for 2 weeks; to exclude from his diet amine-rich foods and beverages (such as bananas, avocados, cheese, coffee, tea, cocoa, beer, and Chianti) for 48 hours; to abstain from smoking for 24 hours (nicotine may alter test results); and to fast for 10 to 12 hours.

Tell the patient that this test requires two blood samples; who will perform the venipunctures and when; and that he may feel some discomfort from the needle punctures. Collecting the samples takes less than 20 minutes, but the laboratory requires at least 1 week to complete the analysis.

If the patient is hospitalized, withhold medications that affect catecholamine levels, such as amphetamines, phenothiazines (chlorpromazine), sympathomimetics, and tricyclic antidepressants, as ordered.

Also, as ordered, insert an indwelling venous catheter (heparin lock) 24 hours before the test. This may be necessary, since the stress of the venipuncture itself may significantly raise catecholamine levels. Make sure the patient is relaxed and recumbent for 45 to 60 minutes before the test. If necessary, provide blankets to keep him warm; low temperatures stimulate catecholamine secretion.

Procedure

Perform a venipuncture between 6 a.m. and 8 a.m. Collect the sample in a 10 ml chilled tube containing EDTA (sodium metabisulfite solution), which can be obtained from Mayo laboratory on request. Then have the patient stand for 10 minutes, and draw a second sample into another tube, exactly like the first. If a heparin lock is used, it may be necessary to discard the first 1 or 2 ml of blood. Check with the laboratory for the preferred procedure.

Precautions

After collecting each sample, roll the tube slowly between your palms to distribute the EDTA without agitating the blood. Then, pack the tube in crushed ice, to minimize deactivation of catecholamines, and send it to the laboratory immediately. Indicate on the laboratory slip whether the patient was supine or standing, and the time the sample was drawn.

Values

In fractional analysis, catecholamine levels range as follows:

□ supine: epinephrine, undetectable to 110 pg/ml; norepinephrine, 70 to 750 pg/

FIGHT OR FLIGHT STRESS REACTION

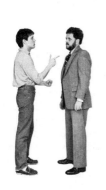

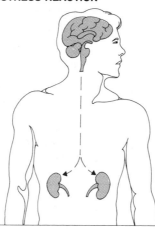

Stress—emotional or physical—initiates the transmission of nerve impulses by way of the sympathetic nervous system to the adrenal medullae.

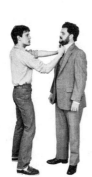

Nerve impulses cause the adrenal medullae to release catecholamines (primarily epinephrine and norepinephrine) into the bloodstream to prepare the body for reaction to stress (fight or flight).

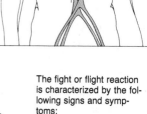

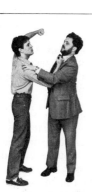

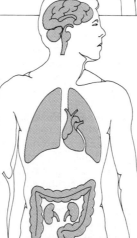

Adapted with permission from *Atlas of the Body and Mind*. Copyright Mitchell Beazley Publishers, 1977. Distributed in the U.S. by Rand McNally & Co

The fight or flight reaction is characterized by the following signs and symptoms:

- increased respiratory rate
- increased blood pressure, pulse rate, and cardiac output
- increased muscle strength
- increased blood supply to major organs: brain, heart, kidneys
- decreased blood supply to periphery (skin) and intestines.

ml; dopamine, undetectable to 30 pg/ml
☐ standing: epinephrine, undetectable to 140 pg/ml; norepinephrine, 200 to 1,700 pg/ml; dopamine, undetectable to 30 pg/ml.

Implications of results

High catecholamine levels may indicate pheochromocytoma, neuroblastoma, ganglioneuroblastoma, or ganglioneuroma. Similar elevations are possible in thyroid disorders, hypoglycemia, or cardiac disease but do not directly confirm these disorders. Electroshock therapy, shock resulting from hemorrhage, endotoxins, or anaphylaxis also causes catecholamine levels to rise.

In the patient with normal or low baseline catecholamine levels, failure to show increased catecholamine levels in the sample taken after standing suggests autonomic nervous system dysfunction. No known dysfunction is associated with insufficiency of the adrenal medulla.

Fractional analysis helps identify the specific abnormality that is producing elevated catecholamine levels. For example, adrenal medullary tumors secrete epinephrine; ganglioneuromas, ganglioblastomas, and neuroblastomas secrete norepinephrine.

Post-test care

☐ If a hematoma develops at the venipuncture site, apply warm soaks.
☐ As ordered, resume diet and medications discontinued before the test.

Interfering factors

☐ Failure to observe pretest restrictions may interfere with accurate determination of test results.
☐ Epinephrine, levodopa, amphetamines, phenothiazines (chlorpromazine), sympathomimetics, decongestants, and tricyclic antidepressants raise plasma catecholamine levels. Reserpine lowers plasma catecholamine levels.
☐ Radioactive scan performed within 1 week before the test may influence results, since plasma catecholamine levels are determined by radioimmunoassay.

CAROL K. BARKER, RN, MSN, MEd

Androstenedione

This test helps identify the causes of various disorders related to altered estrogen levels. Androstenedione, secreted by the adrenal cortex and the gonads, is converted to estrone (an estrogen of relatively low biologic activity) by adipose tissue and the liver. In premenopausal women, the amount of estrogen derived from androstenedione is relatively small compared to the amount of the more potent estrogen, estradiol, secreted by the ovaries. Usually, estrogen derived from androstenedione doesn't interfere with gonadotropin feedback during the menstrual cycle. But in such conditions as obesity, increased adrenal production of androstenedione or increased conversion of androstenedione to estrone may interfere with normal feedback, causing menstrual irregularities.

In children and postmenopausal women, estrone is a major souce of estrogen. Increased androstenedione production or increased conversion to estrone may induce premature sexual development in children; and renewed ovarian stimulation, endometriosis, bleeding, and polycystic ovaries in postmenopausal women. In men, overproduction of androstenedione may cause feminizing signs, such as gynecomastia.

Purpose

☐ To aid in determining the cause of gonadal dysfunction; menstrual or menopausal irregularities; and premature sexual development.

Patient preparation

Explain to the patient that this test helps determine the cause of symptoms. Tell the patient the test requires a blood sample; who will perform the venipuncture and when; and that she may experience transient discomfort from the needle puncture. If appropriate, explain that the test should be done 1 week before or after her menstrual period and that it may have to be repeated. As ordered, withhold steroid and pituitary-based hormones. If these must be continued, note this on the laboratory slip.

Procedure
Perform a venipuncture, and collect a serum sample in a 10-ml *red-top* tube. (Collect a plasma sample in a *green-top* tube.) Label it appropriately and send it to the laboratory immediately.

Precautions
☐ Handle the sample gently to prevent hemolysis. If a plasma sample is taken, refrigerate it or place it on ice.
☐ Record the patient's age, sex, and (if appropriate) phase of menstrual cycle on the laboratory slip.

Values
Females: Premenopausal—0.6 to 3 ng/ml; postmenopausal—0.3 to 8 ng/ml; males: 0.9 to 1.7 ng/ml.

Implications of results
Elevated androstenedione levels are associated with Stein-Levanthal syndrome; Cushing's syndrome; ovarian, testicular, or adrenocortical tumors; ectopic ACTH-producing tumors; late-onset congenital adrenal hyperplasia; and ovarian stromal hyperplasia. Elevated levels result in increased estrone levels, causing premature sexual development (children); menstrual irregularities (premenopausal women); bleeding, endometriosis, or polycystic ovaries (postmenopausal women); or feminizing signs, such as gynecomastia (men). Decreased levels occur in hypogonadism.

Post-test care
☐ If a hematoma develops at the venipuncture site, apply warm soaks.
☐ As ordered, resume medications discontinued before the test.

Interfering factors
☐ Hemolysis due to rough handling of the sample may affect test results.
☐ Ingestion of steroids or pituitary hormones may alter test results.

WENDY BAKER, RN, MS, CCRN

PANCREATIC & GASTRIC HORMONES

Serum Insulin

This radioimmunoassay is a quantitative analysis of serum insulin levels, which are always measured concomitantly with glucose levels, since glucose is the primary stimulus for insulin release from pancreatic islet cells. It helps evaluate patients suspected of having hyperinsulinemia due to pancreatic tumor or hyperplasia.

Insulin, a hormone secreted by beta cells of the islets of Langerhans, regulates the metabolism and transport or mobilization of carbohydrates, amino acids, and lipids. Stimulated by increased plasma levels of glucose, insulin secretion reaches peak levels after meals, when metabolism and food storage are greatest. An insufficient level of insulin or resistance to its effects is the primary abnormality in diabetes mellitus.

Purpose
☐ To aid diagnosis of hypoglycemia resulting from tumor or hyperplasia of pancreatic islet cells, glucocorticoid deficiency, or severe hepatic disease
☐ To aid diagnosis of diabetes mellitus and insulin-resistant states.

Patient preparation
Explain to the patient that this test helps determine if the pancreas is functioning normally. Instruct him to fast for 10 to 12 hours before the test. (Questionable results may make it necessary to repeat the test or, frequently, to perform a glucose tolerance test simultaneously, which requires that the patient drink glucose solution.) Tell him that the test requires

HOW THE PANCREAS PRODUCES INSULIN

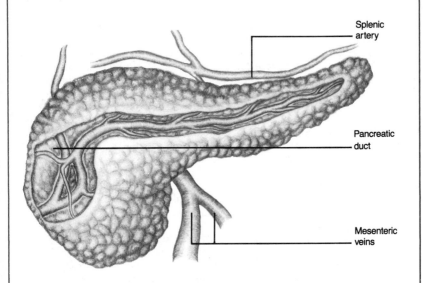

Splenic artery

Pancreatic duct

Mesenteric veins

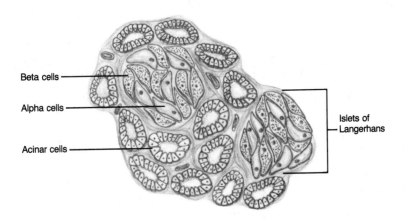

Beta cells

Alpha cells

Acinar cells

Islets of Langerhans

The pancreas (shown magnified directly above) is composed of an exocrine portion—acinar glands that secrete digestive enzymes—and an endocrine portion that secretes insulin and glucagon into the bloodstream in response to changes in blood sugar levels. The islets of Langerhans contain two principal types of cells—beta cells, which produce insulin when blood sugar increases, and alpha cells, which produce glucagon when blood sugar decreases. Splenic arteries transport oxygenated blood to the pancreas; mesenteric veins transport insulin and glucagon, contained in deoxygenated blood, from the pancreas. Insulin lowers blood sugar by increasing the conversion of glucose into liver and muscle glycogen and prevents breakdown of liver glycogen to yield glucose. Glucagon exerts an opposite effect.

blood samples; who will perform the venipuncture and when; and that he may feel transient discomfort from the needle puncture. Reassure him that collecting the samples takes only a few minutes.

As ordered, withhold ACTH, steroids (including oral contraceptives), thyroid supplements, epinephrine, or other medications that may interfere with accurate determination of test results. If these medications must be continued, note this on the laboratory slip.

Make sure the patient is relaxed and recumbent for 30 minutes before the test.

Procedure
Perform a venipuncture, and collect one sample for insulin level in a 7 ml *red-top* tube; collect another sample, for glucose, in a *gray-top* tube.

Precautions
□ Make sure the patient is relaxed before the samples are collected, since agitation or stress may affect insulin levels.
□ Pack the sample for insulin in ice, and send it, along with the glucose sample, to the laboratory immediately.

 □ In the patient with an insulinoma, this test may precipitate dangerously severe hypoglycemia. Keep glucose I.V. (50%) available to combat possible hypoglycemia.
□ Handle the sample gently to prevent hemolysis.

Values
Serum insulin levels normally range from undetectable to 25 μU/ml.

Implications of results
Insulin levels are interpreted in light of the prevailing glucose concentration. A normal insulin level may be inappropriate for the glucose results. High insulin and low glucose levels after a significant fast suggest an insulinoma. Prolonged fasting or stimulation testing may be required to confirm diagnosis. In insulin-resistant diabetic states, insulin levels are elevated; in non–insulin-resistant diabetes, they are low.

Post-test care
□ If a hematoma develops at the venipuncture site, apply warm soaks.
□ Resume diet and medications discontinued before the test, as ordered.

Interfering factors
□ Failure to observe restrictions of diet and activity may affect test results.
□ Use of ACTH, steroids (including oral contraceptives), thyroid hormones, or epinephrine increases insulin requirements by exerting a hyperglycemic effect, thereby raising serum insulin levels.
□ Use of insulin by non-insulin-dependent patients suppresses endogenous insulin secretion, lowering levels.
□ In patients with insulin-dependent diabetes mellitus, high levels of insulin antibodies may interfere with the test.

CONNECTING PEPTIDE

Connecting peptide (C-peptide) is a biologically inactive peptide chain formed during the proteolytic conversion of proinsulin to insulin in the pancreatic beta cells. It has no insulin effect, either biologically or immunologically. This is important, because circulating insulin is measured by immunologic assay. As insulin is released into the bloodstream, the C-peptide chain splits off from the hormone. Except in patients with islet cell tumors and, possibly, in obese patients, serum C-peptide levels generally parallel those of insulin: normal values range between 0.9 and 4.2 ng/ml.

A C-peptide assay may help to:
□ determine the cause of hypoglycemia by distinguishing between endogenous hyperinsulinism or insulinoma (elevated C-peptide levels) or surreptitious insulin injection (decreased C-peptide levels).
□ determine beta cell function in patients with diabetes mellitus. Absence of C-peptide indicates no beta cell function; presence indicates residual beta cell function.
□ indirectly measure insulin secretion in the presence of circulating insulin antibodies, which interfere with insulin assays but not with C-peptide assays.
□ detect residual tissue (some C-peptide present) after total pancreatectomy for carcinoma.
□ indicate the remission phase (some C-peptide present) of diabetes mellitus.

☐ Failure to pack the insulin sample in ice and send it to the laboratory promptly, or hemolysis caused by rough handling of the sample may hinder accurate determination of test results.

THAD C. HAGEN, MD

Serum Glucagon

Glucagon, a polypeptide hormone secreted by the alpha cells of the Islets of Langerhans in the pancreas, acts primarily on the liver to promote glucose production and control glucose storage. Glucagon is secreted in response to hypoglycemia; secretion is inhibited by the other pancreatic hormones, insulin and somatostatin. Normally the coordinated release of glucagon, insulin, and somatostatin ensures an adequate and constant fuel supply while maintaining blood glucose levels within relatively stable limits.

This test, a quantitative analysis of serum glucagon by radioimmunoassay, evaluates patients suspected of having glucagonoma (alpha cell tumor) or hypoglycemia due to idiopathic glucagon deficiency or pancreatic dysfunction. Glucagon is usually measured concomitantly with serum glucose and insulin, since glucose and insulin levels influence glucagon secretion.

Purpose
☐ To aid diagnosis of glucagonoma and hypoglycemia due to chronic pancreatitis or idiopathic glucagon deficiency.

Patient preparation
Explain to the patient that this test helps evaluate pancreatic function. Instruct him to fast for 10 to 12 hours before the test. Tell him that the test requires a blood sample; who will perform the venipuncture and when; and that he may feel transient discomfort from the needle puncture. Reassure him that collecting the sample takes only a few minutes.

As ordered, withhold insulin, catecholamines, and other drugs that could influence test results. If these drugs must be continued, note this on the laboratory slip.

Since exercise and stress elevate serum glucagon levels, make sure the patient is relaxed and recumbent for 30 minutes before the test.

Procedure
Perform a venipuncture, and collect a blood sample in a chilled 10-ml *lavender-top* tube.

Precautions
☐ Make sure the patient is relaxed before sample collection, since stress may elevate glucagon levels.
☐ Place the sample on ice and send it to the laboratory immediately.
☐ Handle the sample gently to prevent hemolysis.

Values
Fasting glucagon levels are normally less than 250 pg/ml.

Implications of results
Markedly elevated fasting glucagon levels occur in glucagonoma; values may range from 900 to 7800 pg/ml. Elevated levels also occur in diabetes mellitus, acute pancreatitis, and pheochromocytoma.

Abnormally low glucagon levels are associated with idiopathic glucagon deficiency and hypoglycemia due to chronic pancreatitis. Stimulation or suppression tests may be necessary to confirm diagnosis.

Post-test care
☐ If a hematoma develops at the venipuncture site, apply warm soaks.
☐ As ordered, resume diet and administration of drugs that were discontinued before the test.

Interfering factors
☐ Prolonged fasting, undue stress, or use of catecholamines or insulin before the collection of blood samples may elevate glucagon levels.

☐ Failure to pack the sample in ice and send it to the laboratory immediately may affect test results.
☐ Hemolysis caused by rough handling of the sample may interfere with accurate determination of test results.

WENDY BAKER, RN, MS, CCRN

Serum Gastrin

Gastrin is a polypeptide hormone produced and stored primarily by specialized G cells in the antrum of the stomach and, to a lesser degree, by the islets of Langerhans, in the pancreas. The main function of gastrin is to facilitate digestion of food by triggering gastric acid secretion in the parietal area of the stomach in response to food—especially proteins—vagal stimulation, or decreased stomach acidity. Secondarily, gastrin stimulates the release of pancreatic enzymes and the gastric enzyme pepsin, increases gastric and intestinal motility, and stimulates bile flow from the liver. Through a strong negative feedback control mechanism, acid in the gastric antrum inhibits gastrin release in response to all stimuli. However, abnormal secretion of gastrin can result from tumors (gastrinomas) and from pathologic disorders affecting the stomach, pancreas, and less commonly, the esophagus and the small bowel.

This radioimmunoassay, a quantitative analysis of gastrin levels, has significant diagnostic usefulness in patients suspected of having gastrinomas (Zollinger-Ellison syndrome). In doubtful situations, provocative testing may be necessary. However, gastrin estimation has limited value in persons with duodenal ulcer, as the role of gastrin in peptic ulcers is unclear.

Purpose

☐ To confirm diagnosis of gastrinoma, the gastrin-secreting tumor in Zollinger-Ellison syndrome

☐ To aid differential diagnosis of gastric and duodenal ulcers and pernicious anemia.

Patient preparation

Explain to the patient that this test helps determine the cause of gastrointestinal symptoms. Instruct him to abstain from alcohol for at least 24 hours before the test and to fast for 12 hours before the test (water is permitted). Tell him the test requires a blood sample; who will perform the venipuncture and when; and that he may feel some transient discomfort from the needle puncture. Reassure him that collecting the sample takes only a few minutes.

As ordered, withhold all medications that may interfere with test results, especially anticholinergics, such as atro-

---

GASTRIN STIMULATION TESTS

Since some patients with duodenal or gastric ulcers have normal fasting levels of gastrin, provocative testing is necessary to identify them; a protein-rich test meal serves this purpose. In a patient with duodenal or gastric ulcers, gastrin levels increase markedly after such a meal, while these levels rise only moderately in a healthy person.

Provocative testing is also necessary to distinguish a patient with duodenal or gastric ulcers from one suspected of having Zollinger-Ellison syndrome, since both may show similar baseline gastrin levels. One effective test involves I.V. infusion of calcium gluconate in a dosage of 5 mg/kg body weight over 3 hours. After the infusion, 10 ml of venous blood is drawn and sent to the laboratory. Gastrin levels double, rising to about 500 pg/ml, in a patient with Zollinger-Ellison syndrome; a patient with duodenal or gastric ulcers shows only a moderate rise or no change at all.

A third indication for provocative testing is an abnormally—but not strikingly—high fasting serum gastrin level. This is possible in both Zollinger-Ellison syndrome and in patients with pernicious anemia. To distinguish between the two, hydrochloric acid may be infused into the stomach through a nasogastric tube. Such infusion causes a sharp drop in gastrin levels in patients with pernicious anemia but not in patients with Zollinger-Ellison syndrome.

pine and belladonna, or insulin. If these medications must be continued, note this on the laboratory slip.

Because stress can increase gastrin levels, make sure the patient is relaxed and recumbent for at least 30 minutes before the test.

Procedure
Perform a venipuncture, and collect the sample in a 10 to 15 ml *red-top* tube.

Precautions
□ Handle the sample gently to avoid hemolysis.
□ To prevent destruction of serum gastrin by proteolytic enzymes, immediately send the sample to the laboratory, to have the serum separated and frozen.

Values
Serum gastrin levels are less than 300 pg/ml.

Implications of results
Strikingly high serum gastrin levels (over 1,000 pg/ml) confirm Zollinger-Ellison syndrome. (Levels as high as 450,000 pg/ml have been reported.)

Gastrin levels may be high in various conditions, but the concomitant findings of very low gastric juice pH and a very high serum gastrin level indicate autonomous hormone secretion not governed by a negative feedback mechanism. Increased serum levels of gastrin may occur in a few patients with duodenal ulceration (less than 1%) and in patients with achlorhydria (with or without pernicious anemia) or with extensive stomach carcinoma (because of hyposecretion of gastric juices and hydrochloric acid).

Post-test care
□ If a hematoma develops at the venipuncture site, apply warm soaks.
□ As ordered, resume diet, and administration of medications that were discontinued before the test.

Interfering factors
□ Failure to observe restrictions of diet, medications, or physical activity may interfere with accurate determination of test results.
□ Gastrin secretion is increased by amino acids (especially glycine), calcium carbonate, acetylcholine, calcium chloride, and ethanol; gastrin secretion is decreased by anticholinergics (atropine), hydrochloric acid, or secretin (a strongly basic polypeptide).
□ Insulin-induced hypoglycemia increases gastrin secretion.
□ Hemolysis caused by rough handling of the sample may interfere with accurate determination of test results.

THAD C. HAGEN, MD

GONADAL HORMONES

Serum Estrogens

Estrogens (and progesterone) are secreted by the ovaries under the influence of the pituitary gonadotropins, follicle-stimulating hormone (FSH) and luteinizing hormone (LH). Estrogens—in particular, estradiol, which is the most potent estrogen—interact with the hypothalamic-pituitary axis through both negative and positive feedback mechanisms. Slowly rising or sustained high levels inhibit secretion of FSH and LH (negative feedback), but a rapid rise in estrogen that occurs just before ovulation seems to stimulate LH secretion (positive feedback).

Estrogens are responsible for the development of secondary female sexual characteristics and for normal menstruation; levels are usually undetectable in children. These hormones are secreted by ovarian follicular cells during the first half of the menstrual cycle, and by the corpus luteum during the luteal phase and during pregnancy. In menopause, estrogen secretion drops to a constant, low level.

This radioimmunoassay measures serum levels of estradiol, estrone, and estriol—the only estrogens that appear in serum in measurable amounts—and has diagnostic significance in evaluating female gonadal dysfunction. Tests of hypothalamic-pituitary function may be required to confirm diagnosis.

Purpose
□ To determine sexual maturation and fertility
□ To aid diagnosis of gonadal dysfunction: precocious or delayed puberty, menstrual disorders (especially amenorrhea), or infertility
□ To determine fetal well-being
□ To aid diagnosis of tumors known to secrete estrogen.

Patient preparation
Explain to the patient that this test helps determine if secretion of female hormones is normal, and that the test may be repeated during the various phases of the menstrual cycle. Tell her she needn't restrict food or fluids. Inform her that the test requires a blood sample; who will perform the venipuncture and when; and that she may experience transient discomfort from the needle puncture. Collecting the sample takes only a few minutes. Withhold all steroid and pituitary-based hormones (including estrogens and progestogen), as ordered. If these medications must be continued, note this on the laboratory slip.

Procedure
Procedure may vary slightly, depending on choice of plasma or serum assay.

Perform a venipuncture, and collect the sample in a 10 ml *red-top* tube.

If the patient is premenopausal, indicate the phase of her menstrual cycle on the laboratory slip.

Precautions
To prevent hemolysis, handle the sample gently. Send it to the laboratory immediately for centrifugation.

ESTRIOL: CLUE TO FETAL WELL-BEING

Estriol represents about 90% of the estrogen produced during pregnancy after 20 weeks' gestation. The placenta converts fetal adrenal precursors into estriol, which is then conjugated by the maternal liver and excreted in maternal urine. Because estriol production depends on the fetus and placenta, levels serve as an index of fetal well-being and placental adequacy.

Disagreement exists as to the merits of measuring total plasma estriol, plasma unconjugated estriol (about 10% to 15% of total plasma estriol), and urine estriol. However, plasma estriol has several advantages over urine estriol—samples don't have to be collected at specific times and are less affected by medications. Of the plasma samples, unconjugated estriol appears to be preferred, because the sample is easier to analyze in the laboratory. Despite these differences, all three types of samples are commonly used to assess placental function and fetal well-being.

Values
Normal serum estrogen levels for premenopausal females vary widely during the menstrual cycle:

1 to 10 days	24 to 68 pg/ml
11 to 20 days	50 to 186 pg/ml
21 to 30 days	73 to 149 pg/ml

Serum estrogen levels in males range from 12 to 34 pg/ml. In girls age 6 and older, levels rise gradually to adult female values. In children under age 6, the normal range of serum estrogen is 3 to 10 pg/ml.

Implications of results
Decreased estrogen levels may indicate primary hypogonadism, or ovarian failure, as in Turner's syndrome or ovarian agenesis; secondary hypogonadism, as in hypopituitarism; or menopause. Abnormally high levels can occur with estrogen-producing tumors, in precocious puberty, or in severe hepatic dis-

ease, such as cirrhosis, that prevents clearance of plasma estrogens. High levels may also result from congenital adrenal hyperplasia (increased conversion of androgens to estrogen).

Post-test care
☐ If a hematoma develops at the venipuncture site, apply warm soaks.
☐ As ordered, resume administration of medications discontinued before the test.

Interfering factors
☐ Pregnancy and pretest use of estrogens (oral contraceptives) can increase serum estrogen levels. Clomiphene, an estrogen antagonist, can decrease serum estrogen levels. Ingestion of steroids or pituitary-based hormones can alter test results. For example, dexamethasone may suppress adrenal androgen secretion.
☐ Hemolysis caused by rough handling of the sample may interfere with accurate determination of test results.

SUSAN F. MORROW, RN

Plasma Progesterone

Progesterone, an ovarian steroid hormone secreted by the corpus luteum, causes thickening and secretory development of the endometrium in preparation for implantation of the fertilized ovum. Progesterone levels, therefore, peak during the midluteal phase of the menstrual cycle. Progesterone may prolong the surge of luteinizing hormone after ovulation. If implantation doesn't occur, progesterone (and estrogen) levels drop sharply and menstruation begins about 2 days later.

During pregnancy, the placenta releases about 10 times the normal monthly amount of progesterone to maintain the pregnancy. Increased secretion begins toward the end of the first trimester and continues until delivery. Progesterone causes thickening of the endometrium, which contains large amounts of stored nutrients for the developing ovum (blastocyst). Progesterone also prevents abortion by decreasing uterine contractions and, with estrogen, prepares the breasts for lactation.

This radioimmunoassay is a quantitative analysis of plasma progesterone levels, and provides reliable information about corpus luteum function in fertility studies or placental function in pregnancy. Serial determinations are recommended. Although plasma levels provide accurate information, progesterone can also be monitored by measuring urine pregnanediol, a catabolite of progesterone.

Purpose
☐ To assess corpus luteum function as part of infertility studies
☐ To evaluate placental function during pregnancy
☐ To aid in confirming ovulation. Test results support basal body temperature readings.

Patient preparation
Explain to the patient that this test helps determine if her female sex hormone secretion is normal. Inform her that she needn't restrict food or fluids. Tell her the test requires a blood sample, and who will perform the venipuncture and when. Reassure her that, although she may experience some transient discomfort from the needle puncture, collecting the blood sample takes only a few minutes. Inform her that the test may be repeated at specific times coinciding with phases of her menstrual cycle, or with each prenatal visit.

Procedure
Perform a venipuncture, and collect the sample in a 7 ml *green-top* (heparinized) tube.

Precautions
☐ Handle the sample gently to prevent hemolysis.
☐ Completely fill the collection tube, then invert it gently at least 10 times to mix sample and anticoagulant adequately.

THE ENDOMETRIAL CYCLE

Menstrual	Proliferative	Secretory	Menstrual

| 1 | 2 | 3 | 4 | 5 | 6 | 7 | 8 | 9 | 10 | 11 | 12 | 13 | 14 | 15 | 16 | 17 | 18 | 19 | 20 | 21 | 22 | 23 | 24 | 25 | 26 | 27 | 28 | 1 | 2 | 3 | 4 | 5 |

Days ───►

Each month progesterone, released by the corpus luteum, stimulates endometrial thickening in preparation for implantation of a fertilized ovum. The endometrial layer contains nutrients necessary for growth of the blastocyst. Immediately after menstruation, in the proliferative phase, the endometrium is thin and relatively homogenous. It continuously thickens until the end of the secretory phase, just before the menstrual phase begins again.

☐ Indicate the date of the patient's last menstrual period and the phase of her cycle on the laboratory slip. If the patient is pregnant, also indicate the month of gestation.
☐ Send the sample to the laboratory immediately.

Values
Normal values during menstruation:
☐ follicular phase: less than 150 ng/100 ml
☐ luteal phase: about 300 ng/100 ml (rises daily during periovulation)
☐ midluteal phase: 2,000 ng/100 ml.
Normal values during pregnancy:
☐ first trimester: 1,500 to 5,000 ng/100 ml
☐ second and third trimesters: 8,000 to 20,000 ng/100 ml.

Implications of results
Elevated progesterone levels may indicate ovulation, luteinizing tumors, ovarian cysts that produce progesterone, or adrenocortical hyperplasias and tumors that produce progesterone along with other steroidal hormones.

Low progesterone levels are associated with amenorrhea due to several causes (such as panhypopituitarism or gonadal dysfunction), toxemia of pregnancy, threatened abortion, and fetal death.

Post-test care
If a hematoma develops at the venipuncture site, apply warm soaks.

Interfering factors
☐ Hemolysis caused by rough handling of the sample may affect test results.
☐ Progesterone or estrogen therapy may interfere with accurate determination of test results.

SUSAN F. MORROW, RN

Testosterone

The principal androgen secreted by the interstitial cells of the testes (Leydig cells), testosterone induces puberty in the male and maintains male secondary sex characteristics. Prepubertal levels of testosterone are low. Increased testosterone secretion during puberty stimulates growth of the seminiferous tubules and the production of sperm; it also contributes to the enlargement of external genitalia, accessory sex organs (such as prostate glands), and voluntary muscles, and to the growth of facial, pubic, and axillary hair.

Testosterone production begins to increase at onset of puberty, under the influence of luteinizing hormone (LH) from the anterior pituitary, and continues to rise during adulthood. Testosterone inhibits gonadotropin secretion by a negative feedback mechanism similar to that of ovarian hormones in females. Production begins to taper off at about age 40, eventually dropping to approximately one fifth the peak level by age 80.

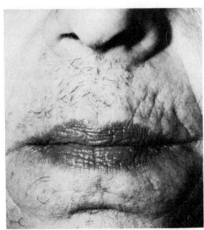

High levels of testosterone produce masculinization, including hirsutism (shown above)—abnormally heavy hair growth in androgen-sensitive areas, such as those around the mouth and on the chin.

In females, the adrenal glands and the ovaries secrete small amounts of testosterone.

This competitive protein-binding test measures plasma or serum testosterone levels and, when combined with plasma gonadotropin levels (follicle-stimulating hormone and LH), reliably aids evaluation of gonadal dysfunction in males and females.

Purpose
☐ To facilitate differential diagnosis of male sexual precocity (before age 10). True precocious puberty must be distinguished from pseudoprecocious puberty.
☐ To aid differential diagnosis of hypogonadism. Primary hypogonadism must be distinguished from secondary hypogonadism.
☐ To evaluate male infertility or other sexual dysfunction
☐ To evaluate hirsutism and virilization in females.

Patient preparation
Explain to the patient that this test helps determine if male sex hormone secretion is adequate. Inform him that he needn't restrict food or fluids. Tell him this test requires a blood sample; who will perform the venipuncture and when; and that he may experience some discomfort from the needle puncture. Reassure him that collecting the sample takes only a few minutes.

Procedure
Perform a venipuncture, and collect the sample in a 7 ml *red-top* tube. Use a *green-top* (heparinized) tube if plasma is to be collected. Indicate the patient's age, sex, and history of hormone therapy on the laboratory slip.

Precautions
Handle the sample gently to prevent hemolysis, and send it to the laboratory. The sample is stable and requires no refrigeration or preservative for up to 1 week. Frozen samples are stable for at least 6 months.

SITES OF TESTOSTERONE SECRETION

CROSS SECTION OF A TESTIS

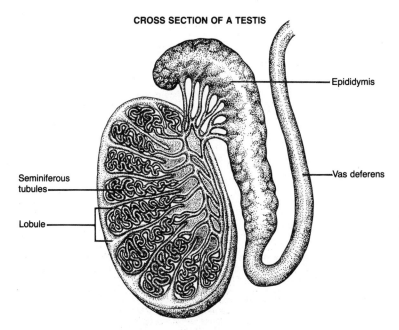

Epididymis

Seminiferous tubules

Lobule

Vas deferens

MICROSCOPIC VIEW OF SEMINIFEROUS TUBULES AND INTERSTITIAL LEYDIG CELLS

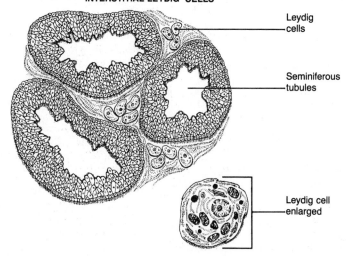

Leydig cells

Seminiferous tubules

Leydig cell enlarged

In the testis, several hundred pyramid-shaped lobules contain one or several seminiferous tubules. Within the tissue connecting the tubules, large polygonal Leydig cells secrete testosterone, the most potent androgenic hormone.

PRODUCTION OF SPERMATOZOA

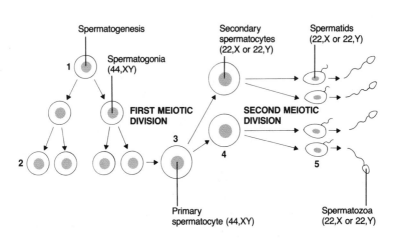

Spermatogenesis, the production of male gametes within the seminiferous tubules of the testes, is basically a five-step process: 1) Diploid spermatogonia, the cells forming the tubule's outer layer, divide mitotically to generate new cells used in spermatozoa production. 2) Some of the spermatogonia move toward the lumen of the tubule and enlarge to primary spermatocytes. 3) Each primary spermatocyte divides meiotically, forming two secondary spermatocytes, one retaining the X chromosome and the other the Y chromosome. 4) Each secondary spermatocyte also divides meiotically, becoming spermatids. 5) After a series of structural changes, the spermatids develop into mature spermatozoa.

Values

Normal levels of testosterone are as follows:

☐ males: 300 to 1,200 ng/dl
☐ females: 30 to 95 ng/dl
☐ prepubertal children: in males, less than 100 ng/dl; in females, less than 40 ng/dl.

Testosterone values vary slightly among laboratories.

Implications of results

Elevated testosterone levels in prepubertal males may indicate true sexual precocity due to excessive gonadotropin secretion, or pseudoprecocious puberty due to male hormone production by a testicular tumor. They can also indicate congenital adrenal hyperplasia, which results in virilization and precocious puberty in males (between ages 2 and 3), and pseudohermaphroditism and milder virilization in females (during and after puberty). Increased levels can also occur with a benign adrenal tumor or cancer, hyperthyroidism, or incipient puberty. In females with ovarian tumors or polycystic ovary syndrome, testosterone levels may rise slightly, leading to hirsutism.

Depressed testosterone levels can indicate primary hypogonadism (testicular failure, as in Klinefelter's syndrome) or secondary hypogonadism (hypogonadotropic eunuchoidism) resulting from hypothalamic-pituitary dysfunction. Depressed testosterone levels can also follow orchiectomy, testicular or prostatic cancer, delayed male puberty, estrogen therapy, or cirrhosis of the liver.

Post-test care

If a hematoma develops at the venipuncture site, apply warm soaks.

Interfering factors

□ Exogenous sources of estrogens or androgens can interfere with test results. Estrogens decrease free testosterone levels by increasing sex hormone–binding globulin (SHBG), which binds testosterone; androgens can elevate these levels.

Both thyroid and growth hormones decrease SHBG and increase free testosterone. Other pituitary-based hormones may also influence test results.

□ Hemolysis due to rough handling of the sample may affect test results.

SUSAN F. MORROW, RN

PLACENTAL HORMONES

Serum Human Chorionic Gonadotropin

Human chorionic gonadotropin (hCG) is a glycoprotein hormone produced by the trophoblastic cells (probably the syn-

cytiotrophoblasts) of the placenta. If conception occurs, a specific assay for hCG—commonly called the beta-subunit assay—may detect this hormone in the blood 9 days after ovulation. This interval coincides with the implantation of the fertilized ovum into the uterine wall. Although the precise function of hCG is still unclear, it appears that hCG, with progesterone, maintains

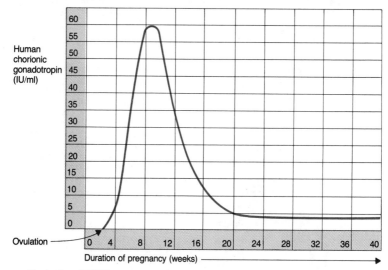

RATE OF HCG PRODUCTION AT DIFFERENT STAGES OF PREGNANCY

Human chorionic gonadotropin (IU/ml)

Ovulation

Duration of pregnancy (weeks)

Production of hCG increases steadily during the first trimester, peaking around the 10th week of gestation. Levels then fall to less than 10% of first trimester levels during the remainder of the pregnancy

Adapted with permission from Arthur C. Guyton, *Textbook of Medical Physiology* (Philadelphia: W.B. Saunders Co., 1981), p.1026.

the corpus luteum during early pregnancy.

Production of hCG increases steadily during the first trimester, peaking around the 10th week of gestation. Levels then fall to less than 10% of first trimester peak levels during the remainder of the pregnancy. At approximately 2 weeks after delivery, the hormone may no longer be detectable.

This serum radioimmunoassay, a quantitative analysis of hCG beta-subunit level, is much more sensitive (and costly) than the routine pregnancy test using a urine specimen.

Purpose

☐ To detect early pregnancy
☐ To determine adequacy of hormonal production in high-risk pregnancies (for example, habitual abortion)
☐ To aid diagnosis of trophoplastic tumors, such as hydatidiform moles or choriocarcinoma, and of tumors that ectopically secrete hCG
☐ To monitor treatment for induction of ovulation and conception.

Patient preparation

Explain to the patient that this test determines if she is pregnant. (If detection

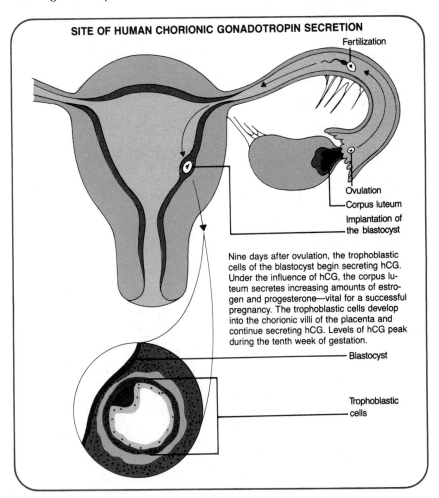

SITE OF HUMAN CHORIONIC GONADOTROPIN SECRETION

Fertilization

Ovulation
Corpus luteum
Implantation of the blastocyst

Nine days after ovulation, the trophoblastic cells of the blastocyst begin secreting hCG. Under the influence of hCG, the corpus luteum secretes increasing amounts of estrogen and progesterone—vital for a successful pregnancy. The trophoblastic cells develop into the chorionic villi of the placenta and continue secreting hCG. Levels of hCG peak during the tenth week of gestation.

Blastocyst

Trophoblastic cells

of pregnancy isn't the diagnostic objective, offer the appropriate explanation.) Inform her she needn't restrict food or fluids. Tell her the test requires a blood sample; who will perform the venipuncture and when; and that she may feel transient discomfort from the needle puncture. Collecting the sample, however, takes only a few minutes.

Procedure
Perform a venipuncture, and collect the sample in a 7 ml *red-top* tube.

Precautions
Handle the sample gently to prevent hemolysis, and send it to the laboratory immediately.

Values
Normal values for hCG are less than 3 mIU/ml. During pregnancy, hCG levels are quite variable and depend partially on the number of days after the last normal menstrual period.

Implications of results
Elevated hCG beta-subunit levels indicate pregnancy; significantly higher concentrations are present in a multiple pregnancy. Increased levels may also suggest hydatidiform mole, trophoblastic neoplasms of the placenta, or nontrophoplastic carcinomas that secrete hCG (including gastric, pancreatic, and ovarian adenocarcinomas). Low hCG beta-subunit levels can occur in ectopic pregnancy or pregnancy of less than 9 days. Beta-subunit levels cannot differentiate between pregnancy and tumor recurrence, because these levels are high in both conditions.

Post-test care
If a hematoma develops at the venipuncture site, apply warm soaks.

Interfering factors
☐ Heparin anticoagulants or EDTA (ethylenediaminotetraacetate) depresses plasma hCG levels and may interfere with accurate determination of test re-

sults. Check with the laboratory to be sure if the test is to be performed on plasma or serum.
☐ Hemolysis due to rough handling of the sample may affect test results.

WILLIAM M. DOUGHERTY, BS

Serum Human Placental Lactogen
[Human chorionic somatomammotropin (hCS)]

A polypeptide hormone secreted by placental syncytial trophoblasts, human placental lactogen (hPL) displays lactogenic and somatotropic (growth hormone) properties in the pregnant female. In combination with prolactin, hPL prepares the breasts for lactation. It also promotes lipolysis, liberating free fatty acids to provide energy for maternal metabolism and fetal nutrition. By exerting an anti-insulin effect, hPL causes the pancreas to secrete more insulin in response to rising blood sugar levels, thus facilitating protein synthesis and mobilization essential to fetal growth. Secretion is autonomous, beginning about the fifth week of gestation and declining rapidly after delivery. According to some evidence, this hormone may not be essential for a successful pregnancy.

This radioimmunoassay measures plasma hPL levels, which are roughly proportional to placental mass, as evidenced by higher levels in a multiple pregnancy. Such assays may be required in high-risk pregnancies (patients with diabetes mellitus, hypertension, or toxemia) or in suspected placental tissue dysfunction. Since values vary widely during the last half of pregnancy, serial determinations over several days provide the most reliable test results. This test, when combined with measurement of estriol levels, is a reliable indicator of placental function as well as fetal well-

being. This test may also be useful as a tumor marker in certain malignant states, such as ectopic tumors that secrete hPL.

Purpose
☐ To assess placental function
☐ To aid diagnosis of hydatidiform mole and choriocarcinoma. However, human chorionic gonadotropin levels are more diagnostic in these conditions.
☐ To aid diagnosis and monitor treatment of nontrophoblastic tumors that ectopically secrete hPL.

Patient preparation
Explain to the patient that this test helps assess placental function and fetal well-being. (If assessing fetal well-being isn't the diagnostic objective, offer an appropriate explanation.) Tell her the test requires a blood sample, and who will perform the venipuncture and when. Although she may experience transient discomfort from the needle puncture, reassure her that collecting the sample takes only a few minutes. Inform the pregnant patient that this test may be repeated during her pregnancy.

Procedure
Perform a venipuncture, and collect the sample in a 7 ml *red-top* tube.

Precautions
Handle the sample gently to prevent hemolysis, and send it to the laboratory without delay.

Values
For pregnant females, values are as follows:

Weeks of gestation	Normal hPL levels
5 to 27	< 4.6 mcg/ml
28 to 31	2.4 to 6.1 mcg/ml
32 to 35	3.7 to 7.7 mcg/ml
36 to term	5 to 8.6 mcg/ml

At term, patients with diabetes mellitus may have mean levels of 9 to 11 mcg/ml.

Normal levels for nonpregnant females are < 0.5 mcg/ml; normal levels for males, < 0.5 mcg/ml.

Implications of results
For reliable interpretation, hPL levels must be correlated with gestational age; for example, after 30 weeks' gestation, levels below 4 mcg/ml may indicate placental dysfunction. Subnormal concentrations of hPL are also associated with trophoblastic neoplastic disease, such as hydatidiform mole or choriocarcinoma. Low hPL concentrations are also characteristically associated with postmaturity syndrome, retardation of intrauterine growth, and toxemia of pregnancy. However, low hPL concentrations don't confirm fetal distress, although declining concentrations may help differentiate incomplete abortion from threatened abortion.

Conversely, concentrations over 4 mcg/ml after 30 weeks' gestation don't guarantee fetal well-being, since elevated levels have been reported after fetal death. An hPL value above 6 mcg/ml after 30 weeks' gestation may suggest an unusually large placenta, commonly occurring in patients with diabetes mellitus, multiple pregnancy, or Rh isoimmunization. Nevertheless, this test has limited use in predicting fetal death in a patient with diabetes or in managing Rh isoimmunization during pregnancy.

Abnormal concentrations of hPL have been found in the sera of patients with various malignancies, including bronchogenic carcinoma, hepatoma, lymphoma, and pheochromocytoma. In these patients, hPL levels are used as tumor markers for evaluation of chemotherapy, for monitoring tumor growth and recurrence, and for detection of residual tissue after excision.

Post-test care
If a hematoma develops at the venipuncture site, ease discomfort by applying warm soaks.

Interfering factors
Hemolysis caused by rough handling of the sample may interfere with accurate determination of test results.

SUSAN F. MORROW, RN

Selected References

Burke, M.D. "Thyroid Function Studies," *Postgraduate Medicine,* December 1980.

Butnaurescu, Glenda F. *Perinatal Nursing: Reproductive Health,* vol. 1. New York: John Wiley & Sons, 1978.

DeGroot, Leslie J. *Endocrinology,* vols. 1 to 3. New York: Grune & Stratton, 1979.

Endocrine Disorders. Nurse's Clinical Library. Springhouse, Pa.: Springhouse Corp., 1984.

Fischbach, Frances. *A Manual of Laboratory Diagnostic Tests,* 2nd ed. Philadelphia: J.B. Lippincott Co., 1984.

Gitnick, Gary L. *Practical Diagnosis: Gastrointestinal and Liver Disease.* New York: John Wiley & Sons, 1979.

Given, Barbara A., and Simmons, Sandra J. *Gastroenterology in Clinical Nursing,* 4th ed. St. Louis: C.V. Mosby Co., 1983.

Guyton, Arthur C. *Textbook of Medical Physiology,* 6th ed. Philadelphia: W.B. Saunders Co., 1981.

Hansten, Philip D. *Drug Interactions,* 5th ed. Philadelphia: Lea & Febiger, 1984.

Henry, John Bernard, ed. *Todd-Sanford-Davidsohn Clinical Diagnosis and Management by Laboratory Methods,* vol. 1, 17th ed. Philadelphia: W.B. Saunders Co., 1984.

Lamb, Jane O. *Laboratory Tests for Clinical Nursing.* Bowie, Md.: Robert J. Brady Co., 1984.

Leavelle, Dennis E., ed. *Mayo Medical Laboratories Test Catalog.* Rochester, Minn.: Mayo Medical Laboratories, 1984.

Luckmann, Joan, and Sorensen, Karen C. *Medical-Surgical Nursing: A Psychophysiologic Approach,* 2nd ed. Philadelphia: W.B. Saunders Co., 1980.

McNeely, Michael D. "Drug Interference with Laboratory Tests of Endocrine Function," *Drug Therapy* 11:1:105-14, 1981.

Nursing Critically Ill Patients Confidently, 2nd ed. New Nursing Skillbook series. Springhouse, Pa.: Springhouse Corp., 1984.

Petersdorf, Robert G., and Adams, Raymond

D., eds. *Harrison's Principles of Internal Medicine,* 10th ed. New York: McGraw-Hill Book Co., 1983.

Price, Sylvia, and Wilson, Lorraine. *Pathophysiology: Clinical Concepts of Disease Processes,* 2nd ed. New York: McGraw-Hill Book Co., 1982.

Pritchard, Jack, and MacDonald, Paul, eds. *Williams Obstetrics,* 16th ed. East Norwalk, Conn.: Appleton-Century-Crofts, 1980.

Ravel, Richard. *Clinical Laboratory Medicine,* 4th ed. Chicago: Year Book Medical Pubs., 1984.

Tilkian, Sarko M., et al. *Clinical Implications of Laboratory Tests,* 3rd ed. St. Louis: C.V. Mosby Co., 1983.

Tucker, Susan M., and Bryant, Sandra. *Fetal Monitoring and Fetal Assessment in High Risk Pregnancy.* St. Louis: C.V. Mosby Co., 1978.

Tulchinsky, Dan, and Ryan, Kenneth J. *Maternal-Fetal Endocrinology.* Philadelphia: W.B. Saunders Co., 1980.

Wallach, Jacques B. *Interpretation of Diagnostic Tests: A Handbook Synopsis of Laboratory Medicine,* 3rd ed. Boston: Little, Brown & Co., 1978.

Watts, Nelson B., and Keffer, Joseph H. *Practical Endocrine Diagnosis,* 3rd ed. Philadelphia: Lea & Febiger, 1982.

Wegener, Lee T., ed. *Mayo Medical Laboratories Interpretive Handbook.* Rochester, Minn.: Mayo Medical Laboratories, 1984.

Widmann, Frances K. *Clinical Interpretation of Laboratory Tests,* 9th ed. Philadelphia: F.A. Davis Co., 1983.

Williams, Robert H. *Textbook of Endocrinology,* 6th ed. Philadelphia: W.B. Saunders Co., 1981.

Wyngaarden, James, and Smith, Lloyd. *Cecil Textbook of Medicine,* 16th ed. Philadelphia: W.B. Saunders Co., 1982.

Vaughan, Victor C. III, et al., eds. *Nelson Textbook of Pediatrics,* 11th ed. Philadelphia: W.B. Saunders Co., 1979.

6 Lipids and Lipoproteins

LEARNING OBJECTIVES

After completing this chapter, the reader will be able to:
- name the four major lipids and the four major lipoproteins.
- describe the lipoprotein characteristics that permit classification by ultracentrifugation density and electrophoretic mobility.
- describe synthesis and metabolism of lipids and lipoproteins.
- list six types of familial hyperlipoproteinemias, their causes, incidences, signs, and laboratory findings.
- state the purpose of each test discussed in the chapter.
- prepare the patient physically and psychologically for each test.
- describe the procedure for performing each test.
- specify appropriate precautions for accurate administration of each test.
- implement appropriate post-test care.
- state the normal values for each test.
- discuss the implications of abnormal test results.
- list factors that may interfere with accurate test results.

Lipids and Lipoproteins

Introduction

Lipids, also called fats, are organic substances with a hydrophobic side chain or a steroid nucleus—or with both of these molecular features—that causes them to be insoluble in water. The major lipids are the triglycerides, free cholesterol, cholesteryl esters, and phospholipids. For transportation through the body, lipids must combine with plasma proteins into a lipid-protein molecular complex called lipoproteins: nonesterified fatty acids (free fatty acids) bind to albumin; other blood lipids (cholesterol [free and esterified], triglycerides, and phospholipids) bind to globulin.

Lipid differences

Lipoproteins can be described as an inner core of hydrophobic lipids (triglycerides and cholesteryl esters) within a membrane of proteins (apoproteins), associated with free cholesterol and phospholipids. Biochemical and physical differences among the lipoproteins depend on the specific apoprotein and the relative amount of the four lipids each contains. These differences permit classification by ultracentrifugation density and electrophoretic mobility:

□ *Chylomicrons*, the lowest density lipoproteins, consist mostly of triglyceride and are the form in which long-chain fats and cholesterol are transported from the intestine to the blood. Eventually, chylomicrons break down into other lip-

ids and nonesterified fatty acids. They are of such low density that they float without centrifugation and fail to migrate on paper electrophoresis.

□ *Very low-density (prebeta) lipoproteins* (VLDL) consist mostly of triglycerides, and smaller amounts of phospholipids, cholesterol, and protein.

□ *Low-density (beta) lipoproteins* (LDL) are approximately half cholesterol, and half protein, phospholipids, and triglycerides.

□ *High-density (alpha) lipoproteins* (HDL) are about half protein, and half phospholipids, cholesterol, and triglycerides.

Clinical implications

Lipoprotein phenotyping—classifying patients by the pattern of their lipoprotein levels—is an important procedure for diagnosing and treating hyper- and hypolipoproteinemias. These disorders produce a variety of symptoms ranging from mild (such as xanthomas) to severe (such as pancreatitis).

Lipoprotein determinations are also useful in evaluating the risk of coronary artery disease (CAD). At one time, total blood cholesterol—the amount of cholesterol in all lipoproteins—was considered the major indicator of CAD for patients under age 50. However, the Framingham Heart Study found that high levels of HDL-cholesterol actually help

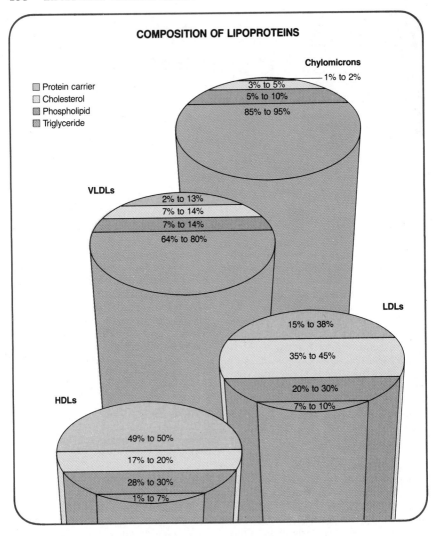

COMPOSITION OF LIPOPROTEINS

☐ Protein carrier
☐ Cholesterol
☐ Phospholipid
☐ Triglyceride

Chylomicrons
1% to 2%
3% to 5%
5% to 10%
85% to 95%

VLDLs
2% to 13%
7% to 14%
7% to 14%
64% to 80%

LDLs
15% to 38%
35% to 45%
20% to 30%
7% to 10%

HDLs
49% to 50%
17% to 20%
28% to 30%
1% to 7%

prevent CAD, whereas high levels of LDL-cholesterol increase the risk. Apparently, HDLs help the enzyme lecithin cholesterol acyltransferase remove cholesterol from arterial walls. Further study has shown that patients with angina pectoris or myocardial infarction generally have lower HDL-cholesterol than healthy persons, and that low HDL-cholesterol levels—which can be hereditary—are not just associated with CAD but precede it. Low HDL-cholesterol levels are also connected with diabetes mellitus, hypertension, cigarette smoking, obesity, and lack of exercise.

Although HDL-cholesterol and LDL-cholesterol are good indicators of risk of CAD, a full lipoprotein profile is a more useful measure. This battery of tests includes total cholesterol, total triglycerides, and lipoprotein phenotyping.

Antilipemic regimen

Care for patients with elevated LDL-cholesterol consists of teaching modification of diet and life-style to reduce the

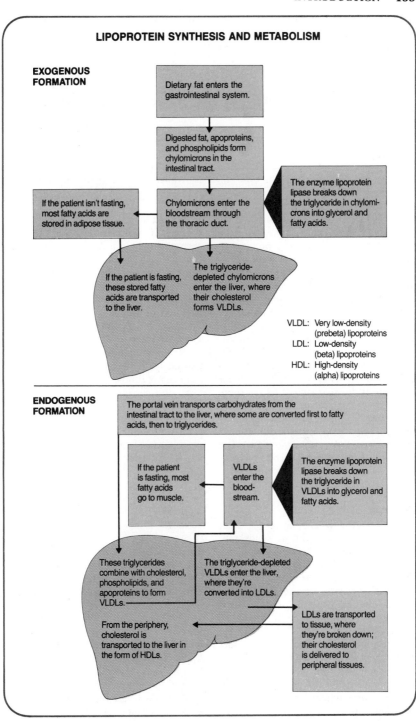

LIPOPROTEIN SYNTHESIS AND METABOLISM

EXOGENOUS FORMATION

Dietary fat enters the gastrointestinal system.

Digested fat, apoproteins, and phospholipids form chylomicrons in the intestinal tract.

The enzyme lipoprotein lipase breaks down the triglyceride in chylomicrons into glycerol and fatty acids.

If the patient isn't fasting, most fatty acids are stored in adipose tissue.

Chylomicrons enter the bloodstream through the thoracic duct.

If the patient is fasting, these stored fatty acids are transported to the liver.

The triglyceride-depleted chylomicrons enter the liver, where their cholesterol forms VLDLs.

VLDL: Very low-density (prebeta) lipoproteins
LDL: Low-density (beta) lipoproteins
HDL: High-density (alpha) lipoproteins

ENDOGENOUS FORMATION

The portal vein transports carbohydrates from the intestinal tract to the liver, where some are converted first to fatty acids, then to triglycerides.

If the patient is fasting, most fatty acids go to muscle.

VLDLs enter the bloodstream.

The enzyme lipoprotein lipase breaks down the triglyceride in VLDLs into glycerol and fatty acids.

These triglycerides combine with cholesterol, phospholipids, and apoproteins to form VLDLs.

The triglyceride-depleted VLDLs enter the liver, where they're converted into LDLs.

From the periphery, cholesterol is transported to the liver in the form of HDLs.

LDLs are transported to tissue, where they're broken down; their cholesterol is delivered to peripheral tissues.

risk of heart disease. For example, exercise (especially running), low blood pressure, and diets that restrict fat intake may raise levels of beneficial HDL-cholesterol.

JOHN J. FENTON, PhD

LIPIDS

Triglycerides

This test provides quantitative analysis of triglycerides—the main storage form of lipids—which constitute about 95% of fatty tissue. Although not in itself diagnostic, serum triglyceride analysis permits early identification of hyperlipemia (characteristic in nephrotic syndrome and other conditions) and risk of coronary artery disease (CAD).

Triglyceride consists of one molecule of glycerol bonded to three molecules of fatty acids (usually some combination of stearic, oleic, and palmitic). Thus, the degradation of triglyceride leads directly to production of fatty acid. Together with carbohydrates, these compounds furnish energy for metabolism. Serum triglycerides are associated with several lipid aggregates, primarily chylomicrons, whose major function is transport of dietary triglycerides. When present in serum, chylomicrons produce a cloudiness that interferes with many laboratory tests.

Purpose
☐ To screen for hyperlipemia
☐ To help identify nephrotic syndrome
☐ To determine the risk of CAD.

Patient preparation
Define triglycerides for the patient, and explain that this test helps detect disorders of fat metabolism. Advise him to abstain from food for 12 to 14 hours before the test and from alcohol for 24 hours before the test; he doesn't need to abstain from water. Tell him the test requires a blood sample; who will perform the venipuncture and when; and that he may experience transient discomfort from the needle puncture and the pressure of the tourniquet. Collecting the sample takes no more than 3 minutes.

As ordered, withhold medications that may alter test results (antilipemics, steroids, estrogen, and some diuretics).

Procedure
Perform a venipuncture, and collect a serum sample in a 7 ml *red-top* tube. A plasma sample is acceptable if a serum sample can't be collected but gives values that are usually slightly lower and that do not correlate reliably with the normal range in serum.

Precautions
Send the sample to the laboratory immediately. Some redistribution may occur among lipids.

Values
Triglyceride values are age-related. Some controversy exists over the most appropriate normal ranges, but the following are fairly widely accepted:

Age	Triglycerides, mg/dl
0 to 29	10 to 140
30 to 39	10 to 150
40 to 49	10 to 160
50 to 59	10 to 190

Implications of results
Increased or decreased serum triglyceride levels merely suggest a clinical abnormality, and additional tests are required for definitive diagnosis. For example, measurement of cholesterol may also be necessary, since cholesterol and triglycerides vary independently. High levels of triglyceride and cholesterol reflect an exaggerated risk of CAD.

Mild-to-moderate increase in serum triglyceride levels indicates biliary obstruction, diabetes, nephrotic syndrome, endocrinopathies, or overconsumption of alcohol. Markedly increased levels without an identifiable cause reflect congenital hyperlipoproteinemia and necessitate lipoprotein phenotyping to confirm diagnosis.

Decreased serum levels are rare, occurring mainly in malnutrition or abetalipoproteinemia. In the latter, serum is virtually devoid of beta-lipoproteins and triglycerides, because the body lacks the capacity to transport preformed triglycerides from the epithelial cells of the intestinal mucosa or from the liver.

Post-test care
□ If a hematoma develops at the venipuncture site, apply warm soaks.
□ As ordered, resume the administration of any medications and diet discontinued before the test.

Interfering factors
□ A plasma sample may produce slightly lower values than a serum sample.
□ Failure to comply with dietary restrictions may interfere with accurate determination of test results.
□ Ingestion of alcohol within 24 hours of the test may cause elevated triglyceride levels. In fact, excessive consumption of alcohol is a common cause of excess concentration of triglycerides. Alcohol is heavily hydrogenated. As a result, this hydrogen has to be disposed of during alcohol metabolism; most of it ultimately ends up in triglyceride. Fatty liver is an early manifestation of this metabolic phenomenon.
□ Certain drugs lower cholesterol levels but raise or may have no effect on triglyceride levels: All antilipemics lower serum lipid concentration in the bloodstream, although their mechanism of action may differ. Cholestyramine lowers cholesterol; it raises or may have no effect on triglycerides. Colestipol lowers cholesterol; it raises or may have no effect on triglycerides.
□ Long-term use of corticosteroids raises triglyceride levels, as does use of oral contraceptives, estrogen, ethyl alcohol, furosemide, and miconazole.

□ Clofibrate, dextrothyroxine, gemfibrozil, and niacin lower cholesterol and triglyceride levels.
□ Certain drugs have a variable effect: Probucol inhibits transport of cholesterol from the intestine and may also affect cholesterol synthesis. It lowers cholesterol but has a variable effect on triglycerides.

JOHN J. FENTON, PhD

Total Cholesterol

This test, the quantitative analysis of serum cholesterol, measures the circulating levels of free cholesterol and cholesterol esters; it reflects the level of the two forms in which this biochemical compound appears in the body. Total cholesterol is the only cholesterol routinely measured.

Cholesterol, a structural component in cell membranes and plasma lipoproteins, is both absorbed from the diet and synthesized in the liver and other body tissues. It's then metabolized to steroid hormones, glucocorticoids, and bile acids.

A diet high in saturated fat raises cholesterol levels by stimulating absorption of lipids, including cholesterol, from the intestine; a low–saturated-fat diet lowers them. High serum cholesterol levels may be associated with an increased risk of coronary artery disease (CAD).

Purpose
□ To assess the risk of CAD
□ To evaluate fat metabolism
□ To aid diagnosis of nephrotic syndrome, pancreatitis, hepatic disease, and hypo- and hyperthyroidism.

Patient preparation
Explain to the patient that this test determines the body's fat metabolism. If the patient is hospitalized, enforce overnight fast and abstention from alcohol for 24 hours before the test. Tell the patient the test will require a blood sample; who

---

CHOLESTEROL AND ESTROGEN

The higher incidence of heart disease among men and postmenopausal women, as compared with premenopausal women, may result from low levels of estrogen, a hormone that helps regulate HDL-cholesterol synthesis. Paradoxically, oral contraceptives and pregnancy elevate serum HDL-cholesterol levels. However, since HDL-cholesterol levels are only 5% to 8% lower in premenopausal women than in men of the same age, the potentially protective action of estrogens against atherosclerosis remains controversial. Moreover, most men would reject estrogen therapy because of its side effects.

---

will perform the venipuncture and when; and that he may experience transient discomfort from the needle puncture and the pressure of the tourniquet. Collecting the sample takes no more than 3 minutes.

As ordered, withhold drugs that influence cholesterol levels.

Procedure

Perform a venipuncture, and collect the sample in a 7 ml *red-top* tube.

Precautions

Send the sample to the laboratory immediately, since cholesterol isn't stable at room temperature.

Values

Total cholesterol concentrations vary with age and sex, and may range from 120 mg/dl to 330 mg/dl.

Implications of results

Elevated serum cholesterol (hypercholesterolemia) may indicate risk of CAD, as well as incipient hepatitis, lipid disorders, bile duct blockage, nephrotic syndrome, obstructive jaundice, pancreatitis, and hypothyroidism. Hypercholesterolemia due to high dietary intake requires modification of eating habits and, possibly, medication to retard absorption of cholesterol.

Low serum cholesterol (hypocholes-

terolemia) is commonly associated with malnutrition, cellular necrosis of the liver, and hyperthyroidism. Abnormal cholesterol levels frequently necessitate further testing to pinpoint the disorder, depending on the type of abnormality and the presence of overt signs. Abnormal levels associated with cardiovascular diseases, for example, may necessitate lipoprotein phenotyping.

Post-test care

□ If a hematoma develops at the venipuncture site, apply warm soaks.
□ As ordered, resume diet and medications discontinued before the test.

Interfering factors

□ Cholesterol levels are lowered by cholestyramine, clofibrate, colestipol, dextrothyroxine, haloperidol, neomycin, niacin, and chlortetracycline. Levels are raised by epinephrine, chlorpromazine, trifluoperazine, oral contraceptives, and trimethadione. Androgens may have a variable effect on cholesterol levels.
□ Failure to follow dietary restrictions may interfere with test results.

JOHN J. FENTON, PhD

Phospholipids

Phospholipid assay was formerly an important test because of the lack of more specific tests and the relative unreliability of other lipid assays. Today, however, this quantitative analysis of phospholipid levels adds minimal information to that provided by cholesterol levels. Phospholipids are not associated with coronary artery disease and are seldom included in routine lipid evaluation.

Phospholipids, the largest and most soluble of the lipid elements, are molecules composed of glycerol, fatty acids, and phosphate. In human plasma, the main phospholipids are lecithins, cephalins, and sphingomyelins. Dietary phospholipids are partially broken down by pancreatic enzymes before absorption by the mucosal cells. Phospholipids fulfill a variety of body functions, including cellular membrane composition and permeability, and some control of enzyme activity within the membrane. They have a tendency to concentrate at cell membranes and aid the transport of fatty acids and lipids across the intestinal barrier, and from the liver and other fat depots to other body tissues. Phospholipids, especially saturated lecithin, are also essential for pulmonary gas exchange, as evidenced by neonatal respiratory distress syndrome in premature infants who lack them.

Purpose
□ To aid in the evaluation of fat metabolism
□ To aid diagnosis of hypothyroidism, diabetes mellitus, nephrotic syndrome, chronic pancreatitis, obstructive jaundice, and hypolipoproteinemia.

Patient preparation
Explain to the patient that this test helps determine how the body metabolizes fats. Instruct him to abstain from ingestion of alcohol for 24 hours before the test, and from food and fluids after midnight before the test. Tell him the test requires a blood sample; who will perform the venipuncture and when; and that he may experience transient discomfort from the needle puncture and the pressure of the tourniquet. Collecting the sample takes about 3 minutes. Withhold antilipemic drugs, as ordered.

Procedure
Perform a venipuncture, and collect the sample in a 10 to 15 ml *red-top* tube.

Precautions
Send the sample to the laboratory immediately, since spontaneous redistribution may occur among plasma lipids.

Values
Normal phospholipid levels range from 180 to 320 mg/dl. Although males usually have higher levels than females, values in pregnant females exceed those of males.

Implications of results
Elevated levels may indicate hypothyroidism, diabetes mellitus, nephrotic syndrome, chronic pancreatitis, or obstructive jaundice. Decreased levels may indicate primary hypolipoproteinemia.

Post-test care
□ If a hematoma develops at the venipuncture site, apply warm soaks.
□ Resume diet and administration of medications that were discontinued before the test, as ordered.

Interfering factors
□ Clofibrate and other antilipemics may lower phospholipid levels; estrogens, epinephrine, and some phenothiazines, such as chlorpromazine, increase levels.
□ Failure to follow dietary restrictions may interfere with accurate determination of test results.

JOHN J. FENTON, PhD

LIPOPROTEINS

Lipoprotein-Cholesterol Fractionation

Cholesterol fractionation tests isolate and measure the cholesterol in serum—low-density lipoproteins (LDL) and high-density lipoproteins (HDL)—by ultracentrifugation or electrophoresis. The cholesterol in LDL and HDL fractions is significant, since the Framingham Heart Study has shown that cholesterol in HDL is inversely related to the incidence of coronary artery disease (CAD)—the higher the HDL level, the lower the incidence of CAD; conversely, the higher the

---

APOLIPOPROTEINS AND CAD

Although measurement of apolipoproteins—the protein fractions of lipoprotein molecules—is primarily a research procedure, mounting evidence suggests that it may have important clinical applications as well. Because apolipoprotein levels can be directly measured in serum, they may more accurately indicate an individual's risk of CAD than HDL or LDL levels, which must be indirectly measured.

Currently, eight apolipoproteins have been identified. Of these, apolipoprotein A (ApoA)—the major protein component of HDL—and apolipoprotein B (ApoB)—the major protein component of LDL—are the most clinically significant. Reduced ApoA levels (below 140 mg/dl) occur in ischemic heart disease, while elevated ApoB levels (above 135 mg/dl) occur in hyperlipemia, angina pectoris, and myocardial infarction.

LDL level, the higher the incidence of CAD.

Purpose
☐ To assess the risk of CAD.

Patient preparation
Tell the patient that this test helps determine the risk of CAD. Instruct him to maintain his normal diet for 2 weeks before the test, to abstain from alcohol for 24 hours before the test, and to fast and avoid exercise for 12 to 14 hours before the test. Tell the patient the test requires a blood sample; who will perform the venipuncture and when; and that he may experience transient discomfort from the needle puncture and the pressure of the tourniquet. Collecting the sample takes less than 3 minutes.

As ordered, withhold thyroid hormones, oral contraceptives, and antilipemics, which alter test results.

Procedure
Perform a venipuncture, and collect the sample in a 7 ml *red-top* tube.

Precautions
Send the sample to the laboratory immediately, since spontaneous redistri-

bution of cholesterol occurs among the lipoproteins. If the sample can't be transported immediately, it should be refrigerated but not frozen.

Values
Since normal cholesterol values vary according to age, sex, geographic region, and ethnic group, check the laboratory for the normal values in your hospital. An alternate method (measuring cholesterol and triglyceride levels, and separating out HDL by selective precipitation and using these values to calculate LDL) provides normal HDL-cholesterol levels that range from 29 to 77 mg/100 ml and normal LDL-cholesterol levels that range from 62 to 185 mg/100 ml.

Implications of results
High LDL levels increase the risk of CAD. Elevated HDL levels generally reflect a healthy state but can also indicate chronic hepatitis, early-stage primary biliary cirrhosis, or alcohol consumption. Rarely, a sharp rise (to as high as 100 mg/dl) in a second type of HDL (alpha$_2$-HDL) may signal CAD. Although cholesterol fractionation provides valuable information about the risk of heart disease, remember that other sources of such risk—diabetes mellitus, hypertension, cigarette smoking—are at least as important.

Post-test care
☐ If a hematoma develops at the venipuncture site, apply warm soaks.
☐ Resume diet and administration of medications withheld, as ordered.

Interfering factors
☐ Values are lowered by antilipemic medications, such as clofibrate, cholestyramine, colestipol, dextrothyroxine, niacin, probucol, and gemfibrozil.
☐ Oral contraceptives, disulfiram, alcohol, miconazole, and high doses of phenothiazines may increase values.
☐ Estrogens usually increase but may decrease values.
☐ Failure to send the sample to the laboratory immediately may allow sponta-

neous redistribution of the lipoproteins and alter test results.

☐ Collecting the sample in a heparinized tube may produce false elevation of values through activation of the enzyme lipase, which, in turn, causes the release of fatty acids from triglycerides.

☐ Presence of bilirubin, hemoglobin, salicylates, iodine, vitamins A and D, and some other substances may affect accurate determination of values. Some procedures (for example, Abell-Kendall) are less susceptible to interference than others.

☐ Concurrent illness, especially if accompanied by fever, recent surgery, or myocardial infarction, may interfere with accurate determination of test results.

JOHN J. FENTON, PhD

Lipoprotein Phenotyping

In lipoprotein phenotyping, ultracentrifugation and electrophoresis of a blood sample determine lipoprotein levels. The density of the four major lipoproteins varies, depending on their relative percentages of triglyceride and protein: chylomicrons, which are very light lipid aggregates, consist of 85% to 95% triglycerides, 5% to 10% phospholipids, 3% to 5% cholesterol, and 1% to 2% protein; very low-density (prebeta) lipoproteins (VLDL) consist of 64% to 80% triglycerides, 7% to 14% phospholipids, 7% to 14% cholesterol, and 2% to 13% protein; low-density (beta) lipoproteins (LDL), consist of 7% to 10% triglycerides, 20% to 30% phospholipids, 35% to 45% cholesterol, and 15% to 38% protein; and high-density (alpha) lipoproteins (HDL), consist of about 1% to 7% triglycerides, 28% to 30% phospholipids, 17% to 20% cholesterol, and 49% to 50% protein.

For transportation through the blood, most lipids must combine with water-soluble proteins (apoproteins) to form lipoproteins. Several types of lipoproteins normally exist in the body, but in certain familial disorders, the blood levels of these types change. Classification of patients by the pattern of their lipoprotein levels identifies hyper- and hypolipoproteinemias.

Purpose

☐ To determine classification of hyper- or hypolipoproteinemia.

Patient preparation

Explain to the patient that this test helps determine how the body metabolizes fats. Instruct him to abstain from alcohol for 24 hours before the test and to fast after midnight before the test. Tell him this test requires a blood sample; who will perform the venipuncture and when; and that he may experience transient discomfort from the needle puncture and the pressure of the tourniquet. Reassure the patient that collecting the sample generally takes no more than 3 minutes. Provide a low-fat meal the night before the test.

Check the patient's drug history for use of heparin. As ordered, withhold antilipemics, such as cholestyramine, about 2 weeks before the test.

Notify the laboratory if the patient is hospitalized for any other condition that might significantly alter lipoprotein metabolism, such as diabetes mellitus, nephrosis, or hypothyroidism.

Procedure

Perform a venipuncture, and collect the sample in a 7 ml *lavender-top* tube.

Precautions

☐ When drawing multiple samples, collect the sample for lipoprotein phenotyping first, since venous obstruction for 2 minutes can affect test results.

☐ Fill the collection tube completely, and invert it gently several times to mix the sample and the anticoagulant.

☐ Handle the sample gently to prevent he-

FAMILIAL HYPERLIPOPROTEINEMIAS

TYPE	CAUSES AND INCIDENCE	CLINICAL SIGNS	LABORATORY FINDINGS
I	• Deficient lipoprotein lipase, resulting in increased chylomicrons • May be induced by alcoholism • Incidence: rare	• Eruptive xanthomas • Lipemia retinalis • Abdominal pain	• Increased chylomicron, total cholesterol, and triglyceride levels • Normal or slightly increased VLDL • Normal or decreased LDL and HDL • Cholesterol-triglyceride ratio under 0.2
IIa	• Deficient cell receptor, resulting in increased LDL and excessive cholesterol synthesis • May be induced by hypothyroidism • Incidence: common	• Premature coronary artery disease (CAD) • Arcus cornea • Xanthelasma • Tendinous and tuberous xanthomas	• Increased LDL • Normal VLDL • Cholesterol-triglyceride ratio over 2.0
IIb	• Deficient cell receptor resulting in increased LDL and excessive cholesterol synthesis • May be induced by dysgammaglobulinemia, hypothyroidism, uncontrolled diabetes mellitus, and nephrotic syndrome • Incidence: common	• Premature CAD • Obesity • Possible xanthelasmas	• Increased LDL, VLDL, total cholesterol, and triglycerides
III	• Unknown cause, resulting in deficient VLDL-to-LDL conversion • May be induced by hypothyroidism, uncontrolled diabetes mellitus, and paraproteinemia • Incidence: rare	• Premature CAD • Arcus cornea • Eruptive tuberous xanthomas	• Increased total cholesterol, VLDL, and triglycerides • Normal or decreased LDL • Cholesterol-triglyceride ratio of VLDL over 0.4 • Broad beta band observed on electrophoresis
IV	• Unknown cause, resulting in decreased levels of lipoprotein lipase (LPL) • May be induced by uncontrolled diabetes mellitus, alcoholism, pregnancy, steroid or estrogen therapy, dysgammaglobulinemia, and hyperthyroidism • Incidence: common	• Possible premature CAD • Obesity • Hypertension • Peripheral neuropathy	• Increased VLDL and triglycerides • Normal LDL • Cholesterol-triglyceride ratio of VLDL under 0.25
V	• Unknown cause, resulting in defective triglyceride clearance • May be induced by alcoholism, dysgammaglobulinemia, uncontrolled diabetes mellitus, nephrotic syndrome, pancreatitis, and steroid therapy • Incidence: rare	• Premature CAD • Abdominal pain • Lipemia retinalis • Eruptive xanthomas • Hepatosplenomegaly	• Increased VLDL, total cholesterol, and triglycerides • Chylomicrons present • Cholesterol-triglyceride ratio under 0.6

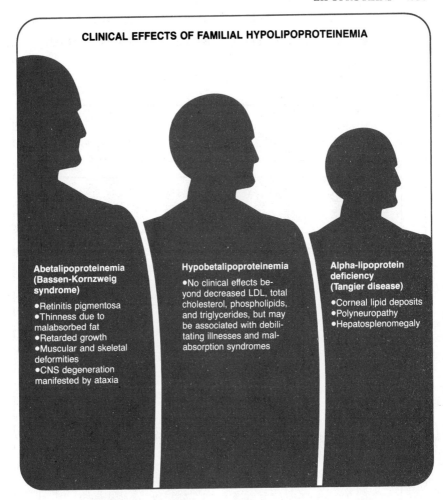

CLINICAL EFFECTS OF FAMILIAL HYPOLIPOPROTEINEMIA

Abetalipoproteinemia (Bassen-Kornzweig syndrome)
- Retinitis pigmentosa
- Thinness due to malabsorbed fat
- Retarded growth
- Muscular and skeletal deformities
- CNS degeneration manifested by ataxia

Hypobetalipoproteinemia
- No clinical effects beyond decreased LDL, total cholesterol, phospholipids, and triglycerides, but may be associated with debilitating illnesses and malabsorption syndromes

Alpha-lipoprotein deficiency (Tangier disease)
- Corneal lipid deposits
- Polyneuropathy
- Hepatosplenomegaly

molysis, which can alter test results.

Values

The types of hyperlipoproteinemias or hypolipoproteinemias are identified by their characteristic electrophoretic patterns. The laboratory reports the type of lipoproteinemia present. (See the chart on page 208 for patterns in the six types of hyperlipoproteinemias.)

Implications of results

Familial lipoprotein disorders are classified as either hyper- or hypolipoproteinemias.

The hyperlipoproteinemias break down into six types—I, IIa, IIb, III, IV, and V. Types IIa, IIb, and IV are relatively common. In contrast, all hypolipoproteinemias are rare, and include hypobetalipoproteinemia, abetalipoproteinemia (Bassen-Kornzweig syndrome), and alpha-lipoprotein deficiency (Tangier disease).

Post-test care

☐ If a hematoma develops at the venipuncture site, apply warm soaks.
☐ Instruct the patient to resume his normal diet.
☐ As ordered, resume administration of medications withheld before the test.

HYPERLIPOPROTEINEMIAS: ELECTROPHORETIC PATTERNS ON PAPER

In electrophoresis, lipoproteins are separated into four bands: chylomicrons, beta, prebeta, and alpha. The migratory patterns of these lipoproteins help identify the six types of familial hyperlipoproteinemias.

A heavy chylomicron band with faint beta and prebeta bands indicates Type I. Type IIa is characterized by heavy beta and negligible prebeta bands; Type IIb, by heavy beta and prebeta bands. In Type III, the two beta bands usually merge. A heavy prebeta band distinguishes Type IV. In Type V, both the chylomicron and prebeta bands are most distinct.

Interfering factors

□ Hemolysis due to rough handling of the sample may affect accurate determination of test results.

□ Failure to observe diet and alcohol restrictions, or recent use of antilipemics, which lower lipid levels, may interfere with accurate determination of values.

□ Administration of heparin (which activates the enzyme lipase, producing fatty acids from triglycerides) or collection of the sample in a heparinized tube may falsely elevate values.

JOHN J. FENTON, PhD

Selected References

Cardiovascular Disorders. Nurse's Clinical Library. Springhouse, Pa.: Springhouse Corp., 1984.

Gilman, Alfred G., et al., eds. *Goodman and Gilman's The Pharmacological Basis of Therapeutics,* 6th ed. New York: Macmillan Publishing Co., 1980.

Guyton, Arthur C. *Textbook of Medical Physiology,* 6th ed. Philadelphia: W.B. Saunders Co., 1981.

Hansten, Philip D. *Drug Interactions,* 5th ed. Philadelphia: Lea & Febiger, 1984.

Hartung, G. Harley, et al. "Relation of Diet to High-Density Lipoprotein Cholesterol in Middle-Aged Marathon Runners, Joggers, and Inactive Men," *New England Journal of Medicine* 302:1357-61, February 14, 1980.

Henry, John Bernard, ed. *Todd-Sanford-Davidsohn Clinical Diagnosis and Management by Laboratory Methods,* vol. 1, 17th ed. Philadelphia: W.B. Saunders Co., 1984.

Mazzaferri, Ernest L., ed. *Endocrinology: A Review of Clinical Endocrinology.* New Hyde Park, N.Y.: Medical Examination Pub. Co., 1980.

Netter, Frank, illus. *The CIBA Collection of Medical Illustrations.* West Caldwell, N.J.: CIBA Pharmaceutical Co., 1974.

Nursing85 Drug Handbook. Springhouse, Pa.: Springhouse Corp., 1985.

Petersdorf, Robert G., and Adams, Raymond D., eds. *Harrison's Principles of Internal Medicine,* 10th ed. New York: McGraw-Hill Book Co., 1983.

Ravel, Richard. *Clinical Laboratory Medicine,* 4th ed. Chicago: Year Book Medical Pubs., 1984.

Stallones, Revel A. "The Rise and Fall of Ischemic Heart Disease," *Scientific American* 243:53-59, November 1980.

Stanbury, John B., and Wyngaarden, James B. *The Metabolic Basis of Inherited Disease,* 5th ed. New York: McGraw-Hill Book Co., 1983.

Tilkian, Sarko M., et al. *Clinical Implications of Laboratory Tests,* 3rd ed. St. Louis: C.V. Mosby Co., 1983.

Widmann, Frances K. *Clinical Interpretation of Laboratory Tests,* 9th ed. Philadelphia: F.A. Davis Co., 1983.

Witzun, Joseph L., et al. "Normalization of Triglycerides in Type IV Hyperlipoproteinemia Fails to Correct Low Levels of High-Density Lipoprotein Cholesterol," *New England Journal of Medicine* 303:907-13, October 16, 1980.

Zilva, Joan F., and Pannall, P.R. *Clinical Chemistry in Diagnosis and Treatment,* 3rd ed. Chicago: Year Book Medical Pubs., 1979.

7 Proteins, Protein Metabolites, and Pigments

LEARNING OBJECTIVES

After completing this chapter, the reader will be able to:
- describe the formation and metabolism of serum proteins.
- identify the five major steps in the formation of bile pigments.
- discuss excretion mechanisms of protein metabolites.
- explain inheritance patterns in phenylketonuria.
- identify the four stages of hepatic coma.
- explain bilirubin metabolism.
- recognize signs of hemolysis in patients with low serum haptoglobin levels.
- state the purpose of each test discussed in the chapter.
- prepare the patient physically and psychologically for each test.
- describe the procedure for performing each test.
- specify appropriate precautions for accurate administration of each test.
- implement appropriate post-test care.
- state the normal values for each test.
- discuss the implications of abnormal test results.
- list factors that may interfere with accurate test results.

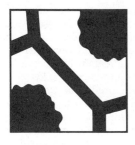

Proteins, Protein Metabolites, and Pigments

Introduction

Serum proteins, the most abundant compounds in serum, function quite differently from tissue proteins. They have great diagnostic significance because of their various and vital functions: binding and detoxifying drugs and other potentially toxic substances; synthesizing antibodies, enzymes, and hormones; sustaining the physical stability of the blood; maintaining acid-base balance through the buffering action; and serving as a reserve source of nutrition for tissues.

One protein—albumin—makes up more than 50% of the total proteins in serum; a group of proteins, collectively

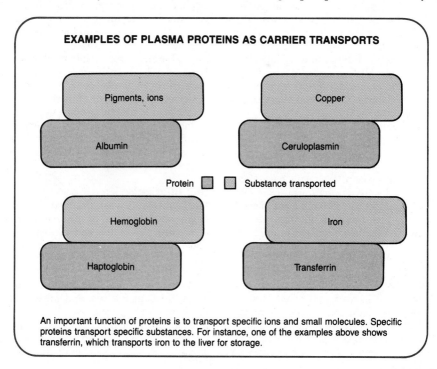

EXAMPLES OF PLASMA PROTEINS AS CARRIER TRANSPORTS

Pigments, ions

Albumin

Copper

Ceruloplasmin

Protein ▢ ▢ Substance transported

Hemoglobin

Haptoglobin

Iron

Transferrin

An important function of proteins is to transport specific ions and small molecules. Specific proteins transport specific substances. For instance, one of the examples above shows transferrin, which transports iron to the liver for storage.

called globulins, accounts for the remainder. Fibrinogen, a major plasma protein, does not appear in serum, because it is converted to fibrin during coagulation.

Serum protein formation

The major serum proteins are albumin and the globulins (alpha$_1$, alpha$_2$, beta, and gamma). The liver forms most of the albumin, and the alpha and beta globulins. The reticuloendothelial system and immature plasma cells in the spleen, lymph nodes, and bone marrow produce gamma globulin. Albumin is primarily responsible for maintaining the oncotic pressure of plasma, which, in turn, maintains normal distribution of water in the various body compartments. Albumin also aids transport of many drugs, dyes, and fatty acids by combining with them in the plasma. Reflecting their heterogeneous composition, globulins have many diverse functions, including binding free hemoglobin and certain hormones, transporting metals, and forming antibodies. For example, ceruloplasmin, an alpha$_2$-globulin, binds most of the circulating copper in the body (persons with Wilson's disease have defective formation of ceruloplasmin); haptoglobin, another alpha$_2$-globulin, binds free plasma hemoglobin; and transferrin, a beta globulin, binds and transports dietary iron.

Nutritional status markedly affects serum protein formation. Thus, inadequate nutrition inhibits formation of plasma proteins. In turn, declining plasma protein levels can have serious clinical consequences. For example, a sharp decline in albumin leads to edema; also, low levels of gamma globulin weaken the host's defense to infection.

Protein metabolism

Unlike carbohydrates and fats, proteins aren't stored by the body. Instead, in the intestinal mucosa and other sites, proteins are continuously broken down into amino acids. These amino acids form a common reserve for the synthesis of new proteins and of hormones, enzymes, or nonprotein nitrogenous compounds like creatine. Certain genetic diseases, such as phenylketonuria, can result in the loss of a specific enzyme or transport activity, which alters the metabolic function of one or more involved amino acids.

The major end product of protein metabolism is *urea,* which is formed in the liver by the deamination of amino acids. Urea is excreted in the urine and is the primary method of nitrogen elimination. Blood levels of urea begin to rise with impaired glomerular excretion and are measured as an important index of renal function.

Another important protein metabolite is *ammonia,* most of which is ultimately metabolized to urea in the liver and then excreted. Failing liver function inhibits such conversion of ammonia. Consequently, serum ammonia levels rise in severe hepatic disease, especially after gastrointestinal bleeding, and can lead to hepatic coma.

Creatine is a nonprotein nitrogenous compound that combines with phosphate to form phosphocreatine, an important storage form of high-energy phosphate. This compound is especially prevalent in muscle tissue. *Creatinine,* the end product of creatine metabolism, is excreted in the urine and, like blood urea nitrogen levels, reflects the efficiency of renal excretory function.

Uric acid is the end product of purine metabolism and is excreted in urine. Serum uric acid levels and urate crystal deposits in synovial fluid are significant in the diagnosis of gout.

Bile pigments

Bile pigments are waste products of heme degradation, initiated by the breakdown of erythrocytes at the end of their life cycle. The five major steps in the metabolism of bile pigments include formation, plasma transport, hepatic uptake, conjugation, and biliary excretion. In humans, the bone marrow and spleen are the main sites of normal red cell destruction and heme degradation. Although bile pigments have no known function, abnormalities in their overall transfor-

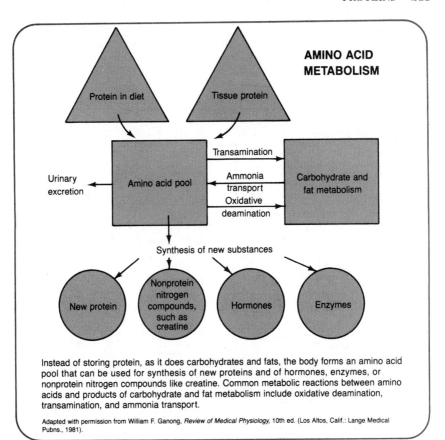

AMINO ACID METABOLISM

Protein in diet

Tissue protein

Transamination

Urinary excretion

Amino acid pool

Ammonia transport

Oxidative deamination

Carbohydrate and fat metabolism

Synthesis of new substances

New protein

Nonprotein nitrogen compounds, such as creatine

Hormones

Enzymes

Instead of storing protein, as it does carbohydrates and fats, the body forms an amino acid pool that can be used for synthesis of new proteins and of hormones, enzymes, or nonprotein nitrogen compounds like creatine. Common metabolic reactions between amino acids and products of carbohydrate and fat metabolism include oxidative deamination, transamination, and ammonia transport.

Adapted with permission from William F. Ganong, *Review of Medical Physiology*, 10th ed. (Los Altos, Calif.: Lange Medical Pubns., 1981).

mation have considerable significance in the diagnosis of hepatobiliary disease and in conditions marked by excessive hemolysis. Conjugated bilirubin is converted into pigments responsible for the characteristic color of bile and feces; un-conjugated bilirubin migrates in normal plasma, largely combined with albumin. Serum bilirubin levels may rise in hemolytic anemia, hepatocellular injury, or biliary duct occlusion.

PATRICIA J. NOONE, RN, BSN, MEd

PROTEINS

Serum Protein Electrophoresis

This test measures serum albumin and globulins, the major blood proteins, in an electric field by separating the pro-teins according to their size, shape, and electric charge at pH 8.6. Because each protein fraction moves at a different rate, this movement separates the fractions into recognizable and measurable patterns.

Albumin, which comprises more than 50% of total serum protein, maintains oncotic pressure (preventing leakage of

SERUM PROTEINS AND THEIR ELECTROPHORETIC VALUES IN VARIOUS DISEASE STATES

In electrophoresis, blood serum is placed on specially treated paper exposed to an electric current. According to their molecular size, shape, and electric charge, albumin and globulins in the serum migrate to form five homogeneous bands that indicate the relative proportions of each protein fraction. As these graphs show, variations in the proportions of these serum proteins can be plotted, making electrophoresis a valuable diagnostic tool.

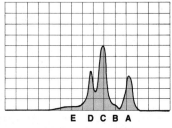

(3) A marked decline in gamma globulins characterizes hypogammaglobulinemia.

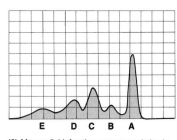

(1) Normal serum pattern

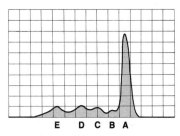

(4) Nephrotic syndrome produces a distinct fall in albumin and gamma globulins, as well as considerable increases in alpha$_2$ and beta globulins.

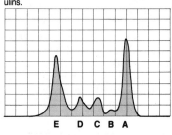

(2) Myocardial infarction causes a relative increase in alpha$_1$ and alpha$_2$ globulins.

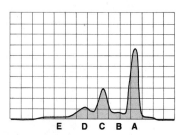

(5) An apparent decrease in albumin and, more importantly, a sharp rise in gamma globulins indicate multiple myeloma.

KEY:
A: Albumin
B: Alpha$_1$ globulin

C: Alpha$_2$ globulin
D: Beta globulin
E: Gamma globulin

capillary plasma), and transports substances that are insoluble in water alone, such as bilirubin, fatty acids, hormones, and drugs. Four types of globulins exist—alpha$_1$, alpha$_2$, beta, and gamma. The first three types act primarily as carrier proteins that transport lipids, hormones, and metals *through the blood. The fourth type, gamma globulin, is an important component in the body's immune system.*

Electrophoresis is the most current method for measuring serum proteins. However, determinations of total protein and albumin/globulin (A/G ratio) are still commonly performed. When the relative percent of each component protein fraction is multiplied by the total protein concentration, the proportions can be converted into absolute values. Regardless of test method, however, a single protein fraction is rarely significant by itself. The usual clinical indication for this test is suspected hepatic disease or protein deficiency.

Purpose
□ To aid diagnosis of hepatic disease, protein deficiency, blood dyscrasias, renal disorders, and gastrointestinal and neoplastic diseases.

Patient preparation
Explain to the patient that this test determines the protein content of blood. Inform him that he needn't restrict food or fluids. Tell him the test requires a blood sample; who will perform the venipuncture and when; and that he may feel some discomfort from the needle puncture and the pressure of the tourniquet. Reassure him that collecting the sample takes only a few minutes and that test results should be available the next day.

Check the patient's medication history for drugs that may influence serum protein levels. If they must be continued, note this on the laboratory slip.

Procedure
Perform a venipuncture, and collect the sample in a 7 ml *red-top* tube.

Precautions
This test must be performed on a serum sample to avoid measuring the fibrinogen fraction.

Values
Normally, total serum protein levels range from 6.6 to 7.9 g/dl. The albumin fraction ranges from 3.3 to 4.5 g/dl. The alpha$_1$-globulin fraction ranges from 0.1 to 0.4 g/dl; alpha$_2$-globulin ranges from 0.5 to 1 g/dl. Beta globulin ranges from 0.7 to 1.2 g/dl; gamma globulin ranges from 0.5 to 1.6 g/dl. (For percentage values, see chart below.)

HOW HEPATIC DISEASES AFFECT PROTEIN FRACTIONS

KEY: 0 = normal
+ = increased
− = decreased

	NORMAL	HEPATITIS	CIRRHOSIS	OBSTRUCTIVE JAUNDICE	METASTATIC LIVER CARCINOMA
Total protein	100%	0	−	0	0
Albumin	53%	0	−	0 / −	−
Alpha$_1$ globulin	14%	−	0	0	+
Alpha$_2$ globulin		−	0	0 / +	+
Beta globulin	12%	+	+	0 / +	0 / +
Gamma globulin	20%	+	+	0	0 / +

Since the liver synthesizes albumin as well as alpha and beta globulins, changes in the concentration of these major plasma proteins can indicate hepatic malfunction or hepatocellular damage. Although total protein—the sum of albumin and globulin fractions—may remain normal, hepatic disease will alter one, several, or all of the protein fractions.

CLINICAL IMPLICATIONS OF ABNORMAL PROTEIN LEVELS

Abnormal levels of albumin or globulin are characteristic in many pathologic states, such as those listed below.

INCREASED LEVELS

TOTAL PROTEINS

- dehydration
- vomiting, diarrhea
- diabetic acidosis
- fulminating and chronic infections
- multiple myeloma
- monocytic leukemia
- chronic inflammatory disease (such as rheumatoid arthritis or early-stage Laennec's cirrhosis)

ALBUMIN

- multiple myeloma

GLOBULINS

- chronic syphilis
- tuberculosis
- subacute bacterial endocarditis
- multiple myeloma
- collagen diseases
- systemic lupus erythematosus
- rheumatoid arthritis
- diabetes mellitus
- Hodgkin's disease

DECREASED LEVELS

TOTAL PROTEINS

- malnutrition
- gastrointestinal disease
- blood dyscrasias
- essential hypertension
- Hodgkin's disease
- uncontrolled diabetes mellitus
- malabsorption
- hepatic dysfunction
- toxemia of pregnancy
- nephrosis
- surgical and traumatic shock
- severe burns
- hemorrhage
- hyperthyroidism
- benzene and carbon tetrachloride poisoning
- congestive heart failure

ALBUMIN

- malnutrition
- nephritis/nephrosis
- diarrhea
- plasma loss from burns
- hepatic disease
- Hodgkin's disease
- hypogammaglobulinemia
- peptic ulcer
- acute cholecystitis
- sarcoidosis
- collagen diseases
- systemic lupus erythematosus
- rheumatoid arthritis
- essential hypertension
- metastatic carcinoma
- hyperthyroidism

GLOBULINS

- Levels are variable in neoplastic and renal diseases, hepatic dysfunction, and blood dyscrasias

Implications of results
For common findings, see *Clinical Implications of Abnormal Protein Levels.*

Post-test care
If a hematoma develops at the venipuncture site, apply warm soaks.

Interfering factors
□ Pretest administration of a contrast dye (such as sulfobromophthalein) falsely elevates total protein test results. Pregnancy and the use of cytotoxic agents may lower serum albumin.
□ Use of plasma instead of serum alters test results.

SUZANNE G. ROTZELL, RN, BSN

ALPHA₁-ANTITRYPSIN TEST

Using immunoelectrophoresis, this test measures fasting serum levels of alpha₁-antitrypsin (AAT), a major component of the alpha₁-globulin. AAT is believed to inhibit release of protease into body fluids by dying cells. Congenital absence or deficiency of AAT increases susceptibility to emphysema. As a result, the serum AAT test provides a useful screening tool for high-risk patients. Such patients must be instructed to refrain from smoking, since irritants in tobacco stimulate leukocytes in the lungs to release protease.

In addition to identifying congenital AAT deficiency, the AAT test is a nonspecific method of detecting inflammation, severe infection, and necrosis.

BARRY L. TONKONOW, MD

Serum Ceruloplasmin

This test measures serum levels of ceruloplasmin, an alpha₂-globulin that binds about 95% of serum copper (little copper exists in a free state), usually in the liver. Because ceruloplasmin catalyzes oxidation of ferrous compounds to ferric ions, it is thought to regulate iron uptake by transferrin, making iron available to reticulocytes for heme synthesis. The usual clinical indications for this assay are Menkes' kinky hair syndrome, suspected copper deficiency from total parenteral nutrition, and suspected Wilson's disease.

Purpose
□ To aid diagnosis of Wilson's disease, Menkes' kinky hair syndrome, and copper deficiency.

Patient preparation
Explain to the patient that this test helps determine the copper content of blood. Tell him the test requires a blood sample; who will perform the venipuncture and when; and that he may feel discomfort from the needle puncture and the tourniquet. Check his history for drugs that may influence ceruloplasmin levels.

Procedure
Perform a venipuncture, and collect the sample in a 7 ml *red-top* tube.

Precautions
Send the sample to the laboratory immediately.

Values
Serum ceruloplasmin levels normally range from 22.9 to 43.1 mg/dl.

Implications of results
Low ceruloplasmin levels usually indicate Wilson's disease; this is confirmed by Kayser-Fleischer rings (copper deposits in the corneas that form green-gold rings) or liver biopsy results that show 250 mcg of copper/g of dry weight. Low ceruloplasmin levels may also occur in Menkes' kinky hair syndrome, nephrotic syndrome, and hypocupremia caused by total parenteral nutrition. Elevated levels may indicate certain hepatic diseases and infections.

Post-test care
If a hematoma develops at the venipuncture site, apply warm soaks.

Interfering factors
Estrogen, methadone, and phenytoin may elevate serum ceruloplasmin levels.

SR. MARY BRIAN KELBER, RN, DNS

Serum Haptoglobin

Using radial immunodiffusion, this test measures serum levels of haptoglobin, a glycoprotein produced in the liver. Haptoglobin binds with free hemoglobin and prevents its accumulation in plasma, permitting clearance by reticuloendothelial cells and conserving body iron. Normally, hemoglobin circulates inside erythrocytes but appears in plasma when bacterial toxins, mechanical disruption (from a prosthetic heart valve, for example), or antibodies cause intravascular hemolysis.

When haptoglobin levels are inadequate to remove all hemoglobin from plasma, hemolysis is severe. After such hemolysis, low haptoglobin levels may persist for 5 to 7 days, until the liver can synthesize more of this glycoprotein.

Purpose
☐ To serve as an index of hemolysis
☐ To distinguish between hemoglobin and myoglobin in plasma, since haptoglobin doesn't bind with myoglobin
☐ To investigate hemolytic transfusion reactions
☐ To establish proof of paternity, using genetic (phenotypic) variations in haptoglobin structure.

Patient preparation
Explain to the patient that this test helps determine the condition of red blood cells. Inform him that he needn't restrict food or fluids. Tell him the test requires a blood sample; who will perform the venipuncture and when; and that he may feel some discomfort from the needle puncture and the pressure of the tourniquet. Reassure him that collecting the sample takes only a few minutes. Check the patient's history for drugs that may influence haptoglobin levels.

Procedure
Draw a venous blood sample into a 10 to 15 ml *red-top* tube.

Precautions
Handle the sample gently to prevent hemolysis.

Values
Normally, serum haptoglobin concentrations, measured in terms of the protein's hemoglobin-binding capacity, are 38 to 270 mg/dl.

Implications of results
Markedly depressed serum haptoglobin levels are characteristic in acute and chronic hemolysis, severe hepatocellular disease, infectious mononucleosis, and transfusion reactions. Hepatocellular disease inhibits the synthesis of haptoglobin. In hemolytic transfusion reactions, haptoglobin levels begin falling after 6 to 8 hours and drop to 40% of pretransfusion levels after 24 hours.

If serum haptoglobin values are very low, watch for symptoms of hemolysis: chills, fever, back pain, flushing, distended neck veins, tachycardia, tachypnea, and hypotension.

Although haptoglobin is absent in 90% of neonates, in most of these infants, levels gradually rise to normal by age 4 months. In about 1% of the population—including 4% of Blacks—haptoglobin is permanently absent; this disorder is known as congenital ahaptoglobinemia.

Strikingly elevated serum haptoglobin levels occur in diseases marked by chronic inflammatory reactions or tissue destruction, such as rheumatoid arthritis and malignant neoplasms.

Post-test care
If a hematoma develops at the venipuncture site, apply warm soaks.

Interfering factors
☐ Steroids and androgens can elevate haptoglobin levels and mask hemolysis in patients with inflammatory disease.
☐ Hemolysis caused by rough handling of the sample can interfere with accurate determination of test results.

SUZANNE G. ROTZELL, RN, BSN

Serum Transferrin
[Siderophilin]

A quantitative analysis of serum transferrin levels, this test evaluates iron metabolism. Transferrin, a glycoprotein that is formed in the liver, transports circulating iron obtained from dietary sources and from the breakdown of RBCs by reticuloendothelial cells. Most of this iron is transported to bone marrow for use in hemoglobin synthesis; some is converted to hemosiderin and ferritin, and is stored in these forms in the liver, the spleen, and bone marrow. Inadequate transferrin levels may therefore lead to impaired hemoglobin synthesis and, possibly, anemia. Transferrin, normally about 30% saturated with iron, is measured directly by immunoelectrophoresis; a serum iron level is usually obtained simultaneously.

Purpose
□ To determine the iron-transporting capacity of the blood
□ To evaluate iron metabolism in iron deficiency anemia.

Patient preparation
Explain to the patient that this test helps determine the cause of anemia. Inform him that he needn't restrict food or fluids. Tell him the test requires a blood sample; who will perform the venipuncture and when; and that he may feel some discomfort from the needle puncture and the pressure of the tourniquet. Reassure him that collecting the sample takes only a few minutes. Check the patient's history for drugs that may influence transferrin levels.

Procedure
Perform a venipuncture, and collect the sample in a 10 to 15 ml *red-top* tube.

Precautions
Handle the sample gently, and send it to the laboratory immediately.

Values
Normal serum transferrin values range from 250 to 390 mcg/dl, of which 65 to 170 mcg/dl are usually bound to iron.

Implications of results
Depressed serum levels may indicate inadequate production of transferrin due to hepatic damage or excessive protein loss from renal disease. Decreased transferrin levels may also result from acute or chronic infection or from cancer.

Elevated serum transferrin levels indicate severe iron deficiency.

Post-test care
If a hematoma develops at the venipuncture site, apply warm soaks.

Interfering factors
□ Late pregnancy or the use of oral contraceptives may raise transferrin levels.
□ Hemolysis due to rough handling of the sample may affect test results.

WILLIAM M. DOUGHERTY, BS

PROTEIN METABOLITES

Plasma Amino Acid Screening

This test is a qualitative but effective screen for inborn errors of amino acid metabolism. Thin-layer chromatography is the method used, since it can profile many amino acids simultaneously.

Amino acids are the chief components of all proteins and polypeptides. The body contains at least 20 amino acids; 10 are considered "essential"—that is, the body doesn't form them, so they must be acquired through diet. Certain congenital enzymatic deficiencies interfere with normal metabolism of one or more amino acids and cause accumulation or deficiency of these amino acids. Excessive accumulation of amino acids typically produces overflow aminoacidurias. Congenital abnormalities of the amino acid transport system in the kidneys produce a second group of disorders called renal aminoacidurias.

Purpose
☐ To screen for inborn errors of amino acid metabolism.

Patient preparation
Explain to the parents of the infant that this test helps determine if their child can metabolize amino acids normally. The infant must fast for 4 hours before the test. Tell the parents the test requires a blood sample, and that a small amount of blood will be drawn from the infant's heel. Advise them that collecting the sample takes only a few minutes.

Procedure
Perform a heelstick, and collect 0.1 ml of blood in a heparinized capillary tube.

Values
Chromatography shows a normal plasma amino acid pattern.

Implications of results
The plasma amino acid pattern is normal in renal amino acidurias and abnormal in overflow aminoacidurias. Comparisons of blood and urine chromatography can help distinguish between the two types of aminoacidurias.

Post-test care
☐ If a hematoma develops at the heelstick site, apply warm soaks.
☐ As ordered, resume diet that was discontinued before the test.

Interfering factors
Failure to observe restrictions of diet may influence amino acid levels.

SUZANNE G. ROTZELL, RN, BSN

Serum Phenylalanine Screening
[Guthrie screening test]

This test is a screening method used to detect elevated serum phenylalanine, an indication of possible phenylketonuria (PKU). Phenylalanine is a naturally occurring amino acid essential to growth and nitrogen balance. At birth, an infant with PKU usually has normal phenylalanine levels, but after milk or formula feeding begins (both contain phenylalanine), levels gradually rise due to a deficiency of the liver enzyme that converts phenylalanine to tyrosine. The serum phenylalanine screening test detects abnormal phenylalanine levels through the growth rate of Bacillus subtilis, an organism that needs phenylalanine to thrive. To ensure accurate results, the test must be performed after 3 full days (preferably 4 days) of milk or formula feeding.

Purpose
☐ To screen infants for PKU.

Patient preparation
Explain to the parents of the infant that the test is a routine screening measure for possible PKU and is a required test in many states. Tell them the test requires a blood sample, and that a small amount of blood will be drawn from the infant's heel.

Procedure
Perform a heelstick, and collect three drops of blood—one in each circle—on the filter paper.

Precautions
Note the infant's name and birth date, and the date of the first milk or formula feeding on the laboratory slip, and send the sample to the laboratory immediately.

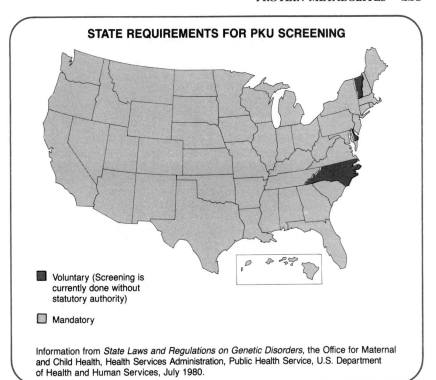

STATE REQUIREMENTS FOR PKU SCREENING

■ Voluntary (Screening is
currently done without
statutory authority)

□ Mandatory

Information from *State Laws and Regulations on Genetic Disorders,* the Office for Maternal
and Child Health, Health Services Administration, Public Health Service, U.S. Department
of Health and Human Services, July 1980.

Values

In the laboratory, the sample is mixed with a culture medium containing a special phenylalanine-dependent strain of *B. subtilis,* and an antagonist to phenylalanine. A negative test, in which the presence of the phenylalanine antagonist inhibits growth of *B. subtilis* around the blood on the filter paper, indicates normal phenylalanine levels (less than 2 mg/dl) and no appreciable danger of PKU.

Implications of results

Growth of *B. subtilis* on the filter paper indicates that serum phenylalanine levels are high enough to overcome the antagonist. Such an abnormal finding, or positive test, suggests the *possibility* of PKU. Diagnosis requires exact serum phenylalanine measurement and urine testing. A positive test may also result from hepatic disease, galactosemia, or delayed development of certain enzyme systems.

Post-test care

Reassure the parents of a child who may have PKU that although this disease is a common cause of congenital mental deficiency, early detection and continuous treatment with a low-phenylalanine diet can prevent permanent mental retardation.

CONFIRMING PKU

After the Guthrie screening test detects the possible presence of PKU, serum phenylalanine and tyrosine levels are measured to confirm diagnosis. Phenylalanine hydroxylase is the enzyme that converts phenylalanine to tyrosine. If this enzyme is absent, increasing phenylalanine levels and falling tyrosine levels indicate PKU. Samples are obtained by venipuncture (femoral or external jugular) and measured by fluorometry. Elevated serum phenylalanine (more than 4 mg/dl) and decreased tyrosine (less than 0.6 mg/dl)—with urinary excretion of phenylpyruvic acid—confirm diagnosis of PKU.

INHERITANCE PATTERNS IN PKU

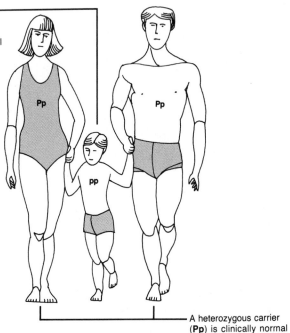

Of the offspring of two heterozygous carriers, 25% will inherit both recessive genes and will require a restricted diet to avoid retardation

A heterozygous carrier (**Pp**) is clinically normal

PKU is inherited as an autosomal recessive trait. A person with the genotype pp will have a deficiency of the liver enzyme phenylalanine hydroxylase that normally converts phenylalanine to tyrosine. The resulting accumulation of phenylalanine, phenylpyruvic acid, and other metabolites hinders the normal development of central nervous system cells, causing mental retardation. Dietary restriction of foods that contain phenylalanine prevents such accumulation of toxic compounds and hence prevents mental retardation.

Interfering factors

Performing the test before the infant has received at least 3 full days of milk or formula feeding yields a false-negative finding.

SUZANNE G. ROTZELL, RN, BSN

Plasma Ammonia

This test measures plasma levels of ammonia, a nonprotein nitrogen compound that helps maintain acid-base balance.

Most ammonia is absorbed from the intestinal tract, where it is produced by bacterial action on protein; a smaller amount of ammonia is produced in the kidneys from hydrolysis of glutamine. Normally, the body uses the nitrogen fraction of ammonia to rebuild amino acids; then it converts the ammonia to urea in the liver, for excretion by the kidneys. In diseases such as cirrhosis of the liver, however, ammonia can bypass the liver and accumulate in the blood. Therefore, plasma ammonia levels, often measured by isothermal diffusion, may help indicate the severity of hepatocellular damage.

Purpose

□ To help monitor the progression of severe hepatic disease and the effectiveness of therapy

□ To recognize impending or established hepatic coma.

Patient preparation

Explain to the patient that this test evaluates liver function. (If the patient is comatose, explain the procedure to a family member.) Inform the conscious patient that he must observe an overnight fast since plasma ammonia levels may vary with protein intake. Tell him the test requires a blood sample; who will perform the venipuncture and when; and that he may feel some discomfort from the needle puncture. Reassure him that collecting the sample takes only a few minutes.

Check the patient's medication history for use of drugs that may influence plasma ammonia levels.

Procedure

Perform a venipuncture, and collect the sample in a 10 ml *green-top* (heparinized) tube.

Precautions

□ Notify the laboratory before performing the venipuncture, so that preliminary preparations can begin before you send the sample.

□ Handle the sample gently to prevent hemolysis. Pack it in ice, and send it to the laboratory immediately. (*Don't* use a chilled container.)

Values

Normally, plasma ammonia levels are less than 50 mcg/dl.

Implications of results

Elevated plasma ammonia levels are common in severe hepatic disease—such as cirrhosis and acute hepatic necrosis—and may lead to hepatic coma. Elevated ammonia levels are also possible in Reye's syndrome, severe congestive heart failure, gastrointestinal hemorrhage, and erythroblastosis fetalis.

Post-test care

□ Make sure bleeding has stopped before removing pressure from the venipuncture site, since hepatic disease can prolong bleeding time. If a hematoma develops, apply warm soaks.

□ Watch for signs of impending or established hepatic coma if levels are high.

Interfering factors

□ Acetazolamide, thiazides, ammonium salts, or furosemide raise ammonia levels, as can hyperalimentation or a portacaval shunt. Lactulose, neomycin, and kanamycin depress ammonia levels.

□ Hemolysis caused by rough handling of the sample may alter test results.

SUZANNE G. ROTZELL, RN, BSN

RECOGNIZING HEPATIC COMA

Patients in hepatic coma progress through the following four stages, with accompanying clinical features:

• *Prodromal:* mild confusion, euphoria or depression, vacant stare, inappropriate laughter, forgetfulness, inability to concentrate, slow mentation, slurred speech, untidiness, lethargy, belligerence, minimal asterixis (flapping tremor).

Watch carefully for these subtle symptoms. These are not necessarily present at the same time.

• *Impending:* obvious obtundation, aberrant behavior, definite asterixis, constructional apraxia.

To test for asterixis (flapping tremor), have the patient raise both arms, with forearms flexed and fingers extended. To test for constructional apraxia, keep a serial record of the patient's handwriting and figure construction, and check it for progressive deterioration.

• *Stuporous* (patient can still be aroused): marked confusion, incoherent speech, asterixis, noisiness, abusiveness, violence, definitely abnormal EEG.

Restraints may be necessary at this stage. *Do not sedate the patient; sedation could be fatal.*

• *Comatose* (patient cannot be aroused, responds only to painful stimuli): no asterixis but positive Babinski's sign, hepatic fetor (breath has musty, sweet odor), and *elevated serum ammonia level.*

Degree of hepatic fetor correlates with the degree of somnolence and confusion.

Blood Urea Nitrogen

This test measures the nitrogen fraction of urea, the chief end product of protein metabolism. Formed in the liver from ammonia and excreted by the kidneys, urea constitutes 40% to 50% of the blood's nonprotein nitrogen. The blood urea nitrogen (BUN) level reflects protein intake and renal excretory capacity, but is a less reliable indicator of uremia than the serum creatinine level. Photometry is a commonly used test method.

Purpose
☐ To evaluate renal function and aid diagnosis of renal disease
☐ To aid assessment of hydration.

Patient preparation
Tell the patient this test evaluates kidney function. Inform him he needn't restrict food or fluids. Tell him the test requires a blood sample; who will perform the venipuncture and when; and that he may feel some discomfort from the needle puncture and the pressure of the tourniquet. Reassure him that collecting the sample takes only a few minutes, and that test results should be available the next day. Check the history for drugs that influence BUN levels.

Procedure
Perform a venipuncture, and collect the sample in a 10 to 15 ml *red-top* tube.

Precautions
Handle the sample gently to prevent hemolysis.

Values
BUN values normally range from 8 to 20 mg/dl.

Implications of results
Elevated BUN levels occur in renal disease, reduced renal blood flow (due to dehydration, for example), urinary tract obstruction, and in increased protein catabolism (as in burns).

Depressed BUN levels occur in severe hepatic damage, malnutrition, and overhydration.

Post-test care
If a hematoma develops at the venipuncture site, apply warm soaks.

Interfering factors
☐ Chloramphenicol can depress BUN levels.
☐ Nephrotoxic drugs, such as aminoglycosides, amphotericin B, and methicillin can elevate BUN levels.
☐ Hemolysis caused by rough handling of the sample may affect test results.
SUZANNE G. ROTZELL, RN, BSN

Serum Creatine

This test measures serum levels of creatine, an end product of protein metabolism. Creatine is formed in the liver, kidneys, small intestinal mucosa, and pancreas, and is distributed to muscle tissues, where it combines with phosphate to form phosphocreatine—a high-energy compound. In the anaerobic stage of muscle contraction, this compound is enzymatically cleaved, and some creatine enters the bloodstream, normally in an amount proportional to the body's muscle mass. However, muscular diseases may greatly increase the amount of creatine released into the blood. Creatine levels are usually measured by the difference in creatinine before and after conversion to creatinine by heat.

Purpose
☐ To aid diagnosis of muscular diseases, including muscular dystrophies.

Patient preparation
Explain to the patient that this test helps evaluate the function of muscles. Instruct him to restrict food, fluids, and exercise for approximately 12 hours before the

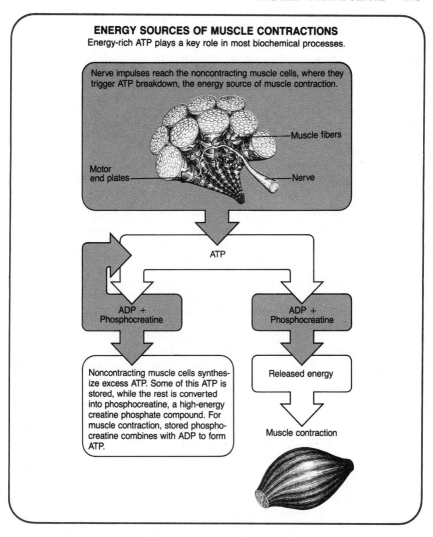

ENERGY SOURCES OF MUSCLE CONTRACTIONS
Energy-rich ATP plays a key role in most biochemical processes.

Nerve impulses reach the noncontracting muscle cells, where they trigger ATP breakdown, the energy source of muscle contraction.

Muscle fibers

Motor end plates

Nerve

ATP

ADP + Phosphocreatine

ADP + Phosphocreatine

Noncontracting muscle cells synthesize excess ATP. Some of this ATP is stored, while the rest is converted into phosphocreatine, a high-energy creatine phosphate compound. For muscle contraction, stored phosphocreatine combines with ADP to form ATP.

Released energy

Muscle contraction

---

test. Tell him the test requires a blood sample; who will perform the venipuncture and when; and that he may feel some discomfort from the needle puncture and the pressure of the tourniquet. Reassure him that collecting the sample takes only a few minutes, and that test results should be available the next day.

Check the patient's medication history for recent use of drugs that may influence creatine levels. If such drugs must be continued, note this on the laboratory slip.

Procedure

Perform a venipuncture, and collect the sample in a 10 to 15 ml *red-top* tube.

Precautions

□ Handle the sample gently to prevent hemolysis, and send the specimen to the laboratory immediately.

Values

Creatine values in males normally range from 0.2 to 0.6 mg/dl; in females, from 0.6 to 1 mg/dl.

Implications of results

Greatly increased serum creatine levels follow necrosis or atrophy of skeletal muscle, as in trauma, amyotrophic lateral sclerosis, dermatomyositis, and the progressive muscular dystrophies. Creatine levels may also rise above normal in hyperthyroidism and pregnancy, and after excessive dietary intake of protein.

Post-test care

☐ If a hematoma develops at the venipuncture site, apply warm soaks.
☐ As ordered, resume medications withheld before the test.

Interfering factors

☐ Testosterone therapy increases creatine synthesis by the liver and can therefore elevate serum creatine levels.
☐ Hemolysis caused by rough handling of the sample may alter test results.

SUZANNE G. ROTZELL, RN, BSN

Serum Creatinine

A quantitative analysis of serum creatinine levels, this test provides a more sensitive measure of renal damage than BUN levels, because renal impairment is virtually the only cause of creatinine elevation. Creatinine is a nonprotein end product of creatine metabolism. Similar to creatine, creatinine appears in serum in amounts proportional to the body's muscle mass; unlike creatine, it is easily excreted by the kidneys, with minimal or no tubular reabsorption. Creatinine levels, therefore, are directly related to the glomerular filtration rate. Since creatinine levels normally remain constant, elevated levels usually indicate diminished renal function. Determination of serum creatinine is commonly based on the Jaffé reaction.

Purpose

☐ To assess renal glomerular filtration
☐ To screen for renal damage.

Patient preparation

Explain to the patient that this test evaluates kidney function. Instruct him to restrict food and fluids for about 8 hours before the test. Tell him the test requires a blood sample; who will perform the venipuncture and when; and that while he may feel some discomfort from the needle puncture and the pressure of the tourniquet, collecting the sample takes only a few minutes. Test results should be available the next day.

Check the patient's medication history for any medications that may interfere with test results.

Procedure

Perform a venipuncture, and collect the sample in a 10 to 15 ml *red-top* tube.

Precautions

Send the sample to the laboratory immediately.

Values

Creatinine concentrations in males normally range from 0.8 to 1.2 mg/dl; in females, from 0.6 to 0.9 mg/dl.

Implications of results

Elevated serum creatinine levels generally indicate renal disease that has seriously damaged 50% or more of the nephrons. Elevated creatinine levels may also be associated with gigantism and acromegaly.

Post-test care

If a hematoma develops at the venipuncture site, apply warm soaks.

Interfering factors

☐ Ascorbic acid, barbiturates, and diuretics may raise serum creatinine levels.
☐ Sulfobromophthalein or phenolsulfonphthalein given within the previous 24 hours can elevate creatinine levels if the test is based on the Jaffé reaction.
☐ Patients with exceptionally large muscle masses, such as athletes, may have above-average creatinine levels, even in the presence of normal renal function.

SUZANNE G. ROTZELL, RN, BSN

Serum Uric Acid

Used primarily to detect gout, this test measures serum levels of uric acid, the major end metabolite of purine. Large amounts of purines are present in nucleic acids and derive from dietary and endogenous sources. Uric acid clears the body by glomerular filtration and tubular secretion. However, uric acid is not very soluble at a pH of 7.4 or lower. Disorders of purine metabolism, rapid destruction of nucleic acids, and conditions marked by impaired renal excretion characteristically raise serum uric acid levels.

Purpose
□ To confirm diagnosis of gout
□ To help detect kidney dysfunction.

Patient preparation
Explain to the patient that this test helps detect gout or kidney dysfunction. Inform him that he needn't restrict food or fluids. Tell him the test requires a blood sample; who will perform the venipuncture and when; and that he may feel some discomfort from the needle puncture and the pressure of the tourniquet. Reassure him that collecting the sample takes only a few minutes, and that test results should be available the next day.

Check the patient's medication history for any drugs that may influence uric acid levels.

Procedure
Perform a venipuncture, and collect the sample in a 10 to 15 ml *red-top* tube.

Precautions
Handle the sample gently to prevent hemolysis.

Values
Uric acid concentrations in men normally range from 4.3 to 8 mg/dl; in women, from 2.3 to 6 mg/dl.

Implications of results
Increased serum uric acid levels may indicate gout or impaired renal function (levels don't correlate with severity of disease). Levels may also rise in congestive heart failure, glycogen storage disease (type I, von Gierke's disease), infections, hemolytic or sickle cell anemia, polycythemia, neoplasms, and psoriasis. Depressed uric acid levels may indicate defective tubular absorption (as in Fanconi's syndrome and Wilson's disease) or acute hepatic atrophy.

Post-test care
If a hematoma develops at the venipuncture site, apply warm soaks.

Interfering factors
□ Loop diuretics, ethambutol, vincristine, pyrazinamide, thiazides, and low doses of aspirin may raise uric acid levels. When uric acid is measured by the colorimetric method, false elevations may be caused by acetaminophen, ascorbic acid, levodopa, and phenacetin. Aspirin in high doses may decrease uric acid levels.
□ Starvation, a high-purine diet, stress, and abuse of alcohol may raise uric acid levels.

SUZANNE G. ROTZELL, RN, BSN

PIGMENTS

Serum Bilirubin

This test measures serum levels of bilirubin, the predominant pigment in bile.

Bilirubin is the major product of hemoglobin catabolism. After being formed in the reticuloendothelial cells, bilirubin is bound to albumin and is transported to the liver, where it is conjugated with

BILIRUBIN METABOLISM

After formation in the reticuloendothelial cells, bilirubin is bound to
albumin and transported to the liver,
where it is conjugated with glucuronic acid to form bilirubin diglucuronide, and is excreted into the
bile. A small portion of conjugated
bilirubin recycles into the reticuloendothelial system.

In the intestine, bacteria converts
the remaining bilirubin diglucuronide
into urobilinogen, a portion of
which is reabsorbed into the portal
blood and carried back to the
liver. Most urobilinogen eventually
travels back through bile into
the intestine, but a small amount
reaches the kidneys and is excreted
in urine. The urobilinogen that
escaped portal reabsorption is excreted in feces. With exposure
to air, urobilinogen in urine oxidizes
to urobilin, and urobilinogen in
feces oxidizes to stercobilin.

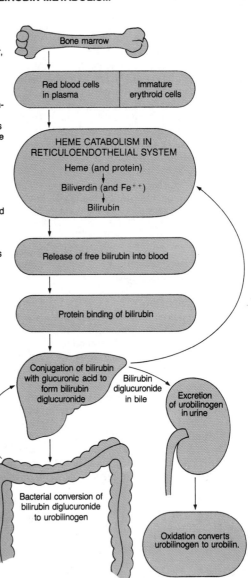

Bone marrow

Red blood cells in plasma | Immature erythroid cells

HEME CATABOLISM IN
RETICULOENDOTHELIAL SYSTEM
Heme (and protein)
Biliverdin (and Fe^{++})
Bilirubin

Release of free bilirubin into blood

Protein binding of bilirubin

Conjugation of bilirubin with glucuronic acid to form bilirubin diglucuronide

Bilirubin diglucuronide in bile

Excretion of urobilinogen in urine

Recirculation of urobilinogen

Excretion of urobilinogen in feces

Bacterial conversion of bilirubin diglucuronide to urobilinogen

Oxidation converts urobilinogen to stercobilin.

Oxidation converts urobilinogen to urobilin.

Adapted with permission from A. McGehee Harvey, et al, eds., *Principles and Practice of Medicine* (New York: Appleton-Century-Crofts, 1980), p. 706.

glucuronide by the enzymatic action of glucuronyl transferase. The resulting compound—bilirubin diglucuronide—is then excreted in bile.

Effective conjugation and excretion of bilirubin depends on a properly functioning hepatobiliary system and a normal RBC turnover rate. Therefore, measurement of unconjugated (indirect) or prehepatic bilirubin, and conjugated (direct) or posthepatic bilirubin can help evaluate hepatobiliary and erythropoietic functions. Serum bilirubin measurements are especially significant in the newborn, since elevated unconjugated bilirubin can accumulate in the brain and cause irreparable tissue damage.

Purpose
□ To evaluate liver function
□ To aid differential diagnosis of jaundice and to monitor the progression of this disorder
□ To aid diagnosis of biliary obstruction and hemolytic anemia
□ To determine whether a newborn requires an exchange transfusion or phototherapy because of dangerously high unconjugated bilirubin levels.

Patient preparation
Explain to the patient that this test evaluates liver function and the condition of red blood cells. If the patient is a newborn infant, explain the importance of this test to his parents. Inform the adult patient that he needn't restrict fluids but should fast for at least 4 hours before the test. (Fasting is not necessary for a newborn.) Tell the patient the test requires a blood sample; who will perform the venipuncture and when; and that he may experience transient discomfort from the needle puncture and the pressure of the tourniquet. If the patient is a newborn, tell his parents that a small amount of blood will be drawn from his heel, and who will perform the heelstick and when. Reassure the patient or the parents that collecting the sample takes only a few minutes. Check the patient's medication history for use of drugs that are known to interfere with serum bilirubin levels.

Procedure
If the patient is an adult, perform a venipuncture, and collect the sample in a 10 to 15 ml red-top tube.

If the patient is an infant, perform a heelstick, and fill the microcapillary tube to the designated level with blood.

Precautions
□ Protect the sample from strong sunlight and ultraviolet light, since bilirubin breaks down when exposed to light.
□ Handle the sample gently to prevent hemolysis, and send it to the laboratory immediately.

Values
Normally in an adult, indirect serum bilirubin measures 1.1 mg/dl or less; direct serum bilirubin, less than 0.5 mg/dl. Total serum bilirubin in the newborn measures 1 to 12 mg/dl.

Implications of results
Elevated indirect serum bilirubin levels often indicate hepatic damage in which the parenchymal cells can no longer conjugate bilirubin with glucuronide. Consequently, indirect bilirubin reenters the bloodstream. High levels of indirect bilirubin are also likely in severe hemolytic anemia, when excessive indirect bilirubin overwhelms the liver's conjugating mechanism. If hemolysis continues, both direct and indirect bilirubin may rise. Other causes of elevated indirect bilirubin levels include congenital enzyme deficiencies, such as Gilbert's disease and Crigler-Najjar syndrome.

Elevated direct serum bilirubin levels usually indicate biliary obstruction, in which direct bilirubin, blocked from its normal pathway from the liver into the biliary tree, overflows into the bloodstream. If the obstruction continues, both direct and indirect bilirubin may be eventually elevated due to hepatic damage. In severe chronic hepatic damage, direct bilirubin concentrations may return to normal or near-normal levels, but elevated indirect bilirubin levels persist.

In newborn infants, total bilirubin levels that reach or exceed 20 mg/dl indicate the need for exchange transfusion.

Post-test care
If a hematoma develops at the venipuncture or heelstick site, apply warm soaks.

Interfering factors
□ Novobiocin raises bilirubin levels.
□ Exposure of the sample to direct sunlight or ultraviolet light may depress bilirubin levels.
□ Hemolysis due to rough handling of the sample may alter test results.

WILLIAM M. DOUGHERTY, BS

Serum Myoglobin

Using radioimmunoassay, this test measures serum levels of myoglobin, an oxygen-binding muscle protein similar to hemoglobin. Myoglobin binds, stores, and transports oxygen to the muscle cells' mitochondria, where oxygen generates energy by converting glucose into carbon dioxide and water. Myoglobin is normally found in skeletal and cardiac muscle, but is released into the blood after muscle injury. Thus, serum myoglobin levels help estimate the severity of muscle damage. However, because myoglobin levels don't indicate the site of injury, they're commonly used to confirm other studies, such as total creatine phosphokinase (CPK) or the myocardial-specific isoenzyme, CPK-MB.

Purpose
□ To estimate damage caused by myocardial infarction or skeletal muscle injury
□ To predict exacerbation of polymyositis, a degenerative muscle disease.

Patient preparation
Explain to the patient that this test helps determine the severity of muscle damage. Inform him that he needn't restrict food or fluids. Tell him the test requires a blood sample; who will perform the venipuncture and when; and that he may feel some discomfort from the needle puncture and the pressure of the tourniquet. Reassure him that collecting the sample takes only a few minutes.

Procedure
Perform a venipuncture and collect the sample in a 10-ml *red-top* tube.

Precautions
□ Don't collect a blood sample from a patient who's recently had an angina attack or undergone cardioversion.
□ Collect a blood sample 4 to 8 hours after the onset of an acute MI, when myoglobin levels peak.

Values
Normal serum myoglobin levels range from 30 to 90 ng/ml.

Implications of results
Elevated serum myoglobin levels help estimate the severity of damage after myocardial infarction or skeletal muscle injury. In a patient with polymyositis, elevated levels may signal exacerbation of the disease. However, elevated myoglobin levels are also associated with dermatomyositis, systemic lupus erythematosus, shock, or severe renal failure. Because test results are nonspecific, elevated serum levels must be correlated with the patient's signs and symptoms.

Post-test care
If a hematoma develops at the venipuncture site, apply warm soaks.

Interfering factors
□ Recent cardioversion or angina attacks may increase myoglobin levels.
□ Performing this test immediately after onset of an acute MI produces misleading results, since myoglobin levels don't peak for 4 to 8 hours.
□ A radioactive scan performed within 1 week before the test may affect results.

TOBIE VIRGINIA HITTLE, RN, BSN, CCRN

Erythrocyte Total Porphyrins

[Erythropoietic porphyrins]

This test measures total erythrocyte porphyrins—mostly protoporphyrin, but also coproporphyrin and uroporphyrin. Porphyrins are pigments that are present in all protoplasm and have a significant role in energy storage and use. Protoporphyrin, coproporphyrin, and uroporphyrin are produced during heme biosynthesis. Small amounts of these porphyrins or their precursors normally appear in blood, urine, and feces. Production and excretion of porphyrins or their precursors increase in porphyrias, which are separated into erythropoietic and hepatic types. This test detects erythropoietic porphyrias.

After an initial screening test for total porphyrins, quantitative fluorometric analysis can identify specific porphyrins and suggest specific disorders.

Purpose

□ To aid diagnosis of congenital or acquired erythropoietic porphyrias
□ To help confirm diagnosis of disorders affecting red blood cell activity.

Patient preparation

Explain to the patient that this test helps detect red blood cell disorders. Inform him that he must fast for 12 to 14 hours before the sample is drawn, but that he may drink water. Tell him who will perform the venipuncture and when, and that he may feel some transient discomfort from the needle puncture and the pressure of the tourniquet.

Procedure

Perform a venipuncture and collect the sample in a 5-ml or larger *green-top* tube. Label the sample, place it on ice, and send it to the laboratory.

Precautions

Handle the sample gently to prevent hemolysis.

Values

Total porphyrin levels range from 16 to 60 mg/dl of packed red blood cells. Protoporphyrin levels range from 16 to 60 mg/dl; coproporphyrins and uroporphyrins each have levels below 2 mg/dl.

Implications of results

Elevated protoporphyrin levels may indicate erythropoietic protoporphyria, infection, increased erythropoiesis, thalassemia, sideroblastic anemia, iron deficiency anemia, or lead poisoning. Elevated coproporphyrin levels may indicate congenital erythropoietic porphyria, erythropoietic protoporphyria or coproporphyria, and sideroblastic anemia. Elevated uroporphyrin levels may indicate congenital erythropoietic porphyria or erythropoietic protoporphyria.

Post-test care

If a hematoma develops at the venipuncture site, apply warm soaks.

Interfering factors

Hemolysis or failure to observe dietary restrictions may alter test results.
TOBIE VIRGINIA HITTLE, RN, BSN, CCRN

Selected References

Bauer, John D., and Ackermann, Philip G. *Clinical Laboratory Methods*, 9th ed. St. Louis: C.V. Mosby Co., 1982.

Brunner, Lillian S., and Suddarth, Doris S. *Lippincott Manual of Nursing Practice*, 3rd ed. Philadelphia: J.B. Lippincott Co., 1982.

Lamb, Jane O. *Laboratory Tests for Clinical Nursing*. Bowie, Md.: Robert J. Brady Co., 1984.

Tilkian, Sarko M., et al. *Clinical Implications of Laboratory Tests*, 3rd ed. St. Louis: C.V. Mosby Co., 1983.

8 Carbohydrates

LEARNING OBJECTIVES

After completing this chapter, the reader will be able to:
- explain carbohydrate metabolism after food intake and after fasting.
- state the effects of abnormal insulin secretion.
- list the signs and symptoms of diabetes mellitus.
- describe how the pancreas functions.
- explain how to administer oral glucose solutions.
- describe the body's response to hypoglycemia and hyperglycemia.
- state the purpose of each test discussed in the chapter.
- prepare the patient physically and psychologically for each test.
- describe the procedure for performing each test.
- specify appropriate precautions for safe administration of each test.
- recognize signs of hypoglycemia and respond appropriately.
- implement appropriate post-test care.
- state the normal values for each test.
- discuss the implications of abnormal test results.
- list factors that may interfere with accurate test results.

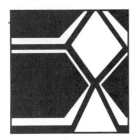

Carbohydrates

Introduction

Tests that measure the body's tolerance for carbohydrates—that is, the capacity to metabolize carbohydrates—have great clinical significance and rank among the most commonly performed laboratory tests. Blood glucose determinations are also useful for evaluating the function of hormone-secreting organs that help regulate blood glucose, for assessing intestinal absorption of glucose, and for evaluating liver function.

Such tests actually measure the capacity for conversion of carbohydrates by insulin. Since direct assay of insulin is technically difficult and costly, the most useful tests measure insulin activity indirectly—by measuring blood concentrations of glucose.

These tests encompass many techniques for measuring blood glucose and differ greatly in specificity and sensitivity. The sample itself varies; many normal values given in common reference sources represent values derived from analysis of whole blood, which includes all reducing substances present in blood, such as fructose and other sugars, and some drugs. Methods using a nonspecific reducing substance are not entirely specific for glucose but yield results fairly close to true glucose. Most current automated laboratory equipment is specific for true glucose. (Normal values listed in this book are for plasma and for true glucose, unless otherwise specified.)

Why measure glucose?

Glucose, a 6-carbon monosaccharide, is the body's major source of energy. Blood glucose derives from the conversion of ingested carbohydrates to glucose and to other simple sugars by enzymatic activity in the digestive tract; from the metabolic conversion of noncarbohydrate sources in the liver and kidneys; and from the breakdown of hepatic glycogen (a major storage form of glucose).

Insulin and glucagon are the two chief regulators of glucose levels, but several other hormones also influence glucose levels and are vital to normal carbohydrate metabolism. Growth hormone and adrenocorticotropic hormone, secreted by the anterior pituitary, raise glucose levels by promoting glucose formation from fat and protein. Cortisol and similar 11-oxysteroids, secreted by the adrenal cortex, produce the same effect. Epinephrine and thyroxine raise blood levels by stimulating the conversion of glycogen to glucose.

Metabolism after food and after fasting

Carbohydrate metabolism is most easily explained by examining the body's response to food and fasting. Ingestion of food causes a modest rise in blood glucose levels, triggering secretion of the hormone insulin by the beta cells in the islets of Langerhans, in the pancreas.

RECOGNIZE SYMPTOMS OF DIABETES

When diabetes is suspected, observe the patient carefully for the following classic symptoms:
• *Polyuria:* Excessive plasma glucose overflows into the urine and exerts an osmotic pressure, due to its concentration. This inhibits normal reabsorption of water by the renal tubules and leads to osmotic diuresis and dehydration.
• *Polydipsia:* Frequent urination leads to dehydration and severe thirst.
• *Weight loss:* Depletion of fat and protein stores to satisfy energy requirements causes severe, unexplained weight loss.
• *Polyphagia:* In some patients, tissue destruction raises metabolic requirements and produces severe hunger.

Insulin, a simple protein, acts as a hypoglycemic by stimulating cellular absorption of glucose and promoting its conversion to storage forms. In the liver, insulin increases the synthesis of glucose to glycogen (glycogenesis) and thus inhibits the breakdown of hepatic glycogen to glucose. Normally, the liver stores 60% or more of ingested glucose as glycogen; peripheral tissues receive the remainder. In the muscles, insulin enhances protein synthesis and the storage of amino acids, and promotes the conversion of glucose to glycogen or fat. In adipose tissue, most of the absorbed glucose acts to synthesize triglyceride, inhibiting its breakdown to free fatty acids and glycerol. The two major determinants of hepatic and peripheral glucose uptake are prompt secretion of insulin and the normal responsiveness of the tissues to insulin.

In the fasting state, the body derives energy from stored sources. In response to diminishing levels of circulating carbohydrates, secretion of insulin falls to a low level and the concentration of glucagon rises. Glucagon is a hyperglycemic, a small protein secreted by the alpha cells of the islets of Langerhans. When dietary carbohydrates, the body's preferred source of energy, are in short supply, glucagon stimulates the formation of glucose from protein and fat catabolized in the liver and kidneys (glyconeogenesis) and from the breakdown of hepatic glycogen stores (glycogenolysis). In adipose tissue, glucagon stimulates the breakdown of triglycerides to free fatty acids and glycerol (lipolysis); in the muscles, glucagon breaks down protein into amino acids (proteolysis).

Effects of abnormal insulin secretion

Insulin deficiency, as in diabetes mellitus, causes profound abnormalities in carbohydrate, lipid, and protein metabolism that ultimately affect all body tissues, especially skeletal muscle, adipose tissue, and the liver. Without adequate insulin, the body cannot use ingested carbohydrates efficiently. The resulting deficiency of carbohydrate energy sources causes the body to metabolize fat. Consequently, ketone bodies—intermediate products of fat metabolism—accumulate in the blood. The end result of this abnormal metabolic pattern is marked hyperglycemia, osmotic diuresis, severe dehydration, electrolyte imbalance, metabolic acidosis, and severe weight loss.

Excessive insulin secretion, as in insulinoma (islet beta cell tumor), causes similarly disruptive metabolic effects. Insulin excess produces hypoglycemia, characterized by low blood glucose levels, diaphoresis, nervousness, weakness, nausea, and tachycardia. In patients without diabetes, insulinoma is one cause of severe episodes of hypoglycemia. Unlike other causes of hypoglycemia, in which excessive insulin secretion immediately follows eating (functional or reactive hypoglycemia), insulin secretion in insulinoma follows no distinct pattern. Hypoglycemia may develop long after eating (fasting hypoglycemia). Although hyperglycemia is usually characteristic of diabetes, *hypo*glycemia may result from kidney failure, hepatic disease, alcoholism, decreased food intake, or excessive administration of insulin. Brain tissue is most vulnerable to hypoglycemia, since it doesn't synthesize

PATIENT TEACHING AID

High-carbohydrate Diet for Glucose Tolerance Test

Dear Patient:
To prepare for the OGTT and ensure accurate results, follow a high-carbohydrate diet like the one below for at least 3 days before the test. If you find the diet too restrictive, follow your regular regimen and eat *12 additional slices of bread* each day.

BREAKFAST
1 serving fruit
Eggs as desired
5 bread exchanges*
1 cup milk
Butter or margarine
Coffee or tea, if desired

LUNCH AND SUPPER
Meat, as desired
5 bread exchanges*
2 vegetables
1 serving fruit
1 cup milk
Butter or margarine
Coffee or tea, if desired

***One* of the following equals one bread exchange:**

1 slice bread, white or whole wheat	1 biscuit
1½ inch cube of cornbread	½ corn muffin
½ hamburger or hot dog roll	1 roll
	5 saltine crackers
	2 graham crackers
½ cup cooked cereal	½ cup grits or rice
¾ cup dry cereal (avoid sugar-coated varieties)	1 small white potato
½ cup noodles, spaghetti, or macaroni	½ cup mashed potato
½ cup cooked dried beans or peas	¼ cup sweet potato
⅓ cup corn or ½ small ear of corn	¼ cup baked beans
	¼ cup pork and beans

glucose or store it in significant amounts. Thus, hypoglycemia is likely to impair cerebral function.

Glucagon imbalance rare

Primary glucagon imbalance is rare. Primary causes of elevated glucagon levels include familial hyperglucagonemia (an autosomal dominant disorder), and glucagonoma (islet alpha cell tumor). Since abnormal islet alpha cells and abnormal beta cells may appear simultaneously, glucagonoma is characteristically associated with mild diabetes.

Most often, elevated glucagon levels are linked to diabetes and to insulin deficiency. Because insulin inhibits glucagon secretion, its absence or deficiency allows secretion of glucagon to continue, even in the presence of hyperglycemia. Another factor that enhances the activity of glucagon is unresponsiveness to in-sulin of the hepatic cells. Thus, glucagon may contribute to hyperglycemia, especially in hypoinsulinemia diabetes.

Carbohydrate metabolism tests

Various tests screen for diabetes mellitus by measuring the body's response to fasting and to carbohydrate ingestion. The *fasting plasma glucose test* measures plasma glucose levels after a 12- to 14-hour fast. A patient with diabetes will have consistently high glucose levels due to insufficient insulin levels.

The *2-hour postprandial plasma glucose test*, performed 2 hours after the patient has eaten a high-carbohydrate meal, measures immediate insulin response to carbohydrate ingestion.

The *oral glucose tolerance test* (OGTT), the most sensitive method for evaluating borderline diabetes in selected patients, measures carbohydrate

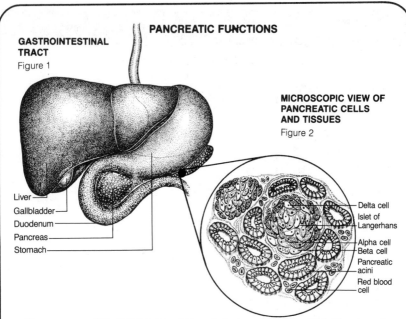

PANCREATIC FUNCTIONS

GASTROINTESTINAL TRACT
Figure 1

MICROSCOPIC VIEW OF PANCREATIC CELLS AND TISSUES
Figure 2

Liver
Gallbladder
Duodenum
Pancreas
Stomach

Delta cell
Islet of Langerhans
Alpha cell
Beta cell
Pancreatic acini
Red blood cell

The pancreas, a 3″ to 4″ (7.5 to 10 cm) triangularly shaped gland, lies behind the stomach (figure 1). Two major tissue types perform its dual functions: the *acini* secrete digestive juices into the duodenum and the *islets of Langerhans* secrete insulin and glucagon into the bloodstream. Specific staining techniques and structural distinctions reveal three major islet cells: *alpha, beta,* and *delta* (figure 2).

Beta cells secrete insulin
The polygonal beta cells contain insulin-bearing capsules. After a carbohydrate meal (and in response to other stimuli, including amino acids, as well as gastrointestinal and pituitary hormones), these cells rapidly secrete insulin.

Insulin is a metabolic hormone that regulates the body's carbohydrate metabolism. One of insulin's primary functions is glycogenesis, whereby the liver stores 60% of the ingested glucose for later use. Insulin also influences synthesis and storage of muscle glycogen, triglycerides, and protein. An insulin deficiency, as in diabetes mellitus, inhibits the body's normal metabolism of glucose. Consequently, glucose accumulates in the blood. In turn, the unavailability of glucose for energy needs causes the increased conversion of stored fats and protein for energy and eventually leads to ketosis and acidosis. At the same time, hyperglycemia increases osmotic pressure and causes dehydration and loss of glucose in the urine. Insulin deficiency also promotes lipid deposits in the vascular cells and leads to atherosclerosis.

Alpha cells secrete glucagon
The alpha cells are larger than the beta cells and contain dark granules that secrete the hormone glucagon. Unlike insulin, glucagon has a hyperglycemic effect. When blood glucose concentration is low (during periods of fasting) and insulin secretion falls, the alpha cells secrete glucagon to maintain body glucose levels (insulin's hypoglycemic role suppresses glucagon secretion). Glucagon breaks down stored liver glycogen and combats hypoglycemia. Since glucose is the brain's only nutrient, it's mandatory that glucose levels be maintained.

Delta cells secrete somatostatin
The delta cells secrete somatostatin, a hormone whose metabolic role isn't completely understood. Since somatostatin can inhibit insulin and glucagon secretion, it might someday be used to control the secretion of one or both of these hormones. Somatostatin is also secreted by the hypothalamus (where it is known as growth hormone inhibitory factor) and by the mucosa of the upper gastrointestinal tract, where its function is unknown.

metabolism after ingestion of a challenge dose of glucose. This test is used to confirm diabetes and to aid diagnosis of hypoglycemia. It has significant limitations, however. Because no universal agreement exists regarding what values indicate an abnormal OGTT curve, the test allows no absolute distinction between a healthy person and one with mild diabetes. Moreover, it has been known to suggest diabetes in a significant percentage of normal persons. This overdiagnosis of diabetes may be related to the release of epinephrine in response to stress resulting from the numerous venipunctures required in the OGTT. Epinephrine stimulates the conversion of glycogen to glucose.

Patients without overt symptoms of diabetes who produce abnormal OGTT curves present an additional difficulty: many patients with abnormal OGTT curves don't subsequently develop overt diabetes. Thus, an OGTT-confirmed diagnosis of latent or asymptomatic diabetes is not necessarily significant.

Another limitation of this test is that different test methods provide different sets of values. Moreover, even when the same values are used for repeated testing, test results aren't consistently reproducible.

Because of these limitations, the trend in laboratory testing is away from the OGTT and towards the fasting plasma glucose test for diagnosing diabetes mellitus.

Variant carbohydrate metabolism tests

The *I.V. glucose tolerance test*, an infrequently used variation of the OGTT, is more specific than the OGTT but less sensitive. The clinical significance of the test is under investigation, and the American Diabetes Association has yet to suggest a standardized procedure.

Another variant of the OGTT is the *cortisone glucose tolerance test*. In this test, the patient is given an oral dose of cortisone acetate 8½ hours and 2 hours before an OGTT is performed. Because cortisone elevates plasma glucose by promoting glyconeogenesis, it is useful in detecting probable diabetes in patients with borderline deficiencies in carbohydrate tolerance or with family histories of diabetes. However, since the sensitivity and specificity of the test has been challenged, it isn't considered a primary tool in diagnosing diabetes.

Other useful tests

The *tolbutamide tolerance test* helps diagnose insulinoma. The hypoglycemic tolbutamide is injected I.V. at a rapid rate, and the patient's blood glucose and serum insulin levels are carefully monitored for several hours. Because this test has two serious drawbacks—it produces false-positive results in patients who are obese and false-negative results in up to 50% of patients with insulinoma—it's used infrequently.

The *glycosolated hemoglobin test* measures the relative amount of glucose in hemoglobin and evaluates carbohydrate status for up to 120 days. This test is useful because patients with diabetes are known to have abnormal concentrations of hemoglobins A_{1a}, A_{1b}, and A_{1c} in the red cells—about twice the level in persons without diabetes. In patients with poorly controlled diabetes, the abnormal concentrations of these hemoglobins may rise to three times the normal levels.

The *oral lactose tolerance test* measures plasma glucose levels after a challenge dose of lactose, and helps diagnose lactose intolerance due to lactase deficiency.

Levels of *blood lactate*, the reduction product of pyruvate, are measured by enzymatic methods using lactate dehydrogenase. These methods are recommended for evaluating patients with symptoms of lactic acidosis, such as Kussmaul's respiration. Arterial or venous blood can be used for this test, but venous samples are easily obtained and so are more commonly used. However, unless the patient rests for 1 hour before testing, venous blood may yield higher values than arterial blood. Comparison of pyruvate and lactate levels reliably indicates tissue oxidation, but measurement of pyruvate is technically difficult and infrequently performed.

Home monitoring of blood glucose

The long-term goal of diabetes therapy is to maintain blood glucose levels at normal or near-normal levels, since persistent hyperglycemia leads to serious complications, such as retinopathy, vascular insufficiency, urinary tract infection, and peripheral neuropathy. Self-testing of blood glucose at home can help the diabetic patient improve blood glucose control by allowing him to record and monitor daily fluctuations. It also has the positive effect of promoting the patient's independence.

The home monitoring systems now available allow rapid, reliable blood glucose determination. These systems use a reagent test strip either alone or in combination with a reflectance meter. After applying a drop of capillary blood to the test strip, the patient compares the test strip to a color-coded key, for an approximate measurement, or inserts the test strip into a reflectance meter, for a precise measurement.

Home monitoring of blood glucose levels is becoming more widely accepted, because findings closely approximate laboratory results if the patient carefully follows directions. Improper timing of the test or overzealous washing of the reagent strip can alter test results.

CHERYL A. WALKER, RN, MSN

CARBOHYDRATE METABOLISM TESTS

Fasting Plasma Glucose

[Fasting blood sugar]

Commonly used to screen for diabetes mellitus, the fasting plasma glucose test measures plasma glucose levels following a 12- to 14-hour fast.

In the fasting state, plasma glucose levels decrease, stimulating release of the hormone glucagon. Glucagon then acts to raise plasma glucose by accelerating glycogenolysis, stimulating glyconeogenesis, and inhibiting glycogen synthesis. Normally, secretion of insulin checks this rise in glucose levels. In diabetes, however, absence or deficiency of insulin allows persistently high glucose levels.

Purpose
□ To screen for diabetes mellitus
□ To monitor drug or dietary therapy in patients with diabetes mellitus.

Patient preparation
Explain to the patient that this test de-

tects disorders of glucose metabolism and aids diagnosis of diabetes. Advise him to fast for 12 to 14 hours before the test. Tell him this test requires a blood sample; who will perform the venipuncture and when; and that he may experience transient discomfort from the needle puncture and the pressure of the tourniquet. Reassure him that collecting the sample takes less than 3 minutes.

Withhold drugs that affect test results, as ordered. If these medications must be continued, note this on the laboratory slip. Advise the patient with diabetes that he will receive his medication after the test.

Alert the patient to the symptoms of hypoglycemia—weakness, restlessness, nervousness, hunger, and sweating—and tell him to report such symptoms immediately.

Procedure
Perform a venipuncture, and collect the sample in a 5 ml *gray-top* tube.

Precautions
□ Send the sample to the laboratory immediately, because blood glucose levels

decrease when the sample is left at room temperature. If transport is delayed, refrigerate the sample.

□ Specify on the laboratory slip the time when the patient last ate, the sample collection time, and the time the last pretest insulin or oral hypoglycemic dose (if applicable) was given.

Values

Normal range for fasting plasma glucose varies according to the laboratory procedure. Generally, normal values after a 12- to 14-hour fast are 70 to 100 mg of "true glucose"/100 ml of blood when measured by the glucose oxidase and hexokinase methods.

Implications of results

Fasting plasma glucose levels of 140 mg/100 ml or more obtained on two or more occasions confirm diabetes mellitus; however, borderline or transient elevated levels require the 2-hour postprandial plasma glucose test or the oral glucose tolerance test to confirm diagnosis. Although increased fasting plasma glucose levels most commonly occur with diabetes, such levels can also result from pancreatitis, recent acute illness (such as myocardial infarction), Cushing's syndrome, acromegaly, and pheochromocytoma. Hyperglycemia may also stem from hyperlipoproteinemia (especially type III, type IV, or type V), chronic hepatic disease, nephrotic syndrome, brain tumor, sepsis, or gastrectomy with dumping syndrome, and is typical in eclampsia, anoxia, and convulsive disorders.

Depressed plasma glucose levels can result from hyperinsulinism, insulinoma, von Gierke's disease, functional or reactive hypoglycemia, myxedema, adrenal insufficiency, congenital adrenal hyperplasia, hypopituitarism, malabsorption syndrome, and some cases of hepatic insufficiency.

Post-test care

□ If a hematoma develops at the venipuncture site, apply warm soaks.
□ Provide a balanced meal or a snack.

As ordered, resume administration of medications withheld before the test.

Interfering factors

□ False-positive findings may be caused by acetaminophen when the glucose oxidase/hexokinase method is used. Other drugs known to elevate plasma glucose levels are chlorthalidone, thiazide diuretics, furosemide, triamterene, oral contraceptives (estrogen-progestogen combination), benzodiazepines, phenytoin, phenothiazines, lithium, epinephrine, arginine, phenolphthalein, dextrothyroxine, diazoxide, large doses of nicotinic acid, corticosteroids, and recent I.V. glucose infusions. Ethacrynic acid may also cause hyperglycemia, but large doses can produce hypoglycemia in patients with uremia.

□ Decreased plasma glucose levels may be caused by beta-adrenergic blockers, ethanol, clofibrate, insulin, oral hypoglycemic agents, and MAO inhibitors.

□ Failure to observe dietary restrictions may elevate plasma glucose levels.

□ Recent illness, infection, or pregnancy can elevate plasma glucose levels; strenuous exercise can depress them.

□ Glycolysis due to failure to refrigerate the sample or to send it to the laboratory immediately can result in false-negative results.

CHERYL A. WALKER, RN, MSN

Two-hour Postprandial Plasma Glucose
[Two-hour postprandial blood sugar]

The 2-hour postprandial test is a valuable screening tool for detecting diabetes mellitus. This procedure is performed when the patient demonstrates symptoms of diabetes (polydipsia and polyuria) or when results of the fasting plasma glucose test suggest diabetes.

In the OGTT, plasma glucose measurements are obtained at regular intervals, but the 2-hour measurement reliably indicates the body's insulin response to carbohydrate ingestion. The postprandial test relies solely on the 2-hour glucose level, avoiding the multiple venipunctures required for the OGTT. If postprandial test results are borderline, the OGTT may confirm diagnosis.

Purpose

☐ To aid diagnosis of diabetes mellitus
☐ To monitor drug or diet therapy in patients with diabetes mellitus.

Patient preparation

Explain to the patient that this test evaluates glucose metabolism and helps detect diabetes. Tell him to eat a balanced meal or one containing 100 g of carbohydrate before the test (recommended by the American Diabetes Association), and then to fast for 2 hours. Instruct him to avoid smoking and strenuous exercise after the meal. Tell him this test requires a blood sample; who will perform the venipuncture and when; and that he may experience transient discomfort from the needle puncture and the pressure of the tourniquet. Reassure him that collecting the sample takes less than 3 minutes.

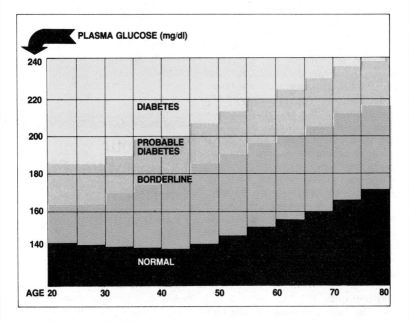

2-HOUR POSTPRANDIAL PLASMA GLUCOSE LEVELS BY AGE

The greatest difference in normal and diabetic insulin responses, and thus in plasma glucose concentration, occurs about 2 hours after a glucose challenge. Values of this test, however, can fluctuate according to the patient's age. After age 50, for example, normal levels rise markedly and steadily, sometimes reaching 160 mg/dl or higher. In younger patients, glucose concentration over 145 mg/dl suggests incipient diabetes and requires further evaluation.

PLASMA GLUCOSE (mg/dl)

DIABETES

PROBABLE DIABETES

BORDERLINE

NORMAL

Adapted with permission from Karl E. Sussman and J.S. Metz, eds., *Diabetes Mellitus* (4th ed.; New York: American Diabetes Association, 1975), p. 63.

Procedure

Perform a venipuncture, and collect the sample in a 5 ml *gray-top* tube.

Precautions

☐ Send the sample to the laboratory immediately or refrigerate it.

☐ Specify on the laboratory slip the time when the patient last ate, the sample collection time, and the time the last pretest insulin or hypoglycemic dose (if applicable) was given. If the sample is to be drawn by a technician, tell him the exact time the venipuncture must be performed.

Values

In a person without diabetes, postprandial glucose values are less than 145 mg/dl by the glucose oxidase or hexokinase method; levels are slightly elevated in persons over age 50.

Implications of results

Two 2-hour postprandial blood glucose values of 200 mg/dl or above indicate diabetes mellitus. High levels may also occur with pancreatitis, Cushing's syndrome, acromegaly, and pheochromocytoma. Hyperglycemia may also be caused by hyperlipoproteinemia (especially type III, type IV, or type V), chronic hepatic disease, nephrotic syndrome, brain tumor, sepsis, gastrectomy with dumping syndrome, eclampsia, anoxia, or convulsive disorders.

Depressed glucose levels occur in hyperinsulinism, insulinoma, von Gierke's disease, functional or reactive hypoglycemia, myxedema, adrenal insufficiency, congenital adrenal hyperplasia, hypopituitarism, malabsorption syndrome, and some cases of hepatic insufficiency.

Post-test care

☐ If a hematoma develops at the venipuncture site, ease discomfort by applying warm soaks.

☐ As ordered, resume diet, normal activity, and administration of medications that were discontinued before the test.

TWO-HOUR POSTPRANDIAL: PREFERRED SCREENING TEST

Because the 2-hour postprandial test is a simpler procedure than the oral glucose tolerance test or the fasting plasma glucose test, it's often the preferred test for diabetes screening in patients with any of the following conditions:

• obesity
• family histories of diabetes
• transient glycosuria or hyperglycemia (especially during pregnancy, surgery, or administration of adrenal steroids), or after trauma, emotional stress, myocardial infarction, or cerebrovascular accident
• unexplained hypoglycemia, neuropathy, retinopathy, nephropathy, or peripheral vascular disease
• pregnancy resulting in abortion, premature labor, stillbirth, neonatal death, or an unusually large infant
• recurrent infection, especially boils and abscesses.

Interfering factors

☐ False-positive results may be caused by acetaminophen when the glucose oxidase or hexokinase method is used. Other drugs known to cause plasma glucose elevations are chlorthalidone, thiazide diuretics, furosemide, triamterene, oral contraceptives (estrogen-progestogen combination), benzodiazepines, phenytoin, phenothiazines, lithium, epinephrine, arginine, phenolphthalein, dextrothyroxine, diazoxide, large doses of nicotinic acid, corticosteroids, and recent I.V. glucose infusions. Ethacrynic acid may also cause hyperglycemia, but large doses can cause hypoglycemia in patients with uremia.

☐ Depressed glucose levels may result from the use of beta-adrenergic blockers, amphetamines, ethanol, clofibrate, insulin, oral hypoglycemics, and MAO inhibitors.

☐ Recent illness, infection, or pregnancy may raise glucose levels; strenuous exercise or stress may depress them.

☐ Glycolysis caused by failure to refrigerate the sample or to send it to the laboratory immediately can depress glucose levels.

CHERYL A. WALKER, RN, MSN

Oral Glucose Tolerance Test

The oral glucose tolerance test, the most sensitive method of evaluating borderline cases of diabetes mellitus in selected patients, measures carbohydrate metabolism after ingestion of a challenge dose of glucose. The body absorbs this dose rapidly, causing plasma glucose levels to rise and peak within 30 minutes to 1 hour. The pancreas responds by secreting more insulin, causing glucose levels to return to normal after 2 to 3 hours. During this period, plasma and urine glucose levels are monitored to assess insulin secretion and the body's ability to metabolize glucose. Occasionally, levels are monitored an additional 2 to 3 hours to aid diagnosis of hypoglycemia and malabsorption syndrome. Such extended testing is contraindicated when insulinoma is strongly suspected, because prolonged fasting in such a patient can lead to fainting and coma.

In a patient with mild or diet-controlled diabetes, fasting plasma glucose levels may be within normal range; however, insufficient secretion of insulin after ingestion of carbohydrates causes plasma glucose to rise sharply and return to normal slowly. This decreased tolerance for glucose helps confirm mild diabetes.

The oral glucose tolerance test is not generally used in patients with fasting plasma glucose values above 140 mg/100 ml or postprandial plasma glucose above 200 mg/100 ml.

Purpose
☐ To confirm diabetes mellitus in selected patients
☐ To aid diagnosis of hypoglycemia and malabsorption syndrome.

Patient preparation
Explain to the patient that this test evaluates glucose metabolism. Instruct him to maintain a high-carbohydrate diet for 3 days and then to fast for 10 to 16 hours before the test. Advise him not to smoke, drink coffee or alcohol, or exercise strenuously for 8 hours before or during the test. Tell him this test requires five blood samples and usually five urine specimens; who will perform the venipunctures and when; and that he may experience transient discomfort from the needle punctures and the pressure of the tourniquet. Reassure him that collecting each blood sample takes less than 3 minutes. Suggest that he bring a book or other quiet diversions with him to the test, since the procedure usually takes 3 hours but can last as long as 6 hours.

Withhold drugs that affect test results, as ordered. If these drugs must be continued, note this on the laboratory slip.

Alert the patient to the symptoms of hypoglycemia—weakness, restlessness, nervousness, hunger, and sweating—and tell him to report such symptoms immediately.

Procedure
Between 7 a.m. and 9 a.m., perform a venipuncture to obtain a fasting blood sample. Draw this sample into a 7 ml gray-top tube. Collect a urine specimen

---

HOW TO ADMINISTER ORAL GLUCOSE SOLUTIONS

How much glucose should the patient receive? The oral glucose load in a glucose tolerance test is variable, ranging from 50 to 100 g. The American Diabetes Association, however, recommends a dose of 40 g of glucose/m² of body surface area, as calculated by a nomogram based on height and weight. Other workers advocate a glucose load of 1.75 g/kg of body weight, which is especially useful in testing pediatric patients.

Since many patients become nauseated after drinking the overly sweet glucose solution, how can the dose be made palatable? One way is to dissolve the glucose in water, flavor it with lemon juice, and chill. Another is to substitute Glucola, a carbonated drink, or Gel-a-dex, a cherry-flavored gelatin, for the appropriate amount of glucose.

INTERPRETING RESULTS OF
THE ORAL GLUCOSE TOLERANCE TEST (OGTT)

METHOD	HOUR	WHOLE BLOOD	PLASMA	POINTS
Wilkerson point system	Fasting	≥ 110 mg/dl	≥ 130 mg/dl	1
	1	≥ 170 mg/dl	≥ 195 mg/dl	½
	2	≥ 120 mg/dl	≥ 140 mg/dl	½
	3	≥ 110 mg/dl	≥ 130 mg/dl	1
Two or more total points confirm diagnosis of diabetes.				
Fajans-Conn	1	≥ 160 mg/dl	≥ 185 mg/dl	
	1½	≥ 140 mg/dl	≥ 165 mg/dl	
	2	≥ 120 mg/dl	≥ 140 mg/dl	
If all levels exceed or equal established values, diagnosis of diabetes is confirmed.				
National Institutes of Health (NIH)	Fasting		> 140 mg/dl	
	2		> 200 mg/dl	
If all levels exceed established values, diagnosis of diabetes is confirmed.				

Since a variety of methods are used to measure OGTT serum levels, inconsistent results, misinterpretations, and confusion are common. Despite the fact that age, race, inactivity, and obesity may also affect established OGTT criteria, the American Diabetes Association recommends using those diagnostic values obtained with the Wilkerson point system, the Fajans-Conn, or the NIH, depending on whether the patient is a child or is pregnant.

at the same time, if your institution includes this as part of the test. After collecting these samples, administer the test load of oral glucose, and record the time of ingestion. Encourage the patient to drink the entire glucose solution within 5 minutes.

Draw blood samples 30 minutes, 1 hour, 2 hours, and 3 hours after giving the loading dose, using 7 ml *gray-top* tubes. Collect urine specimens at the same intervals.

Tell the patient to lie down if he feels faint from the numerous venipunctures. Encourage him to drink water throughout the test, to promote adequate urine excretion.

Precautions

□ Send blood and urine samples to the laboratory immediately, or refrigerate them. Specify when the patient last ate,

and the blood and urine sample collection times. As appropriate, record the time the patient received his last pretest insulin or oral hypoglycemic dose.

□ If the patient develops severe hypoglycemia, notify the doctor. Draw a blood sample, record the time on the laboratory slip, and discontinue the test. Have the patient drink a glass of orange juice with sugar added, or administer glucose I.V. to reverse the reaction.

Values

Normal plasma glucose levels peak at 160 to 180 mg/100 ml within 30 minutes to 1 hour after administration of an oral glucose test dose and return to fasting levels or lower within 2 to 3 hours. Urine glucose tests remain negative throughout.

Implications of results

Depressed glucose tolerance, in which levels peak sharply before falling slowly to fasting levels, may confirm diabetes mellitus, or may result from Cushing's disease, hemochromatosis, pheochromocytomas, or CNS lesions.

Increased glucose tolerance, in which levels may peak at less than normal, may indicate insulinoma, malabsorption syndrome, adrenocortical insufficiency (Addison's disease), hypothyroidism, or hypopituitarism.

Post-test care
□ If a hematoma develops at the venipuncture site, apply warm soaks.
□ Provide a balanced meal or a snack, but observe for hypoglycemic reaction.
□ As ordered, resume administration of medications withheld before the test.

Interfering factors
□ Elevated plasma glucose levels may result from chlorthalidone, thiazide diuretics, furosemide, triamterene, oral contraceptives (estrogen-progestogen combination), benzodiazepines, phenytoin, phenothiazines, lithium, epinephrine, phenolphthalein, caffeine, arginine, dextrothyroxine, diazoxide, large doses of nicotinic acid, corticosteroids, and recent glucose I.V. infusions.
□ Depressed glucose levels may be caused by ingestion of beta-adrenergic blockers, amphetamines, ethanol, clofibrate, insulin, oral hypoglycemics, and MAO inhibitors.
□ Failure to adhere to dietary and exercise restrictions may interfere with accurate determination of test results.
□ Carbohydrate deprivation before the test can produce a diabetic response (abnormal increase in plasma glucose, with a delayed decrease), because the pancreas is unaccustomed to responding to high-carbohydrate load.
□ Recent infection, fever, pregnancy, or acute illness, such as myocardial infarction, may elevate glucose levels.
□ Persons over age 50 tend toward decreasing carbohydrate tolerance, which causes an increase in glucose tolerance, to upper limits of about 1 mg/100 ml for every year over age 50.

CHERYL A. WALKER, RN, MSN

SUPPLEMENTARY GLUCOSE TOLERANCE TESTS

Although the OGTT is the most effective test for detecting diabetes, two other glucose tolerance tests are sometimes used as research tools to sensitize or confirm OGTT findings.

The *I.V. glucose tolerance test (IVGTT)* measures blood glucose after the patient receives an intravenous infusion of 50% glucose over 3 or 4 minutes. Blood samples are then drawn at ½-, 1-, 2-, and 3-hour intervals. After an immediate glucose peak of 300 to 400 mg/dl (accompanied by glycosuria), the normal glucose curve falls steadily, reaching fasting levels within 1 to 1¼ hours. Failure to achieve fasting glucose levels within 2 to 3 hours generally confirms diabetes. A similarly delayed return to fasting glucose levels may result from fever, stress, old age, inactivity, carbohydrate deprivation, neoplasms, cirrhosis, and steroid-producing endocrine diseases. Nevertheless, the IVGTT has the following distinct advantages over the OGTT:

• gastrointestinal hormones causing insulin secretion won't affect IVGTT glucose tolerance curves
• patients afflicted with intestinal absorption syndromes won't present abnormal curves
• the IVGTT provides an alternative to flat OGTT curves resulting from hypopituitarism, hypoparathyroidism, or Addison's disease
• this test avoids the inconvenience to the patient of the unpalatable oral glucose load.

The *cortisone glucose tolerance test (CGTT)* is occasionally used for patients with borderline carbohydrate-tolerance deficiencies and for those with strong familial predisposition to diabetes who produce a normal OGTT curve. Following a 3-day high-carbohydrate diet, oral cortisone acetate is administered 8½ and 2 hours before the standard OGTT. (Cortisone promotes glyconeogenesis and may accentuate carbohydrate intolerance in latent or mild diabetes.) Although this test is used primarily for research, values rising approximately 20 mg/dl above those of standard OGTT after 2 hours demonstrate probable diabetes in some persons with only minimally decreased carbohydrate intolerance.

GLUCOSE TOLERANCE CURVES

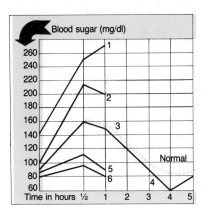

An OGTT measures both blood and urine sugar levels. As shown, various diseases other than diabetes mellitus produce abnormal glucose tolerance curves: (1) diabetes mellitus, myasthenia gravis, brain injury, Cushing's syndrome, acromegaly (early), and hemochromatosis; (2) alimentary glycosuria and glucose infusions; (3) the dotted line indicates the normal curve while the adjoining line (4) shows that persons with insulin shock, spontaneous hypoglycemia, and hypoadrenalism have normal glucose tolerance until 2 hours after ingestion of the sugar load, but then have marked hypoglycemia; (5) pituitary deficiency and myxedema; (6) anorexia nervosa, panhypopituitarism, hyperinsulinism, and Addison's disease.

Adapted from John Bauer, et al, *Clinical Laboratory Methods*, 8th ed. (St. Louis: C.V. Mosby Co., 1974).

Tolbutamide Tolerance Test

I.V. *infusion of tolbutamide stimulates the pancreatic beta cells and certain tumors to secrete insulin, and is used to evaluate patients with pancreatic disorders. (Oral tolbutamide is ineffective for this purpose.) Since plasma glucose levels normally decrease rapidly after such infusion and return to pretest levels in 1½ to 3 hours, abnormal insulin secretion can be demonstrated indirectly by monitoring plasma glucose levels.*

Although this test can help determine the cause of severe hypoglycemia shown in the fasting plasma glucose or 2-hour postprandial glucose test, it's contraindicated in patients with fasting glucose levels that fall below 50 mg/dl. Since tolbutamide depresses plasma glucose to about half the fasting level, it can cause such patients to develop severe hypoglycemia, leading to seizures and coma. The tolbutamide tolerance test is also con- *traindicated in patients with hypersensitivity to tolbutamide or other sulfonylureas, and should also be used cautiously in patients with known hypersensitivity to sulfonamides.*

Purpose
□ To diagnose insulinoma and rule out functional hyperinsulinism.

Patient preparation
Explain to the patient that this test evaluates insulin production. Instruct him to maintain a high-carbohydrate diet (150 to 300 g/day) for 3 days before the test and then to fast overnight, and to avoid smoking during the fast and the test. Inform him who will infuse the tolbutamide and when, and that a doctor will be present or nearby during the infusion. Then, tell him how many blood samples are required; who will perform the venipunctures and when; and that he may experience transient discomfort from the needle punctures and the pressure of the tourniquet. Reassure him that collecting each sample takes less than 3 minutes.

Withhold drugs that affect test results,

PHYSIOLOGIC RESPONSE TO HYPOGLYCEMIA

Various body organs respond to hypoglycemic states. Describe to the patient the symptoms he is most likely to notice, such as headache, sweating, and nausea.

Brain
Headache, aphasia, twitching, dizziness, depression, blurred vision, drowsiness, loss of consciousness, convulsions

Heart
Hypotension, tachycardia

Stomach
Vomiting, hunger, belching, nausea

Adrenal gland
Increased epinephrine secretion causes sweating, shakiness, trembling, weakness, anxiety, pallor, increased respirations.

KEY: Parasympathetic system =====
Sympathetic system ═══

---

as ordered, but report such drugs to the laboratory if use is continued.

NURSING ALERT To avoid the multiple venipunctures required for this test, maintain the patency of the vein through a KVO (keep-vein-open) I.V. infusion with normal saline solution or by insertion of a heparin lock. Alert the patient to the symptoms of hypoglycemia—weakness, restlessness, nervousness, hunger, and sweating—and tell him to report such symptoms immediately. Provide books, games, or puzzles for diversion, if necessary, since the procedure takes about 3 hours.

Check patient history for previous adverse reactions to tolbutamide, other sulfonylureas, and sulfonamides.

Procedure

Perform a venipuncture to obtain a fasting blood sample, and collect the sample in a 10 ml *gray-top* tube. A mixture of 1 g tolbutamide and 20 ml sterile water is prepared; the solution should be shaken to dissolve any crystals. This solution is infused I.V. over 2 or 3 minutes. After the infusion, if insulinoma or hyperinsulinism is suspected, draw blood samples at 15, 30, 45, 60, 90, 120, 150, and 180 minutes.

Precautions

□ The tolbutamide solution must be used within 1 hour of preparation. Specify the collection time of each sample on the laboratory slip, and send each sample to the laboratory immediately.

NURSING ALERT □ If the patient develops severe hypoglycemia, notify the doctor. Record on the laboratory slip the time when symptoms developed, draw a blood sample, and discontinue the test. Give glucose I.V. to reverse this reaction.
□ If the patient develops anaphylaxis, administer epinephrine subcutaneously or I.M., as ordered, to reverse the reaction, and notify the doctor promptly.

Values

After tolbutamide infusion in normal

subjects, plasma glucose levels promptly drop to about half the fasting level, remain low for 30 minutes, and then gradually rise to pretest levels in 1½ to 3 hours.

Implications of results

The degree and duration of hypoglycemia help establish the diagnosis. In hyperinsulinism, plasma glucose levels mirror those found in normal persons. In insulinoma, however, glucose levels drop markedly and may take 3 hours or more to return to pretest levels.

Post-test care

□ If phlebitis develops at the I.V. site, notify the doctor. Elevate the arm, and apply warm soaks.

□ If a hematoma develops at the venipuncture site, apply warm soaks.

□ Provide the patient with a balanced meal or a snack. As ordered, administration of medications withheld before the test may begin again, and the patient may resume his regular diet and normal activities.

Interfering factors

□ Hypoglycemic action of tolbutamide may be enhanced by salicylates, chloramphenicol, phenylbutazone, MAO inhibitors, and sulfonamides.

□ False-positive test results may result from hepatic dysfunction, the ingestion of excessive amounts of alcohol, malnutrition, azotemia, sarcoma, and some nonpancreatic tumors.

CHERYL A. WALKER, RN, MSN

Glycosylated Hemoglobin

[Total fasting hemoglobin, glycohemoglobin]

The glycosylated hemoglobin test is a relatively new diagnostic tool for monitoring diabetes therapy. The three minor hemoglobins measured in this test—hemoglobins (Hgb) A_{1a}, A_{1b}, and A_{1c}—are variants of Hgb A formed by glycosylation, a nearly irreversible molecular process in which glucose becomes chemically incorporated in Hgb A. Since glycosylation occurs at a constant rate during the 120-day life span of an erythrocyte, glycosylated hemoglobin levels reflect the average blood glucose level during the preceding 2 to 3 months, and therefore can be used for evaluating long-term effectiveness of diabetes therapy.

Since the goal of diabetes therapy is to establish and maintain near-normal carbohydrate metabolism to prevent sequelae, the glycosylated hemoglobin test has distinct advantages compared with traditional blood or urine glucose tests. Determination of blood glucose levels requires repeated venipunctures; each measurement reflects glucose control only at the moment the sample was taken. Measuring urinary glucose excretion also reflects glucose control only at the time of collection. In contrast, measuring glycosylated hemoglobin requires only one venipuncture every 6 to 8 weeks and reflects diabetes control over several months. In addition, since this test measures glucose within an erythrocyte, levels are more stable than with plasma glucose, which is affected by metabolic processes within the body.

Glycosylated hemoglobin is measured by processing red cell hemolysates through a cation exchange chromatography column, to separate glycosylated hemoglobins from Hgb A.

Purpose

□ To assess control of diabetes mellitus.

Patient preparation

Explain to the patient that this test evaluates the effectiveness of diabetes therapy. Advise him he need not restrict food or fluids, and instruct him to maintain his prescribed medication or diet regimen. Tell him the test requires a blood sample; who will perform the venipuncture and when; and that he may experience transient discomfort from the needle puncture and the pressure of the tourniquet. Reassure him that collecting the sample generally will take less than 3 minutes.

Procedure

Perform a venipuncture, and collect the sample in a 5 ml *lavender-top* tube.

MONITORING DIABETES THERAPY WITH GLYCOSYLATED HEMOGLOBIN

The glycosylated hemoglobin test measures glucose levels chemically incorporated within three minor hemoglobins (all variants of hemoglobin A) over a 120-day period. Since glycosylated hemoglobin, unlike other test measures, represents a 120-day process—the life span of the erythrocytes containing glucose—this test provides stable values that may help assess average daily glucose levels over long periods in patients with diabetes. This valuable diagnostic tool may also help prevent serious complications of diabetes that occur even in patients whose insulin regimen, ingestion of hypoglycemic agents, and diet are strictly controlled. Without proper diabetes therapy and management, the chronic complications listed below can affect all the body's organs:

- cardiovascular disease, such as atherosclerosis, resulting in strokes and myocardial infarction
- peripheral vascular disorders, such as gangrene, intermittent claudication, and microangiopathy
- renal failure, specifically intercapillary glomerulosclerosis (Kimmelstiel-Wilson syndrome)
- urinary tract infections
- neuropathies ranging from extraocular muscle palsies to more common peripheral nerve problems
- neuropathies of the bladder, gastrointestinal tract, and reproductive system
- skin lesions and infections, such as candidiasis and necrobiosis lipoidica diabeticorum
- periodontal disease resulting in tooth loss
- cataracts and retinopathy leading to impaired vision and blindness
- diabetic acidosis, possibly resulting in coma

Precautions

Completely fill the collection tube, and invert it gently several times to mix the sample and anticoagulant adequately.

Values

Glycosylated hemoglobin values are reported as a percentage of the total hemoglobin within an erythrocyte. Since Hgb A_{1c} is present in a larger quantity than the other minor hemoglobins, it's commonly measured and reported separately. Hgbs A_{1a} and A_{1b} account for about 1.6% and 0.8%, respectively; Hgb A_{1c} accounts for approximately 5%; and total glycosylated hemoglobin accounts for 5.5% to 9%.

Implications of results

In diabetes, Hgbs A_{1a} and A_{1b} constitute approximately 2.5% to 3.9% of total hemoglobin; Hgb A_{1c} constitutes 8% to 11.9%; and total glycosylated hemoglobin, 10.9% to 15.5%. As effective therapy brings diabetes under control, glycosylated hemoglobin levels approach normal range.

Post-test care

☐ If a hematoma develops at the venipuncture site, ease discomfort by applying warm soaks.
☐ Schedule the patient for an appointment in 6 to 8 weeks for appropriate follow-up testing.

Interfering factors

Failure to mix the sample and anticoagulant adequately may influence and interfere with accurate determination of test results.

KAREN E. DYER, RN, BSN

Oral Lactose Tolerance Test

This test measures plasma glucose levels after ingestion of a challenge dose of lac-

tose. It's used to screen for lactose intolerance due to lactase deficiency.

Lactose, a disaccharide, is found in milk and other dairy products. The intestinal enzyme lactase splits lactose into the monosaccharides glucose and galactose, for absorption by the intestinal epithelium. Absence or deficiency of lactase causes undigested lactose to remain in the intestinal lumen, producing such symptoms as abdominal cramps and watery diarrhea. True congenital lactase deficiency is rare. Usually, lactose intolerance is acquired, as lactase levels generally fall with age.

Purpose
To detect lactose intolerance.

Patient preparation
Explain to the patient that this test determines if his symptoms are due to an inability to digest lactose. Instruct him to fast and to avoid strenuous activity for 8 hours before the test. Tell him this test may require a stool sample. Also tell him this test requires four blood samples; who will perform the venipunctures and when; and that he may feel transient discomfort from the needle punctures and the pressure of the tourniquet. Reassure him that collecting each blood sample takes less than 3 minutes, but explain that the entire procedure may take as long as 2 hours. As ordered, withhold drugs that may affect plasma glucose levels. If these drugs must be continued, note this on the laboratory slip.

Procedure
After the patient has fasted for 8 hours, perform a venipuncture and collect a blood sample in a 7-ml *gray-top* tube. Then, administer the test load of lactose—for an adult, 50 g of lactose dissolved in 400 ml of water; for a child, 50 g per square meter of body surface area. Record the time of ingestion.

Draw a blood sample 30, 60, and 120 minutes after giving the loading dose, using 7-ml *gray-top* tubes. Collect a stool sample 5 hours after the loading dose, if ordered.

Precautions
□ Send blood and stool samples to the laboratory immediately, or refrigerate them if transport is delayed. Specify the time of collection on the laboratory slips.
□ Watch for symptoms of lactose intolerance—abdominal cramps, nausea, bloating, flatulence, and watery diarrhea—caused by the loading dose.

Values
Normally, plasma glucose levels rise more than 20 mg/dl over fasting levels within 15 to 60 minutes after ingestion of the lactose loading dose. Stool sample analysis shows normal pH (7 to 8) and low glucose content (less than 1 + on a glucose-indicating dipstick).

Implications of results
A rise in plasma glucose of less than 20 mg/dl indicates lactose intolerance, as does stool acidity (pH of 5.5 or less) and high glucose content (greater than 1 + on the dipstick). Accompanying signs and symptoms provoked by the test also suggest but do not confirm it because such symptoms may develop for patients with normal lactase activity after a loading dose of lactose. Small-bowel biopsy with lactase assay may be done to confirm the diagnosis.

Post-test care
□ If a hematoma develops at the venipuncture site, apply warm soaks.
□ As ordered, instruct the patient to resume diet, activity, and medications withheld before the test.

Interfering factors
□ Drugs that affect plasma glucose levels—such as thiazide diuretics, oral contraceptives, benzodiazepines, propranolol, and insulin—may alter test results.
□ Delayed emptying of stomach contents can cause depressed glucose levels.
□ Failure to follow diet and exercise restrictions may alter test results.
□ Glycolysis may cause false-negative results.

CLARKE LAMBE, MD
LAUREL LAMBE, MS, RD

TISSUE OXIDASE TEST

Lactic Acid and Pyruvic Acid

[Lactate and pyruvate]

Lactic acid, present in blood as lactate ion, is derived primarily from muscle cells and erythrocytes. It is an intermediate product of carbohydrate metabolism and is normally metabolized by the liver. Blood lactate concentration depends on the rate of production and on the rate of metabolism; lactate levels may rise significantly during exercise.

Lactate is the reduction product of pyruvate, a by-product of carbohydrate metabolism. Together these compounds form a reversible reaction that's regulated by oxygen supply. When oxygen levels are deficient, pyruvate converts to lactate; when they are adequate, lactate converts to pyruvate. When the hepatic system fails to metabolize lactate sufficiently, or when excess pyruvate converts to lactate due to tissue hypoxia and circulatory collapse, lactic acidosis (lactate levels more than 2 mEq/liter, with a pH lower than 7.37) may result. Measurement of blood lactate levels by enzymatic methods, using lactic dehydrogenase, is recommended for all patients with

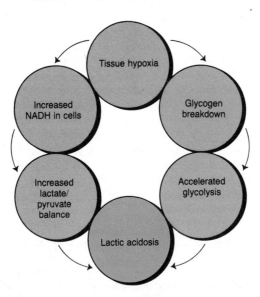

TISSUE HYPOXIA AND LACTIC ACIDOSIS

Tissue hypoxia

Glycogen breakdown

Accelerated glycolysis

Lactic acidosis

Increased lactate/pyruvate balance

Increased NADH in cells

When cells lack oxygen, glucose metabolism malfunctions. Nicotinamide-adenine dinucleotide bound with hydrogen (NADH), a facilitator in the energy-release process, builds up and cannot oxidize normally. The lactate/pyruvate balance, which depends on NADH, tilts to create a lactate overload. Simultaneously, glycogen stored in the cells converts back to glucose and degrades, further increasing cell and then blood concentrations of lactate. The liver cells, which usually filter and recycle lactate, now mimic other cells and become a lactate producer.

symptoms of lactic acidosis, such as Kussmaul's respiration.

Although arterial or venous blood can be used for lactate analysis, a venous sample is more convenient to obtain. However, unless the patient rests for 1 hour before the test, venous blood may yield higher values than arterial blood. Comparison of pyruvate and lactate levels reliably mirrors tissue oxidation, but measurement of pyruvate is technically difficult and infrequently performed.

Purpose
☐ To assess tissue oxidation
☐ To help determine the cause of lactic acidosis.

Patient preparation
The patient with acidosis is likely to be comatose or extremely lethargic. Nevertheless, explain to him that this blood test evaluates the oxygen level in tissues. Tell him who will perform the venipuncture and when; and that he may experience transient discomfort from the needle puncture and the tourniquet pressure. Reassure him that collecting the sample takes less than 3 minutes. Withhold food overnight, and make sure he rests for at least 1 hour before the test.

Procedure
Perform a venipuncture, and collect the sample in a 5 ml *gray-top* tube.

Precautions
☐ Since venostasis may raise blood lactate levels, tell the patient he must not clench his fist during the venipuncture.
☐ Because lactate and pyruvate are extremely unstable, place the sample container in an ice-filled cup, and send it to the laboratory immediately.

Values
Blood lactate values range from 0.93 to 1.65 mEq/liter; pyruvate levels, from 0.08 to 0.16 mEq/liter. Normally, the lactate-pyruvate ratio is less than 10:1.

Implications of results
Elevated blood lactate levels associated with hypoxia may result from strenuous muscle exercise, shock, hemorrhage, septicemia, myocardial infarction, pulmonary embolism, and cardiac arrest. When no reason for diminished tissue perfusion is apparent, increased lactate levels may result from systemic disorders—such as diabetes mellitus, leukemias and lymphomas, hepatic disease, and renal failure—and from enzymatic defects—such as in von Gierke's disease (glycogen storage disease) and fructose 1,6-diphosphatase deficiency.

Lactic acidosis can follow ingestion of large doses of acetaminophen and ethanol, and I.V. infusion of epinephrine, glucagon, fructose, and sorbitol. Because phenformin causes severe lactic acidosis, the Food and Drug Administration has removed it from clinical use as an antidiabetic agent.

Post-test care
☐ If a hematoma develops at the venipuncture site, apply warm soaks.
☐ As ordered, instruct the patient to resume his normal diet.

Interfering factors
☐ Failure to adhere to restrictions of diet and activity may interfere with accurate determination of test results.
☐ Failure to pack the sample in ice and to transport it to the laboratory immediately may elevate blood lactate levels.
CHERYL A. WALKER, RN, MSN

Selected References

American Diabetes Association. *The Physician's Guide to Type II Diabetes (NIDDM)—Diagnosis and Treatment,* 1984.

Petersdorf, Robert G., and Adams, Raymond D., eds. *Harrison's Principles of Internal Medicine,* 10th ed. New York: McGraw-Hill Book Co., 1983.

Stock-Barkman, Patricia. "Confusing Concepts: Is It Diabetic Shock or Diabetic Coma?" *Nursing83* 13:32-41, June 1983.

9 Vitamins and Trace Elements

LEARNING OBJECTIVES

After completing this chapter, the reader will be able to:
- explain why proper intake of vitamins and trace elements is necessary to maintain health.
- identify food sources of major vitamins and minerals.
- name and define the two classes of vitamins.
- describe how vitamin A deficiency can result in night blindness.
- list the principal properties and actions of vitamins and trace elements.
- state the purpose of each test discussed in the chapter.
- prepare the patient physically and psychologically for each test.
- describe the procedure for performing each test.
- specify appropriate precautions for accurate administration of each test.
- implement appropriate post-test care.
- state the normal values for each test.
- discuss the implications of abnormal test results.
- list factors that may interfere with accurate test results.

Vitamins and Trace Elements

Introduction

Vitamins and trace elements—organic and inorganic nutrients, respectively—are indispensable to normal metabolism and proper nutrition. Since the body can't synthesize most of these compounds, their normal concentrations within the body depend on adequate intake from nutritional sources. Except in persons with severely inadequate diets, this rarely presents a problem, however, because generous amounts of vitamins and trace elements are prevalent throughout the four basic food groups. Although food processing and cooking can reduce or destroy some of the nutrient value, a balanced diet usually provides sufficient amounts to maintain health. Supplements are recommended only for severely inadequate diet or a known deficiency.

Today, a far greater danger than trace element deficiency is toxic excess—through industrial exposure to potentially toxic levels of trace elements. Fortunately, sophisticated diagnostic techniques have been developed to detect minute concentrations of trace elements in serum. One such technique is atomic absorption spectroscopy. Equally sensitive tests are available to investigate vitamin toxicity or deficiency, using bioassays or chemical assays. Radioisotopes, for example, have been used to measure minute amounts of a specific vitamin, such as vitamin B_{12}, in serum.

Vitamins support life

Originally classified as "vital amines," vitamins differ in chemical composition and are not, in fact, all amines. However, they are vital for body maintenance, growth, and reproduction. Laboratory animals fed vitamin-depleted diets of carbohydrates, fats, minerals, and proteins failed to survive; only the animals fed diets containing adequate vitamins survived.

Because vitamins are generously prevalent in so many foods, absence of a vitamin, or *avitaminosis*, is rare indeed. A more common condition is hypovitaminosis, in which serum levels of a particular vitamin are below normal and may produce adverse clinical effects.

Fat soluble or water soluble

Vitamins are classified as fat soluble or water soluble. *Fat-soluble vitamins*, which include vitamins A, D, E, and K, are associated with lipids in food sources and are similarly absorbed. Although these vitamins are necessary for survival, excessive or prolonged ingestion of most fat-soluble vitamins—especially in doses that exceed the recommended daily allowance—can have toxic effects, since the body stores these vitamins in varying amounts and does not readily excrete them.

Fat-soluble vitamins have different functions that are only partially under-

WHAT TO LOOK FOR IN VITAMIN OR TRACE ELEMENT IMBALANCES

VITAMIN/TRACE ELEMENT	DEFICIENCY	TOXICITY
Vitamin A and carotene	• Night blindness • Xerophthalmia • Bitot's spots • Skin and mucous membrane infections • Follicular hyperkeratosis	• Hyperirritability • Yellow skin • Alopecia • Bone and joint pain • Headaches, vertigo • Hepatosplenomegaly • Malaise • Abdominal pain, anorexia • Transient hydrocephalus and vomiting in infants
Vitamin B$_{12}$	Megaloblastic anemia with: • Yellow skin • Anorexia and weight loss • Dyspnea • Prolonged bleeding time • Abdominal pain, constipation, anorexia, and weight loss • Glossitis • Peripheral neuropathy • Ataxia • Weakness	Nontoxic (even in high doses)
Vitamin C	• Bleeding gums, loose teeth • Joint pain • Irritability • Retarded growth • Dyspnea • Poor wound healing • Increased susceptibility to infection • Weight loss • Fever • Vomiting and diarrhea	Only after prolonged ingestion of massive doses (5,000 to 15,000 mg daily): • Nausea and vomiting • Possible formation of urinary tract stones, especially uric acid stones
Folic acid	Megaloblastic anemia with: • Yellow skin • Dyspnea • Prolonged bleeding • Abdominal pain, anorexia, and weight loss • Peripheral neuropathy • Ataxia • Weakness	Nontoxic (even in high doses)

WHAT TO LOOK FOR IN VITAMIN OR TRACE ELEMENT IMBALANCES *(continued)*

VITAMIN/TRACE ELEMENT	DEFICIENCY	TOXICITY
Vitamin D₃	Rickets in infants and children: • In early stages, profuse sweating, restlessness, and irritability • In late stages, bony malformations due to bone softening, delayed closing of fontanelles, poorly developed muscles, and tetany Osteomalacia in adults: • Bony malformation due to softening of bones in pelvis, spine, legs, and thorax • Rheumatic pain in lower back and legs • Spontaneous fractures	Early: • Anorexia • Nausea • Vomiting • Diarrhea • Headache Late: • Hypercalcemia leading to metastatic calcification, renal failure • Osteoporosis due to increased mobilization from bone
Chromium	• Possible impaired glucose tolerance	• Dermatitis and persistent ulcertion • Vertigo • Abdominal pain • Anuria • Shock, convulsions, coma
Manganese	• Retarded growth • Bone abnormalities • Reproductive dysfunction • Ataxia	• Pulmonary infiltrates • Early-stage, encephalitis-like syndrome: weakness, anorexia, apathy, headache, impotence • Late-stage, Parkinson-like syndrome: masklike face, monotone voice, tremor, muscle rigidity, spastic gait, clonus
Zinc	• Sparse hair growth • Hepatosplenomegaly • Severe anemia • Impaired taste and smell acuity • Unpleasant odor in nasopharynx • Anorexia • Pica (in children) • Retarded growth • Testicular atrophy • Hyperpigmentation	From accidental ingestion: • Gastrointestinal irritation with fever, cramps, diarrhea, nausea, and vomiting • Metallic taste in mouth From accidental inhalation: • Metal fume fever • Dry throat, cough, chest discomfort • Tachycardia and hypertension • Pulmonary edema due to inhalation

stood: vitamin A maintains night vision and the integrity of epithelial cells; vitamin D regulates calcium and phosphorus metabolism, and is thus primarily associated with bone maintenance; vitamin E, an antioxidant of polyunsaturated fatty acids, is associated with various synthetic processes in the body; and vitamin K is necessary for formation of certain blood-clotting factors.

Unlike fat-soluble vitamins, which tend to be stored and accumulate in the body, *water-soluble vitamins,* including vitamin C and the B complex vitamins, are readily excreted in the urine. Consequently, excessive dietary ingestion doesn't produce toxicity, and deficiency of these vitamins is more common. Water-soluble vitamins have many important functions. The B complex vitamins prevent certain diseases (vitamin B_1 [thiamine], for example, is an antiberi-beri factor), serve as coenzymes in energy metabolism (vitamin B_6 [pyridoxine], for example, is essential to protein metabolism), contribute to cell growth and the development of blood-forming factors (vitamin B_{12} is essential for normal hematopoiesis, as is folic acid). Vitamin C is necessary for collagen synthesis and for the maintenance of healthy bone and cartilage.

The vitamins and trace elements that will be discussed in detail in this chapter are vitamins A (and carotene), B_{12}, C, D_3, and folic acid, and the trace elements chromium, manganese, and zinc.

Trace elements

Trace elements are minerals found in the body in minute quantities. Vital to health, many trace elements are an integral part

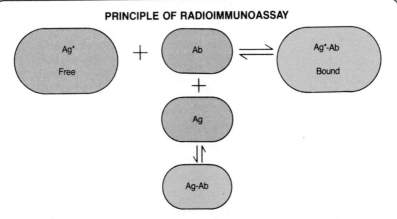

PRINCIPLE OF RADIOIMMUNOASSAY

Radioimmunoassay, a collection of laboratory procedures based on displacement reactions, allows sensitive and specific measurement of vitamins, hormones, and other compounds.

The laboratory technician radioactively tags a specific quantity of the subject substance, or antigen (Ag* in diagram) and then combines it with an equal amount of its specific antibody (Ab). This forms the bound complex (Ag*-Ab). When the technician introduces a patient's serum specimen containing the subject substance, this new and untagged antigen (Ag) displaces the tagged antigen in the complex and itself combines with the antibody until all the untagged antigen is bound. Since the amount of the freed radioactive antigen equals the amount of bound antigen, measurement of the tagged substance gives a clear accounting of the amount of nonradioactive antigen present in the serum sample.

Although antibodies are the most widely used binding reagents, certain naturally occurring binding proteins and receptors are also used. Binding proteins need little preparation and are stable, inexpensive, and of uniform consistency. However, they're available for only a limited number of compounds, have lower affinity constants, and don't always have good specificity. Receptors measure biologic rather than immunologic activity. They're uniformly consistent, but unstable and difficult to isolate.

of intracellular enzyme systems necessary for energy metabolism and other important biologic processes. Although more than 20 trace elements have been identified, only a handful (including manganese, cobalt, chromium, and zinc) are known to be essential to body functions. Manganese and zinc, for example, figure prominently in enzyme activation; cobalt is a critical factor in hematopoiesis; chromium is essential in amino acid transport. (Copper, another essential trace element, is often measured indirectly [see SERUM CERULOPLASMIN in Chapter 7] or in urine [see URINE COPPER in Chapter 17].)

Trace elements are found throughout nature in water, plants, and soil. Their concentrations in plant and animal food sources can lead to deficiencies or intoxication. However, since amounts required are so small and available from so many food sources, trace element deficiencies are rare. Deficiencies are most likely to develop during long-term hyperalimentation, unless the hyperalimentation solution contains trace element supplements. Excessive accumulations and toxicity are becoming a more common problem. For example, heavy industrial use of such minerals as chromium or zinc can result in overexposure through inhalation, skin contact, or accidental ingestion. Similarly, contamination of drinking water and of edible plants by dispersal of industrial wastes through soil can also cause overexposure to trace elements.

Managing imbalance

A patient suspected of having a vitamin or trace element deficiency or toxicity requires close observation for characteristic clinical features that may aid diagnosis (see pages 254-255). Accurate assessment of the patient's nutritional status is essential for identification of dietary needs and appropriate intervention. The hospitalized patient with nutritional imbalance requires careful monitoring of his diet to replace deficient nutrients; he may also need dietary supplements, as appropriate. To maintain correction of the imbalance after he leaves the hospital, the patient needs thorough teaching about good nutrition to make it an integral part of his life.

WILLIAM M. DOUGHERTY, BS

VITAMINS

Serum Vitamin A and Carotene

This test measures serum levels of vitamin A (retinol) and its precursor, carotene. A fat-soluble vitamin normally supplied by diet, vitamin A is important for reproduction, vision (especially night vision), and epithelial tissue and bone growth. It also maintains cellular and subcellular membranes and synthesis of mucopolysaccharides (the ground substance of collagenous tissue). Vitamin A is found mostly in fruits, vegetables, eggs, poultry, meat, and fish. Carotene is present in leafy green vegetables and in yellow fruits and vegetables. The body absorbs vitamin A from the intestines as a fatty acid ester; chylomicrons in the lymphatic system then transport it to the liver, where nearly 90% is stored. Absorption of vitamin A requires the presence of adequate amounts of dietary fat and bile salts. Thus, impaired fat absorption or biliary obstruction inhibits vitamin A absorption, causing a deficiency of this vitamin. Serum levels of vitamin A can remain normal as long as the liver retains even a low reserve of vitamin A.

In this serum test, the color reactions produced by vitamin A and related compounds with various reagents provide both quantitative and qualitative determinations.

COLORIMETRIC TESTING

Colorimetry, the analysis of a liquid's capacity to absorb light of a specific wavelength, refers to a variety of procedures that determine the amount of a test element, such as vitamin A, present in a liquid, such as serum.

In colorimetry, a lamp provides light of multiple wavelengths that is filtered to allow only a single predetermined color, or wavelength, to strike the sample liquid. Each element has just such a unique absorbance band, and the test solution absorbs this monochromatic light energy in proportion to the amount of the element present in the sample. Surplus light continues on to the detector, where it converts to electric current and registers on the readout dial. When compared with a standard gradient, the degree of light transmission through a sample liquid inversely indicates the degree of light absorption and reveals the amount of test element present in the liquid.

Purpose

□ To investigate suspected vitamin A deficiency or toxicity
□ To aid diagnosis of visual disturbances, especially night blindness and xerophthalmia
□ To aid diagnosis of skin diseases, such as keratosis follicularis or ichthyosis
□ To screen for malabsorption.

Patient preparation

Explain to the patient that this test measures the level of vitamin A in the blood. Instruct him to observe an overnight fast; advise him he needn't restrict water before the test. Tell him this test requires a blood sample; who will perform the venipuncture and when; and that he may feel some discomfort from the needle puncture and the pressure of the tourniquet. Reassure him that collecting the sample takes only a few minutes.

Procedure

Perform a venipuncture, and collect the sample in a 15 ml *red-top* tube (this test requires 6 ml of serum).

Precautions

□ Protect the sample from light, since vitamin A characteristically absorbs light.
□ Handle the sample gently to prevent hemolysis, and send it to the laboratory immediately.

Values

Using colorimetry, serum vitamin A values normally range from 125 to 150 IU/dl; carotene, from 48 to 200 mcg/dl.

Implications of results

Low serum levels of vitamin A (hypovitaminosis A) may indicate impaired fat absorption, as in celiac disease, infectious hepatitis, cystic fibrosis of the pancreas, or obstructive jaundice. These disorders interfere with intestinal absorption of vitamin A and thus lower serum levels. Low levels are also associated with protein-calorie malnutrition (marasmic kwashiorkor); this condition is rare in the United States but is a major nutritional disorder worldwide, especially among children. Similar decreases in vitamin A levels may also result from chronic nephritis, due to excessive loss of vitamin A in urine.

Elevated vitamin A levels (hypervitaminosis A) usually indicate chronically excessive intake of vitamin A supplements or of foods high in vitamin A. Increased levels are also associated with hyperlipemia and hypercholesterolemia of uncontrolled diabetes mellitus.

Decreased serum carotene levels may indicate impaired fat absorption or, rarely, insufficient dietary intake of carotene. Carotene levels may also be suppressed during pregnancy, due to the body's increased metabolic demand for carotene. Elevated carotene levels indicate grossly excessive dietary intake.

Post-test care

□ If a hematoma develops at the venipuncture site, apply warm soaks.
□ As ordered, remove diet restrictions.

Interfering factors

□ Patient failure to observe overnight fast

may influence test results.
☐ Hemolysis caused by rough handling of the sample may alter test results.

WILLIAM M. DOUGHERTY, BS

Serum Vitamin B₂
[Riboflavin]

This test evaluates the nutritive status and metabolism of vitamin B₂, helping to detect vitamin B₂ deficiency. Absorbed from the intestinal tract and excreted in the urine, vitamin B₂ is essential for growth and tissue function. In the tissues, this vitamin combines with phosphate to produce the coenzymes flavin mononucleotide and flavin adenine dinucleotide (FAD); these coenzymes subsequently participate in oxidation-reduction reactions with oxidative enzymes, such as glutathione reductase.

In this test, glutathione reductase activity is measured before and after administration of exogenous FAD. Normally, glutathione reductase binds with FAD. If vitamin B₂ supply is inadequate, glutathione reductase activity and the degree of FAD unsaturation will markedly increase, inversely proportional to vitamin B₂ concentration.

This serum test is considered more reliable than the urine vitamin B₂ test, which can produce artificially high values in patients after surgery or prolonged fasting.

Purpose
☐ To detect vitamin B₂ deficiency.

Patient preparation
Explain to the patient that this test evaluates vitamin B₂ levels. Instruct him to maintain a normal diet before the test. Inform him that the test requires a blood sample; who will perform the venipuncture and when; and that he may experience some discomfort from the needle puncture and the pressure of the tourniquet. Reassure him that collecting the sample takes only a few minutes.

Procedure
Perform a venipuncture and collect the sample in a 7-ml *red-top* tube. Mix the blood immediately with an equal amount of Alsever's solution, a preservative.

Precautions
☐ Handle the sample gently and send it to the laboratory immediately; do not refrigerate or freeze the sample.

Values
Normally, glutathione reductase has an activity index of 0.9 to 1.3.

Implications of results
An index of 1.4 or greater indicates vitamin B₂ deficiency. Such deficiency can result from insufficient dietary intake of vitamin B₂, malabsorption syndrome, or conditions that increase metabolic demands, such as stress.

Post-test care
☐ If a hematoma develops at the venipuncture site, apply warm soaks.
☐ Inform the patient with vitamin B₂ deficiency that good dietary sources of vitamin B₂ are milk products, organ meats (liver and kidneys), fish, green leafy vegetables, and legumes.

Interfering factors
☐ Hemolysis caused by rough handling of the sample may alter test results.
☐ Failure to add Alsever's solution to the sample may cause vitamin B₂ to deteriorate before testing.

WILLIAM M. DOUGHERTY, BS

Serum Vitamin B₁₂
[Cyanocobalamin, antipernicious anemia factor, extrinsic factor]

This radioisotopic assay of competitive binding is a quantitative analysis of

COBALT: CRITICAL TRACE ELEMENT

A trace element found mainly in the liver, cobalt is an essential component of vitamin B_{12} and therefore is a critical factor in hematopoiesis. A balanced diet supplies sufficient cobalt to maintain hematopoiesis, primarily through foods containing vitamin B_{12}. However, excessive ingestion of cobalt may have toxic effects. Toxicity has occurred, for example, in persons who consumed large quantities of beer containing cobalt as a stabilizer, resulting in congestive heart failure from cardiomyopathy. Since quantitative analysis of cobalt alone is difficult because of the minute amount found in the body, cobalt is often measured by bioassay as part of vitamin B_{12}.

The normal cobalt concentration of human plasma is about 60 to 80 pg/ml.

serum vitamin B_{12} levels. This test is usually performed concurrently with measurement of serum folic acid levels, since deficiencies of vitamin B_{12} and folic acid are the two most common causes of megaloblastic anemia. A water-soluble vitamin containing cobalt, vitamin B_{12} is essential to hematopoiesis, DNA synthesis and growth, and myelin synthesis and nervous system integrity. Ingested almost exclusively in animal products, such as meat (also shellfish), milk, and eggs, vitamin B_{12} is absorbed from the ileum, after forming a complex with intrinsic factor, and is stored in the liver. A clinical vitamin B_{12} deficiency takes years to develop, since almost total conservation is provided by a cyclic pathway (enterohepatic circulation) that allows reabsorption of the vitamin B_{12} normally excreted in bile. Deficiency of intrinsic factor, however, causes malabsorption of vitamin B_{12} and may result in pernicious anemia.

Purpose

☐ To aid differential diagnosis of megaloblastic anemia, which may be due to a deficiency of vitamin B_{12} or folic acid
☐ To aid differential diagnosis of CNS disorders that are affecting peripheral and spinal myelinated nerves.

Patient preparation

Explain to the patient that this test determines the amount of vitamin B_{12} in the blood. Instruct him to observe an overnight fast before the test. Tell him this test requires a blood sample; who will perform the venipuncture and when; and that he may feel some discomfort from the needle puncture and the pressure of the tourniquet. Reassure him that collecting the sample takes only a few minutes.

Check patient history for use of drugs—such as para-aminosalicylic acid, phenytoin, neomycin, and colchicine—that may alter test results.

Procedure

Perform a venipuncture, and collect the sample in a 7 ml *red-top* tube.

Precautions

Handle the sample gently to prevent hemolysis, and send it to the laboratory immediately.

Values

Normally, serum vitamin B_{12} values range from 200 to 1,100 pg/ml.

Implications of results

Decreased serum levels may indicate inadequate dietary intake of vitamin B_{12}, especially if the patient is a strict vegetarian. Low levels are also associated with malabsorption syndromes (such as celiac disease), isolated malabsorption of vitamin B_{12}, hypermetabolic states (such as hyperthyroidism), pregnancy, and CNS damage (posterolateral sclerosis or funicular degeneration, for example).

Elevated levels of serum vitamin B_{12} may result from excessive dietary intake; hepatic disease, such as cirrhosis, or acute or chronic hepatitis; or myeloproliferative disorders, such as myelocytic leukemia. These conditions raise levels of serum vitamin B_{12}–binding proteins, causing high serum levels of vitamin B_{12}.

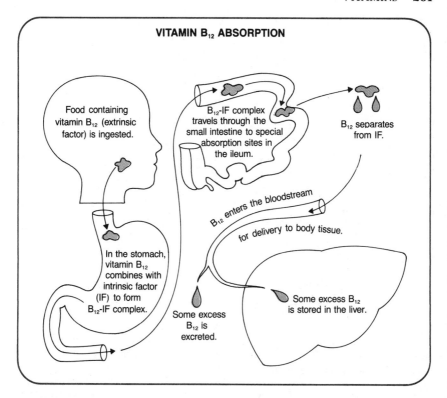

VITAMIN B₁₂ ABSORPTION

Food containing vitamin B₁₂ (extrinsic factor) is ingested.

B₁₂-IF complex travels through the small intestine to special absorption sites in the ileum.

B₁₂ separates from IF.

B₁₂ enters the bloodstream for delivery to body tissue.

In the stomach, vitamin B₁₂ combines with intrinsic factor (IF) to form B₁₂-IF complex.

Some excess B₁₂ is excreted.

Some excess B₁₂ is stored in the liver.

Post-test care
☐ If a hematoma develops at the venipuncture site, apply warm soaks.
☐ As ordered, resume diet.

Interfering factors
☐ The patient's failure to observe the overnight fast, or administration of substances that decrease absorption of vitamin B₁₂ may alter test results.
☐ Hemolysis caused by rough handling of the sample may alter test results.

WILLIAM M. DOUGHERTY, BS

Plasma Vitamin C
[Ascorbic acid]

This chemical assay measures plasma levels of vitamin C, a water-soluble vitamin required for collagen synthesis, and cartilage and bone maintenance. Vitamin C also promotes iron absorption, influences folic acid metabolism, and may be necessary for withstanding the stresses of injury and infection.

After vitamin C is absorbed from the small intestine, it's transported in the blood to the kidneys and oxidized to dehydroascorbic acid. Then, it's stored in the adrenal and salivary glands, pancreas, spleen, testes, and brain. However, because the adrenal glands contain high concentrations of vitamin C, stimulation of these glands by adrenocorticotropic hormone may deplete stores of vitamin C.

This vitamin is present in generous amounts in citrus fruits, berries, tomatoes, raw cabbage, green peppers, and green leafy vegetables. Severe vitamin C deficiency, or scurvy, causes capillary fragility, joint abnormalities, and multiple systemic symptoms.

RISKS OF HIGH-DOSE VITAMIN C

In the early 1970s, Nobel Laureate Linus Pauling sparked interest in vitamin C when he suggested that megadoses of this vitamin may increase resistance to viral and bacterial infection, increase resistance to malignancy, and lower serum cholesterol levels. Pauling recommended daily doses of vitamin C two to five times the RDA (60 mg daily for adults), and much higher doses during times of stress or illness. In particular, he advocated very high doses to treat cancer and to relieve common cold symptoms.

To date, clinical studies haven't supported Pauling's theories. In fact, a recent study has proved definitively that high-dose vitamin C is no more effective than a placebo in the treatment of cancer. Other studies have shown that high-dose vitamin C has little or no effect on the severity of colds. But despite this, many people supplement their diets with high doses of vita-

min C. And, in addition to delaying proper treatment, some of them experience severe side effects.

The most common side effects of vitamin C are diarrhea and vomiting. However, in some people, high-dose vitamin C promotes formation of uric acid crystals, which may trigger or intensify gout, and causes oxalic acid accumulation in the kidneys, which may lead to formation of calculi. Vitamin C also promotes iron absorption, which can possibly lead to iron toxicity.

Additional risks include interference with drug metabolism and diagnostic tests. For example, high-dose vitamin C impairs the effectiveness of warfarin and other anticoagulants and can cause rapid excretion of other drugs by acidifying urine pH. And it interferes with fecal occult blood testing and produces false-positive test results for glycosuria.

Purpose
☐ To aid diagnosis of scurvy, scurvy-like conditions, and metabolic disorders, such as malnutrition and malabsorption syndromes.

Patient preparation
Explain to the patient that this test detects the amount of vitamin C in the blood. Instruct him to observe an overnight fast before the test. Tell him this test requires a blood sample; who will perform the venipuncture and when; and that he may feel some discomfort from the needle puncture and the pressure of the tourniquet. Reassure him that collecting the sample takes only a few minutes.

Procedure
Perform a venipuncture, and collect the sample in a 15 ml *black-top* tube containing oxalate.

Precautions
Handle the sample gently to prevent hemolysis, and send it to the laboratory immediately.

If transport is delayed, place the sample on ice.

Values
Normally, plasma vitamin C values range from 0.2 to 2 mg/dl.

Implications of results
Vitamin C levels diminish during pregnancy, reaching their lowest point immediately postpartum. Depressed levels are also associated with infection, fever, and anemia. Severe deficiencies result in scurvy.

High plasma levels can indicate increased ingestion of vitamin C in amounts far exceeding the recommended daily allowances. Excess vitamin C is converted to oxalate, which is excreted in the urine. Excessive concentration of oxalate can produce urinary calculi.

Post-test care
☐ If a hematoma develops at the venipuncture site, ease discomfort by applying warm soaks.
☐ As ordered, resume diet that was discontinued before the test.

Interfering factors
Failure to follow dietary restrictions or to transport the sample to the laboratory promptly, or hemolysis due to rough han-

dling of the sample may alter test results.
WILLIAM M. DOUGHERTY, BS

Serum Vitamin D₃
[Cholecalciferol]

Vitamin D₃, the major form of vitamin D, is endogenously produced in the skin by the sun's ultraviolet rays and occurs naturally in fish liver oils, egg yolks, liver, and butter. Like all other fat-soluble vitamins, vitamin D₃ is absorbed from the intestine in the presence of bile salts and is stored in the liver. To become active, this vitamin must undergo conversion to 25-hydroxycholecalciferol, its circulating metabolite; and then to 1,25-dihydroxycholecalciferol, a potent compound—often called a hormone—which controls bone mineralization.

The hormonal function of vitamin D₃ closely parallels that of parathyroid hormone in maintaining calcium and phosphorus homeostasis. Low serum calcium and phosphorus levels stimulate production of parathyroid hormone, which then stimulates renal secretion of 1,25-dihydroxycholecalciferol to promote intestinal absorption of calcium and phosphate. Together the two hormones stimulate renal absorption of calcium and mobilization of calcium from bone.

This test, a competitive protein binding assay, determines serum levels of 25-hydroxycholecalciferol after chromatography has separated it from other vitamin D metabolites and contaminants. Clinically useful in evaluating nutritional status and biologic activity of vitamin D₃, this test is commonly combined with measurement of serum calcium and alkaline phosphatase levels.

Purpose
□ To evaluate skeletal disease, such as rickets and osteomalacia
□ To aid diagnosis of hypercalcemia
□ To detect vitamin D toxicity

□ To monitor therapy with vitamin D₃.

Patient preparation
Explain that this test measures vitamin D in the body. Tell the patient he needn't restrict food or fluids, that the test requires a blood sample, who will perform the venipuncture and when, and that he may feel discomfort from the needle puncture and the pressure of the tourniquet. Collecting the sample takes less than 3 minutes. Check for drugs that alter test results (corticosteroids or anticonvulsants). If they must be continued, note this on the laboratory slip.

Procedure
Perform a venipuncture, and collect the sample in a 7 ml *red-top* tube.

Precautions
Handle the sample carefully to prevent hemolysis.

Values
The normal range for serum 25-hydroxycholecalciferol is 10 to 55 ng/ml.

Implications of results
Low or undetectable levels may result from vitamin D deficiency, which can cause rickets or osteomalacia. Such deficiency may stem from poor diet, decreased exposure to the sun, or impaired absorption of vitamin D (secondary to hepatobiliary disease, pancreatitis, celiac disease, cystic fibrosis, or gastric or small bowel resection). Low levels may also be related to various hepatic diseases that directly affect vitamin D metabolism. Elevated levels (over 100 ng/ml) may indicate toxicity due to excessive self-medication or prolonged therapy. Elevated levels associated with hypercalcemia may be due to hypersensitivity to vitamin D, as in sarcoidosis.

Post-test care
If a hematoma develops at the venipuncture site, apply warm soaks.

Interfering factors
□ Anticonvulsants and corticosteroids

may lower serum levels by inhibiting formation of vitamin D_3 metabolites.

☐ Hemolysis may alter test results.

LENORA R. HASTON, RN, MSN

Serum Folic Acid

[Pteroylglutamic acid, folacin, folate]

A quantitative analysis of serum folic acid levels by radioisotopic assay of competitive binding, this test is often performed concomitantly with serum vitamin B_{12} determinations. Like vitamin B_{12}, folic acid is a water-soluble vitamin that influences hematopoiesis, DNA synthesis, and overall body growth. The parent compound of folate vitamins, folic acid is biologically inactive and requires enzymatic breakdown in the small intestine for absorption into the bloodstream. Once in the bloodstream, folic acid is rapidly absorbed into the tissues. Normally, diet supplies folic acid in liver, kidney, yeast, fruits, leafy vegetables, eggs, and milk. Because the body stores only small amounts of folic acid (mostly in the liver), inadequate dietary intake causes a deficiency, especially during pregnancy, when the metabolic demand for folic acid rises. Because of folic acid's vital role in hematopoiesis, the usual indication for this test is a suspected hematologic abnormality.

Purpose

☐ To aid differential diagnosis of megaloblastic anemia, which may result from deficiency of folic acid or vitamin B_{12}

☐ To assess folate stores in pregnancy.

Patient preparation

Explain to the patient that this test determines the folic acid level in the blood. Instruct him to observe an overnight fast before the test. Tell him the test requires a blood sample; who will perform the venipuncture and when; and that he may experience some discomfort from the needle puncture and the pressure of the tourniquet. Reassure him that collecting the sample takes only a few minutes.

Check the patient's medication history for drugs that may affect test results.

Procedure

Perform a venipuncture, and collect the sample in a 7 ml *red-top* tube.

Precautions

Handle the sample gently to prevent hemolysis and send it to the laboratory immediately.

Values

Normally, serum folic acid values range from 2 to 14 ng/ml.

Implications of results

Low serum levels (less than 2 ng/ml) may indicate hematologic abnormalities, such as anemia (especially megaloblastic anemia), leukopenia, and thrombocytopenia. The Schilling test is often performed to rule out vitamin B_{12} deficiency, which also causes megaloblastic anemia (pernicious anemia). Decreased folic acid levels can also result from hypermetabolic states (such as hyperthyroidism), inadequate dietary intake, chronic alcoholism, small-bowel malabsorption syndrome, or pregnancy.

High serum levels (more than 20 ng/ml) may indicate excessive dietary intake of folic acid or folic acid supplements. This vitamin is nontoxic in humans, even when taken in large doses.

Post-test care

☐ If a hematoma develops at the venipuncture site, apply warm soaks.

☐ As ordered, resume diet.

Interfering factors

☐ Alcohol and phenytoin interfere with folic acid absorption and lower serum folic acid. Pyrimethamine can induce folate deficiency and low folic acid levels.

☐ Hemolysis caused by rough handling of the sample may alter test results.

WILLIAM M. DOUGHERTY, BS

TRACE ELEMENTS
Serum Chromium

This analysis by atomic absorption spectroscopy measures serum levels of chromium, a trace element found in most body tissues. Chromium aids the transport of amino acids to the liver and heart cells, and appears to enhance the effects of insulin in glucose utilization. In fact, when combined in a complex with nicotinic acid, trivalent chromium (the biologically active form) is known as the glucose tolerance factor because of its special role in glucose metabolism. The effect of impaired chromium metabolism on diabetes mellitus is under investigation. The primary natural sources of chromium are dairy products, meats, and fish. Chromium toxicity can result from industrial overexposure to the metal, such as in the tanning, electroplating, and steelmaking industries.

Purpose
☐ To detect chromium toxicity.

Patient preparation
Explain to the patient that this test helps detect excessive levels of chromium. Inform him he needn't restrict food or fluids. Tell him this test requires a blood sample; who will perform the venipuncture and when; and that he may feel some discomfort from the needle puncture and the pressure of the tourniquet. Reassure him that collecting the sample takes only a few minutes.

Check the patient's history for diagnostic tests performed during the previous 3 months in which radioactive

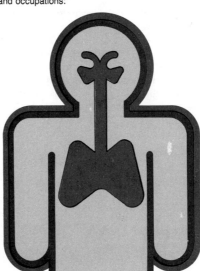

INDUSTRIAL EXPOSURE TO CHROMIUM VI

Approximately 175,000 industrial workers risk toxic exposure to chromium VI, the most toxic form of chromium. Such overexposure can result from inhalation or skin contact in the following industries and occupations:

- Abrasives manufacturing
- Cement manufacturing
- Diesel locomotive repair
- Electroplating
- Explosives manufacturing
- Furniture polishing
- Fur processing

- Glassmaking
- Jewelrymaking
- Metal cleaning
- Oil drilling
- Photography
- Textile dyeing
- Wood preservative manufacturing

Information from *NIOSH Criteria for a Recommended Standard Occupational Exposure to Chromium VI* (Washington, D.C.: Department of Health, Education and Welfare, 1975), #76129

hexavalent chromium was used (such as in RBC survival studies).

Procedure
Perform a venipuncture, and collect the sample in a metal-free collection tube. Laboratories provide special kits for this test on request.

Precautions
Handle the sample gently to prevent hemolysis, and send it to the laboratory immediately.

Values
Normally, serum chromium values range from 0.30 to 0.85 ng/ml.

Implications of results
High chromium levels are normal at birth but steadily decrease with age. Significant elevations indicate chromium toxicity, which usually causes dermatitis, and liver and kidney impairment.

Low chromium levels may diminish protein synthesis, due to decreased utilization of amino acids, but little evidence exists to verify clinical chromium deficiency.

Post-test care
If a hematoma develops at the venipuncture site, apply warm soaks.

Interfering factors
□ Recently performed diagnostic tests in which radioactive hexavalent chromium was used may interfere with accurate determination of test results.
□ Failure to use a metal-free collection tube may interfere with accurate determination of test results.

WILLIAM M. DOUGHERTY, BS

Serum Manganese

This test, an analysis by atomic absorption spectroscopy, measures serum levels of manganese, a trace element.

Manganese is found throughout the body but concentrates mainly in the pituitary, the pineal, and lactating mammary glands, as well as in the liver and bones. Although the function of this element in humans is only partially understood, manganese is known to activate several enzymes—including cholinesterase and arginase—that are essential to metabolism. Arginase, for example, is necessary for the formation of urea during protein catabolism.

Because of poor intestinal absorption, the body retains only a fraction of the manganese supplied by foods such as unrefined cereals, green leafy vegetables, and nuts. Industrial workers exposed to potentially dangerous levels of manganese may require testing for toxicity. Such toxicity can follow inhalation of manganese dust or fumes—a constant hazard in the steel and dry-cell battery industries—or ingestion of contaminated water.

Purpose
□ To detect manganese toxicity.

Patient preparation
Explain to the patient that this test determines the manganese level in the blood. Inform him he needn't restrict food or fluids. Tell him this test requires a blood sample; who will perform the venipuncture and when; and that he may feel some discomfort from the needle puncture and the pressure of the tourniquet. Reassure him that collecting the sample takes only a few minutes.

Check patient history for use of medications that may influence serum manganese levels.

Procedure
Perform a venipuncture, and collect the sample in a metal-free collection tube. Laboratories will supply a special kit for this test on request.

Precautions
Handle the sample gently to prevent hemolysis, and send it to the laboratory immediately.

ATOMIC ABSORPTION SPECTROPHOTOMETRY
(USED FOR MEASURING CHROMIUM, MANGANESE, AND ZINC)

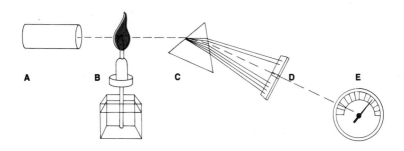

A   B   C   D   E

The term "photometry" originally meant measuring the intensity of light without regard to wavelength, while the newer technique of "spectrophotometry" meant measurement in a narrowed wavelength range.

Since most equipment today can isolate particular wave bands of the spectrum for study, "photometer" has come to mean an instrument that uses filters to accomplish this, while "spectrophotometer" refers to instruments using prisms or prismlike gratings, or both. Often, too, the old terms "colorimeter/colorimetry" substitute for "photometer/photometry."

Atomic absorption spectrophotometry measures the amount of light of a specific wavelength that a given substance absorbs when applied heat makes its atoms receptive. The technique uses a hollow cathode lamp (A) whose cathode is made of the test element, such as chromium, manganese, or zinc. The lamp emits a monochromatic light beam in the wavelength of the test element. An aspirator sprays the test sample (for example, serum containing zinc) up through the flame (B), where the heat releases the test element's atoms from their normal chemical bonds. In this free state, the element's atoms will absorb energy of their own wavelength, the same wavelength as the light beam emanating from the cathode tube. Light from the cathode tube that the atoms in the flame do not absorb passes on to a prism or other monochromator (C) and diffracts. The monochromator and the focus slit (D) act to refine the light beam so that only the very narrow, desired wavelength registers on the detector readout (E).

The net decrease in intensity of the beam from the lamp is an inverse measure of light absorbed in the flame by the test element, and hence the amount of the element (such as zinc) present in the (serum) sample. The greater the amount of element in the sample, the more light absorbed in the flame, and the less light transmitted to the detector.

Adapted with permission from Beckman Instruments, Inc., Fullerton, Calif.

Values

Normally, serum manganese values range from 0.4 to 0.85 ng/ml.

Implications of results

Significantly elevated serum levels indicate manganese toxicity, which requires prompt medical attention since it can lead to CNS deterioration. Depressed serum manganese levels may indicate deficient dietary intake, although such deficiency has not been linked to human disease.

Post-test care

If a hematoma develops at the venipuncture site, apply warm soaks.

Interfering factors

☐ High dietary intake of calcium and phosphorus can interfere with intestinal absorption of manganese and subsequently decrease serum levels.

☐ Serum manganese levels are influenced by estrogen, which increases levels, and by glucocorticoids, which alter its distribution in the body.

□ Hemolysis caused by rough handling of the sample may alter test results.

□ Failure to use a metal-free collection tube can interfere with accurate determination of test results.

WILLIAM M. DOUGHERTY, BS

Serum Zinc

This test, an analysis by atomic absorption spectroscopy, measures serum levels of zinc, an important trace element. Zinc is found throughout the body but concentrates primarily in the blood cells, especially in leukocytes. This element is an integral component of more than 80 enzymes and proteins, and plays a critical role in enzyme catalytic reactions. For example, zinc is closely linked to the activity of carbonic anhydrase, the enzyme that catalyzes the elimination of carbon dioxide.

Zinc occurs naturally in water and in most foods; high concentrations are found in meat, seafood, dairy products, whole grains, nuts, and legumes. Zinc deficiency (hypozincemia) can seriously impair body metabolism, growth, and development. This defect is most apt to develop in patients with certain diseases, such as chronic alcoholism or renal disease, that tend to deplete its body stores. Zinc toxicity is rare but can occur after inhalation of zinc oxide during industrial exposure.

Purpose
□ To detect zinc deficiency or toxicity.

Patient preparation
Explain to the patient that this test determines the concentration of zinc in the blood. Inform him he needn't restrict food or fluids. Tell him the test requires

---

INDUSTRIAL EXPOSURE TO ZINC OXIDE

Approximately 50,000 industrial workers risk toxic exposure to zinc oxide. Such overexposure can result from inhalation of dust or fumes in the following industries and occupations:

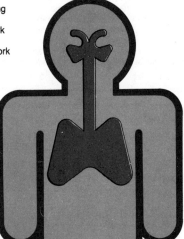

- Alloy manufacturing
- Brass foundry work
- Bronze foundry work
- Electric fuse manufacturing
- Gas welding
- Electroplating
- Galvanizing

- Junk metal refining
- Paint manufacturing
- Metal cutting
- Metal spraying
- Rubber manufacturing
- Roof making
- Zinc manufacturing

Information from *NIOSH Criteria for a Recommended Standard Occupational Exposure to Zinc Oxide* (Washington,D.C.: Department of Health, Education and Welfare, 1975), #76104.

a blood sample; who will perform the venipuncture and when; and that he may feel some discomfort from the needle and the pressure of the tourniquet. Collecting the sample takes only a few minutes.

Check the patient's recent drug history for zinc-chelating agents and other medications that may interfere with the test results.

Procedure

Perform a venipuncture, and collect the sample in a metal-free collection tube. Laboratories provide special kits for this test on request.

Precautions

Handle the sample gently to prevent hemolysis, and send it to the laboratory immediately. Reliable analysis must begin before platelet disintegration can alter test results.

Values

Normally, serum zinc values range from 0.75 to 1.4 mcg/ml.

Implications of results

Decreased serum zinc levels may indicate an acquired deficiency (due to insufficient dietary intake or to an underlying disease) or a hereditary deficiency. Markedly depressed levels are common in leukemia and may be related to impaired zinc-dependent enzyme systems. Low serum zinc levels are commonly associated with alcoholic cirrhosis of the liver, myocardial infarction, ileitis, chronic renal failure, rheumatoid arthritis, and anemia (such as hemolytic or sickle cell anemia).

Elevated and potentially toxic serum zinc levels may result from accidental ingestion or industrial exposure.

Post-test care

If a hematoma develops at the venipuncture site, apply warm soaks.

Interfering factors

☐ Zinc-chelating agents (such as penicillinase) and corticosteroids decrease serum zinc levels and may interfere with determination of results.
☐ Hemolysis caused by rough handling of the sample, or failure to use metal-free collection tube or to send the sample to the laboratory immediately can alter test results.

WILLIAM M. DOUGHERTY, BS

Selected References

Borhani, N.O. "Exposure to Trace Elements and Cardiovascular Disease," *Circulation* 63(1):260A-63A, January 1981.

David, Juan. "Vitamin D Metabolism," *Postgraduate Medicine* 68(5):210-18, November 1980.

Goldstein, D.A., et al. "Vitamin D Metabolites and Calcium Metabolism in Patients with Nephrotic Syndrome and Normal Renal Function," *Journal of Clinical Endocrinology and Metabolism* 52(1):116-21, January 1981.

Goodhart, Robert, and Shils, Maurice E., eds. *Modern Nutrition in Health and Disease*, 6th ed. Philadelphia: Lea & Febiger, 1980.

Guyton, Arthur C. *Textbook of Medical Physiology*, 6th ed. Philadelphia: W.B. Saunders Co., 1981.

Henry, John Bernard, ed. *Todd-Sanford-Davidsohn Clinical Diagnosis and Management by Laboratory Methods*, vol. 1, 17th ed. Philadelphia: W.B. Saunders Co., 1984.

Lamb, Jane O. *Laboratory Tests for Clinical Nursing*. Bowie, Md.: Robert J. Brady Co., 1984.

Petersdorf, Robert G., and Adams, Raymond D., eds. *Harrison's Principles of Internal Medicine*, 10th ed. New York: McGraw-Hill Book Co., 1983.

Ravel, Richard. *Clinical Laboratory Medicine*, 3rd ed. Chicago: Year Book Medical Pubs., 1978.

Tietz, Norbert W., ed. *Fundamentals of Clinical Chemistry*, 2nd ed. Philadelphia: W.B. Saunders Co., 1976.

Williams, Sue Rodwell. *Mowry's Basic Nutrition and Diet Therapy*, 7th ed. St. Louis: C.V. Mosby Co., 1984.

10 Immunohematology

LEARNING OBJECTIVES

After completing this chapter, the reader will be able to:
- explain the ABO and the RH blood group systems.
- list the health standards required of prospective blood donors.
- name the compatibility tests commonly performed on donor blood.
- state the causes and major characteristics of nine transfusion reactions and complications.
- discuss safety precautions for transfusing blood.
- state the purpose of each test discussed in the chapter.
- prepare the patient physically and psychologically for each test.
- describe the procedure for performing each test.
- specify appropriate precautions for safe administration of each test.
- implement appropriate post-test care.
- state the normal findings for each test.
- discuss the implications of abnormal test results.
- list factors that may interfere with accurate test results.

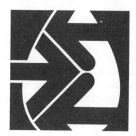

Immunohematology

Introduction

Immunohematology is the study of antigen-antibody reactions and their effect on blood. An *antigen* is a substance that can initiate an immune response and induce the formation of a corresponding antibody. The established major antigens found in blood are inherited, such as those in the ABO system and the Rh-Hr system; others can be introduced into the body from exogenous sources, such as blood transfusions or drugs. An *antibody* can be defined as an immunoglobulin molecule synthesized in response to a specific antigen. Successful blood transfusions require tests that identify these naturally occurring or acquired antigens and antibodies to make possible correct matching of donor and recipient blood. Among the most important of these tests are ABO blood typing, Rh typing, crossmatching, direct antiglobulin test, and antibody screening test. If a transfusion reaction occurs despite correct transfusion of compatible blood, tests for other antibodies (such as leukoagglutinins) help identify the cause and prevent further reactions.

ABO blood group

All blood group classifications are based on the types of antigens present or absent on the surfaces of RBCs. Karl Landsteiner, Austrian immunologist and winner of the 1930 Nobel prize for his work in physiology, created the most important

of these classifications—the ABO blood group system. Landsteiner classified human RBCs as A, B, AB, or O, depending on the presence or absence of these antigens on the surface of RBCs. Persons with group A blood have RBCs with A antigens; those with group B blood have B antigens. AB blood contains both A and B antigens; group O blood contains neither. In the ABO system, one or both of two naturally occurring antibodies, anti-A and anti-B, are found in the serum. Thus, a person with group A blood has anti-B antibodies, rather than anti-A antibodies, because the latter would destroy his RBCs. Similarly, a person with group B blood has anti-A antibodies. The person with group O blood, has both anti-A and anti-B antibodies; with AB blood, neither type of antibody.

Because group O blood lacks both A and B antigens, it can be transfused in limited amounts to any recipient in an emergency, regardless of the recipient's blood type, with little risk of agglutination. For this reason, a person with group O blood is called a *universal donor*. However, such transfusion should be given as packed RBCs, from which the plasma has been removed. Because a person with AB blood has neither anti-A nor anti-B antibodies, he can receive A, B, or O blood (packed cells) and is called a *universal recipient*.

Typing and crossmatching of donor

and recipient blood are required before transfusion, to establish compatibility. These tests minimize the risk of a hemolytic reaction—the greatest danger with blood transfusions. A hemolytic reaction is the immune reaction that occurs when the donor's and recipient's blood types are mismatched—that is, when blood containing anti-A antibodies is mixed with blood containing A antigens or when blood containing anti-B antibodies is mixed with blood containing B antigens. When mismatching happens, the antibodies attach to the surface of the foreign RBCs, causing the cells to clump together. This clumping can eventually plug small blood vessels and arterioles. Such an antibody-antigen reaction activates the body's complement system—a group of enzymatic proteins—which promotes and accelerates RBC hemolysis and phagocytosis by the reticuloendothelial cells. RBC hemolysis releases free hemoglobin into the bloodstream, which can damage the renal tubules and lead to renal failure and death.

Rh blood group

In 1940, Landsteiner and immunoserologist Alexander S. Wiener developed the Rh blood group system after discovering a certain antigen on the surface of RBCs in virtually all rhesus monkeys. Among humans, about 85% of Caucasians and an even higher percentage of Blacks, American Indians, and Orientals carry this Rh antigen, $Rh_o(D)$ factor, on their RBCs. Such blood is therefore classified Rh-positive. The remaining 15% or less of the population lack this factor, and their blood is typed Rh-negative. The Rh antigen is highly immunogenic—that is, it is more likely to stimulate formation of an antibody than other known antigens.

Consequently, then, a person with Rh-positive blood does not carry anti-Rh antibodies in his serum, because they would destroy his RBCs. However, a person with Rh-negative blood develops anti-Rh antibodies following exposure to Rh-positive blood (by transfusion or pregnancy). A transfusion reaction usually does not occur after the initial exposure to Rh-positive blood. Rather, anti-Rh antibodies generally develop slowly, over several months, causing the transfusion recipient to become sensitized to the Rh antigen. Subsequent exposure to Rh-positive blood then provokes a transfusion reaction and hemolysis, as in hemolytic disease of the newborn (HDN).

An important variant in the Rh system is the D^u antigen. This antigen, considered Rh-positive, is somewhat less immunogenic than $Rh_o(D)$ and may not provoke antibody production in persons lacking this antigen. Thus, all prospective donors must be screened for this antigen, which is more commonly found in Blacks than in Caucasians. Persons whose blood contains this antigen are considered Rh-positive donors but are generally transfused as Rh-negative recipients. This precaution is taken to protect persons with a D^u variant whose blood may not be distinguished serologically from that of D^u blood.

Other clinically significant Rh antigens have been discovered since Landsteiner's and Wiener's work; these additional antigens, such as rh' (C), rh" (E), hr' (c), and hr" (e) are much less immunogenic and not so likely to provoke an antibody reaction. Tests for these antigens are done only in special cases, as for establishing paternity, determining family studies, or distinguishing between heterozygous and homozygous Rh-positive factors.

Selection and screening of blood donors

To qualify for selection, prospective blood donors must meet strict criteria established by the Scientific Committee of the Joint Blood Council and the Standards Committee of the American Association of Blood Banks. The purpose of these guidelines is to protect the donor and the recipient and to ensure a safe, therapeutic blood transfusion.

Before donation, a detailed medical history must be obtained from the prospective donor, to detect abnormalities or conditions that may exclude or defer the donation. Such conditions include any disease that can be transmitted by blood transfusion (such as viral hepatitis, malaria, or acquired immunodeficiency syndrome [AIDS]), active tuberculosis, alcoholism, drug addiction or drug therapy, pregnancy, and recent immunizations or dental surgery.

A physical examination and laboratory tests must then be done to determine if the prospective donor meets the following minimum health standards:

□ *age:* should be between 17 and 65 years
□ *weight:* should be at least 110 lbs (50k)
□ *blood pressure:* systolic pressure between 90 and 180 mmHg; diastolic pressure between 50 and 100 mmHg
□ *pulse:* between 50 and 100 beats per minute and regular
□ *oral temperature:* should not exceed 99.6° F. (37.5° C.)
□ *skin:* should be free of all lesions at the venipuncture site; should show no

TRANSFUSION REACTIONS AND COMPLICATIONS

REACTION	CAUSE	SIGNS AND SYMPTOMS
Acute intravascular hemolysis	ABO donor-recipient incompatibility (rare)	Rapid onset of hemolysis with chills, fever, low back or chest pain, hypotension, nausea, vomiting, and bleeding disorders
Delayed extravascular hemolysis	Immunogenicity (as in Rh incompatibility); previous immunization through pregnancy	Slow onset of hemolysis with symptoms listed above
Allergy	Sensitivity to foreign plasma protein very common in transfused blood	Onset of pruritis and urticaria, possibly with facial swelling, dyspnea, and wheezing
Circulatory overload	Rapid or excessive blood infusion over a short time	Onset of dyspnea and enlarged neck veins, leading to congestive heart failure or pulmonary edema
Febrile nonhemolytic	Sensitization to leukocyte, platelet, or protein antigens (very common); bacterial contamination (rare)	Onset of chills and fever; later symptoms resemble a hemolytic reaction

COMPLICATION	CAUSE	SIGNS AND SYMPTOMS
Hepatitis	Blood transfusion containing hepatitis surface antigen or core antibody	Delayed onset of hepatitis B with fatigue, nausea, and yellow scleras
Potassium toxicity	Potassium leakage (out of RBCs into plasma) during blood storage (rare)	Immediate onset of hyperkalemia with tachycardia and later bradycardia, nausea, and muscle weakness
Citrate toxicity	Massive transfusion of citrated blood; citrate binds with plasma calcium because the liver can't metabolize it (rare)	Onset of hypocalcemia after several hours with tingling in fingers, cramps, and convulsions
Syphilis	Blood contaminated with *T. pallidum* (rare)	Onset of syphilis after 4 to 6 weeks with painless genital chancres, rash, and headache
AIDS	Transfusion of blood contaminated with AIDS virus (rare)	Insidious onset of AIDS with fever, adenopathy, and skin nodules

evidence of intravenous drug abuse
□ *hemoglobin:* 12.5 g/dl for females; 13.5 g/dl for males
□ *hematocrit:* 38% or more for females; 41% or more for males.

Testing of donor blood

Except in the case of identical twins or of a recipient being his own donor (autologous transfusion), testing for blood compatibility between donor and recipient can never be foolproof. However, certain tests on donor blood can ensure the best possible blood selection for the recipient. These include:
□ determining ABO and Rh blood groups
□ detecting unexpected antibodies that can coat, hemolyze, or agglutinate RBCs
□ crossmatching of donor blood and recipient blood (usually done while testing for unexpected antibodies)
□ detecting hepatitis B$_s$ antigen, syphilis, and AIDS.

Nursing considerations

After testing to establish the compatibility of donor and recipient blood, the most important nursing consideration is to make sure you match the *right* blood with the *right* patient. Hemolytic reactions are most often caused by giving blood to the wrong person and mislabeling the specimen. Double-check the patient's name, medical record number, and ABO and Rh status, preferably with another nurse or a doctor. If there is a discrepancy—no matter how slight—*don't* administer the blood. Instead, notify the blood bank immediately, so a substitution can be made without delay. Preventing potentially fatal hemolytic reactions from mismatched blood transfusions ranks among the most critical of nursing responsibilities. Uncompromising thoroughness and strict adherence to protocol ensures the safety of your patients in this regard.

After blood is administered, another important nursing consideration is to watch for signs and symptoms of a transfusion reaction. Check the patient's vital signs before and during the blood transfusion. For the first 15 minutes, transfuse the blood slowly to lessen the severity of any reaction that may occur, and stay with the patient. Notify the doctor immediately at the first signs of a transfusion reaction.

DEBORAH S. PARZIALE, RN, MS

AGGLUTINATION TESTS

ABO Blood Typing

This test classifies blood according to the presence of major antigens A and B on red cell surfaces and according to serum antibodies anti-A and anti-B. ABO blood typing, using both forward and reverse methods, is required before transfusion, to prevent a lethal reaction—even if the patient is carrying an ABO blood group identification card.

In forward typing, the patient's red cells are mixed with anti-A serum, then with anti-B serum; the presence or absence of agglutination determines the blood group. In reverse typing, the results of the forward method are verified by mixing the patient's serum with known group A and group B cells. Blood group determination is confirmed when the results of forward and reverse typing match perfectly.

Purpose

□ To establish blood group according to the ABO system
□ To check compatibility of donor and recipient blood before transfusion.

Patient preparation

Tell the patient this test determines blood group. If he's scheduled for a transfusion, explain that once his blood group is known, it can be matched with the

ABO BLOOD TYPES

ABO RECIPIENT-DONOR COMPATIBILITY

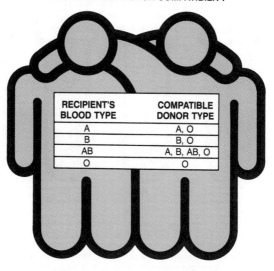

RECIPIENT'S BLOOD TYPE	COMPATIBLE DONOR TYPE
A	A, O
B	B, O
AB	A, B, AB, O
O	O

ABO FREQUENCY IN U.S. POPULATION

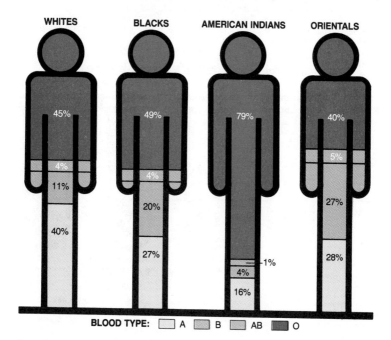

WHITES · BLACKS · AMERICAN INDIANS · ORIENTALS

BLOOD TYPE: ☐ A ☐ B ☐ AB ☐ O

Figures taken with permission from *Technical Methods and Procedures of the American Association of Blood Banks* (Washington, D.C.: American Association of Blood Banks, 1977).

ROUTINE ABO TYPING

FORWARD TYPING: CELLS TESTED WITH ANTI-A AND ANTI-B SERUM ANTIBODIES

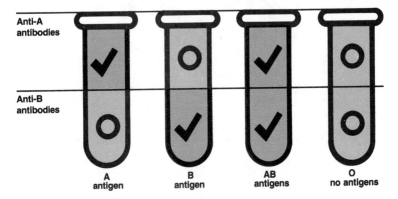

Blood types correspond to the antigens present or absent in red blood cells (RBCs). Almost everyone produces antibodies that work against foreign antigens, thereby protecting RBCs. Thus, a person with type A blood has A antigens and forms anti-B antibodies. Conversely, a person with type B blood has B antigens and forms anti-A antibodies. Type AB blood contains both antigens and neither antibody. Type O blood contains no antigens, thereby allowing the body to form both anti-A and anti-B antibodies.

To avert a hemolytic reaction—the greatest danger with blood transfusions—blood typing and crossmatching are routinely performed. In forward typing, a saline solution of RBCs with specific antigens is mixed first with anti-A antiserum, and then with anti-B antiserum. Agglutination occurs when A antigens and anti-A antibodies, or B antigens and anti-B antibodies are tested together.

REVERSE TYPING: SERUM TESTED AGAINST A, B, AND O CELLS

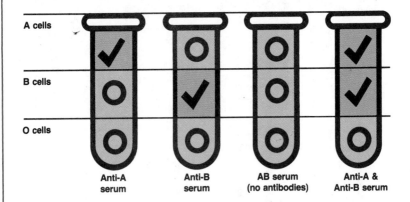

To confirm the results of forward typing, serum is tested against A, B, and O cells. (O cells serve as a control and help detect agglutinizing materials unrelated to antigen-antibody reactions.) In this typing procedure, agglutination occurs when serum and cells are mismatched.

KEY **Agglutination** **No agglutination**

right donor blood. Inform him he needn't fast. Tell him the test requires a blood sample; who will perform the venipuncture and when; and that he may feel transient discomfort from the needle puncture and the pressure of the tourniquet. Reassure him that collecting the sample takes only a few minutes. Check his history for recent administration of blood, dextran, or I.V. contrast media.

Before the patient receives a transfusion, compare current and past ABO typing and crossmatching to detect mistaken identification and prevent transfusion reaction.

Procedure

Perform a venipuncture, and collect the sample in a 10 ml *lavender-top* tube or *red-top* tube, as ordered (one tube per three units of blood).

Precautions

Handle the sample gently, and send the sample to the lab immediately, with a properly completed request form.

Findings and implications of results

In forward typing, if agglutination occurs when the patient's red cells are mixed with anti-A serum, the A antigen is present and the blood is typed A. If agglutination occurs when the patient's red cells are mixed with anti-B serum, the B antigen is present and the blood is typed B. If agglutination occurs in both mixes, both A and B antigens are present and the blood is typed AB. If it does not occur in either mix, no antigens are present and the blood is typed O.

In reverse typing, if agglutination occurs when B cells are mixed with the patient's serum, anti-B is present and the blood is typed A. If agglutination occurs when A cells are mixed, anti-A is present and the blood is typed B. If agglutination occurs when both A and B cells are mixed, anti-A and anti-B are present and the blood is typed O. If agglutination does not occur when both A and B cells are mixed, neither anti-A nor anti-B is present and the blood is typed AB.

Post-test care

If a hematoma develops at the venipuncture site, apply warm soaks.

Interfering factors

□ Recent administration of dextran or I.V. contrast media causes cellular aggregation that resembles agglutination.
□ Hemolysis due to rough handling of the sample may affect test results.
□ If a patient has received blood in the past three months, antibodies to this donor blood may develop and linger, interfering with the patient's compatibility testing.

DEBORAH S. PARZIALE, RN, MS

Rh Typing

The Rh system classifies blood by the presence or absence of the $Rh_o(D)$ antigen on the surface of RBCs. In this test, a patient's RBCs are mixed with serum containing anti-$Rh_o(D)$ antibodies and are observed for agglutination. If agglutination occurs, the $Rh_o(D)$ antigen is present, and the patient's blood is typed Rh-positive; if agglutination doesn't occur, the antigen is absent, and the patient's blood is typed Rh-negative.

Rh typing is performed routinely on prospective blood donors and on recipients before transfusion. Only prospective blood donors are fully tested to exclude the D^u variant of the $Rh_o(D)$ antigen before being classified as having Rh-negative blood. Persons who have this antigen are considered Rh-positive donors but are generally transfused as Rh-negative recipients.

Purpose

□ To establish blood type according to the Rh system
□ To help determine the compatibility of donor before transfusion
□ To determine if the patient needs a RhoGam (Rh immunoglobulin) injection.

Patient preparation

Explain to the patient that the test determines or verifies blood group—an important step in ensuring safe transfusion. Inform him he needn't fast before the test. Tell him the test requires a blood sample; who will perform the venipuncture and when; and that he may experience transient discomfort from the needle puncture and the pressure of the tourniquet. Reassure him that collecting the sample takes only a few minutes.

Check patient history for recent administration of dextran, I.V. contrast media, or drugs that may alter results.

Rh TYPING

Positive Reaction
In Rh-positive blood, agglutination occurs (drawn below) when serum containing anti-D antibodies is added.

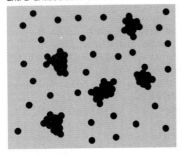

Negative Reaction
Since the Rh(D) antigen is absent in Rh-negative blood, agglutination does not occur (drawn below) when serum containing anti-D antibodies is added.

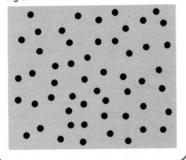

Procedure

Perform a venipuncture, and collect the sample in a 10 to 15 ml *lavender-top* tube or *red-top* tube, as ordered (one tube per three units of blood).

Precautions

☐ Label the sample with the patient's name, room number, and hospital or blood bank number, and send it to the laboratory immediately, since the test must be performed within 48 hours.

☐ If a transfusion is ordered, a transfusion request form must accompany the sample to the laboratory.

Findings and implications of results

Classified as Rh-positive, Rh-negative, or Rh-positive D^u, donor blood may be transfused only if compatible with the recipient's blood (see chart).

If an Rh-negative woman delivers an Rh-positive baby or aborts a fetus whose Rh-type is unknown, she should receive a RhoGam (Rh immunoglobulin) injection within 72 hours, to prevent hemolytic disease of the newborn (HDN) in future births.

Post-test care

☐ If a hematoma develops at the venipuncture site, apply warm soaks.

☐ Encourage the patient to carry a blood group identification card in his wallet to protect him in an emergency. Most laboratories will provide such a card on request.

Interfering factors

☐ Recent administration of dextran or I.V. contrast media results in cellular aggregation resembling antibody-mediated agglutination.

☐ If the patient has received blood in the past three months, antibodies to this donor blood may develop and linger, interfering with compatibility testing.

☐ Methyldopa, cephalosporins, or levodopa may cause false-positive results of the direct antiglobulin test (Coombs') for the D^u antigen.

DEBORAH S. PARZIALE, RN, MS

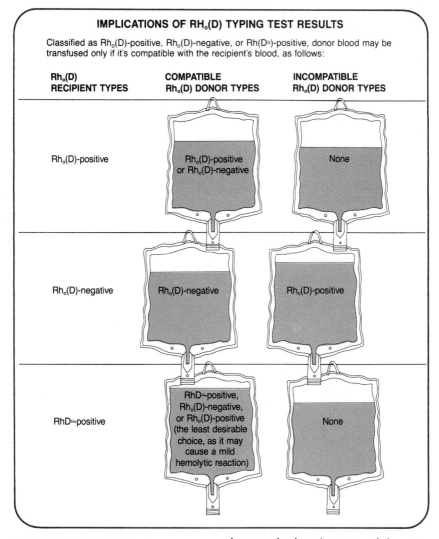

IMPLICATIONS OF RH₀(D) TYPING TEST RESULTS

Classified as Rh_o(D)-positive, Rh_o(D)-negative, or Rh(D^u)-positive, donor blood may be transfused only if it's compatible with the recipient's blood, as follows:

Rh_o(D) RECIPIENT TYPES	COMPATIBLE Rh_o(D) DONOR TYPES	INCOMPATIBLE Rh_o(D) DONOR TYPES
Rh_o(D)-positive	Rh_o(D)-positive or Rh_o(D)-negative	None
Rh_o(D)-negative	Rh_o(D)-negative	Rh_o(D)-positive
RhD^u-positive	RhD^u-positive, Rh_o(D)-negative, or Rh_o(D)-positive (the least desirable choice, as it may cause a mild hemolytic reaction)	None

Crossmatching

Crossmatching establishes compatibility or incompatibility of the donor's and the recipient's blood. It's the best antibody detection test available for avoiding lethal transfusion reactions. After the donor's and the recipient's ABO blood type and Rh factor type are determined, major crossmatching tests for compatibility between the donor's RBCs and the recipient's serum. They're compatible if the recipient's serum has no antibodies that would destroy transfused cells and possibly cause an acute hemolytic reaction. Minor crossmatching tests for compatibility between the donor's serum and the recipient's RBCs. This crossmatch is less important, however, because the donor's antibodies are greatly diluted in the recipient's plasma. Indeed, since the antibody-screening test is routinely performed on all blood donors, minor *crossmatching is often omitted.*

Blood is always crossmatched before transfusion, except in extreme emergencies. Because a complete crossmatch may take from 45 minutes to 2 hours, an incomplete (10-minute) crossmatch may be acceptable in these emergencies, such as severe blood loss due to trauma. In such an emergency, transfusion can begin with limited amounts of group O packed RBCs while crossmatching is completed. An emergency transfusion must proceed with special awareness of the complications that may arise because of incomplete typing and crossmatching. After crossmatching, compatible units of blood are labeled, and a compatibility record is completed.

Purpose
□ To serve as the final check for compatibility between the donor's blood and the recipient's blood.

Patient preparation
Explain to the patient that this test ensures that the blood he receives correctly matches his own to prevent a transfusion reaction. Inform him that he needn't fast. Tell him the test requires a blood sample; who will perform the venipuncture and when; and that he may experience some discomfort from the needle puncture and the pressure of the tourniquet. Collecting the sample takes only a few minutes. Check the patient's history for recent administration of blood, dextran, or I.V. contrast media.

Procedure
Perform a venipuncture, and collect the sample in a 10 ml *red-top* tube (one tube per three units of blood). If ABO typing, Rh typing, and crossmatching will be done together, collect the sample in a *red-top* tube.

Precautions
□ Handle the sample gently to prevent hemolysis, which can mask hemolysis of the donor RBCs.
□ Label the sample with the patient's name, room number, and hospital or

blood bank number. Also include history of transfusions, pregnancies, and drug therapy, and the amount and type of blood component desired.
□ Send the sample to the laboratory immediately. (Crossmatching must be performed on the sample within 48 hours).
□ If more than 48 hours have elapsed since the previous transfusion, previously crossmatched donor blood must be recrossmatched with a new recipient serum sample to detect newly acquired incompatibilities before transfusion.
□ If the patient is scheduled for surgery and has received blood during the previous three months, his blood will need to be crossmatched again if his surgery is rescheduled, to detect recently acquired incompatibilities.

Findings
Absence of agglutination indicates compatibility between the donor's and the recipient's blood, which means the transfusion of donor blood *can* proceed.

Implications of results
A *positive* crossmatch indicates incompatibility between the donor's blood and the recipient's blood, which means the donor's blood can't be transfused to the recipient. The sign of a positive crossmatch is agglutination, or clumping, when the donor's red cells and the recipient's serum are correctly mixed and incubated. Agglutination indicates an undesirable antigen-antibody reaction. The donor's blood must be withheld and the crossmatch continued, to determine the cause of the incompatibility and to identify the antibody.

A *negative* crossmatch—the absence of agglutination—indicates probable compatibility between the donor's blood and the recipient's blood, which means the transfusion of donor blood *can* proceed. It doesn't guarantee a safe transfusion, but it's the best method available to prevent an acute hemolytic reaction.

Post-test care
□ If hematoma develops at the venipuncture site, apply warm soaks.

□ Encourage the patient to carry an ABO group identification card. Such identification is helpful but doesn't replace crossmatching before a transfusion.

Interfering factors
□ Previous administration of dextran or I.V. contrast media causes aggregation resembling agglutination. Previous blood administration may produce antibodies to the donor blood that may interfere with compatibility testing.
□ Hemolysis due to rough handling of the sample may interfere with accurate determination of test results.

DEBORAH S. PARZIALE, RN, MS

Direct Antiglobulin Test

[Direct Coombs' test]

The direct antiglobulin test detects immunoglobulins (antibodies) on the surfaces of RBCs. These immunoglobulins coat RBCs when they become sensitized to an antigen, such as the Rh factor.

In this test, antiglobulin (Coombs') serum added to saline-washed RBCs results in agglutination if immunoglobulins or complement is present. This test is "direct" because it requires only one step—the addition of Coombs' serum to washed cells.

Purpose
□ To diagnose hemolytic disease of the newborn (HDN)
□ To investigate hemolytic transfusion reactions
□ To aid differential diagnosis of hemolytic anemias, which may result from an autoimmune reaction or drugs or may be congenital.

Patient preparation
If the patient is a newborn, explain to the parents that the test helps diagnose HDN. If the patient is suspected of having hemolytic anemia, explain that the test determines whether the condition results from an abnormality in the body's immune system, from the use of certain drugs, or from some unknown cause. Inform the adult patient he needn't fast. Tell the patient (or the neonate's parents) that the test requires a blood sample; who will collect the blood or perform the venipuncture and when; and that the procedure may cause transient discomfort. Collecting the sample, however, takes only a few minutes.

As ordered, withhold medications that can induce autoimmune hemolytic anemia.

Procedure
□ For an adult, perform a venipuncture and collect the sample in two 5 ml *red-top* tubes. For a neonate, draw 5 ml of cord blood into a *red-top* or *lavender-top* tube, as ordered, after the cord is clamped and cut.

Precautions
□ Handle the sample gently to prevent hemolysis, and send it to the laboratory immediately. The test must be performed within 24 hours after the sample is drawn.
□ Label the sample with the patient's full name, hospital identification number, age, and history of transfusions, pregnancy, and drug therapy.

Findings
A negative test, in which neither antibodies nor complement appears on the RBCs, is normal.

Implications of results
A positive test on umbilical cord blood indicates that maternal antibodies have crossed the placenta and have coated fetal RBCs, causing HDN. Transfusion of compatible, Rh-negative blood may be necessary to prevent anemia.

In other patients, a positive test result may indicate hemolytic anemia and help differentiate between autoimmune and secondary hemolytic anemia, which can be drug-induced or associated with an underlying disease, such as lymphoma. A positive test can also indicate sepsis.

A weakly positive test may suggest a transfusion reaction in which the patient's antibodies react with transfused RBCs containing the corresponding antigen.

Post-test care
□ If a hematoma develops at the venipuncture site, apply warm soaks.
□ As ordered, resume administration of medications withheld before the test.
□ Tell the patient or the parents of an infant with HDN that further testing will be necessary to monitor anemia.

Interfering factors
□ Hemolysis caused by rough handling of the sample may interfere with accurate determination of test results.
□ False-positive results may follow use of quinidine, methyldopa, cephalosporins, sulfonamides, chlorpromazine, diphenylhydantoin, dipyrone, ethosuximide, hydralazine, levodopa, mefenamic acid, melphalan, penicillin, procainamide, rifampin, streptomycin, tetracyclines, and isoniazid.

DEBORAH S. PARZIALE, RN, MS

Antibody Screening Test
[Indirect Coombs' test, indirect antiglobulin test]

This test detects unexpected circulating antibodies in the patient's serum. After incubating the serum with group O red cells, which are unaffected by anti-A or anti-B antibodies, an antiglobulin (Coombs') serum is added. Agglutination occurs if the patient's serum contains an antibody to one or more antigens on the red cells.

The antibody screening test detects 95 to 99% of the circulating antibodies. After this screening procedure detects them, the antibody identification test can determine the specific identity of the antibodies present.

Purpose
□ To detect unexpected circulating antibodies to red cell antigens in the recipient's or donor's serum before transfusion
□ To determine the presence of anti-$Rh_o(D)$ (Rh-positive) antibody in maternal blood
□ Evaluate the need for $Rh_o(D)$ immune globulin administration
□ To aid diagnosis of acquired hemolytic anemia.

Patient preparation
Explain to the prospective blood recipient that the antibody screening test helps evaluate the possibility of a transfusion reaction. If the test is being performed because the patient is anemic, explain to him that it helps identify the specific type of anemia.

Inform the patient that he needn't fast before the test. Tell him the test requires a blood sample; who will perform the venipuncture and when; and that he may feel transient discomfort from the needle puncture and the pressure of the tourniquet. Reassure him that collecting the sample takes only a few minutes.

Check patient history for recent administration of blood, dextran, or I.V. contrast media. Be sure to note such administration on the laboratory slip to prevent spurious interpretation of test results.

Procedure
Perform a venipuncture, and collect the sample in two 10 ml *red-top* tubes. Some laboratories require 20 ml of clotted blood to perform this test.

Precautions
□ Handle the sample gently to prevent hemolysis.
□ Label the sample with patient's name, room number, and hospital or blood bank number. Be sure to include the pa-

tient's diagnosis, and any history of transfusions, pregnancy, and drug therapy.

□ Send the sample to the laboratory immediately. (The antibody screening must be done within 48 hours after the sample is drawn.)

Findings

Normally, agglutination does not occur, indicating that the patient's serum contains no circulating antibodies (other than anti-A and anti-B).

Implications of results

A positive result indicates the presence of unexpected circulating antibodies to red cell antigens. Such a reaction demonstrates donor and recipient incompatibility.

A positive result in a pregnant patient with Rh-negative blood may indicate the presence of antibodies to the Rh factor from previous transfusion with incompatible blood or from a previous pregnancy with an Rh-positive fetus.

A positive result above a titer of 1:8 indicates that the fetus may develop hemolytic disease of the newborn. As a result, repeated testing throughout the patient's pregnancy is necessary for evaluating progressive development of circulating antibody levels.

Post-test care

If a hematoma develops at the venipuncture site, ease discomfort by applying warm soaks.

Interfering factors

□ Previous administration of blood, dextran, or I.V. contrast media causes aggregation that resembles agglutination.

□ Hemolysis caused by rough handling of the sample may interfere with accurate determination of test results.

□ If a patient has received blood transfusions within the past 3 months, antibodies to this donor blood may develop and linger, thereby interfering with the patient's compatibility testing.

DEBORAH S. PARZIALE, RN, MS

ANTIBODY IDENTIFICATION TEST

This test identifies unexpected circulating antibodies detected by the antibody screening test (indirect Coombs' test). Group O red cells—at least three with and three without a specific antigen—are combined with serum containing unknown antibodies and are observed for agglutination. If the serum contains the corresponding antibody to the red cell antigen, a positive reaction occurs with RBCs that have the antigen but not with those that lack the antigen. Serum that reacts with Rh-positive cells, for example, but not with Rh-negative cells, probably contains the anti-Rh_o(D) antibody. At least three red cells containing the antigen and three without it are used in each test to reduce error. Serum that contains rare or multiple antibodies requires more complicated procedures.

Leukoagglutinin Test
[White cell antibodies]

This test detects leukoagglutinins—antibodies that react with white blood cells and may cause a transfusion reaction. These antibodies usually develop after exposure to foreign white cells through transfusions, pregnancies, or allografts.

If a blood recipient has these antibodies, a febrile nonhemolytic reaction may occur 1 to 4 hours after the start of whole blood, red blood cell, platelet, or granulocyte transfusion. (All these blood products contain some granulocytes, which react with the antibodies.) This nonhemolytic reaction (marked by fever and severe chills, sometimes with nausea, headache, and transient hypertension) must be distinguished from a true hemolytic reaction before further transfusion can proceed.

If a blood donor has these antibodies, the recipient may develop acute, noncardiogenic pulmonary edema after transfusion of the donor's blood. In this case, the donor's blood must be tested for leukoagglutinins to determine if these have caused the recipient's reaction.

Two methods can detect leukoagglutinins. The older method detects white cell agglutination by microscopic examination of the patient's serum after it's combined with a suspension of granulocytes and lymphocytes. A new method uses a special fluorescence microscope to detect antibodies attached to normal granulocytes that have been incubated with recipient or donor serum. The immunofluorescent method is more sensitive and is now more widely used.

Purpose
□ To detect leukoagglutinins in blood recipients who develop transfusion reactions, thus differentiating between hemolytic and febrile nonhemolytic transfusion reactions

□ To detect leukoagglutinins in blood donors after transfusion of donor blood causes a reaction.

Patient preparation
If a blood recipient is being tested, explain that this test helps determine the cause of his transfusion reaction. If a blood donor is being tested, explain that this test determines if his blood caused a transfusion reaction and predicts whether he'll have a reaction if he receives blood in the future.

A pretransfusion blood sample taken from the blood bank's crossmatch sample is preferred for this test. If such a sample isn't available, tell the patient that the test requires a blood sample. Inform him who will perform the venipuncture and when. Advise him that he may feel some discomfort from the needle puncture and the pressure of the tourniquet. Reassure him that collecting the sample takes only a few minutes.

Note recent administration of blood or dextran or testing with I.V. contrast media on the laboratory slip.

Procedure
If a pretransfusion sample isn't available from the blood bank, perform a venipuncture and collect a blood sample in a 10-ml *red-top* tube. (The laboratory will require 3 to 4 ml of serum for testing.)

Precautions
Label the sample with the patient's name, room number, and hospital or blood bank number. Be sure to include on the laboratory slip the patient's suspected diagnosis and any history of blood transfusions, pregnancies, and drug therapy.

Findings
Normally, test results are negative: agglutination doesn't occur because serum contains no antibodies.

Implications of results
In a recipient's blood, a positive result indicates the presence of leukoagglutinins, identifying his transfusion reaction as a febrile nonhemolytic reaction to these antibodies.

In a donor's blood, a positive result indicates the presence of leukoagglutinins, identifying the cause of a recipient's reaction as an acute, noncardiogenic pulmonary edema.

Post-test care
□ If a hematoma develops at the venipuncture site, ease discomfort by applying warm soaks.

 □ If a transfusion recipient has a positive leukoagglutinin test, continued transfusions require premedication with acetaminophen 1 to 2 hours before the transfusion; specially prepared leukocyte-poor blood; or both, to prevent further reactions.

□ If a donor has a positive leukoagglutinin test, explain to him the meaning of this result to help prevent future transfusion reaction.

Interfering factors
Previous administration of dextran or I.V. contrast media causes aggregation resembling agglutination.

S. BREANNDAN MOORE, MD, DCH, FCAP

Selected References

Bryant, Neville J. *An Introduction to Immunohematology,* 2nd ed. Philadelphia: W.B. Saunders Co., 1982.

Circular of Information for the Use of Human Blood and Blood Components by Physicians. Washington, D.C.: American Association of Blood Banks, September 1978.

Dickason, Elizabeth Jean, and Schultz, Martha. *Maternal and Infant Care,* 2nd ed. New York: McGraw-Hill Book Co., 1979.

Diseases, 2nd ed. Nurse's Reference Library. Springhouse, Pa.: Springhouse Corp., 1986.

French, Ruth M. *Guide to Diagnostic Procedures,* 5th ed. New York: McGraw-Hill Book Co., 1980.

Giving Medications. Nursing Photobook series. Springhouse, Pa.: Springhouse Corp., 1982.

Hansten, Philip D. *Drug Interactions,* 5th ed. Philadelphia: Lea & Febiger, 1984.

Henry, John Bernard, ed. *Todd-Sanford-Davidsohn Clinical Diagnosis and Management by Laboratory Methods,* vol. 1, 17th ed. Philadelphia: W.B. Saunders Co., 1984.

Lamb, Jane O. *Laboratory Tests for Clinical Nursing.* Bowie, Md.: Robert J. Brady Co., 1984.

Leavelle, Dennis E., ed. *Mayo Medical Laboratories Test Catalog.* Rochester, Minn.: Mayo Medical Laboratories, 1984.

Luckmann, Joan, and Sorensen, Karen C. *Basic Nursing: A Psychophysiologic Approach.* Philadelphia: W.B. Saunders Co., 1979.

Miller, William V., ed. *Technical Manual of the American Association of Blood Banks,* 7th ed. Philadelphia: J.B. Lippincott Co., 1977.

Miller, William V., et al. *Technical Methods and Procedures of the American Association of Blood Banks.* Washington, D.C.: American Association of Blood Banks, 1974.

Nursing85 Drug Handbook. Springhouse, Pa.: Springhouse Corp., 1985.

Petersdorf, Robert G., and Adams, Raymond D., eds. *Harrison's Principles of Internal Medicine,* 10th ed. New York: McGraw-Hill Book Co., 1983.

Phipps, Wilma J., et al. *Medical-Surgical Nursing: Concepts and Clinical Practice.* St. Louis: C.V. Mosby Co., 1979.

Reeder, Sharon R., and Mastroianni, Luigi, Jr. *Maternity Nursing,* 15th ed. New York: J.B. Lippincott Co., 1983.

Rose, Noel R., and Friedman, Herman, eds. *Manual of Clinical Immunology,* 2nd ed. Washington, D.C.: American Society for Microbiology, 1980.

Stites, Daniel P., et al., eds. *Basic and Clinical Immunology,* 4th ed. Los Altos, Calif.: Lange Medical Publishers, 1982.

Tietz, Norbert W., ed. *Fundamentals of Clinical Chemistry,* 2nd ed. Philadelphia: W.B. Saunders Co., 1976.

Tilkian, Sarko M., et al. *Clinical Implications of Laboratory Tests,* 3rd ed. St. Louis: C.V. Mosby Co., 1983.

Wegener, Lee T., ed. *Mayo Medical Laboratories Interpretive Handbook.* Rochester, Minn.: Mayo Medical Laboratories, 1984.

Wyngaarden, James, and Smith, Lloyd. *Cecil Textbook of Medicine,* 16th ed. Philadelphia: W.B. Saunders Co., 1982.

11 Immune Response

LEARNING OBJECTIVES

After completing this chapter, the reader will be able to:
- explain how the immune system protects the body.
- describe seven common techniques used in immunologic tests.
- define the term *autoimmunity*.
- explain the purpose and procedure of each test discussed in this chapter.
- prepare the patient physically and psychologically for each test.
- state the normal values or findings for each test.
- discuss the implications of abnormal test results.
- list factors that may interfere with accurate test results.

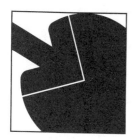

Immune Response

Introduction

A normally functioning immune system provides continuous physiologic surveillance. It protects the body from the effects of invasion by microorganisms and maintains homeostasis by governing the degradation and removal of damaged cells. It also discovers and disposes of abnormal cells that continually arise within the body. Abnormal immune function causes serious physiologic disruptions. For example, immune hyperreactivity leads to allergic symptoms; immunodeficiency may lead to exaggerated vulnerability to infection; misdirected immune response leads to autoimmune disorders; failure of surveillance may allow uncontrolled growth of tumor cells. Thus, tests for immune dysfunction have great clinical significance.

The range of immunologic tests to study antigen-antibody reactions has expanded rapidly since the mid-1970s. Existing tests have been modified or replaced to reflect new data and technology. New tests of the cell-mediated immunologic response and of its components have been developed from the application of immunopotentiation, immunosuppression, and immunomodulation to clinical therapeutic medicine. New tests of the autoimmune response and of tumors have been developed using cell sorter technology and monoclonal antibodies.

Both nonspecific and specific defense mechanisms protect the body against "nonself" attack. Nonspecific mechanisms—such as skin, mucous membranes and their secretions, and various enzymes, secretions, and cellular activities—protect the body from foreign invasion. However, when a foreign agent penetrates the body, a specific immune mechanism takes over, destroying the invading organism through the specialized activity of lymphocytes and macrophages. This specific response is the focus of the tests of the immune system that are described in this chapter.

Lymphoreticular system
The lymphoreticular system—which comprises primary and secondary lymphoid organs (thymus, spleen, and lymph nodes and related areas in the liver, bone marrow, and respiratory and gastrointestinal tracts)—is responsible for specific immune reactions to foreign substances. This system includes both macrophages and T and B lymphocytes. To become properly differentiated, T lymphocytes need an intact, functioning thymus during their development. B lymphocytes mature through action of an unknown primary lymphoid organ, thought to be the bone marrow.

Macrophages recognize and phagocytize an antigen that enters the body, processing the antigen to make it rec-

T AND B LYMPHOCYTES:
THEIR ORIGIN AND ROLE IN THE IMMUNE RESPONSE

When the immune system recognizes an antigen as nonself, two distinct types of immune responses cooperate to protect the body. Both involve lymphocytes that share a common origin in stem cells. However, these lymphocytes differentiate and mature in different microenvironments, producing two populations: B cells and T cells.

In humoral immunity, antigen-stimulated B cells produce immunoglobulins (antibodies) to destroy antigens before they reach host cells. In cell-mediated immunity, antigen-activated T cells destroy antigens by direct cell-to-cell interaction. Macrophages, phagocytic cells of the reticuloendothelial system, affect both types of immune response, by presenting antigens in the proper orientation to B cells and to T cells for recognition and destruction.

Two groups of activated T cells trigger overlapping humoral and cell-mediated immune responses. *T-regulatory cells* (consisting of T-helper and T-suppressor cells) are influenced by interleukin-1 (IL-1), a monokine produced by antigen-stimulated macrophages. IL-1 activates T-helper cells and induces them to produce interleukin-2 (IL-2), B-cell growth factor (BCGF), and B-cell differentiating factor (BCDF); activated B cells then respond to these lymphokines by proliferating into clones of B cells, which differentiate into antibody-secreting plasma cells. The antibodies circulate through the body, find the antigen and bind to it, and assist in its destruction. IL-2 also stimulates effector-T-cell (NK and cytotoxic-T-cell) function and induces the production of immune interferon by T cells. Interferon suppresses B cells and enhances the cell-mediated immune response by *effector T cells*, which destroys antigenic substances. These effector T cells also play a role in graft tissue rejection, delayed hypersensitivity, and graft-versus-host disease. Macrophages activated by macrophage activating factor (MAF), a T-helper lymphokine, regulate the response by producing prostaglandin E_2, which suppresses T-helper lymphokine activity and activates T-suppressor function. They also produce a tumor necrosis factor, which assists in destruction of foreign antigens.

Both humoral and cell-mediated immune responses record the battle by producing B- and T-memory cells. These memory cells can respond again to the same antigen, providing long-term immunity.

lins—IgG, IgM, IgA, IgE, and IgD—are distinguished by the constant portions of their heavy chains. However, each class has a kappa or a lambda light chain, which gives rise to many subtypes and provides almost limitless combinations of light and heavy chains that give immunoglobulins their specificity.

□ *IgG*, the smallest immunoglobulin, appears in all body fluids due to its ability to move across membranes as a single structural unit (a monomer). It comprises 75% of the total immunoglobulins and is the major antibacterial and antiviral antibody.

□ *IgM*, the largest immunoglobulin, appears as a pentamer (five monomers joined by a J-chain). Unlike IgG—which is produced mainly in the secondary, or recall, response—IgM dominates in the primary, or initial, immune response. But like IgG, IgM is involved in classic antibody reactions, including precipitation, agglutination, neutralization, and complement fixation. Because of its size, IgM cannot readily cross membrane barriers and is usually present only in the vascular system. IgM constitutes 5% of total serum immunoglobulin.

□ *IgA* exists in serum primarily as a monomer; in secretory form, IgA exists almost exclusively as a dimer (two monomer molecules joined by a J-chain and a secretory component chain). As a secretory immunoglobulin, IgA defends external body surfaces and is present in colostrum, saliva, tears, nasal fluids, and respiratory, gastrointestinal, and genitourinary secretions. This antibody is considered important in preventing antigenic agents from attaching to epithelial surfaces. IgA makes up 20% of total immunoglobulins.

□ *IgE*, present in trace amounts in serum, is involved in the release of vasoactive amines stored in basophils and tissue mast cell granules. When released, these bioamines cause the allergic effects characteristic of this type of hypersensitivity (erythema, itching, smooth-muscle contraction, secretions, and swelling).

□ *IgD*, present as a monomer in serum in minute amounts, is the predominate antibody found on the surface of B lymphocytes and serves mainly as an antigen receptor. It may function in controlling lymphocyte activation or suppression.

Complement system

Complement is the collective term for a system of plasma proteins—labeled C1 through C9—circulating in the blood as inactive precursors of enzymes. The complement system is activated by the coupling of antigen and antibody on the surface of a cell, with a subsequent bonding of C1 to the Fc portion of the immunoglobulin heavy chain. The complement cascade that follows this ac-

---

HOW IMMUNOLOGIC RESPONSES DIFFER

CELL-MEDIATED RESPONSES	HUMORAL RESPONSES
Transplant rejection	Bacterial phagocytosis and lysis
Delayed hypersensitivity-tuberculin reaction, contact dermatitis	Viral and toxin neutralization
Graft-vs-host reactions	Anaphylaxis
Tumor surveillance and/or destruction	Allergic hay fever and asthma
Intracellular infections	Immune complex disease

Adapted with permission from Lillian S. Brunner and Doris S. Suddarth, *Textbook of Medical-Surgical Nursing* (4th ed.; Philadelphia: J.B. Lippincott Co., 1980).

cytes and activate them. Once activated, these T lymphocytes destroy the presenting antigen, either directly by cytotoxicity or indirectly by secreting lymphokines—soluble substances that stimulate proliferation of lymphocytes and cytotoxic macrophages. Thus, T lymphocytes respond differently than B lymphocytes. For example, B lymphocytes are not required to be present at the antigen site, whereas T lymphocytes must be present and must actively participate in destroying the offending antigen.

Two subsets of regulatory T lymphocytes—helper and suppressor cells—function in both humoral and cell-mediated responses and regulate the magnitude, intensity, and duration of the immune response. A balance of helper and suppressor T lymphocytes is required for a normally functioning immune response. An excess of either helper or suppressor cells can change the intensity and the outcome of the immune response. T-helper cells appear to enhance the immune response. Alternatively, T-suppressor cells seem to prevent an excessive immune response.

Activated by interleukin-1 (a soluble monokine produced by macrophages), T-helper cells secrete the lymphokine interleukin-2, which induces the growth and differentiation of B lymphocytes into antibody-secreting plasma cells and potentiates T-cell proliferation with subsequent cytotoxicity of effector cells. T-suppressor cells are also activated by interleukin-1 to produce interferon, a soluble protein that suppresses the growth and the differentiation of B lymphocytes.

T-cell interferon enhances cell-mediated immune destruction by activating effector T cells—cytotoxic T lymphocytes and natural killer (NK) cells. Interferon can also promote the production of natural killer cells. These cells have the capacity to respond to an antigen immediately and without differentiation when they're targeting tumor cells, certain microbially infected cells, and perhaps other cells.

tivation causes cell membranes to undergo lysis. Activated complement fragments also cause chemotaxis of neutrophils and macrophages, initiate release of histamine from mast cells, neutralize viruses, and enhance phagocytosis and other nonspecific inflammatory effects. Alternately, the complement system can be activated by foreign polysaccharides and bacterial endotoxins.

Cell-mediated immune response

In cell-mediated immune response, macrophages present antigens to T lymphocytes and activate them. Once activated,

Misdirected response

Autoimmunity is the one form of hypersensitivity in which the immune response is misdirected against the body's own tissues. Disorders thought to be autoimmune include rheumatoid arthritis, systemic lupus erythematosus, scleroderma, Sjögren's syndrome, and hemolytic anemia. Autoantibodies usually attack intracellular "self-antigens" normally not exposed to the lymphoreticular system, including inner layers of cell membranes, nucleoprotein, nucleic acids, and cytoplasmic structures, such as mitochondria.

Viruses or haptens attached to the body's own cells also provoke autoimmune cell and tissue destruction. In many instances, tissue destruction results when intracellular antigens escape to form immune complexes, which are then deposited in the kidneys or blood vessels, activating complement and causing cytotoxic damage (type III hypersensitivity). Depletion of T-suppressor cells is believed to cause autoimmune disease by allowing unregulated T-helper-cell function.

In other hypersensitive states, excessive amounts of immunoglobulins, T-helper cells, T-suppressor cells, B lymphocytes, or complement, or a combination of any of these, are present. In such conditions, overproduction of one immune response component retards the production of others. In multiple myeloma, for example, the excessive production of a single clone of plasma cells can result in a single type of immunoglobulin that completely inhibits the production of other types. In this respect, hypersensitivity reactions can lead to immunodeficiency.

Immunodeficiency is a congenital or acquired deficiency of the immune response. Congenital deficiencies include Bruton's agammaglobulinemia (B-cell deficiency) and DiGeorge's syndrome (thymic parathyroid aplasia). Acquired immunodeficiency disorders can result from chemotherapy or from radiation or corticosteroid therapy. They're related to a change in the ratio of T-helper to T-suppressor cells and/or macrophages. An imbalance of these regulatory cells may also result from infection, stress, drug use, old age, malnutrition, and malignancy.

Immunologic test methods

Most immunologic tests use combinations of techniques to evaluate humoral and cell-mediated immune responses or their individual components. The most commonly used laboratory methods include precipitation, immunodiffusion, agglutination, immunofluorescence, radioimmunoassay, enzyme-linked immunosorbent assay, complement fixation, histochemical techniques, and, most recently, monoclonal antibody assays.

Precipitation

When a soluble antibody reacts with a soluble antigen, cross-linking occurs between the antibody and the antigen. This phenomenon, known as the *lattice hypothesis,* results from the presence of multiple receptor sites on the surfaces of the antibody and the antigen, allowing cross-linkage between them. As more antigen and antibody complex, they create an insoluble lattice structure and precipitate out of solution.

The quantity of antibody and antigen in solution determines the precipitation reaction. When a small amount of antigen is added to a large amount of antibody, all antigen sites are satisfied, and the resultant complexes contain much antibody and little antigen. Optimal cross-linking occurs when antigen and antibody are present in equal proportions; this point of optimal proportion is called the *zone of equivalence.* An excess of antigen or antibody may produce false-negative test results.

Immunodiffusion

Immunodiffusion relies on the tendency of antigen and antibody particles to diffuse in an agar matrix and to form a precipitin line where they meet. This test may be performed using one of three methods:

THREE METHODS OF IMMUNODIFFUSION

Immunodiffusion is an important laboratory method for identifying antigen-antibody complexes. Three variants of this method are single diffusion, double diffusion, and immunoelectrophoresis. All three rely on the tendency of antigen (AG) and antibody (AB) particles to diffuse in an agar matrix and to form a precipitin line where the two fronts meet.

Single diffusion

1A (Side view)

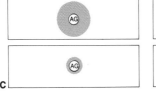

Precipitin line

1B (Top view)

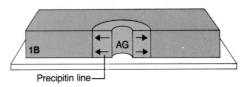

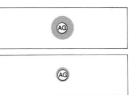

1C

1. The single diffusion method uses agar gel containing antibodies specific to the antigen to be tested. A well is formed in the agar gel and filled with the antigen (serum) sample. In 24 hours, the antigen diffuses around the well and forms a ring of precipitate at a point of equivalence where maximal binding of antigen and antibody takes place (**1A**). The intensity of the ring and its distance from the well are directly proportional to concentration of the test antigen in the serum sample, with maximum concentration demonstrated as the most intense and farthest removed line (**1B**).

Double diffusion

Precipitin line

2A (Side view)

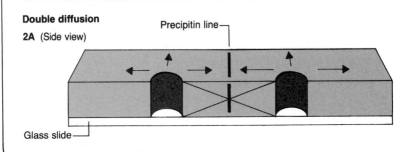

Glass slide

---

1. *Single diffusion* (radial immunodiffusion) uses an agar slide containing antibody specific to a certain antigen. A well is punched in the agar and is filled with the specific antigen. After 24 hours, a precipitation ring forms around the well. The distance between the precipitin line and the well is directly proportional to the antigen concentration.

Clinically, single diffusion is used to measure serum immunoglobulin concentrations. However, interference with diffusion (molecular size or weight) or precipitation (excess antigen or antibody) affects accurate determination of findings.

2. *Double diffusion,* a similar method, uses an agar-filled slide or a Petri dish

2B (Top view)

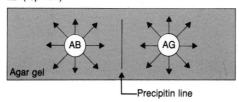

Precipitin line

2. The double diffusion method also uses agar gel. Two wells are formed in it: one well holds antibody, the other holds antigen. Diffusion of the two substances creates a precipitin line at the point of equivalence (**2A** and **2B**). More than one precipitin line indicates the presence of more than one type of antigen-antibody complex. As with the single diffusion method, the intensity and relative location of the precipitin line indicate concentrations of the reactant.

Immunoelectrophoresis
(Top view)

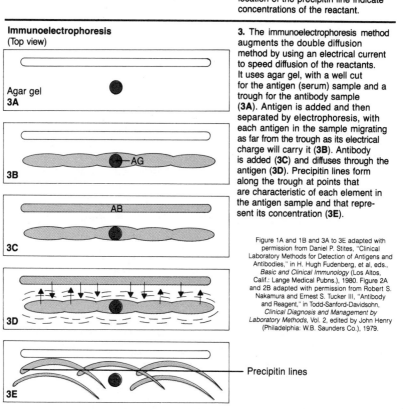

3A — Agar gel

3B — AG

3C — AB

3D

3E — Precipitin lines

3. The immunoelectrophoresis method augments the double diffusion method by using an electrical current to speed diffusion of the reactants. It uses agar gel, with a well cut for the antigen (serum) sample and a trough for the antibody sample (**3A**). Antigen is added and then separated by electrophoresis, with each antigen in the sample migrating as far from the trough as its electrical charge will carry it (**3B**). Antibody is added (**3C**) and diffuses through the antigen (**3D**). Precipitin lines form along the trough at points that are characteristic of each element in the antigen sample and that repre- sent its concentration (**3E**).

Figure 1A and 1B and 3A to 3E adapted with permission from Daniel P. Stites, "Clinical Laboratory Methods for Detection of Antigens and Antibodies," in H. Hugh Fudenberg, et al, eds., *Basic and Clinical Immunology* (Los Altos, Calif.: Lange Medical Pubns.), 1980. Figure 2A and 2B adapted with permission from Robert S. Nakamura and Ernest S. Tucker III, "Antibody and Reagent," in Todd-Sanford-Davidsohn, *Clinical Diagnosis and Management by Laboratory Methods*, Vol. 2, edited by John Henry (Philadelphia: W.B. Saunders Co.), 1979.

with small wells. After the addition of antigen to one well and antibody to the other, precipitin lines form where op- timal proportions of antigen and anti- body meet. The number of precipitin lines indicates the number of different antigen-antibody complexes present. Formation of a single precipitin line pro- vides a rough quantitative estimate of antigen or antibody purity. Although double diffusion is a simple, useful method for detecting unknown antigens or antibodies, it lacks sensitivity and thus has limited practical application.
3. *Immunoelectrophoresis* combines electrophoresis and immunodiffusion to identify and measure serum immuno- globulins and other proteins. A direct

electric current is applied to an agar slide, causing each protein to migrate at a different speed, according to its size and net electrical charge. After the proteins are separated, addition of antigen to each one results in diffusion and the formation of precipitin lines; these lines may be photographed or stained for a permanent record. Clinically, immunoelectrophoresis aids diagnosis of monoclonal and polyclonal gammopathies, and immunodeficiency diseases.

Agglutination

Agglutination occurs when large, insoluble particles, such as bacteria or RBCs, are clumped together by antibodies to the particles, or to the antigens attached to the particles. Unlike precipitation, agglutination employs high–molecular-weight antigens for rough quantitation of antibody levels.

Direct agglutination results from the addition of antibody to a cell or to insoluble particulate native antigen. If the antigen is added to increasing dilutions of antiserum in tubes or wells with rounded bottoms, the reciprocal of the dilution of antiserum in the last tube to show visible agglutination is the titer (relative concentration) of antibody.

Indirect or *passive agglutination* refers to the agglutination of soluble antigen attached to blood cells, bacteria, or latex particles, which are inert carrier particles.

Agglutination is clinically useful to detect specific antibodies, such as those causing rheumatoid arthritis, syphilis, or salmonella infections.

Immunofluorescence

In immunofluorescence, a histochemical technique, fluorescent dyes are attached to antibody molecules. When complexed with antigen, the antibody appears as a colored fluorescence when viewed under an ultraviolet microscope. Both direct and indirect immunofluorescence allow precise detection and demonstration of

---

SCREENING BLOOD FOR A.I.D.S. ANTIBODIES

Tests that measure serum antibodies for human T-cell lymphotrophic virus type III (HTLV-III), the AIDS virus, have been licensed by the Food and Drug Administration and are now commercially available. The tests are used to screen donated blood for AIDS, preventing contamination of the nation's blood supply. However, these tests only confirm the presence of antibodies to the AIDS virus. They do not confirm that an individual has AIDS or is likely to develop it. The initial screening test is an enzyme-linked immunosorbent assay, commonly called by its acronym ELISA.

Drawbacks
The ELISA test isn't 100% accurate, though, and sometimes gives false results. For instance, because test sensitivity varies among laboratories, a negative result doesn't necessarily mean that HTLV-III antibodies are absent. Also, in an asymptomatic patient, a positive result may result from immunity, subclinical infection, or cross-reactivity with other viral antigens. Or a false-positive result may reflect a laboratory error. As a result, the U.S. Public Health Service recommends confirmation of any positive result *before* the patient is notified, using the Western blot test to detect antibodies for viral proteins. This test is more reliable than the ELISA test, but it's technically more difficult and is used primarily for research.

Clinical implications of a positive test for an asymptomatic patient are currently unknown.

Your role
Encourage the patient with positive screening tests to seek medical follow-up care, even if he is asymptomatic. Instruct him to report early signs of AIDS, such as fever, weight loss, axillary or inguinal lymphadenopathy, rash, and persistent cough or diarrhea.

Assume that he can transmit AIDS to others, until further or more conclusive evaluation proves otherwise. To prevent possible contagion, instruct him not to share razors, toothbrushes, or utensils (which may be contaminated with blood) and to cleanse such items with household bleach diluted 1:10 in water. Advise the patient to avoid donating blood, tissues, or an organ. If you suspect I.V. drug abuse, warn the patient not to share needles.

Encourage the patient to inform his doctor and dentist about his condition, so they can take proper precautions.

BASIA BELZA TACK, RN, MSN, ANP

human tissue antigens and of bacterial, viral, and protozoan antigens. In the *direct* method, the fluorescein-labeled antibody reacts with an antigen specific to it. In the *indirect* method, a fluorescein-labeled antiglobulin reacts with an unlabeled antigen-antibody complex; the antiglobulin then binds to the unlabeled antibody. Both methods are widely used to detect autoantibodies, immunoglobulins of cell surfaces, components of complement, T and B lymphocytes, tumor-specific antigens, and microorganisms.

Radioimmunoassay

Radioimmunoassay relies on the competition between radiolabeled and unlabeled antigens for binding sites on antibody to determine the amount of antigen in a serum sample. Specifically, radioimmunoassay measures small quantities of a substance by combining a radiolabeled antigen with a particular antibody. Radiolabeled antigen is added to the sample, and it binds with about 70% of antibody. Various amounts of unlabeled antibody are then added to the mixture; the radiolabeled and unlabeled antigens compete for binding sites on the antibody. A curve is then constructed from the amount of radiolabeled antigen at various unlabeled antigen concentrations, to determine the amount of antigen already present in the serum sample.

Enzyme-linked immunosorbent assay

Enzyme-linked immunosorbent assay (ELISA) can identify antibody or antigen, and is replacing or supplementing radioimmunoassay and immunofluorescence. This method is safe, sensitive, and simple to perform, and provides reproducible results at a low cost. To measure a specific antibody, antigen is fixed to a solid-phase medium, incubated with a serum sample, and then incubated with an anti-immunoglobulin–tagged enzyme. Excess unbound enzyme is washed from the system and a substrate is added. To measure a specific antigen, antibody instead of antigen is fixed to a solid-phase medium. Hydrolysis of the substrate produces a color change, quantified by a spectrophotometer. The amount of substrate hydrolyzed is directly proportional to the amount of antigen or antibody in the serum sample.

Complement fixation

Used to determine the presence and extent of antigen-antibody reaction, complement fixation is performed by adding a known antigen or antibody, directed against an unknown antibody or antigen, to a patient's serum and incubating the sample. Then, RBCs coated with this same known antigen or antibody are added. If hemolysis doesn't occur, complement must have been depleted in the original reaction; in other words, the unknown antibody or antigen was present in the sample. The unknown antibody or antigen is then assayed.

Monoclonal antibody assays

B lymphocytes respond to antigen stimulation by rapidly proliferating and producing antibodies against the antigen. Laboratory production of monoclonal antibodies takes advantage of B-lymphocyte reaction to an antigen, to create unlimited numbers of completely homogenous antibodies. Typically, a selected antigen is injected into a mouse, stimulating its immune response to develop antibody-secreting plasma cells. These cells are then harvested from the mouse's spleen and fused with myeloma cells—malignant cells that secrete an infinite amount of the single antibody specific to the antigen that's been injected. The resulting hybridomas are grown in culture, cloned, and tested for the desired antibody. Finally, selected hybridomas are grown in culture or injected into a mouse to produce monoclonal antibodies, which are purified for future use.

Monoclonal antibodies have been used extensively for typing cells and cell subsets, detecting specific antigens, and differentiating malignant from nonmalignant cells.

BEVERLY A. ZENK WHEAT, RN, MA
SR. REBECCA FIDLER, MT(ASCP), PhD

GENERAL CELLULAR TESTS

T- and B-Lymphocyte Assays

Lymphocytes—key cells in the immune system—have the capacity to recognize antigens through special receptors found on their surfaces. The two main kinds of lymphocytes, T and B cells, originate in the bone marrow. The T cells mature under the influence of the thymus gland; B cells evolve without thymic influence.

Cell separation is used to isolate lymphocytes from other cellular blood elements. In this method, a whole blood sample is layered on Ficoll-Hypaque in a narrow tube, which is then centrifuged. Granulocytes and erythrocytes form a sediment at the bottom of the tube, and lymphocytes, monocytes, and platelets form a distinct band at the Ficoll-Hypaque–plasma interface. This procedure recovers approximately 80% of the lymphocytes but doesn't differentiate between T and B cells. The percent of T and B cells is determined by attaching a label or marker and by using different identification techniques. The E rosette test identifies T cells, which tend to form unstable clusterlike shapes (or rosettes) after exposure to sheep RBCs at 39.2° F. (4° C.). Direct immunofluorescence detects B cells, which have monoclonal immunoglobulin on their surfaces; unlike T cells, B cells present receptors for complement as well as for Fc portions of immunoglobulin.

Null cells, which make up the remainder of the lymphocytes, possess Fc receptors but no other detectable surface markers, and presently have no diagnostic significance. Null cells are usually determined by subtracting the sum of T and B cells from total lymphocytes.

Purpose
□ To aid diagnosis of primary and secondary immunodeficiency diseases
□ To distinguish benign from malignant lymphocytic proliferative diseases
□ To monitor response to therapy.

Patient preparation
Explain to the patient that this test measures certain WBCs. Tell him the test requires a blood sample; who will perform the venipuncture and when; and that he may experience transient discomfort from the needle puncture and the pressure of the tourniquet. Reassure him that collecting the sample takes less than 3 minutes.

Procedure
Perform a venipuncture, and collect the sample in a 7-ml *green-top* tube.

Precautions
□ Completely fill the collection tube, and invert it gently several times to mix the sample and anticoagulant adequately.
□ Send the sample to the laboratory immediately, to ensure viable lymphocytes.
□ If antilymphocyte antibodies are suspected, as in autoimmune disease, notify the laboratory.

Values
Currently, T-cell and B-cell assays are being standardized, and values may differ from one laboratory to another, depending on test technique. Generally, T cells comprise 68% to 75% of total lymphocytes; B cells, 10% to 20%; and null cells, 5% to 20%. The total lymphocyte count ranges from 1,500 to 3,000/mm³; the T-cell count varies from 1,400 to 2,700/mm³; and the B-cell count ranges from 270 to 640/mm³. These counts are higher in children.

Implications of results
An abnormal T-cell or B-cell count suggests but doesn't confirm specific diseases. The B-cell count is elevated in chronic lymphocytic leukemia (thought

to be a B-cell malignancy), multiple myeloma, Waldenström's macroglobulinemia, and DiGeorge's syndrome (a congenital T-cell deficiency). B cells decrease in acute lymphocytic leukemia and in certain congenital or acquired immunoglobulin deficiency diseases. In other immunoglobulin deficiency diseases, especially if only one immunoglobulin class is deficient, the B-cell count remains normal.

The T-cell count rises occasionally in infectious mononucleosis; it rises more often in multiple myeloma and acute lymphocytic leukemia. T cells decrease in congenital T-cell deficiency diseases, such as DiGeorge's, Nezelof's, and Wiskott-Aldrich syndromes, and in certain B-cell proliferative disorders, such as chronic lymphocytic leukemia, Waldenström's macroglobulinemia, and AIDS.

Normal T-cell and B-cell counts don't necessarily assure a competent immune system. In autoimmune diseases, such as SLE and rheumatoid arthritis, T and B cells, though present in normal numbers, may not be functionally competent.

Post-test care

Because many patients with T- and B-cell changes have a compromised immune system, keep the venipuncture site clean and dry. If a hematoma develops at the site, apply warm soaks.

Interfering factors

□ Failure to use the proper collection tube, to mix the sample and anticoagulant adequately, or to send the sample to the laboratory immediately can interfere with accurate testing.

□ T- and B-cell counts can change rapidly with changes in health status, from the effects of stress, or after surgery, chemotherapy, steroid or immunosuppressive therapy, and X-rays.

□ The presence of immunoglobulins, such as autologous antilymphocyte antibodies that sometimes occur in autoimmune disease, can alter test results.

BEVERLY A. ZENK WHEAT, RN, MA
SR. REBECCA FIDLER, MT(ASCP), PhD

Lymphocyte Transformation Tests

Transformation tests evaluate lymphocyte competency without injection of antigens into the patient's skin. These in vitro tests eliminate the risk of adverse effects but can still accurately assess the ability of lymphocytes to proliferate and to recognize and respond to antigens.

The mitogen assay, performed using nonspecific plant lectins, evaluates the mitotic response of T and B lymphocytes to a foreign antigen. The mitogens phytohemagglutinin (PHA) and concanavalin A (Con-A) stimulate T lymphocytes preferentially, whereas pokeweed primarily stimulates B lymphocytes, and T lymphocytes to a lesser extent. In the mitogen assay, a purified culture of lymphocytes from the patient's blood is incubated with a nonspecific mitogen for 72 hours—the interval during which the greatest effect on deoxyribonucleic acid (DNA) synthesis usually occurs. The culture is then pulse-labeled with tritiated thymidine, which is incorporated in the newly formed DNA of dividing cells. The uptake of radioactive thymidine can be measured by a liquid scintillation spectrophotometer in counts per minute (cpm), which parallels the rate of mitosis. Lymphocyte responsiveness, or the extent of mitosis, is then reported as a stimulation index, determined by dividing the cpm of the stimulated culture by the cpm of a control culture. The antigen assay uses specific antigens, such as PPD, Candida, mumps, tetanus toxoid, and streptokinase, to stimulate lymphocyte transformation. After incubation of 4½ to 7 days, transformation is measured by the same method used in the mitogen assay.

The mixed lymphocyte culture (MLC) assay tests the response of lymphocytes to histocompatibility antigens determined by the D locus of the sixth chromosome. The MLC assay is useful in matching transplant recipients and donors and in testing immunocompetence. In this assay, lymphocytes from a recipient and potential donor are cultured together for 5 days to test compatibility.

Recipient and potential donor lymphocytes (if viable and unaltered) will recognize any genetic differences and undergo transformation, demonstrating incompatibility. In the one-way MLC, one

LYMPHOCYTE MARKER ASSAYS

A normal immune response requires a balance between the regulatory activities of several interacting cell types—most notably, T-helper and T-suppressor cells. By using highly specific monoclonal antibodies, levels of lymphocyte differentiation can be defined, and both normal and malignant cell populations can be analyzed. Direct and indirect immunofluorescence, microcytotoxicity, and immunoperoxidase immunoassay techniques are used most frequently: these employ an anticoagulated blood sample combined with monoclonal antibodies that react with specific T- and B-cell markers. The chart below lists some commonly ordered lymphocyte marker assays and their indications.

LYMPHOCYTE MARKER ASSAY	PURPOSE
Pan T-cell marker	• To measure mature T-cells in immune dysfunction
T-helper/inducer subset marker	• To identify and characterize the proportion of T-helper cells in autoimmune or immunoregulatory disorders • To detect immunodeficiency disorders, such as AIDS • To differentiate T-cell acute lymphoblastic leukemia from T-cell lymphomas and other lymphoproliferative disorders
T-suppressor/cytotoxic subset marker	• To identify and characterize the proportion of T-suppressor cells in autoimmune and immunoregulatory disorders • To characterize lymphoproliferative disorders.
T-cell/E-Rosette receptor	• To differentiate lymphoproliferative disorders of T-cell origin, such as T-cell lymphocytic leukemia and lymphoblastic lymphoma, from those of non-T-cell origin
Pan-B (B-1) marker	• To differentiate lymphoproliferative disorders of B-cell origin, such as B-cell chronic lymphocytic leukemia, from those of T-cell origin
Pan-B (BA-1) marker	• To identify B-cell lymphoproliferative disorders, such as B-cell chronic lymphocytic leukemia
CALLA (common acute lymphocytic leukemia antigen) marker	• To identify bone marrow regeneration • To identify non-T-cell acute lymphocytic leukemia
Lymphocyte subset panel (B, pan-T, T-helper/inducer, T-suppressor/cytotoxic, and T-helper/T-suppressor ratio)	• To evaluate immunodeficiencies • To identify immunoregulation associated with autoimmune disorders • To characterize lymphoid malignancies
Lymphocytic leukemia marker panel (T-cell markers [E-Rosette receptor and Leu-9], B-cell markers [B-1 and BA-1], and CALLA)	• To characterize lymphocytic leukemias as T, B, non-T, or non-B, regardless of the stage of differentiation of the malignant cells

group of lymphocytes is pretreated with radiation or mitomycin C, so it can't divide but can still stimulate the other group of lymphocytes. Lymphocyte transformation is identified by an increased incorporation of radioactive thymidine labeling and reported as the stimulation index. After the culture is labeled with radioactive thymidine, the MLC stimulation index is then determined.

Purpose
□ To assess and monitor genetic and acquired immunodeficiency states
□ To provide histocompatibility typing of both tissue transplant recipients and donors
□ To detect exposure to various pathogens, such as those causing malaria, hepatitis, and mycoplasmal pneumonia.

Patient preparation
Explain to the patient that this test evaluates lymphocyte function, which is the keystone of the immune system. If appropriate, inform him that the test monitors his response to therapy. For histocompatibility typing, explain that this test helps determine the best match for a transplant. Advise the patient he needn't restrict food or fluids. Tell him the test requires a blood sample; who will perform the venipuncture and when; and that he may experience transient discomfort from the needle puncture and the pressure of the tourniquet. Reassure him that collecting the sample takes less than 3 minutes. If a radioisotope scan is scheduled, be sure the serum sample for this test is drawn first.

Procedure
Perform a venipuncture. If the patient is an adult, collect the sample in a 7 ml *green-top* (heparinized) tube; for a child, use a 5 ml *green-top* tube.

Precautions
Completely fill the collection tube, and invert it gently several times to mix the sample and anticoagulant. Send the sample to the laboratory immediately.

NEUTROPHIL FUNCTION TESTS

Normal neutrophils—the body's primary defense against bacterial invasion—engulf and destroy bacteria and foreign particles by a process known as phagocytosis. In patients who suffer from repeated bacterial infections, neutrophil function tests may reveal the inability of neutrophils to kill a target bacteria or to migrate to the bacterial site (chemotaxis).

Neutrophil killing ability can be evaluated by the *nitroblue tetrazolium (NBT) test*, which relies on neutrophil generation of bactericidal enzymes and toxins during killing. This action results in increased oxygen consumption and glucose metabolism, which reduces colorless NBT to blue formazan. The reduced dye is then extracted with pyridine and measured photometrically; the level of reduction indicates phagocytic activity.

Neutrophil killing activity can also be evaluated by noting the *chemiluminescence*—or ability to emit light—of neutrophils. After a neutrophil phagocytizes a microorganism, oxygen-containing substances form within phagocytic vacuoles. As the cell is stimulated, it emits light in proportion to the amount of oxygen-containing substances that are formed, providing an indirect measurement of phagocytosis.

Chemotaxis can be assessed in vitro by placing bacteria in the lower half of a two-part chamber and phagocytic neutrophils in the upper half. After incubation, migrating cells are counted microscopically and compared to standard values.

Values
In the mitogen assay, the normal stimulation index exceeds 10; in the antigen assay, the normal stimulation index exceeds 3. In the MLC assay, unresponsiveness indicates histocompatibility for the D locus antigens.

Implications of results
In the mitogen and antigen assays, a low stimulation index or unresponsiveness indicates a depressed or defective immune system. Serial testing can be performed to monitor the effectiveness of therapy in a patient with an immunodeficiency disease.

In the MLC test, the stimulation index is a measure of compatibility. A high index indicates poor compatibility. Conversely, a low stimulation index indicates good compatibility.

A high stimulation index, in response to the relevant pathogen, can also demonstrate exposure to malaria, hepatitis, mycoplasmal pneumonia, periodontal disease, and certain viral infections in patients who no longer have detectable serum antibodies.

Post-test care
Because many of these patients may have a compromised immune system, take special care to keep the venipuncture site clean and dry. If a hematoma develops at the venipuncture site, apply warm soaks.

Interfering factors
☐ Pregnancy or the use of oral contraceptives depresses lymphocyte response to PHA and thus causes a low stimulation index.
☐ Chemotherapy may hinder accurate determination of test results unless pretherapy baseline values are available for comparison.
☐ A radioisotope scan performed within 1 week before test, and failure to send the sample to the laboratory immediately can affect accuracy of test results.

BEVERLY A. ZENK WHEAT, RN, MA
SR. REBECCA FIDLER, MT(ASCP), PhD

Terminal Deoxynucleotidyl Transferase Test

Using indirect immunofluorescence, this test measures levels of terminal deoxynucleotidyl transferase (TdT), an intranuclear enzyme found in certain primitive lymphocytes in the normal thymus and bone marrow. Since TdT acts as a biochemical marker for these lymphocytes, it can help classify the origin of a particular tissue. Thus, the TdT test is useful in differentiating certain types of leukemias and lymphomas marked by primitive cells that can't be identified by histology alone. Measurement of TdT may also help determine prognosis for these diseases and may provide early diagnosis of a relapse.

Purpose
☐ To help differentiate acute lymphocytic leukemia (ALL) from acute non-lymphocytic leukemia
☐ To help differentiate lymphoblastic lymphomas from non-Hodgkin's lymphomas
☐ To monitor response to therapy.

Patient preparation
Explain to the patient that this test detects an enzyme that can help classify tissue origin. If the patient is scheduled for a blood test, tell him to fast for 12 to 14 hours before the test. Tell him the test requires a blood sample; who will perform the venipuncture and when; and that he may experience transient discomfort from the pressure of the tourniquet. Reassure him that collecting the sample takes less than 3 minutes.

If the patient is scheduled for a bone marrow aspiration, describe the procedure to him and answer any questions. Inform the patient that he needn't restrict food or fluids before the test. Tell him who will perform the biopsy and where, and that it usually takes only 5 to 10 minutes to perform. Make sure the patient or a responsible family member has signed a consent form. Check the patient's history for hypersensitivity to the local anesthetic. After checking with the doctor, tell the patient which bone will be the biopsy site. Inform him that he will receive a local anesthetic but will feel pressure on insertion of the biopsy needle and a brief, pulling pain when the marrow is withdrawn. As ordered, administer a mild sedative 1 hour before the test.

Procedure
If a blood test is scheduled, perform a

venipuncture and collect the sample in two 7-ml *green-top* tubes. Wrap the tubes in a paper towel, refrigerate them on cold packs or wet ice, and send them to the laboratory immediately.

If assisting with a bone marrow aspiration, inject 1 ml of bone marrow into a 7-ml *green-top* tube and dilute it with 5 ml of sterile saline. Wrap the tube in a paper towel, refrigerate it on cold packs or wet ice, and send it to the laboratory immediately.

Precautions
☐ Contact the laboratory before performing the venipuncture to ensure that they are able to process the sample and to find out how much blood to draw.
☐ Since patients with leukemia are more susceptible to infection, cleanse the skin thoroughly before performing the venipuncture.
☐ Send the sample to the laboratory immediately.

Values
Normal serum TdT levels range from 0 to 10 IU/10^{13} cells. Normal TdT levels in bone marrow have not been established but are similar to serum TdT levels.

Implications of results
TdT levels are elevated in ALL, the blastic phase of chronic myelogenous leu-kemia, lymphoblastic lymphoma, acute lymphoblastic leukemia, and in a small percentage of acute nonlymphocytic leukemias. TdT-positive cells are absent in patients with ALL who are in remission.

Post-test care
☐ Since patients with leukemia may bleed excessively, apply pressure to the venipuncture site until bleeding stops. If a hematoma develops at the venipuncture site, apply warm soaks.
☐ Check the bone marrow aspiration site for bleeding and inflammation, and observe the patient for signs of hemorrhage and infection.

Interfering factors
☐ Failure to obtain a representative sample may interfere with accurate determination of bone marrow aspiration results.
☐ Performing a bone marrow aspiration on a child may produce false-positive results, since TdT is normally present in bone marrow during proliferation of prelymphocytes.
☐ Bone marrow regeneration, idiopathic thrombocytopenic purpura, and neuroblastoma may produce false-positive bone marrow aspiration results, since these conditions cause TdT-positive bone marrow.

BARRY L. TONKONOW, MD

GENERAL HUMORAL TESTS

Immunoglobulins G, A, and M

Immunoglobulins, proteins that can function as specific antibodies in response to antigen stimulation, are responsible for the humoral aspects of immunity. They are classified into five groups—IgG, IgA, IgM, IgD, and IgE— that are normally present in serum in predictable percentages. IgG comprises about 75% of serum immunoglobulins and includes the warm-temperature type; IgA, about 15% of the total; IgM, 5% to 7% and includes cold agglutinins, rheumatoid factor, and ABO blood group isoagglutinins; IgD and allergen-specific IgE comprise less than 2%. Deviations from these normal immunoglobulin percentages are characteristic in many immune disorders—cancer, hepatic disorders, rheumatoid arthritis, and systemic lupus erythematosus, to mention a few.

Immunoelectrophoresis identifies IgG,

INSULIN ANTIBODIES TEST

Using radioimmunoassay, this test detects insulin antibodies in the blood of patients who receive insulin for treatment of diabetes mellitus. Most insulin preparations are derived from beef and pork pancreases and contain insulin-related peptides, impurities that are the major immunogenic components in insulin. IgG antibodies that form in response to these peptides complex with subsequent insulin injections and neutralize the insulin so it cannot regulate glucose metabolism. Detection of insulin antibodies confirms this process as the cause of insulin resistance and suggests the need for alternate therapy to control hyperglycemia.

Detection of insulin antibodies may also confirm "factitious hypoglycemia," an unusual condition that results from insulin injection rather than from a disorder, such as insulinoma.

IgA, and IgM in a serum sample; the level of each is measured by radial immunodiffusion or nephelometry. Some laboratories detect immunoglobulin by indirect immunofluorescence and radioimmunoassay.

In immunoelectrophoresis, serum is placed in a well on a slide containing agar gel, and an electric current is passed through the gel. Immunoglobulins (and other serum proteins) separate according to their different electric charges. Then antiserum is deposited in a shallow trough alongside the separated proteins, from which it diffuses into the agar. Distinct precipitin arcs form wherever the antiserum reacts with specific serum proteins, allowing identification of the immunoglobulins and other proteins. In radial immunodiffusion, addition of a class-specific antiserum diffuses the serum to form a precipitation ring that is proportional to the immunoglobulin concentration. In nephelometry, photometric measurement of the degree of light scattering caused by the immunoprecipitation reaction provides the relative immunoglobulin concentration.

Purpose
☐ To diagnose paraproteinemias, such as multiple myeloma and Waldenström's macroglobulinemia

☐ To detect hypo- and hypergammaglobulinemia, as well as nonimmunologic diseases, such as cirrhosis and hepatitis, that are associated with abnormally high immunoglobulin levels

☐ To assess the effectiveness of chemotherapy or radiation therapy.

Patient preparation
Explain to the patient that this test measures antibody levels. If appropriate, tell the patient that the test evaluates the effectiveness of treatment. Instruct him to restrict food and fluids, except for water, for 12 to 14 hours before the test. Tell him the test requires a blood sample; who will perform the venipuncture and when; and that he may experience transient discomfort from the needle puncture and the pressure of the tourniquet. Reassure him that collecting the sample takes less than 3 minutes.

Check the patient's medication history for drugs that may affect test results. If these medications must be continued, note this on the laboratory slip.

Procedure
Perform a venipuncture, and collect the sample in a 7 ml *red-top* tube.

Precautions
Send the sample to the laboratory immediately to prevent deterioration of immunoglobulins.

Values
Using nephelometry, serum immunoglobulin levels for adults range as follows:

IgG: 6.4 to 14.3 mg/ml
IgA: 0.3 to 3 mg/ml
IgM: 0.2 to 1.4 mg/ml.

Implications of results
The accompanying chart shows IgG, IgA, and IgM levels in various disorders. In congenital and acquired hypogammaglobulinemias, myelomas, and macro-

SERUM IMMUNOGLOBULIN LEVELS IN VARIOUS DISORDERS

DISORDER	IgG	IgA	IgM
Immunoglobulin disorders			
Lymphoid aplasia	D	D	D
Agammaglobulinemia	D	D	D
Type I dysgammaglobulinemia (selective IgG and IgA deficiency)	D	D	N or I
Type II dysgammaglobulinemia (absent IgA and IgM)	N	D	D
IgA globulinemia	N	D	N
Ataxia-telangiectasia	N	D	N
Multiple myeloma, macroglobulinemia, lymphomas			
Heavy chain disease (Franklin's disease)	D	D	D
IgG myeloma	I	D	D
IgA myeloma	D	I	D
Macroglobulinemia	D	D	I
Acute lymphocytic leukemia	N	D	N
Chronic lymphocytic leukemia	D	D	D
Acute myelocytic leukemia	N	N	N
Chronic myelocytic leukemia	N	D	N
Hodgkin's disease	N	N	N
Hepatic disorders			
Hepatitis	I	I	I
Laennec's cirrhosis	I	I	N
Biliary cirrhosis	N	N	I
Hepatoma	N	N	D
Other disorders			
Rheumatoid arthritis	I	I	I
Systemic lupus erythematosus	I	I	I
Nephrotic syndrome	D	D	N
Trypanosomiasis	N	N	I
Pulmonary tuberculosis	I	N	N

KEY: N = Normal; I = Increased; D = Decreased

Adapted with permission from Jacques B. Wallach, *Interpretation of Diagnostic Tests: A Handbook Synopsis of Laboratory Medicine* (3rd ed.; Boston: Little, Brown & Co., 1978), p. 71.

globulinemia, the findings confirm diagnosis. In hepatic and autoimmune diseases, leukemias, and lymphomas, such findings are less important but can support diagnosis based on other tests, such as biopsies and WBC differential, and on physical examination.

Post-test care

□ Advise the patient with abnormally low immunoglobulin levels (especially of IgG or IgM) to protect himself against bacterial infection. When caring for such a patient, watch for signs of infection, such as fever, chills, rash, or skin ulcers.
□ Instruct the patient with abnormally high immunoglobulin levels and symptoms of monoclonal gammopathies to report bone pain and tenderness. Such a patient has numerous antibody-producing malignant plasma cells in bone marrow, which hamper production of other blood components. When caring for such a patient, watch for signs of hypercalcemia, renal failure, and spontaneous pathologic fractures.

☐ If a hematoma develops at the venipuncture site, apply warm soaks.

☐ The patient may resume his normal diet.

☐ As ordered, resume administration of medications withheld before the test.

Interfering factors

☐ Radiation therapy or chemotherapy—for example, with methotrexate—may reduce immunoglobulin levels, due to the suppressive effects of these treatments on bone marrow.

☐ Aminophenazone, anticonvulsants, asparaginase, hydralazine, hydantoin derivatives, oral contraceptives, and phenylbutazone may raise all immunoglobulin levels. Methotrexate and severe hypersensitivity to BCG (bacille Calmette-Guérin) vaccine may lower all levels. Dextrans, phenytoin, and high doses of methylprednisolone lower IgG and IgA levels; dextrans and methylprednisolone lower IgM levels. Methadone raises IgG levels; alcoholism raises IgA; narcotics addiction may raise IgM.

BEVERLY A. ZENK WHEAT, RN, MA
SR. REBECCA FIDLER, MT(ASCP), PhD

Serum Immune Complex Assays

When immune complexes are produced faster than they can be cleared by the lymphoreticular system, immune complex disease may occur; for example, postinfectious syndromes, serum sickness, drug sensitivity, rheumatoid arthritis, and systemic lupus erythematosus (SLE). Immune complexes can develop when a certain ratio of antigen reacts with antibody of isotypes IgG 1, 2, 3, or IgM in tissues. These complexes can fix the first component of complement (C1) and activate the complement cascade. Subsequent complement-mediated activity leads to inflammation and local tissue necrosis. In the blood, *soluble circulating immune complexes may also activate complement and eventually cause damage, usually in the renal glomeruli, the aorta, and other large blood vessels.*

Histologic examination of tissue obtained by biopsy and the use of fluorescence or peroxidase staining with antibodies specific for immunologic types generally detect immune complexes. However, since tissue biopsies cannot provide information about titers of complexes still in circulation, serum assays, which detect circulating immune complexes indirectly, may be required. Because of the inherent variability of these complexes, several serum test methods may be appropriate, using C1, the rheumatoid factor (RF), or cellular substrates, such as Raji cells, as reagents.

Since most immune complex assays haven't been standardized, more than one test may be required to achieve accurate results.

Purpose

☐ To demonstrate circulating immune complexes in serum

☐ To monitor response to therapy

☐ To estimate severity of disease.

Patient preparation

Explain to the patient that these tests help evaluate his immune system. If appropriate, inform him that the test will be repeated to monitor his response to therapy. Advise him he needn't restrict food or fluids before the test. Tell him the test requires a blood sample; who will perform the venipuncture and when; and that he may experience transient discomfort from the needle puncture and the pressure of the tourniquet. Reassure him that collecting the sample takes less than 3 minutes.

If the patient is scheduled for C1q assays, check his history for recent heparin therapy. Report such therapy to the laboratory, since it may affect test results.

Procedure

Perform a venipuncture, and collect the

IMMUNE COMPLEX ASSAY METHODS

In the **C1q precipitin assay,** a subunit of C1q binds with IgG 1, 2, or 3, or IgM. This binding increases greatly in the presence of aggregated IgG. If enough C1q-bound immunoglobulin is present, a visible precipitation appears in gel diffusion. Because of the test's relative insensitivity, it can evaluate only such conditions as systemic lupus erythematosus, in which there are numerous circulating immune complexes.

In the **complement binding radioimmunoassay,** addition of radiolabeled C1q to a serum sample and to a standard solution of aggregated IgG allows comparison of the binding in each. Polyethylene glycol precipitates the complexes (including bound C1q), and its radioactivity is measured. This radioimmunoassay technique is more sensitive than the C1q precipitin assay, but it's subject to error from possible binding of C1q to substances other than IgG.

Rheumatoid factor (RF) techniques may also be used to determine immune complexes. In the solid-phase radioimmunoassay, addition of the serum sample to RF-bound insoluble cellulose or polystyrene blocks binding of a standardized radiolabeled immunoglobulin aggregate if immune complexes are present. Comparison of this blocking with that of an unlabeled control immunoglobulin aggregate provides the test finding. In another RF method, incubation of the serum sample with RF takes place before addition of IgG-coated latex particles. If immune complexes are present, they bind with RF and inhibit the aggregation of IgG-coated

latex particles; this inhibition can be quantitated. RF tests are sensitive and may detect smaller complexes than other methods; however, the results of such tests are misleading, since different rheumatoid factors vary in their affinity for immune complexes.

The remaining tests involve cellular substrate techniques. **Immunofluorescence** or **radioimmunoassay** can estimate immune complexes bound to the surface of Raji cells (a lymphoblastoid B-cell line derived from a Burkitt's lymphoma), which possess low-avidity Fc receptors and many C3 receptors but lack surface immunoglobulins. This technique is sensitive to relatively large complexes. However, its extreme sensitivity produces many false-positive results. Similarly, since B cells have surface receptors for C3, to which complement-fixing immune complexes can attach, the B cell assay can also detect these complexes, using direct immunofluorescence. Since immune complexes cause platelet aggregation, a sensitive but difficult to standardize test based on this principle compares the amount of aggregation between serial dilutions of a test serum and a positive control serum containing immune complexes.

The **phagocytosis inhibition test** uses peritoneal macrophages to phagocytize immune complexes; after incubation of radiolabeled aggregated IgG with macrophages and test serum, the presence of immune complexes causes decreased uptake of the labeled IgG aggregates when compared with a control where incubation takes place with aggregates alone.

sample in a 7 ml *red-top* tube.

Precautions
Send the sample to the laboratory immediately to prevent deterioration of immune complexes.

Findings
Normally, immune complexes are not detectable in serum.

Implications of results
The presence of detectable immune complexes in serum has etiologic importance in many autoimmune diseases, such as SLE and rheumatoid arthritis. However,

for definitive diagnosis, the presence of these complexes must be considered with the results of other studies. For example, in SLE, immune complexes are associated with high titers of antinuclear antibodies and circulating antinative deoxyribonucleic acid antibodies.

Because of their filtering function, renal glomeruli seem most vulnerable to immune complex deposition, although blood vessel walls and choroid plexuses (vascular folds in the ventricles of the brain) can be affected. Renal biopsy to detect immune complexes can provide conclusive evidence for immune complex (Type III) glomerulonephritis, differentiating it from other types of glomerulonephritis.

Post-test care
Since many patients with immune complexes have compromised immune systems, take special care to keep the venipuncture site clean and dry. If a hematoma develops at the site, ease discomfort by applying warm soaks.

Interfering factors
□ Failure to send the serum sample to the laboratory immediately can result in the deterioration of immune complexes and therefore can interfere with accurate determination of test results.
□ The presence of cryoglobulins in the patient's serum can interfere with accurate determination of test results.
□ Inability to standardize RF inhibition tests and platelet aggregation assays can interfere with accurate determination of test results.

BEVERLY A. ZENK WHEAT, RN, MA
SR. REBECCA FIDLER, MT(ASCP), PhD

Complement Assays

Complement is a collective term for a system of at least 20 serum proteins designed to destroy foreign cells and to help remove foreign materials. The system may be triggered by contact with antigen-antibody complexes or by clotting factor XIIa. A cascade of events follows, which results in the formation of a complex that ruptures cell membranes. Complement components are numerically designated as C1 through C9, with C1 having three subcomponents: C1q, C1r, and C1s. It comprises 3% to 4% of total serum globulins and plays a key role in antibody-mediated immune reactions. Complement can function as a defense by promoting removal of infectious agents, or as a threat by triggering destructive reactions in host tissues. Therefore, complement deficiency can increase susceptibility to infection and can predispose to other diseases. Complement assays are thus indicated in patients with known or suspected immunomediated disease or repeatedly abnormal response to infection.

Normally, complement is present in serum in an inactive state until "fixed," or activated, in the classic pathway by binding to an antibody-coated surface. In the classic pathway, a specific antibody identifies and coats an antigen that enters the body. C1 then recognizes and binds with this specific antibody, activating the complement cascade—a series of enzymatic reactions involving all complement components—producing a coordinated inflammatory response, and usually resulting in cell lysis or some other damaging outcome.

In the alternate pathway, substances such as polysaccharides, bacterial endotoxins, and aggregated immunoglobulins react with properdin and Factors B, D, H, and I, producing an enzyme that activates C3. In turn, C3 activates the remainder of the complement cascade.

In both pathways, specific inhibitors regulate the sequential activation of complement components. The C1 esterase inhibitor, the most commonly studied inhibitor, regulates the classic pathway; the C3b inhibitor can regulate either pathway, since C3 is a pivotal component of both.

Although various laboratory methods are used to evaluate and measure total complement and its components, hemolytic assay, laser nephelometry, and radial immunodiffusion are the most common. Hemolytic assay evaluates the lytic capacity of complement and is expressed as hemolytic units per millimeter, which is the dilution of serum needed to lyse 50% of the erythrocytes in the assay. In the hemolytic assay, sheep RBCs are mixed with a specific antiserum that lacks complement. Antibody-antigen complexes form, but since complement is absent, lysis can't occur. After the patient's serum sample is serially diluted, equal volumes of these

COMPLEMENT CASCADE: TWO PATHWAYS

CLASSICAL PATHWAY

Initiated by antigen-antibody complexes

▼

C1$\overline{qrs}$ generates an enzyme that cleaves C4 and C2

▼

C$\overline{142}$ is formed, which cleaves C3

▼

C3a (anaphylatoxin) and C3b are formed; C3a is released and functions in inflammation; C3b is an opsonin and is active in the enzyme C1$\overline{423b}$

▼

C$\overline{1423b}$ induces cleavage of C5

ALTERNATIVE PATHWAY

Initiated by IgA, some IgG, and certain polysaccharides, lipopolysaccharides, and trypsin-like enzymes

▼

Factor B combines with C3b in the presence of Factor D

▼

C3bBb (stabilized by properdin) is formed, which acts on C3

▼

C3bBbC3b (stabilized by properdin) is formed, which induces cleavage of C5

Forms C5a (anaphylatoxin) and C5b; C5a is released and functions in inflammation; C5b binds to C6,7

▼

C5b,6,7 binds to C8

▼

C5b,6,7,8 binds to C9

▼

C5b,6,7,8,9 causes cell lysis

The complement system plays an indispensable role in the humoral immune response. Activation of this system, the complement cascade, follows one of two pathways: the *classical pathway*, initiated by antigen-antibody complexes, or the *alternative pathway*, triggered by IgA; some IgG molecules; and certain polysaccharides, lipopolysaccharides, and trypsin-like enzymes.

Classical: Upon activation of the classical pathway by antigen-antibody complexes, C1$\overline{qrs}$ generates an enzyme that cleaves C4 and C2, producing C$\overline{142}$ (the classical pathway C3 convertase). C$\overline{142}$ then cleaves C3 into C3a (anaphylatoxin) and C3b. This forms C$\overline{1423b}$, the classical pathway C5 convertase.

Alternative: C3b, spontaneously cleaved from C3 continuously in the blood, is inactivated by Factors I and H. However, in the presence of certain activators (such as polysaccharides), Factors I and H are less able to inactivate C3b. This initiates the alternative pathway. Factor B combines with C3b in the presence of Factor D to form the alternative pathway C3 convertase, C3bBb. C3bBb, in turn, acts on C3 to form C3bBbC3b, the alternative pathway C5 convertase. Properdin stabilizes both C3bBb and C3bBbC3b, causing cleavage of C3 into C3a and C3b. C3bBbC3b induces cleavage of C5, producing C5a and C5b.

The binding of C5b to C6,7 initiates the membrane attack phase. C5b,6,7 causes leakage of intracellular fluid. Leakage increases dramatically when C5b,6,7 binds with C8. Rapid cytolysis occurs when the final complement component, C9, binds to C5b,6,7,8.

sensitized sheep RBCs are added to each dilution. Complement activity, reported in CH_{50} units, is the dilution capable of lysing 50% of available RBCs.

Laser nephelometry measures C1 esterase inhibitor; immunodiffusion measures C3, C4, C5, properdin, Factor B, and C1 inhibitor. In laser nephelometry, the serum sample is mixed with monospecific antiserum for C1 esterase inhibitor. They react to form a precipitate that scatters light from a laser beam directed through it. The amount of light scattered reflects the amount of C1 esterase inhibitor in the serum.

In radial immunodiffusion, an agar slide is impregnated with monospecific antibody for the factor to be studied. Known standards of complement and the patient's serum are placed in appropriate wells punched in the agar. Within 24 hours, a precipitation ring forms around this well where antigen and antibody react; its diameter is proportional to the concentration of complement component.

Although complement assays provide valuable information about the patient's immune system, the results must be considered in light of serum immunoglobulin and autoantibody tests for definitive diagnosis of immunomediated disease or abnormal response to infection.

Purpose

□ To help detect immunomediated disease and genetic complement deficiency
□ To monitor effectiveness of therapy.

Patient preparation

Explain to the patient that this test measures a group of proteins that fight infection. Advise him he needn't restrict food or fluids. Tell him the test requires a blood sample; who will perform the venipuncture and when; and that he may experience transient discomfort from the needle puncture and the pressure of the tourniquet. Reassure the patient that collecting the sample usually takes less than 3 minutes. If the patient is scheduled for C1q assay, check his history for recent heparin therapy. Report such therapy to the laboratory, since it may affect test results.

Procedure

Perform a venipuncture, and collect the sample in a 7 ml *red-top* tube.

Precautions

Handle the sample gently to prevent hemolysis, and send it to the laboratory immediately, since complement is heat labile and deteriorates rapidly.

Values

Normal values for complement range as follows:
total complement: 41 to 90 hemolytic units
C1 esterase inhibitor: 16 to 33 mg/dl
C3: in males, 88 to 252 mg/dl; in females, 88 to 206 mg/dl
C4: in males, 12 to 72 mg/dl; in females, 13 to 75 mg/dl.

Implications of results

Complement abnormalities may be genetic or acquired; acquired abnormalities are most common. Depressed total complement levels (which are clinically more significant than elevations) may result from excessive formation of antigen-antibody complexes, insufficient synthesis of complement, inhibitor formation, or increased complement catabolism, and are characteristic in conditions such as systemic lupus erythematosus (SLE), acute poststreptococcal glomerulonephritis, and acute serum sickness. Low levels may also occur in some patients with advanced cirrhosis of the liver, multiple myeloma, hypogammaglobulinemia, and rapidly rejecting allografts.

Elevated total complement may occur in obstructive jaundice, thyroiditis, acute rheumatic fever, rheumatoid arthritis, acute myocardial infarction, ulcerative colitis, and diabetes.

C1 esterase inhibitor deficiency is characteristic in hereditary angioedema, the most common genetic abnormality associated with complement; C3 deficiency is characteristic in recurrent pyogenic infection; C4 deficiency is characteristic in SLE.

Post-test care
Because many patients with complement defects have a compromised immune system, keep the venipuncture site clean and dry. If a hematoma develops at the venipuncture site, apply warm soaks.

Interfering factors
□ Hemolysis caused by rough handling of the sample, or failure to send the sample to the laboratory immediately may interfere with accurate determination of test results.
□ A history of recent heparin therapy can affect test results.

BEVERLY A. ZENK WHEAT, RN, MA
SR. REBECCA FIDLER, MT(ASCP), PhD

Radioallergosorbent Test

The radioallergosorbent test (RAST) measures IgE antibodies in serum by radioimmunoassay and identifies specific allergens that cause rashes, asthma, hay fever, drug reactions, or other atopic complaints. Before RAST was developed, skin testing was the only reliable method for identifying allergens. RAST is easier to perform and more specific than skin testing; it is also less painful for and less dangerous to the patient. However, careful selection of specific allergens, based on the patient's clinical history, is crucial for effective testing. Although skin testing is still the preferred means of diagnosing IgE-mediated hypersensitivities, RAST may be more useful when a skin disorder makes accurate reading of skin tests difficult, when a patient requires continual antihistamine therapy, or when skin tests are negative but the patient's clinical history supports IgE-mediated hypersensitivity.

In RAST, a sample of the patient's serum is exposed to a panel of allergen particle complexes (APCs) on cellulose disks. The patient's IgE complexes with those APCs to which it is sensitive. Radiolabeled anti-IgE antibody is then added, and this binds to the IgE-APC complexes. After centrifugation, the amount of radioactivity in the particulate material is directly proportional to the amount of IgE antibodies present. Test results are compared with control values and represent the patient's reactivity to a specific allergen.

Purpose
□ To identify allergens to which the patient has an immediate (IgE-mediated) hypersensitivity
□ To monitor response to therapy.

Patient preparation
Explain to the patient that this test may detect the cause of allergy or, when appropriate, that it monitors the effectiveness of treatment. Inform him he needn't restrict food or fluids. Tell him the test requires a blood sample; who will perform the venipuncture and when; and that he may experience transient discomfort from the needle puncture and the pressure of the tourniquet. Reassure him that collecting the sample takes less than 3 minutes. If the patient is scheduled for a radioactive scan, be sure the sample is collected before the scan.

Procedure
Perform a venipuncture, and collect the sample in a 7 ml *red-top* tube. Generally, 1 ml of serum is sufficient for five allergen assays. Be sure to note on the laboratory slip the specific allergens to be tested.

Precautions
None.

Findings
RAST results are interpreted in relationship to a control or reference serum that differs among laboratories.

Implications of results
Elevated serum IgE levels suggest hy-

persensitivity to the specific allergen or allergens used.

Post-test care
If a hematoma develops at the venipuncture site, apply warm soaks.

Interfering factors
Radioactive scan within 1 week before sample collection may affect the accuracy of test results.

BEVERLY A. ZENK WHEAT, RN, MA
SR. REBECCA FIDLER, MT(ASCP), PhD

Ham Test
[Acidified serum lysis test]

The Ham test is performed to determine the cause of undiagnosed hemolytic anemia, hemoglobinuria, and bone marrow aplasia. It helps establish a diagnosis of paroxysmal nocturnal hemoglobinuria (PNH), a rare hematologic disease.

The Ham test relies on the susceptibility of red blood cells (RBCs) to lysis: RBCs from patients with PNH are unusually susceptible to lysis by complement. To perform the test, washed RBCs are mixed with ABO-compatible normal serum and acid. After incubation at 37°C., the cells are examined for hemolysis. In the presence of acidified human serum, a substantial portion of PNH cells are lysed, whereas normal RBCs show no hemolysis.

Purpose
□ To help establish a diagnosis of PNH.

Patient preparation
Explain to the patient that this test helps determine the cause of his anemia or other signs. Advise him he needn't restrict food or fluids. Tell him the test requires a blood sample; who will perform the venipuncture and when; and that he may experience transient discomfort from the needle puncture and the pressure of the tourniquet. Reassure him that collecting the sample takes less than 3 minutes.

Procedure
Because the blood sample must be defibrinated immediately, laboratory personnel will perform the venipuncture and collect the sample.

Precautions
None.

Findings
Normally, RBCs do not undergo hemolysis.

Implications of results
Hemolysis of RBCs indicates PNH.

Post-test care
If a hematoma develops at the venipuncture site, apply warm soaks.

Interfering factors
□ Blood containing large numbers of spherocytes may produce false-positive results.
□ Blood from patients with congenital dyserythropoietic anemia or HEM-PAS (a rare hematologic disorder) will show false-positive results.

BARRY L. TONKONOW, MD

Human Leukocyte Antigen Test

The human leukocyte antigen (HLA) test identifies a group of antigens present on the surfaces of all nucleated cells but most easily detected on lymphocytes. These antigens are essential to immunity and determine the degree of histocompatibility between transplant recipients and donors. Numerous antigenic determinants (over 60, for instance, at the HLA-B locus) are present for each site; one set of each antigen is inherited from each parent.

Three types of HLA (HLA-A, HLA-B, and HLA-C) are measured with a lymphocyte microcytotoxicity assay. A lymphocyte sample is mixed with known antisera to these antigens and complement. Lymphocytes that react with a specific antiserum lyse and allow a dye to enter; they may then be detected by phase microscopy.

A fourth type of HLA, HLA-D, is measured by a mixed leukocyte reaction. Leukocytes from recipient and donor are combined in culture to determine HLA-D compatibility. If the leukocytes are incompatible, the culture will demonstrate blast formation, DNA synthesis, and proliferation.

High incidences of specific HLA types have been linked to specific diseases, such as rheumatoid arthritis and multiple sclerosis, but these findings have little diagnostic significance. Thus, HLA testing is best used as an adjunct to diagnosis. It is useful in genetic counseling and paternity testing.

Purpose
☐ To provide histocompatibility typing of tissue recipients and donors
☐ To aid genetic counseling
☐ To aid paternity testing.

Patient preparation
Explain to the patient that this test detects antigens on white blood cells. Advise him he needn't restrict food or fluids before the test.

Tell the patient that this test requires a blood sample; who will perform the venipuncture and when; and that he may experience transient discomfort from the needle puncture and the pressure of the tourniquet. Reassure him that collecting the blood sample usually takes less than 3 minutes.

Check the patient's history for recent blood transfusions, and report such transfusions to the doctor. He may want to postpone HLA testing.

Procedure
Perform a venipuncture and collect the sample in an ACD collection tube.

Precautions
Handle the sample gently to avoid hemolysis.

Findings
In HLA-A, HLA-B, and HLA-C testing, lymphocytes that react with the test antiserum undergo lysis; they're detected by phase microscopy. In HLA-D testing, leukocyte incompatibility is marked by blast formation, DNA synthesis, and proliferation.

Implications of results
Incompatible HLA-A, HLA-B, HLA-C, or HLA-D groups may cause unsuccessful tissue transplantation.

Many diseases have a strong association with certain types of HLAs. For example, HLA-DR5 is associated with Hashimoto's thyroiditis. B8 and Dw3 are associated with Graves' disease, whereas B8 alone is associated with chronic autoimmune hepatitis, celiac disease, and myasthenia gravis. Dw3 alone is associated with Addison's disease, Sjögren's syndrome, dermatitis herpetiformis, and systemic lupus erythematosus.

In paternity testing, a putative father who presents a phenotype (two haplotypes: one from the father and one from the mother) with no haplotype or antigen pair identical to one of the child's is excluded as the father. A putative father with one haplotype identical to one of the child's *may* be the father; the probability varies with the incidence of the haplotype in the population.

Post-test care
If a hematoma develops at the venipuncture site, ease discomfort by applying warm soaks.

Interfering factors
☐ Hemolysis caused by rough handling of the sample may interfere with accurate determination of test results.
☐ HLA from blood transfused within 72 hours before collection of a blood sample may interfere with accurate determination of test results.

BARRY L. TONKONOW, MD

AUTOANTIBODY TESTS

Antinuclear Antibodies

In conditions such as systemic lupus erythematosus (SLE), scleroderma, and certain infections, the body's immune system may perceive portions of its own cell nuclei as foreign and may produce antinuclear antibodies (ANA). Specific ANA include antibodies to DNA, nucleoprotein, histones, nuclear ribonucleoprotein, and other nuclear constituents. Although ANA are harmless in themselves, since they don't penetrate living cells, they sometimes form antigen-antibody complexes that cause tissue damage (as in SLE). Because of multiorgan involvement, test results are not diagnostic and can only partially confirm clinical evidence.

This test measures the relative concentration of ANA in a serum sample, through indirect immunofluorescence. Serial dilutions of serum are mixed with cell nuclei (usually taken from a rat). If the serum contains ANA, it forms antigen-antibody complexes with the cell nuclei. This preparation is then mixed with fluorescein-labeled antihuman serum and is examined under an ultraviolet microscope. If ANA are present, the nuclei fluoresce. Titer is taken as the greatest dilution that shows the reaction. About 99% of patients with SLE exhibit ANA; a large percentage of these persons do so at high titers. Although this test is not specific for SLE, it is a useful screening tool. Failure to detect ANA essentially rules out active SLE.

Purpose
☐ To screen for SLE
☐ To monitor the effectiveness of immunosuppressive therapy for SLE.

Patient preparation
Explain to the patient that this test evaluates the immune system, and that further testing is commonly required for accurate diagnosis. If appropriate, inform him that the test will be repeated to monitor his response to therapy. Advise him he needn't restrict food or fluids. Tell him the test requires a blood sample;

COMPARATIVE INCIDENCE OF ANTINUCLEAR ANTIBODIES (ANA)	
DISEASE	**INCIDENCE OF POSITIVE ANA**
Systemic lupus erythematosus (SLE)	95% to 100%
Lupoid hepatitis	95% to 100%
Felty's syndrome	95% to 100%
Progressive systemic sclerosis (scleroderma)	75% to 80%
Drug-associated SLE-like syndrome: (hydralazine, procainamide, isoniazid)	~50%
Sjögren's syndrome	40% to 75%
Normal old age	~40%
Rheumatoid arthritis	25% to 60%
Healthy family member of SLE patient	~25%
Chronic discoid lupus erythematosus	15% to 50%
Juvenile arthritis	15% to 30%
Polyarteritis nodosa	15% to 25%
Miscellaneous diseases	10% to 50%
Dermatomyositis, polymyositis	10% to 30%
Rheumatic fever	~5%
Normal persons (general population)	~5%

From Henry J. Smith and Robert G. Blaker, *Laboratory Aids for the Diagnosis of Autoimmune Disorders* (Van Nuys, Calif.: Bio-Science Laboratories, 1975), p. 7. Used by permission of the publisher.

who will perform the venipuncture and when; and that he may experience transient discomfort from the needle puncture and the pressure of the tourniquet. Reassure him that collecting the sample takes less than 3 minutes.

Check the patient's medication history for drugs that may affect test results, such as isoniazid, hydralazine, and procainamide. Note such drug use on the laboratory slip.

Procedure
Perform a venipuncture, and collect the sample in a 7 ml *red-top* tube.

Precautions
None.

Values
The test for ANA is negative at a titer of 1:32 or below.

Implications of results
Although the test is a sensitive indicator of ANA, it is not specific for SLE. Low titers may occur in patients with viral diseases, chronic hepatic disease, collagen vascular disease, and autoimmune diseases, and in some healthy adults; incidence increases with age. Consequently, the higher the titer, the more specific the test is for SLE (titer often exceeds 1:256).

The pattern of nuclear fluorescence helps identify the type of immune disease present. A peripheral pattern is almost exclusively associated with SLE, since it indicates the presence of anti-deoxyribonucleic acid (DNA) antibodies; anti-DNA antibodies are sometimes measured by radioimmunoassay if ANA titers are high or a peripheral pattern is observed. A homogeneous, or diffuse, pattern is also associated with SLE, as well as with related connective tissue disorders; a nucleolar pattern, with scleroderma; and a speckled, irregular pattern, with infectious mononucleosis and mixed connective tissue disorders (for example, SLE and scleroderma).

A single serum sample, especially one collected from a patient with collagen

---

PATTERNS OF IMMUNOFLUORESCENT STAINING FOR ANTINUCLEAR ANTIBODIES

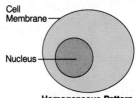

Cell Membrane —

Nucleus —

Homogeneous Pattern
(Diffuse)

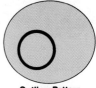

Outline Pattern
(Peripheral)

Speckled Pattern

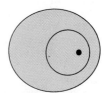

Nucleolar Pattern

Antinuclear antibodies are present in many connective-tissue disorders but display certain patterns of fluorescence in specific ones. For example, systemic lupus erythematosus (SLE) allies strongly with peripheral staining, which outlines the nucleus, and with homogeneous or uniform staining of the nucleus. The speckled pattern, with many fluorescent points throughout the nucleus, is characteristic of scleroderma and is less common in SLE. Homogeneous staining of the nucleolus causes the nucleolar pattern, common in scleroderma (54%), less common in SLE (24%), and relatively rare in rheumatoid arthritis (9%).

From H. Hugh Fudenberg, et al, eds., *Basic and Clinical Immunology* (3rd ed.; Los Altos, Calif.: Lange Medical Pubns., 1980), p. 445. Used by permission of the publisher.

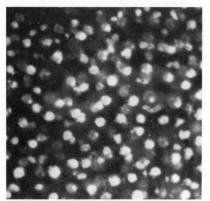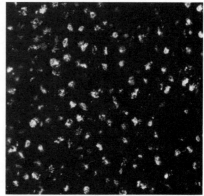

Homogeneous staining of rat liver nuclei (photograph at left) indicates the presence of antinuclear antibodies (ANA). This characteristic fluorescent pattern is often found in patients with systemic lupus erythematosus. The photograph at right shows the speckled pattern of ANA staining (rat liver substrate) typical of scleroderma.

vascular disease, may contain antibodies to several parts of the cell's nucleus. In addition, as serum dilution increases, the fluorescent pattern may change, because different antibodies are reactive at different titers.

Post-test care

□ Since a patient with an autoimmune disease has a compromised immune system, observe the venipuncture site for signs of infection, and report any changes to the doctor immediately. Keep a clean, dry bandage over the site for at least 24 hours.

□ If a hematoma develops at the venipuncture site, ease discomfort by applying warm soaks.

Interfering factors

Certain drugs—most commonly isoniazid, hydralazine, and procainamide—can produce a syndrome resembling SLE; other such drugs include para-aminosalicylic acid, chlorpromazine, clofibrate, phenytoin, griseofulvin, ethosuximide, gold salts, methyldopa, oral contraceptives, penicillin, propylthiouracil, phenylbutazone, methysergide, streptomycin, sulfonamides, tetracyclines, mephenytoin, quinidine, primidone, reserpine, and trimethadione.

BEVERLY A. ZENK WHEAT, RN, MA
SR. REBECCA FIDLER, MT(ASCP), PhD

Anti-Deoxyribonucleic Acid Antibodies

This test measures antinative deoxyribonucleic acid (DNA) antibody levels in a serum sample, using radioimmunoassay or a less sensitive technique, such as agglutination, complement fixation, or immunoelectrophoresis. For radioimmunoassay, the sample is mixed with radio-labeled native DNA. If antinative DNA antibodies are in the serum sample, they combine with the native DNA, forming complexes that are too large to pass through a membrane filter. If such antibodies are not present, the radiolabeled DNA is able to pass through the filter. The DNA that does not pass through the membrane filter is then counted.

In autoimmune diseases, such as systemic lupus erythematosus (SLE), native DNA is thought to be the antigen that complexes with antibody and complement, and causes local tissue damage where these complexes are deposited. Serum antinative DNA levels are directly related to the extent of renal damage caused by the disease.

Two different types of anti-DNA an-

tibodies are present in patients with SLE: *anti–single-stranded (denatured) DNA and anti–double-stranded (native) DNA. Antibodies to native DNA, however, are more specific for SLE. Determination of these antibodies, with serum complement, also proves useful in monitoring immunosuppressive therapy.*

Purpose
☐ To confirm SLE after a positive antinuclear antibody test
☐ To monitor response to therapy.

Patient preparation
Explain to the patient that the test detects certain antibodies, and that test results help determine diagnosis and appropriate therapy; or, when indicated, tell the patient the test assesses the effectiveness of present treatment. Advise him he needn't restrict food or fluids. Tell him the test requires a blood sample; who will perform the venipuncture and when; and that he may experience transient discomfort from the needle puncture and the pressure of the tourniquet. Reassure him that collecting the sample takes less than 3 minutes.

If the patient is scheduled for a radionuclide scan, make sure the sample is collected before the scan.

Procedure
Perform a venipuncture, and collect the sample in a 7 ml *red-top* tube. (Some laboratories may specify a *lavender* or *gray-top* tube.)

Precautions
Handle the sample gently to prevent hemolysis.

Values
Normal values are less than 1 mcg of native DNA bound/ml of serum.

Implications of results
Elevated antinative DNA levels may indicate SLE. A value of 1 to 2.5 mcg/ml suggests a remission phase of SLE or the presence of other autoimmune disorders. A value of 10 to 15 mcg/ml indicates active SLE. Depressed levels following immunosuppressive therapy demonstrate effective treatment of SLE.

Post-test care
If a hematoma develops at the venipuncture site, apply warm soaks.

Interfering factors
☐ Hemolysis caused by rough handling of the sample may interfere with accurate determination of test results.
☐ Radioactive scan performed within 1 week of collecting the sample may alter the test results.

BEVERLY A. ZENK WHEAT, RN, MA
SR. REBECCA FIDLER, MT(ASCP), PhD

Extractable Nuclear Antigen Antibodies
[Ribonucleoprotein antibodies; anti-Smith antibodies; Sjögren's antibodies]

Extractable nuclear antigen (ENA) is a complex of at least two and possibly three antigens. One of these—ribonucleoprotein (RNP)—is susceptible to degradation by ribonuclease. The second—Smith (Sm) antigen—is an acidic nuclear protein that resists ribonuclease degradation. The third antigen sometimes included in this group—Sjögren's (SS-B) antigen—forms a precipitate when antibody is present. Antibodies to these antigens are associated with certain autoimmune disorders.

Tests to detect ENA antibodies help differentiate autoimmune disorders with similar signs and symptoms. The RNP antibody test detects RNP autoantibodies, which are associated with systemic lupus erythematosus (SLE), progressive systemic sclerosis, and other rheumatic disorders. This test aids in the differential diagnosis of systemic rheumatic disease and is a useful follow-up test for collagen vascular autoimmune disease. The Anti-Sm antibody test *detects Sm autoantibodies, which are a specific marker for SLE; positive results are thus highly diagnostic of SLE. This test, too, helps monitor collagen vascular autoimmune disease. The* Sjögren's antibody test *detects the SS-B autoantibodies produced in Sjögren's syndrome, an immunologic abnormality sometimes associated with rheumatoid arthritis and SLE. However, this test is not diagnostic for Sjögren's syndrome.*

To perform these tests, sheep red blood cells are sensitized with ENA extracted from rabbit thymus, and then incubated with serum samples; ENA antibodies present in the serum will agglutinate the cells. If the serum sample shows agglutination, differential double immunoassays are performed to determine which of the antibodies are present. Anti-ENA tests are most useful in tandem with anti-DNA, serum complement, and antinuclear antibody tests.

Purpose
□ To aid differential diagnosis of autoimmune disease
□ To distinguish between anti-RNP and anti-Sm antibodies
□ To screen for anti-RNP antibodies (common in mixed connective tissue disease)
□ To screen for anti-Sm antibodies (common in SLE)
□ To support diagnosis of collagen vascular autoimmune diseases
□ To monitor response to therapy.

Patient preparation
Explain to the patient that this test detects certain antibodies and that test results help determine diagnosis and treatment; or, when indicated, explain that the test assesses the effectiveness of treatment. Advise him he needn't restrict food or fluids. Tell him the test requires a blood sample; who will perform the venipuncture and when; and that he may experience transient discomfort from the needle puncture and the pressure of the tourniquet. Reassure him that collecting the sample takes less than 3 minutes.

Procedure
Perform a venipuncture, and collect the sample in a 7-ml red-top tube.

Precautions
Send the sample to the laboratory immediately.

Findings
Normally, serum is negative for anti-RNP, anti-Sm, and SS-B antibodies.

Implications of results
The presence of anti-Sm antibodies is highly diagnostic of SLE. A high level of anti-RNP antibodies with a low titer of anti-Sm antibodies suggests mixed connective tissue disease. Although SS-B antibodies are associated with primary Sjögren's disease, their presence is not considered diagnostic of this disorder; however, a positive test for SS-B antibodies mandates further testing.

Post-test care
□ Since a patient with an autoimmune disease has a compromised immune system, check the venipuncture site for infection, and report any change promptly. Keep a clean, dry bandage over the site for at least 24 hours.
□ If a hematoma develops at the venipuncture site, ease discomfort by applying warm soaks.

Interfering factors
Failure to send the sample to the laboratory immediately may interfere with accurate determination of test results.

SR. REBECCA FIDLER, MT(ASCP), PhD

Antimitochondrial Antibodies

This test for antimitochondrial antibodies, which is usually performed with the test for anti–smooth-muscle antibodies, detects antibodies in serum by indirect immunofluorescence. Antimitochondrial antibodies react with mitochondria in the renal tubules, gastric mucosa, and other organs in which cells expend large amounts of energy. These autoantibodies are present in several hepatic diseases, although their etiologic role is unknown, and there's no evidence that they cause hepatic damage. Most commonly, they are associated with primary biliary cirrhosis and, sometimes, chronic active hepatitis and drug-induced jaundice. Antimitochondrial antibodies are also associated with autoimmune diseases, such as systemic lupus erythematosus, rheumatoid arthritis, pernicious anemia, and idiopathic Addison's disease.

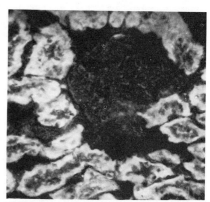

The photograph above shows a positive reaction to the antimitochondrial antibody test (rat kidney substrate). This reaction is common in patients with primary biliary cirrhosis. The site of the reaction is the cytoplasm (white areas) of the mitochondria-rich renal tubules. Large, dark, C-shaped area is a glomerulus, one of the millions of principal filtration units in the kidneys.

Purpose
☐ To aid diagnosis of primary biliary cirrhosis
☐ To distinguish between extrahepatic jaundice and biliary cirrhosis.

Patient preparation
Explain to the patient that this test helps evaluate liver function. Advise him he needn't restrict food or fluids. Tell him the test requires a blood sample; who will perform the venipuncture and when; and that he may experience transient discomfort from the needle puncture and the pressure of the tourniquet. Reassure him that collecting the sample takes less than 3 minutes. Check the patient's medication history for oxyphenisatin. Report such drug usage to the laboratory, since it may produce antimitochondrial antibodies.

Procedure
Perform a venipuncture, and collect the sample in a 7 ml *red-top* tube.

Precautions
None.

Findings
Normally, serum is negative for antimitochondrial antibodies at a 1:5 dilution.

Implications of results
Although antimitochondrial antibodies appear in 79% to 94% of patients with primary biliary cirrhosis, this test alone doesn't confirm diagnosis. Further tests, such as serum alkaline phosphatase, serum bilirubin, SGOT, SGPT, or possibly, liver biopsy or cholangiography, may also be necessary. The autoantibodies also appear in some patients with chronic active hepatitis, drug-induced jaundice, and cryptogenic cirrhosis. However, antimitochondrial antibodies rarely appear in patients with extrahepatic biliary obstruction, and a positive test helps rule out this condition.

Post-test care
Since patients with hepatic disease may bleed excessively, apply pressure to the venipuncture site until bleeding stops. If a hematoma develops at the venipuncture site, apply warm soaks.

Interfering factors
☐ Confusion of antimitochondrial antibodies with heterophil antibodies, cardiolipin antibodies to syphilis, ribosomal antibodies, or microsomal hepatic or renal autoantibodies can cause in-

INCIDENCE OF SERUM ANTIBODIES IN VARIOUS CONDITIONS

DISEASE OR CONDITION	PERCENTAGE OF PATIENTS SHOWING ANTIBODIES TO:	
	Mitochondria	Smooth Muscle
Primary biliary cirrhosis	75% to 95%	0% to 50%[a]
Chronic active hepatitis	0% to 30%	50% to 80%
Extrahepatic biliary obstruction	0% to 5%	0%
Cryptogenic cirrhosis	0% to 25%	0% to 1%
Viral (infectious) hepatitis	0%	1% to 2%[b]
Drug-induced jaundice	50% to 80%	
Intrinsic asthma		20%
Rheumatoid arthritis and other collagen diseases	1% to 2%	
Systemic lupus erythematosus	3% to 5%[c]	0%
Normal	0% to 1%	

[a]In chronic disease, values fall at upper end of range.
[b]Much higher incidence occurs with hepatic damage.
[c]Much higher incidence occurs with renal involvement.

From *Bio-Science Handbook* (12th ed.; Van Nuys, Calif.: Bio-Science Laboratories, 1979), p. 181. Used by permission of the publisher.

accurate determination of test results.
□ Oxyphenisatin can produce antimitochondrial antibodies in patients taking this drug.

BEVERLY A. ZENK WHEAT, RN, MA
SR. REBECCA FIDLER, MT(ASCP), PhD

Anti–Smooth-Muscle Antibodies

Using indirect immunofluorescence, this test measures the relative concentration of anti–smooth-muscle antibodies in serum, and is usually performed with the test for antimitochondrial antibodies. The serum sample is exposed to a thin section of smooth muscle and incubated; then, a fluorescent-labeled antiglobulin is added. This antiglobulin binds only to antibodies that have complexed with smooth-muscle and appears fluorescent when viewed through the microscope under ultraviolet light.

Anti–smooth-muscle antibodies appear in several hepatic diseases, especially chronic active hepatitis and, less often, primary biliary cirrhosis. Although anti–smooth-muscle antibodies are most commonly associated with hepatic diseases, their etiologic role is unknown, and there's no evidence that they cause hepatic damage.

Purpose
□ To aid diagnosis of chronic active hepatitis and primary biliary cirrhosis.

Patient preparation
Explain to the patient that this test helps evaluate liver function. Inform him that he needn't restrict food or fluids. Tell him that this test requires a blood sample; who will perform the venipuncture and when; and that he may experience transient discomfort from the needle puncture and the pressure of the tourniquet. Reassure the patient that collecting the blood sample usually takes less than 3 minutes.

Procedure
Perform a venipuncture, and collect the sample in a 7 ml *red-top* tube.

Precautions
None.

Values
Normal titer of anti–smooth-muscle antibodies is less than 1:20.

Implications of results
The test for anti–smooth-muscle antibodies is not very specific; these antibodies appear in about 66% of patients with chronic active hepatitis and 30% to 40% of patients with primary biliary cirrhosis.

Anti–smooth-muscle antibodies may also be present in patients with infectious mononucleosis, acute viral hepatitis, malignant tumor of the liver, and intrinsic asthma.

Post-test care
Since patients with hepatic disease may bleed excessively, apply pressure to the venipuncture site until bleeding stops. If a hematoma develops at the site, apply warm soaks.

Interfering factors
None.

BEVERLY A. ZENK WHEAT, RN, MA
SR. REBECCA FIDLER, MT(ASCP), PhD

Antithyroid Antibodies

In autoimmune disorders such as Hashimoto's thyroiditis and Graves' disease (hyperthyroidism), thyroglobulin, the major colloidal storage compound, is released into the blood. Because thyroxine usually separates from thyroglobulin before its release into the blood, thyroglobulin doesn't normally enter the circulation. When it does, antithyroglobulin

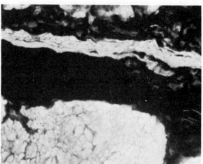

Anti–smooth-muscle antibodies are demonstrated in smooth-muscle cells (white areas covering lower half of photograph) by fluorescing brightly, a characteristic reaction in chronic active hepatitis. Shadowy nuclei are visible in many of the smooth-muscle cells (rat-kidney substrate). The dark area that laterally bisects the photograph contains cells of the gastric mucosa.

antibodies come into existence to attack this foreign substance; the ensuing autoimmune response damages the thyroid gland. The serum of a patient whose autoimmune system produces antithyroglobulin antibodies usually contains antimicrosomal antibodies, which react with the microsomes of the thyroid epithelial cells.

The tanned red cell hemagglutination test detects antithyroglobulin and antimicrosomal antibodies. In this assay, sheep RBCs that have been pretreated with tannic acid and coated with thyroglobulin or with microsomal fragments are mixed with a serum sample. The mixture agglutinates in the presence of these specific antibodies, and serial dilutions can quantify the antibody concentration. Another laboratory technique, indirect immunofluorescence, can detect antimicrosomal antibodies.

Purpose
□ To detect circulating antithyroglobulin antibodies when clinical evidence indicates Hashimoto's thyroiditis, Graves' disease, or other thyroid diseases.

Patient preparation
Explain to the patient that this test evaluates thyroid function. Advise him that he needn't restrict food or fluids. Tell him

INCIDENCE OF THYROID AUTOANTIBODIES IN VARIOUS DISEASES

DISORDER	PRESENCE OF ANTI-THYROGLOBULIN	PRESENCE OF ANTIMICRO-SOMAL ANTIBODIES
Hashimoto's disease	60% to 95%	70% to 90%
Idiopathic myxedema	75%	65%
Graves' disease	30% to 40%	50% to 85%
Adenomatous goiter	20% to 30%	20%
Thyroid carcinoma	40%	15%
Pernicious anemia	25%	10%

Adapted with permission from Burton Zweiman and Robert P. Lisak, "Autoimmunity and Autoimmune Diseases." In John Bernard Henry, ed., *Todd-Sanford-Davidsohn Clinical Diagnosis and Management by Laboratory Methods* (16th ed.; Philadelphia: W.B. Saunders Co., 1979), p. 1279.

the test requires a blood sample; who will perform the venipuncture and when; and that he may experience transient discomfort from the needle puncture and the pressure of the tourniquet. Reassure him that collecting the sample takes less than 3 minutes.

Procedure
Perform a venipuncture, and collect the sample in a 7 ml *red-top* tube.

Precautions
None.

Values
The normal titer is less than 1:100 for both antithyroglobulin and antimicrosomal antibodies. (Low levels of these antibodies are normal in 10% of the general population and in 20% or more of persons aged 70 or older.)

Implications of results
The presence of antithyroglobulin or antimicrosomal antibodies in serum can indicate subclinical autoimmune thyroid disease, Graves' disease, or idiopathic myxedema. High titers (which may be in the millions) strongly suggest Hashimoto's thyroiditis. The accompanying chart shows the approximate incidence

of antithyroglobulin antibodies in selected diseases. Such antibodies may also occur in some patients with other autoimmune disorders, such as SLE, rheumatoid arthritis, and autoimmune hemolytic anemia.

Post-test care
If a hematoma develops at the venipuncture site, apply warm soaks.

Interfering factors
None.

RICHARD EDWARD HONIGMAN, MD

Lupus Erythematosus Cell Preparation

Lupus erythematosus (LE) cell preparation is an in vitro procedure used in the diagnosis of systemic lupus erythematosus (SLE). Although this test is less sensitive and reliable than either the antinuclear antibody (ANA) or the antideoxyribonucleic acid (DNA) antibody test, it's often used because it requires minimal equipment and reagents.

In this test, a blood sample is mixed with laboratory-treated nucleoprotein (the antigen). If the sample contains ANA, the ANA reacts with the nucleoprotein, causing swelling and rupture. Phagocytes from the serum then engulf the extruded nuclei, forming LE cells, which are then detected by microscopic examination of the sample.

Purpose

□ To aid diagnosis of SLE
□ To monitor treatment of SLE (about 60% of successfully treated patients fail to show LE cells after 4 to 6 weeks of therapy).

Patient preparation

Explain to the patient that this test helps detect antibodies to his own tissue. If appropriate, inform him that the test will be repeated to monitor his response to therapy. Advise him that he needn't restrict food or fluids. Tell him the test requires a blood sample; who will perform the venipuncture and when; and that he may experience transient discomfort from the needle puncture and the pressure of the tourniquet. Reassure him that collecting the sample takes less than 3 minutes.

Check the patient's medication history for drugs, such as isoniazid, hydralazine, and procainamide, that may affect test results. If such drugs must be continued, be sure to note this on the laboratory slip.

Procedure

Perform a venipuncture, and collect the sample in a 7 ml *red-top* tube.

Precautions

Handle the sample gently to prevent hemolysis.

Findings

Normally, no LE cells are present.

ALL ABOUT SLE: WHO, WHAT, WHEN, AND WHY?

Who? Systemic lupus erythematosus (SLE) develops in 10 times as many women as men (15 times as many women of childbearing age), and most often in Blacks.

What? SLE is a chronic inflammatory disease of the connective tissue that produces biochemical and structural changes in skin, joints, and muscles, usually with multiple organ involvement. It may eventually cause death from failure of vital organs, especially the kidneys. However, the course is variable and not always fatal; it may be controlled in some patients. Four or more of the following criteria help support the diagnosis:
- facial erythema (butterfly rash)
- alopecia
- photosensitivity
- Raynaud's phenomenon
- pleuritis or pericarditis
- hemolytic anemia, leukopenia, or thrombocytopenia
- positive antinuclear antibody or LE cell test
- chronic false-positive serologic test for syphilis
- profuse proteinuria
- cellular casts
- discoid lupus erythematosus
- nondeforming arthritis
- oral or nasopharyngeal ulcerations
- psychosis or convulsions.

When? Onset of SLE is most common between ages 15 and 30, but occurs in all age groups.

Why? The cause is unknown. SLE is believed to stem from autoimmune malfunction, triggered by viral, drug, environmental, or genetic stimulus.

From *Primer on the Rheumatic Diseases*, pp. 139-140. Used with permission of the American Rheumatism Association.

UNDERSTANDING AUTOANTIBODIES IN AUTOIMMUNE DISEASE

When the immune system produces autoantibodies against the antigenic determinants on and in cells, two types of autoimmune disease can result. *Organ-specific disease,* such as pernicious anemia, occurs when the targeted antigenic determinants are specific to an organ or tissue, or to certain cells or cell types. Lymphocytes invade the target organ, tissue, or cell and destroy targeted cells. *Non-organ-specific disease,* such as myasthenia gravis, occurs when the targeted antigenic determinants are shared with other cells (self-antigens). This causes deposition of immune complexes (Type III hypersensitivity), with subsequent lesions anywhere in the body.

Various diagnostic techniques are used to detect antibodies in autoimmune disease, including radioimmunoassay, hemagglutination, complement fixation, and immunofluorescence. The chart below lists common test methods and findings in various autoimmune diseases.

DISEASE	AFFECTED AREA	ANTIGEN	ANTIBODY	DIAGNOSTIC TECHNIQUE
Hashimoto's thyroiditis	Thyroid gland	Thyroglobulin, second colloid antigen, cytoplasmic microsomes, cell-surface antigens	Antibodies to thyroglobulin and to microsomal antigens	Radioimmunoassay, hemagglutination, complement fixation, immunofluorescence
Pernicious anemia	Hematopoietic system	Intrinsic factor	Antibodies to gastric parietal cells and vitamin B_{12} binding site of intrinsic factor	Immunofluorescence, radioimmunoassay
Pemphigus vulgaris	Skin	Desmosomes between prickle cells in the epidermis	Antibodies to intercellular substances of the skin and mucous membranes	Immunofluorescence
Myasthenia gravis	Neuromuscular system	Acetylcholine receptors of skeletal and heart muscle	Anti-acetylcholine antibody	Immunoprecipitation radioimmunoassay
Autoimmune hemolytic anemia	Hematopoietic system	Red blood cells (RBCs)	Anti-RBC antibody	Direct and indirect Coombs' test

Implications of results

The presence of at least two LE cells may indicate SLE. Although these cells occur primarily in SLE, they may also form in chronic active hepatitis, rheumatoid arthritis, scleroderma, and drug reactions. Also, up to 25% of patients with SLE demonstrate no LE cells. Apart from supportive clinical signs, definitive diagnosis of SLE may necessitate a confirming ANA or anti-DNA test. The ANA test detects autoantibodies in the sera of many SLE patients with negative LE cell tests.

Anti-DNA antibodies appear in two thirds of all SLE patients but are rare in other conditions; the presence of such antibodies is strong evidence of SLE.

Post-test care

□ Since many patients with SLE have compromised immune systems, keep a clean, dry bandage over the venipuncture site for at least 24 hours, and check for infection.

□ If a hematoma develops at the venipuncture site, apply warm soaks.

UNDERSTANDING AUTOANTIBODIES IN AUTOIMMUNE DISEASE *(continued)*

DISEASE	AFFECTED AREA	ANTIGEN	ANTIBODY	DIAGNOSTIC TECHNIQUE
Primary biliary cirrhosis	Small bile ducts in liver	Mitochondria	Mitochondrial antibody	Immunofluorescence of mitochondrial-rich cells (kidney biopsy)
Rheumatoid arthritis	Joints, blood vessels, skin, muscles, lymph nodes	IgG	Antigammaglobulin antibody	Sheep RBC agglutination, latex immunoglobulin agglutination, radioimmunoassay, immunofluorescence, immunodiffusion
Goodpasture's syndrome	Lungs and kidneys	Glomerular and lung basement membranes	Anti-basement membrane antibody	Immunofluorescence of kidney biopsy sample, radioimmunoassay
Systemic lupus erythematosus	Skin, joints, muscles, lungs, heart, kidneys, brain, eyes	DNA, nucleoprotein, blood cells, clotting factors, IgG, Wasserman antigen	Antinuclear antibody, anti-DNA antibody, anti-ds-DNA antibody, anti-SS-DNA antibody, anti-ribonucleoprotein antibody, antigammaglobulin antibody, anti-RBC antibody, antilymphocyte antibody, anti-platelet antibody, antineuronal cell antibody, anti-Sm antibody	Counterelectrophoresis, hemagglutination, radioimmunoassay, immunofluorescence, Coombs' test

☐ If test results indicate SLE, tell the patient further diagnostic tests may be required to monitor treatment.

Interfering factors

☐ Hemolysis caused by rough handling of the sample may interfere with accurate determination of test results.

☐ Certain drugs—most commonly isoniazid, hydralazine, and procainamide—can produce a syndrome resembling SLE. Other such drugs include para-aminosalicylic acid, chlorpromazine, clofibrate, phenytoin, griseofulvin, ethosuximide, gold salts, methyldopa, oral contraceptives, penicillin, propylthiouracil, phenylbutazone, methysergide, streptomycin, sulfonamides, tetracyclines, mephenytoin, quinidine, primidone, reserpine, and trimethadione.

BEVERLY A. ZENK WHEAT, RN, MA
SR. REBECCA FIDLER, MT(ASCP), PhD

Rheumatoid Factor

The rheumatoid factor (RF) test is the most useful immunologic test for con-

> ## PRESENCE OF RHEUMATOID FACTOR (RF) IN VARIOUS DISEASES WHEN BOTH SCAT AND LATEX TEST USED
>
> | DISEASE | RF |
> | --- | --- |
> | Classic rheumatoid arthritis (RA) | 80% |
> | Early or atypical RA | 50% |
> | Juvenile RA | 20% |
> | Infectious diseases | 10% |
> | Healthy adults | 5% |
> | Elderly persons | 25% |
>
> Adapted with permission from Henry J. Smith and Robert G. Blaker, *Laboratory Aids for the Diagnosis of Autoimmune Disorders* (Van Nuys, Calif.: Bio-Science Laboratories, 1975), p. 13. Used by permission of the publisher.

firming rheumatoid arthritis (RA). In this disease, "renegade" IgG antibodies, produced by lymphocytes in the synovial joints, react with other IgG or IgM to produce immune complexes, complement activation, and tissue destruction. How IgG molecules become antigenic is still unknown, but they may be altered by aggregating with viruses or other antigens. These immune complexes can migrate from the synovial fluid to other areas of the body, causing vasculitis, subcutaneous nodules, or lymphadenopathy. The IgG or IgM molecules that react with altered IgG are called rheumatoid factors. Agglutination and flocculation tests can detect RF: the sheep cell agglutination test and the latex fixation test. In the sheep cell test, rabbit IgG adsorbed onto sheep RBCs is mixed with the patient's serum in serial dilutions; in the latex fixation test, human IgG adsorbed onto latex particles is mixed with the patient's serum. Visible agglutination indicates the presence of RF. The last tube dilution to show visible agglutination is used as the titer. The sheep cell agglutination test is the better diagnostic method for confirming RA; the latex fixation test is the better screening method.

Purpose
□ To confirm RA, especially when clinical diagnosis is doubtful.

Patient preparation
Explain to the patient that this test helps confirm RA. Advise him he needn't restrict food or fluids before the test. Tell him that the test requires a blood sample; who will perform the venipuncture and when; and that he may experience transient discomfort from the needle puncture and the pressure of the tourniquet. Reassure him that collecting the blood sample usually takes less than 3 minutes.

Procedure
Perform a venipuncture, and collect the sample in a 7-ml *red-top* tube.

Precautions
None.

Values
Normal RF titer is < 1:20; normal rheumatoid screening test is nonreactive.

Implications of results
Positive RF titers are found in 80% of patients with RA. Titers above 1:80 are usually considered diagnostic for RA; titers between 1:20 and 1:80 are difficult to interpret, since they occur in many other diseases, such as systemic lupus erythematosus, scleroderma, polymyositis, tuberculosis, infectious mononucleosis, leprosy, syphilis, sarcoidosis, chronic hepatic disease, subacute bacterial endocarditis, and chronic pulmonary interstitial fibrosis. In addition, 5% of the general population, including as many as 25% of the elderly, have positive RF titers.

Conversely, a negative RF titer doesn't rule out RA; 20% to 25% of patients with RA lack reactive RF titers, and RF itself isn't reactive until 6 months after onset of active disease. Repeating the test is sometimes useful. However, correlation between RF and RA is inconclusive, and positive diagnosis always requires correlation with clinical status.

Post-test care
□ Since a patient with RA may be immunologically compromised from the disease or from corticosteroid therapy,

keep the venipuncture site covered with a clean, dry bandage for 24 hours. Check regularly for signs of infection.
□ If a hematoma develops at the venipuncture site, apply warm soaks.

Interfering factors
□ Inadequately activated complement may cause false-positive results.
□ Serum with high lipid or cryoglobulin levels may cause false-positive test results and requires repetition of the test after restriction of fat intake.
□ Serum with high IgG levels may cause false-negative results through competition with IgG on the surface of latex particles or sheep RBCs used as substrate.

BEVERLY A. ZENK WHEAT, RN, MA
SR. REBECCA FIDLER, MT(ASCP), PhD

Cold Agglutinins

Cold agglutinins are antibodies (usually of the IgM type) that cause RBCs to aggregate at low temperatures, and may occur in small amounts in healthy persons. Transient elevations of these antibodies develop during certain infectious diseases, notably primary atypical pneumonia. This test reliably detects such pneumonia within 1 to 2 weeks after onset. Although cold agglutinins are inert at inner body temperatures, some become active in exposed areas of skin at 82.4° to 89.6° F. (28° to 32° C.), producing pallor and acrocyanosis (Raynaud's phenomenon), and numbness of hands and feet. Intense agglutination of a whole blood sample occurs on cooling to temperatures between 32° and 68° F. (0° and 20° C.), peaking at 39.2° F. (4° C.), and is reversible by rewarming to 98.6° F. (37° C.). However, after rewarming, complement remains on the cell and may produce hemolysis. Consequently, patients with high cold agglutinin titers, such as those with primary atypical pneumonia, may develop acute transient hemolytic anemia after repeated expo-

sure to cold; patients with persistently high titers may develop chronic hemolytic anemia.

Purpose
□ To help confirm primary atypical pneumonia
□ To provide additional diagnostic evidence for cold agglutinin disease associated with many viral infections or lymphoreticular malignancy.

Patient preparation
Explain to the patient that this test detects antibodies in the blood that attack RBCs after exposure to low temperatures. If appropriate, inform him that the test will be repeated to monitor his response to therapy. Advise him he needn't restrict food or fluids. Tell him the test requires a blood sample; who will perform the venipuncture and when; and that he may experience transient discomfort from the needle puncture and the pressure of the tourniquet. Reassure him that collecting the sample takes less than 3 minutes.

If the patient is receiving antibiotics, note this on the laboratory slip, since such drugs may interfere with the development of cold agglutinins.

Procedure
Perform a venipuncture, and collect the sample in a 7 ml *red-top* tube that has been *prewarmed* to 98.6° F. (37° C.).

Precautions
 Handle the sample gently to prevent hemolysis, and send it to the laboratory immediately. Don't refrigerate the sample; cold agglutinins will coat the RBCs, leaving none in the serum for testing.

Values
Normal titers are less than 1:16 but may be higher in elderly persons.

Implications of results
High titers may occur as primary phenomena, or secondary to infections or

lymphoreticular malignancy. They may be present in infectious mononucleosis, cytomegalovirus infection, hemolytic anemia, multiple myeloma, scleroderma, malaria, cirrhosis, congenital syphilis, peripheral vascular disease, pulmonary embolism, trypanosomiasis, tonsillitis, staphylococcemia, scarlatina, influenza, and, occasionally, in pregnancy. Chronically elevated titers are most commonly associated with pneumonia and lymphoreticular malignancy; an acute transient elevation commonly accompanies many viral infections.

In primary atypical pneumonia, cold agglutinins appear in serum in one half to two thirds of all patients during the first week of acute infection, even before antimycoplasmal antibodies can be detected by complement fixation or metabolic inhibition tests. Thus, titers usually become positive at 7 days, peak above 1:32 in 4 weeks, and commonly disappear rapidly after 6 weeks. When sequential titers verify this pattern and clinical evidence of pneumonia exists, diagnosis is confirmed.

Extremely high titers (1:1,000 to 1:1,000,000) can occur with idiopathic cold agglutinin disease that precedes development of lymphoma. Patients with titers this high are susceptible to intravascular agglutination, which causes significant clinical problems.

Post-test care
□ If cold agglutinin disease is suspected, keep the patient warm. If the patient is exposed to low temperatures, agglutination may occur within peripheral vessels, possibly leading to frostbite, anemia, Raynaud's phenomenon, or, rarely, focal gangrene.
□ Watch for signs of vascular abnormalities, such as mottled skin, purpura, jaundice, or pallor; pain or swelling of extremities; and cramping of fingers and toes. Hemoglobinuria may result from severe intravascular hemolysis on exposure to severe cold.
□ If a hematoma develops at the venipuncture site, ease discomfort by applying warm soaks.

Interfering factors
□ Hemolysis caused by rough handling of the sample can falsely depress titers, as can refrigeration of the sample before serum is separated from RBCs.
□ Antibiotics can interfere with the development of cold agglutinins.

BEVERLY A. ZENK WHEAT, RN, MA
SR. REBECCA FIDLER, MT(ASCP), PhD

Cryoglobulins

Cryoglobulins are abnormal serum proteins that precipitate at low laboratory temperatures (39.2° F. [4° C.]) and redissolve after being warmed. Their presence in the blood (cryoglobulinemia) is usually associated with immunologic disease but can also occur in the absence of known immunopathology. Cryoglobulinemia occurs in three forms: Type I, which involves the reaction of a single monoclonal immunoglobulin; Type II, in which a monoclonal immunoglobulin shows antibody activity against a polyclonal immunoglobulin; and Type III, in which both components are polyclonal immunoglobulins. If patients with cryoglobulinemia are subjected to cold, they may experience Raynaud-like symptoms (pain, cyanosis, and coldness of fingers and toes), which generally result from precipitation of cryoglobulins in cooler parts of the body. In some patients, for example, cryoglobulins may precipitate at temperatures as high as 86° F. (30° C.); such temperatures are possible in some peripheral blood vessels.

The cryoglobulin test involves refrigerating a serum sample at 39.2° F. (4° C.) for at least 72 hours and observing for formation of a heat-reversible precipitate. Such a precipitate requires further study by immunoelectrophoresis or double diffusion, to identify cryoglobulin components.

Purpose
□ To detect cryoglobulinemia in patients

CRYOGLOBULIN LEVELS IN ASSOCIATED DISEASES

TYPE OF CRYOGLOBULIN	SERUM LEVEL	ASSOCIATED DISEASES
Type I **Monoclonal cryoglobulin**	> 5 mg/ml	• Myeloma • Waldenström's macroglobulinemia • Chronic lymphocytic leukemia
Type II **Mixed cryoglobulin**	> 1 mg/ml	• Rheumatoid arthritis • Sjögren's syndrome • Mixed essential cryoglobulinemia
Type III **Mixed polyclonal** **cryoglobulin**	< 1 mg/ml (50% below 80 mcg/ml)	• Systemic lupus erythematosus • Rheumatoid arthritis, Sjögren's syndrome • Infectious mononucleosis • Cytomegalovirus infections • Acute viral hepatitis • Chronic active hepatitis • Primary biliary cirrhosis • Poststreptococcal glomerulonephritis • Infective endocarditis • Leprosy • Kala-azar • Tropical splenomegaly syndrome

Adapted with permission from H.H. Fudenberg, et al, eds., *Basic and Clinical Immunology* (3rd ed.; Los Altos, Calif.: Lange Medical Pubns., 1980), p. 362.

with Raynaud-like vascular symptoms.

Patient preparation
Explain to the patient that this test detects antibodies in blood that may cause sensitivity to low temperatures. Instruct him to fast for 4 to 6 hours before the test.

Tell him the test requires a blood sample; who will perform the venipuncture and when; and that he may experience transient discomfort from the needle puncture and the pressure of the tourniquet. Reassure him that collecting the blood sample usually takes less than 3 minutes.

Procedure
Perform a venipuncture, and collect the sample in a prewarmed 10 ml *red-top* tube.

Precautions
☐ Warm the syringe and collection tube to 98.6° F. (37° C.) before venipuncture and keep it at that temperature, to prevent loss of cryoglobulins.

☐ Send the sample to the laboratory immediately.

Findings
Normally, serum is negative for cryoglobulins.

Implications of results
The accompanying chart indicates expected serum levels and diseases associated with the three types of cryoglobulinemia. Although the presence of cryoglobulins in the blood confirms cryoglobulinemia, this finding doesn't always mean the presence of clinical disease.

Post-test care
☐ The patient may resume usual diet.
☐ If the test is positive for cryoglobulins, tell the patient to avoid cold temperatures or contact with cold objects.
☐ If a hematoma develops at the venipuncture site, apply warm soaks.
☐ Observe for intravascular coagulation (decreased color and temperature in distal extremities, and increased pain).

Interfering factors
□ Failure to adhere to dietary restrictions may interfere with accurate determination of test results.
□ Failure to maintain the sample at 98.6° F. (37° C.) before centrifugation may cause loss of cryoglobulins.
□ Reading the sample before the end of the 72-hour precipitation period may cause test results to be reported incorrectly, since some cryoglobulins take several days to precipitate.

BEVERLY A. ZENK WHEAT, RN, MA
SR. REBECCA FIDLER, MT(ASCP), PhD

Acetylcholine Receptor Antibodies

The acetylcholine receptor (AChR) antibodies test is the most useful immunologic test for confirming acquired (autoimmune) myasthenia gravis (MG), a disorder of neuromuscular transmission. In normal muscle contraction, acetylcholine (ACh) is released from the terminal end of the nerve and binds to AChR sites on the muscle motor end plate. In MG, however, antibodies block and destroy AChR sites, causing muscle weakness that can be either generalized or localized to the ocular muscles.

Two test methods—a binding assay and a blocking assay—are now available to determine the relative concentration of AChR antibodies in serum. In the binding assay, purified AChRs are complexed with ^{125}I-labeled α-bungarotoxin (a molecule that binds specifically to AChRs and blocks them). A serum sample is added to this complex; after incubation, antihuman immunoglobulin is added. Antibodies bind to AChR–^{125}I-labeled α-bungarotoxin complexes, which coprecipitate with the total human immunoglobulin. The amount of radioactivity is then measured to assay the available AChR sites. AChR-binding antibodies are found in about 90% of pa-

tients with generalized MG and in about 50% of those with localized MG.

When the AChR-binding assay is negative in a patient with MG symptoms, the AChR-blocking assay may be performed. Here, the patient's serum is incubated with purified AChRs before ^{125}I-labeled α-bungarotoxin is added, to detect antibodies whose antigenic sites would otherwise be blocked. The blocking assay is relatively new, and its clinical significance is not yet fully known. However, it is specific for the autoimmune form of MG and is useful for research. Determination of AChR antibodies by either method also helps monitor immunosuppressive therapy for MG, although antibody levels do not usually parallel the severity of disease.

Purpose
□ To confirm diagnosis of MG
□ To monitor the effectiveness of immunosuppressive therapy for MG.

Patient preparation
Explain to the patient that this test helps confirm MG or, when indicated, tell him the test assesses the effectiveness of treatment. Advise him he needn't restrict food or fluids. Tell him the test requires a blood sample, who will perform the test and when, and that he may experience transient discomfort from the needle puncture and the pressure of the tourniquet. Reassure him that collecting the sample takes less than 3 minutes.

Check patient history for immunosuppressive drugs that may affect test results. Note such use on the laboratory slip.

Procedure
Perform a venipuncture, and collect the sample in a 7-ml red-top tube.

Precautions
Keep the sample at room temperature, and send it to the laboratory immediately.

Values
Normal serum is negative or ≤0.03 nmol/

liter for AChR-binding antibodies and is negative for AChR-blocking antibodies.

Implications of results

Positive AChR antibodies in symptomatic adults confirm diagnosis of MG. Patients who have only ocular symptoms of MG tend to have lower antibody titers than those who have generalized symptoms.

Post-test care

☐ Since a patient with an autoimmune disease has a compromised immune system, check the venipuncture site for infection, and report any changes promptly. Keep a clean, dry bandage over the site for at least 24 hours.

☐ If a hematoma develops at the venipuncture site, ease discomfort by applying warm soaks.

Interfering factors

☐ Failure to maintain the sample at room temperature and to send it to the laboratory immediately may affect the accurate determination of test results.

☐ Patients undergoing thymectomy, thoracic duct drainage, immunosuppressive therapy, or plasmapheresis may show reduced AChR-antibody levels.

☐ Patients with amyotrophic lateral sclerosis may show false-positive test results.

SR. REBECCA FIDLER, MT (ASCP), PhD

VIRAL, BACTERIAL, & FUNGAL TESTS

Rubella Antibodies

Although rubella (German measles) is generally a mild viral infection in children and young adults, it can produce severe infection in the fetus, resulting in spontaneous abortion, stillbirth, or birth defects. Generally, the earlier the infection occurs during pregnancy, the greater the damage to the fetus. When rubella infection occurs during the first trimester, cataracts, deafness, and cardiac defects—congenital rubella syndrome—can result. Low birth weight, microcephaly, and mental retardation are other common manifestations.

Since rubella infection normally induces IgG and IgM antibody production, measuring rubella antibodies can determine present infection and immunity resulting from past infection. The hemagglutination inhibition (HI) test, the most commonly used serologic test for rubella antibodies, is indicated to diagnose rubella in pregnant women and others possibly exposed to the infection, and to determine susceptibility to it in children and women of childbearing age.

In this test, serial dilutions of the patient's serum are mixed with rubella virus antigen and goose erythrocytes, and then incubated. If rubella antibodies are present, they inhibit hemagglutination. The antibody titer is the highest dilution of serum that totally inhibits hemagglutination. The test for rubella requires two serum samples: one 3 days after onset of rash (acute titer); another, 2 to 3 weeks later (convalescent titer). The test for immunity requires one sample.

Purpose

☐ To diagnose rubella infection, especially congenital infection

☐ To determine susceptibility to rubella in children and in women of childbearing age.

Patient preparation

Explain to the patient that this test diagnoses or evaluates susceptibility to German measles. Inform her that she needn't restrict food or fluids. Tell the patient that this test requires a blood sample (if a current infection is suspected, a second blood sample will be needed in 2 to 3 weeks to identify a rise in the titer). Inform her who will perform the venipuncture and when; and that she may experience transient discomfort from the needle puncture and the pressure of the tourniquet. Reassure her that collecting the sample should take less than 3 minutes.

Provide emotional support, as needed, to parents when congenital rubella is suspected.

Procedure
Perform a venipuncture, and collect the sample in a 7 ml *red-top* tube.

Precautions
Handle the specimen gently to prevent hemolysis.

Values
Titer of < 1:8 or 1:10 (depending on the test) indicates susceptibility to rubella; titer of > 1:10 indicates adequate protection against rubella.

Implications of results
The HI antibodies normally appear 2 to 4 days after the onset of the rash, peak in 2 to 3 weeks, then slowly decline but remain detectable for life. In rubella infection, acute serum titers range from 1:8 to 1:16; convalescent serum titers, from 1:64 to 1:1,024+. A fourfold rise or greater from the acute to the convalescent titer indicates a recent rubella infection.

Since maternal antibodies cross the placenta and persist in the infant's serum for up to 6 months, congenital rubella can be detected only after this period. An antibody titer greater than 1:8 in an infant aged 6 months or older, who hasn't been exposed to rubella postnatally, confirms congenital rubella.

Post-test care
☐ If a hematoma develops at the venipuncture site, ease discomfort by applying warm soaks.
☐ When appropriate, instruct the patient to return for an additional blood test.
☐ If a woman of childbearing age (or a child) is found susceptible to rubella (titer of 1:8 or less), explain to the patient (or to the patient's parents) that vaccination can prevent rubella, and that she must wait at least 3 months after the vaccination before becoming pregnant, or risk permanent damage or death to the fetus.
☐ If the patient who is pregnant is found susceptible to rubella, instruct her to return for follow-up rubella antibody tests, as ordered, to detect possible subsequent infection.
☐ If the test confirms rubella in a pregnant patient, provide emotional support. As needed, refer her for appropriate counseling.

Interfering factors
Hemolysis caused by rough handling of the specimen may interfere with accurate determination of test results.

JANICE SELEKMAN, RN, MSN, DNSc

Hepatitis B Surface Antigen
[Hepatitis-associated antigen, Australia antigen]

Hepatitis B surface antigen (HB$_S$Ag) appears in the sera of patients with hepatitis B virus (formerly called serum hepatitis or long-incubation hepatitis). It can be detected by radioimmunoassay or, less commonly, by reverse passive hemagglutination during the extended incubation period and usually during the first 3 weeks of acute infection or if the patient is a carrier.

Since transmission of hepatitis is one of the gravest complications associated with blood transfusion, all donors must be screened for hepatitis B before their blood is stored. This screening, required by the Food and Drug Administration's Bureau of Biologics, has helped reduce the incidence of hepatitis. However, this test does not screen for hepatitis A virus (infectious hepatitis).

VIRAL HEPATITIS TEST PANEL

The three types of viral hepatitis produce similar symptoms but differ in terms of transmission, course of treatment, prognosis, and carrier status. When clinical history is insufficient for differentiation, serologic tests can aid diagnosis. Hepatitis A and hepatitis B antigens induce type-specific antibodies detectable by radioimmunoassay. The third hepatitis virus—non-A, non-B—is identified only by distinguishing it from A and B types. All tests require only a small sample of blood.

TYPICAL SEQUENCE OF HEPATITIS A MARKERS AFTER EXPOSURE

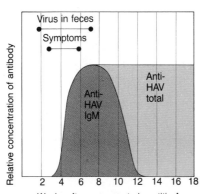

Testing for Hepatitis A: Present in blood and feces only briefly before symptoms appear, hepatitis A virus may elude detection. However, anti-HAV, the antibody to hepatitis A virus, appears early in the acute phase of the disease, persists for many years after recovery, and ultimately gives the patient immunity. A single positive anti-HAV test may indicate previous exposure to the virus, but because this antibody persists so long in the bloodstream, only evidence of *rising* anti-HAV titers confirms hepatitis A as the cause of current or very recent infection. Determining recent infection relies on identifying the antibody as IgM (associated with recent infection). A negative anti-HAV test rules out hepatitis A.

Courtesy of Abbott Laboratories, Abbott Park, Ill., *Serodiagnostic Assessment of Acute Viral Hepatitis.*

TYPICAL SEQUENCE OF HEPATITIS B MARKERS AFTER EXPOSURE

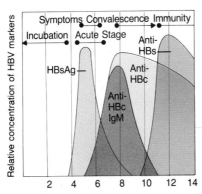

Testing for Hepatitis B: Hepatitis B viral cells are composed of a core protein and a surface protein. The surface antigen (HBsAg) appears in serum during the long incubation period (up to 26 weeks) or during the early acute phase of infection (2 to 3 weeks) and normally peaks after symptoms begin. High levels of HBsAg, continuing 3 or more months after onset of acute infection, suggest the development of chronic hepatitis or carrier status. Potential blood donors are screened for this antigen to prevent transmission of hepatitis B to recipients.

Another antibody to develop after exposure to hepatitis B is anti-HBc, induced by the core component of the B antigen. An early indicator of acute infection, antibody (IgM) to core antigen (anti-HBc IgM) is rarely detected in chronic infection. Thus, it's also useful in distinguishing acute from chronic infection and hepatitis B from non-A, non-B.

Courtesy of Abbott Laboratories, Abbott Park, Ill., *Serodiagnostic Assessment of Acute Viral Hepatitis.*

Anti-HBs, antibody to the surface component of the B virus, appears long after symptoms have subsided and after the antigen itself (HBsAg) has disappeared from blood. Detection of the antibody signals late convalescence or recovery from infection. Anti-HBs remains in the blood to provide immunity to reinfection.

SERODIAGNOSIS OF ACUTE VIRAL HEPATITIS

TEST RESULTS			INTERPRETATION
HBsAg	Anti-HBc IgM	Anti-HAV IgM	
–	–	+	Recent acute hepatitis A infection
+	+	–	Acute hepatitis B infection
+	–	–	Early acute hepatitis B infection or chronic hepatitis B
–	+	–	Confirms acute or recent infection with hepatitis B virus
–	–	–	Possible non-A, non-B hepatitis infection, other viral infection, or liver toxin
+	+	+	Recent probable hepatitis A infection and superimposed acute hepatitis B infection; uncommon profile

KEY: + positive   – negative

Courtesy of Abbott Laboratories, North Chicago, Ill.

Purpose
□ To screen blood donors for hepatitis B
□ To screen persons at high risk for contacting hepatitis B (such as hemodialysis nurses)
□ To aid differential diagnosis of viral hepatitis.

Patient preparation
Explain to the patient that this test helps identify a type of viral hepatitis. Inform him he needn't restrict food or fluids before the test. Tell the patient that the test requires a blood sample; who will perform the venipuncture and when; and that he may experience transient discomfort from the needle puncture and the pressure of the tourniquet. Reassure him that collecting the sample takes less than 3 minutes.

If the patient is giving blood, be sure to explain the donation procedure to him.

Procedure
Perform a venipuncture, and collect the sample in a 7 ml *red-top* tube.

Precautions
Wash your hands carefully after the procedure (or wear gloves when drawing blood). Dispose of the needle properly.

Findings
Normal serum is negative for HB_SAg.

Implications of results
Presence of HB_SAg in a patient with hepatitis confirms hepatitis B. In chronic carriers and persons with chronic active hepatitis, HB_SAg may be present in serum several months after onset of acute infection. HB_SAg may also occur in more than 5% of patients with certain diseases other than hepatitis, such as hemophilia, Hodgkin's disease, and leukemia. If the antigen is found in donor blood, this

blood must be discarded, because it carries a 40% to 70% risk of transmitting hepatitis. Blood samples that test positive should be retested, since inaccurate results do occur. For related tests to diagnose viral hepatitis, see the viral hepatitis test panel on page 333.

Post-test care
Notify the blood donor if test results are positive for the antigen. Report confirmed viral hepatitis to public health authorities. This is a reportable disease in most states.

Interfering factors
None.

DEBORAH S. PARZIALE, RN, MS

Heterophil Agglutination Tests

Heterophil agglutination tests detect and identify two IgM antibodies in human serum that react against foreign RBCs.

In the Paul-Bunnell test—also called the "presumptive" test—Epstein-Barr virus (EBV) antibodies, found in the sera of patients with infectious mononucleosis, agglutinate with sheep RBCs in a test tube. However, Forssman antibodies, present in some normal serum as well as in conditions such as serum sickness, also agglutinate with sheep RBCs, thus rendering test results inconclusive for infectious mononucleosis.

If the Paul-Bunnell test establishes a presumptive titer, Davidsohn's differential absorption test can then distinguish between EBV antibodies and Forssman antibodies. This differential test uses beef red cell antigens and Forssman antigens from guinea pig kidney cells as reagents. If the serum sample contains Forssman antibodies, the guinea pig cells absorb and remove them; these cells have little effect on EBV antibodies. If the sample contains EBV an-

tibodies, the beef red cells absorb them.

Purpose
☐ To aid differential diagnosis of infectious mononucleosis.

Patient preparation
Explain that this test helps detect infectious mononucleosis. Tell him the test requires a blood sample; who will perform the venipuncture and when; and that he may experience transient discomfort from the needle puncture and the pressure of the tourniquet. Collecting the sample takes less than 3 minutes.

Procedure
Perform a venipuncture, and collect the sample in a 7 ml *red-top* tube.

Precautions
None.

Values
Normally, the titer is less than 1:56 but

---

may be higher in elderly persons. Some laboratories refer to a normal titer as "negative" or as having "no reaction."

Implications of results

Although heterophil antibodies are present in the sera of approximately 80% of patients with infectious mononucleosis 1 month after onset, a positive finding—a titer higher than 1:56—does not confirm this disorder; for example, a high titer can result from systemic lupus erythematosus, syphilis, cryoglobulinemia, or the presence of antibodies to nonsyphilitic treponemata (yaws, pinta, bejel). A gradual increase in titer to about 1:224 during week 3 or 4, followed by a gradual decrease during weeks 4 to 8, proves most conclusive for infectious mononucleosis. However, a negative titer doesn't always rule out this disorder; occasionally, the titer becomes reactive 2 weeks later. Therefore, if symptoms persist, the test should be repeated in 2 weeks.

Confirmation of infectious mononucleosis depends on heterophil agglutination tests and hematologic tests that show absolute lymphocytosis, with 10% to 30% or more atypical lymphocytes.

Post-test care

☐ If a hematoma develops at the venipuncture site, ease discomfort by applying warm soaks.
☐ If the titer is positive and infectious mononucleosis is confirmed, instruct the patient in the treatment plan. If the titer is positive but infectious mononucleosis isn't confirmed, or if the titer is negative but symptoms persist, explain that additional testing will be necessary in a few days or weeks to confirm diagnosis and plan effective treatment.

Interfering factors

☐ If treatment for mononucleosis begins before development of heterophil antibodies, the titer is usually negative.
☐ Patients addicted to narcotics may have high titers.

BEVERLY A. ZENK WHEAT, RN, MA
SR. REBECCA FIDLER, MT(ASCP), PhD

Antistreptolysin-O Test

[Streptococcal antibody test]

Because streptococcal infections are often overlooked, serologic testing is valuable in patients with glomerulonephritis and acute rheumatic fever to confirm antecedent infection by showing serologic response to streptococcal antigen. The antistreptolysin-O (ASO) test measures the relative serum concentrations of the antibody to streptolysin O, an oxygen-labile enzyme produced by group A beta-hemolytic streptococci. In this test, a serum sample is diluted with a commercial preparation of streptolysin O and incubated. After the addition of rabbit or human RBCs, the tube is reincubated and examined visually. If hemolysis fails to develop, ASO has complexed with the antigen, inactivated it, and prevented RBC destruction, indicating recent beta-hemolytic streptococcal infection. The end point is read in Todd units, the reciprocal of the highest dilution (titer) that inhibits hemolysis. Very high ASO titers occur in poststreptococcal diseases, such as rheumatic fever or glomerulonephritis. ASO titers may also be elevated in patients with uncomplicated streptococcal disease; however, the incidence is lower and the titers are lower than in poststreptococcal diseases. Micro methods for detecting ASO, such as the Rapi/tex ASO latex agglutination test, currently screen for beta-hemolytic streptococcal infection.

Purpose

☐ To confirm recent or ongoing infection with beta-hemolytic streptococci
☐ To help diagnose rheumatic fever and poststreptococcal glomerulonephritis in the presence of clinical symptoms
☐ To distinguish between rheumatic fever and rheumatoid arthritis when joint pains are present.

Patient preparation

Explain to the patient that this test detects an immunologic response to certain bacteria (streptococci). Inform him he needn't restrict food or fluids. Tell him the test requires a blood sample; who will perform the venipuncture and when; and that he may experience transient discomfort from the needle puncture and the pressure of the tourniquet. Reassure him that collecting the sample takes less than 3 minutes.

If the test is to be repeated at regular intervals to identify active and inactive states of rheumatic fever or to confirm acute glomerulonephritis, tell the patient that measuring changes in antibody levels helps determine the effectiveness of therapy.

Check the patient's medication history for drugs that may suppress the streptococcal antibody response. If such drugs must be continued, note this on the laboratory slip.

Procedure

Perform a venipuncture, and collect the sample in a 7 ml *red-top* tube.

Precautions

Handle the sample gently to prevent hemolysis.

Values

Even healthy persons have some detectable ASO titer from previous minor streptococcal infections. For adults, normal ASO titer is less than 85 Todd units/ml; for school-age children, less than 170 Todd units/ml; and for preschoolers, less than 85 Todd units/ml.

Implications of results

High ASO titers usually occur only after prolonged or recurrent infections. Roughly 15% to 20% of patients with poststreptococcal disease don't have elevated ASO titers. Titers ranging to 250 Todd units may indicate inactive rheumatic fever. Higher titers of 500 to 5,000 Todd units suggest acute rheumatic fever or acute poststreptococcal glomerulonephritis.

TEST FOR ANTI-DNASE B

The antideoxyribonuclease B (anti-DNase B) test, a process similar to the antistreptolysin-O (ASO) test, detects antibodies to DNase B, a potent antigen produced by all group A streptococci.

For adults, normal anti-DNase B titer is less than 85 Todd units/ml; for school-age children, less than 170 Todd units/ml; and for preschoolers, less than 60 Todd units/ml. Elevated anti-DNase B titers appear in 80% of patients with acute rheumatic fever, in 75% of those with poststreptococcal glomerulonephritis (following streptococcal pharyngitis), and 60% of those with glomerulonephritis (following group A streptococcal pyoderma). This is a much higher percentage than those with ASO titer elevations (25%), making the test for anti-DNase B especially valuable in detecting a reaction to group A streptococcal pyoderma. Other streptococcal antigens are of limited diagnostic value, or their use is controversial.

Serial titers, determined at 10- to 14-day intervals, provide more reliable information than a single titer. A rise in titer 2 to 5 weeks after the acute infection, which peaks 4 to 6 weeks after the initial rise, confirms poststreptococcal disease.

Post-test care

If a hematoma develops at the venipuncture site, ease discomfort by applying warm soaks.

Interfering factors

□ Since patients with streptococcal skin infections rarely have abnormal ASO titers, even with poststreptococcal disease, false-negative results are likely in such patients.

□ Antibiotic or corticosteroid therapy may suppress the streptococcal antibody response and may interfere with accurate determination of test results.

□ Hemolysis due to rough handling of the sample may interfere with accurate determination of test results.

BEVERLY A. ZENK WHEAT, RN, MA
SR. REBECCA FIDLER, MT(ASCP), PhD

C-Reactive Protein

Absent in the sera of healthy persons, C-reactive protein (CRP) is an abnormal specific glycoprotein produced by the liver and excreted into the bloodstream during the acute phase of inflammation of any cause. CRP was initially discovered in the sera of patients with pneumococcal pneumonia, where it was shown to react with the C-mucopolysaccharide of the bacterial capsule—hence the name C-reactive protein. The major function of CRP is its interaction with the complement system.

Antiserum is used to detect CRP in several immunoassays—radioimmunoassay, capillary precipitation, gel diffusion, and latex agglutination. Although the presence of CRP strongly suggests active inflammation, the test is nonspecific for any disorder. Nevertheless, early detection of inflammation allows prompt treatment, possibly with anti-inflammatory agents, to prevent tissue damage from the disorder.

Purpose
☐ To detect the acute phase of inflammatory disease, such as exacerbations of rheumatoid arthritis and rheumatic fever
☐ To monitor response to therapy, especially in acute rheumatic fever and rheumatoid arthritis.

Patient preparation
Explain to the patient that this test detects generalized inflammation. If appropriate, explain that this test is a nonspecific method used to evaluate the severity and course of inflammatory diseases, and to monitor the effectiveness of treatment. Instruct him to fast (except for water) for at least 4 hours before the test. Tell him the test requires a blood sample; who will perform the venipuncture and when; and that he may experience transient discomfort from the needle puncture and the pressure of the tourniquet. Reassure the patient that collecting the sample should take less than 3 minutes.

Procedure
Perform a venipuncture, and collect the sample in a 7 ml *red-top* tube.

Precautions
None.

Findings
Normal serum is negative for CRP.

Implications of results
The presence of CRP in serum indicates an acute inflammatory condition (tissue reaction to injury resulting from infectious or noninfectious causes), and an elevation in CRP levels usually occurs before the erythrocyte sedimentation rate (ESR) rises. CRP disappears when treatment with corticosteroids or salicylates suppresses inflammation. A positive test for CRP commonly occurs in bacterial infections, such as tuberculosis and pneumococcal pneumonia, and in many noninfectious inflammatory conditions, such as acute rheumatic fever, acute rheumatoid arthritis, systemic lupus erythematosus, malignancy, and myocardial infarction.

Positive CRP occurs during the last half of pregnancy and also accompanies the use of oral contraceptives, making detection of concomitant inflammation difficult.

Post-test care
☐ If a hematoma develops at the venipuncture site, ease discomfort by applying warm soaks.
☐ The patient may resume the diet that was discontinued before the test.

Interfering factors
Pregnancy, ingestion of oral contraceptives, or use of an intrauterine device may cause positive test results, due to production of CRP because of tissue stress.

BEVERLY A. ZENK WHEAT, RN, MA
SR. REBECCA FIDLER, MT(ASCP), PhD

Febrile Agglutination Tests

Bacterial infections (such as tularemia, brucellosis, and the disorders caused by salmonella) and rickettsial infections (such as Rocky Mountain spotted fever and typhus) sometimes cause puzzling fevers (fever of undetermined origin [FUO]). In these infections and others in which microorganisms are difficult to isolate from blood or excreta, febrile agglutination tests can provide important diagnostic information.

The Weil-Felix reaction for rickettsial disease, Widal's test for Salmonella, and tests for brucellosis and tularemia are essentially the same. In these tests, a serum sample is mixed with a few drops of prepared antigens in normal saline solution on a slide; the reaction is observed with the unaided eye. If agglutination occurs, antigen is added to serial dilutions of the patient's serum. Antibody titer is expressed as the reciprocal of the last dilution showing visible agglutination.

The Weil-Felix reaction establishes rickettsial antibody titers. Unlike other febrile agglutination tests, the Weil-Felix reaction doesn't use the causal agent as the antigen, but uses instead three forms of Proteus *antigens (OX-19, OX-2, and OX-K) that cross-react with the various strains of rickettsiae. The accompanying chart shows that antibodies to certain rickettsial strains react with more than one* Proteus *antigen, while antibodies to other strains fail to react with any* Proteus *antigens.*

In Salmonella *infection—gastroenteritis and extraintestinal focal infections, both caused by* Salmonella enteritidis, *and in enteric (typhoid) fever, caused by* Salmonella typhosa—*the* Salmonella *organism presents flagellar (H) and somatic (O) antigens;* Widal's *test establishes their titers. Antibodies that agglutinate with H antigens form coarse,*

unstable aggregates that return to solution easily; those that agglutinate with O antigens form finer, more stable aggregates. The O antigens are considered more specific for Salmonella *than H antigens. A third antigen—Vi, or envelope, antigen—may indicate typhoid carrier status, which often tests negative for H and O antigens, but results so far have been difficult to standardize.* Widal's *test isn't recommended for diagnosing* Salmonella *gastroenteritis, since symptoms subside before the titer rises.*

Slide-agglutination and tube dilution tests, using killed suspensions of the disease organisms as antigens, establish titers for the gram-negative coccobacilli Brucella *and* Francisella tularensis, *which cause brucellosis and tularemia, respectively.*

Purpose

□ To support clinical findings in diagnosis of disorders caused by *Salmonella*, rickettsiae, *F. tularensis*, or *Brucella* organisms

□ To identify the cause of FUO.

Patient preparation

Explain to the patient that this test detects and quantitates microorganisms that may cause fever and other symptoms. Inform him that he needn't restrict food or fluids. Tell him the test requires a blood sample; who will perform the venipuncture and when; and that he may experience transient discomfort from the needle puncture and the pressure of the tourniquet. Reassure him that collecting the blood sample takes less than 3 minutes.

If appropriate, explain to the patient that this test requires a series of blood samples to detect a pattern of titers that is characteristic of the suspected disorder. Reassure him that a positive titer only suggests a disorder.

If the patient is receiving antibiotics, note on the laboratory slip when such therapy began.

Procedure

Perform a venipuncture, and collect the

sample in a 7 ml *red-top* tube.

Precautions
Use standard hospital isolation procedures when collecting and handling samples. Send samples to the laboratory immediately.

Values
Normal dilutions are as follows:
Salmonella antibody: < 1:80
brucellosis antibody: < 1:80
tularemia antibody: < 1:40
rickettsial antibody: < 1:40.

Implications of results
Observed rise and fall of titers are crucial for detecting active infection. If this is not possible, certain titer levels can suggest the disorder.

The Weil-Felix reaction is positive for rickettsiae with antibodies to *Proteus* 6 to 12 days after infection; titers peak in 1 month and usually drop to negative in 5 or 6 months. However, this test cannot be used for diagnosing rickettsialpox or Q fever, since the antibodies of these diseases don't cross-react with *Proteus* antigens; the test shows positive titers in *Proteus* infections and, in such cases, is nonspecific for rickettsiae.

In *Salmonella* infection, H and O agglutinins usually appear in serum after 1 week, and titers continue to rise for 3 to 6 weeks. O agglutinins usually fall to insignificant levels in 6 to 12 months. H agglutinin titers may remain elevated for several years.

In brucellosis, titers usually rise after 2 or 3 weeks, and reach their highest levels between 4 and 8 weeks; nevertheless, absence of *Brucella* agglutinins doesn't rule out brucellosis. In tularemia, titers usually become positive in the second week of infection, exceed 1:320 by the third week, peak in 4 to 7 weeks, and usually decline gradually 1 year after recovery.

For all febrile agglutinins, a fourfold increase in titers is strong evidence of infection.

Post-test care
□ If a hematoma develops at the veni-

WEIL-FELIX REACTIONS IN RICKETTSIAL INFECTION

INFECTION	*PROTEUS* ANTIGENS		
	OX-19	OX-2	OX-K
Epidemic typhus	+ + + +	+	0
Endemic typhus	+ + + +	+	0
Scrub typhus	0	0	+ + +
Rocky Mountain spotted fever	+ + + +	+	0
Rickettsialpox	0	0	0
Q fever	0	0	0

KEY:
+ + + +   strong agglutination
+ + +   moderate agglutination
+   weak agglutination
0   no agglutination

Adapted with permission from Ralph Michael Aloisi, *Principles of Immunodiagnostics* (St. Louis: C.V. Mosby Co., 1979), p. 91.

puncture site, apply warm soaks.

□ In FUO and suspected infection, contact the hospital infection control department. Isolation may be necessary.

Interfering factors

□ Failure to send the sample to the laboratory immediately may affect the accurate determination of test results.

□ Vaccination or continuous exposure to bacterial or rickettsial infection (resulting in immunity) causes high titers.

□ Many antibodies cross-react with bacteria that cause other infectious diseases. For example, tularemia antibodies cross-react with *Brucella* antigens.

□ Immunodeficient patients may show infectious symptoms but be unable to produce antibodies. In such cases, titers remain negative, even during infection.

□ Patients receiving antibiotic therapy show depressed titers early in the course of the disorder.

□ Patients with elevated immunoglobulin levels due to hepatic disease, or those who use drugs excessively, often have high *Salmonella* titers.

□ Patients who have had skin tests with *Brucella* antigen may show elevated *Brucella* titers.

□ Patients with *Proteus* infections may show positive Weil-Felix titers for rickettsial disease.

BEVERLY A. ZENK WHEAT, RN, MA
SR. REBECCA FIDLER, MT(ASCP), PhD

Fungal Serology

[Blastomycosis, coccidioidomycosis, histoplasmosis, aspergillosis, and sporotrichosis antibodies; cryptococcosis antigen]

Most fungal organisms enter the body as spores inhaled into the lungs or infiltrated through wounds in the skin or mucosa. If the body's defenses can't destroy the organisms initially, the fungi multiply to form lesions; blood and lymph vessels may then spread the mycoses throughout the body. Most healthy persons easily overcome initial mycotic infection, but the elderly and others with deficient immune systems are more susceptible to acute or chronic mycotic infection and to disorders secondary to such infection.

Mycosis may be deep-seated or superficial: deep-seated mycosis occurs primarily in the lungs; superficial mycosis, in the skin or the mucosal linings. Although cultures are usually performed to diagnose mycoses by identifying the causative organism, occasionally serologic tests provide the sole evidence for mycosis. Such serologic tests employ immunodiffusion, complement fixation, precipitin, latex agglutination, or agglutination methods to demonstrate the presence of specific mycotic antibodies.

Purpose

□ To rapidly detect the presence of antifungal antibodies, aiding in the diagnosis of mycoses

□ To monitor effectiveness of therapy for mycoses.

Patient preparation

Explain to the patient that this test aids diagnosis of certain fungal infections. If appropriate, explain to the patient that this test monitors his response to mycoses therapy and that it may be necessary to repeat the test during his illness. Instruct him to restrict food and fluids for 12 to 24 hours before the test. Tell him the test requires a blood sample; who will perform the venipuncture and when; and that he may experience brief discomfort from the needle puncture and the pressure of the tourniquet. Reassure him that collecting the sample takes less than 3 minutes.

Procedure

Perform a venipuncture, and collect the sample in a 10 ml sterile *red-top tube.*

Precautions

Send the sample to the laboratory im-

SERUM TEST METHODS FOR FUNGAL INFECTIONS

DISEASE AND NORMAL VALUES	CLINICAL SIGNIFICANCE OF ABNORMAL RESULTS
Blastomycosis Complement fixation: titers < 1:8	Titers ranging from 1:8 to 1:16 suggest infection; titers > 1:32 denote active disease. A rising titer in serial samples taken every 3 to 4 weeks indicates disease progression; a falling titer indicates regression. This test has limited diagnostic value due to high percentage of false-negatives.
Immunodiffusion: negative	A more sensitive test for blastomycosis; detects 80% of infected persons
Coccidioidomycosis Complement fixation: titers < 1:2	Most sensitive test for this fungus. Titers ranging from 1:2 to 1:4 suggest active infection; titers > 1:16 usually denote active disease. Test may remain negative in mild infections.
Immunodiffusion: negative	Most useful for screening, followed by complement fixation test for confirmation
Precipitin: titers < 1:16	Good screening test; titers > 1:16 usually indicate infection. 80% of infected persons show positive titers by 2 weeks: most revert to negative by 6 months. Early primary disease is shown by positive precipitin and negative complement fixation test. A positive complement fixation and negative precipitin test indicate chronic disease.
Histoplasmosis: Complement fixation (histoplasmin): titers < 1:8	Titers ranging from 1:8 to 1:16 suggest infection; titers > 1:32 indicate active disease. Antibodies generally appear 10 to 21 days after initial infection. Test is positive in 10% to 15% of cases.
Complement fixation (yeast): titers < 1:18	More sensitive than histoplasmin complement fixation test; gives positive results in 75% to 80% of cases. (Both histoplasmin and yeast antigens are positive in 10% of cases.) A rising titer in serial samples taken every 2 to 3 weeks indicates progressive infection; a decreasing titer indicates regression. Titers ranging from 1:8 to 1:16 suggest infection; titers > 1:32 indicate active disease.
Immunodiffusion (histoplasmin): negative	Appearance of both H and M bands indicates active infection. If the M band appears first and lasts longer than the H band, the infection may be regressing. The M band alone may indicate early infection, chronic disease, or a recent skin test.
Aspergillosis: Complement fixation: titer < 1:8	Titers of > 1:8 suggest infection. 70% to 90% of patients with known pulmonary aspergillosis and/or aspergillus allergy present antibodies, and so do about 5% of the general population. This test cannot detect invasive aspergillosis, because patients with this disease do not present antibodies; biopsy is required.
Immunodiffusion: negative	One or more precipitin bands suggests infection; precipitins appear in 95% of patients with pulmonary fungus balls and in 50% of those with allergic bronchopulmonary disorders. The number of bands is related to complement fixation titers; the more precipitin bands, the higher the titer.
Sporotrichosis: Agglutination: titers < 1:40	Titers of > 1:80 usually indicate active disease. The test usually is negative in cutaneous infections, positive in extracutaneous infections.
Cryptococcosis: Latex agglutination for cryptococcal antigen: negative	About 90% of patients with cryptococcal meningoencephalitis present capsular antigen in CSF serum. (Serum is less frequently positive than CSF.) Culturing is definitive since false-positives do occur. (Presence of rheumatoid factor may cause a positive reaction.) Serum antigen tests are positive in 33% of patients with pulmonary cryptococcosis; biopsy is usually required.

mediately. If transport to the laboratory is delayed, store the sample at 39.2° F. (4° C.).

Values
Depending on the test method, a negative finding, or normal titer, usually indicates the absence of mycosis. The accompanying chart lists values for specific appropriate organisms.

Implications of results
The accompanying chart summarizes the clinical significance of abnormal serologic test values for complement fixation, immunodiffusion, precipitin, latex agglutination, and agglutination techniques.

Post-test care
If a hematoma develops at the veni-puncture site, ease discomfort by applying warm soaks.

Interfering factors
□ Some antigens, such as the blastomycosis and histoplasmosis antigens, may cross-react to produce false-positive results or high titers.
□ Recent skin testing with fungal antigens may elevate titers.
□ Many mycoses depress the immune system, causing low titers or false-negative test results.
□ Failure to send a sterile sample to the laboratory immediately or to store the sample properly if transport is delayed may interfere with accurate determination of test results.
□ A nonfasting specimen may alter test results.

SR. REBECCA FIDLER, MT(ASCP), PhD

SYPHILIS TESTS

VDRL

[Venereal Disease Research Laboratory test]

The VDRL test is widely used to screen for primary and secondary syphilis. This flocculation test demonstrates the presence of reagin—an antibody relatively specific for Treponema pallidum, *the spirochete that causes syphilis—in a serum sample, after addition of an antigen consisting of cardiolipin and lecithin (two specific and reactive substances in beef heart muscle) and cholesterol. After the antigen complex is mixed with the serum on a slide, the sample is rotated and examined microscopically. If flocculation appears, the sample is diluted until no reaction occurs. The last dilution to show visible flocculation is taken as the titer of the antibody.*

Although the test has diagnostic significance during the first two stages of syphilis, transient or permanent bio-logic false-positive reactions can make accurate interpretation difficult. A biologic false-positive reaction can result from viral or bacterial infection, chronic systemic illness, or nonsyphilitic treponemal disease.

A serum sample is used in the VDRL test, but this test may also be performed on a specimen of CSF, obtained by lumbar puncture, to test for tertiary syphilis. However, the VDRL test of CSF is less sensitive than the fluorescent treponemal antibody absorption test.

Purpose
□ To screen for primary and secondary syphilis
□ To confirm primary or secondary syphilis in the presence of syphilitic lesions
□ To monitor response to treatment.

Patient preparation
Explain to the patient that this test detects syphilis. Inform him that the disease often goes undetected in the general population because infected persons re-

main untreated. Tell the patient he needn't restrict food, fluids, or medications, but should abstain from alcohol for 24 hours before the test. Tell him the test requires a blood sample; who will perform the venipuncture and when; that he may experience transient discomfort from the needle puncture and the tourniquet pressure; and that collecting the sample takes less than 3 minutes.

Procedure

Perform a venipuncture, and collect the sample in a 7 ml *red-top* tube.

Precautions

Handle the specimen carefully to prevent hemolysis.

Findings

Normal serum shows no flocculation and is reported as a nonreactive test.

Implications of results

Definite flocculation is reported as a reactive test; slight flocculation is reported

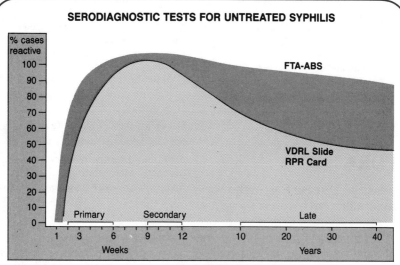

SERODIAGNOSTIC TESTS FOR UNTREATED SYPHILIS

The fluorescent treponemal antibody absorption (FTA-ABS) test—which uses a strain of the *Treponema pallidum* antigen itself as a reagent—is more sensitive than the VDRL (Venereal Disease Research Laboratory) test or the rapid plasma reagin (RPR) test in detecting all stages of untreated syphilis, but its complex testing method and incidence of false-positive results make it an impractical screening tool. The VDRL and RPR tests are preferred for wide-scale screening and also when primary- and secondary-stage disease are suspected. In advanced syphilis, when the VDRL test may be negative for more than one third of infected persons, the FTA-ABS test is preferred for sensitivity and is also the most reliable confirmation of a positive VDRL.

The VDRL test can be used to monitor response to treatment. Untreated syphilis produces titers that are low in the primary stage (<1:32), elevated in the secondary stage (>1:32), and variable in the tertiary stage. Successful therapy markedly reduces titers, with two thirds of patients reverting to a negative VDRL, especially during the first two stages of disease. Third-stage therapy seldom produces a nonreactive VDRL, but maintenance of low-reactive values during the 6- to 12-month post-therapy period indicates success. A subsequent rise signals reinfection. By comparison, FTA-ABS test results usually remain positive following treatment.

A significant number of patients with infectious diseases show temporary false-positive VDRL test results. Chronic false-positive VDRL and FTA-ABS test readings are associated with the immune complex diseases.

Adapted with permission from Allen L. Pusch, "Serodiagnostic Tests," in Todd-Sanford-Davidsohn, *Clinical Diagnosis and Management by Laboratory Methods*, Vol.2, edited by John Bernard Henry (16th ed.; Philadelphia: W.B. Saunders Co., 1979), p. 1890.

as a weakly reactive test. A reactive VDRL test occurs in about 50% of patients with primary syphilis and in nearly all patients with secondary syphilis. If syphilitic lesions exist, a reactive VDRL test is diagnostic. If no lesions are evident, a reactive VDRL test necessitates repeated testing. However, biologic false-positive reactions can be caused by conditions unrelated to syphilis, for example, infectious mononucleosis, malaria, leprosy, hepatitis, systemic lupus erythematosus, rheumatoid arthritis, and nonsyphilitic treponomal diseases, such as pinta or yaws.

A nonreactive test doesn't rule out syphilis, because *T. pallidum* causes no detectable immunologic changes in the serum for 14 to 21 days after infection. However, dark-field microscopic examination of exudate from suspicious lesions can provide early diagnosis by identifying the causative spirochetes.

A reactive VDRL test using a CSF specimen indicates neurosyphilis, which can follow the primary and secondary stages in persons who remain untreated.

Post-test care
□ If a hematoma develops at the venipuncture site, apply warm soaks.
□ If the test is nonreactive or borderline but syphilis hasn't been ruled out, instruct the patient to return for follow-up testing. Explain that borderline test results don't necessarily mean he is free of the disease.
□ If the test is reactive, explain the importance of proper treatment. Provide the patient with further information about venereal disease and how it is spread, and stress the need for antibiotic therapy. Also, prepare him for mandatory inquiries from public health authorities. If the test is reactive but the patient shows no clinical signs of syphilis, explain that many uninfected persons show false-positive reactions. However, stress the need for further specific tests to rule out syphilis.

Interfering factors
□ Ingestion of alcohol within 24 hours

RAPID PLASMA REAGIN (RPR) CARD TEST

This rapid, macroscopic serologic test is an acceptable substitute for the VDRL test in diagnosis of syphilis. The RPR test, available as a kit, employs a cardiolipin antigen to detect reagin, the antibody relatively specific to the causative agent of syphilis. In the RPR test, the patient's serum is mixed with cardiolipin on a plastic-coated card, rotated mechanically, and examined with the unaided eye. If flocculation occurs, the test sample is diluted until no visible reaction occurs. The last dilution to show visible flocculation is the titer of the reagin antibody.

In the RPR test, like the VDRL test, normal serum shows no flocculation.

---

of the test can produce transient, nonreactive results.
□ A faulty immune system can cause nonreactive results.
□ Hemolysis of the sample can interfere with test results.

BEVERLY A. ZENK WHEAT, RN, MA
SR. REBECCA FIDLER, MT(ASCP), PhD

Fluorescent Treponemal Antibody Absorption Test

The fluorescent treponemal antibody absorption (FTA-ABS or simply FTA) test uses indirect immunofluorescence to detect antibodies to the cause of syphilis— the spirochete Treponema pallidum—*in serum. In this test, prepared* T. pallidum *is fixed on a slide, and the patient's serum is added, after addition of an absorbed preparation of Reiter treponema. This addition to the test serum prevents interference by antibodies from nonsyphilitic treponemas; Reiter treponema combines with most nonsyphilitic antibodies, making the FTA-ABS test specific for* T. pallidum.

If syphilitic antibodies are present in the test serum, they will coat the trepone-

mal organisms. The slide is then stained with fluorescein-labeled antiglobulin. This antiglobulin attaches to the coated spirochetes, which fluoresce when viewed under a microscope with ultraviolet light.

Although the FTA-ABS test is generally performed on a serum sample to detect primary or secondary syphilis, it exclusively requires a CSF specimen to detect tertiary syphilis. Because antibody levels remain constant for long periods, the FTA-ABS test is not recommended for monitoring response to therapy.

Purpose
□ To confirm primary or secondary syphilis
□ To screen for suspected false-positive results of VDRL tests.

Patient preparation
Explain to the patient that this test can confirm or rule out syphilis. Inform him that he needn't restrict food or fluids. Tell him the test requires a blood sample; who will perform the venipuncture and when; and that he may experience transient discomfort from the needle puncture and the pressure of the tourniquet. Reassure the patient that collecting the blood sample usually takes less than 3 minutes.

TWO NEW TESTS FOR
TREPONEMA PALLIDUM

The recently developed microhemagglutination assay for *Treponema pallidum* antibody increases the specificity of syphilis testing by eliminating methodologic interference. In this assay, tanned sheep RBCs are coated with *T. pallidum* antigen and are combined with absorbed test serum. Hemagglutination occurs in the presence of specific anti–*T. pallidum* antibodies in the serum.

In the enzyme-linked immunosorbent assay (ELISA), tubes coated with *T. pallidum* are washed and then treated with enzyme-labeled antihuman globulin. After the substrate for the enzymes is added to the tubes, the enzymatic activity is measured by quantitating the reaction product formed.

Procedure
Perform a venipuncture, and collect the sample in a 7-ml *red-top* tube.

Precautions
Handle the sample gently to prevent hemolysis.

Findings
Normally, reaction to the FTA-ABS test is negative (no fluorescence).

Implications of results
The presence of treponemal antibodies in the serum—a reactive test result—does not indicate the stage or the severity of infection. (However, the presence of these antibodies in CSF is strong evidence of tertiary neurosyphilis.) Elevated antibody levels appear in 80% to 90% of patients with primary syphilis and in 100% of patients with secondary syphilis. Higher antibody levels persist for several years, with treatment or without treatment.

The absence of treponemal antibodies—a nonreactive test—doesn't necessarily rule out syphilis. *T. pallidum* causes no detectable immunologic changes in the blood for 14 to 21 days after initial infection. Organisms may be detected earlier by examining suspicious lesions with a dark-field microscope. Low antibody levels or other nonspecific factors produce borderline findings. In such cases, repeated testing and a thorough review of patient history may be productive.

Although the FTA-ABS test is specific, some patients with nonsyphilitic conditions—such as systemic lupus erythematosus, genital herpes, or increased or abnormal globulins—or those who are pregnant may show minimally reactive levels. In addition, the FTA-ABS test doesn't always distinguish between *T. pallidum* and certain other treponemas, such as those that cause pinta, yaws, and bejel.

Post-test care
□ If a hematoma develops at the venipuncture site, apply warm soaks.

□ If the test is reactive, explain the nature of syphilis, and stress the importance of proper treatment and the need to find and treat the patient's sexual contacts. If appropriate, provide the patient with additional information about syphilis and how it is spread; emphasize the need for antibiotic therapy. Also, prepare him for inquiries from the public health authorities.

□ If the test is nonreactive or findings are borderline but syphilis has not been ruled out, instruct the patient to return for follow-up testing; explain that inconclusive results don't necessarily indicate he is free of the disease.

Interfering factors
Hemolysis caused by rough handling of the sample may alter test results.

BEVERLY A. ZENK WHEAT, RN, MA
SR. REBECCA FIDLER, MT(ASCP), PhD

FETAL ANTIGEN TESTS

Carcinoembryonic Antigen

Carcinoembryonic antigen (CEA), a glycoprotein secreted onto the glycocalyx surface of cells lining the gastrointestinal tract, appears during the first or second trimester of fetal life. Normally, production of CEA is halted before birth but may begin again later, if a neoplasm develops. Since CEA levels are raised by biliary obstruction, alcoholic hepatitis, chronic heavy smoking, and other conditions, as well as by benign or malignant neoplasms, this test can't be used as a general indicator of cancer. However, it is useful for staging, assessing the adequacy of surgical resection, and monitoring colorectal cancer therapy, since serum CEA levels, measured by enzyme immunoassay, usually return to normal within 6 weeks if cancer treatment is successful.

Purpose
□ To monitor the effectiveness of cancer therapy
□ To assist in preoperative staging of colorectal cancers and to test for recurrence of colorectal cancers.

Patient preparation
Explain to the patient that this test detects and measures a special protein that's not normally present in adults. If appropriate, inform him that the test will be repeated to monitor the effectiveness of therapy.

Advise the patient that he needn't restrict food, fluids, or medications before the test. Tell him the test requires a blood sample; who will perform the venipuncture and when; and that he may experience transient discomfort from the needle puncture and the pressure of the tourniquet. Reassure the patient that collecting the blood sample normally takes less than 3 minutes.

Procedure
Perform a venipuncture, and collect the sample in a 7 ml *red-top* tube.

Precautions
Handle the sample gently to prevent hemolysis, and send it to the laboratory immediately to ensure integrity of test results.

Values
Normal serum CEA values are less than 5 ng/ml in healthy nonsmokers.

Implications of results
If serum CEA levels exceed normal before surgical resection, chemotherapy, or radiation therapy, their return to normal within 6 weeks suggests successful treatment. Persistent elevation of CEA levels, however, suggests residual or recurrent tumor.

USING CEA TO MONITOR CANCER TREATMENT

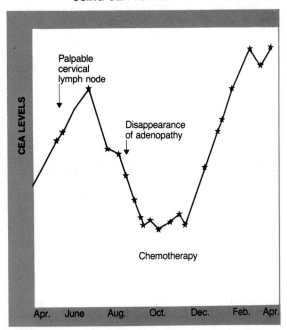

CEA LEVELS

Palpable
cervical
lymph node

Disappearance
of adenopathy

Chemotherapy

Apr.   June   Aug.   Oct.   Dec.   Feb.   Apr.

CEA LEVELS

Negative clinical and
radiologic evaluation

Obstructed
ureters
detected

Sigmoid
colectomy

Mar.   May   July   Sept.   Nov.   Jan.   Mar.   May

Because many patients in the early stages of colorectal cancer have normal or low values for carcinoembryonic antigen (CEA), the CEA test does not screen successfully for early malignancy. It is a good tool, however, for monitoring response to cancer therapy.

Once a patient's serum CEA level has dropped following surgery, chemotherapy, or other treatment, any increase suggests recurrence of cancer or diminished effectiveness of treatment.

Both charts (left) illustrate CEA levels in patients during and after treatment for colorectal cancer. Initial results show the usual dramatic drop in response to treatment. In the top chart, the subsequent rise in CEA indicates a diminishing response to chemotherapy. In the bottom chart, the progressive rise in CEA signaled recurrence of cancer 8 months before clinical symptoms or radiologic evidence.

Adapted with permission from P.H. Sugarbaker, et al, "Patterns of Serial CEA Assays and Their Clinical Use in Management of Colorectal Cancer," *Journal of Surgical Oncology*, 8:523-537, 1976.

High CEA levels are characteristic in various malignant conditions, particularly endodermally derived neoplasms of the gastrointestinal organs and the lungs, and in certain nonmalignant conditions, such as benign hepatic disease, hepatic cirrhosis, alcoholic pancreatitis, and inflammatory bowel disease.

Elevated CEA concentrations may also be associated with nonendodermal carcinoma; for example, breast cancer and ovarian cancer typically elevate CEA levels.

Post-test care

If a hematoma develops at the venipuncture site, ease discomfort by applying warm soaks.

Interfering factors

□ Chronic cigarette smoking may elevate serum CEA levels, causing inaccurate interpretation of test results.
□ Hemolysis caused by rough handling of the sample may elevate serum CEA levels, thereby altering test results.

> BEVERLY A. ZENK WHEAT, RN, MA
> SR. REBECCA FIDLER, MT(ASCP), PhD

Alpha-fetoprotein

Alpha-fetoprotein (AFP) is a glycoprotein produced by fetal tissue and tumors that differentiate from midline embryonic structures. During fetal development, AFP levels in serum and amniotic fluid rise; since this protein crosses the placenta, it also appears in maternal serum. In late stages of pregnancy, AFP concentrations in fetal and maternal serum and in amniotic fluid begin to diminish. During the first year of life, serum AFP levels continue to decline and characteristically persist at a low level thereafter.

High maternal serum AFP levels at 16 to 18 weeks' gestation may suggest fetal neural tube defects, such as spina bifida or anencephaly, but positive con-

firmation necessitates amniocentesis and ultrasonography. Other congenital anomalies may also be associated with high maternal serum AFP concentrations. Elevated AFP levels in those persons who aren't pregnant may occur in malignancy, such as hepatocellular carcinoma, or in certain nonmalignant conditions, such as ataxia-telangiectasia; in these conditions, AFP assays are more useful for monitoring response to therapy than for establishing diagnosis.

AFP levels are best determined by enzyme-immunoassay on plasma or serum and should be used only as a tumor marker.

Purpose

□ To monitor the effectiveness of therapy in malignant conditions, such as hepatomas and germ cell tumors, and in certain nonmalignant conditions, such as ataxia-telangiectasia.

Patient preparation

Explain to the patient that this test monitors response to therapy by measuring a special blood protein. Advise him that further testing may be required if levels of this protein are elevated. Inform him he needn't restrict food, fluids, or medications before the test.

Tell the patient that this test requires a blood sample; who will perform the venipuncture and when; and that he may experience transient discomfort from the needle puncture and the pressure of the tourniquet. Reassure the patient that collecting the blood sample normally takes less than 3 minutes.

Procedure

Perform a venipuncture, and collect the sample in a 7 ml *red-top* tube.

Precautions

Handle the sample gently to prevent hemolysis.

Values

In persons who aren't pregnant, serum AFP values normally are less than 15 ng/ml.

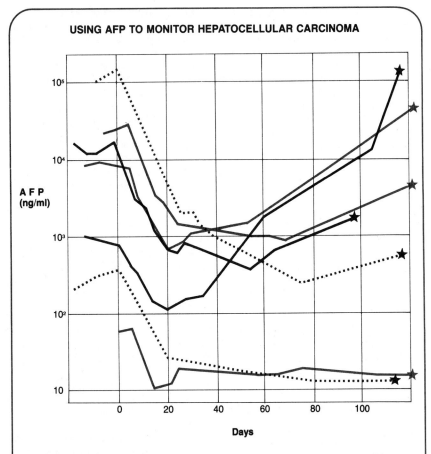

USING AFP TO MONITOR HEPATOCELLULAR CARCINOMA

Serial determinations of serum alpha-fetoprotein (AFP) in seven patients with hepatocellular car-cinomas show a dramatic immediate drop in AFP levels after surgical resection (day 0). Subse-quent rise in five patients indicates recurrent tumor; such an increase commonly precedes clinical evidence of recurrence by 1 to 6 months. All these patients had incomplete resections, but two showed no sign of tumor during follow-up testing. The wide range of AFP values among individuals is common.

Adapted with permission from Noel R. Rose and Herman Friedman, eds., *Manual of Clinical Immunology* (2nd ed.; Washington: American Society for Microbiology, 1980), p. 939.

Implications of results

Elevated maternal serum AFP levels may suggest neural tube defect or other tube anomalies after 14 weeks' gestation. AFP levels rise sharply in approximately 90% of fetuses with anencephaly and in 50% of those with spina bifida. However, de-finitive diagnosis necessitates ultraso-nography and amniocentesis. High AFP levels may also indicate intrauterine death. Occasionally, such levels indicate other anomalies; for example, duodenal atresia, omphalocele, tetralogy of Fallot, and Turner's syndrome.

Elevated serum AFP levels in persons who aren't pregnant may indicate he-patocellular carcinoma (although low AFP levels don't rule it out) or germ cell tumor of gonadal, retroperitoneal, or mediastinal origin. Serum AFP rises in ataxia-telangiectasia and, occasionally, in cancer of the pancreas, the stomach, or the biliary system. Transient modest elevations sometimes occur in nonneoplastic hepatocellular disease, such as acute or chronic hepatitis and alcoholic cirrhosis.

In hepatocellular carcinoma, a gradual decrease in serum AFP levels indicates a favorable response to therapy. In germ cell tumors, serum AFP levels and serum human chorionic gonadotropin levels should be measured concurrently to assess therapy.

Post-test care

If a hematoma develops at the venipuncture site, ease discomfort by applying warm soaks.

Interfering factors

□ Hemolysis caused by rough handling of the sample may alter serum AFP levels, thereby interfering with accurate determination of test results.

□ Multiple pregnancy may cause false-positive test results.

BEVERLY A. ZENK WHEAT, RN, MA
SR. REBECCA FIDLER, MT(ASCP), PhD

Selected References

Bauer, John D., and Ackerman, Philip G. *Clinical Laboratory Methods*, 9th ed. St. Louis: C.V. Mosby Co., 1982.

Berkow, Robert, ed. *The Merck Manual of Diagnosis and Therapy*, 14th ed. Rahway, N.J.: Merck, Sharp, and Dohme Research Laboratories, 1982.

Brunner, Lillian S., and Suddarth, Doris S. *Textbook of Medical-Surgical Nursing*, 5th ed. Philadelphia: J.B. Lippincott Co., 1984.

Byrne, C. Judith, et al. *Laboratory Tests: Implications for Nurses and Allied Health Professionals*. Reading, Mass.: Addison-Wesley Publishing Co., 1981.

Diseases, 2nd ed. Nurse's Reference Library. Springhouse, Pa.: Springhouse Corp., 1986.

Fischbach, Frances. *A Manual of Laboratory Diagnostic Tests*, 2nd ed. Philadelphia: J.B. Lippincott Co., 1984.

Guyton, Arthur C. *Textbook of Medical Physiology*, 6th ed. Philadelphia: W.B. Saunders Co., 1981.

Harvey, A. McGehee, ed. *The Principles and Practice of Medicine*, 21st ed. East Norwalk, Conn.: Appleton-Century-Crofts, 1984.

Henry, John Bernard, ed. *Todd-Sanford-Davidsohn Clinical Diagnosis and Management by Laboratory Methods*, vol. 1, 17th ed. Philadelphia: W.B. Saunders Co., 1984.

Immune Disorders, Nurse's Clinical Library. Springhouse, Pa.: Springhouse Corp., 1985.

Lamb, Jane O. *Laboratory Tests for Clinical Nursing*. Bowie, Md.: Robert J. Brady Co., 1984.

Leavelle, Dennis E., ed. *Mayo Medical Laboratories Test Catalog*. Rochester, Minn.: Mayo Medical Laboratories, 1984.

McNeeley, M.D. "Drug Interference with Laboratory Tests of Immunologic Status," *Drug Therapy*. 73-76, March 1981.

Milgrom, Felix, et al., eds. *Principles of Immunological Diagnosis in Medicine*. Philadelphia: Lea & Febiger, 1981.

Nursing85 Drug Handbook. Springhouse, Pa.: Springhouse Corp., 1985.

Petersdorf, Robert G., and Adams, Raymond D., eds. *Harrison's Principles of Internal Medicine*, 10th ed. New York: McGraw-Hill Book Co., 1983.

Ravel, Richard. *Clinical Laboratory Medicine*, 4th ed. Chicago: Year Book Medical Pubs., 1984.

Rose, Noel R., and Friedman, Herman, eds. *Manual of Clinical Immunology*, 2nd ed. Washington, D.C.: American Society for Microbiology, 1980.

Stites, Daniel P., et al., eds. *Basic and Clinical Immunology*, 5th ed. Los Altos, Calif.: Lange Medical Publications, 1985.

Tilkian, Sarko M., et al. *Clinical Implications of Laboratory Tests*, 3rd ed. St. Louis: C.V. Mosby Co., 1983.

Wegener, Lee T., ed. *Mayo Medical Laboratories Interpretive Handbook*. Rochester, Minn.: Mayo Medical Laboratories, 1984.

Widmann, Frances K. *Clinical Interpretation of Laboratory Tests*, 9th ed. Philadelphia: F.A. Davis Co., 1983.

12 Urinalysis

LEARNING OBJECTIVES

After completing this chapter, the reader will be able to:
- identify the components of the nephron unit and explain their functions.
- describe the three mechanisms by which nephrons form urine.
- list the common components of urine.
- define the terms polyuria, oliguria, nocturia, and anuria.
- state the causes, symptoms, and incidence of urinary calculi.
- explain the importance of routine urinalysis.
- state the purpose of each test discussed in the chapter.
- prepare the patient physically and psychologically for each test.
- describe the procedure for performing each test.
- specify appropriate precautions for safe administration of each test.
- implement appropriate post-test care.
- state the normal values or findings for each test.
- discuss the implications of abnormal test results.
- list factors that may interfere with accurate test results.

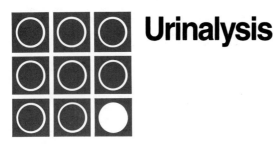

Urinalysis

Introduction

Routine urinalysis and special studies of renal function provide valuable information about the integrity of renal and urinary functions, and also serve as sensitive indicators of overall health. To understand the significance of such tests and their clinical applications, you need to know how urine is normally formed, what elements it contains, and the mechanisms that regulate urine volume.

Urine formation

The kidneys, through the activity of the nephrons, continuously remove metabolic wastes, drugs and other foreign substances, excess fluids, inorganic salts, and acid and base substances from the blood for eventual excretion in the urine. Each kidney has approximately 1 million nephrons; in turn, each nephron consists of a vascular ultrafilter called a *glomerulus* and a *renal tubule*, an epithelial-lined conduit for reabsorption of recyclable matter and secretion of foreign and waste substances. The nephrons form urine through three mechanisms—*glomerular filtration, tubular reabsorption,* and *tubular secretion.*

Blood enters each kidney through the renal artery, passing through progressively smaller vascular channels and eventually entering the glomeruli through the afferent glomerular arterioles. These arterioles subdivide into clusters of capillary loops, each of which is partly enclosed in a membranous covering called Bowman's capsule. The walls of the capillaries are semipermeable, so dissolved substances can pass by simple filtration from the plasma through the glomerular capillaries and into the capsule space.

Blood leaves the glomeruli through the efferent glomerular arterioles and travels to a network of peritubular capillaries, which encircle the renal tubules. Glomerular filtrate leaves the Bowman's capsules and enters the proximal convoluted tubules, where approximately 65% is selectively reabsorbed by the peritubular capillaries. (Reabsorbed substances include water, glucose, some proteins, amino acids, acetoacetate ions, vitamins, and hormones.) The remaining 35% of the filtrate proceeds through the loops of Henle and the distal convoluted tubules, where sodium and water are reabsorbed as needed.

During secretion, fluid and solutes such as potassium, uric acid, exogenous substances (such as drugs), and other waste material move from the peritubular capillaries back into the glomerular filtrate. As the liquid filtrate evolves, it's continuously modified by filtration, reabsorption, and secretion. The end product is urine.

Urine composition

Although the actual composition of normal urine changes—depending on diet, physical activity, and emotional stress—it always includes water, urea, uric acid, and sodium chloride. Urine also usually contains other nonprotein nitrogen compounds, citric acid, other organic acids,

COMPONENTS OF THE NEPHRON UNIT

Each kidney has about 1 million functional units called nephrons. In turn, each nephron contains a vascular ultrafilter called the *glomerulus*, and a *renal tubule*, an epithelial-lined conduit made up of four sections (proximal convoluted tubule, Loop of Henle, distal convoluted tubule, and collecting tubule). As the filtrate from the glomerulus travels through the renal tubules, resorption and secretion modify it to meet the body's needs. The end result is urine.

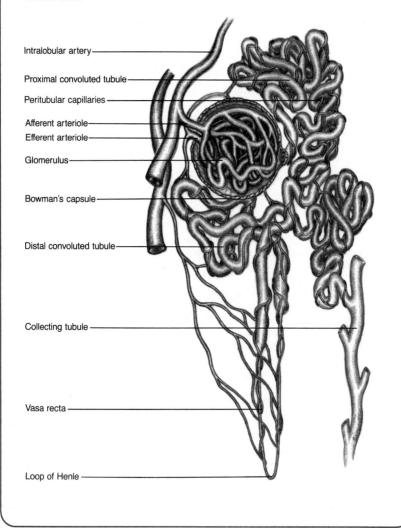

Intralobular artery

Proximal convoluted tubule

Peritubular capillaries

Afferent arteriole

Efferent arteriole

Glomerulus

Bowman's capsule

Distal convoluted tubule

Collecting tubule

Vasa recta

Loop of Henle

catecholamines, sulfur-containing compounds, phosphate, potassium, calcium, magnesium, reducing substances, mucoproteins, vitamins, and hormones.

In the presence of disease, urine may contain protein, glucose, ketone bodies, hemoglobin, lipids, bacteria, pus, urobilinogen, or calculi. Microscopic examination of centrifuged urine sediment can detect cells, casts, crystals, bacteria, yeasts and parasites, spermatozoa, or contaminants and artifacts.

Urine volume varies

Urine volume, closely regulated by the kidneys, reflects overall fluid homeostasis. Actual volume depends on fluid intake, the concentration of solutes in the filtrate, cardiac output, hormonal influences, and fluid loss through the lungs, the large bowel, and the skin. In adults, urine volume normally ranges from 800 to 2,000 ml/day, and averages 1,200 to 1,500 ml/day. In children, volume ranges from 300 to 1,500 ml/day; however, a child's urine output is three to four times greater per kilogram of body weight than that of an adult.

Polyuria, urine volume that exceeds 2,000 ml/day, is typical of many abnormal conditions. For example, polyuria is a common effect of osmotic diuresis in diabetes mellitus, hyperparathyroidism, and infections. Polyuria can also result from insufficient secretion of antidiuretic hormone (ADH) as in pituitary diabetes insipidus, or from inability to respond to ADH, as in nephrogenic diabetes insipidus. Urine volume also increases due to a lack of aldosterone, as in Addison's disease, which decreases renal resorption of sodium and water and decreases plasma volume. Polyuria follows the shift of interstitial fluid to plasma after burns or excessive intake or infusion of fluid. It also results from renal diseases in which the kidneys fail to concentrate urine, and from use of diuretics, alcohol, and caffeine.

Oliguria is the excretion of less than 500 ml of urine volume/day; *anuria,* the absence of urine excretion. Oliguria can result from depressed sodium concentration in the filtrate, since sodium normally promotes water excretion. It also follows any condition that decreases plasma volume: for example, when fluid shifts from plasma to the interstitial spaces, as in congestive heart failure; when fluid intake decreases; and when excess fluid escapes through extrarenal routes. Falling plasma volume and oliguria can follow dehydration due to prolonged vomiting, diarrhea, or profuse diaphoresis. Oliguria may occur with transfusion reactions, acute glomerulonephritis or pyelonephritis, and terminal chronic nephritis; these conditions can impair renal plasma flow and nephron function.

Anuria can follow oliguria in shock. It can follow acute tubular necrosis caused by exposure to toxic agents, such as mercury bichloride, sulfonamides, and carbon tetrachloride, and can also result from obstruction in bilateral hydronephrosis.

Nocturia, urine volume greater than 500 ml at night, with a specific gravity of less than 1.018, is characteristic of chronic glomerulonephritis, or of heart or liver failure.

Clearance principle

Abnormal findings from routine urinalysis suggest renal disease or dysfunction, but tests for filtration, reabsorption, and secretion permit more precise evaluation. Clearance, the volume of plasma that can be cleared of a substance per unit of time, is the principle used to assess urine-forming mechanisms; it's also a measure of renal plasma flow, which, if diminished, impairs renal function.

Clearance depends on how efficiently the renal tubular cells handle the substance that has been filtered by the glomerulus. If the tubules don't reabsorb or secrete the substance, clearance equals the glomerular filtration rate (GFR). If the tubules reabsorb it, clearance is less than the GFR. If the tubules secrete it, clearance is greater than the GFR. If the tubules reabsorb and secrete the substance, clearance is less than, equal to, or greater than the GFR.

DRUGS THAT INFLUENCE ROUTINE URINALYSIS RESULTS

DRUGS THAT CHANGE URINE COLOR:

Alcohol (light, due to diuresis)
Chlorpromazine hydrochloride (dark)
Chlorzoxazone (orange to purple-red)
Deferoxamine mesylate (red)
Fluorescein sodium I.V. (yellow-orange)
Furazolidone (brown)
Iron salts (black)
Levodopa (dark)
Metronidazole (dark)
Methylene blue (blue-green)
Nitrofurantoin (brown)
Oral anticoagulants, indandione derivatives (orange)
Phenazopyridine (orange-red, orange-brown, or red)
Phenolphthalein (red to purple-red)
Phenolsulfonphthalein (pink or red)
Quinacrine (deep yellow)
Riboflavin (yellow)
Rifampin (red-orange)
Sulfasalazine (orange-yellow)
Sulfobromophthalein (red)

DRUGS THAT CAUSE URINE ODOR:

Antibiotics
Paraldehyde
Vitamins

DRUGS THAT INCREASE SPECIFIC GRAVITY:

Albumin
Dextran
Glucose
Radiopaque contrast media

DRUGS THAT DECREASE pH:

Ammonium chloride
Ascorbic acid

pH (continued)

Diazoxide
Methenamine
Metolazone

DRUGS THAT INCREASE pH:

Acetazolamide
Amphotericin B
Mafenide
Sodium bicarbonate
Potassium citrate

DRUGS THAT SHOW A FALSE-POSITIVE RESULT FOR PROTEINURIA:

Acetazolamide (Combistix or Labstix)
Aminosalicylic acid (sulfosalicylic acid or Extons method)
Cephalothin in large doses (sulfosalicylic acid method)
Nafcillin (sulfosalicylic acid method)
Sodium bicarbonate (all methods)
Tolbutamide (sulfosalicylic acid method)
Tolmetin (sulfosalicylic acid method)

DRUGS THAT CAUSE TRUE PROTEINURIA:

Amikacin
Amphotericin B
Bacitracin
Gentamicin
Gold preparations
Kanamycin
Neomycin
Netilmicin
Phenylbutazone
Polymyxin B
Streptomycin
Tobramycin
Trimethadione

DRUGS THAT CAN CAUSE EITHER TRUE PROTEINURIA OR FALSE-POSITIVE RESULTS:

Penicillin in large doses

PROTEINURIA (continued)

(except with Ames Reagent Strips); however, some penicillins cause true proteinuria.
Sulfonamides (sulfosalicylic acid method)

DRUGS THAT CAUSE FALSE-POSITIVE GLYCOSURIA:

Aminosalicylic acid (Benedict's test)
Ascorbic acid (Clinistix, Diastix, or Tes-Tape)
Ascorbic acid in large doses (Clinitest tablets)
Cephalosporins (Clinitest tablets)
Chloral hydrate (Benedict's test)
Chloramphenicol (Benedict's test or Clinitest tablets)
Isoniazid (Benedict's test)
Levodopa (Clinistix, Diastix, or Tes-Tape)
Levodopa in large doses (Clinitest tablets)
Methyldopa (Tes-Tape)
Nalidixic acid (Benedict's test or Clinitest tablets)
Nitrofurantoin (Benedict's test)
Penicillin G in large doses (Benedict's test)
Phenazopyridine (Clinistix, Diastix, or Tes-Tape)
Probenecid (Benedict's test or Clinitest tablets)
Salicylates in large doses (Clinitest tablets, Clinistix, Diastix, or Tes-Tape)
Streptomycin (Benedict's test)
Tetracycline (Clinistix, Diastix, Tes-Tape)
Tetracyclines, due to ascorbic acid buffer (Benedict's test or Clinitest tablets)

DRUGS THAT CAUSE TRUE GLYCOSURIA:

Ammonium chloride
Asparaginase

DRUGS THAT INFLUENCE ROUTINE URINALYSIS RESULTS (continued)

GLYCOSURIA (continued)
Carbamazepine
Corticosteroids
Dextrothyroxine
Lithium carbonate
Nicotinic acid (large doses)
Phenothiazines (long-term)
Thiazide diuretics

DRUGS THAT INCREASE WBC:

Allopurinol
Ampicillin
Aspirin toxicity
Kanamycin
Methicillin

DRUGS THAT CAUSE HEMATURIA:

Amphotericin B
Coumarin derivatives
Methenamine in large doses
Methicillin
Para-aminosalicylic acid
Phenylbutazone
Sulfonamides

DRUGS THAT CAUSE FALSE-POSITIVE RESULTS FOR KETONURIA:

Levodopa (Ketostix or Lab-stix)
Phenazopyridine (Ketostix or Gerhardt's reagent strip shows atypical color)
Phenolsulfonphthalein (Rothera's test)
Phenothiazines (Gerhardt's reagent strip shows atypical color)
Salicylates (testing with Gerhardt's reagent strip shows reddish color)
Sulfobromophthalein (Bili-Labstix)

DRUGS THAT CAUSE TRUE KETONURIA:

Ether—anesthesia
Isoniazid—intoxication
Isopropyl alcohol—intoxication
Insulin—excessive doses

DRUGS THAT CAUSE CASTS:

Amphotericin B
Aspirin toxicity
Bacitracin
Ethacrynic acid
Furosemide
Gentamicin
Griseofulvin
Isoniazid
Kanamycin
Neomycin
Penicillin
Radiographic agents
Streptomycin
Sulfonamides

DRUGS THAT CAUSE CRYSTALS (IF URINE IS ACIDIC):

Acetazolamide
Aminosalicylic acid
Ascorbic acid
Nitrofurantoin
Theophylline
Thiazide diuretics

The clearance tests described in this chapter determine excretion of exogenous substances infused into the blood, including inulin, para-aminohippuric acid (PAH), and phenolsulfonphthalein (PSP). Inulin clearance measures the GFR; PAH and PSP excretion measure tubular secretion and renal plasma flow. Urine concentration and dilution tests, and the test for tubular reabsorption of phosphate assess tubular function.

ELAINE GILLIGAN WHELAN, RN, BS, MA

PHYSICAL AND CHEMICAL TESTS

Routine Urinalysis

Routine urinalysis is an important, commonly used screening test for urinary and systemic pathologies. Normal urine findings suggest the absence of major disease, while abnormal findings suggest its presence and mandate further urine or blood tests to identify a specific disorder. The elements of routine urinalysis include the evaluation of physical characteristics (color, odor, and opacity); the determination of specific gravity and pH; the detection and rough measurement of protein, glucose, and ketone bodies; and the examination of sediment for red and white blood cells, casts, and crystals.

Laboratory methods for detecting or measuring these elements include visual

NORMAL FINDINGS IN ROUTINE URINALYSIS

	ELEMENT	FINDINGS
MACROSCOPIC	Color	Straw
	Odor	Slightly aromatic
	Appearance	Clear
	Specific gravity	1.005 to 1.020
	pH	4.5 to 8.0
	Protein	None
	Glucose	None
	Ketones	None
	Other sugars	None
	ELEMENT	FINDINGS
MICROSCOPIC	RBCs	0 to 3/high-power field
	WBCs	0 to 4/high-power field
	Epithelial cells	Few
	Casts	None, except occasional hyaline casts
	Crystals	Present
	Yeast cells	None
	Parasites	None

examination for appearance; reagent strip screening for pH, protein, glucose, and ketone bodies; refractometry for specific gravity; and microscopic inspection of centrifuged sediment for cells, casts, and crystals.

Purpose
□ To screen for renal or urinary tract disease
□ To help detect metabolic or systemic disease unrelated to renal disorders.

Patient preparation
Explain to the patient that this test aids diagnosis of renal or urinary tract disease and helps evaluate overall body function. Advise him he needn't restrict food or fluids before the test. Tell him the test requires a urine specimen. Check the history for recent ingestion of medications that may affect test results.

Procedure
Collect a random urine specimen of at least 15 ml. If possible, obtain a first-voided morning specimen, since this contains the greatest concentration of solutes.

Precautions
□ If the patient is being evaluated for renal colic, strain the specimen to catch stones or stone fragments. Place an unfolded 4″ x 4″ gauze pad or a fine-mesh sieve over the specimen container, and carefully pour the urine through the gauze or sieve.
□ Send the specimen to the laboratory immediately, or refrigerate it if analysis will be delayed longer than 1 hour.

Values
The chart above lists normal findings for elements of a routine urinalysis.

Implications of results

Nonpathologic variations in these values may result from diet, nonpathologic conditions, specimen collection time, and other factors. For example, specific gravity influences urine color and odor: as specific gravity increases, urine becomes darker and its odor becomes stronger; as specific gravity decreases, urine lightens. Specific gravity is highest in the first-voided morning specimen.

Urine pH, which is greatly affected by diet and medications, influences the appearance of urine and the composition of crystals. An alkaline pH (above 7.0)—characteristic of a diet high in vegetables, citrus fruits, and dairy products but low in meat—causes turbidity, and formation of phosphate, carbonate, and amorphous crystals. An acid pH (below 7.0)—typical of a high-protein diet—produces turbidity, and formation of oxalate, cystine, amorphous urate, and uric acid crystals.

Although protein is normally absent from the urine, it can appear in urine in a benign condition known as orthostatic (postural) proteinuria. This condition is most common during the second decade of life, is intermittent, appears after prolonged standing, and disappears after recumbency.

Transient benign proteinuria can also occur with fever, exposure to cold, emotional stress, or strenuous exercise. Sugars, also usually absent from the urine, may appear under normal conditions. The most common sugar in urine is glucose. Transient, nonpathologic glycosuria may result from emotional stress or pregnancy and may follow ingestion of a high-carbohydrate meal. Other sugars—fructose, lactose, and pentose—rarely appear in urine under nonpathologic conditions. (Lactosuria, however, can occur during pregnancy and lactation.)

The three important elements present in centrifuged urine sediment are cells, casts, and crystals. Red cells don't commonly appear in urine without pathologic significance, but hematuria may occasionally follow strenuous exercise.

The following abnormal findings generally suggest pathologic conditions.

□ *Color:* Changes in color can result from diet, drugs, and many metabolic, inflammatory, or infectious diseases.

□ *Odor:* In diabetes mellitus, starvation, and dehydration, a fruity odor accompanies formation of ketone bodies. In urinary tract infection, a fetid odor is common, especially if *Escherichia coli* is present. Maple syrup urine disease and phenylketonuria also cause distinctive odors.

□ *Turbidity:* Turbid urine may contain red or white cells, bacteria, fat, or chyle, and may reflect renal infection.

□ *Specific gravity:* Low specific gravity (< 1.005) is characteristic of diabetes insipidus, nephrogenic diabetes insipidus, acute tubular necrosis, and pyelonephritis. Fixed specific gravity, in which values remain 1.010 regardless of fluid intake, occurs in chronic glomerulonephritis with severe renal damage. High specific gravity (> 1.020) occurs in nephrotic syndrome, dehydration, acute glomerulonephritis, congestive heart failure, liver failure, and shock.

□ *pH:* Alkaline urine pH may result from Fanconi's syndrome, urinary tract infection, and metabolic or respiratory alkalosis. Acid urine pH is associated with renal tuberculosis, pyrexia, phenylketonuria and alkaptonuria, and all forms of acidosis.

□ *Protein:* Proteinuria suggests renal diseases, such as nephrosis, glomerulosclerosis, glomerulonephritis, nephrolithiasis, polycystic kidney disease, and renal failure. Proteinuria can also result from multiple myeloma.

□ *Sugars:* Glycosuria usually indicates diabetes mellitus but may also result from pheochromocytoma, Cushing's syndrome, and increased intracranial pressure. Fructosuria, galactosuria, and pentosuria generally suggest rare hereditary metabolic disorders. However, an alimentary form of pentosuria and fructosuria may follow excessive ingestion of pentose or fructose, resulting in hepatic failure to metabolize the sugar. Since the renal tubules fail to reabsorb pentose or

URINE CYTOLOGY

Epithelial cells line the urinary tract and exfoliate easily into the urine. So a simple cytologic examination of these cells can aid diagnosis of urinary tract disease. Although urine cytology is not done routinely, it's particularly useful for detecting cancer and inflammatory diseases of the renal pelvis, ureters, bladder, and urethra. In fact, it's especially useful for detecting bladder cancer in high-risk groups, such as smokers, people who work with aniline dyes, and patients who have received treatment for bladder cancer. Urine cytology can also determine whether bladder lesions that appear on X-rays are benign or malignant. This test can also detect cytomegalovirus infection and other viral diseases.

To perform the test, the patient must collect a 100 to 300 ml clean-catch urine specimen 3 hours after his last voiding. (He should not use the first-voided specimen of the morning.) Then the urine specimen is sent to the cytology laboratory immediately so that it can be examined before the cells begin to degenerate.

The specimen is prepared in one of the following ways and stained with Papanicolaou stain:

• *Centrifuge:* After the urine is spun down, the sediment is smeared on a glass slide and stained for examination.

• *Filter:* Urine is poured through a filter, which traps the cells so that they can be stained and examined directly.

• *Cytocentrifuge:* After the urine is centrifuged, the sediment is resuspended and placed on slides, which are spun in a cytocentrifuge and stained for examination.

Normal urine is relatively free of cellular debris, but should have some epithelial and squamous cells that appear normal under a microscope. Identification of malignant cells or any other signs of malignancy may indicate cancer of the kidney, renal pelvis, ureters, bladder, or urethra. It could also indicate a metastatic tumor. An overgrowth of epithelial cells, an excess of red blood cells, or the presence of leukocytes or atypical cells may indicate a lower urinary tract inflammation, which can result from prostatic hyperplasia, urinary calculi, bladder diverticula, strictures, or malformations. Large intranuclear inclusions may indicate a cytomegalovirus infection, which usually affects the renal tubular epithelium. This viral infection generally occurs in cancer patients undergoing chemotherapy and transplant patients receiving immunosupressive drugs. Cytoplasmic inclusion bodies may also indicate measles and may precede the characteristic Koplick's spots.

ELLEN SHIPES, RN, MN, ET, MEd

fructose, these sugars spill over into the urine.

□ *Ketones:* Ketonuria occurs in diabetes mellitus when cellular energy needs exceed available cellular glucose. In the absence of glucose, cells metabolize fat, an alternate energy supply. Ketone bodies—the end products of incomplete fat metabolism—accumulate in plasma and are excreted in the urine. Ketonuria may also occur in starvation states and in conditions of acutely increased metabolic demand associated with decreased food intake, such as diarrhea or vomiting.

□ *Cells:* Hematuria indicates bleeding within the genitourinary tract and may result from infection, obstruction, inflammation, trauma, tumors, glomerulonephritis, renal hypertension, lupus nephritis, renal tuberculosis, renal vein thrombosis, hydronephrosis, pyelone-

phritis, scurvy, malaria, parasitic infection of the bladder, subacute bacterial endocarditis, polyarteritis nodosa, and hemorrhagic disorders. Numerous white cells in urine usually imply urinary tract inflammation, especially cystitis or pyelonephritis. White cells and white cell casts in urine suggest renal infection. An excessive number of epithelial cells suggests renal tubular degeneration.

□ *Casts* (plugs of gelled proteinaceous material [high–molecular-weight mucoprotein]): Casts form in the renal tubules and collecting ducts by agglutination of protein cells or cellular debris, and are flushed loose by urine flow. Excessive numbers of casts indicate renal disease. Hyaline casts are associated with renal parenchymal disease, inflammation, and trauma to the glomerular capillary membrane; epithelial casts, with renal tubular damage, nephrosis, eclampsia, amyloidosis, and heavy metal poisoning; coarse and fine granular casts, with acute or chronic renal failure, pyelonephritis, and chronic lead intoxication; fatty and waxy casts, with nephrotic syndrome, chronic renal disease, and diabetes mellitus; RBC casts, with renal parenchymal disease (especially glomerulonephritis), renal infarction, subacute bacterial endocarditis, vascular disorders, sickle cell anemia, scurvy, blood dyscrasias, malignant hypertension, collagen disease, and acute inflammation; and WBC casts, with acute pyelonephritis and glomerulonephritis, nephrotic syndrome, pyogenic infection, and lupus nephritis.

□ *Crystals:* Some crystals normally appear in urine, but numerous calcium oxalate crystals suggest hypercalcemia. Cystine crystals (cystinuria) reflect an inborn error of metabolism.

□ *Other components:* Yeast cells and parasites in urinary sediment reflect genitourinary tract infection, as well as contamination of external genitalia. Yeast cells, which may be mistaken for red cells, can be identified by their ovoid shape, lack of color, variable size, and frequently, signs of budding. The most common parasite in sediment is *Trichomonas vaginalis,* a flagellated protozoan that commonly causes vaginitis, urethritis, and prostatovesiculitis.

Post-test care
None.

Interfering factors
□ Failure to follow proper collection procedure, to send the specimen to the laboratory immediately, or to refrigerate the specimen may interfere with accurate determination of test results.
□ Strenuous exercise before routine urinalysis may cause transient myoglobinuria, producing misleading results and inaccurate diagnosis.
□ Many drugs can influence the results of this test. (See chart on pages 356 and 357 for a list of such drugs and their effect on routine urinalysis.)
ELAINE GILLIGAN WHELAN, RNC, BS, MSN

Urinary Calculi
[Urinary stones]

Urinary calculi are insoluble substances—most commonly formed of the mineral salts calcium oxalate, calcium phosphate, magnesium ammonium phosphate, urate, or cystine—that may appear anywhere in the urinary tract. They range in size from microscopic to several centimeters. Calculi usually possess well-defined nuclei composed of bacteria, fibrin, blood clots, or epithelial cells, enclosed in a protein matrix. Mineral salts accumulate around this matrix in layers, causing progressive enlargement.

Formation of calculi can result from reduced urinary volume, increased excretion of mineral salts, urinary stasis, pH changes, and decreased protective substances. Calculi commonly form in the kidney, pass into the ureter, and are excreted in the urine. Since not all calculi pass spontaneously, they may require surgical extraction. Calculi don't always cause symptoms; but when they do, hematuria is most common. If calculi obstruct the ureter, they may cause severe flank pain, dysuria, and urinary retention, frequency, and urgency.

To test for urinary calculi, the patient must have all his urine carefully strained to remove any calculi. Qualitative chemical analysis then reveals their composition to help identify their causes.

Purpose
□ To detect and identify calculi in the urine.

Patient preparation
Explain to the patient that this test detects urinary stones, and that, if such stones are found, laboratory analysis will reveal their composition. Tell him the test requires that his urine be collected and strained. Advise him that he need not

CAUSES AND INCIDENCE OF CALCULI

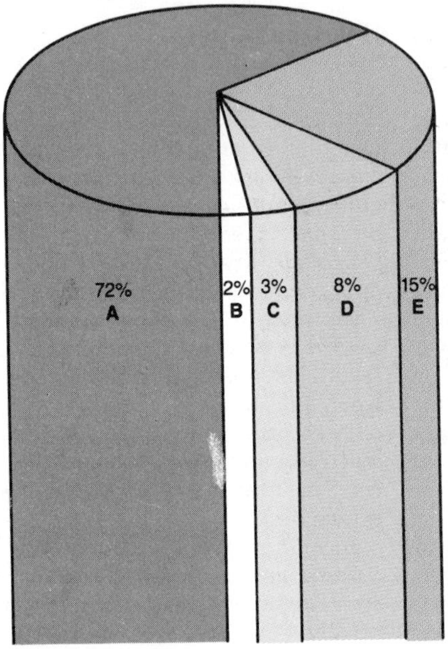

A
Calcium oxalate calculi usually result from idiopathic hypercalciuria, a condition that reflects absorption of calcium from the bowel.

B
Calcium phosphate calculi usually result from primary hyperparathyroidism, which causes excessive resorption of calcium from bone.

C
Cystine calculi result from primary cystinuria, an inborn error of metabolism that prevents renal tubular reabsorption of cystine.

D
Urate calculi result from gout, dehydration (causing elevated uric acid levels), acidic urine (pH 5.0), or hepatic dysfunction.

E
Magnesium ammonium phosphate calculi result from the presence of urea-splitting organisms, such as *Proteus*, which raises ammonia concentration and makes urine alkaline.

72% A   2% B   3% C   8% D   15% E

restrict food or fluids before the test. Reassure him that symptoms will subside immediately after excretion of any stones. Administer medication to control pain, as ordered.

Equipment
Strainer (an unfolded 4" x 4" dressing or a fine-mesh sieve)/specimen container.

Procedure
After the patient voids into the strainer, inspect the strainer carefully, since calculi may be minute. Calculi may look like gravel or sand. Document the appearance of the calculi and the number, if possible. Then, place the calculi in a properly labeled container, and send the container to the laboratory immediately for prompt analysis.

Precautions
If patient has received analgesics, be sure to keep the strainer and urinal or bedpan within his reach, as he may be drowsy and unable to get out of bed to void.

Findings
Normally, calculi are not present in the urine.

Implications of results
More than half of all calculi in urine are of mixed composition, containing two or more mineral salts; calcium oxalate is the most common component. Determination of the composition of calculi helps identify various metabolic disorders (see chart above).

Post-test care
□ Observe for severe flank pain, dysuria, and urinary retention, frequency, or urgency. Hematuria should subside.
□ Inform the patient of dietary limits, to prevent formation of calculi.

Interfering factors
None.

MALINDA S. MITCHELL, RN, MS

Inulin Clearance

Inulin, a polysaccharide of fructose obtained from dahlias and artichokes, is metabolically inert within the body. When injected I.V., inulin is almost entirely filtered by the glomeruli but is reabsorbed by the tubules. Inulin clearance is, therefore, practically an exact measure of the glomerular filtration rate (GFR).

Despite its sensitivity and low incidence of side effects, the inulin clearance test is time-consuming, complex, and uncomfortable for the patient, and thus is infrequently performed. Less accurate tests, such as urea and creatinine clearance, are used instead. Iothalamate ^{125}I can be substituted for inulin and usually follows the same procedure as inulin clearance. Because the iodine content is negligible, ^{125}I can be given to patients with iodine hypersensitivity but is contraindicated during pregnancy, lactation, and periods of growth.

Purpose
☐ To measure GFR
☐ To evaluate renal function.

Patient preparation
Explain to the patient that this test evaluates kidney function. Instruct him to fast for 4 hours before the test, to abstain from exercise the morning of the test, and to drink 1 liter of water 1 hour before the test. Encourage liquids during the test to maintain adequate urine flow. Tell him who will perform the test, that five blood samples and five urine specimens are required, and that he will receive an I.V. infusion of inulin, with a doctor in attendance. Reassure him that although he may experience transient discomfort from the venipunctures, collecting each sample takes less than 3 minutes. Advise him that he may feel bloated or have the urge to void during urine collection,

since a catheter will be in place for 2 hours.

Equipment
25 ml of 10% inulin and 500 ml of 1.5% inulin/five 10 ml *green-top* (heparinized) tubes/equipment for venipuncture/equipment for Foley catheterization/clamp/five urine specimen containers/I.V. pump/I.V. solution (250 ml of 5% dextrose in water/I.V. tubing with a Y-port.

Procedure
Perform a venipuncture, and collect 10 ml of blood in a *green-top* (heparinized) tube, to be used as a control sample. Then, catheterize the patient. Make sure the bladder is empty, and save the urine for a baseline specimen.

Infuse the recommended priming dose of 25 ml of 10% inulin by I.V. bolus over 4 minutes. Allow 30 minutes for distribution. Then, using an I.V. pump, infuse the maintenance solution of 500 ml of 1.5% inulin at a constant rate of 4 ml/minute. Tell the patient not to exert pressure on the arm with the I.V. site or to touch the control, and to notify you if he feels a burning sensation.

Collect a urine specimen 30 minutes after starting the I.V., and three additional specimens at 20-minute intervals thereafter. Clamp the catheter between collections. Draw a blood sample at the midpoint of each 20-minute period and at the end of the test.

Record the inulin dosage on the laboratory slip. Properly label each specimen, and include the collection time.

Precautions
☐ Inulin clearance should be used cautiously in patients with cardiac disease, since increased fluid intake may cause congestive heart failure.
☐ Use the solution for I.V. bolus within 1 hour of preparation. Before administration, shake the ampul and heat it in

boiling water to dissolve all crystals. Then, cool to body temperature.

□ If the patient already has a catheter in place, don't use the urine in the drainage bag. Empty the bag, and clamp the catheter for 1 hour before obtaining a baseline specimen.

□ Handle blood samples gently to prevent hemolysis, and send specimens to the laboratory immediately after each collection. If more than 10 minutes will elapse before transport, refrigerate the urine specimen.

Values

Inulin clearance is normally 90 to 130 ml/minute for age 21 and older; 86 to 126 ml/minute for ages 11 to 20; and 82 to 122 ml/minute from birth to age 10. Clearance may decrease as much as 45% after age 70.

Implications of results

Depressed clearance is characteristic in congestive heart failure, decreased renal blood flow, acute tubular necrosis, acute and chronic glomerulonephritis, advanced chronic bilateral pyelonephritis, nephrosclerosis, advanced bilateral renal lesions, bilateral ureteral obstruction, and dehydration.

Post-test care

□ If a hematoma develops at the venipuncture site, apply warm soaks. If phlebitis develops at the I.V. site, elevate the arm, and apply warm soaks.

□ Be sure the patient voids within 8 to 10 hours after the catheter is removed.

□ As ordered, resume diet and activity restricted before the test.

Interfering factors

□ Failure to infuse inulin at a constant rate, to collect blood and urine specimens at the proper intervals, or to adhere to dietary and exercise restrictions may interfere with accurate determination of test results.

□ Hemolysis caused by rough handling of the blood samples may influence test results.

MALINDA S. MITCHELL, RN, MS

Para-aminohippuric Acid Excretion

When plasma para-aminohippuric acid (PAH) levels are maintained at 10 to 20 mcg/ml by I.V. infusion, the kidneys clear almost all PAH in one passage through the kidneys by glomerular filtration and by tubular secretion. However, since a small fraction of this flow normally fails to perfuse the proximal tubules and a corresponding fraction of PAH fails to be excreted, PAH clearance merely approximates the actual renal plasma flow. Consequently, PAH excretion measures the effective renal plasma flow (ERPF) and is indicated for patients in whom impaired renal function is suspected. Because this test is technically complex and is uncomfortable for the patient, it is infrequently used.

Purpose

□ To evaluate renal function by determining the effective renal plasma flow (ERPF).

Patient preparation

Explain to the patient that this test evaluates kidney function. Instruct him to fast for at least 4 hours before the test, if ordered, and to abstain from exercise the morning of the test. Tell him who will perform the test, that it takes about 2 hours to perform, and that it requires frequent collection of blood and urine specimens and an I.V. infusion. Reassure him that although he may experience transient discomfort from the needle puncture and the pressure of the tourniquet, collecting each sample takes less than 3 minutes. Inform him that he may feel bloated or have the urge to void during urine collection, since a catheter will be in place for 2 hours; however, he won't experience pain. Mention that he may feel a cool sensation in his arm during I.V. infusion.

Withhold drugs that affect test results, as ordered. Encourage fluid intake before and during the test to maintain adequate urine flow.

Tell the patient to watch for and report possible side effects of PAH administration—nausea, vomiting, cramping, vasomotor disturbances, and flushing.

Equipment
25 ml of 10% PAH and 500 ml of 1.5% PAH/five 10 ml *green-top* (heparinized) tubes/equipment for Foley catheterization/clamp/five urine specimen containers/equipment for venipuncture/I.V. pump/I.V. solution (250 ml of 5% dextrose in water)/I.V. tubing with Y-port.

Procedure
Perform a venipuncture, and collect 10 ml of blood in a *green-top* (heparinized) tube, to be used as a baseline sample. Then, catheterize the patient. Make sure the bladder is empty, and save the urine for a baseline specimen.

Infuse the recommended priming dose of 25 ml of 10% PAH by I.V. bolus over 4 minutes, allowing 30 minutes for distribution. Then, using an I.V. pump, infuse the maintenance solution of 500 ml of 1.5% PAH at a constant rate of 4 ml/minute. Tell the patient not to exert pressure on the arm with the I.V. site or to touch the control, and to notify you if he feels a burning sensation.

Collect a urine specimen 30 minutes after the I.V. is started and three additional specimens at 20-minute intervals thereafter. Clamp the catheter between collections. Draw a blood sample at the midpoint of each 20-minute period and at the end of the test.

Record the PAH dosage on the laboratory slip. Properly label each specimen, and include the collection time.

Precautions
□ This test is used cautiously in patients with cardiac dysfunction, since the increased blood volume accompanying enforced hydration and PAH infusion may precipitate congestive heart failure.
□ If the patient already has a catheter

in place, don't use the urine in the drainage bag. Empty the bag, and clamp the catheter for 1 hour before obtaining a baseline specimen.
□ Administer the priming dose of PAH slowly and cautiously, observing the patient closely for adverse reactions. Be sure to record the amount of PAH administered. Wrap the I.V. bottle of maintenance solution in foil, to protect it from light.
□ Handle blood samples gently to prevent hemolysis, and send all specimens to the laboratory immediately. If more than 10 minutes will elapse before transport, refrigerate the urine specimen.

Values
PAH excretion, or ERPF, is normally 400 to 700 ml/minute at age 20; excretion decreases 17 ml/minute each decade thereafter.

Implications of results
Depressed PAH excretion is characteristic of decreased cardiac output or arterial blood pressure, organic disease of the renal vascular system, increased resistance to blood flow resulting from early essential hypertension or systemic arterial hypotension, and diminished functional renal tissue.

Post-test care
□ Continue to observe the patient for adverse reactions to PAH.
□ If a hematoma develops at the venipuncture site, apply warm soaks. If phlebitis develops at the I.V. site, elevate the arm, and apply warm soaks.
□ Be sure the patient voids within 8 to 10 hours after the catheter is removed.
□ As ordered, resume medications, diet, and activity discontinued before the test.

Interfering factors
□ Pyrogenic agents or a high-protein diet can increase PAH excretion; diuretics, penicillin, phenolsulfonphthalein, probenecid, and salicylates can depress excretion; procaine and sulfonamides interfere with the laboratory methodology.

□ Failure to infuse PAH at a constant rate, to collect blood and urine specimens at the proper intervals, or to adhere to dietary and exercise restrictions may interfere with accurate determination of test results.

□ Hemolysis caused by rough handling of the blood samples may influence test results.

MALINDA S. MITCHELL, RN, MS

Phenolsulfonphthalein Excretion

Although the phenolsulfonphthalein (PSP) excretion test is less accurate than the para-aminohippuric acid excretion test or the inulin clearance test, it's a simpler method for evaluating kidney function. This test is indicated in a patient with abnormal results in the urine concentration test, one of the earliest signs of renal dysfunction. When PSP is administered I.V., the kidneys normally clear 70% of the dose in one passage, primarily by proximal tubular excretion. Glomerular filtration removes 5%, and the liver removes an additional 10% to 20%. The PSP excretion rate, which equals 70% of renal plasma flow, is determined by alkalinizing the urine, diluting the samples to equal volumes, and comparing the results with a normal colorimetric graph.

Purpose
□ To determine renal plasma flow
□ To evaluate tubular function.

Patient preparation
Explain to the patient that this test evaluates kidney function. Inform him he needn't restrict food, and encourage him to take fluids before and during the test, to maintain adequate urine flow. Tell him the test requires an I.V. injection and collection of urine specimens 15 minutes, 30 minutes, 1 hour, and if ordered, 2 hours after the I.V. injection. Inform him who will administer the I.V. injection and when; that he may feel transient discomfort from the needle puncture and the pressure of the tourniquet; and that the dye temporarily turns the urine red. If the patient is unable to void and requires catheterization, tell him that he may have the urge to void when the catheter is in place.

Withhold drugs that affect test results, as ordered. If they must be continued, note this on the laboratory slip.

Equipment
6 mg of PSP dye in 1 ml solution/equipment for Foley catheterization/four urine specimen containers.

Procedure
Instruct the patient to empty his bladder, and discard the urine. Then, the doctor will administer exactly 1 ml of PSP (6 mg of dye) I.V.

Collect a urine specimen at 15 minutes, 30 minutes, 1 hour, and if ordered, 2 hours after the injection. Since 40 ml is required for each specimen, encourage fluid intake. If the patient is catheterized, be sure to clamp the catheter between collections.

Record the PSP dosage on the laboratory slip. Properly label each specimen, and include the collection time.

Precautions
□ This test should be used cautiously in a patient with cardiac dysfunction or renal insufficiency, since the increased fluid intake necessary for proper hydration may precipitate congestive heart failure.

□ Keep epinephrine available, since allergic reactions to PSP develop occasionally.

□ If the patient already has a catheter in place, don't use the urine in the drainage bag. Empty the bag, and clamp the catheter for 1 hour before the test.

□ Send specimens to the laboratory immediately after each collection. If more than 10 minutes will elapse before transport, refrigerate the specimen.

Values

Normally, 25% of the PSP dose is excreted in 15 minutes; 50% to 60% in 30 minutes; 60% to 70% in 1 hour; and 70% to 80% in 2 hours. Normal excretion for children (excluding infants) is 5% to 10% higher than for adults.

Implications of results

The 15-minute value is the most sensitive indicator of both tubular function and renal plasma flow, since depressed excretion at this interval but normal excretion at later ones suggests relatively mild or early-stage bilateral renal disease. However, a depressed 2-hour value may reveal moderate-to-severe renal impairment. Depressed PSP excretion is also characteristic in renal vascular disease, urinary tract obstruction, congestive heart failure, and gout. Elevated PSP excretion is characteristic in hypoalbuminemia, hepatic disease, and multiple myeloma.

Post-test care

☐ If phlebitis develops at the I.V. site, elevate the arm and apply warm soaks.
☐ Be sure the patient voids within 8 to 10 hours after the catheter is removed.
☐ As ordered, resume administration of medications that were discontinued before the test.

Interfering factors

☐ Inexact measurement of PSP dosage may alter test results.
☐ Failure to collect urine specimens at the designated times, the patient's inability to void at specified intervals, or collection of insufficient specimens (less than 40 ml) may alter test results.
☐ Decreased PSP excretion may result from administration of I.V. pyelography radiopaque fluid, or from chlorothiazide, aspirin, phenylbutazone, penicillin, sulfonamides, and probenecid.
☐ Azo dyes and sulfobromophthalein interfere with colorimetric measurement of PSP.
☐ Abnormal drainage sites, such as fistulas, or hematuria may interfere with accurate determination of test results.

MALINDA S. MITCHELL, RN, MS

TUBULAR FUNCTION TESTS

Urine Concentration and Dilution Tests

The kidneys normally concentrate or dilute urine according to fluid intake. When such intake is excessive, the kidneys excrete more water in the urine; when intake is limited, they excrete less. To make such variation possible, the distal segment of the renal tubules varies its permeability to water in response to antidiuretic hormone (ADH), which, with renal blood flow, determines urine concentration or dilution.

This test measures specific gravity or osmolality; it evaluates renal capacity to concentrate urine in response to fluid deprivation, or to dilute it in response to fluid overload. Specific gravity, the ratio of urine mass to an equal volume of water, is usually high in small volumes of output (concentrated urine) and low in large volumes (dilute urine). Osmolality, a more sensitive index of renal function, measures the number of osmotically active ions or particles present per kilogram of water. Osmolality is high in concentrated urine and low in dilute urine. Specific gravity is measured by a urinometer or urine refractometer; osmolality, by the effect of solute particles on the freezing point of a fluid.

Purpose

☐ To evaluate renal tubular function
☐ To detect renal impairment.

Patient preparation

Explain to the patient that this test eval-

DEHYDRATION TEST FOR DIABETES INSIPIDUS

The dehydration test measures urine osmolality, which reflects renal concentrating capacity after a period of dehydration and after subcutaneous injection of the pituitary hormone vasopressin. Comparison of the two osmolalities permits reliable diagnosis of diabetes insipidus, a metabolic disorder characterized by vasopressin (antidiuretic hormone) deficiency. Simply measuring urine osmolality after a period of water deprivation doesn't itself confirm vasopressin deficiency; however, subsequent injection of vasopressin raises urine osmolality beyond normal limits only in patients with diabetes insipidus.

To achieve dehydration, withhold fluids the evening before and the morning of the test. Collect a urine sample at hourly intervals in the morning for osmolality measurement. At noon, or after osmolality increases less than 30 mOsm/kg each hour for 3 consecutive hours, draw a blood sample for osmolality measurement. If serum osmolality exceeds 288 mOsm/kg, the level of adequate dehydration, inject 5 units of vasopressin subcutaneously. Within an hour, collect a urine specimen for osmolality measurement.

Clinical Alert: During dehydration, weigh the patient and monitor vital signs every 2 hours; a 1-kg weight loss normally accompanies adequate dehydration. In a patient with polyuria exceeding 10 liters/day, withhold fluids only the morning of the test; if his weight loss exceeds 2 kg, discontinue the test.

In a patient with normal neurohypophyseal function, urine osmolality after vasopressin injection doesn't rise more than 9% of the maximum dehydration osmolality. A larger increase indicates diabetes insipidus. In a patient with polyuria caused by renal disease, potassium depletion, or nephrogenic diabetes insipidus, urine osmolality increases slightly during dehydration but not at all after vasopressin injection.

fluid the night before the test. Then, instruct the patient to restrict food and fluids for at least 14 hours. (Some concentration tests require that water be withheld for 24 hours but permit relatively normal food intake.) Limit salt intake at the evening meal, to prevent excessive thirst. Emphasize to the patient that his cooperation is necessary to obtain accurate results.

For the dilution test: Generally, this test directly follows the concentration test and necessitates no additional patient preparation. However, if it's performed alone, simply withhold breakfast.

Procedure

Concentration test: Collect urine specimens at 6 a.m., 8 a.m., and 10 a.m.

Dilution test: Instruct the patient to void and discard the urine. Then, give him 1,500 ml of water to drink within 30 minutes. Collect urine specimens every half hour or every hour, as ordered, for 4 hours thereafter.

Precautions

□ Concentration and dilution tests should be used cautiously in patients with advanced renal disease or cardiac dysfunction, because fluid overload can precipitate water intoxication, sodium diuresis, or congestive heart failure.
□ Send each specimen to the laboratory immediately after collection.
□ If the patient is unable to urinate into the specimen containers, provide him with a clean bedpan, urinal, or toilet specimen pan. Rinse the collection device after each use.
□ If the patient is catheterized, empty the drainage bag before the test. Obtain the specimens from the catheter, and clamp the catheter between collections.

Values

Concentration test: Specific gravity ranges from 1.025 to 1.032, and osmolality rises above 800 mOsm/kg of water, in patients with normal renal function.

Dilution test: Normally, specific gravity falls below 1.003 and osmolality below 100 mOsm/kg for at least one

uates kidney function. Tell him the test requires urine specimens, and how many specimens will be collected and when. Instruct him to discard any urine voided during the night.

Withhold diuretics, as ordered.

For the concentration test: Provide a high-protein meal and only 200 ml of

specimen; 80% or more of the ingested water is eliminated in 4 hours. In elderly persons, depressed values can be associated with normal renal function.

Implications of results

Decreased renal capacity to concentrate urine in response to fluid deprivation, or to dilute urine in response to fluid overload, may indicate tubular epithelial damage, decreased renal blood flow, loss of functional nephrons, or pituitary or cardiac dysfunction.

Post-test care

□ After collecting the final specimen, provide a balanced meal or a snack.
□ Be sure the patient voids within 8 to 10 hours after the catheter is removed.

Interfering factors

□ Failure to adhere to dietary and fluid restrictions may interfere with accurate determination of test results.
□ Diuretics increase urine volume and dilution, thereby lowering specific gravity; nephrotoxic drugs cause tubular epithelial damage, thereby decreasing renal concentrating ability.
□ Patients who have been markedly overhydrated for several days before the test may have depressed concentration values; those who are dehydrated or have electrolyte imbalances may retain fluids, leading to inaccurate results.

MALINDA S. MITCHELL, RN, MS

Tubular Reabsorption of Phosphate

Since tubular reabsorption of phosphate is closely regulated by parathyroid hormone (PTH), measuring urine and plasma phosphate, with creatinine clearance, provides an indirect method of evaluating parathyroid function. PTH helps maintain optimum blood levels of ionized calcium and controls renal excretion of calcium and phosphate. Specifically, PTH stimulates reabsorption of calcium and inhibits reabsorption of phosphate from the glomerular filtrate. A regulatory feedback mechanism causes PTH secretion to diminish as ionized calcium levels return to normal. In primary hyperparathyroidism, excessive secretion of PTH disrupts this calcium-phosphate balance.

This test is indicated to detect hyperparathyroidism in persons with clinical signs of this disorder, and borderline or normal values for serum calcium, phosphate, and alkaline phosphatase.

Purpose

□ To evaluate parathyroid function
□ To aid diagnosis of primary hyperparathyroidism
□ To aid differential diagnosis of hypercalcemia.

Patient preparation

Explain to the patient that this test evaluates the function of the parathyroid glands, and requires a blood sample and a 24-hour urine collection. Tell him who will perform the venipuncture and when, and that he may experience transient discomfort from the needle puncture and the pressure of the tourniquet. Reassure him that collecting the blood sample generally takes less than 3 minutes.

Instruct the patient to maintain a normal phosphate diet for 3 days before the test, since low phosphate intake (less than 500 mg/day) may elevate tubular reabsorption values and a high-phosphate diet (3,000 mg/day) may lower them. Common nutritional sources of phosphorus include legumes, nuts, milk, egg yolks, meat, poultry, fish, cereals, and cheese. These foods should be eaten in moderate amounts. Instruct the patient to fast from midnight the night before the test.

As ordered, withhold drugs, such as amphotericin B, chlorothiazide diuretics, furosemide, and gentamicin, that are known to influence test results. If these medications must be continued through-

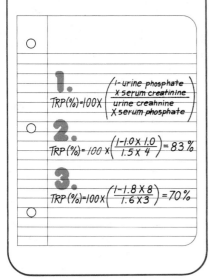

EQUATION FOR TUBULAR REABSORPTION OF PHOSPHATE (TRP)

Using the equation in figure 1, phosphate reabsorption is calculated by comparing creatinine clearance with phosphate clearance. Figure 2 is an example of a normal value for TRP; figure 3 is an example of an abnormal value.

$$TRP(\%) = 100 \times \frac{1 - urine\ phosphate \times serum\ creatinine}{urine\ creatinine \times serum\ phosphate}$$

$$TRP(\%) = 100 \times \left(1 - \frac{1.0 \times 1.0}{1.5 \times 4} \right) = 83\%$$

$$TRP(\%) = 100 \times \left(1 - \frac{1.8 \times 8}{1.6 \times 3} \right) = 70\%$$

out the test period, note this on the laboratory slip.

Procedure

First, perform a venipuncture, and collect the sample in a 10 ml *red-top* tube. Then, instruct the patient to empty his bladder, and discard the urine; record this as time zero. Collect a 24-hour urine specimen. (Occasionally, a 4-hour collection is ordered instead.)

After the venipuncture, allow the patient to eat, and encourage fluid intake to maintain adequate urine flow.

Precautions

□ Handle the collection tube gently to prevent hemolysis, and send it to the laboratory immediately.

□ Keep the urine specimen container refrigerated or on ice during the collection period. Tell the patient to avoid contaminating the specimen with toilet paper or stool.

At the end of the collection period, label the specimen and send it to the laboratory immediately.

Findings

Renal tubules normally reabsorb 80% or more of phosphate.

Implications of results

Reabsorption of less than 74% of phosphate strongly suggests primary hyperparathyroidism, but requires additional studies to confirm primary hyperparathyroidism as the cause of hypercalcemia. Chest and bone X-rays and bone scans should be performed, since bony metastasis is the most common cause of hypercalcemia. Depressed reabsorption occurs in a small number of patients with renal calculi but without parathyroid tumor. However, normal reabsorption occurs in roughly one fifth of patients with parathyroid tumor. Increased reabsorption of phosphate may result from uremia, renal tubular disease, osteomalacia, sarcoidosis, and myeloma.

Post-test care

□ If a hematoma develops at the venipuncture site, apply warm soaks.

□ As ordered, resume administration of medications that were discontinued before the test.

□ The patient may resume his diet.

Interfering factors

□ Hemolysis caused by rough handling of the sample may alter test results.

□ Failure to collect all urine during the test period may interfere with accurate determination of test results.

□ The patient's failure to follow guidelines for diet restrictions and phosphate intake may alter test results.

□ Amphotericin B and chlorothiazide diuretics may diminish reabsorption; furosemide and gentamicin may enhance it.

MALINDA S. MITCHELL, RN, MS

Selected References

Brunner, Lillian S., and Suddarth, Doris S. *Textbook of Medical-Surgical Nursing*, 5th ed. Philadelphia: J.B. Lippincott Co., 1984.

Byrne, C. Judith, et al. *Laboratory Tests: Implications for Nurses and Allied Health Professionals*. Reading, Mass.: Addison-Wesley Publishing Co., 1981.

Cameron, Stewart, et al. *Nephrology for Nurses—A Modern Approach to the Kidney*, 2nd ed. New Hyde Park, N.Y.: Medical Examination Pub. Co., 1977.

Duarte, Cristobal G. *Renal Function Tests*. Boston: Little, Brown & Co., 1980.

Fischbach, Frances. *A Manual of Laboratory Diagnostic Tests*, 2nd ed. Philadelphia: J.B. Lippincott Co., 1984.

French, Ruth M. *Guide to Diagnostic Procedures*. New York: McGraw-Hill Book Co., 1980.

Guyton, Arthur C. *Textbook of Medical Physiology*, 6th ed. Philadelphia: W.B. Saunders Co., 1981.

Hansten, Philip D. *Drug Interactions*, 5th ed. Philadelphia: Lea & Febiger, 1984.

Henry, John Bernard, ed. *Todd-Sanford-Davidsohn Clinical Diagnosis and Management by Laboratory Methods*, vol. 1, 17th ed. Philadelphia: W.B. Saunders Co., 1984.

Kaplan, Alex, and Szabo, LaVerne L. *Clinical Chemistry: Interpretation and Techniques*. Philadelphia: Lea & Febiger, 1979.

Koepke, John A. *Guide to Clinical Laboratory Diagnosis*, 2nd ed. East Norwalk, Conn.: Appleton-Century-Crofts, 1979.

Kozier, Barbara B., and Erb, Glenora L. *Fundamentals of Nursing: Concepts and Procedures*. Reading, Mass.: Addison-Wesley Publishing Co., 1979.

Kunin, Calvin M. *Detection, Prevention and Management of Urinary Tract Infections*, 3rd ed. Philadelphia: Lea & Febiger, 1979.

Luckmann, Joan, and Sorenson, Karen C. *Medical-Surgical Nursing: A Psychophysiologic Approach*, 2nd ed. Philadelphia: W.B. Saunders Co., 1980.

Malasanos, Lois. *Health Assessment*, 2nd ed. St. Louis: C.V. Mosby Co., 1981.

McConnell, Edwina A. "Urinalysis: A Common Test, But Never Routine," *Nursing82* 12:108-11, February 1982.

Petersdorf, Robert G., and Adams, Raymond D., eds. *Harrison's Principles of Internal Medicine*, 10th ed. New York: McGraw-Hill Book Co., 1983.

Price, Sylvia, and Wilson, Lorraine. *Pathophysiology: Clinical Concepts of Disease Processes*, 2nd ed. New York: McGraw-Hill Book Co., 1982.

Ravel, Richard A. *Clinical Laboratory Medicine*, 4th ed. Chicago: Year Book Medical Pubs., 1984.

Smith, Donald R. *General Urology*, 10th ed. Los Altos, Calif.: Lange Medical Publications, 1981.

Tilkian, Sarko M., et al. *Clinical Implications of Laboratory Tests*, 3rd ed. St. Louis: C.V. Mosby Co., 1983.

Wallach, Jacques B. *Interpretation of Diagnostic Tests: A Handbook Synopsis of Laboratory Medicine*, 3rd ed. Boston: Little, Brown & Co., 1978.

Whaley, Lucille F., and Wong, Donna. *Nursing Care of Infants and Children*, 2nd ed. St. Louis: C.V. Mosby Co., 1983.

Widmann, Frances K. *Clinical Interpretation of Laboratory Tests*, 9th ed. Philadelphia: F.A. Davis Co., 1983.

Wood, Lucille A., and Rambo, Beverly J., eds. *Nursing Skills for Allied Health Services*, 2nd ed., vols. 1 and 2. Philadelphia: W.B. Saunders Co., 1980.

13 Urine Enzymes

LEARNING OBJECTIVES

After completing this chapter, the reader will be able to:
- explain the importance of measuring urine enzyme levels.
- define the term *enzyme*.
- discuss the role of cyclic AMP as an intracellular mediator.
- state the purpose of each test discussed in the chapter.
- prepare the patient physically and psychologically for each test.
- describe the procedure for performing each test.
- list conditions that contraindicate the test for cyclic AMP.
- implement appropriate post-test care.
- state the normal values for each test.
- discuss the implications of abnormal test results.
- list factors that may interfere with accurate test results.

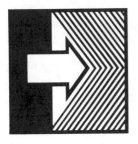

Urine
Enzymes

Introduction

Enzymes are protein molecules that promote chemical reactions in the body without being themselves destroyed or permanently changed. They're present in all body tissues and fluids: tears, saliva, sweat, blood, urine, and digestive juices. Because enzyme actions are quite specific to tissue sites, deviations from normal enzyme levels often can identify and locate tissue damage or disease; cellular damage or necrosis is likely to cause the release of a large aggregation of enzymes into the blood. When such enzymes saturate the serum, they exceed the renal threshold, and a significant quantity spills over into the urine.

Because enzymes that circulate in the blood are normally reabsorbed by the renal tubules, with only small amounts excreted in the urine, increased enzyme concentration in the urine may also signal renal dysfunction, especially impaired tubular reabsorption.

Since elevated urine levels may persist longer than serum levels (for example, of amylase), urine enzyme measurements can provide delayed or retrospective diagnosis. Such measurements also help monitor the progression of illness or the effectiveness of treatment in patients with confirmed diseases.

Urine amylase, the most frequently requested urine enzyme test, can confirm acute pancreatitis and can aid diagnosis of chronic pancreatitis and

salivary gland disorders. Arylsulfatase A, a rarely requested test, aids diagnosis of colorectal or bladder cancer, myeloid leukemia, and metachromatic leukodystrophy. Lysozyme, another rarely requested test, evaluates renal function, helps detect rejection or infarction of kidney transplants, and aids diagnosis of acute monocytic and granulocytic leukemia. (Serum measurements are probably more useful in tracking the levels of lysozyme and some other enzymes.) Cyclic adenosine monophosphate, another enzyme detectable in urine, is measured after injection of parathyroid hormone to aid differential diagnosis of pseudohypoparathyroidism.

Because enzymes are especially affected by pH, specific gravity, and bacteria, reliable enzyme measurement requires certain precautions during urine collection. Such testing requires an uncontaminated timed urine specimen and an adequate patient intake of fluid. For a valid specimen, the collection container must contain the proper preservative, if one is designated by the laboratory, to maintain the required pH. Finally, the specimen must be refrigerated or packed in ice throughout the collection period to inhibit bacterial growth. Failure to meet any of these requirements in preparing the specimen may invalidate the test results.

DEBORAH L. DALRYMPLE, RN, BSN

GENERAL TESTS

Urine Amylase

Amylase is a starch-splitting enzyme produced primarily in the pancreas and salivary glands, usually secreted into the alimentary tract, and absorbed into the blood; small amounts of amylase are also absorbed into the blood directly from these organs. Following glomerular filtration, amylase is excreted in the urine. In the presence of adequate renal function, serum and urine levels usually rise in tandem. However, within 2 or 3 days of onset of acute pancreatitis, serum amylase levels fall to normal, but elevated urine amylase persists for 7 to 10 days. One method for determining urine amylase levels is the dye-coupled starch method.

Purpose
☐ To diagnose acute pancreatitis when serum amylase levels are normal or borderline
☐ To aid diagnosis of chronic pancreatitis and salivary gland disorders.

Patient preparation
Explain to the patient that this test evaluates the function of the pancreas and the salivary glands. Inform him he needn't restrict food or fluids. Tell him the test requires urine collection for 2, 6, 8, or

SERUM AND URINE AMYLASE VALUES IN ACUTE PANCREATITIS		
	SERUM	**URINE**
Normal	• 138 to 404 amylase units/liter (Mayo Clinic)	• 10 to 80 amylase units/hour (Mayo Clinic)
Elevation	• Rises rapidly within 3 to 6 hours after onset of attack • May rise to 40 times normal value • Increase is not proportional to severity of attack.	• Reflects rise in serum level, but lags 6 to 10 hours
Duration	• Peaks 20 to 30 hours after onset • Returns to normal level within 2 or 3 days, although active inflammation of pancreas may persist • Persistent elevation suggests pseudocyst, necrosis, or renal disease that inhibits amylase excretion.	• Elevation persists for 7 to 10 days. • Allows retrospective diagnosis of acute or relapsing pancreatitis when serum level registers in normal range • Persistent elevation in the absence of renal disease suggests pseudocyst formation.

24 hours, and teach him how to collect a timed specimen. The laboratory requires 2 days to complete the analysis.

Withhold morphine, meperidine, codeine, pentazocine, bethanechol, thiazide diuretics, indomethacin, and alcohol, as ordered, for 24 hours before the test. If these medications must be continued, note this on the laboratory slip.

If the female patient is menstruating, the test may have to be rescheduled.

Procedure
Collect a 2-, 6-, 8-, or 24-hour specimen.

Precautions
□ Cover and refrigerate the specimen during the collection period. If the patient is catheterized, keep the collection bag on ice.
□ Instruct the patient not to contaminate the specimen with toilet tissue or stool.
□ Send the specimens to the laboratory immediately when the test is completed.

Values
Because urine amylase is reported in various units of measure, values differ from laboratory to laboratory. The Mayo Clinic reports urinary excretion of 10 to 80 amylase units/hour as normal.

Implications of results
Elevated amylase levels occur in acute pancreatitis; obstruction of the pancreatic duct, intestines, or salivary duct; carcinoma of the head of the pancreas; mumps; acute injury of the spleen; renal disease, with impaired absorption; perforated peptic or duodenal ulcers; and gallbladder disease.

Depressed levels occur in chronic pancreatitis, cachexia, alcoholism, cancer of the liver, cirrhosis, hepatitis, and hepatic abscess.

Post-test care
None.

Interfering factors
□ Heavy bacterial contamination of the specimen or blood in the urine may interfere with test results.

□ Salivary amylase in the urine, caused by coughing or talking over the sample, may raise urine amylase levels.
□ Failure to collect all urine during the test period and improper storage of the specimen may alter test results.
□ Ingestion of morphine, meperidine, codeine, pentazocine, bethanechol, thiazide diuretics, indomethacin, or alcohol within 24 hours of the test may raise urine amylase levels. Fluorides may lower urine amylase levels.

MALINDA S. MITCHELL, RN, MS

Arylsulfatase A

Arylsulfatase A (ARS A), a lysosomal enzyme found in every cell except the mature erythrocyte, is principally active in the liver, the pancreas, and the kidneys, where exogenous substances are detoxified into ester sulfates. When ARS A is present in large amounts, it reverses this process by catalyzing the release of free phenylsulfates, such as benzidine and naphthyline, from the ester sulfates. Although research hasn't resolved whether elevated ARS A levels provoke malignant growths or are simply an enzymatic response to their presence, urine ARS A levels rise in transitional bladder cancer, colorectal cancer, and leukemia. This test measures urine ARS A levels by colorimetric or kinetic techniques.

Purpose
□ To aid diagnosis of cancer of the bladder, the colon, or the rectum; of myeloid (granulocytic) leukemia; and of metachromatic leukodystrophy (an inherited lipid storage disease).

Patient preparation
Tell the patient that this test measures an enzyme that's present throughout the body. Advise him that he needn't restrict food or fluids before the test. Tell him the test requires 24-hour urine collection, and teach him how to collect a

timed specimen. Test results are generally available in 2 or 3 days.

If the female patient is menstruating, the test may have to be rescheduled, since increased numbers of epithelial cells in the urine raise ARS A levels.

Procedure
Collect a 24-hour urine specimen.

Precautions
□ Tell the patient not to contaminate the urine specimen with toilet tissue or stool.
□ Keep the collection container refrigerated or on ice during the collection period, and send the specimen to the laboratory immediately at the end of the collection period. If the patient has a Foley catheter in place, keep the collection bag on ice for the duration of the test; it's advisable to change the continuous urinary drainage apparatus before beginning the test.

Values
ARS A values in men normally range from 1.4 to 19.3 u/liter; in women, from 1.4 to 11 u/liter; and in children, over 1 u/liter.

Implications of results
Elevated ARS A levels may result from cancer of the bladder, the colon, or the rectum, or from myeloid leukemia.

Depressed ARS A levels can result from metachromatic leukodystrophy. In patients with this condition, urine studies show metachromatic granules in the urinary sediment.

Post-test care
None.

Interfering factors
□ Failure to collect all urine during the test period may interfere with accurate determination of test results.
□ Contamination of the urine specimen by stool or menses, or by improper storage of the specimen may alter test results.
□ Surgery performed within 1 week before the test may raise ARS A levels.

MALINDA S. MITCHELL, RN, MS

Lysozyme
[Muramidase]

Lysozyme, a low–molecular-weight enzyme, is present in mucus, saliva, tears, skin secretions, and various internal body cells and fluids. This enzyme splits, or lyses, the cell walls of gram-positive bacteria and, with complement and other blood factors, acts to destroy them. Lysozyme seems to be synthesized in granulocytes and monocytes, and it first appears in serum after destruction of such cells. When serum lysozyme levels exceed three times normal, the enzyme appears in the urine. However, since renal tissue also contains lysozyme, renal injury alone can cause measurable excretion of this enzyme.

This test measures urine lysozyme levels turbidimetrically. Serum lysozyme determinations, using the same method, confirm the results of urine testing.

Purpose
□ To aid diagnosis of acute monocytic or granulocytic leukemia, and to monitor the progression of these diseases
□ To evaluate proximal tubular function and to diagnose renal impairment
□ To detect rejection or infarction of kidney transplantation.

Patient preparation
Explain to the patient that this test evaluates renal function and the immune system. Advise him that he needn't restrict food or fluids before the test. Tell him the test requires collection of a 24-hour urine specimen, and instruct him how to collect the specimen correctly. Test results should be available in 1 day.

If the female patient is menstruating, the test may have to be rescheduled for a later date.

Procedure
Collect a 24-hour urine specimen.

Precautions

□ Tell the patient to avoid contaminating the urine specimen with toilet tissue or stool.

□ Cover and refrigerate the specimen throughout the collection period. If the patient has a Foley catheter in place, keep the collection bag on ice.

□ Send the specimens to the laboratory immediately when the test is completed.

Values

Normally, urine lysozyme values are less than 3 mg/24 hours.

Implications of results

Elevated urine lysozyme levels are characteristic of impaired renal proximal tubular reabsorption, acute pyelonephritis, nephrotic syndrome, tuberculosis of the kidney, severe extrarenal infection, rejection or infarction of kidney transplantation (levels normally increase during first few days after transplantation), and polycythemia vera. Urine levels rise markedly after acute onset or relapse of monocytic or myelomonocytic leukemia, and rise moderately after acute onset or relapse of granulocytic (myeloid) leukemia. Urine lysozyme levels remain normal or decrease in lymphocytic leukemia, and remain normal in myeloblastic and myelocytic leukemias.

Post-test care

None.

Interfering factors

□ The presence of bacteria in the specimen decreases urine lysozyme levels; blood or saliva in the specimen increases lysozyme levels.

□ Failure to collect all urine during the test period may interfere with accurate determination of test results.

MALINDA S. MITCHELL, RN, MS

STIMULATION TEST

Cyclic Adenosine Monophosphate

Formed from adenosine triphosphate by the action of the enzyme adenylate cyclase, the nucleotide cyclic adenosine monophosphate (cAMP) influences the protein synthesis rate within cells. Measurement of urinary excretion of cAMP after I.V. infusion of a standard dose of parathyroid hormone can show renal tubular resistance in a patient with hypoparathyroid symptoms and high levels of parathyroid hormone. Such findings suggest Type I pseudohypoparathyroidism. (Urinary cAMP levels respond normally with Type II pseudohypoparathyroidism, since the defect is beyond the level of cAMP generation.) This rare inherited disorder results from tissue resistance to parathyroid hormone, and produces hypocalcemia, hyperphosphatemia, and skeletal and constitutional abnormalities.

This test is contraindicated in patients with high calcium levels (since parathyroid hormone further raises calcium levels). It should be used cautiously in patients receiving digitalis and in those with sarcoidosis or renal or cardiac disease.

Purpose

□ To aid differential diagnosis of pseudohypoparathyroidism.

Patient preparation

Explain to the patient that this test evaluates parathyroid function. Tell him the test requires a 15-minute I.V. infusion of parathyroid hormone and collection of a 3- to 4-hour urine specimen.

Perform a skin test to detect a possible allergy to parathyroid hormone; keep epinephrine readily available in case of an adverse reaction. Just before the procedure is performed, instruct the patient not to touch the I.V. or exert pressure on the arm receiving the infusion. Tell him he may experience transient discomfort from the needle puncture. Ask him to notify you if he feels severe burning or if the site becomes inflamed or swollen.

Equipment
Parathyroid hormone (300 units, in refrigerated ampules)/vial of sterile water (saline solution causes precipitate to form)/urine collection container, to which hydrochloric acid has been added as a preservative.

Procedure
Instruct the patient to empty his bladder. If the patient has a Foley catheter in place, change the collection bag. If ordered, send this specimen to the laboratory; otherwise, discard it. Prepare the parathyroid hormone for infusion, as directed, using sterile water for dilution. Start the I.V. with 5% dextrose in water, and infuse the parathyroid hormone over 15 minutes. Record the start of the I.V. as time zero.

Collect a urine specimen 3 to 4 hours after infusion. Discontinue the I.V., as ordered.

Precautions
□ Tell the patient to avoid contaminating the urine specimen with toilet tissue or stool.
□ Send the specimen to the laboratory immediately; if transport is delayed, refrigerate the specimen. If the patient has a catheter in place, keep the collection bag on ice.

CYCLIC AMP: THE SECOND MESSENGER

Cyclic adenosine monophosphate (cAMP) is an intracellular mediator that relays hormone messages to target cells to effect programmed physiologic responses. It's the "second messenger" after the hormone itself.

Presumably, binding of hormone with a specific receptor on the cell surface activates the enzyme adenyl cyclase in the cell membrane. This then causes adenosine triphosphate (ATP) to convert to cAMP within the cell.

Then, cAMP initiates functions specific to the cell. For example it tells thyroid cells to produce hormone and kidney cells to increase tubule permeability. It also spurs cell enzymes to convert stored glucose into high-energy ATP needed for cell metabolism. Depletion of this ATP triggers formation of more cAMP.

As the messenger for parathyroid hormone, cAMP helps distinguish pseudohypoparathyroidism and hypoparathyroidism. In the patient with the latter and in a healthy person, urine cAMP rises minutes after a parathyroid hormone dose. But it fails to rise in pseudohypoparathyroidism, in which the glands produce sufficient or excessive hormone, but normal end organ response to it is blocked.

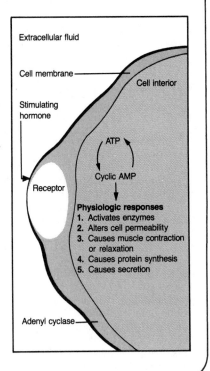

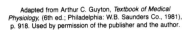
Adapted from Arthur C. Guyton, *Textbook of Medical Physiology*, (6th ed.; Philadelphia: W.B. Saunders Co., 1981), p. 918. Used by permission of the publisher and the author.

Findings and implications of results

A ten- to twentyfold increase (3.6 to 4 micromoles) in cAMP demonstrates a normal response or hypoparathyroidism. Failure to respond to parathyroid hormone, indicated by normal urinary excretion of cAMP, suggests Type I pseudohypoparathyroidism.

Post-test care

☐ Observe the patient for symptoms of hypercalcemia: lethargy, anorexia, nausea, vomiting, vertigo, and abdominal cramps.

☐ If a hematoma or irritation develops at the venipuncture site, apply warm soaks.

Interfering factors

Contamination or improper storage of the specimen, or failure to acidify the urine with hydrochloric acid may alter test results.

THAD C. HAGEN, MD

Selected References

Brunner, Lillian S., and Suddarth, Doris S. *Textbook of Medical-Surgical Nursing,* 5th ed. Philadelphia: J.B. Lippincott Co., 1984.

Byrne, C. Judith, et al. *Laboratory Tests: Implications for Nurses and Allied Health Professionals.* Reading, Mass.: Addison-Wesley Publishing Co., 1981.

DeGroot, Leslie J., ed. *Endocrinology.* New York: Grune & Stratton, 1979.

Fischbach, Frances. *A Manual of Laboratory Diagnostic Tests,* 2nd ed. Philadelphia: J.B. Lippincott Co., 1984.

Guyton, Arthur C. *Textbook of Medical Physiology,* 6th ed. Philadelphia: W.B. Saunders Co., 1981.

Harvey, A. McGehee, ed. *The Principles and Practice of Medicine,* 21st ed. East Norwalk, Conn.: Appleton-Century-Crofts, 1984.

Henry, John Bernard, ed. *Todd-Sanford-Davidsohn Clinical Diagnosis and Management by Laboratory Methods,* vol. 1, 17th ed. Philadelphia: W.B. Saunders Co., 1984.

Jacob, Stanley W., et al. *Structure and Function in Man,* 5th ed. Philadelphia: W.B. Saunders Co., 1982.

Lamb, Jane O. *Laboratory Tests for Clinical Nursing.* Bowie, Md.: Robert J. Brady Co., 1984.

Leavelle, Dennis E., ed. *Mayo Medical Laboratories Test Catalog.* Rochester, Minn.: Mayo Medical Laboratories, 1984.

Petersdorf, Robert G., and Adams, Raymond D., eds. *Harrison's Principles of Internal Medicine,* 10th ed. New York: McGraw-Hill Book Co., 1983.

Phipps, Wilma J., et al. *Medical-Surgical Nursing: Concepts and Clinical Practice.* St. Louis: C.V. Mosby Co., 1979.

Price, Sylvia, and Wilson, Lorraine. *Pathophysiology: Clinical Concepts of Disease Processes,* 2nd ed. New York: McGraw-Hill Book Co., 1982.

Ravel, Richard. *Clinical Laboratory Medicine,* 3rd ed. Chicago: Year Book Medical Publications, 1978.

Smith, Donald R. *General Urology,* 10th ed. Los Altos, Calif.: Lange Medical Publications, 1981.

Sodeman, William A., and Sodeman, Thomas M. *Sodeman's Pathologic Physiology: Mechanisms of Disease,* 6th ed. Philadelphia: W.B. Saunders Co., 1979.

Tilkian, Sarko M., et al. *Clinical Implications of Laboratory Tests,* 3rd ed. St. Louis: C.V. Mosby Co., 1983.

Wallach, Jacques B. *Interpretation of Diagnostic Tests: A Handbook Synopsis of Laboratory Medicine,* 3rd ed. Boston: Little, Brown & Co., 1978.

Wegener, Lee T., ed. *Mayo Medical Laboratories Interpretive Handbook.* Rochester, Minn.: Mayo Medical Laboratories, 1984.

Widmann, Frances K. *Clinical Interpretation of Laboratory Tests,* 9th ed. Philadelphia: F.A. Davis Co., 1983.

Williams, William J., et al. *Hematology,* 2nd ed. New York: McGraw-Hill Book Co., 1977.

Wintrobe, Maxwell M., et al. *Clinical Hematology,* 8th ed. Philadelphia: Lea & Febiger, 1981.

Wyngaarden, James, and Smith, Lloyd. *Cecil Textbook of Medicine,* 16th ed. Philadelphia: W.B. Saunders Co., 1982.

14 Urine Hormones and Metabolites

LEARNING OBJECTIVES

After completing this chapter, the reader will be able to:
- identify the three chemical classes of hormones.
- name the hormones and metabolites that are commonly measured in the urine and describe their principal functions.
- list four common test methods used to measure urine hormone levels.
- discuss the importance of a 24-hour urine specimen in determining urine hormone levels.
- state the purpose of each test discussed in the chapter.
- prepare the patient physically and psychologically for each test.
- describe the procedure for performing each test.
- specify appropriate precautions for accurate administration of each test.
- implement appropriate post-test care.
- state the normal values for each test.
- discuss the implications of abnormal test results.
- list factors that may interfere with accurate test results.

Urine Hormones and Metabolites

Introduction

Hormones are potent, complex chemicals produced and secreted primarily by the endocrine glands to promote and regulate the activity of target organs and tissues. To directly determine circulating levels of hormones, laboratory methods commonly measure hormone concentrations in blood. But many hormones and their metabolites are also conveniently studied in urine.

Measuring urine hormone and metabolite levels provides a reliable estimate of the amount of circulating hormone. Moreover, timed, long-term urine measurements offer an advantage. Unlike a blood sample, which determines hormone levels only at the time of venipuncture, a 24-hour urine specimen reflects total daily secretion, offsets diurnal variations, and masks temporary fluctuations.

Chemical classes

Chemically, hormones can be classified into three groups: *steroids* (such as estrogens and androgens), *amines* (such as dopamine and epinephrine), and *proteins* (such as human chorionic gonadotropin). Each group has a marked structural specificity. This is especially true of steroid hormones—the ones most frequently tested in urine. A single structural change in the composition of a steroid hormone can dramatically alter the hormone's physiologic activity. For ex-

ample, the introduction of a new hydroxyl group is responsible for the conversion of estradiol to estriol.

Hormone metabolites

Although hormones have specific and characteristic functions, they rarely act independently. Quite the contrary, hormones are linked in an intricate series of complex interactions, including positive and negative feedback mechanisms that enable them to function efficiently and maintain homeostasis. Perhaps the most important of these interactions is the formation of hormone metabolites. These metabolites can be degradation products, or essential precursors with individual hormonal effects.

Urine levels of hormone metabolites reflect the secretory rates of the hormones from which these metabolites are derived, and serve as valuable diagnostic indicators when the hormones themselves aren't excreted in measurable quantities. Metabolite levels also provide important information about the integrity of degradation pathways. A case in point is the conversion of 17-OH progesterone to cortisol; when this metabolic process is blocked, as in adrenogenital syndrome (congenital adrenal hyperplasia), excessive amounts of pregnanetriol appear in the urine.

The hormones produced by the endocrine glands and their metabolites that

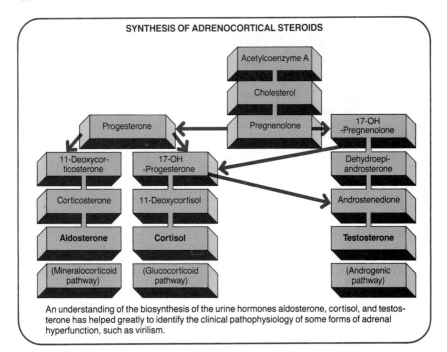

SYNTHESIS OF ADRENOCORTICAL STEROIDS

Acetylcoenzyme A

Cholesterol

Progesterone — Pregnenolone — 17-OH-Pregnenolone

11-Deoxycorticosterone — 17-OH-Progesterone — Dehydroepiandrosterone

Corticosterone — 11-Deoxycortisol — Androstenedione

Aldosterone — **Cortisol** — **Testosterone**

(Mineralocorticoid pathway) — (Glucocorticoid pathway) — (Androgenic pathway)

An understanding of the biosynthesis of the urine hormones aldosterone, cortisol, and testosterone has helped greatly to identify the clinical pathophysiology of some forms of adrenal hyperfunction, such as virilism.

are commonly measured in the urine include the following:

□ *Adrenocortical hormones:* These hormones and metabolites are steroids, synthesized and secreted primarily by the adrenal cortex. Formed from acetylcoenzyme A, cholesterol, and a variety of other precursors, adrenocortical hormones and metabolites fall into three major groups: 1. *Glucocorticoids*—17-hydroxycorticosteroids, particularly cortisol —maintain carbohydrate, protein, and fat metabolism. 2. *Mineralocorticoids,* principally aldosterone, help regulate blood pressure, and fluid and electrolyte balance. 3. *Adrenal androgens* (sex hormones), the most potent of which is dehydroepiandrosterone, aid development of male secondary sex characteristics. Androgens are secreted in minute amounts and are usually measured as part of the 17-ketosteroids. The most inclusive test of adrenocortical hormones, however, measures urine levels of 17-ketogenic steroids.

□ *Adrenal medullary hormones:* The adrenal medullae synthesize and secrete the catecholamines *norepinephrine* and *epinephrine,* which help mediate stress. Although these hormones are less vital to life than the adrenocortical hormones, determinations of urine levels of the catecholamines and their principal metabolite, *vanillylmandelic acid,* can be extremely useful in the detection of catecholamine-producing tumors.

□ *Dopamine and other amines:* A catecholamine secreted primarily by the basal ganglia of the brain, dopamine is the precursor of norepinephrine and epinephrine. When a pheochromocytoma, a catecholamine-secreting tumor, is suspected, measurement of urine levels of dopamine and its major metabolite, homovanillic acid, can aid diagnosis. Urine levels of *serotonin,* an indole amine synthesized by the argentaffin cells of the intestinal mucosa, are reflected by the excretion of 5-hydroxyindoleacetic acid, its primary metabolite, and aid diagnosis of certain carcinoid tumors.

□ *Gonadal and placental hormones:* Urine levels of gonadal and placental hormones, which are principally steroids, are clinically useful for detecting hormone-secreting tumors and pregnancy. Early in pregnancy, the corpus luteum secretes greater amounts of progesterone and estrogen to maintain the pregnancy until the placenta can produce these hormones. Thus, urine levels of total estrogens, estriol, and pregnanediol help evaluate placental status and fetal well-being.

For early diagnosis of pregnancy, human chorionic gonadotropin (hCG) may be measured in the urine. Soon after conception, the trophoblastic cells that develop into the chorionic villi of the placenta secrete hCG. The presence of hCG in urine confirms pregnancy.

Four test methods useful
Quantitative assays of urine hormone levels are usually performed by using one or more of the following methods:

□ *Colorimetry* is based on the principle that some groups of hormones, when combined with certain chemical reagents, take on individual colors; the intensity of color indicates the degree of hormone concentration. A colorimeter or spectrophotometer measures the wavelength of maximum absorption.

□ *Fluorometry* reveals the characteristic fluorescence of hormones on placement in specific media. Under certain laboratory conditions, the wavelengths activated and emitted are specific for a given hormone and can be measured.

□ *Chromatography* determines the adsorption or fractionation of a hormone to a specific medium (solid or liquid). In *gas* chromatography, a urine specimen is mixed with an inert gas to create vapors that are passed over the medium.

KEY FACTS ABOUT URINE HORMONES

HORMONE OR PRINCIPAL METABOLITE	PRINCIPAL SECRETION SITE	METHOD OF QUANTITATION
Aldosterone	Adrenal cortex	Radioimmunoassay
Free cortisol	Adrenal cortex	Radioimmunoassay
Catecholamines	Adrenal medulla	Spectrophotofluorometry
Total estrogens	Gonads, placenta, adrenal glands	Spectrophotofluorometry
Estriol	Placenta, gonads, adrenal cortex	Radioimmunoassay
Human chorionic gonadotropin	Placenta	Hemagglutination inhibition (antigen-antibody reaction)
Pregnanetriol	Adrenal cortex	Spectrophotometry
17-Hydroxycorticosteroids	Adrenal cortex	Chromatography, spectrophotofluorometry
17-Ketosteroids	Adrenal glands, testes	Spectrophotofluorometry
17-Ketogenic steroids	Adrenal cortex	Spectrophotofluorometry
Vanillylmandelic acid	Adrenal medulla	Spectrophotofluorometry
Homovanillic acid	Liver	Chromatography
5-Hydroxyindoleacetic acid	Intestinal wall, stomach	Colorimetry
Pregnanediol	Corpus luteum, adrenal cortex	Gas-liquid chromatography

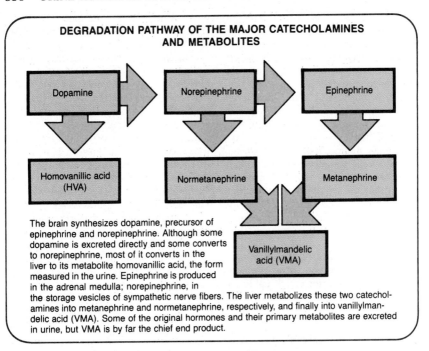

DEGRADATION PATHWAY OF THE MAJOR CATECHOLAMINES AND METABOLITES

Dopamine → Norepinephrine → Epinephrine

Homovanillic acid (HVA)

Normetanephrine

Metanephrine

Vanillylmandelic acid (VMA)

The brain synthesizes dopamine, precursor of epinephrine and norepinephrine. Although some dopamine is excreted directly and some converts to norepinephrine, most of it converts in the liver to its metabolite homovanillic acid, the form measured in the urine. Epinephrine is produced in the adrenal medulla; norepinephrine, in the storage vesicles of sympathetic nerve fibers. The liver metabolizes these two catecholamines into metanephrine and normetanephrine, respectively, and finally into vanillylmandelic acid (VMA). Some of the original hormones and their primary metabolites are excreted in urine, but VMA is by far the chief end product.

Adsorption of the hormone to the medium is measured. In *paper* chromatography, blotting or filter paper replaces the solid or liquid medium.

□ *Radioimmunoassay* involves combining a urine specimen with a radioactively tagged antigen (hormone) and its antibody. The unlabeled hormone being measured displaces the radioactively tagged hormone, which is then measured to determine the urine concentration of the hormone.

Special considerations

In all determinations of urine hormones, 24-hour specimens provide more accurate information than random urine specimens by compensating for diurnal variations in hormonal secretion. For the same reason, urine assays from a 24-hour specimen are often more accurate than serum hormone determinations. However, accurate results require careful attention to certain influential factors. For example, incomplete collection of a 24-hour specimen or impaired renal function can significantly change test results. For accurate test results, keep in mind the following points:

□ Before beginning a 24-hour urine collection, confer with the laboratory to determine if the test method necessitates special collection procedures or precautions. In many cases, you'll need to enforce medication and diet restrictions to ensure accurate determinations. Many of these tests require dark collection containers and the addition of a preservative to the specimen. The specimen may have to be refrigerated or kept on ice during the collection period.

□ Make sure all urine voided during the 24-hour test period is collected. If a voiding is discarded accidentally, note this on the laboratory slip, so the laboratory can take this lost specimen into consideration when determining the results of the test.

□ Since strenuous physical exercise and emotional stress can significantly alter the patient's hormone levels, try to promote an atmosphere of rest and relaxation before the test.

PATRICE M. HARMAN, RN

URINE HORMONES

Urine Aldosterone

This test measures urine levels of aldosterone, the principal mineralocorticoid secreted by the zona glomerulosa of the adrenal cortex. Aldosterone promotes retention of sodium and excretion of potassium by the renal tubules, thereby helping to regulate blood pressure, and fluid and electrolyte balance. In turn, aldosterone secretion is controlled by the renin-angiotensin system. Renin, an enzyme released in the kidneys in response to low plasma volume, stimulates production of angiotensin I, which is converted to angiotensin II, a powerful vasopressor that directly stimulates the adrenal cortex to secrete aldosterone. Potassium levels also influence aldosterone secretion: increased potassium concentration stimulates the adrenal cortex, triggering a substantial increase in aldosterone secretion to promote potassium excretion. This feedback mechanism is vital to maintaining fluid and electrolyte balance.

Urine aldosterone levels, measured through radioimmunoassay, are usually evaluated after measurement of serum electrolyte and renin levels.

Purpose
☐ To aid diagnosis of primary and secondary aldosteronism.

Patient preparation
Explain to the patient that this test evaluates hormonal balance. Instruct him to maintain a normal sodium diet (3 g/day) before the test; to avoid sodium-rich foods, such as bacon, barbeque sauce, corned beef, bouillon cubes or powder, and olives; and to avoid strenuous physical exercise and stressful situations during the collection period. Tell him the test requires collection of a 24-hour urine specimen, and teach him the proper collection technique.

Check the patient's medication history for drugs that may affect aldosterone levels. Review your findings with the laboratory, then notify the doctor; he may want to restrict these medications before the test.

Procedure
Collect a 24-hour specimen in a bottle containing a preservative to keep the specimen at a pH of 4.0 to 4.5.

Precautions
Refrigerate the specimen or place it on ice during the collection period. When the collection is completed, send the specimen to the laboratory immediately.

Values
Normally, urine aldosterone levels range from 2 to 16 mcg/24 hours.

Implications of results
Elevated urine aldosterone levels suggest primary or secondary aldosteronism. The primary form usually arises from an aldosterone-secreting adenoma of the adrenal cortex but may also result from adrenocortical hyperplasia. Secondary aldosteronism, the more common form, results from external stimulation of the adrenal cortex, such as that produced when the renin-angiotensin system is activated by hypertensive and edematous disorders. The major systemic pathologies that result in secondary aldosteronism are malignant hypertension, congestive heart failure, cirrhosis of the liver, nephrotic syndrome, and idiopathic cyclic edema.

Low urine aldosterone levels may result from Addison's disease, salt-losing syndrome, and toxemia of pregnancy. These levels normally rise during pregnancy but rapidly decline following parturition.

Post-test care
☐ If medications were discontinued be-

NORMAL AND ABNORMAL URINE ALDOSTERONE LEVELS ON 135 mEq SODIUM INTAKE (3 G Na) PER DAY

When hypertension and hypokalemia suggest hyperaldosteronism, the urine aldosterone test reveals characteristic elevations. Since salt depletion triggers production of aldosterone, the patient is instructed to maintain his normal diet before the test.

Adapted with permission from an original painting by Frank H. Netter, MD, from *The CIBA Collection of Medical Illustrations*, copyright by CIBA Pharmaceutical Co., Division of CIBA-GEIGY Corp.

fore the test, resume administration, as ordered.

□ Patient may resume normal physical activity restricted before the test.

Interfering factors

□ Antihypertensive drugs promote sodium and water retention, and may suppress urine aldosterone levels. Diuretics and most steroids promote sodium excretion and may raise aldosterone levels. Some corticosteroids, such as fludrocortisone, mimic mineralocorticoid activity and consequently may lower aldosterone levels.

□ Patient failure to maintain a normal dietary intake of sodium can influence test results. Failure to collect *all* urine during the 24-hour specimen collection period or to store the urine specimen properly can interfere with accurate determination of test results.

□ Patient failure to avoid strenuous physical exercise and emotional stress before the test stimulates adrenocortical secretions and thus increases aldosterone levels.

□ Radioactive scan performed within 1 week before the test may interfere with the accurate determination of aldosterone levels using this radioimmunoassay method.

CATHERINE E. KIRBY, RN, BSN

Urine Free Cortisol

Used as a screen for adrenocortical hyperfunction, this test measures urine levels of the portion of cortisol not bound to the corticosteroid-binding globulin transcortin. It is one of the best diagnostic tools for detecting Cushing's syndrome. The major glucocorticoid secreted by the adrenal cortex in response to adrenocorticotropic hormone (ACTH) stimulation, cortisol helps regulate fat, carbohydrate, and protein metabolism; it also helps promote glyconeogenesis, anti-inflammatory response, and cellular permeability. Only about 10% of this hormone is unbound and physiologically active; this small portion is known as free cortisol. Urine cortisol concentrations increase significantly when the amount secreted exceeds the binding capacity of transcortin, which is normally almost saturated.

Radioimmunoassay determinations of free cortisol levels in a 24-hour urine specimen—unlike a single measurement of plasma cortisol—reflect overall secretion levels instead of diurnal variations. Concurrent measurements of plasma cortisol and ACTH, with urine 17-hydroxycorticosteroids and the dexamethasone suppression test, may be used to confirm diagnosis.

Purpose
□ To aid diagnosis of Cushing's syndrome.

Patient preparation
Explain to the patient that this test helps evaluate adrenal gland function. Advise him he should maintain food and fluid intake before the test, but should avoid stressful situations and excessive physical exercise during the collection period. Tell him the test requires collection of a 24-hour urine specimen.

Teach the patient the proper collection technique for a 24-hour urine specimen.

Check the patient's recent drug history for medications (such as those listed below) that may interfere with test results. Review your findings with the laboratory, then notify the doctor; he may want to restrict such medications before the test.

Procedure
Collect a 24-hour urine specimen in a bottle containing a preservative to keep the specimen at a pH of 4.0 to 4.5.

Precautions
Refrigerate the specimen or place it on ice during the collection period.

Values
Normally, free cortisol values range from 24 to 108 mcg/24 hours.

Implications of results
Elevated free cortisol levels may indicate Cushing's syndrome resulting from adrenal hyperplasia, adrenal or pituitary tumor, or ectopic ACTH production. Hepatic disease and obesity, which can raise plasma cortisol levels, generally don't appreciably raise urine levels of free cortisol.

This test is designed to screen for excessive secretion of free cortisol. Low levels have little diagnostic significance and don't necessarily indicate adrenocortical hypofunction.

Post-test care
□ Patient may resume normal activity restricted during test.
□ As ordered, resume administration of medications discontinued before the test.

Interfering factors
□ Prolonged steroid therapy, and drugs such as reserpine, phenothiazines, morphine, and amphetamines may elevate free cortisol levels.
□ Failure to collect all urine during the test period or to store the specimen properly may interfere with accurate determination of test results.
□ Failure to observe drug restrictions may interfere with accurate determination of test results.

CATHERINE E. KIRBY, RN, BSN

Urine Catecholamines

This test uses spectrophotofluorometry to measure urine levels of the major catecholamines—epinephrine, norepinephrine, and dopamine. Epinephrine is secreted by the adrenal medulla; dopamine, by the central nervous system; and norepinephrine, by both. Catecholamines help regulate metabolism and prepare the body for the fight-or-flight response to stress. Certain tumors can also secrete catecholamines. One of the most common of these tumors is a pheochromocytoma, which usually causes intermittent or persistent hypertension.

The specimen of choice for this test is a 24-hour urine specimen, since catecholamine secretion fluctuates diurnally and in response to pain, heat, cold, emotional stress, physical exercise, hypoglycemia, injury, hemorrhage, asphyxia, and drugs. However, a random specimen may be useful for evaluating catecholamine levels after a hypertensive episode.

URINE METANEPHRINE AND NORMETANEPHRINE

Determination of urine levels of metanephrine and normetanephrine—metabolites of epinephrine and norepinephrine, respectively—aids diagnosis of catecholamine-secreting tumors. These metabolites—commonly measured concurrently with catecholamines—are analyzed by spectrophotofluorometry, using a 24-hour urine specimen acidified to a pH of 4.0 to 4.5. Total excretion is normally less than 1.3 mg/24 hours.

Before performing this test, review the patient's drug history, and check with a laboratory technician for medications that may interfere with test results. Imipramine may raise levels of metanephrine and normetanephrine. Phenothiazines and methyldopa may raise or suppress levels.

For a complete diagnostic workup of catecholamine secretion, urine levels of catecholamine metabolites are measured concurrently. These metabolites—metanephrine, normetanephrine, homovanillic acid (HVA), and vanillylmandelic acid (VMA)—normally appear in the urine in greater quantities than the catecholamines.

Purpose
☐ To aid diagnosis of pheochromocytoma in a patient with unexplained hypertension
☐ To aid diagnosis of neuroblastoma, ganglioneuroma, and dysautonomia.

Patient preparation
Explain to the patient that this test evaluates adrenal function. Inform him that he needn't restrict food or fluids before the test, but should avoid stressful situations and excessive physical activity during the collection period. Tell him that either a 24-hour or a random specimen is required, and explain the collection procedure.

Check the patient's drug history for medications (such as those listed below) that may affect catecholamine levels. Review your findings with a laboratory technician, then notify the doctor. He may want to restrict such medications before the test.

Procedure
Collect a 24-hour urine specimen in a bottle containing a preservative to keep the specimen acidified to a pH of 3.0 or less. (If a random specimen is ordered, collect it immediately after a hypertensive episode.)

Precautions
Refrigerate a 24-hour specimen or place it on ice during the collection period. At the end of the collection period, send the specimen to the laboratory immediately.

Values
Normally, urine catecholamine values range from undetectable to 135 mcg/24 hours, or from undetectable to 18 mcg/dl in a random specimen.

Implications of results
In a patient with undiagnosed hypertension, elevated urine catecholamine levels following a hypertensive episode usually indicate a pheochromocytoma. With the exception of HVA—a metabolite of dopamine—catecholamine metabolites may also be elevated. Abnormally high HVA levels rule out a pheochromocytoma, because this tumor mainly secretes epinephrine, whose primary metabolite is VMA, not HVA. If tests indicate a pheochromocytoma, the patient may also be tested for multiple endocrine neoplasia.

Elevated catecholamine levels, without marked hypertension, may be due to a neuroblastoma or a ganglioneuroma, although HVA levels reflect these conditions more accurately. Neuroblastomas and ganglioneuromas primarily composed of immature cells secrete large quantities of dopamine and HVA. Myasthenia gravis and progressive muscular dystrophy commonly cause urine catecholamine levels to rise above normal, but this test is rarely performed to diagnose these disorders.

Consistently low-normal catecholamine levels may indicate dysautonomia, marked by orthostatic hypotension.

Post-test care

□ Patient may resume activity restricted during the test.

□ As ordered, resume administration of medications withheld before the test.

Interfering factors

□ Caffeine, insulin, nitroglycerin, aminophylline, ethanol, sympathomimetics, methyldopa, tricyclic antidepressants, chloral hydrate, quinidine, quinine, tetracycline, B-complex vitamins, isoproterenol, levodopa, and monoamine oxidase inhibitors may raise urine catecholamine levels.

□ Clonidine, guanethidine, reserpine, and iodine-containing contrast media may suppress the levels of urine catecholamine.

□ Phenothiazines, erythromycin, and methenamine compounds may raise or suppress levels.

□ Failure to comply with drug restrictions, to collect all urine during the test period, or to store the specimen properly may interfere with test results.

□ Excessive physical exercise or emotional stress raises catecholamine levels.

CATHERINE E. KIRBY, RN, BSN

Total Urine Estrogens

This test is a quantitative analysis of total urine levels of estradiol, estrone, and estriol—the major estrogens present in significant amounts in urine. In females who are past puberty, these estrogens are secreted by the theca interna cells of the ovarian follicle and by the corpus luteum; in pregnancy, by the placenta; and after menopause, primarily by the adrenal glands. In males, two thirds of estradiol and of estrone are derived from testosterone; the remaining third of estradiol and smaller quantities of estrone are secreted by the testes. In both sexes, the liver, which oxidizes or converts hormones to glucuronide and sulfate conjugates, is the major organ of estrogen metabolism.

Clinical indications for this test include tumors of ovarian, adrenocortical, or testicular origin. A common method for measuring total urine estrogen levels involves purification by gel filtration, followed by spectrophotofluorometry. Supplementary tests that may provide further information about ovarian function include cytologic examination of vaginal smears, measurement of urine levels of pregnanediol and follicle-stimulating hormone, and evaluation of response to an injection of progesterone.

Purpose

□ To evaluate ovarian activity and help determine the cause of amenorrhea and female hyperestrogenism

□ To aid diagnosis of testicular tumors

□ To assess fetoplacental status.

Patient preparation

Explain to the female patient that this test helps evaluate ovarian function; to the patient who is pregnant that this test helps evaluate fetal development and placental function; and to the male patient that this test helps evaluate testicular function. Inform all patients that the test requires collection of a 24-hour urine specimen, and that no pretest restrictions of food or fluids are necessary. If the 24-hour specimen is to be collected at home, teach the patient the proper collection technique. Check the patient's medication history for use of drugs (such as those listed below) that may influence estrogen levels.

Procedure

Collect a 24-hour specimen in a bottle containing a preservative to keep the specimen at a pH of 3.0 to 5.0. If the patient is pregnant, note the approximate week of gestation on the laboratory slip. If the patient is a nonpregnant female, note the stage of her menstrual cycle.

Precautions

Refrigerate the specimen or keep it on ice during the collection period.

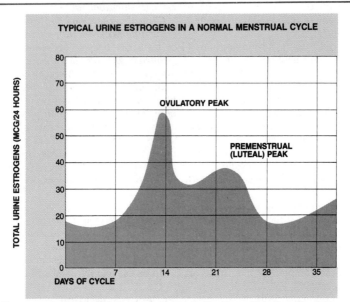

TYPICAL URINE ESTROGENS IN A NORMAL MENSTRUAL CYCLE

(y-axis) TOTAL URINE ESTROGENS (MCG/24 HOURS)

OVULATORY PEAK

PREMENSTRUAL
(LUTEAL) PEAK

DAYS OF CYCLE

Estrogen excretion levels during a normal menstrual cycle are biphasic, with a primary peak at midpoint in the cycle (ovulatory phase), and another smaller increase (luteal or premenstrual phase) occurring just before onset of menses.

Quantitation of total estrogens in the urine provides information for a clinical evaluation of ovarian function.

Urine estrogens rise slowly in the first trimester of pregnancy, and then increase rapidly to reach high levels as term approaches. With menopause, the cyclical pattern fluctuates and eventually flattens out to a constant low level.

From Daniel R. Mishell, et al, "Serum Gonadotropin and Steroid Patterns During the Normal Menstrual Cycle," *American Journal of Obstetrics and Gynecology,* 111:60, September 1, 1971. Used by permission of the publisher and the authors.

Values

In nonpregnant females, total urine estrogen levels rise and fall during the menstrual cycle, peaking shortly before midcycle, decreasing immediately following ovulation, increasing through the life of the corpus luteum, and decreasing greatly as the corpus luteum degenerates and menstruation begins (see illustration above).

Normal values for nonpregnant females are as follows: *preovulatory phase:* 5 to 25 mcg/24 hours; *ovulatory phase:* 24 to 100 mcg/24 hours; *luteal phase:* 12 to 80 mcg/24 hours.

In postmenopausal females, values are less than 10 mcg/24 hours; in males, from 4 to 25 mcg/24 hours.

Implications of results

Decreased total urine estrogen levels may reflect ovarian agenesis, primary ovarian insufficiency (due to Stein-Leventhal syndrome, for example), or secondary ovarian insufficiency (due to pituitary or adrenal hypofunction, or metabolic disturbances).

Elevated total estrogen levels in nonpregnant females may indicate tumors of ovarian or adrenocortical origin, adrenocortical hyperplasia, or a metabolic or hepatic disorder. In males, elevated total estrogen levels are associated with testicular tumors.

Elevated total urine estrogen levels are normal during pregnancy; serial determinations should show a rising titer (see also URINE PLACENTAL ESTRIOL).

Post-test care

As ordered, resume administration of medications withheld before the test.

Interfering factors

☐ Drugs that may influence total urine estrogen levels include steroids (such as estrogens, progesterone, and high-dose corticosteroids), methenamine mandelate, phenazopyridine hydrochloride, phenothiazines, tetracyclines, phenolphthalein, ampicillin, meprobamate, senna, cascara sagrada, and hydrochlorothiazide.

☐ Failure to collect all urine during the 24-hour period and to refrigerate the specimen or keep it on ice, and improper pH control may affect test results.

CATHERINE E. KIRBY, RN, BSN
SUSAN F. MORROW, RN

Urine Placental Estriol

This test monitors fetal viability by measuring urine levels of placental estriol, the predominant estrogen excreted in urine during pregnancy. Toward the end of the first trimester, placental constituents combine with estriol precursors from the fetal adrenal cortex and liver to steadily increase estriol production. This steady rise in estriol reflects a properly functioning placenta and, in most cases, a healthy, growing fetus. Normally, estriol is secreted in much smaller amounts by the ovaries in nonpregnant females, by the testes in males, and by the adrenal cortex in both sexes.

The usual clinical indication for this test is high-risk pregnancy, such as one complicated by maternal hypertension, diabetes mellitus, preeclampsia, toxemia, or a history of stillbirth. Serial testing is necessary to plot the expected rise in estriol levels, or to show the absence of such a rise. The specimen of choice for this test is a 24-hour urine specimen, since estriol levels fluctuate diurnally. Radioimmunoassay is the usual test method. Generally, serum estriol levels are considered more reliable

than urine levels. Serum levels aren't influenced by maternal glomerular filtration rate (GFR), nor are they as readily affected by drugs, some of which actually destroy urinary estriol.

Purpose

☐ To assess fetoplacental status, especially in high-risk pregnancy.

Patient preparation

Explain to the patient that this test helps determine if the placenta is functioning properly, which is essential to the health of the fetus. Tell her she needn't restrict food or fluids. Advise her that a 24-hour urine specimen is required for this test, and instruct her how to collect the specimen. Emphasize that proper collection technique is necessary for test results to be valid.

Check the patient's medication history for use of drugs that may affect urine estriol levels.

Procedure

Collect a 24-hour urine specimen in a bottle containing a preservative to keep the specimen at a pH of 3.0 to 5.0. Note the week of gestation on the laboratory slip, and send the specimen to the laboratory.

Precautions

Refrigerate the specimen or keep it on ice during the collection period.

Values

Normal values vary considerably, but serial measurements of urine estriol levels, when plotted on a graph, should describe a steadily rising curve (see illustration, page 392).

Implications of results

A 40% drop from baseline values that occurs on 2 consecutive days strongly suggests placental insufficiency and impending fetal distress. A 20% drop over 2 weeks, or failure of consecutive estriol levels to rise in a normal curve similarly indicates inadequate placental function and undesirable fetal status. These de-

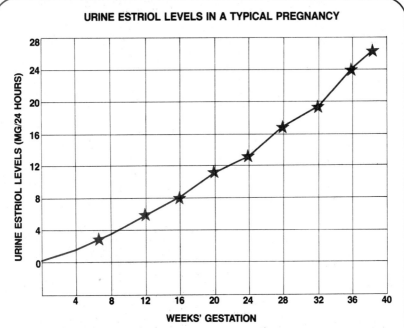

URINE ESTRIOL LEVELS IN A TYPICAL PREGNANCY

Since urine estriol rises as normal gestation proceeds, any significant changes in serial urine determinations suggest abnormal conditions that may require prompt medical intervention.

velopments may necessitate cesarean section, depending on the patient's condition and other apparent signs of fetal distress.

A chronically low urine estriol curve may result from fetal adrenal insufficiency, congenital anomalies (such as anencephaly), Rh isoimmunization, or placental sulfatase deficiency. A high-risk pregnancy in which maternal GFR decreases, as in hypertension or diabetes mellitus, may cause a low-normal estriol curve. In such a case, the pregnancy may continue, so long as no complications develop and estriol levels continue to rise. However, falling estriol levels or a sudden drop from baseline values indicates severe fetal distress.

High urine estriol levels are possible in multiple pregnancy.

Post-test care

As ordered, resume administration of medications discontinued before the test.

Interfering factors

□ Administration of the following drugs may influence urine estriol levels: steroid hormones (including estrogens, progesterone, and corticosteroids), methenamine mandelate, phenothiazines, ampicillin, phenazopyridine hydrochloride, tetracyclines, cascara sagrada, senna, phenolphthalein, hydrochlorothiazide, and meprobamate.

□ Maternal hemoglobinopathy, anemia, malnutrition, or hepatic or intestinal disease characteristically decreases estriol levels.

□ Failure to collect all urine during the 24-hour period may interfere with accurate determination of test results.

□ Failure to refrigerate the specimen or keep it on ice may alter test results.

□ Failure to maintain the prescribed pH level in the specimen may interfere with the accurate determination of test results.

SUSAN F. MORROW, RN

Urine Human Chorionic Gonadotropin

[Pregnancy test]

As a qualitative analysis of urine levels of human chorionic gonadotropin (hCG), this test can detect pregnancy as early as 10 days after a missed menstrual period. Quantitative measurements can evaluate suspected hydatidiform mole or hCG-secreting tumors. After conception, placental trophoblastic cells start to produce hCG, a glycoprotein, which prevents degeneration of the corpus luteum at the end of the normal menstrual cycle. The corpus luteum then secretes large quantities of progesterone and estrogen, promoting early development of the endometrium, placenta, and fetus. During the first trimester, hCG levels rise steadily and rapidly, peaking around the 10th week of gestation, subsequently tapering off to less than 10% of peak levels.

The most common method of evaluating hCG in urine is hemagglutination inhibition. This laboratory procedure based on an antigen-antibody reaction can provide both qualitative and quantitative information. The qualitative urine test is easier and less expensive than the serum hCG test (beta-subunit assay); so it's used more frequently to detect pregnancy. The earliest possible determination of pregnancy (as early as 7 days after conception) can be achieved only through the serum hCG test.

Purpose
□ To detect and confirm pregnancy
□ To aid diagnosis of hydatidiform mole or hCG-secreting tumors.

Patient preparation
Explain to the patient that this test determines whether she is pregnant (if this isn't the test's purpose, offer an appro-priate explanation). Tell her she needn't restrict food or fluids before the test. Inform her that the test requires a first-voided morning specimen or a 24-hour urine collection, depending on whether the test is qualitative or a quantitative. Check the patient's recent medication history for use of drugs that may affect hCG levels.

Procedure
For verification of pregnancy (qualitative analysis), collect a first-voided morning specimen. If this is not possible, collect a random specimen.

For quantitative analysis of hCG, collect a 24-hour urine specimen.

Specify the date of the patient's last menstrual period on the laboratory slip.

Precautions
Refrigerate the 24-hour specimen or keep it on ice during the collection period.

Values
In qualitative analysis, if agglutination fails to occur, test results are positive, indicating pregnancy.

In quantitative analysis, urine hCG levels in the first trimester of a normal pregnancy may be as high as 500,000 IU/24 hours; in the second trimester, they range from 10,000 to 25,000 IU/24 hours; and in the third trimester, from 5,000 to 15,000 IU/24 hours. After delivery, hCG levels decline rapidly and within a few days are undetectable.

Measurable hCG shouldn't be found in the urine of males or nonpregnant females.

Implications of results
During pregnancy, elevated urine hCG levels may indicate multiple pregnancy or erythroblastosis fetalis; depressed urine hCG levels may indicate threatened abortion or ectopic pregnancy. Measurable levels of hCG in males and non-pregnant females may indicate choriocarcinoma, ovarian or testicular tumors, melanoma, multiple myeloma, or gastric, hepatic, pancreatic, or breast cancer.

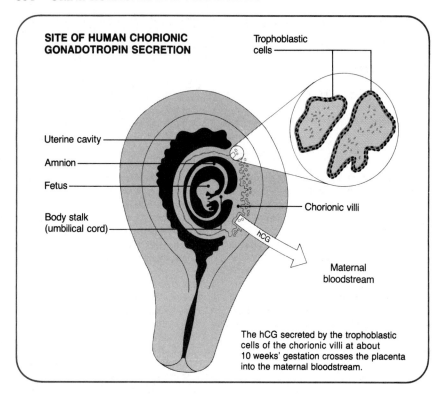

SITE OF HUMAN CHORIONIC GONADOTROPIN SECRETION

Trophoblastic cells

Uterine cavity

Amnion

Fetus

Body stalk (umbilical cord)

Chorionic villi

hCG

Maternal bloodstream

The hCG secreted by the trophoblastic cells of the chorionic villi at about 10 weeks' gestation crosses the placenta into the maternal bloodstream.

Post-test care
As ordered, resume administration of medications discontinued before the test.

Interfering factors
☐ Gross proteinuria (in excess of 1 g/ 24 hours), hematuria, or an elevated ESR may produce false-positive results, depending on laboratory method used.

☐ Early pregnancy, ectopic pregnancy, or threatened abortion may produce false-negative test results.
☐ Phenothiazines may cause false-negative or false-positive test results.
☐ Tap water or soap in the specimen may produce false-positive test results.

CATHERINE E. KIRBY, RN, BSN
SUSAN F. MORROW, RN

URINE METABOLITES

Urine Pregnanetriol

Using spectrophotometry, this test determines urine levels of pregnanetriol, the metabolite of the cortisol precursor 17-hydroxyprogesterone. Pregnanetriol is normally excreted in the urine in minute amounts. However, when cortisol

biosynthesis is impaired at the point of 17-hydroxyprogesterone conversion, urinary excretion of pregnanetriol rises significantly. Such impairment results from the absence or deficiency of particular biosynthetic enzymes that convert 17-hydroxyprogesterone to cortisol; in turn, low plasma cortisol levels interfere with the negative feedback mechanism that inhibits secretion of adrenocorti-

cotropic hormone (ACTH). Consequently, excessive 17-hydroxyprogesterone accumulates in the plasma, leading to increased formation and excretion of pregnanetriol in urine.

Urine pregnanetriol levels may be measured concomitantly with urine 17-ketosteroids and urine 17-ketogenic steroids, to assess androgen levels, which also rise with impairment of cortisol biosynthesis. Elevated androgen levels, which occur in adrenogenital syndrome (congenital adrenal hyperplasia), result from conversion of excessive 17-hydroxyprogesterone to androgens and from hypersecretion of adrenal androgens in response to excessive ACTH stimulation.

Purpose
□ To aid diagnosis of adrenogenital syndrome
□ To monitor cortisol replacement.

Patient preparation
Explain to the patient (or to his parents if the patient is a child) that this test evaluates hormonal secretion. Inform him that he need not restrict food or fluids before the test. Tell him the test requires collection of a 24-hour urine specimen, and teach him the proper collection technique.

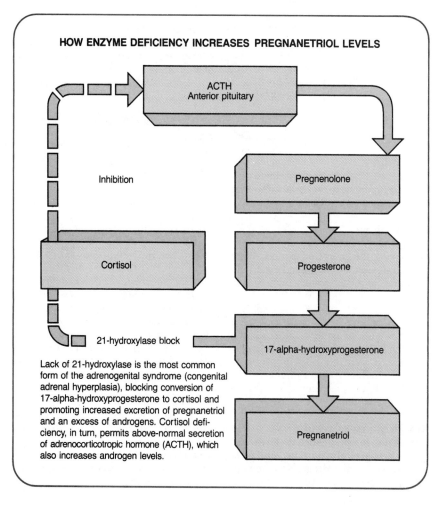

HOW ENZYME DEFICIENCY INCREASES PREGNANETRIOL LEVELS

Lack of 21-hydroxylase is the most common form of the adrenogenital syndrome (congenital adrenal hyperplasia), blocking conversion of 17-alpha-hydroxyprogesterone to cortisol and promoting increased excretion of pregnanetriol and an excess of androgens. Cortisol deficiency, in turn, permits above-normal secretion of adrenocorticotropic hormone (ACTH), which also increases androgen levels.

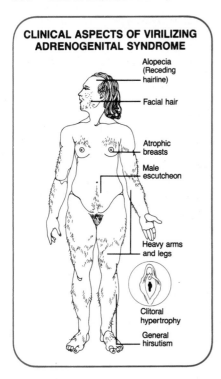

CLINICAL ASPECTS OF VIRILIZING ADRENOGENITAL SYNDROME

- Alopecia (Receding hairline)
- Facial hair
- Atrophic breasts
- Male escutcheon
- Heavy arms and legs
- Clitoral hypertrophy
- General hirsutism

Procedure

Collect a 24-hour urine specimen in a bottle containing a preservative to keep the specimen at a pH of 4.0 to 4.5.

Precautions

Refrigerate the specimen or keep it on ice during the collection period. When the collection is completed, send the specimen to the laboratory immediately.

Values

The normal rate of pregnanetriol excretion for adults is less than 3.5 mg/ 24 hours; for children aged 7 to 16, the rate ranges from 0.3 to 1.1 mg/24 hours; and for children younger than age 6 (including infants), the excretion rate is up to 0.2 mg/24 hours.

Implications of results

Elevated urine pregnanetriol levels suggest adrenogenital syndrome, marked by excessive adrenal androgen secretion and resulting virilization. Females with this

condition fail to develop normal secondary sex characteristics and show marked masculinization of external genitalia at birth. Males usually appear normal at birth but later develop signs of somatic and sexual precocity.

In monitoring treatment with cortisol replacement, elevated urine pregnanetriol levels indicate insufficient dosage of cortisol. When cortisol replacement adequately inhibits hypersecretion of ACTH and subsequent overproduction of 17-hydroxyprogesterone, pregnanetriol levels fall within the normal range.

Post-test care

None.

Interfering factors

Failure to collect all urine during the test period, or to store the specimen properly may interfere with test results.

CATHERINE E. KIRBY, RN, BSN

Urine 17-Hydroxy-corticosteroids

This test measures urine levels of 17-hydroxycorticosteroids (17-OHCS)— metabolites of the hormones that regulate gluconeogenesis. More than 80% of all urinary 17-OHCS are metabolites of cortisol, the primary adrenocortical steroid. Test findings thus reflect cortisol secretion and, indirectly, adrenocortical function. Since cortisol secretion varies diurnally and in response to stress and many other factors, urine 17-OHCS levels are most accurately determined from a 24-hour specimen. Column chromatography and spectrophotofluorometry with the Porter-Silber reagent are used to measure 17-OHCS levels. Levels of plasma cortisol, urine free cortisol, and urine 17-ketosteroids may be measured, and adrenocorticotropic hormone stimulation and suppression testing performed to confirm results of this test.

Purpose

☐ To assess adrenocortical function.

Patient preparation

Explain to the patient that this test evaluates how his adrenal glands are functioning. Inform him he needn't restrict food or fluids, but should avoid excessive physical exercise and stressful situations during the testing period. Tell him the test requires collection of a 24-hour urine specimen, and instruct him in the proper collection technique.

Check the patient's medication history for drugs that may affect 17-OHCS levels. Review your findings with the laboratory, then notify the doctor; he may restrict medications before the test.

Procedure

Collect a 24-hour urine specimen in a bottle containing a preservative, to prevent deterioration of the specimen.

Precautions

Refrigerate the specimen or place it on ice during the collection period.

Values

Normally, urine 17-OHCS values range from 4.5 to 12 mg/24 hours in males, and from 2.5 to 10 mg/24 hours in females. Children aged 8 to 12 years normally excrete less than 4.5 mg/24 hours; younger children excrete less than 1.5 mg/24 hours. Levels normally increase slightly during the first trimester of pregnancy. Patients who are obese or very muscular may excrete slightly higher amounts of 17-OHCS, due to increased cortisol catabolism.

Implications of results

Elevated urine 17-OHCS levels may indicate Cushing's syndrome, adrenal carcinoma or adenoma, or pituitary tumor. Increased levels may also occur in patients with virilism, hyperthyroidism, and severe hypertension. Extreme stress induced by conditions such as acute pancreatitis and eclampsia, also cause urine 17-OHCS levels to elevate above normal.

Low urine 17-OHCS levels may indicate Addison's disease, hypopituitarism, or myxedema.

Post-test care

☐ Patient may resume activity restricted during the test.
☐ If medications are restricted before the test, resume administration, as ordered.

Interfering factors

☐ Drugs such as the following may elevate urine 17-OHCS levels: meprobamate, phenothiazines, spironolactone, ascorbic acid, chloral hydrate, glutethimide, chlordiazepoxide, penicillin G, hydroxyzine, quinidine, quinine, iodides, and methenamine.
☐ Drugs such as the following may suppress urine 17-OHCS levels: hydralazine, phenytoin, thiazide diuretics, ethinamate, nalidixic acid, and reserpine.
☐ Failure to follow drug restrictions, to collect all urine during the test period, or to store the specimen properly may interfere with test results.

CATHERINE E. KIRBY, RN, BSN

Urine 17-Ketosteroids

This test uses the spectrophotofluorometric technique to measure urine levels of 17-ketosteroids (17-KS). Steroids and steroid metabolites characterized by a ketone group on carbon 17 in the steroid nucleus, 17-KS originate primarily in the adrenal glands but also in the testes, which produce one third of 17-KS in males, and in the ovaries, which produce a minimal amount of 17-KS in females. Although not all 17-KS are androgens, they cause androgenic effects. For example, excessive secretion of 17-KS may result in hirsutism and may increase clitoral or phallic size; in utero, elevated 17-KS levels may cause a female fetus to develop a male urogenital tract. Because 17-KS do not include all the androgens (testosterone, for example, the

17-KETOSTEROID FRACTIONATION NORMAL TEST VALUES (MG/24 HOURS)

STEROID	ADULT MALE	ADULT FEMALE	MALE (AGE 10 TO 15)	FEMALE (AGE 10 TO 15)	BOTH SEXES (AGE 0 TO 9)
ANDROSTERONE	2.2 to 5	0.5 to 2.4	0.2 to 2	0.2 to 2.5	≤ 1
DEHYDROEPIANDROS-TERONE	0 to 2.3	0 to 1.2	< 0.4	< 0.4	< 0.2
ETIOCHOLANOLONE	1.9 to 4.7	1.1 to 3	0.1 to 1.6	0.7 to 3.1	≤ 1
11-HYDROXYANDROS-TERONE	0.5 to 1.3	0.2 to 0.6	0.1 to 1.1	0.2 to 1	≤ 1
11-HYDROXYETIOCHO-LANOLONE	0.3 to 0.7	0.2 to 0.6	< 0.3	0.1 to 0.5	≤ 0.5
11-KETOANDROSTERONE	0 to 0.1	0 to 0.2	< 0.1	< 0.1	< 0.1
11-KETOETIOCHOLANO-LONE	0.2 to 0.7	0.2 to 0.6	0.2 to 0.6	0.1 to 0.6	≤ 0.7
PREGNANEDIOL	0.6 to 1.6	0.2 to 2.4	0.1 to 0.7	0.1 to 1.2	< 0.5
PREGNANETRIOL	0.6 to 1.3	0.1 to 1	0.2 to 0.6	0.1 to 0.6	< 0.3
5-PREGNANETRIOL	0 to 0.3	0 to 0.3	< 0.3	< 0.3	< 0.2
11-KETOPREGNANE-TRIOL	0 to 0.2	0 to 0.4	< 0.3	< 0.2	< 0.2

Through gas-liquid chromatography, this fractionation test shows which specific steroids in the 17-KS group are elevated or suppressed, and thus aids differential diagnosis of conditions suggested by abnormal 17-KS levels.

most potent androgen, is not a 17-KS), these levels provide only a rough estimate of androgenic activity. To provide additional information about androgen secretion, plasma testosterone levels may be measured concurrently; 17-KS fractionation may also be appropriate.

Purpose
□ To aid diagnosis of adrenal and gonadal dysfunction
□ To aid diagnosis of adrenogenital syndrome (congenital adrenal hyperplasia)
□ To monitor cortisol therapy in the treatment of adrenogenital syndrome.

Patient preparation
Explain to the patient that this test evaluates hormonal balance. Inform him he needn't restrict food or fluids before the test, but should avoid excessive physical exercise and stressful situations during the collection period. Tell him the test requires 24-hour urine collection, and instruct him in the proper collection technique.

If the female patient is menstruating, the urine collection may have to be postponed, since presence of blood in the specimen interferes with test findings.

Check the patient's medication history for drugs that may affect test results. Review your findings with the laboratory, then notify the doctor; he may want to restrict such drugs before the test.

Procedure
Collect a 24-hour urine specimen in a bottle containing a preservative to keep the specimen at a pH of 4.0 to 4.5.

Precautions
Refrigerate the specimen or place it on ice during the collection period. When

the collection is completed, send the specimen to the laboratory immediately.

Values

Normally, urine 17-KS values range from 6 to 21 mg/24 hours in men, and from 4 to 17 mg/24 hours in women. Children between ages 11 and 14 excrete 2 to 7 mg/24 hours; younger children and infants excrete 0.1 to 3 mg/24 hours.

Implications of results

Elevated urine 17-KS levels may result from adrenal hyperplasia, carcinoma or adenoma, or adrenogenital syndrome. In women, elevated levels may also indicate ovarian dysfunction—such as polycystic ovarian disease (Stein-Leventhal syndrome)—or lutein cell tumor of the ovary or androgenic arrhenoblastoma. In men, elevated 17-KS may indicate interstitial cell tumor of the testis. Characteristically, 17-KS levels also rise during pregnancy, severe stress, chronic illness, or debilitating disease.

Depressed urine 17-KS levels may result from Addison's disease, panhypopituitarism, eunuchoidism, or castration, and may occur in cretinism, myxedema, and nephrosis. When this test is used to monitor cortisol therapy for adrenogenital syndrome, 17-KS levels typically return to normal with adequate cortisol administration.

Post-test care

☐ Patient may resume activity restricted during the test.

☐ As ordered, resume administration of medications withheld before the test.

Interfering factors

☐ Meprobamate, phenothiazines, spironolactone, and oleandomycin may elevate urine 17-KS levels. Estrogens, penicillin, ethacrynic acid, and phenytoin may suppress 17-KS levels. Nalidixic acid and quinine may elevate or suppress 17-KS levels.

☐ Failure to observe drug restrictions, collect all urine, or to store the specimen properly may interfere with test results.

CATHERINE E. KIRBY, RN, BSN

Urine 17-Ketogenic Steroids

Using spectrophotofluorometry, this test determines urine levels of 17-ketogenic steroids (17-KGS), which consist of the 17-hydroxycorticosteroids—cortisol and its metabolites, for example—and other adrenocortical steroids, such as pregnanetriol, that can be oxidized in the laboratory to 17-ketosteroids. Because 17-KGS represent such a large group of steroids, this test provides an excellent overall assessment of adrenocortical function. For accurate diagnosis of specific disease, 17-KGS must be compared with results of other tests, including plasma ACTH, plasma cortisol, ACTH stimulation, single-dose metyrapone, and dexamethasone suppression.

Purpose

☐ To evaluate adenocortical function

☐ To aid diagnosis of Cushing's syndrome and Addison's disease.

Patient preparation

Explain to the patient that this test evaluates adrenal function. Inform him he needn't restrict food or fluids before the test, but should avoid excessive physical exercise and stressful situations during the collection period. Tell him the test requires 24-hour urine collection, and teach him how to collect such a specimen correctly. Check the history for drugs that may affect 17-KGS levels. Review your findings with the laboratory, then notify the doctor; he may want to withhold medications before the test.

Procedure

Collect a 24-hour urine specimen in a bottle containing a preservative to keep the specimen at a pH of 4.0 to 4.5.

Precautions

Refrigerate the specimen or keep it on

ice during the collection period. When the collection is completed, send the specimen to the laboratory immediately.

Values

Normally, urine 17-KGS levels range from 4 to 14 mg/24 hours in men, and from 2 to 12 mg/24 hours in women. Children aged 11 to 14 excrete 2 to 9 mg/24 hours; younger children and infants excrete 0.1 to 4 mg/24 hours.

Implications of results

Elevated urine 17-KGS levels reflect hyperadrenalism, as in Cushing's syndrome; some cases of adrenogenital syndrome (congenital adrenal hyperplasia); and adrenal carcinoma or adenoma. Levels rise with severe physical or emotional stress.

Low levels may reflect hypoadrenalism, as in Addison's disease, and may also be associated with panhypopituitarism, cretinism, and general wasting.

Post-test care

□ Patient may resume activity restricted before the test.

□ As ordered, resume administration of drugs withheld before the test.

Interfering factors

□ Urine 17-KGS levels may be elevated by ACTH therapy and by drugs such as meprobamate, phenothiazines, spironolactone, penicillin, oleandomycin, and hydralazine. Levels may be suppressed by estrogens, quinine, reserpine, and thiazides, as well as by long-term corticosteroid therapy. Nalidixic acid and dexamethasone may elevate or suppress urine 17-KGS levels.

□ Failure to observe drug restrictions, to collect all urine, or to store the specimen properly may alter test results.

CATHERINE E. KIRBY, RN, BSN

Urine Vanillylmandelic Acid

Using spectrophotofluorometry, this test determines urine levels of vanillylmandelic acid (VMA), a phenolic acid. VMA is the catecholamine metabolite that is normally most prevalent in the urine, and is the product of hepatic conversion of epinephrine and norepinephrine; urine VMA levels reflect endogenous production of these major catecholamines. Like the test for urine total catecholamines, this test helps detect catecholamine-secreting tumors—most prominently pheochromocytoma—and helps evalu-

URINARY VALUES IN PHEOCHROMOCYTOMA

METABOLITE	NORMAL EXCRETION RATE (MG/24HOURS)	USUAL RANGE IN PHEOCHROMOCYTOMA (MG/24 HOURS)
Free catecholamines	< 0.1	0.2 to 4
Metanephrines (normetanephrine plus metanephrine)	< 1.3	2.5 to 40
Vanillylmandelic acid	< 6.8	10 to 250

Adapted with permission from Karl Engelman, *Textbook of Medicine*, Vol. 2, edited by Paul B. Beeson and Walsh McDermott (15th ed.; Philadelphia: W.B. Saunders Co., 1979), p. 2204.

ate the function of the adrenal medulla, the primary site of catecholamine production. This test is performed preferably on a 24-hour urine specimen (not a random specimen) to overcome the effects of diurnal variations in catecholamine secretion. Other catecholamine metabolites—metanephrine, normetanephrine, and homovanillic acid (HVA)—may be measured at the same time.

Purpose
□ To help detect pheochromocytoma, neuroblastoma, and ganglioneuroma
□ To evaluate the function of the adrenal medulla.

Patient preparation
Explain to the patient that this test evaluates hormonal secretion. Instruct him to restrict foods and beverages containing phenolic acid, such as coffee, tea, bananas, citrus fruits, chocolate, and vanilla, for 3 days before the test, and to avoid stressful situations and excessive physical activity during the urine collection period. Tell him the test requires collection of a 24-hour urine specimen, and teach him the proper collection technique.

Check the patient's medication history for drugs that may affect test results. Review your findings with the laboratory, then notify the doctor; he may want to withhold these drugs before the test.

Procedure
Collect a 24-hour urine specimen in a bottle containing a preservative, to keep the specimen at a pH of 3.0.

Precautions
Refrigerate the specimen or keep it on ice during the collection period. When the collection is completed, send the specimen to the laboratory immediately.

Values
Normally, urine VMA values range from 0.7 to 6.8 mg/24 hours.

Implications of results
Elevated urine VMA levels may result

URINE DETERMINATIONS IN DIAGNOSIS OF CATECHOLAMINE-SECRETING TUMORS

Although a pheochromocytoma is a catecholamine-producing tumor, causing hypersecretion of epinephrine and norepinephrine by the adrenal medulla, not every patient shows elevations of catecholamines in the urine. Moreover, hypertension, a prime clue in this condition, is sometimes absent. Thus, an analysis of one or more catecholamine metabolites offers diagnostic support to an analysis of total catecholamines.

When catecholamines remain normal in the presence of hypertension, elevated vanillylmandelic acid (VMA) may signal a tumor. Or metanephrine may be high, when VMA and catecholamines are essentially unchanged. VMA assay is also an alternate method, when catecholamine analysis has been compromised by interfering food or drugs. Elevated excretion of homovanillic acid (HVA) typically indicates malignant pheochromocytoma, although the incidence of malignancy is very low.

Measurement of urine VMA is diagnostically useful in two neurogenic tumors—neuroblastoma, a common soft-tissue tumor that's a leading cause of death in infants and young children, and ganglioneuroma, a well-defined tumor of the sympathetic nervous system that occurs in older children and young adults. Both tumors primarily produce dopamine and give the expected high readings of dopamine's metabolite HVA, especially in their malignant forms. But both disorders also show abnormal increases in urine VMA.

---

from a catecholamine-secreting tumor. Further testing, such as measurement of urine HVA levels to rule out pheochromocytoma, is necessary for precise diagnosis. If pheochromocytoma is confirmed, the patient may be tested for multiple endocrine neoplasia, an inherited condition commonly associated with pheochromocytoma. (Family members of a patient with confirmed pheochromocytoma should also be carefully evaluated for multiple endocrine neoplasia.)

Post-test care
As ordered, resume administration of medications withheld before the test. Also, as appropriate, the patient may resume his normal diet and activity.

Interfering factors

□ Epinephrine, norepinephrine, lithium carbonate, and methocarbamol may raise urine VMA levels. Chlorpromazine, guanethidine, reserpine, monoamine oxidase inhibitors, and clonidine may lower VMA levels. Levodopa and salicylates may raise or lower VMA levels.

□ Failure to observe drug and dietary restrictions, to collect all urine during the test period, or to store the specimen properly may interfere with test results.

□ Excessive physical exercise or emotional stress may raise VMA levels.

CATHERINE E. KIRBY, RN, BSN

Urine Homovanillic Acid

This test is a quantitative analysis of urine levels of homovanillic acid (HVA), which is a metabolite of dopamine, one of the three major catecholamines. Synthesized primarily in the brain, dopamine is a precursor to epinephrine and norepinephrine, the other principal catecholamines. The liver breaks down most dopamine into HVA, for eventual excretion; a minimal amount of dopamine appears in the urine.

Using two-dimensional chromatography, urine HVA levels are usually measured simultaneously with the major catecholamines and other catecholamine metabolites—metanephrine, normetanephrine, and vanillylmandelic acid. The principal indication for this test is suspected neuroblastoma or ganglioneuroma, which usually affects children and adolescents.

Purpose

□ To aid diagnosis of neuroblastoma and ganglioneuroma
□ To rule out pheochromocytoma.

Patient preparation

Explain to the patient that this test assesses hormone secretion. Inform him that he needn't restrict food or fluids before the test, but should avoid stressful situations and excessive physical exercise during the collection period. Tell him the test requires collection of a 24-hour urine specimen, and teach him the proper collection technique.

Check the patient's history for drugs that may affect test results. Review your findings with the laboratory, then notify the doctor; he may want to withhold these medications before the test.

Procedure

Collect a 24-hour urine specimen in a bottle containing a preservative, to keep the specimen at a pH of 2.0 to 4.0.

Precautions

Refrigerate the specimen or keep it on ice during the collection period. When the collection is completed, send the specimen to the laboratory immediately.

Values

Normally, the urine HVA value for adults is less than 8 mg/24 hours. The range of normal urine HVA (mcg/mg creatinine) values in children varies with age:

Age (years)	HVA
15 to 17	0.5 to 2
10 to 15	0.25 to 12
5 to 10	0.5 to 9
2 to 5	0.5 to 13.5
1 to 2	4 to 23
0 to 1	1.2 to 35.

Implications of results

Elevated urine HVA levels suggest neuroblastoma, a malignant soft-tissue tumor that develops in infants and young children, or ganglioneuroma, a tumor of the sympathetic nervous system that develops in older children and adolescents and rarely metastasizes. HVA levels don't usually rise in patients with pheochromocytoma, because this tumor secretes mainly epinephrine, which metabolizes primarily into vanillylmandelic acid. Thus, an abnormally high urine HVA level generally rules out pheochromocytoma.

Post-test care

As ordered, resume administration of medications withheld before the test. The patient may also resume activity restricted during the test.

Interfering factors

☐ Monoamine oxidase inhibitors decrease urine HVA levels by inhibiting dopamine metabolism. Aspirin, methocarbamol, and levodopa may raise or lower HVA levels.

☐ Failure to observe drug restrictions, to collect all urine during the test period, or to store the specimen properly may interfere with test results.

☐ Excessive physical exercise or emotional stress during the collection period may raise HVA levels.

CATHERINE E. KIRBY, RN, BSN

Urine 5-Hydroxyindoleacetic Acid

This quantitative analysis of urine levels of 5-hydroxyindoleacetic acid (5-HIAA) is used mainly to screen for carcinoid tumors (argentaffinomas). Urine 5-HIAA levels reflect plasma concentrations of serotonin (5-hydroxytryptamine). This powerful vasopressor is produced by argentaffin cells, primarily in the intestinal mucosa, and is metabolized through oxidative deamination into 5-HIAA. Carcinoid tumors, found generally in the intestine or appendix, secrete an excessive amount of serotonin, which is reflected by high 5-HIAA levels. This test measures 5-HIAA levels by the colorimetric technique, and is most accurately performed with a 24-hour urine specimen, which can detect small or intermittently secreting carcinoid tumors.

Purpose

☐ To aid diagnosis of carcinoid tumors (argentaffinomas).

Patient preparation

Explain to the patient what serotonin is and why this test is important. Instruct him not to eat foods containing serotonin, such as bananas, plums, pineapples, avocados, eggplants, tomatoes, or walnuts, for 4 days before the test. Tell him the test requires collection of a 24-hour urine specimen, and teach him the proper collection technique.

Check the patient's history for recent use of drugs that may affect test results. Review your findings with the laboratory, then notify the doctor; he may want to withhold these drugs before the test.

Procedure

Collect a 24-hour urine specimen in a bottle containing a preservative, to keep the specimen at a pH of 2.0 to 4.0.

Precautions

Refrigerate the specimen or keep it on ice during the collection period. When the collection is completed, send the specimen to the laboratory immediately.

Values

Normally, urine 5-HIAA values are less than 6 mg/24 hours.

Implications of results

Marked elevation of urine 5-HIAA levels, possibly as high as 200 to 600 mg/24 hours, indicates a carcinoid tumor. However, since these tumors vary in their capacity to store and secrete serotonin, some patients with carcinoid syndrome (metastatic carcinoid tumors) may not show elevated levels. Repeated testing is often necessary.

Post-test care

As ordered, resume administration of medications withheld before the test. The patient may resume his normal diet restricted before the test.

Interfering factors

☐ Melphalan, reserpine, and fluorouracil raise urine 5-HIAA levels. Ethanol, tricyclic antidepressants, monoamine oxidase inhibitors, methyldopa, and iso-

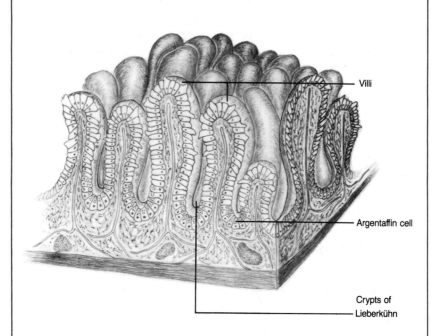

ARGENTAFFIN CELLS: SITE OF SEROTONIN SECRETION

Villi

Argentaffin cell

Crypts of Lieberkühn

Argentaffin cells in the crypts of Lieberkühn, the indentations between the villi in the mucosa of the small intestine, produce serotonin, which metabolizes into 5-hydroxyindoleacetic acid. High urine levels of this acid can signal the presence of serotonin-secreting argentaffinomas—carcinoid tumors that arise from the argentaffin cells.

Adapted from Myrin Borysenko, et al, *Functional Histology: A Core Text* (Boston: Little, Brown & Co., 1979), p. 144. Used by permission of the author.

niazid characteristically suppress 5-HIAA levels.

□ Methenamine compounds, phenothiazines, salicylates, guaifenesin, mephenesin, methocarbamol, and acetaminophen may raise or lower 5-HIAA levels.

□ Failure to observe drug and dietary restrictions, to collect all urine during the test period, or to store the specimen properly may interfere with accurate determination of test results.

□ Severe gastrointestinal disturbance or diarrhea may interfere with accurate determination of test results.

WILLIAM M. DOUGHERTY, BS

Urine Pregnanediol

Using gas chromatography or radioimmunoassay, this test measures urine levels of pregnanediol, the chief metabolite of progesterone. Although biologically inert, pregnanediol has diagnostic significance because it reflects about 10% of the endogenous production of its parent hormone. Progesterone is produced in nonpregnant females by the corpus luteum during the latter half of each menstrual cycle, preparing the uterus for implantation of a fertilized ovum. If implantation doesn't occur, progesterone secretion drops sharply; if implantation does occur, the corpus luteum secretes more progesterone, to further prepare the uterus for pregnancy and to begin development of the placenta. Toward the end of the first trimester, the placenta becomes the primary source of progesterone secretion, producing the progressively larger amounts needed to maintain pregnancy.

Normally, urine levels of pregnanediol reflect variations in progesterone secretion during the menstrual cycle and during pregnancy. Direct measurement of plasma progesterone levels by radioimmunoassay may also be done. Pregnanediol is present in the urine as a metabolite of progesterone and is produced in small amounts by the adrenal cortex, the principal site of secretion in males, postmenopausal women, and menstruating females before ovulation.

Purpose
□ To evaluate placental function in pregnant females
□ To evaluate ovarian function in nonpregnant females.

Patient preparation
Explain to the patient that this test evaluates placental or ovarian function. Inform her she needn't restrict food or fluids. Tell her the test requires a 24-hour urine specimen, and teach her the proper collection technique.

Check the patient's medication history for recent use of drugs that may affect pregnanediol levels.

Procedure
Collect a 24-hour urine specimen.

Precautions
□ Refrigerate the specimen or keep it on ice during the collection period.
□ If the patient is pregnant, note the approximate week of gestation on the laboratory slip. For other premenopausal females, note the stage of the menstrual cycle on the laboratory slip.

Values
In nonpregnant females, urine pregnanediol values normally range from 0.5 to 1.5 mg/24 hours during the proliferative phase of the menstrual cycle. Within 24 hours after ovulation, pregnanediol levels begin to rise and continue to rise for 3 to 10 days, as the corpus luteum develops. During this luteal phase, normal urine pregnandiol values range from 2 to 7 mg/24 hours. In the absence of fertilization, levels drop sharply, as the corpus luteum degenerates and menstruation begins.

During pregnancy, urine pregnanediol levels rise markedly (see graph on page 406), peaking around the 36th week of gestation and returning to prepregnancy levels by day 5 to 10 postpartum.

Normal postmenopausal values range from 0.2 to 1 mg/24 hours. In males, urine pregnanediol levels rarely rise above 1.5 mg/24 hours.

Implications of results
During pregnancy, a marked decrease in urine pregnanediol levels based on a single 24-hour urine specimen, or a steady decrease in pregnanediol levels in serial measurements may indicate placental insufficiency and necessitates immediate investigation. A precipitous drop in pregnanediol values may suggest fetal distress, as in threatened abortion or preeclampsia, or fetal death. However, pregnanediol measurements are not reliable indicators of fetal viability, since levels can remain normal even after fetal death, as long as maternal circulation to the placenta remains adequate.

In nonpregnant females, abnormally low urine pregnanediol levels may occur with anovulation, amenorrhea, or other menstrual abnormalities. Low to normal pregnanediol levels may be associated with hydatidiform mole. Elevations may indicate luteinized granulosa or theca cell tumors, diffuse thecal luteinization, or metastatic ovarian cancer.

Adrenal hyperplasia or biliary tract obstruction may elevate urine pregnane-

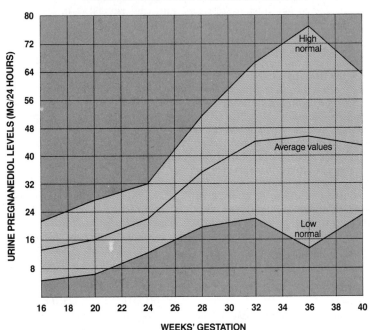

URINE PREGNANEDIOL IN NORMAL PREGNANCY

Serial determinations of the *average* levels (middle line on chart) of pregnanediol rise steadily until about 32 weeks' gestation, then level off. Excretion decreases 24 hours postpartum and drops to prepregnancy levels within 5 to 10 days. A wide range of normal values is possible—high normal, low normal, and average levels.

Adapted with permission from R. P. Sherman, *Journal of Obstetrics and Gynecology.* 66:1, 1959.

diol values in males or females. Some forms of primary hepatic disease produce abnormally low levels in both sexes.

Post-test care
□ As ordered, resume administration of drugs withheld before the test.
□ Advise the pregnant patient that this test may be repeated several times to obtain serial measurements.

Interfering factors
□ Methenamine mandelate, methena-mine hippurate, and drugs containing adrenocorticotropic hormone elevate urine pregnanediol levels. Progestogens and combination oral contraceptives characteristically lower pregnanediol levels.

□ Failure to collect all urine during the collection period may influence the test results.

□ Failure to refrigerate the specimen or to keep it on ice during the collection period may alter test results.

CATHERINE E. KIRBY, RN, BSN

Selected References

Bondy, Philip K., and Rosenberg, Leon E. *Diseases of Metabolism,* 8th ed. Philadelphia: W.B. Saunders Co., 1980.

Danforth, David N., ed. *Obstetrics and Gynecology,* 4th ed. Philadelphia: J. B. Lippincott Co., 1982.

DeGroot, Leslie J., ed. *Endocrinology,* vols. 1 and 2. New York: Grune & Stratton, 1979.

Endocrine Disorders, Nurse's Clinical Library. Springhouse, Pa.: Springhouse Corp., 1984.

Gold, Jay J., and Iosinovich, John B. *Gynecologic Endocrinology,* 3rd ed. New York: Harper & Row Publishers, 1980.

Green, Thomas H., Jr. *Gynecology: Essentials of Clinical Practice,* 3rd ed. Boston: Little, Brown & Co., 1977.

Guyton, Arthur C. *Textbook of Medical Physiology,* 6th ed. Philadelphia: W.B. Saunders Co., 1981.

Halsted, Charles H., and Halsted, James A. *The Laboratory in Clinical Medicine.* Philadelphia: W.B. Saunders Co., 1981.

Hansten, Philip D. *Drug Interactions,* 4th ed. Philadelphia: Lea & Febiger, 1979.

Harrison, J., et al., eds. *Campbell's Urology,* 4th ed. Philadelphia: W.B. Saunders Co., 1978.

Henry, John Bernard, ed. *Todd-Sanford-Davidsohn Clinical Diagnosis and Management by Laboratory Methods,* vol. 1, 17th ed. Philadelphia: W.B. Saunders Co., 1984.

Jensen, David. *The Principles of Physiology,* 2nd ed. East Norwalk, Conn.: Appleton-Century-Crofts, 1980.

Jensen, Margaret, et al. *Maternity Care: The Nurse and the Family,* 2nd ed. St. Louis: C.V. Mosby Co., 1981.

Lamb, Jane O. *Laboratory Tests for Clinical Nursing.* Bowie, Md.: Robert J. Brady Co., 1984.

Olds, Sally B. *Obstetric Nursing.* Reading, Mass.: Addison-Wesley Publishing Co., 1980.

Petersdorf, Robert G., and Adams, Raymond D., eds. *Harrison's Principles of Internal Medicine,* 10th ed. New York: McGraw-Hill Book Co., 1983.

Price, Sylvia, and Wilson, Lorraine. *Pathophysiology: Clinical Concepts of Disease Processes,* 2nd ed. New York: McGraw-Hill Book Co., 1982.

Pritchard, Jack A., and MacDonald, Paul C. *Williams Obstetrics,* 16th ed. East Norwalk, Conn.: Appleton-Century-Crofts, 1980.

Ravel, Richard. *Clinical Laboratory Medicine,* 3rd ed. Chicago: Year Book Medical Pubs., 1978.

Tilkian, Sarko M., et al. *Clinical Implications of Laboratory Tests,* 3rd ed. St. Louis: C.V. Mosby Co., 1983.

Vander, A.J., et al. *Human Physiology: The Mechanisms of Body Function,* 2nd ed. New York: McGraw-Hill Book Co., 1980.

Wallach, Jacques B. *Interpretation of Diagnostic Tests: A Handbook Synopsis of Laboratory Medicine,* 3rd ed. Boston: Little, Brown & Co., 1978.

Widmann, Frances K. *Clinical Interpretation of Laboratory Tests,* 9th ed. Philadelphia: F.A. Davis Co., 1983.

Williams, Robert H. *Textbook of Endocrinology,* 6th ed. Philadelphia: W.B. Saunders Co., 1981.

15 Urine Proteins, Protein Metabolites, and Pigments

LEARNING OBJECTIVES

After completing this chapter, the reader will be able to:
- explain the function of urine proteins, protein metabolites, and pigments.
- describe the process of glomerular filtration.
- state the formula for calculating plasma clearance for any substance.
- discuss how the differential diagnosis of jaundice is made.
- know the bedside methods for detecting blood pigments in urine.
- state the purpose of each test discussed in the chapter.
- prepare the patient physically and psychologically for each test.
- describe the procedure for performing each test.
- implement appropriate post-test care.
- state the normal values for each test.
- discuss the implications of abnormal test results.
- list factors that may interfere with accurate test results.

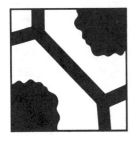

Urine Proteins, Protein Metabolites, and Pigments

Introduction

Laboratory analysis of urine specimens for abnormal levels of proteins, protein metabolites, and pigments is a significant factor in the detection and management of renal disease and in the diagnosis of certain extrarenal or systemic diseases. For example, abnormalities easily detected by analytical techniques include proteinuria and the presence of the pigments hemoglobin, bilirubin, urobilinogen, and the porphyrins. Examination of urine for protein metabolites is especially useful in evaluating renal function, since healthy kidneys excrete these nonprotein nitrogenous (NPN) end products of protein metabolism.

Proteins

Normally, the protein content of urine is too small to be detected by routine screening procedures. Urine contains minute amounts of plasma proteins of low molecular weight or renal mucoproteins derived from the tubular cells. Benign proteinuria can result from changes in body position, as in orthostatic proteinuria, or can be associated with stress, exposure to cold, or fever.

Unusually high levels of proteins in urine, detectable by screening tests, nearly always indicate renal disease. Pathologic proteinuria can result from increased glomerular permeability due to a variety of causes, including glomerulonephritis,

congestive heart failure, or renal tubular damage with defective reabsorption of protein. Infections of the lower urinary tract (cystitis, for example) can also cause proteinuria.

In most forms of renal disease marked by proteinuria, the predominant protein found in the urine is albumin, because it's the smallest, the most easily filterable, and the most prevalent of all proteins. As kidney damage progresses, however, proteins of higher molecular weight—including the larger globulins—escape into the urine. The presence of certain abnormal proteins in urine has special diagnostic significance; for example, Bence Jones protein in urine strongly suggests multiple myeloma.

Protein metabolites

Plasma contains more than 15 different NPN compounds, predominantly urea; amino acids, creatine, creatinine, and uric acid are also important NPN constituents of plasma. The kidneys normally excrete these nitrogenous waste products of protein metabolism, but diminished renal function causes these substances (including urea, uric acid, and creatinine) to accumulate in plasma. Consequently, renal dysfunction lowers the urine levels of these substances. However, urine levels of urea and of uric acid may change as a result of conditions other than renal disease—an important

ANALYZING PROTEIN AND METABOLITE SPECIMENS

SUBSTANCE	NORMAL LEVELS IN URINE	IMPLICATIONS OF ABNORMAL LEVELS
PROTEINS		
Protein	Less than 150 mg/24 hr	▲ Increased glomerular permeability; urinary tract disorders; acute or chronic renal disease; other diseases, such as leukemia and toxemia
Bence Jones protein	Negative	▲ Multiple myeloma
PROTEIN METABOLITES		
Amino acids	50 to 200 mg/24 hr	▲ Defective tubular reabsorption, resulting in increased renal excretion; congenital enzyme deficiencies, leading to metabolic disorders, such as phenylketonuria and cystinuria
Hydroxyproline	14 to 45 mg/24 hours for adults (higher for children and women in the third trimester of pregnancy)	▲ Increased bone resorption caused by such disorders as Paget's disease, myeloma, or hyperthyroidism ▼ Drug treatment that decreases bone resorption
Creatinine	Clearance in men (age 20): 90 ml/min/1.73m^2 Clearance in women (age 20): 84 ml/min/1.73m^2 (Concentrations decrease 6 ml/min/decade in older patients)	▼ Reduced renal blood flow, acute tubular necrosis, acute or chronic glomerulonephritis, advanced bilateral chronic pyelonephritis, advanced bilateral renal lesions, nephrosclerosis, severe dehydration, congestive heart failure
Urea	Maximal clearance: 64 to 99 ml/min	▼ Reduced renal blood flow, acute or chronic glomerulonephritis, advanced bilateral chronic pyelonephritis, acute tubular necrosis, nephrosclerosis, advanced bilateral renal lesions, bilateral ureteral obstruction, congestive heart failure, dehydration
Uric acid	250 to 750 mg/24 hr (varies with purine intake)	▲ Chronic myeloid leukemia, polycythemia vera, multiple myeloma, pernicious anemia, lymphosarcoma and lymphatic leukemia during radiotherapy, defective tubular reabsorption, Wilson's disease ▼ Chronic glomerulonephritis, diabetic glomerulosclerosis, collagen disorders

diagnostic consideration. Excessive purine catabolism, for example—which may be caused by a pathologic condition, such as leukemia, or simply by a high-purine diet—can raise both serum and urine uric acid levels, since uric acid is a product of purine metabolism. Several factors, including dehydration, dietary ingestion of protein, and hepatic disease, can cause alterations in the levels of blood urea nitrogen (BUN) and urine urea.

Because formation and urinary excretion of creatinine are more constant than urea and uric acid levels, serum and urine creatinine determinations provide a more reliable index of renal function. By comparing serum creatinine concentration with the total amount of creatinine excreted within a specified period, the creatinine clearance test shows how efficiently the kidneys are removing this substance from the blood. Values for this extremely important diagnostic test typically decrease when renal function is impaired.

Urinary excretion of amino acids is fairly constant in a healthy adult. However, metabolic disturbances can cause amino acids to accumulate in plasma and, when they exceed the renal threshold, to appear in the urine in excessive amounts. Urine amino acid screening can detect these overflow aminoacidurias.

Testing for the amino acid hydroxyproline helps detect disorders that affect bone metabolism.

Urine pigments

Pigments are involved in the biosynthesis of hemoglobin and its subsequent breakdown. A conjugated protein comprising an iron-containing pigment (heme) and a protein (globin), *hemoglobin* normally appears in RBCs, where its primary function is to carry oxygen from the lungs to body tissues. Hemoglobin is *not* a normal component of urine. However, when the amount of free hemoglobin in plasma exceeds the binding capacity of haptoglobin, as in severe intravascular hemolysis, hemoglobinuria results.

Myoglobin, which is closely related to hemoglobin in chemical composition, usually appears in cardiac and skeletal muscle, and like hemoglobin, it doesn't usually appear in urine. Consequently, the presence of myoglobin in urine may indicate extensive muscle damage.

Porphyrins may be considered metabolic intermediates in heme synthesis, which takes place mainly in the marrow of the long bones and in the liver.

Biosynthesis of heme begins with formation of delta-aminolevulinic acid and progresses through porphobilinogen to the precursors uroporphyrinogen, coproporphyrinogen, protoporphyrinogen, and finally, protoporphyrin, which chelates iron to form heme. Porphyrinogens are hematologically active. The inactive end products are normally excreted in small quantities: protoporphyrin is excreted exclusively in feces, and coproporphyrin and uroporphyrin, in feces or urine.

Metabolic defects in heme biosynthesis may cause inherited or acquired porphyrin disorders. Increased urinary excretion of specific porphyrins may aid diagnosis of a particular porphyrin disorder, perhaps assisted by results of fecal and erythrocyte porphyrin testing.

The breakdown of the heme fraction of hemoglobin results in the formation of *bilirubin.* In the liver, free bilirubin conjugates with glucuronic acid, which allows bilirubin to be filtered by the glomeruli (unconjugated bilirubin is not filterable). Bilirubin is normally excreted in bile as its principal pigment, but it is an abnormal element of urine. Conjugated bilirubin is present in urine when serum levels are elevated, as in biliary tract obstruction or hepatocellular damage, and is accompanied by jaundice.

Urobilinogen is formed in the intestine by bacterial action on conjugated bilirubin. Most urobilinogen is eventually excreted in feces, producing its characteristic color. A small amount of urobilinogen is reabsorbed by the portal system and is mainly reexcreted in bile, although the kidneys do excrete some. Therefore, elevated urine urobilinogen levels may be an early indication of hepatic damage. In biliary obstruction, since bilirubin doesn't reach the intestines, urine urobilinogen levels decrease.

Melanin, the main pigment of the hair, skin, and choroid of the eye, is formed from the metabolism of tyrosine and is not normally present in urine. However, melanin-producing tumors (melanomas) may produce sufficient amounts of this pigment to be detected in urine. In liver metastasis, melanins and their precursors—melanogens—commonly appear in urine.

PATRICIA J. NOONE, RN, BSN, MEd
MARY GYETVAN, RN, BSED

PROTEINS

Urine Protein

This is a quantitative test for proteinuria. Normally, the glomerular membrane allows only proteins of low molecular weight to enter the filtrate. The renal tubules then reabsorb most of these proteins, normally excreting a small amount that's undetectable by a screening test. A damaged glomerular capillary membrane and impaired tubular reabsorption allow excretion of proteins in the urine.

A qualitative screening often precedes this test. A positive result requires quantitative analysis of a 24-hour urine specimen by acid precipitation tests. Electrophoresis can detect Bence Jones protein, hemoglobins, myoglobins, or albumin.

Purpose
□ To aid diagnosis of pathologic states characterized by proteinuria, primarily renal disease.

Patient preparation
Explain to the patient that this test detects proteins in the urine. Inform him he needn't restrict food or fluids. Tell him the test usually requires a 24-hour urine collection.

Check the patient's history for drugs that may affect test results. Review your findings with the laboratory, and then notify the doctor; he may want to restrict medications before the test.

Procedure
Collect a 24 hour urine specimen. A special specimen container can be obtained from the laboratory.

Precautions
□ Tell the patient not to contaminate the urine with toilet tissue or stool.
□ Refrigerate the specimen or place it on ice during the collection period.

POSTURAL PROTEINURIA: A SPECIAL CASE

A benign form of proteinuria, postural (orthostatic) proteinuria occurs when a patient stands but not when he's recumbent. It can also happen when he assumes a lordotic position—from bending backward over a chair, for example. Generally, this condition is found in healthy children or young adults and has no pathologic significance, although it causes heavy proteinuria.

Postural proteinuria probably results from obstruction of renal venous outflow, which causes renal congestion and ischemia. To confirm this condition, diagnostic tests must rule out renal disease and clearly establish the absence of proteinuria during recumbency. In one test, the patient voids before retiring and remains recumbent for 12 hours. A urine specimen is collected as soon as he awakens and, for comparison, at specific times during the next 12 hours, while he is ambulatory. In postural proteinuria, the specimen collected at the end of recumbency is free of proteins, but proteins do appear in the ones collected during the ambulatory period.

Values

Normal values show up to 150 mg of protein excreted in 24 hours.

Implications of results

Proteinuria is pathognomonic of renal disease. When proteinuria is present in a single specimen, 24-hour urine collection is subsequently required to identify specific renal abnormalities.

Proteinuria can result from glomular leakage of plasma proteins (a major cause of protein excretion), from overflow of filtered proteins of low molecular weight (when these are present in excessive concentrations), from impaired tubular reabsorption of filtered proteins, and from the presence of renal proteins derived due to the breakdown of kidney tissue.

Persistent proteinuria indicates renal disease resulting from increased glomerular permeability. *Minimal* proteinuria (less than 0.5 g/24 hours), however, is most often associated with renal diseases in which glomerular involvement is not a major factor, such as chronic pyelonephritis.

Moderate proteinuria (0.5 to 4 g/24 hours) occurs in several types of renal disease—acute or chronic glomerulonephritis, amyloidosis, toxic nephropathies—or in diseases in which renal failure often develops as a late complication (diabetes or heart failure, for example). *Heavy proteinuria* (more than 4 g/24 hours) is commonly associated with nephrotic syndrome.

When accompanied by an elevated WBC count, proteinuria indicates urinary tract infection; with hematuria, proteinuria indicates local or diffuse urinary tract disorders. Other pathologic states (infections and lesions of the central nervous system, for example) can also result in detectable amounts of proteins in the urine.

Many drugs (such as amphotericin B, gold preparations, aminoglycosides, polymyxins, and trimethadione) inflict renal damage, causing true proteinuria. This makes the routine evaluation of urine proteins essential during such treatment.

In all forms of proteinuria, fractionation results obtained by electrophoresis provide more precise information than the screening test. For example, excessive hemoglobin in the urine indicates intravascular hemolysis; elevated myoglobin suggests muscle damage; albumin, increased glomerular permeability; and Bence Jones protein, multiple myeloma.

Not all forms of proteinuria have

RANDOM SPECIMEN SCREENING FOR PROTEIN

Qualitative screening tests for proteinuria include reagent strips (dipsticks) and acids that precipitate proteins (sulfosalicylic acid, or acetic acid with heat).

To perform such a test, collect a clean-catch urine specimen, preferably in the morning, when the urine is most concentrated and yields the most reliable information. Commonly, a reagent strip (such as Combistix) is used. Dip the strip into the urine; remove excess urine by taping the strip against a clean surface or the edge of the container; hold the strip in a horizontal position to prevent mixing of chemicals from adjacent areas. Immediately place the strip close to the color block on the bottle and carefully compare colors. The results correspond to mg/dl of protein (usually albumin, since strips are most sensitive to albumin).

Negative	=	0 to 5 mg/dl
Trace	=	5 to 20 mg/dl
1 +	=	30 mg/dl
2 +	=	100 mg/dl
3 +	=	300 mg/dl
4 +	=	1,000 mg/dl

Normally, no detectable protein is present in a random specimen, although normal kidneys do excrete a minute amount. A positive result requires quantitative analysis of a 24-hour urine specimen.

Phenazopyridine can alter the color reaction of certain brands of reagent strips; so can high salt or alkaline content of the urine specimen. Acetazolamide and sodium bicarbonate can cause false-positive results with some reagent strips.

GLOMERULAR FILTRATION: FIRST STEP IN URINE FORMATION

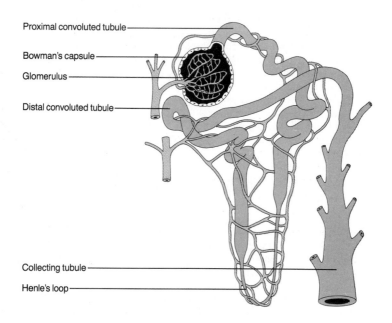

Proximal convoluted tubule

Bowman's capsule

Glomerulus

Distal convoluted tubule

Collecting tubule

Henle's loop

The nephron, the functional unit of the kidney, is the site of glomerular filtration and tubular reabsorption and secretion. Filtration begins when an afferent arteriole carries blood to the glomeruli, extremely porous capillaries enclosed by Bowman's capsules, in the nephron's outer cortex. High hydrostatic pressure in the glomeruli forces small molecules of water, glucose, and other nutrients; sodium, potassium, chloride, urea, and other metabolites; and amino acids through an afferent arteriole into Bowman's capsules; erythrocytes and proteins of high molecular weight (such as albumin) remain unfiltered. The glomerular filtrate joins organic wastes and excess salts secreted from surrounding renal tissues and flows through the convoluted proximal and distal tubules comprising Henle's loop into the straight collecting tubule.

pathologic significance. *Benign* proteinuria can result from changes in body position. *Functional* proteinuria is associated with emotional or physiologic stress, and is usually transient.

Post-test care
As ordered, resume administration of medications withheld before the test.

Interfering factors
□ Administration of tolbutamide, para-aminosalicylic acid, acetazolamide, sodium bicarbonate, penicillin, sulfonamides, iodine contrast media, and cephalosporins may cause false-positive results in acid precipitation tests.
□ Contamination of the urine specimen with heavy mucus, vaginal or prostatic secretions, or the presence of numerous WBCs can alter test results, regardless of laboratory method.
□ Very dilute urine (which may result from forcing fluids) may depress protein values and cause false-negative results.

DEBRA C. BROADWELL, RN, MN, ET

Urine Bence Jones Protein

Bence Jones proteins are abnormal light-chain immunoglobulins of low molecular weight that are derived from the clone of a single plasma cell (monoclonal). This globulin appears in the urine of 50% to 80% of patients with multiple myeloma and in most patients with Waldenström's macroglobulinemia.

In most cases, these proteins—thought to be synthesized by malignant plasma cells in the bone marrow—are rapidly cleared from the plasma and don't usually appear in serum. When these proteins exceed renal tubular capacity to break down and reabsorb them, they overflow and are excreted in the urine (overflow proteinuria). Eventually, the renal tubular cells degenerate from the effort to reabsorb excess amounts of protein. Consequently, protein precipitates and inclusions occur in the renal tubular cells. If renal failure results from such precipitation or from hypercalcemia, increased uric acid, or infiltration by abnormal plasma cells, more Bence Jones proteins and other proteins then appear in the urine, since the dysfunctional nephrons no longer control protein excretion.

Urine screening tests, such as thermal coagulation and Bradshaw's test, can detect Bence Jones proteins, but urine immunoelectrophoresis is usually the method of choice for quantitative studies. Serum immunoelectrophoresis, which is sometimes used, is less sensitive than the urine tests. Nevertheless, both urine and serum studies are frequently used for patients suspected of having multiple myeloma.

Purpose
□ To confirm the presence of multiple myeloma in patients with characteristic clinical signs, such as bone pain (especially in the back and thorax) and persistent anemia and fatigue.

Patient preparation
Explain to the patient that this test can detect an abnormal protein in the urine. Tell him the test requires an early-morning urine specimen, and teach him how to collect a clean-catch specimen.

Procedure
Collect an early-morning urine specimen of at least 50 ml.

Precautions
□ Instruct patient not to contaminate urine specimen with toilet tissue or stool.
□ Send the specimen to the laboratory immediately. If transport is delayed, refrigerate the specimen.

Values
Normal urine should contain no Bence Jones proteins.

Implications of results
The presence of Bence Jones proteins in urine suggests multiple myeloma or Waldenström's macroglobulinemia. Very low levels, in the absence of other symptoms, may result from benign monoclonal gammopathy. However, clinical evidence figures prominently in diagnosis of multiple myeloma.

Post-test care
None.

Interfering factors
□ False-positive results may occur in connective tissue disease, renal insufficiency, or certain malignancies.
□ Contamination of the specimen with menstrual blood, prostatic secretions, or semen may cause false-positive results.
□ Failure to send the specimen to the laboratory immediately or to keep the specimen refrigerated may cause a false-positive result, because heat-coagulable protein denatures or decomposes at room temperature.

BEVERLY ZENK WHEAT, RN, MA
SR. REBECCA FIDLER, MT(ASCP), PHD

PROTEIN METABOLITES

Urine Amino Acid Screening

This test screens for aminoaciduria— elevated urine amino acid levels—a condition that may result from inborn errors of metabolism, due to the absence of specific enzymatic activities. (Normally, up to 200 mg of amino acids may be excreted in the urine in 24 hours.) Abnormal metabolism causes an excess of one or more amino acids to appear in plasma and, as the renal threshold is exceeded, in urine. Aminoacidurias may be classified as either primary (overflow) aminoacidopathies or as secondary (renal) aminoacidopathies. The latter type is associated with conditions marked by defective tubular reabsorption from congenital disorders. A more specific defect, such as cystinuria, may cause one or more amino acids to appear in urine.

To screen newborns, children, and adults for congenital aminoacidurias, plasma or urine specimens may be used. The plasma test is the better indicator of overflow aminoacidurias; urine testing is used to confirm or monitor certain amino acid disorders and to screen for renal aminoacidurias.

Various laboratory techniques are available to screen for aminoacidurias, but chromatography is the preferred method. Positive findings on chromatography can be elaborated by fractionation, showing specific amino acid levels. Testing for specific amino acid levels is also necessary for infants or young children with acidosis, severe vomiting and diarrhea, and abnormal urine odor. Such testing is especially important in newborns, because early diagnosis of certain aminoacidurias may prevent mental retardation by allowing prompt treatment.

Purpose
☐ To screen for renal aminoacidurias
☐ To follow up plasma test findings when results of these tests suggest certain overflow aminoacidurias.

Patient preparation
Explain to the patient (or to his parents if the patient is an infant or a child) that this test helps detect amino acid disorders, and that additional tests may be

CHROMATOGRAPHIC IDENTIFICATION OF AMINO ACID DISORDERS

Chromatographic Band No.	Amino Acids
1	Leucine, isoleucine
2	Phenylalanine
3	Valine, methionine
4	Tryptophan, beta-amino isobutyric acid
5	Tyrosine
6	Proline
7	Alanine, ethanolamine
8	Threonine, glutamic acid
9	Homocitrulline, glycine, serine, hydroxyproline, aspartic acid, glutamine, citrulline
10	Homocystine, asparagine
11	Argininosuccinic acid, histidine, arginine, lysine, ornithine, cystathionine, cystine, cysteine, hydroxylysine

Reproduced with permission from *The Bio-Science Handbook* (Van Nuys, Calif.: Bio-Science Enterprises).

necessary. Inform him he needn't restrict food or fluids before the test. Tell him the test requires a urine specimen.

Check the patient's medication history for drugs that may interfere with test results. If such drugs must be continued, note this on the laboratory slip. (If the patient is a breast-fed infant, record any drugs the mother is receiving.)

Procedure

If the patient is an infant, clean and dry the genital area, attach the collection device, and observe for voiding. Transfer urine—at least 20 ml—to a specimen container. If the patient is an adult or a child, collect a fresh random specimen.

Precautions

☐ For an infant, apply the adhesive flanges of the collection device securely to the skin, to prevent leakage.
☐ Send the specimen to the laboratory immediately.

Values

Patterns on thin-layer chromatography are reported as normal.

METABOLIC AMINO ACID DISORDERS

PKU		Maple Syrup Urine Disease		Cystinuria		Homocystinuria		Hartnup Disease		Argininosuccinic-aciduria		Histidinemia		Hyperprolin-emia Type A		Citrullin-uria	
Plasma	Urine	Plasma	Urine	Plasma	Urine	Plasma	Urine	Plasma	Urine	Plasma	Urine	Plasma	Urine	Plasma	Urine	Plasma	Urine
		+	+						+								
+	+								+								
		+	+			+			+							+	
									+								
									+								
		+												+	+		
									+				+				+
													+				+
		+							+	+						+	+
								+									
					+				+	+		+	+				+

KEY: + = Increased amino acids in the plasma and/or urine

In chromatography—the preferred method for screening aminoacidurias—amino acids migrate into multicolored bands. (The sequence of amino acids and their corresponding band numbers, as listed above, reflect these standard migratory patterns.) When congenital enzyme deficiencies and subsequent metabolic disorders increase plasma and urine amino acid levels, these bands intensify.

Implications of results

If thin-layer chromatography shows gross changes or abnormal patterns, blood and 24-hour urine quantitative column chromatography are performed to identify specific amino acid abnormalities and to differentiate overflow and renal aminoacidurias (see chart, pages 416 and 417).

Post-test care

Remove the collection device carefully from an infant, to prevent skin irritation.

Interfering factors

□ Failure to send the urine specimen to the laboratory immediately may interfere with the accurate determination of test results.

□ Results are invalid in a newborn who has not ingested dietary protein in the 48 hours preceding the test.

DEBRA C. BROADWELL, RN, MN, ET

Urine Hydroxyproline

This test measures total urine levels of hydroxyproline, an amino acid found mainly in collagen (a component of skin and bone). Urine hydroxyproline levels are a good index of bone matrix turnover, because levels increase when collagen breaks down during bone resorption. Bone matrix turnover and hydroxyproline levels normally rise in children during periods of rapid skeletal growth. However, they also rise in disorders that increase bone resorption, such as Paget's disease, metastatic bone tumors, and certain endocrine disorders. This test helps diagnose these disorders, but it's more commonly used to monitor response to drug therapy in conditions marked by rapid bone resorption.

Hydroxyproline levels are most often determined colorimetrically on a timed urine sample; they may also be determined by ion-exchange or gas-liquid chromatography. A collagen-restricted diet is essential for this test, because hydroxyproline levels reflect collagen intake. Free hydroxyproline, a small component of total hydroxyproline and a sensitive indicator of dietary collagen intake, may be measured to validate results.

Purpose

□ To monitor treatment for disorders characterized by bone resorption, primarily Paget's disease

□ To aid diagnosis of disorders characterized by bone resorption.

Patient preparation

Explain to the patient that this test helps monitor treatment or detect an amino acid disorder related to bone formation. Inform him that he must not eat meat, fish, poultry, jelly, or any foods containing gelatin for 24 hours before the test and during the test period itself. Tell him the test requires a 2-hour or 24-hour urine specimen, as appropriate, and teach him the correct collection technique.

Note the patient's age and sex on the laboratory slip. Check his history for drugs that may alter test results. Restrict such drugs as ordered.

Procedure

Collect a 2-hour or 24-hour urine specimen, as ordered, in a container that has a preservative to prevent degradation of hydroxyproline.

Precautions

Refrigerate the specimen or keep it on ice during the collection period, and send it to the laboratory immediately.

Values

Normal values for adults are 14 to 45 mg/24 hours; or 0.4 to 5 mg/2-hour specimen (males) and 0.4 to 2.9 mg/2-hour specimen (females). Normal values for children are much higher, and peak between ages 11 and 18. Values also rise during the third trimester of pregnancy, reflecting fetal skeletal growth.

Implications of results

Hydroxyproline levels should decrease slowly during therapy for bone resorption disorders. Elevated levels may indicate bone disease; metastatic bone tumors; or endocrine disorders that stimulate hormonal secretion.

Post-test care

As ordered, resume foods and drugs withheld before the test.

Interfering factors

□ Ascorbic acid, vitamin D, aspirin, and glucocorticoids, as well as calcitonin and mithramycin (used to treat Paget's disease), can decrease levels.
□ Failure to observe restrictions, to collect all urine during the test period, or to store the specimen correctly may alter test results.
□ Psoriasis and burns can promote collagen turnover, elevating urine hydroxyproline levels.

TOBIE VIRGINIA HITTLE, RN, BSN, CCRN

Urine Creatinine

This test measures urine levels of creatinine, the chief metabolite of creatine. Produced in amounts proportional to total body muscle mass, creatinine is removed from the plasma primarily by glomerular filtration and is excreted in the urine. Since the body doesn't recycle it, creatinine has a relatively high, constant clearance rate, making it an efficient indicator of renal function. However, the creatinine clearance test, which measures both urine and plasma creatinine clearance, is a more precise index than this test. A standard method for determining urine creatinine levels is based on Jaffé's reaction, in which creatinine treated with an alkaline picrate solution yields a bright orange-red complex.

Purpose

□ To help assess glomerular filtration

□ To check the accuracy of 24-hour urine collection, based on the relatively constant levels of creatinine excretion.

Patient preparation

Explain to the patient that this test helps evaluate kidney function. Inform him he need not restrict fluids but should not eat an excessive amount of meat before the test, and should avoid strenuous physical exercise during the collection period. Tell him the test usually requires a 24-hour urine specimen, and teach him the proper collection technique.

Check the patient's medication history for drugs that may affect creatinine levels. Review your findings with the laboratory, then notify the doctor; he may restrict such drugs before the test.

Procedure

Collect a 24-hour urine specimen in a specimen bottle that contains a preservative to prevent the degradation of creatinine.

Precautions

Refrigerate the specimen or keep it on ice during the collection period. When the collection is completed, send the specimen to the laboratory immediately.

Values

Normally, urine creatinine levels range from 1 to 1.9 g/24 hours for men, and from 0.8 to 1.7 g/24 hours for women.

Implications of results

Decreased urine creatinine levels may result from impaired renal perfusion (associated with shock, for example) or from renal disease due to urinary tract obstruction. Chronic bilateral pyelonephritis, acute or chronic glomerulonephritis, and polycystic kidney disease may also depress creatinine levels. Increased urine creatinine levels generally have little diagnostic significance.

Post-test care

□ As ordered, resume medications.
□ The patient may resume his diet and normal activity.

Interfering factors
☐ Drugs that may affect urine creatinine levels include corticosteroids, gentamicin, tetracyclines, diuretics, and amphotericin B.
☐ Failure to observe pretest restrictions, to collect all urine during the test period, or to store the specimen properly may interfere with test results.

MALINDA S. MITCHELL, RN, MS

Creatinine Clearance

Creatinine, an anhydride of creatine, is formed and excreted in constant amounts by an irreversible reaction, and functions solely as the main end product of creatine. Creatinine production is proportional to total muscle mass and is relatively unaffected by normal physical activity, diet, or urine volume.

An excellent diagnostic indicator of renal function, the creatinine clearance test determines how efficiently the kidneys are clearing creatinine from the blood. The rate of clearance is expressed in terms of the volume of blood (in ml) that can be cleared of creatinine in 1 minute. To arrive at this determination, the equation $C = (U x V) \div P$ is used; C represents the clearance rate; U equals the urine concentration of creatinine; V, the volume of urine collected during the test period (converted to ml/minute); and P, the plasma concentration of creatinine. Naturally, urine and plasma concentrations of creatinine must be expressed in the same units (usually mg/dl), so they cancel each other in the equation.

A final adjustment must be made to allow for renal parenchymal mass, which differs in each patient. To do this, the clearance rate established in the above equation is multiplied by $(1.73 \div A)$, where 1.73 equals the body surface area (in square meters) of the average person, and A equals the patient's surface area. Creatinine levels become abnormal when

more than 50% of the total nephron units have been damaged.

Purpose
☐ To assess renal function (primarily glomerular filtration)
☐ To monitor progression of renal insufficiency.

Patient preparation
Explain to the patient that this test assesses kidney function. Inform him he needn't restrict fluids but should not eat an excessive amount of meat before the test, and should avoid strenuous physical exercise during the collection period. Tell him the test requires a timed urine specimen and at least one blood sample. Tell him how the urine specimen will be collected; who will perform the venipuncture and when; and that he may feel some discomfort from the needle puncture. Reassure him that collecting the blood sample takes less than 3 minutes. Explain that more than one venipuncture may be necessary.

Check the patient's medication history for drugs that may affect creatinine clearance. Review your findings with the laboratory, then notify the doctor; he may want to restrict these medications before the test.

Procedure
Collect a timed urine specimen at 2, 6, 12, or 24 hours, in a bottle containing a preservative to prevent degradation of the creatinine.

Perform a venipuncture anytime during the collection period, and collect the sample in a 7 ml *red-top* tube.

Precautions
Refrigerate the urine specimen or keep it on ice during the collection period. When the collection is completed, send the specimen to the laboratory immediately.

Values
For men (age 20), normal creatinine clearance is 90 ml/minute/1.73 m² of body surface; for women (age 20), 84 ml/

CLEARANCE PRINCIPLE

Clearance refers to renal capacity to remove various substances from the plasma. Although plasma clearance values of certain substances (inulin, creatinine) can parallel their glomerular filtration rate, tubular reabsorption and/or secretion of other measured substances (sodium, para-aminohippurate, and uric acid) disqualify clearance tests as an assessment of glomerular filtration.

To calculate plasma clearance for *any* substance, use this formula:

Plasma clearance (ml/min) = urinary concentration (mg/dl) × urinary volume (ml/min)
———
Plasma concentration (mg/dl)

---

minute/1.73 m². For older patients, concentrations normally decrease by 6 ml/minute/decade.

Implications of results

Low creatinine clearance may result from reduced renal blood flow (associated with shock or renal artery obstruction), acute tubular necrosis, acute or chronic glomerulonephritis, advanced bilateral chronic pyelonephritis, advanced bilateral renal lesions (as in polycystic kidney disease, renal tuberculosis, and malignancy), or nephrosclerosis. Congestive heart failure and severe dehydration may also cause creatinine clearance to fall below normal.

High creatinine clearance rates generally have little diagnostic significance.

Post-test care

☐ If a hematoma develops at the venipuncture site, apply warm soaks to ease discomfort.
☐ As ordered, resume administration of medications withheld before the test.
☐ The patient may resume his diet and normal activity.

Interfering factors

☐ Drugs that may affect creatinine clearance include amphotericin B, thiazide diuretics, furosemide, and aminoglycosides.
☐ A high-protein diet before the test and strenuous physical exercise during the collection period may increase creatinine excretion.
☐ Failure to observe pretest restrictions, to collect all urine during the test period,

or to store the specimen properly may interfere with accurate determination of test results.

MALINDA S. MITCHELL, RN, MS

Urea Clearance

The urea clearance test is a quantitative analysis of urine levels of urea, the main nitrogenous component in urine and the end product of protein metabolism. After filtration by the glomeruli, roughly 40% of the urea is reabsorbed by the renal tubules. Because of this reabsorption, urea clearance was once considered a precise fraction (60%) of the glomerular filtration rate (GFR). However, since the reabsorption rate of urea varies with the amount of water reabsorbed, this test actually assesses overall renal function; the creatinine clearance test provides a more accurate evaluation of the GFR. In urea clearance, blood urea content and the total amount of urea excreted in the urine are proportional only when the rate of urine flow is 2 ml/minute or higher (maximal clearance). At lower flow rates, the accuracy of the test decreases. The equation for determining urea clearance is $C = (U \times V) \div P$; it's similar to the equation used for creatinine clearance (see also CREATININE CLEARANCE).

Purpose

☐ To assess total renal function.

HOW UREA IS FORMED

Urea, the main nitrogenous component in urine, is the final product of protein metabolism. Amino acids absorbed by the intestinal villi pass from the portal vein into the liver. Since the liver stores only small amounts of amino acids—which are later returned to the blood for use in the synthesis of enzymes, hormones, or new protoplasm—the excess is converted into other substances, such as glucose, glycogen, or fat.

Before this conversion, the amino acids are deaminated—they lose their nitrogenous amino groups (NH_2^-). These amino groups are then converted to ammonia. Since ammonia is very toxic, especially to the brain, it must be removed as quickly as it's formed. (Serious liver disease causes elevated blood ammonia levels and eventually leads to hepatic coma.) In the liver, ammonia combines with carbon dioxide to form urea, which is released into the blood and ultimately secreted in urine.

Patient preparation

Explain to the patient that this test evaluates kidney function. Instruct him to fast from midnight before the test and to abstain from exercise before and during the test. Tell him the test requires two timed urine specimens and one blood sample. Tell him how the urine specimens will be collected; who will perform the venipuncture and when; and that he may experience transient discomfort from the needle puncture. Reassure him that collecting the blood sample takes less than 3 minutes.

Check the patient's medication history for drugs that may affect urea clearance. Review your findings with the laboratory, then notify the doctor; he may want to restrict medications before the test.

Procedure

Instruct the patient to empty his bladder and discard the urine. Then give him water to drink to assure adequate urine output. Collect two specimens 1 hour apart, and mark the collection time on the laboratory slip. Perform a venipuncture anytime during the collection pe-

riod, and collect the sample in a 7 ml *red-top* tube.

Precautions

☐ Since this is a clearance test, make sure the patient empties his bladder, and that the total amount of urine is collected from each hour's specimen.
☐ Send each specimen to the laboratory as soon as it is collected.
☐ If the patient is catheterized, empty the drainage bag before beginning the specimen collection.
☐ Handle the blood sample gently to prevent hemolysis, and send it to the laboratory immediately.

Values

Normally, the urea clearance rate ranges from 64 to 99 ml/minute with maximal clearance. If the flow rate is less than 2 ml/minute, normal clearance is 41 to 68 ml/minute. (If the urine flow rate is less than 1 ml/minute, this test should not be performed.)

Implications of results

Low urea clearance values may indicate decreased renal blood flow (due to shock or renal artery obstruction), acute or chronic glomerulonephritis, advanced bilateral chronic pyelonephritis, acute tubular necrosis, or nephrosclerosis. Diminished clearance rates may also result from advanced bilateral renal lesions (as in polycystic kidney disease, renal tuberculosis, or malignancy), bilateral ureteral obstruction, congestive heart failure, or dehydration.

High urea clearance usually is not diagnostically significant.

Post-test care

☐ If a hematoma develops at the venipuncture site, apply warm soaks.
☐ As ordered, resume administration of medications that were withheld before the test.
☐ The patient may resume his diet and normal activity.

Interfering factors

☐ The patient's failure to empty his bladder completely—the most common error in this test—and to observe pretest restrictions interfere with the accurate determination of test results.

□ Caffeine, milk, or small doses of epinephrine increase urea clearance; antidiuretic hormone or large doses of epinephrine decrease urea clearance. Corticosteroids, amphotericin B, thiazide diuretics, and streptomycin may also affect test results.

□ Hemolysis caused by rough handling of the blood sample may interfere with accurate determination of test results.

MALINDA S. MITCHELL, RN, MS

Urine Uric Acid

A quantitative analysis of urine uric acid levels, this test supplements serum uric acid testing for identifying disorders that alter production or excretion of uric acid (such as leukemia, gout, and renal dysfunction). Derived from dietary purines in organ meats (liver, kidney, and sweetbread) and from endogenous nucleoproteins, uric acid (as urate) is found normally in the blood and in other tissues in amounts totaling about 1 g. Its primary site of formation is the liver, although the intestinal mucosa is also involved in urate production. As the chief end product of purine catabolism, urate passes from the liver through the bloodstream to the kidneys, where roughly 50% is excreted daily in the urine. Renal urate metabolism is complex, involving glomerular filtration, tubular secretion, and a second reabsorption by the renal tubules.

The most specific laboratory method for detecting uric acid is spectrophotometric absorption, after treatment of the specimen with the enzyme uricase.

Purpose

□ To detect enzyme deficiencies and metabolic disturbances that affect uric acid production

□ To help measure the efficiency of renal clearance.

Patient preparation

Explain to the patient that this test measures the body's production and excretion of a waste product known as uric acid. Inform him that he needn't restrict food or fluids before the test. Tell him the test requires a 24-hour urine specimen, and teach him the proper collection technique.

Check the patient's medication history for recent use of drugs that may influence uric acid levels. If these medications must be continued, note this on the laboratory slip.

Procedure

Collect a 24-hour urine specimen.

Precautions

Send the specimen to the laboratory immediately at the end of the collection period.

Values

Normal urine uric acid values vary with diet but generally range from 250 to 750 mg/24 hours.

Implications of results

Elevated urine uric acid levels may result from chronic myeloid leukemia, polycythemia vera, multiple myeloma, and early remission in pernicious anemia, and may occur in lymphosarcoma and lymphatic leukemia during radiotherapy. High levels also result from tubular reabsorption defects, such as Fanconi's syndrome and hepatolenticular degeneration (Wilson's disease).

Low urine uric acid levels occur in gout (when associated with normal uric acid production but inadequate excretion), and in severe renal damage, such as that resulting from chronic glomerulonephritis, diabetic glomerulosclerosis, and collagen disorders.

Post-test care

As ordered, resume administration of medications withheld before the test.

Interfering factors

☐ Drugs that decrease urine uric acid excretion include diuretics, such as benzthiazide, furosemide, and ethacrynic acid, as well as pyrazinamide. Low doses of salicylates, phenylbutazone, and probenecid also lower uric acid levels; high doses of these drugs cause levels to rise above normal. Allo-purinol, a drug used to treat gout, increases uric acid excretion.

☐ Urine uric acid concentrations rise with a high-purine diet and fall with a low-purine diet.

☐ Failure to observe drug restrictions or to collect all urine during the test period may alter test results.

MALINDA S. MITCHELL, RN, MS

PIGMENTS

Urine Hemoglobin

Free hemoglobin in the urine—an abnormal finding—may occur in hemolytic anemias or in severe intravascular hemolysis resulting from a transfusion reaction. Contained within RBCs, hemoglobin consists of heme—an iron-protoporphyrin complex—and globin—a polypeptide. Hemoglobin combines with oxygen and carbon dioxide, to allow RBCs to deliver these gases between the lungs and the tissues. Aging RBCs are constantly being destroyed by normal mechanisms within the reticuloendothelial system. However, when RBC destruction occurs within the circulation, as in intravascular hemolysis, free hemoglobin enters the plasma and binds with haptoglobin, a plasma alpha$_2$-globulin. If the plasma level of hemoglobin exceeds that of haptoglobin, the excess of unbound hemoglobin is excreted in the urine (hemoglobinuria).

This test is based on the fact that heme proteins act like enzymes that catalyze oxidation of organic substances, such as guaiac or orthotolidine. This reaction produces a blue coloration; the intensity of color varies with the amount of hemoglobin present. Microscopic examination is required to identify intact RBCs in urine (hematuria), which can occur in the presence of unbound hemoglobin.

Purpose

☐ To aid diagnosis of hemolytic ane-

mias, or severe intravascular hemolysis from a transfusion reaction.

Patient preparation

Explain to the patient that this test detects excessive RBC destruction. Inform him he needn't restrict food or fluids. Tell him the test requires a random urine specimen, and teach him the proper collection technique. If the female patient is menstruating, reschedule the test, since contamination of the specimen with menstrual blood alters test results.

Check the patient's medication history for drugs that may affect free hemoglobin levels. Review your findings with the laboratory, then notify the doctor; he may want to restrict these medications before the test.

Procedure

Collect a random urine specimen.

Precautions

Send the specimen to the laboratory immediately.

Values

Normally, hemoglobin is not present in the urine.

Implications of results

Hemoglobinuria may result from severe intravascular hemolysis due to a blood transfusion reaction, burns, or a crushing injury; from acquired hemolytic anemias caused by chemical or drug intoxication or malaria; or from the hemolytic anemia known as paroxysmal nocturnal hemoglobinuria. Hemoglobinuria may also result from congenital hemolytic anemias, as in hemoglobinopathies or enzyme defects, and, less commonly, is associated with cystitis, ureteral calculi, or urethritis.

Hemoglobinuria and hematuria occur in renal epithelial damage (as in acute glomerulonephritis or pyelonephritis), renal tumor, and tuberculosis.

Post-test care

As ordered, resume administration of medications discontinued before the test.

Interfering factors

☐ Lysis of RBCs in stale or alkaline urine and contamination of the specimen with menstrual blood alter test results.

☐ Bacterial peroxidases in highly infected specimens can produce false-positive test results.

☐ Large doses of vitamin C or of drugs that contain vitamin C as a preservative (such as certain antibiotics) can inhibit reagent activity, producing false-negative results. Nephrotoxic drugs (such as amphotericin B) or anticoagulants (such as warfarin) may cause a positive result for hemoglobinuria or hematuria.

WILLIAM M. DOUGHERTY, BS

Urine Myoglobin

This test detects the presence of myoglobin—a red pigment found in the cytoplasm of cardiac and skeletal muscle cells—in the urine. Myoglobin probably serves as a reservoir of oxygen, facilitating its movement within muscle. When muscle cells are extensively damaged, as by disease or severe crushing trauma, myoglobin is released into the blood, quickly cleared by renal glomerular filtration, and eliminated in the urine (myoglobinuria). For example, myoglobin appears in the urine within 24 hours after myocardial infarction. Because of the marked structural similarities of

urine myoglobin and urine hemoglobin, they are not satisfactorily differentiated by qualitative assays.

The test method most commonly used to detect myoglobinuria is the differential precipitation test. Hemoglobin—bound to haptoglobin—precipitates when urine is mixed with ammonium sulfate. Myoglobin, however, remains soluble and can be measured.

Purpose

☐ To aid diagnosis of muscular disease
☐ To detect extensive infarction of muscle tissue

BEDSIDE TESTING FOR URINE BLOOD PIGMENTS

To test a patient's urine for blood pigments at bedside, use one of the following methods:

Dipstick (Hemastix):
• Collect a urine specimen.
• Dip the stick into the specimen, and withdraw it.
• After 30 seconds, compare the stick with the color chart. Blue indicates a positive reaction; the intensity of color indicates pigment concentration.

Occult tablet:
• Collect a urine specimen.
• Put one drop of urine on the filter paper. Place the tablet on the urine, and then put two drops of water on the tablet.
• After 2 minutes, inspect the filter paper around the tablet. Blue indicates a positive reaction; the intensity of color indicates pigment concentration.

Occult solution:
• Collect a urine specimen.
• After placing one drop of urine on the filter paper, close the package and turn it over. Open the opposite side, and place two drops of solution on the filter paper.
• After 30 seconds, inspect the filter paper. Blue indicates a positive reaction; the intensity of color indicates pigment concentration.

Because these methods detect only blood pigments, immunochemical studies are necessary to differentiate hemoglobin from other blood pigments, such as myoglobin.

□ To assess the extent of muscular damage from crushing trauma.

Patient preparation

Explain to the patient that this test detects a red pigment found in muscle cells and helps evaluate muscle injury or disease. Inform him he needn't restrict food or fluids before the test. Tell him that this test requires a random urine specimen, and teach him the proper technique for collecting the specimen. Advise him that test results are generally available in 1 day.

Procedure

Collect a random urine specimen.

Precautions

Send the specimen to the laboratory immediately.

Values

Normally, myoglobin does not appear in the urine.

Implications of results

Myoglobinuria occurs in acute or chronic muscular disease, alcoholic polymyopathy, familial myoglobinuria, and extensive myocardial infarction. Myoglobinuria also results from severe trauma to the skeletal muscles (as in a crushing injury, extreme hyperthermia, or severe burns). Transient myoglobinuria ("march" myoglobinuria) may follow strenuous or prolonged exercise. This form of myoglobinuria disappears after a period of rest.

Post-test care

None.

Interfering factors

□ If this test is performed with reagent strips—Hemastix, for example—the recent ingestion of large amounts of vitamin C can inhibit the test reaction, thereby interfering with accurate determination of test results.

□ Extremely dilute urine can reduce test sensitivity.

WILLIAM M. DOUGHERTY, BS

Urine Porphyrins

This test is a quantitative analysis of urine porphyrins (most notably, uroporphyrins and coproporphyrins) and their precursors (porphyrinogens, such as porphobilinogen [PBG]). Porphyrins are red-orange fluorescent compounds, consisting of four pyrrole rings, that are produced during heme biosynthesis. They are present in all protoplasm, figure in energy storage and utilization, and are normally excreted in urine in small amounts. Elevated urine levels of porphyrins or porphyrinogens, therefore, reflect impaired heme biosynthesis. Such impairment may result from inherited enzyme deficiencies (congenital porphyrias) or from defects caused by disorders such as hemolytic anemias and hepatic disease (acquired porphyrias).

Determination of the specific porphyrins and porphyrinogens found in a urine specimen can help identify the impaired metabolic step in heme biosynthesis. Occasionally, a preliminary qualitative screening is performed on a random specimen; a positive finding on the screening test must be confirmed by the quantitative analysis of a 24-hour specimen. For correct diagnosis of a specific porphyria, urine porphyrin levels should be correlated with plasma and fecal porphyrin levels.

Purpose

□ To aid diagnosis of congenital or acquired porphyrias.

Patient preparation

Explain to the patient that this test detects abnormal hemoglobin formation. Inform him he needn't restrict food or fluids before the test. Tell him the test requires a 24-hour urine specimen, and teach him the proper collection technique.

Check the patient's history for current pregnancy, menstruation, or drug use; such conditions may interfere with ac-

27PIGMENTS

P

curate determination of test results. Inform the laboratory and the doctor, who may reschedule the test or restrict drugs before the test.

Procedure

Collect a 24-hour urine specimen in a light-resistant specimen bottle containing a preservative to prevent degradation

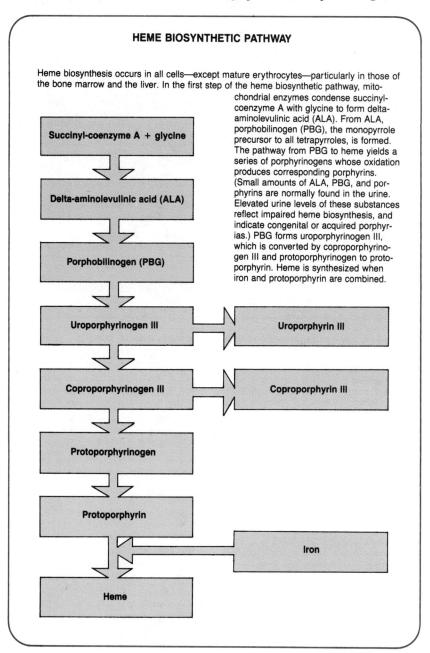

HEME BIOSYNTHETIC PATHWAY

Heme biosynthesis occurs in all cells—except mature erythrocytes—particularly in those of the bone marrow and the liver. In the first step of the heme biosynthetic pathway, mitochondrial enzymes condense succinyl-coenzyme A with glycine to form delta-aminolevulinic acid (ALA). From ALA, porphobilinogen (PBG), the monopyrrole precursor to all tetrapyrroles, is formed. The pathway from PBG to heme yields a series of porphyrinogens whose oxidation produces corresponding porphyrins. (Small amounts of ALA, PBG, and porphyrins are normally found in the urine. Elevated urine levels of these substances reflect impaired heme biosynthesis, and indicate congenital or acquired porphyrias.) PBG forms uroporphyrinogen III, which is converted by coproporphyrinogen III and protoporphyrinogen to protoporphyrin. Heme is synthesized when iron and protoporphyrin are combined.

Succinyl-coenzyme A + glycine

Delta-aminolevulinic acid (ALA)

Porphobilinogen (PBG)

Uroporphyrinogen III → Uroporphyrin III

Coproporphyrinogen III → Coproporphyrin III

Protoporphyrinogen

Protoporphyrin

Iron

Heme

URINE PORPHYRIN LEVELS IN PORPHYRIA

PORPHYRIA	PORPHYRIN PRECURSORS	
	ALA	PBG
Erythropoietic porphyria	Normal	Normal
Erythropoietic protoporphyria	Normal	Normal
Acute intermittent porphyria	Highly increased	Highly increased
Variegate porphyria	Highly increased during acute attack	Normal or slightly increased; highly increased during acute attack
Coproporphyria	Increased during acute attack	Increased during acute attack
Porphyria cutanea tarda (assumed to be acquired in association with other hepatic diseases; genetic causes possible)	Variable	Variable

Defective heme biosynthesis increases urinary porphyrins and their corresponding precursors.

of the light-sensitive porphyrins and their precursors.

Precautions
□ Refrigerate the specimen or keep it on ice during the collection period. Then send it to the laboratory immediately.
□ If a light-resistant container isn't available, protect the specimen from light exposure. If a Foley catheter is in place, put the collection bag in a dark plastic bag.

Values
Normal porphyrin and precursor values for urine fall in these ranges:
   Uroporphyrins: in women, from 1 to 22 mcg/24 hours; in men, from undetectable to 42 mcg/24 hours
   Coproporphyrins: in women, from 1 to 57 mcg/24 hours; in men, from undetectable to 96 mcg/24 hours
   PBG: in both sexes, up to 1.5 mg/24 hours.

Implications of results
The accompanying chart shows typical findings for uroporphyrins, coproporphyrins, and PBG. Because heme synthesis occurs primarily in bone marrow and the liver, porphyrias are classified as erythropoietic or hepatic.

Infectious hepatitis, Hodgkin's disease, CNS disorders, cirrhosis, and heavy metal, benzene, or carbon tetrachloride toxicity can also increase porphyrin levels.

Post-test care
As ordered, resume medications.

Interfering factors
□ Elevated urine urobilinogen levels can interfere with test results by affecting the reagent used in the PBG screening test.
□ Oral contraceptives and griseofulvin can elevate levels; rifampin turns urine red-orange, interfering with results.
□ Pregnancy and menstruation may increase porphyrin levels.

PORPHYRINS	
Uroporphyrins	**Coproporphyrins**
Highly increased	Increased
Normal	Normal
Variable	Variable
Normal or slightly increased; may be highly increased during acute attack	Normal or slightly increased; may be highly increased during acute attack
Not applicable	May be highly increased during acute attack
Highly increased	Increased

□ Barbiturates, chloral hydrate, chlorpropamide, sulfonamides, meprobamate, and chlordiazepoxide generally induce porphyria or porphyrinuria, and should be discontinued at least 10 or 12 days before the test, if possible.
□ If the urine specimen is left standing for a few hours, PBG levels decline.

WILLIAM M. DOUGHERTY, BS

Urine Delta-aminolevulinic Acid

Using the colorimetric technique, this quantitative analysis of urine delta-aminolevulinic acid (ALA) levels helps diagnose porphyrias, hepatic disease, and lead poisoning. (In an emergency, a simple qualitative screening test can be performed.) ALA, the basic precursor of the porphyrins, normally converts to porphobilinogen through the action of the enzyme ALA-dehydrase during heme synthesis. Impaired conversion, as in porphyrias and lead poisoning, causes urine ALA levels to rise before other chemical or hematologic changes occur.

Purpose
□ To screen for lead poisoning
□ To aid diagnosis of porphyrias and certain hepatic disorders, such as hepatitis and hepatic carcinoma.

Patient preparation
Explain to the patient that this test detects abnormal hemoglobin formation. If lead poisoning is suspected, tell the patient (or parents, since the patient is usually a child) that the test helps detect the presence of excessive lead in the body. Inform the patient (or parents) he needn't restrict food or fluids. Tell him that the test requires a 24-hour urine specimen, and teach him (or his parents) the proper collection technique.

Check the patient's medication history for recent administration of drugs that may alter ALA levels. Review your findings with the laboratory, then notify the doctor; he may want to restrict medications before the test.

Procedure
Collect a 24-hour urine specimen in a light-resistant bottle containing a preservative (usually glacial acetic acid) to prevent degradation of ALA.

Precautions
□ Refrigerate the specimen or keep it on ice during the collection period. When the collection is completed, send the specimen to the laboratory immediately.
□ Protect the specimen from direct sunlight. If the patient has a Foley catheter in place, insert the drainage bag in a dark plastic bag.

Values
Normally, urine ALA values range from 1.5 to 7.5 mg/dl/24 hours.

Implications of results

Elevated urine ALA levels occur in lead poisoning, acute porphyria, hepatic carcinoma, and hepatitis.

Post-test care

Resume administration of medications, as ordered.

Interfering factors

☐ Barbiturates and griseofulvin cause porphyrins to accumulate in the liver and thus raise urine ALA levels. Vitamin E in pharmacologic doses may lower urine ALA levels.

☐ Failure to observe medication restrictions, to collect all urine during the test period, or to store the specimen properly may interfere with accurate determination of test results.

WILLIAM M. DOUGHERTY, BS

Urine Bilirubin

This screening test, based on a color reaction with a specific reagent, detects abnormally high urine concentrations of direct (conjugated) bilirubin. The reticuloendothelial system produces bilirubin from hemoglobin breakdown. The pigment bilirubin then combines with albumin, a plasma protein, and is transported to the liver as indirect (unconjugated) bilirubin. In the liver, most indirect bilirubin joins with glucuronic acid to form bilirubin glucuronide and bilirubin diglucuronide— water-soluble compounds almost totally excreted into the bile. In the intestine, bacterial action converts direct bilirubin to urobilinogen. Normally, only a small amount of direct bilirubin—unbound, or bound to albumin—returns to plasma. The kidneys filter the unbound portion, which may appear in trace amounts in the urine. Fat-soluble indirect bilirubin can't be filtered by the glomeruli and is never present in urine. Bilirubin in the urine may indicate liver disease caused by infections, biliary disease, or hepatotoxicity.

When combined with urobilinogen measurements, this test helps identify disorders that can cause jaundice. The analysis can be performed at bedside, using a bilirubin reagent strip, or in the laboratory. Highly sensitive spectrophotometric assays may be needed to detect trace amounts of urine bilirubin. This screening test doesn't detect such minute amounts.

Purpose

☐ To help identify the cause of jaundice.

Patient preparation

Explain to the patient that this test helps determine the cause of jaundice. Inform him he needn't restrict food or fluids before the test. Tell him the test requires a random urine specimen and whether the specimen will be tested at bedside or in the laboratory. Bedside analysis can be performed immediately; laboratory analysis is completed in 1 day.

Procedure

Collect a random urine specimen in the container provided. For bedside analysis, use one of the following procedures:

☐ Dipstrip: Dip the reagent strip into the specimen and remove it immediately. After 20 seconds, compare the strip color with the color standards. Record the test results on the patient's chart.

☐ Ictotest: This test is easier to read and more sensitive than the dipstrip method. Place five drops of urine on the asbestos-cellulose test mat. If bilirubin is present, it will be absorbed into the mat. Next, put a reagent tablet on the wet area of the mat, and place two drops of water on the tablet. If bilirubin is present, a blue to purple coloration will develop on the mat. Pink or red indicates absence of bilirubin—a negative test.

Precautions

☐ Use only a freshly voided specimen. Bilirubin disintegrates after 30 minutes' exposure to room temperature or light.

☐ If the specimen is to be analyzed in

the laboratory, send it to the laboratory immediately. Record the time of collection on the patient's chart.

□ If the specimen is tested at bedside, make sure 20 seconds elapse before interpreting the color change on the dip-strip. Be sure lighting is adequate to make this color determination.

□ If hepatitis is suspected, affix the correct biohazard label to the specimen.

COMPARATIVE VALUES OF BILIRUBIN AND UROBILINOGEN

CAUSES OF JAUNDICE	SERUM		URINE		FECES
	Indirect bilirubin	Direct bilirubin	Bilirubin	Urobilinogen	Urobilinogen
Unconjugated hyperbilirubinemia					
• *Hemolytic disorders* (hemolytic anemia, erythroblastosis fetalis)	↑	N	O	N↑	↑
• *Gilbert's disease* (constitutional hepatic dysfunction)	↑↑	N	O	N↓	N↓
• *Crigler-Najjar syndrome* (congenital hyperbilirubinemia)	↑↑↑	N	O	N↓	N↓
Conjugated hyperbilirubinemia					
• *Extrahepatic obstruction* (calculi, tumor, scar tissue in common bile duct or hepatic excretory duct)	N	↑	+	↓O	↓O
• *Hepatocellular disorders* (viral, toxic, or alcoholic hepatitis; cirrhosis; parenchymal injury)	↑	↑	+	↓N↑	N↓
• *Hepatocanalicular disorders or intrahepatic obstruction* (drug-induced cholestasis; some familial defects, such as Dubin-Johnson and Rotor's syndromes; viral hepatitis; primary biliary cirrhosis)	↑	↑	+	↓N↑	N↓

KEY

↑	Increased
N↑	May be increased
↑↑	Moderately increased
↑↑↑	Markedly increased
N	Normal
O	Absent
+	Present
N↓	Normal or reduced
↓O	Decreased or absent
↓N↑	Variable

Findings

Normally, bilirubin is not found in urine in a routine screening test.

Implications of results

High concentrations of direct bilirubin in urine may be evident from the specimen's appearance (dark, with a yellow foam). To diagnose jaundice, however, the presence or absence of direct bilirubin in urine must be correlated with serum test results, and with urine and fecal urobilinogen levels (see chart).

Post-test care

None.

Interfering factors

☐ Dipstrip testing, such as with Chemstrip or N-Multistix, is affected by large amounts of ascorbic acid and nitrite, which may lower bilirubin levels and cause false-negative test results.

☐ Phenazopyridine and phenothiazine derivatives, such as chlorpromazine and acetophenazine maleate, can cause false-positive results.

☐ Exposure of the specimen to room temperature or light can lower bilirubin levels, due to bilirubin degradation.

WILLIAM M. DOUGHERTY, BS

Urine Urobilinogen

This test detects impaired liver function by measuring urine levels of urobilinogen, the colorless, water-soluble products that result from the reduction of bilirubin by intestinal bacteria. Up to 50% of intestinal urobilinogen returns to the liver, where some of it is resecreted into bile and, eventually, into the intestine through enterohepatic circulation. Small amounts of this reabsorbed urobilinogen also enter general circulation, for ultimate excretion in the urine (urobilinogenuria).

Eliminated in large amounts in the feces (50 to 250 mg/day) and in small amounts in the urine (1 to 4 mg/day), urobilinogen reflects bile pigment metabolism. Consequently, absent or altered urobilinogen levels can indicate hepatic damage or dysfunction. Urine urobilinogen can also indicate hemolysis of RBCs, which increases bilirubin production and causes increased production and excretion of urobilinogen. Quantitative analysis of urine urobilinogen involves addition of Ehrlich's reagent to a 2-hour urine specimen. The resulting color reaction is read promptly by spectrophotometry.

Purpose
□ To aid diagnosis of extrahepatic obstruction, such as blockage of the common bile duct
□ To aid differential diagnosis of hepatic and hematologic disorders.

Patient preparation
Explain to the patient that this test helps assess liver and biliary tract function. Inform him he needn't restrict fluids or food, except for bananas, which he should avoid for 48 hours before the test. Tell him that the test requires a 2-hour urine specimen, and teach him how to collect it.

Check the patient's history for drugs that may affect urine urobilinogen levels. Review your findings with the laboratory and the doctor, who may restrict such drugs before the test.

Procedure
Most laboratories request a random urine specimen; others prefer a 2-hour specimen, usually during the afternoon (ideally, between 1 p.m. and 3 p.m.), when urobilinogen levels peak.

Precautions
Send the specimen to the laboratory *immediately*. This test must be performed within 30 minutes of collection, since urobilinogen quickly oxidizes to an orange compound called urobilin.

Values
Normally, urine urobilinogen values in women range from 0.1 to 1.1 Ehrlich units/2 hours; in men, from 0.3 to 2.1 Ehrlich units/2 hours.

Implications of results
Absence of urine urobilinogen may result

RANDOM SPECIMEN FOR UROBILINOGEN

Quantitative tests for urinary urobilinogen excretion can also be done with reagent strips, such as Bili-Labstix or N-Multistix (dip-and-read test).

To perform such tests, collect a clean-catch urine specimen in a clean, dry container—preferably during the afternoon when urine urobilinogen levels peak—and test the specimen immediately. A fresh urine specimen is essential for reliable results, because urobilinogen is very unstable when exposed to room temperature and light. Dip the strip into the urine, and as you remove it, start timing the reaction. Carefully remove excess urine by tapping the edge of strip against the container or a clean, dry surface, to prevent color changes along the edge of the test area. When using N-Multistix (or a similar product for multiple testing), hold the strip in a horizontal position to prevent mixing of chemicals from adjacent reagent areas. Place the strip near the color block on the bottle, and carefully compare the colors. Read the results at 45 seconds. The results correspond to Ehrlich units/dl of urine.

(Normal)
yellow-green
to yellow = 0.1 to 1 Ehrlich unit/dl of urine

(Positive)
yellow-orange = 2 Ehrlich units/dl of urine

(Positive)
medium
yellow-orange = 4 Ehrlich units/dl of urine

(Positive)
light
brown-orange = 8 Ehrlich units/dl of urine

(Positive)
brown-orange = 12 Ehrlich units/dl of urine

Normally, a random specimen contains small amounts of urobilinogen. This test cannot determine the *absence* of urobilinogen in the specimen being tested.

Para-aminosalicylic acid may cause unreliable results with this reagent strip test. Drugs containing azo dyes (phenazopyridine), such as Azo Gantrisin, mask test results by causing a golden color.

from complete obstructive jaundice or treatment with broad-spectrum antibiotics, which destroy the intestinal bacterial flora. Low urine urobilinogen levels may result from congenital enzymatic jaundice (hyperbilirubinemia syndromes) or from treatment with drugs that acidify urine, such as ammonium chloride or ascorbic acid.

Elevated levels may indicate hemolytic jaundice, hepatitis, or cirrhosis.

Post-test care
As ordered, resume diet and drugs.

Interfering factors
□ The following drugs affect the test reagent and may interfere with accurate determination of urobilinogen levels: para-aminosalicylic acid, phenazopyridine, procaine, mandelate, phenothiazines, and sulfonamides.
□ Highly alkaline urine, which may be caused by acetazolamide or sodium bicarbonate, may elevate urobilinogen levels.
□ Bananas eaten up to 48 hours before the test may increase urobilinogen levels.

WILLIAM M. DOUGHERTY, BS

Urine Melanin

This relatively rare test measures urine levels of melanin, the brown-black pigment that colors the skin, hair, and eyes. An end product of tyrosine metabolism, melanin is normally elaborated by specialized cells called melanocytes. Cutaneous melanomas—malignant tumors that produce excessive amounts of melanin—develop most often around the head and neck but may also originate in mucous membranes (as in the rectum), the retinas, or the central nervous system, where melanocytes appear. Patients with these tumors may excrete melanin precursors—melanogens—in their urine. If the urine is left standing, exposure to air converts the melanogens to melanin in about 24 hours.

Thormählen's test uses sodium nitroprusside (nitroferricyanide) to detect melanogens or melanin in urine, based on characteristic color changes. More specific tests for melanin, such as chromatography, isolate and measure the pigment.

Purpose
□ To aid diagnosis of malignant melanomas.

Patient preparation
Explain to the patient what melanin is, and tell him this test detects its presence in urine. Inform him he needn't restrict food or fluids before the test. Tell him the test requires a random urine specimen, and teach him the correct collection technique. Advise the patient that test results are generally available on the same day.

Procedure
Collect a random urine specimen.

Precautions
Send the specimen to the laboratory immediately.

Findings
Normally, urine does not contain melanogens or melanin.

Implications of results
In the presence of a visible skin tumor, large quantities of melanin or melanogens in urine indicate advanced internal metastasis. Since malignant melanomas may also develop in internal organs, large quantities of melanin or melanogens in a urine specimen, in the absence of a visible skin tumor, indicate an internal melanoma.

Post-test care
None.

Interfering factors
Failure to send the urine specimen to the laboratory immediately may interfere with test results.

WILLIAM M. DOUGHERTY, BS

Selected References

Beyers, Marjorie, and Dudas, Susan. *The Clinical Practice of Medical-Surgical Nursing*. Boston: Little, Brown & Co., 1977.

Burgess, A. *Nurse's Guide to Fluid and Electrolyte Balance*, 2nd ed. New York: McGraw-Hill Book Co., 1979.

Eastham, R.D. *A Laboratory Guide to Clinical Diagnosis*. 5th ed. Littleton, Mass.: John Wright Publishing, 1983.

Henry, John Bernard, ed. *Todd-Sanford-Davidsohn Clinical Diagnosis and Management by Laboratory Methods*, vol. 1, 17th ed. Philadelphia: W.B. Saunders Co., 1984.

Kurtzman, Neil A., and Rogers, Philip W. *A Handbook of Urinalysis and Urinary Sediment*. Springfield, Ill.: Charles C. Thomas Pub., 1974.

Lamb, Jane O. *Laboratory Tests for Clinical Nursing*. Bowie, Md.: Robert J. Brady Co., 1984.

Miale, John B. *Laboratory Medicine: Hematology*, 6th ed. St. Louis: C.V. Mosby Co., 1982.

Papper, Solomon, and Williams, G. Rainey. *Manual of Medical Care of the Surgical Patient*. 2nd ed. Boston: Little, Brown & Co., 1981.

Petersdorf, Robert G., and Adams, Raymond D., eds. *Harrison's Principles of Internal Medicine*, 10th ed. New York: McGraw-Hill Book Co., 1983.

Race, George J., and White, Martin G. *Basic Urinalysis*. Philadelphia: J.B. Lippincott Co., 1979.

Ravel, Richard. *Clinical Laboratory Medicine*, 4th ed. Chicago: Year Book Medical Pubs., 1984.

Smith, Donald R. *General Urology*, 10th ed. Los Altos, Calif.: Lange Medical Publications, 1981.

Stark, June L. "BUN/Creatinine: Your Keys to Kidney Function," *Nursing80* 10:33-38, May 1980.

Strand, Marcella M., and Elmer, Lucille A. *Clinical Laboratory Tests: A Manual for Nurses*, 2nd ed. St. Louis: C.V. Mosby Co., 1980.

Tilkian, Sarko M., et al. *Clinical Implications of Laboratory Tests*, 3rd ed. St. Louis: C.V. Mosby Co., 1983.

Vaughan, Victor C., III, et al. *Nelson Textbook of Pediatrics*, 11th ed. Philadelphia: W.B. Saunders Co., 1979.

Wallach, Jacques B. *Interpretation of Diagnostic Tests: A Handbook Synopsis of Laboratory Medicine*, 3rd ed. Boston: Little, Brown & Co., 1978.

Wyngaarden, James, and Smith, Lloyd. *Cecil Textbook of Medicine*, 16th ed. Philadelphia: W.B. Saunders Co., 1982.

Zilva, Joan F., and Pannall, P.R. *Clinical Chemistry in Diagnosis and Treatment*, 3rd ed. Chicago: Year Book Medical Pubs., 1979.

16 Urine Sugars, Ketones, and Mucopolysaccharides

LEARNING OBJECTIVES

After completing this chapter, the reader will be able to:

- describe the physiologic changes that cause excretion of glucose, ketone bodies, and mucopolysaccharides.
- identify the laboratory methods used to screen for glycosuria, ketonuria, and mucopolysaccharides.
- detect the pass-through phenomenon and understand its significance for glucose concentration.
- state the purpose of each test discussed in the chapter.
- prepare the patient physically and psychologically for each test.
- describe the procedure for performing each test.
- specify appropriate precautions for accurate administration of each test.
- implement appropriate post-test care.
- state the normal values for each test.
- discuss the implications of abnormal test results.
- list factors that may interfere with accurate test results.

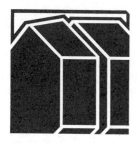

Urine Sugars, Ketones, and Mucopolysaccharides

Introduction

This group of tests, used to detect excessive urinary excretion of glucose, ketones, and mucopolysaccharides, has great clinical significance, because it encompasses some of the most common tests for diabetes. Several of these tests are sufficiently reliable and accessible to have become commonplace as screening procedures for detecting diabetes and for monitoring its response to therapy.

Glycosuria significant

Since the renal tubules normally reabsorb glucose completely and return it to the blood, the presence of glucose in the urine (glycosuria) is abnormal and usually indicates a pathologic condition. Rarely, transient urinary traces of glucose and other reducing sugars (galactose, lactose, and pentoses) reflect a benign state, such as hyperalimentation, the third trimester of pregnancy, or lactation. Characteristically, however, glycosuria reflects decreased glucose reabsorption in the renal tubules or increased amounts of glucose entering the renal tubules per minute—almost invariably the result of blood sugar concentration above the threshold level (160 to 170 mg/dl of venous blood). Such glycosuria with hyperglycemia is suggestive of diabetes mellitus, one of the most common metabolic disorders. The severity and prevalence of diabetes mandates routine screening of urine specimens for sugar in newborns and in persons suspected of having diabetes, and routine determinations of sugar to monitor treatment with exogenous insulin in patients with controlled diabetes.

Testing for glycosuria

Methods for detecting glucose in the urine include copper reduction tests (Benedict's test and Clinitest) and glucose oxidase tests (dip-and-read reagent strips). Several procedures are used to detect glucose in urine, usually through the reduction of copper in hot alkaline solution with formation of a chromatic precipitate, or through sequential enzymatic oxidation of glucose. In both reactions, a color change in the resulting solution indicates the presence of glucose or another reducing substance.

In *Benedict's test,* traditionally the diagnostic test of choice, a solution of cupric sulfate, sodium carbonate, and sodium citrate is added to a urine specimen and heated. After the solution cools, color change indicates the presence of a reducing substance—probably glucose. Although this sensitive test can give a positive reaction to as little as 0.1% glucose concentration, it has important drawbacks: it's time-consuming, inconvenient (because of the need for a water bath and other laboratory apparatus), and nonspecific for glucose. Consequently, newer techniques using tablets and reagent strips have largely replaced Benedict's test.

In the *test tablet procedure* (Clinitest), a simplified version of Benedict's test, a commercially prepared tablet compounded of cupric sulfate, citric acid, sodium carbonate, and sodium hydroxide is added to a test tube containing water and urine. The reaction of the water and sodium hydroxide releases sufficient heat to activate the reduction of cupric ions in the presence of glucose. Comparing the resulting color change with reference color blocks provides the approximate level of the glucose in the specimen. This procedure is more convenient than Benedict's reaction, but it's less sensitive (0.2%) and is also reactive to substances other than glucose.

Reagent test strips (Clinistix, Diastix, Chemstrip G strips, and Tes-Tape) are specific for glucose. The commercially prepared plastic strip is impregnated with a mixture of enzymes and a chromogen, and undergoes a chemical reaction that, in the presence of glucose, produces an oxidized form of the chromogen. A combination strip (such as Combistix) simultaneously tests for glucose, pH, and protein. Despite the possibility of false-negative and false-

positive results, dip-and-read reagent strips are the most common screening method for routine qualitative checks for glycosuria.

Combining the Clinitest tablet test with one of the reagent strip tests offers a semi-quantitative determination of glucose in urine. If a specimen tested with a Clinistix, Diastix, or Tes-Tape paper gives a positive reaction, testing another specimen with a Clinitest tablet can approximately define the glucose concentration by the intensity of the color change.

Ketone bodies

Substances designated ketone bodies (acetone bodies) include acetoacetic (diacetic) acid, acetone (formed by the spontaneous decarboxylation of acetoacetic acid), and beta-hydroxybutyric acid. Formed in the liver during fatty acid metabolism, ketone bodies circulate through the blood to the tissues for further oxidation. Normally, on the usual carbohydrate-protein-fat diet, less than 125 mg of such substances are excreted daily in the urine. Under conditions of absolute or relative carbohydrate deprivation, the metabolism of fat greatly accelerates. Such acceleration overloads the capacity of the liver to metabolize the fragments of acetylcoenzyme A derived from the fatty acids, causing formation and release of significant quantities of ketone bodies into the blood.

The extrahepatic tissues (kidneys, for example) have a great capacity for the utilization of ketone bodies (ketolysis). However, when the rate of ketogenesis by the liver exceeds the rate of ketolysis in peripheral tissues, the blood concentration of ketone bodies rises (ketonemia), causing these bodies to appear in the urine (ketonuria). Ketonuria is characteristic in starvation and uncontrolled diabetes mellitus, and offers clues to metabolic acidosis of various causes; it's usually unrelated to intrinsic urinary system disease.

Screening for ketonuria

Ketonuria is usually nonspecific, and means urinary excretion of acetoacetic

---

RENAL THRESHOLD AND GLUCOSE TESTING

Generally, a patient with diabetes tests his urine for sugars and ketones four times a day—before breakfast, lunch, dinner, and bedtime snack—using a second-voided specimen. A positive result usually indicates elevated blood glucose levels. However, in some patients with diabetes (especially the elderly, and young, well-controlled patients), urine levels don't reflect blood concentration, since glycosuria depends not only on the blood glucose level but also on the renal threshold (blood glucose concentration above which the kidneys excrete glucose). Thus, a patient with a low renal threshold may have a positive urine test, even though his blood glucose is low or normal. Consequently, to ensure the accuracy of urine test results, simultaneous blood and urine glucose tests are sometimes necessary.

acid, acetone, and beta-hydroxybutyric acid. Consequently, a test that identifies any one of the three ketones generally confirms ketonuria. Commercially prepared *dip-and-read reagent strips* (Ketostix) are available for use as a screening procedure. These reagent strips are impregnated with sodium nitroprusside, and are specific for acetoacetic acid and sensitive to 10 mg/dl. When the strip is dipped into the specimen, the presence of acetoacetic acid produces a color change that can be compared with a standard color block to determine approximate concentrations.

A *tablet test* (Acetest) is another convenient screening procedure that is widely used because it works equally well with plasma or urine and reacts to concentrations as low as 5 mg/dl of acetone. (It's not specific for acetoacetic acid.) The Acetest tablet contains glycine, sodium nitroprusside, disodium phosphate, and lactose. Acetoacetic acid or acetone, in the presence of glycine, turns the tablet lavender-purple.

Two other tests, Rothera's test and Gerhardt's ferric chloride test, have been largely replaced by reagent strip and tablet tests. *Rothera's test* detects ketones through the reaction of a mixture of sodium nitroprusside and ammonium sulfate to a urine specimen. If the test is positive, a pink-purple ring develops at the interface of the reactants. This test is sensitive to acetoacetic acid levels of 1 to 5 mg/dl and to acetone levels of 10 to 25 mg/dl but is nonspecific for acetoacetic acid. It requires fresh preparations of the reagents daily and can't be readily performed outside the laboratory. In *Gerhardt's ferric chloride test,* a ferric chloride solution is added to a test tube of urine. If acetoacetic acid is present, the solution turns deep red. Although this test was popular for many years, it is neither specific (salicylates give a false-positive reaction) nor sensitive (25 to 50 mg/dl approaches the lower limit of sensitivity).

Hart's test is an analytical method, the only one other than chromatography, that's specific for beta-hydroxybutyric acid. After acidified urine is boiled to half its original volume, hydrogen peroxide is added (boiling also removes volatile fractions of acetoacetic acid and acetone). If beta-hydroxybutyric acid is present in the solution, a red ring develops on addition of hydrogen peroxide.

Mucopolysaccharides: Large polymers

These compounds are present in various body tissues and fluids, including the ground substance of connective tissue, fetal and adult mucous membranes, and blood group substances. Mucopolysaccharides occur in the free state or are bound to small quantities of proteins. The most important mucopolysaccharides include dermatan sulfate (also known as chondroitin sulfate B), derived from fibroblasts; heparan sulfate (heparitin sulfate), derived from mast cells; keratosulfate (keratan sulfate), distributed in costal cartilage and cornea; and hyaluronic acid, present in synovial fluid, the umbilical cord, and vitreous humor.

Normally, the mucopolysaccharides contribute viscosity and permeability to the tissues, controlling the intercellular migration of small molecules. Hyaluronic acid, for example, decreases fluid viscosity and enhances the lubricating property of synovial fluid. Ordinarily, only minute quantities (10 to 15 mg/day) of these compounds are excreted in the urine. In certain hereditary disorders, however, excessive quantities of these glycoproteins can accumulate in the tissues, eventually resulting in abnormal urinary excretion levels (100 to 500 mg/day). In such patients, the primary defect seems to be the genetically determined absence of the target enzymes that catabolize the mucopolysaccharides. These genetic disorders, the mucopolysaccharidoses, are marked by severe clinical abnormalities including mental retardation, aortic insufficiency, and pronounced skeletal derangements—which usually become apparent during the first decade of life. The most common mucopolysaccharidoses are Hurler's, Hunter's, and Sanfilippo's syndromes.

Screening for mucopolysaccharidoses

Screening tests for mucopolysaccharidoses use an organic dye (toluidine blue) that changes color in the presence of large amounts of acid mucopolysaccharides. One convenient method uses litmus paper impregnated with the dye: a drop of urine is placed on the paper and treated with acidified methyl alcohol. If a blue dye spot persists, acid mucopolysaccharides are present. If the specimen's normal, no dye remains. However, up to 30% of spot tests may have false-negative results.

Another primarily qualitative test uses turbidimetry. Buffered urine is mixed with albumin at acid pH. If acid mucopolysaccharides are present, the solution grows uniformly turbid. (False-negative results occur in about 10% of these tests.) If spot or turbidity tests are positive, paper chromatography can identify the specific mucopolysaccharide. If the patient has Hurler's, Hunter's, or Sanfilippo's syndrome and his initial screening was negative, further tests are needed (paper or column chromatography, or electrophoresis).

DEBRA C. BROADWELL, RN, PhD, ET

CARBOHYDRATE & FAT METABOLISM TESTS

Copper Reduction Test

[Clinitest tablet test]

The copper reduction test measures the concentration of reducing substances in the urine through the reaction of reducing substances in the urine with a commercially prepared tablet—Clinitest. Clinitest, which reacts to glucose and to other reducing substances (mostly sugars), has almost replaced the Benedict's test. This test is most valuable for providing the patient with overt or latent diabetes a simple, at-home method of monitoring urine sugar level. However, it is sometimes used as a rapid laboratory screening tool.

Purpose
☐ To detect mellituria
☐ To monitor urine glucose levels during insulin therapy, after determination that the sugar in the urine is glucose.

Patient preparation
Explain to the patient that this test determines urine sugar level. If he has been recently diagnosed as diabetic, teach him how to perform the Clinitest tablet test.

Have the patient void; then give him a drink of water. After 30 to 45 minutes, collect a second-voided urine specimen.

Check the patient's history for drugs that may interfere with test results.

Equipment
Specimen container/10 ml test tube/medicine dropper/Clinitest tablets/Clinitest color chart.

Procedure
After collecting a second-voided specimen, perform the five-drop Clinitest tablet test: Hold the medicine dropper vertically, and instill five drops of urine from the specimen container into the test tube. Rinse the dropper with water, and add 10 drops of water to the test tube. Add one Clinitest tablet, and observe the color change, especially during effervescence—the pass-through phase. Wait 15 seconds after effervescence subsides, and gently agitate the test tube. If color develops at the 15-second interval, read the color against the Clinitest color chart, and record the results. Ignore any changes that develop after 15 seconds.

If rapid color changes occur in the pass-through phase of the five-drop test, record the results as over 2% without comparison to the color chart. Or, perform a two-drop Clinitest tablet test: Hold

IDENTIFYING REDUCING SUGARS IN URINE

TEST	Glucose	Fructose	Pentose	Galactose	Lactose	Maltose	CLINICAL SIGNIFICANCE
Yeast fermentation	+	+	−	−	−	+	Glycosuria (diabetes), hereditary fructosuria (hepatic disorders), maltosuria (benign condition)
Selivanoff	−	+	−	−	−	−	Essential fructosuria (rare benign condition), hereditary fructosuria
Galactose oxidase	−	−	−	+	−	−	Galactosuria (genetic disorders of galactose metabolism)
Bial's orcinol	−	−	+	+	−	−	Alimentary pentosuria (benign condition), galactosuria (inborn error of metabolism)
Glucose oxidase	+	−	−	−	−	−	Glycosuria (diabetes)

Paper or thin-layer chromatography (TCL) can differentiate one reducing sugar from another by migration rate and solubility.

+ = positive test (presence of sugar)

the medicine dropper vertically, and instill two drops of urine into the test tube. Flush urine residue from the dropper with water, then add ten drops of water to the test tube. Add one Clinitest tablet, and observe the color change during the pass-through phase. Wait 15 seconds after effervescence stops; compare the color with the appropriate color reference chart; and record results.

Rapid color changes (bright orange to dark brown or green-brown) in the pass-through phase in a five-drop Clinitest reaction indicate glycosuria of 2% or more; in a two-drop Clinitest reaction, glycosuria up to 5% can be measured.

Precautions

□ Instruct the patient not to contaminate the specimen with toilet tissue or stool.
□ Make sure hands are dry when handling Clinitest tablets and avoid contact with eyes, mucous membranes, gastrointestinal tract, and clothing, since sodium hydroxide and moisture produce caustic burns.
□ Store tablets in well-marked, child-proof bottle to prevent accidental ingestion.
□ Don't use discolored tablets (dark blue). The normal color of fresh tablets is light blue, with darker blue flecks.
□ During effervescence, hold the test tube near the top to avoid burning your hand; it becomes boiling hot.

REDUCING SUBSTANCES THAT GIVE FALSE-POSITIVE RESULTS

Aminosalicylic acid	Levodopa
Ascorbic acid	Maltose
Cephalosporins	Metolazone
Chloral hydrate	Nalidixic acid
Chloramphenicol	Nitrofurantion
Creatinine	Penicillin G
Cysteine	Pentoses
Fructose	Probenecid
Galactose	Salicylates
Isoniazid	Streptomycin
Ketone bodies	Tetracycline
Lactose	Uric acid

"PASS-THROUGH" PHENOMENON

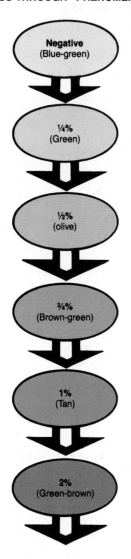

Negative
(Blue-green)

¼%
(Green)

½%
(olive)

¾%
(Brown-green)

1%
(Tan)

2%
(Green-brown)

Remember, color changes during the boiling or effervescent stage are important. If the color of the specimen in the five-drop test goes from blue-green to green to olive to orange to brick red to green-brown, don't compare the color of the specimen with the reference chart: the glucose concentration is 4⁺ (2 g/dl or more). Proceed with the two-drop test. Similar results with the two-drop test mean glycosuria greater than 10 g/dl.

Values
Normally, no glucose is present in urine.

Implications of results
Glycosuria occurs in diabetes mellitus, adrenal and thyroid disorders, hepatic and CNS diseases, Fanconi's syndrome and other conditions involving low renal threshold, toxic renal tubular disease, heavy metal poisoning, glomerulonephritis, nephrosis, pregnancy, and hyperalimentation, with administration of large amounts of glucose and some drugs, such as asparaginase, corticosteroids, carbamazepine, ammonium chloride, thiazide diuretics, dextrothyroxine, large amounts of nicotinic acid, lithium carbonate, and long-term phenothiazines.

Post-test care
☐ Provide written guidelines and a flow sheet to help the patient record the Clinitest results and insulin therapy at home.
☐ Tell the patient when the next urine specimen is needed.

Interfering factors
☐ Cephalosporins, nalidixic acid, ascorbic acid, and large doses of probenecid may produce false-positive results. Tetracycline and ascorbic acid may produce false-positive or false-negative results, depending on the test method. See also ROUTINE URINALYSIS for drugs that may affect urine glucose levels.
☐ Failure to use freshly voided urine or to flush urine residue from the medicine dropper may affect test results.
☐ Failure to detect the pass-through phenomenon or to use the correct reference chart for color comparison of the specimen may influence test results.
☐ Low renal threshold for glucose may alter test results.
☐ Failure to use whole or fresh Clinitest tablets or to keep tablet container tightly closed to prevent absorption of light or moisture may interfere with accurate determination of test results.
☐ Presence of reducing substances other than glucose may influence test results.

DEBRA C. BROADWELL, RN, PhD, ET

Glucose Oxidase Test

The glucose oxidase test—which involves the use of commercial, plastic-coated reagent strips (Clinistix, Diastix), or Tes-Tape—is a specific, qualitative test for glycosuria. Although indicated in routine urinalysis, the test is used primarily to monitor urine glucose in patients with diabetes. Because of this test's simplicity and convenience, patients can perform it at home.

Purpose
□ To detect glycosuria
□ To monitor urine glucose levels during insulin therapy.

Patient preparation
Explain to the patient that this test determines urine glucose concentration. If he's a newly diagnosed patient with diabetes, teach him how to perform a reagent strip test. Have the patient void; then give him a drink of water. After 30 to 45 minutes, collect a second-voided specimen.

If the patient is receiving levodopa, ascorbic acid, phenazopyridine, salicylates, peroxides, or hypochlorites, use Clinitest tablets instead.

Equipment
Specimen container/glucose test strips/reference color blocks.

Procedure
Collect a second-voided specimen.

GLUCOSE OXIDASE TESTS FOR GLYCOSURIA

TEST	0%	1/10%	1/4%	1/2%	1%	≧2%
Diastix	Negative	100 mg/dl	250 mg/dl	500 mg/dl	1,000 mg/dl	≧2,000 mg/dl
Tes-Tape	Negative	**+**	**++**	**+++**		**++++**

Until recently, all glucose oxidase tests used the plus (+) symbol to indicate glycosuria. Lack of standardization in the use of this symbol made it difficult to regulate insulin dosages. Therefore, some manufacturers have stopped using the plus. As the chart above shows, Diastix doesn't use symbols; Tes-Tape, however, still uses the plus. These tests are semiquantitative. Clinistix (not shown above)—another commonly used glucose oxidase test—has no quantitative value; it is strictly qualitative. Results for Clinistix are reported as negative, light, medium, or dark.

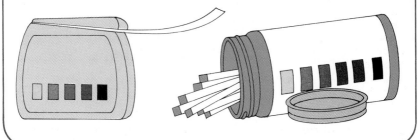

□ *Clinistix test:* Dip the test area of the reagent strip in the specimen for 2 seconds. Remove excess urine by tapping the strip against a clean surface or the side of the container, and begin timing. Hold the strip in the air, and "read" the color *exactly 10 seconds* after taking the strip out of the urine by comparing it with the reference color blocks on the label of the container. Record the results. Ignore color changes that develop after 10 seconds.

□ *Diastix test:* Dip the reagent strip in the specimen for 2 seconds. Remove excess urine by tapping the strip against the container, and begin timing. Hold the strip in the air, and compare the color to the color chart *exactly 30 seconds* after taking the strip out of the urine. Record the results. Ignore color changes that develop after 30 seconds.

□ *Tes-Tape:* Withdraw about 1½" (3.8 cm) of the reagent tape from the dispenser; dip ¼" (0.6 cm) in the specimen for 2 seconds. Remove excess urine by tapping the strip against the side of the container, and begin timing. Hold the tape in the air, and compare the color of the darkest part of the tape to the color chart *exactly 60 seconds* after taking the strip out of the urine. If the tape indicates 0.5% or higher, wait an additional 60 seconds to make the final color comparison. Record the results.

Precautions

□ Instruct the patient not to contaminate the urine specimen with toilet tissue or stool.

□ Keep the test strip container tightly closed to prevent deterioration of strips by exposure to light or moisture. Store it in a cool place (under 86° F. [30° C.]) to avoid heat degradation.

□ Don't use discolored or darkened Clinistix or Diastix, or dark yellow or yellow-brown Tes-Tape.

Values

Normally, no glucose is present in urine.

Implications of results

Glycosuria occurs in diabetes mellitus, adrenal and thyroid disorders, hepatic and CNS diseases, Fanconi's syndrome and other conditions involving low renal threshold, toxic renal tubular disease, heavy metal poisoning, glomerulonephritis, nephrosis, pregnancy, and hyperalimentation, and with administration of large amounts of glucose and of certain drugs, such as asparaginase, corticosteroids, carbamazepine, ammonium chloride, thiazide diuretics, dextrothyroxine, large doses of nicotinic acid, lithium carbonate, and prolonged use of phenothiazines.

Post-test care

□ Provide written guidelines and a flow sheet so the patient can record the Clinitest results and insulin taken at home.

□ Tell the patient when the next specimen is needed.

Interfering factors

□ Dilute, stale urine or bacterial contamination of the specimen may interfere with the determination of test results.

□ Reducing substances, such as levodopa, ascorbic acid, phenazopyridine, methyldopa, or salicylates may cause false-negative results.

□ Tetracyclines also produce false-negative test results. (Parenteral tetracyclines may produce false-positive test results with the copper reduction test [Benedict's test and Clinitest].)

□ Using reagent strips after the expiration date, or failure to keep the reagent strip container tightly closed or to record the reagent strip method used may interfere with accurate determination of test results.

DEBRA C. BROADWELL, RN, PhD, ET

Urine Ketone Test

In this routine, semiquantitative screening test—which has largely replaced Rothera's and Gerhardt's tests—the action of urine on a commercially prepared product *(Acetest tablet, Chemstrip K, Ketostix, or Keto-Diastix) measures the urine level of ketone bodies. Each product measures a specific ketone body. For example, Acetest measures acetone, while Ketostix measures acetoacetic acid. Urine determinations reflect serum concentration.*

Excess amounts of ketone bodies (acetoacetic acid, acetone, and betahydroxybutyric acid)—the by-products of fat metabolism—follow carbohydrate deprivation, such as with starvation or diabetic ketoacidosis.

Purpose
□ To screen for ketonuria
□ To identify diabetic ketoacidosis and carbohydrate deprivation
□ To distinguish between a diabetic and a nondiabetic coma
□ To monitor control of diabetes mellitus, ketogenic weight reduction, and treatment of diabetic ketoacidosis.

Patient preparation
Explain to the patient that this test evaluates fat metabolism. If he is a newly diagnosed patient with diabetes, tell him how to perform the test. Instruct the patient to void; then give him a drink of water. About 30 minutes later, ask him to give a second-voided specimen.

If the patient is taking levodopa or phenazopyridine, or has recently received sulfobromophthalein, Acetest tablets must be used, since reagent strips will give inaccurate results.

Procedure
Collect a second-voided midstream specimen, and use one of these procedures:
□ *Acetest:* Lay the tablet on a piece of white paper, and place one drop of urine on the tablet. After 30 seconds, compare the tablet color (white, lavender, or purple) with the color chart.
□ *Ketostix:* Dip the reagent stick into the specimen and remove it immediately. After 15 seconds, compare the stick color (buff or purple) with the color chart. Record the results as negative, small, moderate, or large amounts of ketones.

□ *Keto-Diastix:* Dip the reagent strip into the specimen, and remove it immediately. Tap the edge of the strip against the container or a clean, dry surface to remove excess urine. Hold the strip horizontally to prevent mixing the chemicals from the two areas. Interpret each area of the strip separately. After exactly 15 seconds, compare the color of the ketone section (buff or purple) with the appropriate color chart; after 30 seconds, compare the color of the glucose section. Ignore color changes that occur after the specified waiting periods. Record the results as negative, or positive for small, moderate, or large amounts of ketones.

Precautions
□ The specimen must be tested within 60 minutes after it is obtained, or it must be refrigerated. Allow refrigerated specimens to return to room temperature before testing.
□ Don't use tablets or strips that have become discolored or darkened.

Values
Normally, no ketones are present in urine.

Implications of results
Ketonuria is present in uncontrolled diabetes mellitus, starvation, and as a metabolic complication of hyperalimentation.

Post-test care
□ If the test is to be performed at home, provide written guidelines and a flow sheet to help the patient record results.
□ Tell the patient when the next specimen is needed.

Interfering factors
□ Failure to keep the reagent container tightly closed to prevent absorption of light or moisture, or bacterial contamination of the specimen causes false-negative results.
□ Levodopa, phenazopyridine, and sulfobromophthalein produce false-positive test results when Ketostix or Keto-Diastix is used.

DEBRA C. BROADWELL, RN, PhD, ET

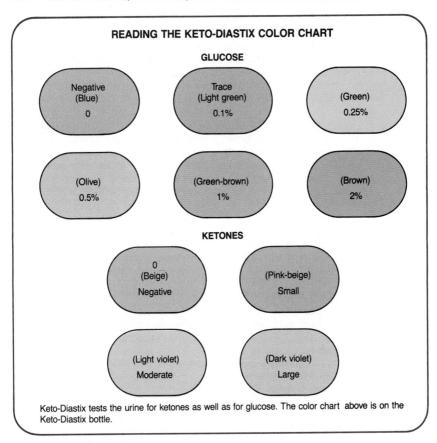

READING THE KETO-DIASTIX COLOR CHART

GLUCOSE

Negative (Blue) 0

Trace (Light green) 0.1%

(Green) 0.25%

(Olive) 0.5%

(Green-brown) 1%

(Brown) 2%

KETONES

0 (Beige) Negative

(Pink-beige) Small

(Light violet) Moderate

(Dark violet) Large

Keto-Diastix tests the urine for ketones as well as for glucose. The color chart above is on the Keto-Diastix bottle.

Acid Mucopolysaccharides

This quantitative test for mucopolysaccharidoses measures the urine level of acid mucopolysaccharides (AMPs), a group of polysaccharides or carbohydrates, in infants with family histories of the disease. When an inborn error of metabolism causes enzymatic deficiencies, AMPs—especially dermatan sulfate and heparitin sulfate—accumulate in the tissues, producing a rare disorder called mucopolysaccharidosis. Its severest form, Hurler's syndrome (gargoylism), results from deposition of these macromolecular complexes in several organs, particularly the heart and kidneys, and excretion of large amounts of mucopolysaccharides in the urine. To measure acid mucopolysaccharides, these compounds are precipitated out of the urine specimen with cetyltrimethylammonium bromide (CTAB). The CTAB is then extracted with ethanol. The glucuronic acid in the now isolated AMPs is measured by the Dische carbazole reaction. The AMP value is then expressed as mg glucuronic acid. This number, divided by the amount of creatinine in the same specimen (which reflects GFR), is a ratio that is used to overcome irregularities in the 24-hour urine collection. The values vary with age.

Purpose
□ To diagnose mucopolysaccharidoses.

Patient preparation
Explain to the parents of the infant that this test helps determine the efficiency of carbohydrate metabolism. Inform them that they needn't restrict the child's food or fluids. Tell the parents that the test requires urine collection for 24 hours, and instruct them on the proper way to collect the specimen at home.

If the child is receiving therapy with heparin and must continue it, note this on the laboratory slip.

Equipment
Pediatric urine collectors/24-hour collection container/20 ml toluene (usually obtained from the laboratory).

Procedure
Obtain a 24-hour urine specimen. Add 20 ml toluene as a preservative at the start of the collection. Indicate the patient's age on the laboratory slip, and send the specimen to the laboratory immediately at the end of the 24-hour collection period.

Precautions
During the collection period, refrigerate the specimen or place it on ice.

Values
Normal AMP values vary with age.

Age	AMPs (mg glucuronic acid) g creatinine / 24 hours
2	8 to 30
4	7 to 27
6	6 to 24
8	4 to 22
10	2 to 18
12	0 to 15
14	0 to 12

Implications of results
Elevated AMP levels reliably indicate mucopolysaccharidosis. Supplementary quantitative analysis and detailed blood studies can identify the defective enzyme.

Post-test care
Be sure to remove all adhesive from the urine collector from the infant's perineum. Wash the area gently with soap and water, and watch for irritation.

Interfering factors
□ Failure to collect all urine during the test period, and improper specimen storage may interfere with accurate determination of test results.
□ Heparin elevates urine levels of AMPs.
WILLIAM M. DOUGHERTY, BS

Selected References

Blevins, Dorothy. *The Diabetic and Nursing Care*. New York: McGraw-Hill Book Co., 1979.

Endocrine Disorders. Nurse's Clinical Library. Springhouse, Pa.: Springhouse Corp., 1984.

Gilman, Alfred G., et al., eds. *Goodman and Gilman's The Pharmacological Basis of Therapeutics*, 6th ed. New York: Macmillan Publishing Co., 1980.

Henry, John Bernard, ed. *Todd-Sanford-Davidsohn Clinical Diagnosis and Management by Laboratory Methods*, 17th ed. Philadelphia: W.B. Saunders Co., 1984.

Lamb, Jane O. *Laboratory Tests for Clinical Nursing*. Bowie, Md.: Robert J. Brady Co., 1984.

Nursing85 Drug Handbook. Springhouse, Pa.: Springhouse Corp., 1985.

Race, George J., and White, Martin G. *Basic Urinalysis*. Philadelphia: J.B. Lippincott Co., 1979.

Ravel, Richard. *Clinical Laboratory Medicine*, 4th ed. Chicago: Year Book Medical Pubs., 1984.

Tietz, Norbert W., ed. *Fundamentals of Clinical Chemistry*, 2nd ed. Philadelphia: W.B. Saunders Co., 1976.

17 Vitamins and Minerals

LEARNING OBJECTIVES

After completing this chapter, the reader will be able to:
- identify the class of vitamins most frequently measured in the urine.
- describe the actions of five major minerals and three trace minerals usually measured in the urine.
- identify food sources of major vitamins and minerals.
- name the disorders associated with deficiency of two or more of the major vitamins and minerals.
- explain the feedback mechanism between sodium and aldosterone.
- state the influence of sodium ions on neuromuscular function.
- recognize the danger signs of severe potassium imbalance.
- state the signs and symptoms of calcium, sodium, and magnesium imbalance.
- state the purpose of each test discussed in the chapter.
- prepare the patient physically and psychologically for each test.
- describe the procedure for performing each test.
- specify appropriate precautions for accurate administration of each test.
- implement appropriate post-test care.
- state the normal values for each test.
- discuss the implications of abnormal test results.
- list factors that may interfere with accurate test results.

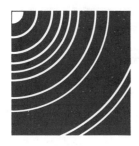

Vitamins and Minerals

Introduction

Vitamins are organic compounds vital to growth and normal metabolism. Vitamins are classified as water soluble (B complex and C) or fat soluble (A, D, E, and K). Water-soluble vitamins are not synthesized within the body and must be absorbed from nutritional sources. Generally, a well-balanced diet provides daily vitamin requirements; however, an inadequate diet or exaggerated metabolic demand may cause depletion and clinical deficiency.

Fat-soluble vitamins

Fat-soluble vitamins require bile salts and lipids for intestinal absorption; much of the amount absorbed is stored—mainly in the liver; the rest is excreted in stool. Storage of these vitamins promotes excessive accumulation; for this reason, toxicity is more common than deficiency. Because fat-soluble vitamins aren't readily excreted in the urine, serum assay is the preferred method for measuring their concentrations within the body (see Chapter 9).

Water-soluble vitamins

Water-soluble vitamins are present in all living cells and act primarily as coenzymes or their precursors. Because water-soluble vitamins are easily absorbed, readily excreted, and stored only briefly (or not at all), they are characteristically vulnerable to deficiency.

Deficiency may result from inadequate diet, malabsorption, chronic alcoholism, or increased metabolic demands, such as result from stress, pregnancy, lactation, or chronic illness. When correlated with clinical features, determining the level of water-soluble vitamins in urine helps evaluate metabolic disorders, malabsorption, and nutritional deficiency. For example, the urine test for vitamin B_1 helps detect neurologic disorders.

Minerals

Minerals are inorganic elements that are necessary for metabolism. Essential minerals—such as calcium, magnesium, and copper—participate in enzymatic catalysis directly and by binding with substrates to form metalloenzymes. Generally, since minerals are stored in the body and tend to accumulate, toxicity is more common than deficiency. Minerals are classified according to their prevalence in the body: major minerals are present in large amounts; trace elements are present in small amounts.

The following major minerals are commonly measured in the urine:

□ *Sodium* helps maintain osmotic pressure, and water, electrolyte, and acid-base balance; it also, with potassium, aids transmission of nerve impulses and muscle contractility. Sodium excretion is usually regulated by adrenocortical hor-

SOURCES OF VITAMINS AND TRACE ELEMENTS

MICRONUTRIENT	FOOD SOURCES	DISORDERS
Thiamine (vitamin B₁)	Pork, liver, dried yeast, whole-grain cereals, enriched cereals, nuts, legumes, potatoes	Deficiency: beriberi
Pyridoxine (vitamin B₆)	Dried yeast, liver, whole-grain cereals, fish, legumes	Deficiency: pellagra
Ascorbic acid (vitamin C)	Citrus fruits, tomatoes, potatoes, cabbage, green peppers	Deficiency: scurvy
Sodium	Table salt, beef, pork, sardines, cheese, milk, eggs	Toxicity: hypernatremia Deficiency: hyponatremia
Chloride	Table salt, seafood, milk, meat, eggs	Toxicity: hyperchloremia Deficiency: hypochloremia
Potassium	Potatoes, dried beans, squash, scallops, veal, dried figs, cantaloupes, bananas	Toxicity: hyperkalemia Deficiency: hypokalemia
Calcium	Milk, milk products, meat, fish, eggs, cereals, beans, fruit, vegetables	Toxicity: hypercalcemia Deficiency: hypocalcemia
Phosphorus	Milk, cheese, meat, poultry, fish, whole-grain cereals, nuts, legumes	Toxicity: hyperphosphatemia Deficiency: hypophosphatemia
Magnesium	Seafood, soybeans, nuts, cocoa, whole-grain cereals, peas, dried beans, meat, milk	Toxicity: hypermagnesemia Deficiency: hypomagnesemia
Copper	Liver, shellfish, nuts, dried legumes, poultry, whole-grain cereals	Toxicity: Wilson's disease Deficiency: anemia
Iron	Liver, meat, egg yolks, beans, clams, peaches, whole or enriched grains, legumes	Toxicity: hemochromatosis Deficiency: anemia
Oxalic acid	Strawberries, tomatoes, rhubarb, spinach	Toxicity: hyperoxaluria

mones, especially aldosterone.

☐ *Chloride* helps control water, electrolyte, and acid-base balance, and osmotic pressure, and is excreted mainly through the kidneys. Chloride levels usually parallel sodium levels.

☐ *Potassium*, the major intracellular cation, helps maintain normal acid-base balance and neuromuscular function. Potassium excretion and concentration is regulated by the kidneys.

☐ *Magnesium* activates several enzyme systems, aids cell metabolism, influences nucleic acid and protein metabolism, and enhances neuromuscular integration. Magnesium and calcium levels may be inversely related. Parathyroid hormone reduces magnesium excretion, but excessive secretion of aldosterone increases it.

☐ *Calcium*, a vital component of bones and teeth, supports blood coagulation, muscle contractility, nerve impulse transmission, and cell wall permeability. It's excreted in urine as a result of excessive mobilization of bone calcium.

☐ *Phosphorus* is necessary for mineralization of bones and teeth, energy metabolism, and fatty acid transport. Urine concentration of phosphorus is regulated by the renal tubules.

The following trace minerals may be measured in the urine:

☐ *Iron* is needed for hemoglobin and myoglobin formation, and cellular oxidation. It's stored in the body as hemosiderin and ferritin, and is excreted in urine, stool, sweat, and menstrual flow.

☐ *Copper* aids formation of hemoglobin and absorption of iron from the gastrointestinal tract. It is a component of several enzymes for energy production, and is mainly excreted in stool.

☐ *Oxalate*, a salt of oxalic acid, combines with calcium in the digestive tract to form calcium oxalate, a component of urinary calculi.

Tests that determine serum or urine concentrations of vitamins and minerals help assess nutritional status, and detect metabolic disorders that cause deficiency or excessive accumulations. Less common uses include assessing the effects of I.V. therapy or therapy with megavitamins or oral contraceptives, and monitoring the progression of debilitating diseases. Serum analysis is generally preferred for determining mineral concentrations. In some cases, however, urine levels are more significant; for instance, in detecting primary oxalosis.

WILLIAM M. DOUGHERTY, BS

VITAMINS

Urine Vitamin B_1

[Thiamine]

This test is used to detect a deficiency of vitamin B_1 (beriberi). This water-soluble vitamin, which requires folic acid (folate) for effective uptake, is absorbed in the duodenum and excreted in the urine. Urine levels of vitamin B_1 reflect dietary intake and metabolic storage of thiamine. A coenzyme in decarboxylase reactions with citric acids, vitamin B_1 helps metabolize carbohydrates, fats, and proteins.

Rare in the United States, vitamin B_1 deficiency is most common in Orientals, in whom it results from subsistence on polished rice. Vitamin B_1 deficiency may result from inadequate dietary intake (usually associated with alcoholism), impaired absorption (malabsorption syndrome), impaired utilization (hepatic disease), or conditions that increase the metabolic demand (pregnancy, lactation, fever, exercise, hyperthyroidism, surgery, and high carbohydrate intake). High dietary intake of fats and protein spares the vitamin B_1 necessary for tissue respiration.

Vitamin B_1 deficiency produces variable clinical effects. Early deficiency pro-

duces variable, nonspecific symptoms that may include fatigue, irritability, sleep disturbances, and abdominal and precordial discomfort. Severe deficiency states vary in several distinct patterns: infantile beriberi produces abdominal pain, edema, irritability, vomiting, pallor, and possibly, convulsions; wet, or edematous, beriberi (a complication of chronic alcoholism) produces severe neurologic symptoms—which may lead to Wernicke/Korsakoff syndrome and Korsakoff's psychosis—emaciation, and edema that rises from the legs; beriberi also causes arrhythmias, cardiomegaly, and circulatory collapse.

Purpose
☐ To help confirm vitamin B_1 deficiency (beriberi) and to distinguish it from other causes of polyneuritis.

Patient preparation
Explain that this test evaluates the body's stores of vitamin B_1. Tell him the test requires a 24-hour urine specimen. Check diet history to rule out deficiency, from inadequate intake. If the patient is to collect the specimen, teach him proper technique.

Procedure
Collect a 24-hour urine specimen.

Precautions
☐ Tell the patient not to contaminate the urine specimen with toilet tissue or stool.
☐ Refrigerate the specimen, or place it on ice during the collection period.

Values
Normal urinary excretion ranges from 100 to 200 mcg/24 hours.

Implications of results
Deficient urine levels of vitamin B_1 can result from inadequate dietary intake, hyperthyroidism, alcoholism, severe hepatic disease, chronic diarrhea, and prolonged diuretic therapy. Negative results indicate neuritis unrelated to deficiency.

Post-test care
Advise patients who are deficient in vi-

tamin B_1 of good dietary sources of this vitamin: beef, pork, organ meats, fresh vegetables (especially peas and beans), and wheat and other whole grains.

Interfering factors
Failure to collect all urine during the test period, or improper specimen storage may alter test results.

WILLIAM M. DOUGHERTY, BS

Tryptophan Challenge Test

Since direct assay of vitamin B_6 isn't currently available, measurement of urine xanthurenic acid after a challenge dose of tryptophan can confirm deficiency long before symptoms appear.

Although vitamin B_6 isn't directly involved in energy metabolism, it is essential for reactions that occur in protein metabolism and for amino acid synthesis. Vitamin B_6 comprises three compounds—pyridoxine, pyridoxal, and pyridoxamine—that function as coenzymes in many biochemical reactions, including the conversion of tryptophan to niacin. Normally, this conversion prevents formation of xanthurenic acid; however, when vitamin B_6 is deficient, xanthurenic acid levels rise. Vitamin B_6 deficiency can cause hypochromic microcytic anemia without iron deficiency and CNS disturbances. When normal magnesium levels accompany a vitamin B_6 deficiency, urinary citrate and oxalate solubility may decrease, causing formation of urinary calculi.

Purpose
☐ To detect vitamin B_6 deficiency.

Patient preparation
Explain to the patient that this test determines the body's stores of vitamin B_6. Tell him he'll receive an oral dose of medication, and then collect a 24-hour urine

specimen. Check his medication history for current use of drugs that may cause vitamin B_6 deficiency.

Procedure
Administer L-tryptophan P.O. (usually, 50 mg/kg for children and up to 2 g/kg for adults). Have the patient void, discard the urine, and immediately begin collection of a 24-hour urine specimen.

Precautions
□ Make sure the specimen bottle contains a crystal of thymol, a preservative.
□ Tell the patient not to contaminate the urine specimen with toilet tissue or stool.
□ Refrigerate the specimen, or place it on ice during the collection period.

Values
Normal excretion of xanthurenic acid after a tryptophan challenge dose is less than 50 mg/24 hours.

Implications of results
Urine levels of xanthurenic acid exceeding 100 mg/24 hours indicate vitamin B_6 deficiency. This rare disorder may result from malnutrition, malignancy, pregnancy; use of oral contraceptives, hydralazine, D-penicillamine, or isoniazid; or familial xanthurenic aciduria.

Post-test care
Inform the patient with vitamin B_6 deficiency that yeast, wheat, corn, liver, and kidneys are good sources of pyridoxine.

Interfering factors
Failure to collect all urine during the test period or improper specimen storage may interfere with test results.
WILLIAM M. DOUGHERTY, BS

Urine Vitamin C
[Ascorbic acid]

Through colorimetric measurement of urinary levels, this test determines body stores of vitamin C. This water-soluble vitamin, which is easily absorbed by the intestine, acts as a reversible reducing agent in metabolic processes, aids collagen formation, and helps maintain connective and osteoid tissues. This analysis is particularly useful in diagnosing scurvy, an extreme deficiency of vitamin C characterized by the degeneration of connective and osteoid tissues, dentin, and endothelial membranes. Scurvy is considered uncommon in the United States today. However, it may appear in alcoholics, persons who are on low-residue or low-citrus diets, and infants who have been weaned to cow's milk that does not contain a vitamin C supplement.

Purpose
□ To aid diagnosis of scurvy, scurvy-like conditions, and metabolic disorders, such as malnutrition, that interfere with oxidative processes.

Patient preparation
Explain to the patient that this test detects vitamin C deficiency. Inform the patient that he should maintain a normal

---

HISTORY OF SCURVY

Scurvy was probably the first disease to be recognized as a dietary deficiency. Rare now, in the past scurvy was common in places where fresh fruits and vegetables—major sources of vitamin C—weren't accessible in the winter. Known as the "plague of the seas," scurvy was most prevalent in sailors because perishable foods couldn't be stored aboard ship. This deficiency also occurred in conjunction with famine or as a result of war-induced food scarcity.

When Vasco da Gama took his first trip around the Cape of Good Hope, in 1497, more than half his crew died of scurvy. Several centuries later, in 1747, Scottish naval surgeon James Lind found he could cure sailors with scurvy by giving them lemons and oranges. In an effort to duplicate Dr. Lind's success, in 1797, lime juice was distributed to the crews of British navy ships during long sea voyages, which explains the nickname limeys, for British sailors.

CLINICAL SIGNS OF SCURVY

(INFANT IN CHARACTERISTIC SCORBUTIC POSITION)

The illustration below shows an infant in characteristic scorbutic position. This infant shows signs of infantile scurvy, such as sunken sternum (scorbutic rosary), weight loss, purpura and ecchymoses, and painful swelling, which cause the infant to lie with his legs flexed. Other signs and symptoms include gum lesions, increased pulse and respiration rates, anemia, anorexia, diarrhea, and vomiting.

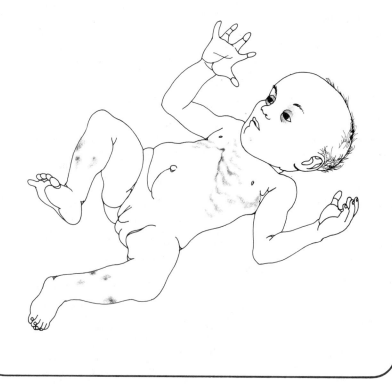

diet. Tell him the test requires urine collection for 24 hours.

If the specimen is to be collected at home, instruct the patient on proper collection technique.

Procedure
Collect a 24-hour urine specimen.

Precautions
□ Tell the patient not to contaminate the specimen with toilet tissue or stool.
□ Refrigerate the specimen, or place it on ice during the collection period.

Values
Normal urine vitamin C excretion is 30 mg/24 hours.

Implications of results
Depressed urine vitamin C levels are common in patients with infection, cancer, burns, or other stress-producing conditions. Decreased vitamin C levels may also indicate malnutrition, malabsorption, renal deficiencies, or pro-

longed I.V. therapy without vitamin C replacement. Severe vitamin C deficiency causes scurvy.

Post-test care
Advise the patient with vitamin C deficiency that citrus fruits, tomatoes, potatoes, cabbage, and strawberries are good dietary sources of vitamin C.

Interfering factors
Improper specimen collection may interfere with accurate determination of test results.

WILLIAM M. DOUGHERTY, BS

> **RANDOM SAMPLE SCREENING**
>
> The laboratory first performs a dip-and-read test, to determine whether or not a 24-hour urine test is necessary to measure vitamin C excretion. Collect a random specimen, label the container, and send it to the laboratory.
>
> A C-Stix reagent strip is dipped into the urine and removed; after 10 seconds, the strip is compared with the color chart on the strip container. A positive result indicates the need for a 24-hour specimen.
>
> Gentisic acid (a metabolite of the breakdown of salicylates) and levodopa cause false-positive results through their reducing action.

MINERALS

Urine Sodium and Chloride

This test determines urine levels of sodium, the major extracellular cation, and of chloride, the major extracellular anion. Less significant than serum levels (and, consequently, performed less frequently), measurement of urine sodium and urine chloride concentrations is used to evaluate renal conservation of these two electrolytes and to confirm serum sodium and chloride values.

Sodium and chloride help maintain osmotic pressure, and water and acid-base balance. After these ions are absorbed by the intestinal tract, they are regulated by the kidneys, and rise and fall in tandem. The kidneys conserve constant serum levels of sodium and of chloride—even at the risk of dehydration or edema—or excrete excessive amounts. Normal ranges of sodium and chloride in the urine vary greatly with dietary salt intake and perspiration.

Purpose
□ To help evaluate fluid and electrolyte imbalance
□ To monitor the effects of a low-salt diet
□ To help evaluate renal and adrenal disorders.

Patient preparation
Explain to the patient that this test helps determine the balance of salt and water in the body. Advise him that no special restrictions are necessary. Tell him the test requires a 24-hour urine specimen, and that the laboratory requires 1 day to complete the analysis. If the specimen is to be collected at home, instruct the patient on proper collection technique.

Check the patient's history for medications that may influence test results.

Procedure
Collect a 24-hour urine specimen.

Precautions
Tell the patient not to contaminate the specimen with toilet tissue or stool.

Values
Normal urine sodium excretion is 30 to 280 mEq/24 hours; normal urine chloride excretion, 110 to 250 mEq/24 hours; and normal urine sodium-chloride excretion, 5 to 20 g/24 hours.

Implications of results
Usually, urine sodium and urine chloride levels are parallel, rising and falling

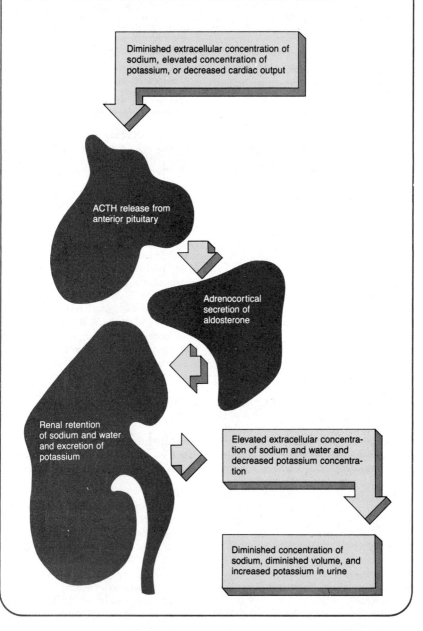

FEEDBACK MECHANISM BETWEEN SODIUM AND ALDOSTERONE

Diminished extracellular concentration of sodium, elevated concentration of potassium, or decreased cardiac output stimulates adrenocorticotropic hormone (ACTH) release from the anterior pituitary, which, in turn, increases aldosterone secretion from the adrenal cortex. Aldosterone promotes renal retention of sodium and water and excretion of potassium to elevate extracellular sodium and water and diminish extracellular potassium.

Diminished extracellular concentration of sodium, elevated concentration of potassium, or decreased cardiac output

ACTH release from anterior pituitary

Adrenocortical secretion of aldosterone

Renal retention of sodium and water and excretion of potassium

Elevated extracellular concentration of sodium and water and decreased potassium concentration

Diminished concentration of sodium, diminished volume, and increased potassium in urine in tandem. Abnormal sodium and chloride levels may indicate the need for more specific determination. Elevated urine sodium levels may reflect increased salt intake, adrenal failure, salicylate toxicity, diabetic acidosis, salt-losing nephritis, and water-deficient dehydration. Decreased urine sodium levels suggest decreased salt intake, primary aldosteronism, acute renal failure, and congestive heart failure.

Elevated urine chloride levels may result from water-deficient dehydration, salicylate toxicity, diabetic acidosis, adrenocortical insufficiency (Addison's disease), and salt-losing renal disease. Decreased levels may result from excessive diaphoresis, congestive heart failure, or hypochloremic metabolic alkalosis, after prolonged vomiting or gastric suctioning.

To evaluate fluid-electrolyte imbalance, results must be correlated with findings of serum electrolyte studies.

Post-test care
None.

Interfering factors
□ Failure to collect all urine during the test period may interfere with accurate determination of test results.
□ Ammonium chloride and potassium chloride elevate urine chloride levels.
□ Sodium bicarbonate and thiazide diuretics raise urine sodium levels; steroids suppress them.

WILLIAM M. DOUGHERTY, BS

Urine Potassium

This quantitative test measures urine levels of potassium, a major intracellular cation that helps regulate acid-base balance and neuromuscular function. Potassium imbalance may cause such signs and symptoms as muscle weakness, nausea, diarrhea, confusion, hypotension, and EKG changes; severe

**SODIUM AND NERVE
CONDUCTION**

1. RESTING CELL

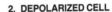

2. DEPOLARIZED CELL

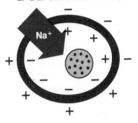

3. REPOLARIZED CELL

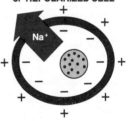

Sodium plays a crucial role in neuromuscular function through the process of depolarization and repolarization.

In the resting cell (Fig. 1) anions accumulate along the outer surface of the cell membrane as cations accumulate along the inner surface. Various stimuli—such as heat, cold, electricity, mechanical damage, or any other factor that temporarily disrupts the normal resting state—cause the cell membrane to become very permeable to sodium. Sodium rushes into the cell, reversing the original resting potential and potassium moves out. This ionic shift is called depolarization (Fig. 2).

Within a few milliseconds, sodium moves out of the cell again and potassium returns to its cellular compartment. This shift is called repolarization (Fig. 3). Repolarization returns the cell to its electric resting potential.

imbalance may lead to cardiac arrest.

Most commonly, a serum potassium test is performed to detect hyperkalemia (abnormally high levels) or hypokalemia (abnormally low levels). A urine potassium test may be performed to evaluate hypokalemia when a history and physical examination fail to uncover the cause. Since the kidneys regulate potassium balance through potassium excretion in the urine, measuring urine potassium levels can determine whether hypokalemia results from a renal disorder, such as renal tubular acidosis, or an extrarenal disorder, such as malabsorption syndrome. If results suggest a renal disorder, additional renal function tests may be ordered.

Purpose
☐ To determine whether hypokalemia is caused by renal or extrarenal disorders.

Patient preparation
Explain to the patient that this test evaluates his kidney function. Advise him that no special dietary restrictions are necessary. Tell him that the test requires a 24-hour urine specimen. If the specimen is to be collected at home, teach him the correct collection technique. Check his history for drugs that may alter test results. If they must be continued, note this on the laboratory slip.

Procedure
Collect a 24-hour urine specimen.

Precautions
☐ Tell the patient not to contaminate the specimen with toilet tissue or stool.
☐ Refrigerate the specimen or place it on ice during the collection period.
☐ After collection, send the specimen to the laboratory immediately or refrigerate it.

Values
Normal potassium excretion is 25 to 125 mEq/24 hours, with an average potassium concentration of 25 to 100 mEq/L. In a patient with hypokalemia and normal kidney function, potassium concentration will be less than 10 mEq/L, indicating that potassium loss is most likely the result of a gastrointestinal disorder, such as malabsorption syndrome.

Implications of results
In a patient with hypokalemia lasting more than 3 days, urine potassium levels above 10 mEq/L indicate renal losses that may result from such disorders as aldosteronism, renal tubular acidosis, or chronic renal failure. However, extrarenal disorders, such as dehydration, starvation, Cushing's disease, or salicylate intoxication, may also elevate urine potassium levels.

Post-test care

☐ Monitor the hypokalemic patient for diminished reflexes; rapid, weak, irregular pulse; mental confusion; hypotension; anorexia; muscle weakness; and paresthesias. Watch for EKG changes, especially a flattened T wave, S-T depression, and U-wave elevation. Severe potassium imbalance may lead to ventricular fibrillation, respiratory paralysis, and cardiac arrest.
☐ Administer potassium supplements and monitor serum levels, as ordered.
☐ Provide dietary supplements and nutritional counseling, as ordered.
☐ Replace volume loss with I.V. or oral fluids, as ordered.
☐ Resume drugs, as ordered.

Interfering factors
☐ Excess dietary potassium raises urine potassium levels.
☐ Excessive vomiting or stomach suctioning produces urine potassium levels that don't reflect actual potassium depletion.
☐ Potassium-wasting medications, such as ammonium chloride, thiazide diuretics, and acetazolamide, raise potassium levels.
☐ Failure to collect all urine during the test period, or incorrect storage of the specimen, may alter test results.

CLARKE LAMBE, MD

Urine Calcium and Phosphates

This test measures the urine levels of calcium and phosphates, elements essential for the formation and resorption of bone. Urine calcium and phosphate levels generally parallel serum levels.

Normally absorbed in the upper intestine and excreted in feces and urine, calcium and phosphates help maintain tissue and fluid pH, electrolyte balance in cells and extracellular fluids, and permeability of cell membranes. Calcium promotes enzymatic processes, aids blood coagulation, and lowers neuromuscular irritability; phosphates aid carbohydrate metabolism. Factors that affect the calcium level and, indirectly, the phosphate level include parathyroid hormone level, calcitonin, and plasma proteins.

PATIENT TEACHING AID

Negative
(Clear urine with no precipitate)

Normal calcium levels
+1
(Slightly cloudy against black background)

Normal calcium levels
+2
(Slightly cloudy to cloudy against black background)

Elevated calcium levels
+3
(Very cloudy)

Elevated calcium levels
+4
(Frank precipitate)

Monitoring calcium levels at home by Sulkowitch's test

Dear Patient:
Sulkowitch's test is a simple, qualitative method that you can use to monitor urine calcium levels. Have ready a clean collection container, 5 ml Sulkowitch reagent, 5 ml 10% glacial acetic acid, test tube, filter paper, and distilled water. Then, do the following:

• Collect a urine specimen in the clean container, and pour 5 ml into the test tube.

• Add acetic acid, and boil the mixture for several minutes to remove any protein. Then add distilled water to restore the original volume, and filter.

• Add the Sulkowitch reagent, mix, let stand for 2 or 3 minutes, and evaluate the specimen (see chart at left).

• Notify your doctor if you detect urine levels higher than +2.

DISORDERS THAT AFFECT URINE CALCIUM AND URINE PHOSPHORUS LEVELS

DISORDER	URINE CALCIUM LEVEL	URINE PHOSPHATE LEVEL
Hyperparathyroidism	Elevated	Elevated
Vitamin D intoxication	Elevated	Suppressed
Metastatic carcinoma	Elevated	Normal
Sarcoidosis	Elevated	Suppressed
Renal tubular acidosis	Elevated	Elevated
Multiple myeloma	Elevated or normal	Elevated or normal
Paget's disease	Normal	Normal
Milk-alkali syndrome	Suppressed or normal	Suppressed or normal
Hypoparathyroidism	Suppressed	Suppressed
Acute nephrosis	Suppressed	Suppressed or normal
Chronic nephrosis	Suppressed	Suppressed
Acute nephritis	Suppressed	Suppressed
Renal insufficiency	Suppressed	Suppressed
Osteomalacia	Suppressed	Suppressed
Steatorrhea	Suppressed	Suppressed

Purpose

□ To evaluate calcium and phosphate metabolism and excretion
□ To monitor treatment of calcium or phosphate deficiency.

Patient preparation

Explain to the patient that this test measures the amount of calcium and phosphates in the urine. Encourage him to be as active as possible before the test. Tell him the test requires 24-hour urine specimen collection. If the patient is to collect the specimen, teach him the proper technique.

As ordered, provide the Albright-Reifenstein diet (which contains about 130 mg of calcium/24 hours) for 3 days before the test, or provide a copy of the diet for the patient to follow at home. Note recent use of thiazide diuretics, sodium phosphate, or glucocorticoids on the laboratory slip.

Procedure

Collect a 24-hour urine specimen.

Precautions

Tell the patient not to contaminate the specimen with toilet tissue or stool.

Values

Normal values depend on dietary intake. Males excrete < 275 mg of calcium/ 24 hours; females, < 250 mg/24 hours. Normal excretion of phosphate is < 1,000 mg/24 hours.

Implications of results

Urine calcium and urine phosphate levels vary (see accompanying chart).

Post-test care

Observe a patient with low urine calcium levels for tetany.

Interfering factors

□ Failure to collect all urine during test period may alter test results.

□ Thiazide diuretics decrease excretion of calcium. Prolonged inactivity and ingestion of corticosteroids, sodium phosphate, and calcitonin increase excretion. Vitamin D increases phosphate absorption and excretion.

□ Parathyroid hormone increases urinary excretion of phosphates and decreases urinary excretion of calcium.

WILLIAM M. DOUGHERTY, BS

Urine Magnesium

This test—which measures the urine level of magnesium, an important cation absorbed in the intestinal tract and excreted in the urine—is especially useful, because magnesium deficiency is detectable in urine before it changes serum magnesium levels. Measurement of urine magnesium was rarely used in the past but is becoming more important, especially in large clinics, to rule out magnesium deficiency as the cause of

SIGNS AND SYMPTOMS OF MAGNESIUM IMBALANCE	
HYPOMAGNESEMIA	**HYPERMAGNESEMIA**
• *Neuromuscular system:* hyperirritability, tetany, leg and foot cramps, Chvostek's sign (facial muscle spasms induced by tapping the area over the branches of the facial nerve)	• *Neuromuscular system:* diminished reflexes, muscle weakness, flaccid paralysis, respiratory muscle paralysis that may cause respiratory distress
• *CNS:* confusion, delusions, hallucinations, convulsions	• *CNS:* drowsiness, flushing, lethargy, confusion, diminished sensorium
• *Cardiovascular system:* arrhythmias, vasomotor changes (vasodilation and hypotension), and occasionally, hypertension	• *Cardiovascular system:* bradycardia, weak pulse, hypotension, heart block, cardiac arrest (common with serum levels of 25 mEq/liter)

neurologic symptoms and to help evaluate glomerular function in suspected renal disease.

Magnesium is found primarily in the bones and in intracellular fluid; a small amount is present in extracellular fluid. This element activates many enzyme systems, helps transport sodium and potassium across cell membranes, affects nucleic acid and protein metabolism, and influences intracellular calcium levels through its effect on secretion of parathyroid hormone. Magnesium deficiency usually results from poor absorption, often related to increased absorption of calcium; magnesium absorption increases as dietary intake of calcium decreases.

Purpose
□ To rule out magnesium deficiency in patients with symptoms of CNS irritation
□ To detect excessive urinary excretion of magnesium
□ To help evaluate glomerular function in renal disease.

Patient preparation
Explain to the patient that this test determines urine magnesium levels. Advise him that no special restrictions are necessary. Tell him this test requires a 24-hour urine specimen, and that the laboratory requires at least 1 day to complete the analysis.

If the patient is receiving magnesium-containing antacids, diuretics (for example, ethacrynic acid and spironolactone), or aldosterone, note this on the laboratory slip.

Procedure
Collect a 24-hour urine specimen.

Precautions
Tell the patient to be careful not to contaminate the urine specimen with toilet tissue or stool.

Values
Normal urinary excretion of magnesium is less than 150 mg/24 hours (atomic absorption).

Implications of results
Low urine magnesium levels may result from malabsorption, acute or chronic diarrhea, diabetic acidosis, dehydration, pancreatitis, advanced renal failure, primary aldosteronism, or decreased dietary intake of magnesium.

Elevated urine magnesium levels may result from early chronic renal disease, adrenocortical insufficiency (Addison's disease), chronic alcoholism, or chronic ingestion of magnesium-containing antacids.

Post-test care
None.

Interfering factors
□ Failure to collect all urine during the test period may interfere with accurate determination of test results
□ Ethacrynic acid, thiazide diuretics, aldosterone, or excessive amounts of magnesium-containing antacids elevate urine magnesium levels.
□ Spironolactone lowers urine magnesium levels.
□ Increased calcium intake reduces urinary excretion of magnesium.

WILLIAM M. DOUGHERTY, BS

Urine Copper

This test measures the urine level of copper, an essential trace element and a component of several metalloenzymes and proteins necessary for hemoglobin synthesis and oxidation reduction. Urine normally contains only a small amount of free copper; only trace amounts of free copper exist in plasma. Most copper in plasma is bound to and transported by an alpha$_2$-globulin (plasma protein) called ceruloplasmin. When copper is unbound, the ions can inhibit many enzyme reactions, resulting in copper toxicity.

Determination of urine copper levels is frequently used to detect Wilson's dis-

ease, a rare, inborn metabolic error, most common among persons of eastern European Jewish, southern Italian, or Sicilian ancestry. Wilson's disease is marked by decreased ceruloplasmin, increased urinary excretion of copper, and accumulation of copper in the interstitial tissues of the liver and brain. The cause of this disorder is unclear. Early detection and treatment (low-copper diet and D-penicillamine) are vital to prevent irreversible changes, such as nerve tissue degeneration and cirrhosis of the liver.

Purpose

□ To help detect Wilson's disease
□ To screen infants with family histories of Wilson's disease.

Patient preparation

Explain to the patient that this test determines the amount of copper in urine. Inform him that no special restrictions are necessary. Tell him the test requires a 24-hour urine specimen, and, if it's to be collected at home, describe the proper collection technique.

Procedure

Collect a 24-hour urine specimen.

Precautions

Tell the patient not to contaminate the urine specimen with toilet tissue or stool.

Values

Normal urinary excretion of copper is 15 to 60 mcg/24 hours.

Implications of results

Elevated urine copper levels usually indicate Wilson's disease (a liver biopsy helps establish this diagnosis). High copper levels may also occur in nephrotic syndromes, chronic active hepatitis, biliary cirrhosis, and rheumatoid arthritis.

Post-test care

None.

Interfering factors

□ Failure to collect all urine during the

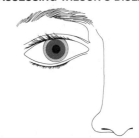

ASSESSING WILSON'S DISEASE

The primary purpose of the copper test is to assess Wilson's disease. Usually, the first symptoms of this rare, inherited disorder are neurologic—rigidity, tremors, incoordination, and ataxia. Later, liver insufficiency with jaundice, ascites, and cirrhosis may develop. Kayser-Fleischer ring, a green or rust-colored ring around the cornea (shown above) caused by copper deposits, confirms Wilson's disease.

test period may alter test results.
□ Administration of D-penicillamine—rarely given before diagnosis—causes elevated urine levels of copper.

WILLIAM M. DOUGHERTY, BS

Urine Hemosiderin

This test measures the urine level of hemosiderin—a colloidal iron oxide and one of the two forms of storage iron deposited in body tissue. When iron storage mechanisms fail to manage iron overload, excess iron may escape to cells unaccustomed to high iron concentrations and may produce toxic effects. Particularly vulnerable to such toxicity are the liver, myocardium, bone marrow, pancreas, kidneys, and skin, which tend to develop tissue damage known as hemochromatosis. This disorder may occur in a rare hereditary form known as primary hemochromatosis, and in exogenous forms. Elevated tissue storage of iron without associated tissue damage is called hemosiderosis and is often confused with hemochromatosis.

Purpose
□ To aid diagnosis of hemochromatosis.

Patient preparation
Explain to the patient that this test helps determine if the body is accumulating excessive amounts of iron. Inform him that no restrictions are necessary and that the test requires a urine specimen.

Procedure
Collect a random urine specimen of approximately 30 ml.

Precautions
Securely seal the container, and send the specimen to the laboratory immediately.

Values
Normally, hemosiderin is not found in urine.

Implications of results
The presence of hemosiderin, appearing as yellow-brown granules in urinary sediment, indicates hemochromatosis; liver or bone marrow biopsy is necessary for confirmation of primary hemochromatosis. Hemosiderin may also suggest pernicious anemia, chronic hemolytic anemia, multiple blood transfusions, and paroxysmal nocturnal hemoglobinuria, the result of excessive iron injections or dietary intake of iron.

Post-test care
None.

Interfering factors
Failure to send the specimen to the laboratory immediately may interfere with accurate determination of test results.

WILLIAM M. DOUGHERTY, BS

Urine Oxalate

This test measures urine levels of oxalate, a salt of oxalic acid. Oxalate is an end product of metabolism and is excreted almost exclusively in the urine. Most important, the test detects hyperoxaluria, a disorder in which oxalate accumulates in the soft and connective tissue, especially in the kidneys and bladder, causing chronic inflammation and fibrosis. Calcium oxalate deposits are the most common cause of renal calculi, which may produce kidney damage.

Purpose
□ To detect primary hyperoxaluria in infants
□ To rule out hyperoxaluria in renal insufficiency.

Patient preparation
Explain to the patient (or to the parents if the patient is a child) that this test determines if the urine contains excess oxalate. Instruct him to restrict intake of tomatoes, strawberries, rhubarb, and spinach for about 1 week before the test. Tell him the test requires a 24-hour urine specimen and that the laboratory requires at least 2 days to complete the analysis.

Procedure
Collect a 24-hour urine specimen in a light-protected container with hydrochloric acid.

Precautions
Tell the patient not to urinate directly into the 24-hour specimen container and not to contaminate the urine specimen with toilet tissue or stool.

Values
Urine oxalate levels up to 40 mg/24 hours are considered normal.

Implications of results
Elevated urine oxalate levels (hyperoxaluria) result from excessive metabolic production of oxalate or increased oxalate intake. Levels as high as 100 to 400 mg/24 hours can occur.

Primary hyperoxaluria, a rare inborn metabolic disorder, causes excessive production and urinary excretion of oxalate. Characteristically, in this type of hyperoxaluria, elevated urine oxalate levels precede elevated serum levels.

Secondary hyperoxaluria can result from pancreatic insufficiency, diabetes mellitus, cirrhosis, pyridoxine deficiency, Crohn's disease, ileal resection, ingestion of antifreeze (ethylene glycol) or stain-remover, or a reaction to a methoxyflurane anesthetic.

Post-test care

None.

Interfering factors

☐ Failure to collect all urine during the test period may interfere with accurate determination of the test results.

☐ Improper storage of the specimen during the collection period may interfere with accurate determination of the test results.

☐ Ingestion of strawberries, tomatoes, rhubarb, or spinach increases urine oxalate levels.

WILLIAM M. DOUGHERTY, BS

Selected References

Diseases, 2nd ed. Nurse's Reference Library. Springhouse, Pa.: Springhouse Corp., 1986.

Endocrine Disorders. Nurse's Clinical Library. Springhouse, Pa.: Springhouse Corp., 1984.

Fischbach, Frances. *A Manual of Laboratory Diagnostic Tests,* 2nd ed. Philadelphia: J.B. Lippincott Co., 1984.

Gilman, Alfred G., et al., eds. *Goodman and Gilman's The Pharmacological Basis of Therapeutics,* 6th ed. New York: Macmillan Publishing Co., 1980.

Goodhart, Robert, and Shils, Maurice E., eds. *Modern Nutrition in Health and Diseases,* 6th ed. Philadelphia: Lea & Febiger, 1980.

Hansten, Philip D. *Drug Interactions,* 5th ed. Philadelphia: Lea & Febiger, 1984.

Henry, John Bernard, ed. *Todd-Sanford-Davidsohn Clinical Diagnosis and Management by Laboratory Methods,* vol. 1, 17th ed. Philadelphia: W.B. Saunders Co., 1984.

Lamb, Jane O. *Laboratory Tests for Clinical Nursing.* Bowie, Md.: Robert J. Brady Co., 1984.

Monitoring Fluid and Electrolytes Precisely, 2nd ed. New Nursing Skillbook series. Springhouse, Pa.: Springhouse Corp., 1983.

Nursing85 Drug Handbook. Springhouse, Pa.: Springhouse Corp., 1985.

Petersdorf, Robert G., and Adams, Raymond D., eds. *Harrison's Principles of Internal Medicine,* 10th ed. New York: McGraw-Hill Book Co., 1983.

Phipps, Wilma J., et al. *Medical-Surgical Nursing: Concepts and Clinical Practice.* St. Louis: C.V. Mosby Co., 1979.

Tilkian, Sarko M., et al. *Clinical Implications of Laboratory Tests,* 3rd ed. St. Louis: C.V. Mosby Co., 1983.

Wallach, Jacques B. *Interpretation of Diagnostic Tests: A Handbook Synopsis of Laboratory Medicine,* 3rd ed. Boston: Little, Brown & Co., 1978.

Widmann, Frances K. *Clinical Interpretation of Laboratory Tests,* 9th ed. Philadelphia: F.A. Davis Co., 1983.

Wyngaarden, James, and Smith, Lloyd. *Cecil Textbook of Medicine,* 16th ed. Philadelphia: W.B. Saunders Co., 1982.

18 Histology

LEARNING OBJECTIVES

After completing this chapter, the reader will be able to:
- state three requirements of accurate histologic diagnosis.
- describe five types of tissue biopsies.
- explain how specimens are prepared for histologic examination.
- describe frozen section tissue analysis.
- explain breast self-examination.
- identify the common sites of bone marrow aspiration and biopsy.
- state the purpose of each test discussed in the chapter.
- prepare the patient physically and psychologically for each test.
- describe the procedure for performing each test.
- specify appropriate precautions for safe administration of each test.
- recognize signs of adverse reaction and respond appropriately.
- implement appropriate post-test care.
- identify the normal findings of each test.
- discuss the implications of abnormal test results.
- list factors that may interfere with accurate test results.

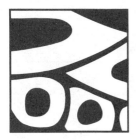

Histology

Introduction

Histology, the study of the microscopic structure of tissues and cells, is vital to confirm malignant disease and has made biopsy—extraction of a living tissue specimen—a common procedure. New tissue preparation techniques and needle designs have made biopsy more accessible—even allowing rapid specimen removal from deep tissues without surgery.

Accurate histologic diagnosis depends on a representative or complete tissue specimen, procured with good technique to prevent damage; proper specimen handling and storage, usually in fixative; and knowledge of the tissue's origin, the suspected diagnosis, previous biopsies at the site, and any current treatments.

Two types of biopsy

In *incisional* biopsy, a scalpel, cutting or aspiration needle, or punch is used to remove a portion of tissue from large, multiple, hidden lesions. Fine needle aspiration differs slightly from traditional needle biopsy. Although the procedure is the same, it provides a smaller specimen, requires cytologic (not histologic) studies, and is usually performed on outpatients for breast biopsies. Incision of a hidden lesion is called a closed, or blind, biopsy. In *excisional* biopsy, a scalpel is used to remove abnormal tissue from the skin or subcutaneous tissue.

When such tissue can be easily and completely removed, excisional biopsy is preferred, because it combines diagnosis and treatment.

Biopsy is commonly performed in a doctor's office or outpatient surgical clinic, or when the patient is already hospitalized, at bedside or in a treatment room. It can also be done in the operating room, using open technique. In open biopsy, a general anesthetic is usually administered, if results from closed biopsy or other tests suggest the need for complete excision of a tissue mass. During open biopsy, a tissue specimen is obtained and sent immediately to the histology laboratory, for rapid analysis. Test results are relayed to the operating room, and a decision is made about subsequent surgery.

Tissue preparation critical

Because a decomposed tissue specimen is diagnostically useless, fixation—a process that arrests cellular structures and prevents decomposition—is very important in slide preparation. Inadequately fixed tissue breaks down immediately after removal from the body, losing one or more components. To prevent this, biopsy specimens are placed immediately in fixing fluid to kill and harden the tissue, and make it resistant to damage by reagents used to process it for microscopic study. The most common

COMMON TISSUE BIOPSIES

BIOPSY TYPE AND TARGET TISSUE	EQUIPMENT
Excision (surgical removal of entire lesion from any tissue; may be excised under local anesthetic)	Scalpel
Shaving (tissue shaved from raised surface lesion on the skin)	Scalpel
Needle (removal of a core of tissue from bone, bone marrow, breast, lung, pleura, lymph node, liver, kidney, prostate, synovial membrane, thyroid)	Cutting needle (such as the Cope or Vim-Silverman cutting needle)
Aspiration (aspiration of tissue sample from bone marrow or breast)	Flexible or fine aspiration needle, needle guide, and aspiration syringe
Punch incision (removal of tissue specimen from core of lesion in skin or cervix)	Punch (such as the Tischler forceps)

ADVANTAGES AND DISADVANTAGES

- Advantage: combines diagnosis and treatment of lesion
- Disadvantage: may require major surgery under general anesthetic

- Advantages: generally safe; combines diagnosis and treatment of benign lesion; yields good cosmetic results
- Disadvantages: may require excision or other treatment if lesion is malignant; may cause seeding of malignant cells

- Advantages: avoids need for surgery; usually furnishes a representative specimen; preserves cell architecture
- Disadvantages: may require excision or other treatment based on histologic results; may be traumatic to surrounding tissues; may not furnish a representative specimen; may cause seeding of malignant cells

- Advantages: avoids need for surgery; aspiration of fluid from a breast cyst combines diagnosis and treatment; fine needle aspiration causes less pain and can be done for outpatients
- Disadvantages: disturbs cell architecture; permits study of individual cells but not of intercellular structure; may not furnish a representative specimen; may cause seeding of malignant cells (less likely with fine needle aspiration)

- Advantages: avoids need for surgery; furnishes a representative specimen
- Disadvantages: may cause seeding of malignant cells when part of mass is removed; may require excision or other treatment based on histologic results

fixative solution is 10% neutral buffered formaldehyde; however, some laboratories require different fixatives and procedures for specimen fixation.

Temperature also influences specimen preservation: cold slows decomposition and heat speeds it. If a fixing fluid isn't immediately available, tissue refrigeration temporarily prevents deterioration. However, even a refrigerated specimen deteriorates significantly after 24 hours.

When a tissue specimen arrives in the histology department, a histologist numbers and labels the specimen, and a pathologist examines it, recording the weight, length, width, color, contents, unusual markings, and hollowness of the specimen. After sectioning, the pathologist selects representative cuts of tissue and places them in numbered capsules, for processing. To prevent loss in processing, small pieces of tissue, such as those obtained from needle biopsies or curettage, are placed in embedding bags, are wrapped in lens paper, or placed between wet sponges before being inserted in the capsules. A histologist then places the capsules in an automatic processor that moves them through a fixing fluid, through ascending strengths of dehydrating fluids, through a clearing fluid, and finally, into melted paraffin, which infiltrates the tissue. This procedure generally takes place overnight. After processing, the tissue, now embedded in paraffin, is ready for cutting and staining. Special stains color various cellular components and permit identification. One stain used routinely—hematoxylin-eosin stain—is an example of this: hematoxylin stains the nucleus, while eosin stains the cytoplasm. After staining, the histologist seals the tissues under labeled coverslips and delivers them to the pathologist for diagnosis. Because of these preparations, a stat tissue report generally takes 24 hours.

Rapid analysis: Frozen sections

Frozen sections, an alternative method of preparing tissue for study, permit rapid, accurate analysis of potentially malignant tissue during surgery. In this method, an individual tissue specimen is sent directly from the operating room to the histology department, where a pathologist grossly examines the tissue, sections it, and selects a representative section for quick freezing. Freezing fixes the tissue, hardening it to allow cutting into microscopic sections. After rapid staining, the pathologist analyzes the tissue for malignancy and tissue margins, which indicate adequate excision, and reports findings to the surgeon, who then closes the wound or begins further excision of malignant tissue. Generally, this technique allows pathologic diagnosis within 10 to 15 minutes after excision. Results from frozen section analysis are usually reliable, but standard analysis on tissue from the same specimen must verify the diagnosis.

Frozen sections can eliminate the need for two separate surgical and anesthetic procedures (one for biopsy, the second for treatment), and can eliminate anxious waiting for the biopsy report.

SHIRLEY GIVEN, HT(ASCP)

GLAND BIOPSIES

Breast Biopsy

Although mammography, thermography, and X-rays aid diagnosis of breast masses, only histologic examination of breast tissue obtained by biopsy can confirm or rule out cancer. Needle biopsy or fine needle biopsy can provide a core of tissue or a fluid aspirate, but needle biopsy should be restricted to fluid-filled cysts and advanced malignant lesions. Both methods have limited diagnostic value because of the small and perhaps unrepresentative specimens they provide. Open biopsy provides a complete tissue specimen, which can be sectioned to allow more accurate evaluation. All three techniques require only a local anesthetic and can often be performed on outpatients; however, open biopsy may require a general anesthetic if the patient is fearful or uncooperative.

Breast biopsy is indicated in patients with palpable masses, suspicious areas in mammography, or persistently encrusted, inflamed, or eczematoid breast lesions or bloody discharge from the nipples. Breast tissue analysis often includes an estrogen and progesterone receptor assay to help select therapy if the mass proves malignant. This assay measures quick-frozen tumor tissue to determine binding capacity of its estrogen and progesterone receptors.

Purpose
□ To differentiate between benign and malignant breast tumors.

Patient preparation
Obtain a complete medical history, including when the patient first noticed the lesion, the presence or absence of pain, a change in the lesion's size, association with the patient's menstrual cycle, nipple discharge, and nipple or skin changes, such as the characteristic "orange-peel" skin that may indicate an underlying inflammatory carcinoma.

Describe the procedure to the patient, and explain that this test permits microscopic examination of a breast tissue specimen. Offer her emotional support, and assure her that breast masses don't always indicate cancer. It may help to mention that 80% of breast lumps aren't malignant. If the patient is to receive a local anesthetic, tell her she needn't restrict food, fluids, or medication. If she's to receive a general anesthetic, advise her to fast from midnight the night before the test. Tell her who will perform the biopsy and where; that it will take 15 to 30 minutes, and that pretest blood studies, urinalysis, and a chest X-ray may be required.

Make sure the patient or an appropriate family member has signed a consent form. Check patient history for hypersensitivity to anesthetics.

Procedure

Needle biopsy: Instruct the patient to undress to the waist. After guiding her to a sitting or recumbent position, with her hands at her sides, tell her to remain still. The biopsy site is prepared, a local anesthetic is administered, and the syringe (Luer-Lok syringe for aspiration, Vim-Silverman needle for tissue specimen) is introduced into the lesion. Fluid aspirated from the breast is expelled into a properly labeled, heparinized tube; the tissue specimen is placed in a labeled specimen bottle containing normal saline solution or formaldehyde. (With fine needle aspiration, a slide is made for cytology and viewed immediately under a microscope.) Pressure is exerted on the biopsy site, and after bleeding stops, an adhesive bandage is applied. (Since breast fluid aspiration is not considered diagnostically accurate, some doctors aspirate fluid only from cysts. If such fluid is clear yellow and the mass disappears, the aspiration procedure is both diagnostic and therapeutic, and the aspirate is discarded. If aspiration yields no fluid, or if the lesion recurs two or three times, an open biopsy is then considered appropriate.)

Open biopsy: After the patient receives a general or local anesthetic, an incision is made in the breast, to expose the mass. The examiner may then *incise* a portion of tissue or *excise* the entire mass. If the mass is smaller than ¾″ (2 cm) and appears benign, it is usually excised; if it is larger or appears malignant, a specimen is usually incised before the mass is excised. (Incisional biopsy generally provides an adequate specimen for histologic analysis.) The specimen is placed in a properly labeled specimen bottle containing 10% formaldehyde solution. Tissue that appears malignant is sent for frozen section and receptor assays. (Receptor assay specimens must not be placed in formaldehyde.) The wound is sutured, and an adhesive bandage is applied.

Precautions

☐ Open breast biopsy is contraindicated in patients with conditions that preclude surgery.

☐ Send the specimen to the laboratory immediately.

Findings

Normally, breast tissue consists of cellular and noncellular connective tissue, fat lobules, and various lactiferous ducts. It's pink, more fatty than fibrous, and shows no abnormal development of cells or tissue elements.

Implications of results

Abnormal breast tissue may exhibit a wide range of malignant or benign pathology. Breast tumors are common in women and account for 27% of female cancers; such tumors are rare in men (0.2% of male cancers). Benign tumors

---

NIPPLE DISCHARGE CYTOLOGY

Nipple discharge occurs normally only during lactation. However, when this discharge can't be attributed to lactation or occurs without breast masses or other signs of breast cancer, cytologic study of the discharge can help determine its cause. (The presence of signs of breast cancer necessitates breast biopsy and other tests.) For example, cytologic study of discharge can differentiate between malignant conditions, such as intraductal papillary carcinoma and intracystic infiltrating carcinoma, and benign conditions, such as mastitis and intraductal papilloma.

Before obtaining a discharge specimen, wash the patient's nipple and pat it dry. Then, show the patient how to "milk" the breast to express the fluid. Discard the first drop and collect the next drop by moving a labeled glass slide across the nipple. (If a larger specimen is required, you'll need to collect it with a breast pump.) Fix the specimen immediately with cytology spray, or place it in 95% ethanol solution. Label the specimen and send it to the laboratory immediately for staining. Note which breast was used to obtain the specimen. Also note if the patient is pregnant, perimenopausal, or taking drugs that alter hormonal balance, such as oral contraceptives, phenothiazines, digitalis, diuretics, or steroids.

PATIENT TEACHING AID

Breast Self-examination

Dear Patient:
Since 90% of breast cancers are discovered by the patients themselves, it's important to learn and practice self-examination. You should examine your breasts at least monthly. If you've not yet reached menopause, the best time is immediately after your menstrual period. If you're past menopause, choose any convenient day.

To examine your breasts: Undress to the waist, and sit or stand in front of a mirror, with your arms at your sides. (1) Carefully observe each breast for asymmetry of size or shape (some difference in size is not unusual); deviation or asymmetry of the nipple; retraction of the skin, nipple, or areola; edema or ulceration of the skin; and any other changes. Since you're most familiar with the structure of your own breasts, you should be the first to notice any changes. Repeat this visual inspection in the following two positions: (2) First, raise your arms and press your hands together behind your head; (3) then, press your palms firmly on your hips. If you see anything unusual, palpate the area carefully for any abnormality.

(4) Next, lie flat on your back. This position flattens and spreads your breasts more evenly over the chest wall. Place a small pillow under your left shoulder, and put your left hand behind your head. (5) Examine your left breast with your right hand, using a circular motion and progressing clockwise, until you've examined every portion. You'll notice a ridge of firm tissue in the lower curve of your breast; this is normal. (6) Check the area under your arm with your elbow slightly bent. (7) Then, gently squeeze your nipple between your thumb and forefinger, and note any discharge. Repeat this examination on your right breast, using your left hand.

(8) Now, examine your breasts while in the shower, lubricating your breasts with soap and water. Using the same circular, clockwise motion, gently inspect both breasts with your fingertips. After you're toweled dry, squeeze each nipple gently, and note any discharge.

If you discover any abnormality, notify the doctor immediately. Although self-examination is important, it's not a substitute for examination by your doctor. Be sure to see your doctor annually or biannually (if you're considered a special risk).

include fibrocystic disease, adenofibroma, intraductal papilloma, mammary fat necrosis, and plasma cell mastitis (mammary duct ectasia). Malignant tumors include adenocarcinoma, cystosarcoma, intraductal carcinoma, infiltrating carcinoma, inflammatory carcinoma, medullary or circumscribed carcinoma, colloid carcinoma, lobular carcinoma, sarcoma, and Paget's disease.

In the receptor assays, a binding capacity of ≥ 3 fmol/mg of protein indicates an estrogen- or progesterone-positive tumor. Over half of all estrogen-positive, protesterone-negative tumors respond to ablative endocrine therapy, such as ovariectomy, adrenalectomy, or hypophysectomy; or additive endocrine therapy, such as administration of estrogen, androgen, progestin, or glucocorticoids. Tumors that are estrogen- *and* progesterone-positive are even more likely to respond to therapy.

Post-test care

☐ If the patient has received a local anesthetic during needle or open biopsy, check vital signs, and provide medication for pain, as ordered. Watch for and report bleeding, tenderness, or redness at the biopsy site.

☐ If the patient has received a general anesthetic, check vital signs every 30 minutes for the first 4 hours, every hour for the next 4 hours, and then every 4 hours. Administer an analgesic, as ordered. Watch for and report bleeding, tenderness, or redness at the biopsy site.

☐ Provide emotional support to the patient who is awaiting diagnosis. If the biopsy confirms cancer, the patient will require follow-up tests, including radiographic tests, blood studies, bone scans, and urinalysis, to determine appropriate treatment.

Interfering factors

Failure to obtain an adequate tissue specimen or to place the specimen in the proper solution container may interfere with test results.

SHIRLEY GIVEN, HT(ASCP)

Prostate Gland Biopsy

Prostate gland biopsy is the needle excision of a prostate tissue specimen for histologic examination. A perineal, transrectal, or transurethral approach may be used; the transrectal approach is usually used for high prostatic lesions. Indications include potentially malignant prostatic hypertrophy and prostatic nodules.

Purpose
□ To confirm prostatic cancer
□ To determine the cause of prostatic hypertrophy.

Patient preparation
Describe the procedure to the patient, answer his questions, and tell him the test provides a tissue specimen for microscopic study. Tell him who will perform the biopsy and where; that he'll receive a local anesthetic; and that the procedure takes less than 30 minutes.

Make sure the patient or an appropriate family member has signed a consent form. Check patient history for hypersensitivity to the anesthetic or to other drugs. For a transrectal approach, prepare the bowel by administration of enemas until the return is clear. And, as ordered, administer an antibacterial to minimize the risk of infection. Just before the biopsy, check vital signs and administer a sedative, as ordered. Tell the patient to remain still during the procedure and to follow instructions.

Procedure
Perineal approach: Place the patient in the proper position (left lateral, knee-chest, or lithotomy), and cleanse the perineal skin. After the local anesthetic is administered, a 2-mm incision may be made into the perineum. The examiner immobilizes the prostate by inserting a finger into the rectum, and introduces the biopsy needle into a prostate lobe.

The needle is rotated gently, pulled out about 5 mm, and reinserted at another angle. The procedure is repeated at several areas. Specimens are placed immediately in a labeled specimen bottle containing 10% formaldehyde solution. Pressure is exerted on the puncture site, which is then bandaged.

Transrectal approach: This approach may be performed on outpatients without an anesthetic. Place the patient in a left lateral position. A curved needle guide is attached to the finger palpating the rectum. The biopsy needle is pushed along the guide, into the prostate. As the needle enters the prostate, the patient may experience pain. The needle is rotated to cut off the tissue and then is withdrawn. The specimen is placed immediately in a labeled specimen bottle containing 10% formaldehyde solution.

Transurethral approach: An endoscopic instrument is passed through the urethra, permitting direct viewing of the prostate and passage of a cutting loop. The loop is rotated to chip away pieces of tissue and is then withdrawn. The specimen is placed immediately in a labeled specimen bottle containing 10% formaldehyde solution.

Precautions
Complications may include transient, painless hematuria and bleeding into the prostatic urethra and bladder.

Findings
Normally, the prostate gland consists of a thin, fibrous capsule surrounding the stroma, which is made up of elastic and connective tissues and smooth-muscle fibers. The epithelial glands, found in these tissues and muscle fibers, drain into the chief excreting ducts.

Implications of results
Histologic examination can confirm cancer, but further tests are required to check for possible extension of the tumor. Bone scans, bone marrow biopsy, and serum acid phosphatase determinations help identify the stage of prostatic carcinoma. Acid phosphatase levels usually

rise in metastatic prostatic carcinoma; they tend to be low in carcinoma that is confined to the prostatic capsule. In the latter case, radical surgery and irradiation, although controversial, can provide a high cure rate. If discovery of cancer is delayed (this is common, because symptoms are generally absent in early stages and most men don't have regular rectal examinations), treatment necessitates estrogen therapy, since continued growth of the tumor depends on secretion of testosterone.

Histologic examination can also detect benign prostatic hyperplasia, prostatitis, tuberculosis, lymphomas, and rectal or bladder carcinomas.

Post-test care
□ Check vital signs immediately after the procedure, every 2 hours for 4 hours, and then every 4 hours.
□ Observe the biopsy site for a hematoma and for signs of infection, such as

redness, swelling, and pain. Watch for urinary retention or frequency, and for hematuria.

Interfering factors
Failure to obtain an adequate tissue specimen or to place the specimen in formaldehyde solution may interfere with accurate determination of test results.

SHIRLEY GIVEN, HT(ASCP)

Thyroid Biopsy

Thyroid biopsy is the excision of a thyroid tissue specimen for histologic examination. This procedure is indicated in patients with thyroid enlargement or nodules (even if serum triiodothyronine [T_3] and serum thyroxine [T_4] levels are normal), breathing and swallowing dif-

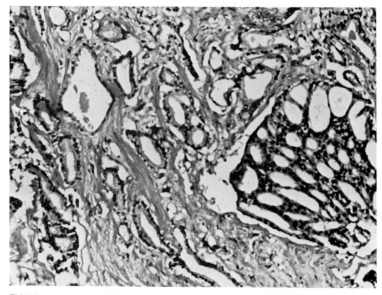

NORMAL PROSTATE TISSUE

This biopsy specimen of a normal prostate shows epithelial glands embedded in connective and elastic tissue, and smooth muscle.

ficulties, vocal cord paralysis, weight loss, hemoptysis, and a sensation of fullness in the neck. It's commonly performed when noninvasive tests, such as thyroid ultrasonography and scans, are abnormal or inconclusive.

Thyroid tissue may be obtained with a hollow needle, under local anesthetic, or during open (surgical) biopsy, under general anesthetic. Open biopsy, performed in the operating room, is obviously more complex and provides more accurate information than needle biopsy. In open biopsy, the surgeon obtains a tissue specimen from the exposed thyroid and sends it to the histology laboratory for rapid analysis. This method also permits direct examination and immediate excision of suspicious thyroid tissue.

Coagulation studies should always precede thyroid biopsy.

Purpose
☐ To differentiate between benign and malignant thyroid disease
☐ To help diagnose Hashimoto's thyroiditis, subacute granulomatous thyroiditis, hyperthyroidism, and nontoxic nodular goiter.

Patient preparation
Describe the procedure to the patient, and answer any questions. Explain that this test permits microscopic examination of a thyroid tissue specimen. Inform the patient that he needn't restrict food or fluids (unless he'll receive a general anesthetic). Tell him who will perform the biopsy and where; that it takes 15 to 30 minutes; and that results should be available in 1 day. Make sure the patient or an appropriate family member has signed a consent form. Check for hypersensitivity to anesthetics or analgesics.

Tell the patient he'll receive a local anesthetic to minimize pain during the procedure, but he may experience some pressure when the tissue specimen is procured. Advise him that he may have a sore throat the day after the test.

Administer a sedative to the patient 15 minutes before biopsy, as ordered.

Procedure
For needle biopsy, place the patient in a supine position, with a pillow under his shoulder blades. (This position pushes the trachea and thyroid forward and allows the neck veins to fall backward.) Prepare the skin over the biopsy site. As the examiner prepares to inject the local anesthetic, warn the patient not to swallow. After the anesthetic is injected, the carotid artery is palpated, and the biopsy needle is inserted parallel to and about 3″ (1 cm) from the thyroid cartilage, to prevent damage to the deep structures and the larynx. When the specimen is obtained, the needle is removed, and the specimen placed immediately in formaldehyde.

Apply pressure to the biopsy site to stop bleeding. If bleeding continues for more than a few minutes, press on the site for up to an additional 15 minutes. Apply an adhesive bandage. Bleeding may persist in a patient with abnormal prothrombin time (PT) or abnormal activated partial thromboplastin time (APTT), or in a patient with a large vascular thyroid, with distended veins.

Precautions
☐ Thyroid biopsy should be used cautiously in patients with coagulation defects—abnormal PT or APTT.
☐ Since cell breakdown in the tissue specimen begins immediately after excision, the specimen must be placed immediately in formaldehyde solution.

Findings
Histologic examination of normal tissue shows fibrous networks dividing the gland into pseudolobules that comprise follicles and capillaries. Cuboidal epithelium lines the follicle walls and contains the protein thyroglobulin, which stores T_4 and T_3.

Implications of results
Malignant tumors appear as well-encapsulated, solitary nodules of uniform but abnormal structure. Papillary carcinoma is the most common thyroid malignancy. Follicular carcinoma, a less

common form, strongly resembles normal cells.

Benign tumors—such as nontoxic nodular goiter—demonstrate hypertrophy, hyperplasia, and hypervascularity. Distinct histologic patterns characterize subacute granulomatous thyroiditis, Hashimoto's thyroiditis, and hyperthyroidism.

Since thyroid malignancies are frequently multicentric and small, a negative histologic report doesn't rule out malignancy.

Post-test care
☐ To make the patient more comfortable, place him in semi-Fowler's position. Tell him he may avoid undue strain on the biopsy site by putting both hands behind his neck when he sits up.
☐ Watch for signs of bleeding, tenderness, or redness at the biopsy site. Observe for difficult breathing due to edema or hematoma, with resultant tracheal collapse. Also check the back of the neck and the patient's pillow for bleeding every hour for 8 hours. Report bleeding immediately.
☐ Keep the biopsy site clean and dry.

Interfering factors
Failure to obtain a representative tissue specimen or to place the specimen in formaldehyde solution may interfere with accurate determination of test results.

SHIRLEY GIVEN, HT(ASCP)

Lymph Node Biopsy

Lymph node biopsy is the surgical excision of an active lymph node or the needle aspiration of a nodal specimen, for histologic examination. Both techniques usually employ a local anesthetic and sample the superficial nodes in the cervical, supraclavicular, axillary, or inguinal region. Excision is the preferred technique, because it provides a larger specimen.

Lymph nodes swell from their usually flat, bean shape during infection but return to normal size as infection clears. When nodal enlargement is prolonged and is accompanied by backache, leg edema, breathing and swallowing difficulties, and later, weight loss, weakness, severe itching, fever, night sweats, cough, hemoptysis, or hoarseness, biopsy is indicated. Generalized or localized lymph node enlargement is typical of diseases such as chronic lymphatic leukemia, Hodgkin's disease, infectious mononucleosis, and rheumatoid arthritis.

Complete blood count, liver function studies, liver and spleen scans, and X-rays should precede this test.

Purpose
☐ To determine the cause of lymph node enlargement
☐ To distinguish between benign and malignant lymph node tumors
☐ To stage metastatic carcinoma.

Patient preparation
Describe the procedure to the patient, and ask if he has any questions. Explain that this test allows microscopic study of lymph node tissue. For excisional biopsy, instruct the patient to restrict food from midnight and to drink only clear liquids on the morning of the test (if general anesthetic is needed for deeper nodes, he must also restrict fluids). For needle biopsy, inform him he needn't restrict food or fluids. Tell him who will perform the biopsy and where; that the procedure takes 15 to 30 minutes; and that the analysis takes 1 day to complete.

Make sure the patient or a responsible family member has signed a consent form. Check patient history for hypersensitivity to the anesthetic.

If the patient will receive a local anesthetic, explain that he may experience discomfort during injection. Just before the biopsy, record baseline vital signs.

Procedure
Excisional biopsy: Prepare the skin over the biopsy site; drape the area for privacy. The anesthetic is then administered.

ABNORMAL LYMPH NODE BIOPSY

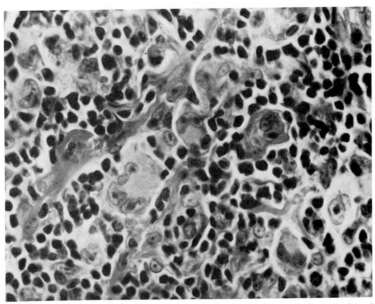

This lymph node biopsy reveals Hodgkin's disease (nodular sclerosing type), which is indicated by the presence of lacunar and polyploid Sternberg-Reed cells, in a matrix of small lymphocytes and collagen bands.

The examiner makes an incision, removes an entire node, and places it in a properly labeled bottle containing normal saline solution. Then the wound is sutured, and a sterile dressing is applied.

Needle biopsy: After preparing the biopsy site and administering a local anesthetic, the examiner grasps the node between his thumb and forefinger, inserts the needle directly into the node, and obtains a small core specimen. The needle is then removed, and the specimen is placed in a properly labeled bottle containing normal saline solution. Pressure is exerted on the biopsy site to control bleeding, and an adhesive bandage is applied.

Precautions

Storing the tissue specimen in normal saline solution instead of in 10% for-maldehyde solution allows part of the specimen to be used for cytologic impression smears, which are studied along with the biopsy specimen.

Findings

The normal lymph node is encapsulated by collagenous connective tissue, and is divided into smaller lobes by tissue strands called *trabeculae.* It has an outer *cortex,* composed of lymphoid cells and nodules or follicles containing lymphocytes, and an inner *medulla,* composed of reticular phagocytic cells that collect and drain fluid.

Implications of results

Histologic examination of the tissue specimen distinguishes between malignant and nonmalignant causes of lymph node enlargement. Lymphatic malignancy accounts for up to 5% of all cancers and is slightly more prevalent in males than in females. Hodgkin's disease, a lymphoma affecting the entire lymph system, is the leading cancer affecting adolescents and young adults. Lymph node malignancy may also result from metastasizing carcinoma.

When histologic results aren't clear or nodular material isn't involved, mediastinoscopy or laparotomy can provide another nodal specimen. Occasionally, lymphangiography can furnish additional diagnostic information.

Post-test care
□ Check vital signs, and watch for bleeding, tenderness, and redness at the biopsy site.
□ Patient may resume usual diet.

Interfering factors
□ Improper specimen storage or failure to obtain a representative tissue specimen may alter test results.
□ Inability to differentiate nodal pathology may interfere with accurate determination of test results.

SHIRLEY GIVEN, HT(ASCP)

ORGAN BIOPSIES
Skin Biopsy

Skin biopsy is the removal of a small piece of tissue, under local anesthetic, from a lesion suspected of malignancy or other dermatoses. A specimen for histologic examination may be secured by one of three techniques—shave, punch, or excision. A shave biopsy cuts the lesion above the skin line and, since it leaves the lower layers of dermis intact, permits further biopsy at the site. The punch biopsy removes an oval core from the center of a lesion. Excision biopsy, the procedure of choice, removes the entire lesion and is indicated for rapidly expanding lesions; for sclerotic, bullous, or atrophic lesions; and for examination of the border of a lesion and surrounding normal skin.

Lesions suspected of harboring malignancy usually have changed color, size, or appearance, or have failed to heal properly after injury. Since fully developed lesions provide more diagnostic information than those that are resolving or in early developing stages, whenever possible such full-blown lesions should be selected for biopsy. For example, if the skin shows blisters, biopsy should include the most mature ones.

Purpose
□ To provide differential diagnosis among basal cell carcinoma, squamous cell carcinoma, malignant melanoma, and benign growths
□ To diagnose chronic bacterial or fungal skin infections.

Patient preparation
Describe the procedure to the patient, and answer any questions he may have. Explain that the biopsy provides a sample of skin for microscopic study. Inform him that he needn't restrict food or fluids. Tell him who will perform the procedure and where; that he'll receive a local anesthetic to minimize pain during the procedure; and that the biopsy takes approximately 15 minutes. Test results are usually available in 1 day.

Make sure the patient or an appropriate relative has signed a consent form. Check patient history for hypersensitivity to the local anesthetic.

Procedure
Position the patient comfortably, and cleanse the biopsy site. Then the local anesthetic is administered.

Shave biopsy: The protruding growth is cut off at the skin line with a #15 scalpel, then the tissue is placed immediately in a properly labeled specimen bottle containing 10% formaldehyde so-

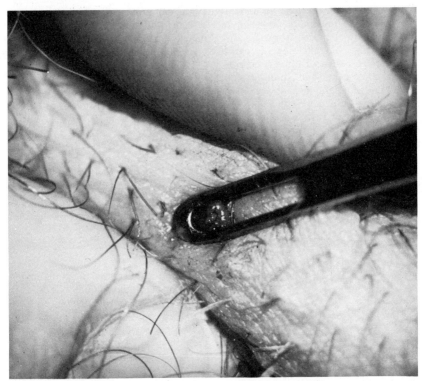

Curettage is another method of removing a skin lesion. This photograph shows a curette cupping a suspected molluscum lesion for biopsy. After the tissue is removed and properly prepared, it's examined microscopically for characteristic molluscum cells, which confirm diagnosis.

lution. Apply pressure to the area to stop the bleeding.

Punch biopsy: The skin surrounding the lesion is pulled taut, and the punch is firmly introduced into the lesion and is rotated to obtain a tissue specimen. The plug is lifted with forceps or a needle, and is severed as deeply into the fat layer as possible. The specimen is placed in a properly labeled specimen bottle containing 10% formaldehyde solution, or in a sterile container, if indicated. The method used to close the wound depends on the size of the punch. A 3-mm punch biopsy requires only an adhesive bandage; a 4-mm punch biopsy requires one suture; and a 6-mm punch biopsy requires two sutures.

Excision biopsy: A #15 scalpel is used to totally excise the lesion; the incision is made as wide and as deep as neces-

sary. After the tissue specimen is removed, it is placed immediately in a properly labeled specimen bottle containing 10% formaldehyde solution. Apply pressure to the site to stop the bleeding. The wound is closed using 4-0 suture. If the incision is large, skin graft may be required.

Precautions
Send the specimen to the laboratory immediately.

Findings
Normal skin consists of squamous epithelium (epidermis) and fibrous connective tissue (dermis).

Implications of results
Histologic examination of the tissue specimen may reveal a benign or malig-

nant lesion. Malignant tumors include basal cell carcinoma, squamous cell carcinoma, and malignant melanoma. Basal cell carcinoma occurs on hair-bearing skin, the most common location being the face—including the nose and its folds. Squamous cell carcinoma most often appears on the lips, mouth, and genitalia. Malignant melanoma, the most deadly skin cancer, can spread throughout the body by way of the lymphatic system and the blood vessels. Benign growths include cysts, seborrheic keratoses, warts, pigmented nevi (moles), keloids, dermatofibromas, and multiple neurofibromas.

Cultures can detect chronic bacterial and fungal infections in which flora are relatively sparse.

Post-test care
☐ Check the biopsy site for bleeding.
☐ If the patient experiences pain at the biopsy site, administer medication, as ordered.
☐ Advise the patient with sutures to keep the area clean and as dry as possible. Tell him the facial sutures will be removed in 3 to 5 days; trunk sutures, in 7 to 14 days. Instruct the patient with adhesive strips to leave them in place for 14 to 21 days.

Interfering factors
☐ Improper selection of biopsy site may interfere with accurate determination of test results.
☐ Failure to use the appropriate fixative or to use a sterile container when it's indicated may alter test results.

SHIRLEY GIVEN, HT(ASCP)

Small Bowel Biopsy

Small bowel biopsy helps evaluate diseases of the intestinal mucosa, which may cause malabsorption or diarrhea. Using a capsule, it produces larger specimens than does endoscopic biopsy, and

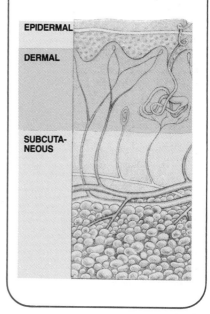

SKIN LAYER BIOPSIES

Epidermal tissue specimens are generally removed by shave biopsy, while both epidermal and dermal specimens may be obtained by punch biopsy. Subcutaneous tissue specimens can be removed by excision.

EPIDERMAL

DERMAL

SUBCUTA-
NEOUS

allows removal of tissue from those areas beyond an endoscope's reach.

Several types of capsules are available, all similar in design and use. The Carey capsule, for example, has a spring-loaded, two-piece capsule, 8 mm in diameter and 2.6 cm long. A mercury-weighted bag is attached to one end of the capsule; a thin polyethylene tube about 150 cm long is attached to the other end. Once the bag, capsule, and tube are in place in the small bowel, suction applied to the tube causes the mucosa to enter the capsule. Continued suction closes the capsule, cutting off the piece of tissue within.

The biopsy sample verifies diagnosis of some diseases, such as Whipple's disease; it may help confirm others, such as tropical sprue. Capsule biopsy is an invasive procedure, but it causes little pain and complications are rare.

Purpose

☐ To help diagnose diseases of the intestinal mucosa.

ENDOSCOPIC BIOPSY OF THE GI TRACT

Endoscopy allows direct visualization of the GI tract and any site that requires biopsy of tissue samples for histologic analysis. This relatively painless procedure helps detect, support diagnosis of, or monitor GI tract disorders. Its complications, notably hemorrhage, perforation, and aspiration, are rare.

Careful patient preparation is vital for this procedure. Describe the procedure to the patient and reassure him that he will be able to breathe with the endoscope in place. Tell him to fast for at least 8 hours before the procedure. (For lower GI biopsy, cleanse the bowel, as ordered.) Make sure the patient or a responsible family member has signed a consent form.

Just before the procedure, sedate the patient, as ordered. He should be relaxed but not asleep, because his cooperation promotes smooth passage of the endoscope. Spray the back of his throat with a local anesthetic, to suppress his gag reflex. Have suction equipment and bipolar cauterizing electrodes available, to prevent aspiration and excessive bleeding.

After the doctor passes the endoscope into the upper or lower GI tract and visualizes a lesion, node, or other abnormal area, he pushes a biopsy forceps through a channel in the endoscope until this, too, can be seen. Then he opens the forceps, positions them at the biopsy site, and closes them on the tissue. The closed forceps and tissue sample are removed from the endoscope, and the tissue is taken from the forceps. The specimen is placed mucosal side up on fine mesh gauze or filter paper and then placed in a labeled biopsy bottle containing fixative. When all samples have been collected, the endoscope is removed. Samples are sent to the laboratory immediately.

Endoscopic biopsy of the GI tract can diagnose cancer, lymphoma, amyloidosis, candidiasis, and gastric ulcers; support diagnosis of Crohn's disease, chronic ulcerative colitis, gastritis, esophagitis, and melanosis coli in laxative abuse; and monitor progression of Barrett's esophagus, multiple gastric polyps, colon cancer and polyps, and chronic ulcerative colitis.

Patient preparation

Describe the procedure to the patient, and ask if he has any questions. Explain that this test helps identify intestinal disorders. Tell him to restrict food and fluids for at least 8 hours before the test; who will perform the biopsy and where; and that the procedure takes 45 to 60 minutes but causes little discomfort.

Make sure the patient or a responsible family member has signed a consent form. Ensure that coagulation tests have been performed and that the results are recorded on the patient's chart.

Withhold aspirin and anticoagulants, as ordered. If these must be continued, note this on the laboratory slip.

Procedure

Check the tubing and the mercury bag for leaks. Lightly lubricate the tube and the capsule with a water-soluble lubricant, and moisten the mercury bag with water. Spray the back of the patient's throat with a local anesthetic, as ordered, to decrease gagging during passage of the tube. Ask the patient to sit upright. The capsule is placed in his pharynx, and he is asked to flex his neck and swallow as the doctor advances the tube about 50 cm. (If a local anesthetic is used to control the gag reflex, the patient must not receive any fluids to help him swallow the capsule. Place the patient on his right side; the doctor then advances the tube another 50 cm. The tube's position must be checked by fluoroscopy or by instilling air through the tube and listening with a stethoscope for air to enter the stomach.

Next, the tube is advanced 5 to 10 cm at a time to pass the capsule through the pylorus. Talk to the patient about food to stimulate the pylorus and help the capsule pass. When fluoroscopy confirms that the capsule has passed the pylorus, keep the patient on his right side to allow the capsule to move into the second and third portions of the small bowel. Tell the patient that he may hold the tube loosely to one side of his mouth, if it makes him more comfortable. Capsule position is checked again by fluoroscopy.

When the capsule is at or beyond the ligament of Trietz, the biopsy sample can be taken. (The doctor will determine the biopsy site.) Place the patient supine, so the capsule's position can be verified fluoroscopically. A 100-ml glass syringe is placed on the end of the tube and steady suction is applied to close the capsule and cut off a tissue specimen. Suction is maintained on the syringe as the tube and capsule are removed; then the suction is released. This opens the capsule and exposes the specimen, mucosal side down. The specimen is gently removed with forceps, placed mucosal side up on a piece of mesh, and placed in a biopsy bottle with required fixative. Send the specimen to the laboratory immediately.

Precautions

□ Keep suction equipment nearby to prevent aspiration if the patient vomits.
□ Do not allow the patient to bite the tubing.
□ Handle the tissue carefully and place it correctly on the slide, as ordered.
□ Biopsy is contraindicated in uncooperative patients, in those taking aspirin or anticoagulants, and in those with uncontrolled coagulation disorders.

Findings

A normal small bowel biopsy sample consists of finger-like villi, crypts, columnar epithelial cells, and round cells.

Implications of results

Small bowel tissue that reveals histologic changes in cell structure may indicate Whipple's disease, abetalipoproteinemia, lymphoma, lymphangiectasia, eosinophilic enteritis, and such parasitic infections as giardiasis and coccidiosis. Abnormal samples may also suggest celiac sprue, tropical sprue, infectious gastroenteritis, intraluminal bacterial overgrowth, folate and B_{12} deficiency, radiation enteritis, and malnutrition, but such disorders require further studies.

Post-test care

□ As ordered, resume diet after confirm-

ing return of gag reflex.
□ Complications are rare. However, watch for signs of hemorrhage, bacteremia with transient fever and pain, and bowel perforation. Tell the patient to report abdominal pain or bleeding.

Interfering factors

□ Mechanical failure of the biopsy capsule or any hole in the tubing can prevent removal of a tissue sample.
□ Incorrect handling or positioning of the specimen may alter test results.
□ Failure to fast before the biopsy may yield a poor specimen or cause vomiting and aspiration.
□ Failure to place specimen in fixative or a delay in transport may alter test results.

KATHERINE FULTON, RN

Percutaneous Liver Biopsy

Percutaneous biopsy of the liver is the needle aspiration of a core of tissue for histologic analysis. This procedure is performed under a local or general anesthetic. Such analysis can identify hepatic disorders after ultrasonography, computerized tomography, and radionuclide studies have failed to detect them. Because many patients with hepatic disorders have clotting defects, testing for hemostasis should precede liver biopsy.

Purpose

□ To diagnose hepatic parenchymal disease, malignancy, and granulomatous infections.

Patient preparation

Describe the procedure to the patient, and ask if he has any questions. Explain that this test helps diagnose liver disorders. Instruct the patient to restrict food and fluids for 4 to 8 hours before

OBTAINING A LIVER BIOPSY USING MENGHINI NEEDLE

A needle attached to a 5-ml syringe containing normal saline solution is introduced through the chest wall and intercostal space (1). Negative pressure is created in the syringe. Then, the needle is pushed rapidly into the liver (2) and pulled out of the body entirely (3), to obtain a tissue specimen.

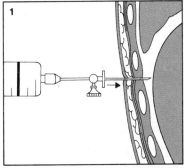

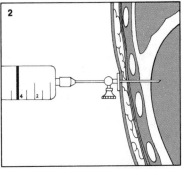

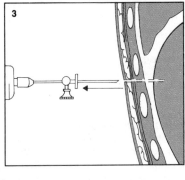

the test, as ordered. Tell him who will perform the biopsy and where; that the biopsy needle remains in the liver about 1 second; and that the entire procedure takes about 10 to 15 minutes. Test results are usually available in 1 day.

Make sure the patient or an appropriate family member has signed a consent form. Check patient history for hypersensitivity to the local anesthetic. Make sure prothrombin time and platelet count tests have been performed and that the results are recorded on the patient's chart.

Just before the biopsy, tell the patient to void. After he does, record vital signs. Inform him that he will receive a local anesthetic but may experience pain similar to that of a punch in his right shoulder, as the biopsy needle passes the phrenic nerve.

Procedure

For aspiration biopsy using the Menghini needle, place the patient in a supine position, with his right hand under his head. Instruct him to maintain this position and remain as still as possible during the procedure. The liver is palpated, the biopsy site is selected and marked, and the anesthetic is then injected. The needle flange is set to control the depth of penetration, and 2 ml of sterile normal saline solution are drawn into the syringe. The syringe is attached to the biopsy needle, and the needle is introduced into the subcutaneous tissue, through the right eighth or ninth intercostal space, between the anterior and posterior axillary lines. One ml of normal saline solution is injected to clear the needle and the plunger, then the plunger is drawn back to the 4-ml mark to create negative pressure. At this point in the procedure, ask the patient to take a deep breath, exhale, and hold his breath at the end of expiration to prevent any movement of the chest wall. As the patient holds his breath, the biopsy needle is quickly inserted into the liver and withdrawn in 1 second. After the needle is withdrawn, tell the patient to resume normal respirations. The tissue specimen is then placed in a properly labeled specimen cup containing 10% formalin solution. This is done by releasing negative pressure while the point of the needle is in the formalin solution. Again, 1 ml of normal saline solution is injected to clear the needle of the tissue specimen. Apply pressure to the biopsy site to halt bleeding.

Precautions
☐ Percutaneous liver biopsy is contraindicated in a patient with a platelet count below 100,000; prothrombin time longer than 15 seconds; empyema of the lungs, pleurae, peritoneum, biliary tract, or liver; vascular tumor; hepatic angiomas; hydatid cyst; or tense ascites. If extrahepatic obstruction is suspected, ultrasonography or subcutaneous transhepatic cholangiography should rule out this condition before the biopsy is considered.
☐ Instruct the patient to hold his breath while the needle is in place.
☐ Send the specimen to the laboratory immediately.

Findings
The normal liver consists of sheets of hepatocytes supported by a reticulin framework.

Implications of results
Examination of the hepatic tissue may reveal diffuse hepatic disease, such as cirrhosis or hepatitis, or granulomatous infections, such as tuberculosis. Primary malignant tumors include hepatocellular carcinoma, cholangiocellular carcinoma, and angiosarcoma, but hepatic metastases are more common.

Nonmalignant findings with a known focal lesion require further studies—laparotomy, or laparoscopy with biopsy, for example.

Post-test care
☐ Position the patient on his right side for 2 hours, with a small pillow or sandbag under the costal margin to provide extra pressure. Advise bed rest for 24 hours.

NORMAL AND ABNORMAL LIVER BIOPSIES

The biopsy specimen shown below (1) is of normal liver tissue. The biopsy specimen at (2) confirms cancer of the liver, indicated by the small, dark malignant cells. The biopsy specimen at (3) confirms alcoholic cirrhosis, indicated by the fibrous septa that divide the liver into nodules.

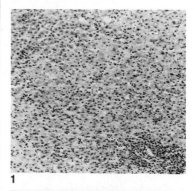

1

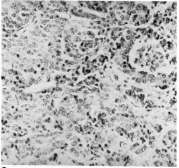

2

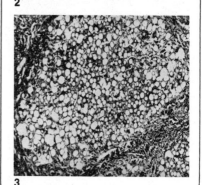

3

☐ Check the patient's vital signs every 15 minutes for 1 hour, then every 30 minutes for 4 hours, and every 4 hours thereafter for 24 hours. Throughout, observe carefully for signs of shock.

☐ Watch for bleeding or signs of bile peritonitis—tenderness and rigidity around the biopsy site. Be alert for symptoms of pneumothorax: rising respiration rate, depressed breath sounds, dyspnea, persistent shoulder pain, and pleuritic chest pain. Report such complications promptly.

☐ If the patient experiences pain, which may persist for several hours after the test, administer analgesic medication, as ordered.

☐ The patient may resume normal diet.

Interfering factors

Failure to obtain a representative specimen or to place the specimen in the proper preservative, and delayed transport of the specimen to the laboratory may interfere with accurate determination of test results.

SHIRLEY GIVEN, HT(ASCP)

Percutaneous Renal Biopsy

Percutaneous renal biopsy is needle excision of a core of kidney tissue to obtain a specimen for histologic examination, using light, electron, and immunofluorescent microscopy. Such examination provides valuable information about glomerular and tubular function. Acute and chronic glomerulonephritis, pyelonephritis, renal vein thrombosis, amyloid infiltration, and systemic lupus erythematosus produce characteristic histologic changes in the kidneys. Complications of percutaneous biopsy may include bleeding, hematoma, arteriovenous fistula, and infection. Despite the risk of these complications, this procedure is considered safer than open biopsy, which is usually the preferred method for removing a tissue specimen from a solid lesion. However, more recent noninvasive procedures, especially renal ultrasonography and CAT scan, have replaced percutaneous renal biopsy in many hospitals.

Purpose

☐ To aid diagnosis of renal parenchymal disease

☐ To monitor progression of renal disease and to assess the effectiveness of treatment.

Patient preparation

Describe the procedure to the patient, and ask him if he has any questions. Explain that this test helps diagnose kidney disorders. Instruct the patient to restrict food and fluids for 8 hours before the test. Tell him who performs the biopsy and where; that the procedure takes only 15 minutes; and that the needle is in the kidney for only a few seconds.

Tell the patient that blood and urine specimens are collected and tested before the biopsy, and that other tests, such as intravenous pyelography, ultrasonography, or an erect film of the abdomen, may be ordered to help determine the biopsy site.

Make sure the patient or an appropriate family member has signed a consent form. Check patient history for hemorrhagic tendencies and hypersensitivity to the local anesthetic. As ordered, 30 minutes to 1 hour before the biopsy administer a mild sedative to help the patient relax. Inform him that he'll receive a local anesthetic but may experience a pinching pain when the needle is inserted through the back into the kidney. Check vital signs, and tell the patient to void just before the test.

Procedure

Place the patient in a prone position on a firm surface, with a sandbag beneath his abdomen. Tell him to take a deep breath while his kidney is being palpated. A 7″ 20G needle is used to inject the local anesthetic into the skin at the biopsy site. Instruct the patient to hold his breath and remain immobile as the needle is inserted just below the angle formed by the intersection of the lowest palpable rib and the lateral border of the sacrospinal muscle. The needle is directed through the back muscles, the deep lumbar fascia, the perinephric fat, and the kidney capsule. After the needle is inserted, tell the patient to take several deep breaths. If the needle swings smoothly during deep breathing, it has penetrated the kidney capsule. After the penetration depth is marked on the needle shaft, instruct the patient to hold his breath and remain as still as possible while the needle is withdrawn, injecting the local anesthetic into the back tissues.

After a small incision is made in the anesthetized skin, instruct the patient to hold his breath and remain immobile while the Vim-Silverman needle with stylet is inserted through the incision, down the tract of the infiltrating needle, to the measured depth. Tell the patient to breathe deeply. If the characteristic needle swing occurs, instruct the patient to hold his breath and remain still while the tissue specimen is obtained. After the tissue is examined immediately under a hand lens to ensure that the specimen contains tissue from both cortex and medulla, the tissue is placed on a saline-soaked gauze pad and placed in a properly labeled container. If an adequate tissue specimen has not been obtained, the procedure is repeated immediately. After an adequate specimen is secured, apply pressure to the biopsy site for 3 to 5 minutes to stop superficial bleeding. Then, apply a pressure dressing.

URINARY TRACT BRUSH BIOPSY

Retrograde brush biopsy of the urinary tract may be used to obtain a renal tissue specimen when X-rays show a lesion in the renal pelvis or calyx. It can also be used to obtain specimens from other areas of the urinary tract. However, retrograde brush biopsy is contraindicated in patients with acute urinary tract infection or an obstruction at or below the biopsy site.

To prepare the patient for brush biopsy, describe the procedure and tell him he may feel some discomfort. Inform him who will perform the biopsy and when. Reassure the patient that the procedure will take only 30 to 60 minutes.

Make sure the patient or a responsible family member has signed an appropriate consent form. Because this procedure requires use of a contrast agent and a general, local, or spinal anesthetic, check the patient's history for hypersensitivity to anesthetics, contrast media, or iodine-containing foods, such as shellfish. Just before the biopsy procedure, administer a sedative to the patient, as ordered.

After the patient has received a sedative and an anesthetic, place him in the lithotomy position. Using a cystoscope, the doctor passes a guide wire up the ureter and passes a urethral catheter over the guide wire. Contrast medium is instilled through the catheter, which is positioned next to the lesion under fluoroscopic guidance. The contrast medium is washed out with normal saline solution to prevent cell distortions from the dye. A nylon or steel brush is passed up the catheter and the lesion is brushed. This procedure is repeated at least six times, using a new brush each time.

As each brush is removed from the catheter, a smear is made for Papanicolaou staining and the brush tip is cut off and placed in formalin for 1 hour. The biopsy material is then removed from the brush tip for histologic examination. When the last brush is withdrawn, the catheter is irrigated with normal saline solution to remove additional cells. These cells are also sent for histologic examination.

Results differentiate between malignant and benign lesions, which may appear the same on X-rays.

Because brush biopsy may cause such complications as perforation, hemorrhage, sepsis, or contrast medium extravasation, carefully monitor the patient's vital signs. Be sure to record the time, color, and amount of voiding, being alert for hematuria and abdominal or flank pain. Report any abnormal findings to the doctor immediately, and administer analgesics and antibiotics, as ordered.

ELLEN SHIPES, RN, MN, ET, MEd

Precautions

□ Percutaneous renal biopsy is contraindicated in a patient with renal tumors, severe bleeding disorder, markedly reduced plasma or blood volume, severe hypertension, hydronephrosis, perinephric abscess, advanced renal failure with uremia, or only one kidney.

 □ Instruct the patient to hold his breath and remain still whenever the needle or prongs are advanced into or retracted from the kidney.

□ Send the tissue specimen to the laboratory immediately.

Findings

Normally, a section of kidney tissue shows Bowman's capsule—the area between two layers of flat epithelial cells—the glomerular tuft, and the capillary lumen. The tubule sections differ depending on the area of tubule involved. The proximal tubule is one layer of epithelial cells with microvilli that form a brush border. The descending Henle's loop has flat squamous epithelial cells, unlike the ascending, distal convoluted and collecting tubules, which are lined with squamous epithelial cells.

Implications of results

Histologic examination of renal tissue can reveal malignancy or renal disease. Malignant tumors include Wilms' tumor, usually present in early childhood, and renal cell carcinoma, most prevalent in persons over age 40. Diseases indicated by characteristic histologic changes include disseminated lupus erythematosus, amyloid infiltration, acute and chronic glomerulonephritis, renal vein thrombosis, and pyelonephritis.

Post-test care

□ Instruct the patient to lie flat on his back without moving for at least 12 hours to prevent bleeding. Check vital signs every 15 minutes for 4 hours, then every 30 minutes for 4 hours, then every hour for 4 hours, and finally every 4 hours. Report any changes.

□ Examine all urine for blood; small amounts may be present after biopsy but should disappear within 8 hours. Occasionally, hematocrit may be monitored after the procedure, to screen for internal bleeding.

□ Encourage fluids, to initiate mild diuresis, which minimizes colic and obstruction from blood clotting within the renal pelvis.

□ The patient may resume normal diet discontinued before the test.

Interfering factors

Failure to obtain an adequate tissue specimen, to store the specimen properly, or to send the specimen to the laboratory immediately may interfere with accurate determination of test results.

SHIRLEY GIVEN, HT(ASCP)

Lung Biopsy

In biopsy of the lung, a specimen of pulmonary tissue is excised by closed or open technique for histologic examination. Closed technique, performed under local anesthetic, includes both needle and transbronchial biopsies; open technique, performed under general anesthetic in the operating room, includes both limited and standard thoracotomies. Needle biopsy is appropriate when the lesion is readily accessible, or when it originates in the lung parenchyma, is confined to it, or is affixed to the chest wall; it provides a much smaller specimen than the open technique. Transbronchial biopsy, the removal of multiple tissue specimens through a fiberoptic bronchoscope, is appropriate for diffuse infiltrative pulmonary disease, tumors, or when severe debilitation contraindicates open biopsy. Open biopsy is appropriate for the study of a well-circumscribed lesion that may require resection.

Generally, a biopsy of the lung is recommended after chest X-ray, computed tomography (CT) scan, and bron-

choscopy have failed to identify the cause of diffuse parenchymal pulmonary disease or of a pulmonary lesion. Complications of lung biopsy include bleeding, infection, and pneumothorax.

Purpose

□ To confirm diagnosis of diffuse parenchymal pulmonary disease and pulmonary lesions.

Patient preparation

Describe the procedure to the patient, and answer any questions. Explain that this test assesses the condition of the lungs. Instruct the patient to fast after midnight before the procedure. (Sometimes the patient is permitted to have clear liquids the morning of the test.) Tell him who will perform the biopsy and where; that the procedure takes 30 to 60 minutes; and that test results should be available in several days.

Tell the patient that a chest X-ray and blood studies (prothrombin time, activated partial thromboplastin time, and platelet count) will be performed before the biopsy.

Make sure the patient or an appropriate family member has signed a consent form. Check patient history for hypersensitivity to the local anesthetic. Administer a mild sedative, as ordered, 30 minutes before the biopsy, to help the patient relax. Tell him he'll receive a local anesthetic but may experience a sharp, transient pain when the biopsy needle touches the lung.

Procedure

After the biopsy site is selected, lead markers are placed on the patient's skin, and X-rays are ordered, to verify their correct placement. Place the patient in a sitting position, with arms folded on a table in front of him, and instruct him to maintain this position, remaining as still as possible, and to refrain from coughing. The skin over the biopsy site is prepared, and the area is draped. With a 25G needle, the local anesthetic is injected just above the lower rib to prevent damage to the intercostal nerves and ves-

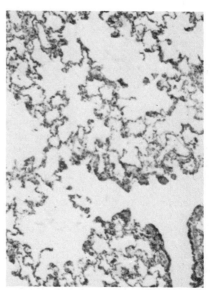

Normal lung parenchyma is a uniformly textured network of bronchioles and blood vessels, honeycombed with alveoli, as shown here. Alveolar walls are composed of a thin epithelial lining, primarily a single layer of attenuated squamous cells on a layer of connective tissue.

Alveoli are separated by interalveolar septa, which have three main tissue components: alveolar epithelium, capillary endothelium, and interstitial spaces. Alveolar epithelium consists of squamous cells and secretory cells that produce and secrete surfactant. Capillary endothelium is a simple layer of continuous-type squamous cells. Interstitial space comprises fibroblasts and pericytes (both with contractile properties), free fluid, collagen, elastic fibers, and various other cell types.

sels. Using a 22G needle, the examiner anesthetizes the intercostal muscles and parietal pleura, makes a small incision (2 to 3 mm) with a scalpel, and introduces the biopsy needle through the incision, chest wall, and pleura, into the tumor or the pulmonary tissue.

If the intercostal space at the incision site is wide, the needle is inserted at a 90° angle; if the ribs overlap and the intercostal space is narrow, at a 45° angle. When the needle is in the tumor or pulmonary tissue, the specimen is obtained and the needle is withdrawn. The specimen is divided immediately: the tissue for histology is placed in a properly labeled bottle containing 10% neutral buffered formaldehyde solution; the tissue for microbiology is placed in a sterile container.

Pressure is exerted on the biopsy site to stop the bleeding, and then a small bandage is applied.

Precautions

□ Needle biopsy is contraindicated in patients with a lesion that's separated from the chest wall or that's accompanied by emphysematous bullae, cysts, or gross emphysema, and in patients with coagulopathy, hypoxia, pulmonary hypertension, or cardiac disease with cor pulmonale.

□ During biopsy, observe for signs of respiratory distress—shortness of breath, elevated pulse, and cyanosis (late sign)—and if they develop, report them immediately.

□ Since coughing or movement during biopsy can cause tearing of the lung by the biopsy needle, keep the patient calm and still.

Findings

Normal pulmonary tissue shows uniform texture of the alveolar ducts, alveolar walls, bronchioles, and small vessels.

Implications of results

Histologic examination of a pulmonary tissue specimen can reveal squamous-cell or oat cell carcinoma, and adenocarcinoma. Such examination supplements the results of microbiologic cultures, deep-cough sputum specimens, chest X-rays, bronchoscopy, and the patient's physical history, in confirming cancer or parenchymal pulmonary disease.

Post-test care

□ Check vital signs every 15 minutes for 1 hour, every hour for 4 hours, then every 4 hours. Watch for bleeding, shortness of breath, elevated pulse, diminished breath sounds on the biopsy side, and eventually, cyanosis. Make sure the chest X-ray is repeated immediately after the biopsy is completed.

□ The patient may resume normal diet.

Interfering factors

Failure to obtain a representative tissue specimen or to store the specimens for histology and microbiology in the appropriate containers may interfere with accurate determination of test results.

SHIRLEY GIVEN, HT(ASCP)

Pleural Biopsy

Pleural biopsy is the removal of pleural tissue, by needle biopsy or open biopsy, for histologic examination. Needle pleural biopsy is performed under local anesthetic. It generally follows thoracentesis—aspiration of pleural fluid—which is performed when the etiology of the effusion is unknown, but it can be performed separately.

Open pleural biopsy, performed in the absence of pleural effusion, permits direct visualization of the pleura and the underlying lung. It's performed in the operating room.

Purpose

□ To differentiate between nonmalignant and malignant disease

□ To diagnose viral, fungal, or parasitic disease, and collagen vascular disease of the pleura.

Patient preparation

Describe the procedure to the patient and answer his questions. Explain that this test permits microscopic examination of pleural tissue. Tell him who will perform the biopsy and where, and that it takes 30 to 45 minutes to perform, although the needle remains in the pleura less than 1 minute. Also tell him that blood studies will precede the biopsy, and that chest X-rays will be taken before and after the biopsy.

Make sure the patient or an appropriate family member has signed a consent form. Check patient history for hypersensitivity to the local anesthetic. Tell him that he'll receive an anesthetic and should experience little pain. Just before the procedure, record vital signs.

Procedure

Seat the patient on the side of the bed, with his feet resting on a stool and his arms supported by the overbed table or upper body. Tell him to hold this position and remain still during the procedure. Prepare the skin and drape the area. The local anesthetic is then administered.

Vim-Silverman needle biopsy: The needle is inserted through the appropriate intercostal space into the biopsy site, with the outer tip distal to the pleura and the central portion pushed in deeper and held in place. The outer case is inserted about ⅜″ (1 cm), the entire assembly rotated 360°, and the needle and tissue specimen are withdrawn.

Cope's needle biopsy: The trocar is introduced through the appropriate intercostal space into the biopsy site. The sharp obturator is then removed and a hooked stylet is inserted through the trocar. The opened notch is directed against the pleura, along the intercostal space, and is slowly withdrawn. While the outer tube is held stationary, the inner tube is twisted to cut off the tissue specimen, and the assembly is withdrawn.

The specimen is immediately put in 10% neutral buffered formaldehyde solution in a labeled specimen bottle.

Cleanse the skin around the biopsy site, and apply an adhesive bandage.

Precautions

☐ Pleural biopsy is contraindicated in patients with severe bleeding disorders.
☐ Send the specimen to the laboratory immediately.

Findings

The normal pleura consists primarily of mesothelial cells, flattened in a uniform layer. Layers of areolar connective tissue—containing blood vessels, nerves, and lymphatics—lie below.

Implications of results

Histologic examination of the tissue specimen can reveal malignant disease; tuberculosis; or viral, fungal, parasitic, or collagen vascular disease. Primary neoplasms of the pleura are generally fibrous and epithelial.

Post-test care

☐ Check vital signs every 15 minutes for 1 hour, then every hour for 4 hours or until stable. Make sure the chest X-ray is repeated immediately after the biopsy.
☐ Watch for signs of respiratory distress (shortness of breath), shoulder pain, and complications, such as pneumothorax

USING COPE'S NEEDLE

Cope's needle, used to obtain a pleural biopsy specimen, has three parts: a sharp obturator (A) and a cannula (B), which, when fitted together, are called a trocar, and a blunt-ended, hooked stylet (C). The trocar is used to gain access to the pleural cavity. Then, the obturator is removed, leaving the cannula in place. The stylet is passed through the cannula to excise a tissue specimen, as shown here.

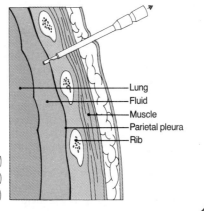

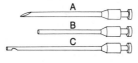

(immediate) and pneumonia (delayed).

Interfering factors
Failure to use proper fixative or obtain adequate specimens may alter results.

SHIRLEY GIVEN, HT(ASCP)

Cervical Punch Biopsy

Cervical punch biopsy is the excision by sharp forceps of a tissue specimen from the cervix for histologic examination. Generally, multiple biopsies are done to obtain specimens from all areas with abnormal tissue, or from the squamo-columnar junction and other sites around the cervical circumference. This procedure is indicated in women with suspicious cervical lesions and should be performed when the cervix is least vascular (usually 1 week after menses). Biopsy sites are selected by direct visualization of the cervix with a colposcope—the most accurate method—or by Schiller's test, which stains normal squamous epithelium a dark mahogany but fails to color abnormal tissue.

Purpose
☐ To evaluate suspicious cervical lesions
☐ To diagnose cervical cancer.

Patient preparation
Describe the procedure to the patient, and explain that it provides a cervical tissue specimen for microscopic study. Tell her who will perform the biopsy and where; and that the procedure takes about 15 minutes. Tell the patient that she may experience mild discomfort during and after the biopsy. Advise the outpatient to have someone accompany her home after the biopsy.

Make sure the patient or a responsible family member has signed a consent form. Just before the biopsy, ask the patient to void.

Procedure
Place the patient in the lithotomy position. Tell her to relax as the unlubricated speculum is inserted.

For *direct visualization,* the colposcope is inserted through the speculum, the biopsy site is located, and the cervix is cleansed with a swab soaked in 3% acetic acid solution. The biopsy forceps are then inserted through the speculum or the colposcope, and tissue is removed from any lesion or from selected sites, starting from the posterior lip to avoid obscuring other sites with blood. Each specimen is immediately put in 10% formaldehyde solution in a labeled bottle. To control bleeding after biopsy, the cervix is swabbed with 5% silver nitrate solution (cautery or sutures may be used instead). If bleeding persists, the examiner may insert a tampon.

For *Schiller's test,* an applicator stick saturated with iodine solution is inserted through the speculum. This stains the cervix to identify lesions for biopsy.

Record the patient's and doctor's names, and biopsy sites on the laboratory slip.

Precautions
Send the specimens to the laboratory immediately.

Findings
Normal cervical tissue is composed of columnar and squamous epithelial cells, loose connective tissue, and smooth-muscle fibers, with no dysplasia or abnormal cell growth.

Implications of results
Histologic examination of a cervical tissue specimen identifies abnormal cells and differentiates the tissue as intraepithelial neoplasia or invasive cancer. If the cause of an abnormal Pap test isn't demonstrated by cervical biopsy, or if the specimen shows advanced dysplasia or carcinoma in situ, a cone biopsy is performed in the operating room, under general anesthetic. Cone biopsy garners a larger tissue specimen and allows a more accurate evaluation of dysplasia.

ENDOMETRIAL AND OVARIAN BIOPSIES

METHOD	PURPOSE	SPECIAL CONSIDERATIONS
ENDOMETRIAL BIOPSY		
• Dilation and curettage (D&C) • Endometrial washing (by jet irrigation, aspiration, or brushing)	• To evaluate uterine bleeding • To diagnose suspected endometrial carcinoma • To diagnose a missed abortion	• Time of menstrual cycle affects accuracy of biopsy results • Type of specimen obtained depends on patient's age and disorder • Endometrial washing requires no anesthesia and can be done in a doctor's office • D&C may follow negative biopsy by endometrial washing • Specimens obtained by D&C may be processed as frozen sections
OVARIAN BIOPSY		
• Transrectal or transvaginal fine needle biopsy • Aspiration biopsy during laparoscopy	• To detect an ovarian tumor • To determine the spread of malignancy	• Fine needle biopsy may follow palpation, laparoscopy, or computed tomography that detects an abnormal ovary • Aspiration during laparoscopy is particularly useful for young women who are infertile or who have lesions that appear benign

SHIRLEY GIVEN, HT(ASCP)

Post-test care

□ Instruct the patient to avoid strenuous exercise for 8 to 24 hours after the biopsy. Encourage the outpatient to rest briefly before leaving the office.

□ If a tampon was inserted after the biopsy, tell the patient to leave it in place for 8 to 24 hours, as ordered. Inform her that some bleeding may occur, but tell her to report heavy bleeding (heavier than menstrual) to the doctor. Warn the patient to avoid using tampons, which can irritate the cervix and provoke bleed-ing, according to her doctor's directions.

□ Tell the patient to avoid douching and intercourse for 2 weeks, or as directed.

□ Inform the patient that a foul-smelling, gray-green vaginal discharge is normal for several days after biopsy and may persist for 3 weeks.

Interfering factors

Failure to obtain representative specimens or to place them in the preservative immediately may alter results.

KAREN DYER VANCE, RN, BSN

SKELETAL BIOPSIES

Bone Biopsy

Bone biopsy is the removal of a piece or a core of bone for histologic examina- *tion. It's performed either by using a special drill needle, under local anesthetic, or by surgical excision, under general anesthetic. Bone biopsy is indicated in patients with bone pain and tenderness, after bone scan, computed tomography*

(CAT) scan, X-ray, or arteriography reveals a mass or deformity. Excision provides a larger specimen than drill biopsy, and permits immediate surgical treatment if quick histologic analysis of the specimen reveals malignancy. In the presence of tumors, bone bows slightly, thickens, and sometimes fractures—the result of increased osteoblastic or osteoclastic activity, or both.

Possible complications of bone biopsy include bone fracture, damage to surrounding tissue, and infection (osteomyelitis).

Purpose
□ To distinguish between benign and malignant bone tumors.

Patient preparation
Describe the procedure to the patient, and answer any questions. Explain that this test permits microscopic examination of a bone specimen. If the patient is to have a drill biopsy, inform him he needn't restrict food or fluids. If the patient is to have open biopsy, instruct him to fast overnight before the test. Tell him who will perform the biopsy and where, and that the procedure should take no longer than 30 minutes.

Tell the patient that he will receive a local anesthetic but will still experience discomfort and pressure when the biopsy needle enters the bone. Explain that a special drill forces the needle into the bone; if possible, show him a photograph of the bone drill to make the biopsy seem less ominous. Stress the importance of his cooperation during the biopsy.

Make sure the patient or a responsible family member has signed a consent form. Check patient history for hypersensitivity to the local anesthetic.

Procedure
For *drill biopsy*, the patient is properly positioned, and the biopsy site is shaved and meticulously prepared. After the local anesthetic is injected, the doctor makes a small incision (usually about 3 mm) and pushes the biopsy needle with pointed trocar into the bone, using

firm, even pressure. Once the needle is engaged in the bone, it is rotated about 180°, while continuing steady pressure. When the bone core is obtained, the trocar is withdrawn by reversing the drilling motion, and the specimen is placed in a properly labeled bottle containing 10% formaldehyde solution. Apply pressure to the site with a sterile gauze pad. When bleeding stops, remove the gauze and apply a topical antiseptic (povidone-iodine ointment) and an adhesive bandage or other sterile covering, to close the wound and prevent infection.

For *open biopsy*, the patient is anesthetized, and the biopsy site is prepared by shaving the area, cleansing it with surgical soap, and then disinfecting it with an iodine wash and alcohol. The doctor makes an incision, removes a piece of bone, and sends it to the histology laboratory immediately for analysis. Further surgery can then be performed, depending on bone specimen findings.

Precautions
□ Bone biopsy should be performed cautiously in patients with coagulopathy.
□ Send the specimen to the laboratory immediately.

Findings
Normal bone tissue consists of fibers of collagen, osteocytes, and osteoblasts.

Normal bone is of two histologic types: compact and cancellous. Compact bone has dense, concentric layers of mineral deposits, or lamellae. Cancellous bone has widely spaced lamellae, with osteocytes and red and yellow marrow lying between them.

Implications of results
Histologic examination of a bone specimen can reveal benign or malignant tumors. Benign tumors, generally well-circumscribed and nonmetastasizing, include osteoid osteoma, osteoblastoma, osteochondroma, unicameral bone cyst, benign giant-cell tumor, and fibroma. Malignant tumors, which spread irregularly and rapidly, most commonly in-

clude both multiple myeloma and osteosarcoma, although the most lethal is Ewing's sarcoma. Most malignant tumors spread to bone through the blood and lymph systems from the breast, lungs, prostate, thyroid, or kidneys.

Post-test care

□ Check vital signs and the dressing at the biopsy site, as ordered. Ask the doctor how much drainage is expected, and notify him if drainage is excessive.

□ If the patient experiences pain at the biopsy site, administer an analgesic, as ordered.

□ For several days after biopsy, watch for indications of bone infection: fever, headache, pain on movement, and tissue redness or abscess at or near the biopsy site. Notify the doctor if these symptoms develop.

□ Advise the patient that he may resume his usual diet.

Interfering factors

Failure to obtain a representative bone specimen, to use the proper fixative, or to send the specimen to the laboratory immediately may interfere with accurate determination of test results

SHIRLEY GIVEN, HT(ASCP)

Bone Marrow Aspiration and Biopsy

Bone marrow, the soft tissue contained in the medullary canals of long bone and in the interstices of cancellous bone, may be removed by aspiration or needle biopsy, under local anesthetic. In aspiration biopsy, a fluid specimen in which pustula of marrow are suspended is removed from the bone marrow. In needle biopsy, a core of marrow—cells, not fluid—is removed. These methods are often used concurrently to obtain the best possible marrow specimens. Because

bone marrow is the major site of hematopoiesis, the histologic and hematologic examination of its contents provides reliable diagnostic information about blood disorders. Marrow removed from the bone may be red or yellow. Red marrow, which comprises about 50% of an adult's marrow, actively produces RBCs; yellow marrow contains fat cells and connective tissue, and is inactive. Because yellow marrow can become active in response to the body's needs, an adult has a large hematopoietic capacity. An infant's marrow is mainly red and, consequently, reflects a small hematopoietic capacity.

Bleeding and infection may result from bone marrow biopsy at any site, but the most serious complications occur at the sternum. Such complications are rare but include puncture of the heart and major vessels—causing severe hemorrhage—and puncture of the mediastinum—causing mediastinitis or pneumomediastinum.

Purpose

□ To diagnose thrombocytopenia, leukemias, granulomas, and aplastic, hypoplastic, and pernicious anemias

□ To diagnose primary and metastatic tumors

□ To determine the cause of infection

□ To aid staging of disease, such as Hodgkin's disease

□ To evaluate the effectiveness of chemotherapy and help monitor myelosuppression.

Patient preparation

Describe the procedure to the patient, and answer any questions. Explain that the test permits microscopic examination of a bone marrow specimen. Inform the patient that he needn't restrict food or fluids before the test. Tell him who will perform the biopsy and where; that it usually takes only 5 to 10 minutes; and that test results are generally available in 1 day.

Inform him that more than one bone marrow specimen may be required, and that a blood sample will be collected before biopsy, for laboratory testing.

Make sure the patient or a responsible family member has signed a consent form. Check patient history for hypersensitivity to the local anesthetic. After checking with the doctor, tell the patient which bone—sternum, anterior or posterior iliac crest, vertebral spinous process, rib, or tibia—will be the biopsy site. Inform him that he will receive a local anesthetic but will feel pressure on insertion of the biopsy needle and a brief, pulling pain on removal of the marrow. As ordered, administer a mild sedative 1 hour before the test.

Procedure

After positioning the patient, instruct him to remain as still as possible. Offer emotional support during the biopsy by talking quietly to the patient, describing what is being done, and answering any questions.

For aspiration biopsy: After the skin over the biopsy site is prepared and the area is draped, the local anesthetic is injected. With a twisting motion, the marrow aspiration needle is inserted through the skin, the subcutaneous tissue, and the cortex of the bone. The stylet is removed from the needle, and a 10- to 20-ml syringe is attached. The examiner aspirates 0.2 to 0.5 ml of marrow, then withdraws the needle. Apply pressure to the site for 5 minutes, while the marrow slides are being prepared. (If the patient has thrombocytopenia, apply pressure to the site for 10 to 15 minutes.) The biopsy site is cleansed again, and a sterile adhesive bandage is applied.

If an adequate marrow specimen has not been obtained on the first attempt, the needle may be repositioned within the marrow cavity, or may be removed and reinserted in another site within the anesthetized area. If the second attempt fails, a needle biopsy may be necessary.

For needle biopsy: After preparing the biopsy site and draping the area, the examiner marks the skin at the site with an indelible pencil or marking pen. A local anesthetic is then injected intradermally, subcutaneously, and at the

BONE MARROW:

CELL TYPES

Normoblasts, total
  Pronormoblasts
  Basophilic
  Polychromatic
  Orthochromatic

Neutrophils, total
  Myeloblasts
  Promyelocytes
  Myelocytes
  Metamyelocytes
  Bands
  Segmented

Eosinophils

Basophils

Lymphocytes

Plasma cells

Megakaryocytes

Myeloid: Erythroid ratio

NORMAL VALUES AND IMPLICATIONS OF ABNORMAL FINDINGS

NORMAL MEAN VALUES			CLINICAL IMPLICATIONS	
Adults	Children	Infants	Elevated Values	Depressed Values
25.6% 0.2% to 1.3% 0.5% to 2.4% 17.9% to 29.2% 0.4% to 4.6%	23.1% 0.5% 1.7% 18.2% 2.7%	8.0% 0.1% 0.34% 6.9% 0.54%	Polycythemia vera	Vitamin B_{12} or folic acid deficiency; hypoplastic or aplastic anemia
56.5% 0.2% to 1.5% 2.1% to 4.1% 8.2% to 15.7% 9.6% to 24.6% 9.5% to 15.3% 6.0% to 12.0%	57.1% 1.2% 1.4% 18.3% 23.3% 0 12.9%	32.4% 0.62% 0.76% 2.5% 11.3% 14.1% 3.6%	Acute myeloblastic or chronic myeloid leukemia	Lymphoblastic, lymphatic, or monocytic leukemia; aplastic anemia
3.1%	3.6%	2.6%	Bone marrow carcinoma, lymphadenoma, myeloid leukemia, eosinophilic leukemia, pernicious anemia (in relapse)	
.01%	0.06%	0.07%	No relationship between basophil count and symptoms	No relationship between basophil count and symptoms
16.2%	16.0%	49.0%	B- and T-cell chronic lymphocytic leukemia, other lymphatic leukemias, lymphoma, mononucleosis, aplastic anemia, macroglobulinemia	
1.3%	.4%	0.02%	Myeloma, collagen disease, infection, antigen sensitivity, malignancy	
0.1%	0.1%	0.05%	Old age, chronic myeloid leukemia, polycythemia vera, megakaryocytic myelosis, infection, idiopathic thrombocytopenic purpura, thrombocytopenia	Pernicious anemia
2.3	2.9	4.4	Myeloid leukemia, infection, leukemoid reactions, depressed hematopoiesis	Agranulocytosis, hematopoiesis after hemorrhage or hemolysis, iron deficiency anemia, polycythemia vera

Adapted with permission from *Pediatric Hematology*, by A.M. Mauer, copyright © 1969, McGraw-Hill Book Company, and from *Clinical Hematology*, by M.M. Wintrobe, copyright © 1981, Lea & Febiger.

COMMON SITES OF BONE MARROW ASPIRATION AND BIOPSY

(1) **Posterior superior iliac spine** is the preferred site, since no vital organs or vessels are located nearby. With the patient in a lateral position with one leg flexed, the doctor inserts the needle several centimeters lateral to the iliosacral junction, entering the bone plane crest with the needle directed downward and toward the anterior inferior spine, or entering a few centimeters below the crest at a right angle to the surface of the bone.

(2) **Sternum** involves the greatest risks but is commonly used for marrow aspiration, because it's near the surface, the cortical bone is thin, and the marrow cavity contains numerous cells and relatively little fat or supporting bone. For this procedure, the patient is supine on a firm bed or examining table with a small pillow beneath the shoulders to elevate the chest and lower the head. The doctor secures the needle guard 3 to 4 mm from the tip of the needle to avoid accidental puncture of the heart or a major vessel. Then, he inserts the needle at the midline of the sternum at the second intercostal space.

(3) **Spinous process** is preferred if multiple punctures are necessary, marrow is absent at other sites, or the patient objects to sternal puncture. In this procedure, the patient sits on the edge of the bed, leaning over the bedside stand; or, if the patient is uncooperative, he may be placed in the prone position with restraints. The doctor selects the spinous process of the third or fourth lumbar vertebrae and inserts the needle at the crest or slightly to one side, advancing the needle in the direction of the bone plane.

(4) **Tibia** is the site of choice for infants younger than age 1. The infant is placed in a prone position on a bed or examining table with a sandbag beneath the leg. The foot is taped to the surface of the table, or an assistant holds the leg stationary by placing a hand under it. The doctor inserts the needle about ⅜″ (1 cm) below the tibial tuberosity and slightly toward the medial side, being careful to angle the needle point toward the foot to avoid epiphyseal injury.

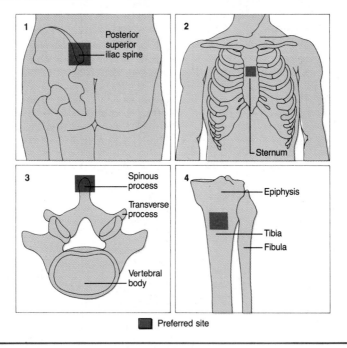

Preferred site

surface of the bone. Then the biopsy needle is inserted into the periosteum, and the needle guard is set, as indicated. The needle is advanced with a steady boring motion, until the outer needle passes through the cortex of the bone.

The inner needle with trephine tip is inserted into the outer needle, and the stylet is removed. By alternately rotating the inner needle clockwise and counter-clockwise, the examiner directs the needle into the marrow cavity and then removes a tissue plug. The needle assembly is withdrawn, and the marrow is expelled into a labeled bottle containing Zenker's acetic acid solution. After the biopsy site is cleansed, a sterile adhesive bandage or a pressure dressing is applied.

Precautions

☐ Bone marrow biopsy is contraindicated in patients with severe bleeding disorders.

☐ Send the tissue specimen or slides to the laboratory immediately.

Findings

Yellow marrow contains fat cells and connective tissue; red marrow contains hematopoietic cells, fat cells, and connective tissue. (See chart on pages 496 and 497 for values of components.)

In addition, special stains that detect hematologic disorders produce these normal findings: the iron stain, which measures hemosiderin (storage iron), has a $+2$ level; the Sudan Black B (SBB) stain, which shows granulocytes, is negative; and the periodic acid-Schiff (PAS) stain, which detects glycogen reactions, is negative.

Implications of results

Histologic examination of a bone marrow specimen can help detect myelofibrosis, granulomas, lymphoma, or cancer. Hematologic analysis, including the differential count and myeloid-erythroid ratio, can implicate a wide range of disorders (see chart).

In an iron stain, decreased hemosiderin levels may indicate a true iron deficiency. Increased levels may accompany other types of anemias or blood disorders. A positive SBB stain can differentiate acute granulocytic leukemia from acute lymphocytic leukemia (SBB negative) or may indicate granulation in myeloblasts. A positive PAS stain may

---

BONE MARROW BIOPSY IN CHILDREN

To prepare a child for a bone marrow biopsy, give him his own biopsy kit: a syringe without a needle, cotton balls, and adhesive bandages. Illustrate the procedure by using a doll or a stuffed animal as a model. In this way, you can gain the child's confidence and answer any questions he may have. Be sure to prepare him by describing the kinds of pressure and discomfort he will feel during the procedure.

Before the biopsy, explain the equipment on the tray to the child. Ask the parents to get involved: they can help you hold the child still and reassure him. Tell the child he will feel some pain when the doctor aspirates the bone marrow, and it's OK to cry or yell if he wants to, but the pain will go away quickly.

---

indicate acute or chronic lymphocytic leukemia, amyloidosis, thalassemia, lymphomas, infectious mononucleosis, iron-deficiency anemia, or sideroblastic anemia.

Post-test care

☐ Check the biopsy site for bleeding and inflammation.

☐ Observe the patient for signs of hemorrhage and infection, such as rapid pulse rate, low blood pressure, and fever.

Interfering factors

Failure to obtain a representative specimen, to use a fixative (for histologic analysis), or to send the specimen immediately may alter test results.

SHIRLEY GIVEN, HT(ASCP)
MARYLOU K. MCHUGH, RN, MSN

Synovial Membrane Biopsy

Biopsy of the synovial membrane is needle excision of a tissue specimen for histo-

logic examination of the thin epithelium lining the diarthrodial joint capsules. In a large joint, such as the knee, preliminary arthroscopy can aid selection of the biopsy site. Synovial membrane biopsy is performed when analysis of synovial fluid—a viscous, lubricating fluid contained within the synovial membrane—proves nondiagnostic or when the fluid itself is absent.

Purpose

□ To diagnose gout, pseudogout, bacterial infections and lesions, and granulomatous infections

□ To aid diagnosis of rheumatoid arthritis, systemic lupus erythematosus (SLE), or Reiter's disease, and to monitor joint pathology.

Patient preparation

Describe the procedure to the patient, and ask if he has any questions. Explain that this test provides a tissue specimen from the membrane that lines the affected joint. Advise him he needn't restrict food or fluids. Tell him who will perform the procedure and where, and that he'll receive a local anesthetic to minimize discomfort but will experience transient pain when the needle enters the joint. Advise him that the procedure takes about 30 minutes and that test results are usually available in 1 or 2 days. Inform the patient that complications may include infection and bleeding into the joint, but that these are rare.

Make sure the patient or an appropriate family member has signed a consent form. Check patient history for hypersensitivity to the local anesthetic.

Inform the patient which site—knee (most common), elbow, wrist, ankle, or shoulder—has been chosen for this biopsy (usually, the most symptomatic joint is selected). Administer a sedative, if ordered, to help him relax.

Procedure

Place the patient in the proper position, cleanse the biopsy site, and drape the area. After the local anesthetic is injected into the joint space, the trocar is

forcefully thrust into the joint space, away from the site of anesthetic infiltration, to minimize the possibility of artifacts. The biopsy needle is inserted through the trocar. The hooked notch side of the biopsy needle is positioned against the synovium, and suction is applied with a 50-ml Luer-Lok syringe. While the trocar is held stationary, the biopsy needle is twisted to cut off a tissue segment. Then the biopsy needle is withdrawn, and the specimen is placed in a properly labeled sterile container or a specimen bottle containing absolute ethyl alcohol, as indicated. By changing the angle of the biopsy needle, several specimens can be obtained without reinserting the trocar. The trocar is then removed, the biopsy site cleaned, and a pressure bandage is applied.

Precautions

Send the container with absolute ethyl alcohol to the histology laboratory immediately. Send the sterile container to the microbiology laboratory.

Findings

The synovial membrane contains cells that are identical to those found in other connective tissue. The membrane surface is relatively smooth, except for villi, folds, and fat pads that project into the joint cavity. The membrane tissue produces synovial fluid, and contains a capillary network, lymphatic vessels, and a few nerve fibers. Pathology of the synovial membrane also affects the cellular composition of the synovial fluid.

Implications of results

Histologic examination of synovial tissue can diagnose coccidioidomycosis, gout, pseudogout, hemochromatosis, tuberculosis, sarcoidosis, amyloidosis, pigmented villonodular synovitis, synovial tumors, or synovial malignancy (rare). Such examination can also aid diagnosis of rheumatoid arthritis, SLE, and Reiter's disease.

Post-test care

□ Watch for signs of bleeding into the

joint (swelling and tenderness) every hour for 4 hours, then every 4 hours for 12 hours.

☐ Administer medication, as ordered, if the patient experiences pain at the biopsy site.

☐ Instruct the patient to rest the joint from which the tissue specimen was removed for 1 day before resuming normal activity.

Interfering factors

Failure to obtain several biopsy specimens, to obtain these specimens away from the infiltration site of the anesthetic, to store the specimens in the appropriate solution, or to send the tissue specimen to the laboratory immediately may interfere with accurate determination of test results.

SHIRLEY GIVEN, HT(ASCP)

Selected References

Arndt, Kenneth A. *Manual of Dermatologic Therapeutics,* 2nd ed. Boston: Little, Brown and Co., 1978.

Berkow, Robert, ed. *The Merck Manual of Diagnosis and Therapy,* 14th ed. Rahway, N.J.: Merck, Sharp and Dohme, 1982.

Bordow, Richard A., et al., eds. *Manual of Clinical Problems in Pulmonary Medicine.* Boston: Little, Brown & Co., 1980.

Brunner, Lillian S., and Suddarth, Doris S. *Textbook of Medical-Surgical Nursing,* 5th ed. Philadelphia: J.B. Lippincott Co., 1984.

Conn, Howard F., and Conn, Rex B., eds. *Current Diagnosis,* 6th ed. Philadelphia: W.B. Saunders Co., 1980.

Diseases, 2nd ed. Nurse's Reference Library. Springhouse, Pa.: Sprinhouse Corp., 1986.

Guyton, Arthur F. *Textbook of Medical Physiology,* 6th ed. Philadelphia: W.B. Saunders Co., 1981.

Harvey, A. McGehee, ed. *The Principles and Practice of Medicine,* 21st ed. East Norwalk, Conn.: Appleton-Century-Crofts, 1984.

Henry, John Bernard, ed. *Todd-Sanford-Davidsohn Clinical Diagnosis and Management by Laboratory Methods,* 17th ed. Philadelphia: W.B. Saunders Co., 1984.

Markus, Susan. "Taking the Fear Out of Bone Marrow Examinations," *Nursing81* 11:64-67, April 1981.

Morel, Alice, and Wise, Gilbert J. *Urologic Endoscopic Procedures,* 2nd ed. St. Louis: C.V. Mosby Co., 1979.

Neoplastic Disorders. Nurse's Clinical Library. Springhouse, Pa.: Springhouse Corp., 1985.

Petersdorf, Robert G., and Adams, Raymond D., eds. *Harrison's Principles of Internal Medicine,* 10th ed. New York: McGraw-Hill Book Co., 1983.

Price, Sylvia, and Wilson, Lorraine. *Pathophysiology: Clinical Concepts of Disease Processes,* 2nd ed. New York: McGraw-Hill Book Co., 1982.

Sabiston, D.C., Jr., ed. *Davis-Christopher Textbook of Surgery: The Biological Basis of Modern Surgical Practice,* 12th ed. Philadelphia: W.B. Saunders Co., 1981.

Sheehan, Dezna C., and Hrapchak, Barbara B. *Theory and Practice of Histotechnology,* 2nd ed. St. Louis: C.V. Mosby Co., 1980.

Tannebaum, Myron, ed. *Urologic Pathology: The Prostate.* Philadelphia: Lea & Febiger, 1977.

Tilkian, Sarko M., et al. *Clinical Implications of Laboratory Tests,* 3rd ed. St. Louis: C.V. Mosby Co., 1983.

Wallach, Jacques B. *Interpretation of Diagnostic Tests: A Handbook Synopsis of Laboratory Medicine,* 3rd ed. Boston: Little, Brown & Co., 1978.

Widmann, Frances K. *Clinical Interpretation of Laboratory Tests,* 9th ed. Philadelphia: F.A. Davis Co., 1983.

Williams, William J., et al. *Hematology,* 2nd ed. New York: McGraw-Hill Book Co., 1977.

Wintrobe, Maxwell M., et al. *Clinical Hematology,* 8th ed. Philadelphia: Lea & Febiger, 1981.

Wyngaarden, James, and Smith, Lloyd. *Cecil Textbook of Medicine,* 16th ed. Philadelphia: W.B. Saunders Co., 1982.

19

Microbes and Parasites

LEARNING OBJECTIVES

After completing this chapter, the reader will be able to:
- discuss the importance of staining procedures.
- describe culture and sensitivity testing.
- define four classes of protozoa.
- explain how protozoa are transmitted.
- state the characteristics of helminths.
- explain the anatomy and physiology of the lymphatic system.
- explain the purpose of each test discussed in the chapter.
- prepare the patient physically and psychologically for each test.
- describe the procedure for performing each test.
- specify appropriate precautions for safe administration of each test.
- recognize signs of adverse reaction and respond appropriately.
- implement appropriate post-test care.
- identify the normal findings of each test.
- discuss the implications of abnormal test results.
- list factors that may interfere with accurate test results.

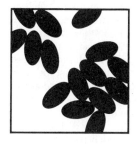

Microbes and Parasites

Introduction

Microbiology is the study of microorganisms—bacteria, fungi, viruses, and protozoa—that are so small they require special techniques, such as staining or electron microscopy, to reveal their sizes, shapes, and cellular structures.

Gram's stain

Gram's staining method, the most common and useful staining procedure, separates bacteria into two classifications, according to the composition of their cell walls: Gram-positive organisms, which retain crystal violet stain after decolorization, and Gram-negative organisms, which lose the purple stain but counterstain red with safranine. Microscopic examination of a Gram stain frequently allows tentative identification of the suspected organism.

This method of staining can also give clues to the type of infection present and consequent mobilization of the immune system, by examining a direct Gram smear of the specimen for inflammatory cells, such as neutrophils and macrophages. For example, a large number of segmented neutrophils in a smear of cerebrospinal fluid suggests bacterial meningitis; a large number of mononuclear cells suggests viral, fungal, or tubercular meningitis.

Acid-fast stain

Another staining procedure, the acid-fast method, helps identify organisms of the genus *Mycobacterium*. Since mycobacteria (including pathogens of tuberculosis and leprosy) are acid-fast, they retain carbolfuchsin stain after treatment with an acid-alcohol solution. This technique is particularly useful for identifying mycobacteria in sputum specimens, which may contain many different organisms.

Culture confirms smears

Although stained smears provide rapid, valuable diagnostic leads, they only tentatively identify a pathogen. For example, detection of acid-fast organisms in sputum doesn't conclusively diagnose tuberculosis; nor does a negative acid-fast smear preclude the possibility of tuberculosis. Generally, visualization of an acid-fast microorganism requires the presence of 10,000 to 100,000 microbes per gram of sputum or per milliliter of body fluid.

Confirmation requires culturing and identifying the microbes. Since this process depends on a particular organism's growth rate and nutritional requirements, growing microbes in culture takes longer than microscopic examination of a stained smear. For instance, the slow-growing mycobacteria may need weeks of incubation before growth appears. Nevertheless, sufficient growth must take place before further micro-

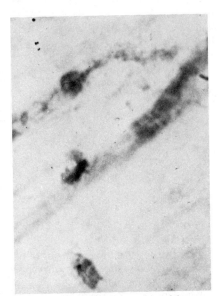

Acid-fast stains distinguish members of the genus Mycobacterium *from other microorganisms. Like all mycobacteria, the tuberculosis bacillus retains a carbolfuchsin stain even after treatment with an acid-alcohol solution. In the photograph above, the slender, acid-fast, slightly beaded curved rods in sputum from a patient with pulmonary tuberculosis typify tubercle bacilli.*

scopic and biochemical studies can identify the organism.

Sensitivity testing

After a microbe is isolated, its susceptibility to specific antibiotics and the extent of infection must be determined, to guide selection of antimicrobial therapy. Some pathogens—*Streptococcus pneumoniae (pneumococcus), Streptococcus pyogenes,* and *Neisseria meningitidis,* for example—usually have predictable sensitivity patterns; other pathogens—such as most Gram-negative bacilli (*Escherichia coli, Enterobacter* species, *Salmonella, Shigella, Klebsiella, Proteus,* and *Pseudomonas*), enterococci (such as *Streptococcus faecalis*), and *Staphylococcus* species—require testing to determine antibiotic susceptibility.

These tests also help determine the dosage needed to inhibit or kill an organism in vivo. However, in vitro tests can't account for pharmacologic prop-

erties of the selected antibiotic, such as toxicity, protein-binding, absorption, and excretion; nor can they establish the immune status of the host or the nature of the underlying pathologic process. Thus, in vitro antibiotic susceptibility studies give only an approximate guide; the patient's clinical response determines the precise dosage of the selected agent. In the Kirby-Bauer disk-diffusion method, the most widely used qualitative test, disks of filter paper are impregnated with exact amounts of different antibiotics and are added to an agar plate that has been seeded with the test organism. After overnight incubation, zones of inhibition around the antibiotics demonstrate the sensitivity patterns of the organism. A *resistant* strain isn't inhibited by a therapeutic amount of an antibiotic; a *moderately susceptible* strain may be inhibited by high dosages of the antibiotic; a *sensitive* strain is inhibited or killed by the recommended dosage of an antibiotic; and an *intermediate* or *indeterminate* strain is equivocally susceptible.

Quantitative sensitivity testing may be necessary for patients with bacterial endocarditis, bacteremias, or impaired renal function; for those who fail to respond to antibiotic therapy; or for those who relapse during therapy. Quantitative testing requires the dilution technique, in which serial dilutions are inoculated with the organism and incubated to determine the minimal inhibitory concentration (MIC) and the minimum lethal concentration (MLC) for the tested isolate.

The antibacterial serum level determination test can help evaluate the effectiveness of antibiotic therapy. This test consists of titrating serum drawn at peak levels (when antibacterial level is highest) or at trough levels (when antibacterial level is lowest, before the next antibiotic dose) against dilutions of the infecting organism.

Parasitology

Transmission of parasites—organisms that live in or on other biological species

FOUR PATHOGENIC PROTOZOA

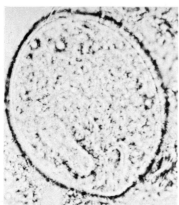

Balantidium coli: *This is the largest intestinal protozoan found in humans and the only pathogenic ciliate. In this photograph of an unstained B. coli trophozoite taken from a stool specimen, food vacuoles and an anterior cytostome are visible.*

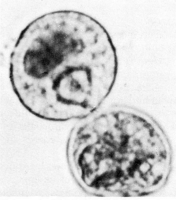

Entamoeba histolytica: *This is the only human pathogen of the six species of Entamoeba protozoa. Notice the large chromatoid bodies, diffused glycogen, and the delicate chromatin beads on the inner surface of the nuclear membrane that distinguish these infective cysts from nonpathogenic amoeba.*

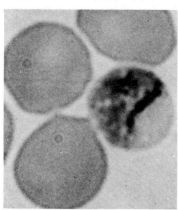

Plasmodium malariae: *This organism attacks mature erythrocytes. The trophozoite shown in the photograph displays the granular band of dark brown or black pigment acquired during growth of this sporozoa.*

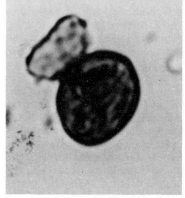

Giardia lamblia: *These flagellates commonly infest the intestinal tract. The photograph shows an ellipsoid cyst with a smooth well-defined wall and multiple nuclei. Notice the trophozoites—forms in the feeding stage—within the cyst.*

to take nourishment from them—is affected by such factors as sanitation, diet, and climate. In countries with good sanitation and effective infection control, the incidence of parasitic disease is relatively low. The clinically important groups of parasites are protozoa (single-cell organisms), helminths (worms), and arthropods (insects and arachnids, such as spiders, mites, and ticks).

Protozoa

Protozoa are classified according to their means of locomotion:

□ *Sarcodina* (amebae) move on temporary cytoplasmic protrusions called pseudopodia. Most species of amebae appear in humans in the motile, feeding stage (trophozoite form) and the infective stage (cyst form). Of these species, only *Entamoeba histolytica* causes significant disease.

□ *Mastigophora* (flagellates) propel themselves by long filamentous appendages called flagella. The most common pathogenic species of flagellates in the United States are *Giardia lamblia*, which infests the intestinal tract, and *Trichomonas vaginalis*, which infests the genital tract. Hemoflagellates, an important subgroup, include the genera *Trypanosoma* and *Leishmania*.

□ *Ciliophora* (ciliates and suctorians) move on hundreds of hairlike projections that cover their bodies. The only pathogenic ciliate is *Balantidium coli*, the largest protozoan parasite affecting humans and the cause of balantidial dysentery.

□ *Sporozoa* are immobile in the adult stages, and include tissue and blood parasites, such as *Toxoplasma gondii*, *Pneumocystis carinii*, *Cryptosporidium*, and *Plasmodium* (the cause of malaria).

Transmission of protozoa usually results from ingestion of parasitic cysts contained in fecally contaminated food, water, or soil; other modes of transmission include sexual intercourse *(Trichomonas vaginalis)*, mechanical vectoring by flies and other insects *(Entamoeba histolytica, Giardia lamblia)*, or the bites of blood-sucking insects (the genera *Trypanosoma*, *Plasmodium*, and *Leishmania*).

Helminths

Both types of helminths—Platyhelminthes (flatworms) and Nemathelminthes (roundworms)—are usually visible to the naked eye, but confirmation of infestation requires microscopic examination of ova, since the worms themselves are rarely passed. Flatworms include tapeworms, which inhabit the intestinal tract, and leaf-shaped flukes, which appear in the intestinal tract, bile ducts, and blood. While some species of tapeworms, such as *Taenia saginata* and *Diphyllobothrium latum* are common in the United States, all fluke infections are rare. Pathogenic species of the slender roundworms include blood and tissue parasites, such as *Wuchereria bancrofti* and *Onchocerca volvulus*—which rarely cause infection in the United States—and intestinal parasites, such as *Ascaris lumbricoides, Necator americanus, Enterobium vermicularis, Trichuris trichiura,* and *Strongyloides stercoralis*—which are indigenous to the United States.

Arthropods

Arthropods include flies, spiders, mites, ticks, crayfish, crabs, lice, fleas, beetles, gnats, and mosquitoes. Although some arthropods, such as lice and the itch mite *Sarcoptes scabiei*, are true parasites, most are vectors (carriers) of parasitic disease. Two kinds of vectors transmit such infections: a mechanical vector, such as an insect, simply carries parasites from one person or object to another; a biological vector, such as a mosquito, acts as a host, allowing parasites to develop and multiply before passing them to another host.

Testing procedures

All protozoan parasites, helminth eggs and larvae, and some arthropods require microscopic identification. Wet films of unstained material can detect various stages of intestinal parasites; the addition of iodine stains protozoan cysts. Permanent stains, such as Giemsa's stain, help identify species of blood and tissue parasites, and reveal the cytologic detail necessary to identify protozoan parasites. Preservation with formalin, followed by concentration procedures, can detect small numbers of ova, as in helminth infections. Serologic tests are available for detecting at least 24 protozoan and helminth infections, especially those that cause high antibody levels (such as amebiasis, trichinosis, echinococcosis, and toxoplasmosis) or clinically occult infections (such as filariasis or cysticercosis). The degree of sensitivity and specificity of such testing varies with the disease and the serologic method.

Culturing, a sometimes time-consuming and difficult process, is available only for a few protozoan parasites and larvae, and is mainly performed for research purposes. A culture may be performed if infection with *Entamoeba histolytica*, *Trichomonas vaginalis*, *Trypanosoma cruzi*, or *Leishmania* is suspected and conventional methods fail to confirm it.

SUSAN A. KAYES, BS, SM(ASCP)

CULTURES FOR BACTERIA AND VIRUSES

Urine Culture

Laboratory examination and culture of urine are necessary for evaluation of urinary tract infections, most commonly of bladder infections. Although urine in the kidneys and bladder is normally sterile, a small number of bacteria are usually present in the urethra. Consequently, urine may contain a variety of organisms. Nevertheless, bacteriuria generally results from prevalence of a single type of bacteria. Indeed, the presence in a urine specimen of more than two distinct bacterial species strongly suggests contamination during collection. However, a single negative culture doesn't always rule out infection, as in chronic, low-grade pyelonephritis.

Thus, isolation of known pathogenic bacteria doesn't necessarily confirm urinary tract infection, since specimens are commonly contaminated by organisms from the urethra and external genitalia. Significant results of urine culture are possible only after quantitative examination. To distinguish between true bacteriuria and contamination, it is necessary to know the number of organisms in a milliliter of urine, estimated by a culture technique called a colony count. Clean-voided midstream collection is now considered the method of choice rather than collection by su-

prapubic aspiration or catheterization.

Purpose
☐ To diagnose urinary tract infection
☐ To monitor microorganism colonization after urinary catheter insertion.

Patient preparation
Explain to the patient that this test helps detect urinary tract infection. Advise him that the test requires a urine specimen, and that no restriction of food or fluids is necessary. Provide instruction on how to collect a clean-voided midstream specimen; emphasize that external genitalia must be cleansed thoroughly. Or, if appropriate, explain catheterization or suprapubic aspiration to the patient, and inform him that he may experience discomfort during specimen collection. Tell the patient with suspected tuberculosis that specimen collection may be necessary on three consecutive mornings.

Check patient history for current antibiotic therapy.

Equipment
Sterile specimen cup/towelettes, or sterile water, cleansing solution (such as aqueous green soap), and cotton balls or sterile gauze sponges. Commercial clean-catch urine kits are available; many include instructions in several languages.

Procedure
Collect a urine specimen as ordered. Re-

QUICK CENTRIFUGATION TEST

A new test for determining whether the source of urinary tract infection is in the lower tract (bladder) or the upper tract (kidneys) is centrifugation of urine in a test tube, followed by staining the sediment with fluorescein. Viewed under a fluorescent microscope, the sediment fluoresces in upper tract infection; it doesn't fluoresce in lower tract infection.

---

cord the suspected diagnosis, the collection time and method, current antibiotic therapy, and fluid- or drug-induced diuresis on the laboratory slip.

Precautions
□ Collect at least 3 ml of urine, but don't fill the specimen cup more than halfway.
□ Seal the cup with a sterile lid, and send the specimen to the laboratory immediately. If transport is delayed longer than 30 minutes, store the specimen at 39.2° F. (4° C.) or place it on ice.

Findings
Culture results of sterile urine are normally reported as "no growth." Usually, this finding indicates the absence of urinary tract infection.

Implications of results
Bacterial counts of 100,000 or more organisms/ml of a single microbe species indicate probable urinary tract infection. Counts under 100,000/ml may be significant, depending on the patient's age, sex, history, and other individual factors. However, counts under 10,000/ml usually suggest that the organisms are contaminants, except in symptomatic patients, those with urologic disorders, or those whose urine specimens were collected by suprapubic aspiration. A special test for acid-fast bacteria isolates *M. tuberculosis*, thus indicating tuberculosis of the urinary tract.

Isolation of more than two species of organisms, or of vaginal or skin organisms, usually suggests contamination and requires a repeat culture. However, polymicrobial infection may occur after prolonged catheterization or urinary diversion, such as an ileal conduit.

Post-test care
None.

Interfering factors
□ Improper collection technique may contaminate the specimen.
□ Fluid- or drug-induced diuresis and antibiotic therapy may lower bacterial counts.
□ Failure to refrigerate the specimen or to send it to the laboratory immediately may lead to inaccurate counts.

SUSAN A. KAYES, BS, SM(ASCP)

Stool Culture

Bacteriologic examination of feces is valuable for identifying pathogens that cause overt gastrointestinal disease— such as typhoid and dysentery—and carrier states. Normal bacterial flora in feces include many species and several potentially pathogenic organisms. The most common pathogenic organisms of the gastrointestinal tract are Shigella, Salmonella, *and* Campylobacter jejuni; *less common pathogenic organisms include* Vibrio cholerae, Clostridium botulinum, Clostridium difficile, Clostridium perfringens, Staphylococcus aureus, *enterotoxigenic* Escherichia coli, Bacillus cereus, Yersinia enterocolitica, Aeromonas hydrophila, *and* Vibrio parahaemolyticus. *Identification of these organisms is vital not only to treatment and to prevention of possibly fatal complications—especially in a debilitated patient—but also to confinement of these severe infectious diseases. A sensitivity test may follow isolation of the pathogen.*

Some virus groups, such as rotavirus and parvovirus, may also cause gas-

trointestinal symptoms. However, these viruses can only be detected by immunoassay or electron microscopy. Stool culture may detect other viruses, such as enterovirus, which can cause aseptic meningitis.

Purpose
□ To identify pathogenic organisms causing gastrointestinal disease
□ To identify carrier states.

Patient preparation
Explain to the patient that this test helps determine the cause of gastrointestinal distress or may establish whether or not he is a carrier of infectious organisms. Inform him he needn't restrict food or fluids. Tell him the test may require the collection of a stool specimen on 3 consecutive days.

Check patient history for dietary patterns and recent antibiotic therapy, and for recent travel that might suggest endemic infections or infestations.

Equipment
Half-pint, waterproof container with tight-fitting lid, or sterile swab and commercial sterile collection and transport system/tongue blade/bedpan (if needed).

Procedure
Collect a stool specimen directly into the container or, if the patient isn't ambulatory, into a clean, dry bedpan. Then, using a tongue blade, transfer the specimen to the container. If you must collect the specimen by rectal swab, insert the swab past the anal sphincter, rotate it gently, and withdraw it. Then, place the swab in the appropriate container.

If the specimen is to be processed for a viral test, check with the laboratory for the proper collection procedure before obtaining a specimen.

Label the specimen with the patient's name and room number (if applicable), the doctor's name, and the date and time of collection.

Precautions
□ If the patient uses a bedpan or a dia-

per, avoid contaminating the stool specimen with urine.
□ Send the specimen to the laboratory immediately; be sure to include mucoid and bloody portions. The specimen should always be representative of the first, middle, and last portion of the feces passed.
□ Use aseptic technique when handling the specimen. Place the specimen container in a leakproof bag before transporting it to the laboratory.
□ Indicate the suspected cause of enteritis and current antibiotic therapy on the laboratory slip.

Findings
Approximately 96% to 99% of normal fecal flora consist of anaerobes, including non-sporeforming bacilli, clostridia, and anaerobic streptococci. The remaining 1% to 4% consist of aerobes, including gram-negative bacilli (predominant-

---

PATHOGENS OF THE GASTROINTESTINAL TRACT

Presence of the following pathogens in a stool culture may indicate certain disorders:
Shigella: shigellosis, bacillary dysentery
Salmonella: gastroenteritis, typhoid fever, nontyphoidal salmonellosis, paratyphoid fever
Campylobacter jejuni: gastroenteritis
Vibrio cholerae: cholera
Vibrio parahaemolyticus: food poisoning, especially seafood
Toxin-producing *Clostridium difficile:* pseudomembranous enterocolitis
Yersinia enterocolitica: gastroenteritis, enterocolitis (resembles appendicitis), mesenteric adenitis, ileitis
Enterotoxigenic *Escherichia coli:* gastroenteritis (resembles cholera or shigellosis)
Staphylococcus aureus: food poisoning; suppression of normal bowel flora from antimicrobial therapy
Bacillus cereus: food poisoning, acute gastroenteritis (rare)
Clostridium perfringens: food poisoning
Clostridium botulinum: food poisoning and infant botulism, a possible cause of sudden infant death syndrome
Aeromonas hydrophila: gastroenteritis, which causes diarrhea, especially in children.

ly *E. coli* and other Enterobacteriaceae, plus small amounts of *Pseudomonas*), gram-positive cocci (mostly enterococci), and a few yeasts.

Implications of results

Isolation of some pathogens (such as *Salmonella, Shigella, Campylobacter, Yersinia,* and *Vibrio*) indicates bacterial infection in patients with acute diarrhea and may require antibiotic sensitivity tests. Since normal fecal flora may include *Clostridium difficile, E. coli,* and other organisms, isolation of these may require further tests to demonstrate invasiveness or toxin production. Isolation of pathogens such as *Clostridium botulinum* indicates food poisoning; however, the pathogens must also be isolated from the contaminated food. In a patient undergoing long-term antibiotic therapy, isolation of large numbers of *Staphylococcus aureus* or yeast, such as *Candida,* may indicate infection. (Asymptomatic carrier states are also indicated by these enteric pathogens.) Isolation of enteroviruses may indicate aseptic meningitis.

If a stool culture shows no unusual growth, detection of viruses by immunoassay or electron microscopy may diagnose nonbacterial gastroenteritis. Highly increased polymorphonuclear leukocytes in fecal material may indicate an invasive pathogen.

Post-test care

None.

Interfering factors

□ Improper collection technique or the presence of urine may injure or destroy some enteric pathogens.
□ Antibiotic therapy may decrease bacterial growth in the specimen.
□ Failure to transport the specimen promptly or, if delivery is delayed, to use a transport medium that stabilizes pH (such as a buffered glycerol medium) may result in loss of some enteric pathogens or overgrowth of nonpathogenic organisms.

SUSAN A. KAYES, BS, SM(ASCP)

Throat Culture

A throat culture is used primarily to isolate and identify group A beta-hemolytic streptococci (Streptococcus pyogenes)—*allowing early treatment of pharyngitis—and to prevent sequelae, such as rheumatic heart disease or glomerulonephritis. This test is also used to screen for carriers of* Neisseria meningitidis. *Rarely, throat culture may be used to identify* Corynebacterium diphtheriae *or* Bordetella pertussis. *Although a throat culture may also be used to identify* Candida albicans, *direct potassium hydroxide preparation usually provides the same information faster.*

This test requires swabbing the throat, streaking a culture plate, and allowing the organisms to grow, for isolation and identification of pathogens. A smear of the specimen is gram-stained to provide preliminary identification, which may be helpful for clinical management and for determining further examinations. Culture results necessitate correlation with clinical status, recent antibiotic therapy, and amount of normal flora.

Purpose

□ To isolate and identify pathogens, particularly group A beta-hemolytic streptococci
□ To screen asymptomatic carriers of pathogens, especially *N. meningitidis.*

Patient preparation

Explain to the patient that this test helps identify the microorganisms that could be causing his symptoms or a carrier state. Inform him that he needn't restrict food or fluids before the test. Tell him who will perform the procedure and when. Reassure him that the test takes less than 30 seconds and that test results should be available in 2 or 3 days.

Describe the procedure, and warn him that he may gag during the swabbing.

Check patient history for recent antibiotic therapy. Determine immunization history if pertinent to preliminary diagnosis. Procure the throat specimen before beginning any ordered antibiotic therapy.

Equipment
Sterile swab and culture tube with transport medium, or commercial collection and transport system.

Procedure
Tell the patient to tilt his head back and close his eyes. With the throat well illuminated, check for inflamed areas, using a tongue depressor. Swab the tonsillar areas from side to side; include any inflamed or purulent sites. *Don't* touch the tongue, cheeks, or teeth with the swab. Immediately place the swab in the culture tube. If a commercial sterile collection and transport system is used, crush the ampule and force the swab into the medium, to keep the swab moist.

Note recent antibiotic therapy on the laboratory slip. Label the specimen with the patient's name, the doctor's name, date and time of collection, and the origin of the specimen. Also indicate the suspected organism, especially *Corynebacterium diphtheriae* (requires two swabs and special growth medium), *B. pertussis* (requires a nasopharyngeal culture and a special growth medium), and *N. meningitidis* (requires enriched selective media).

Precautions
☐ Send the specimen to the laboratory immediately to prevent growth or deterioration of microbes. Unless a commercial sterile collection and transport system is used, keep the container upright during transport.
☐ To protect the specimen and prevent its exposure to pathogens, use aseptic technique during the procedure, and observe proper precautions when sending the specimen to the laboratory.

Findings
Normal throat flora includes nonhemolytic and alpha-hemolytic streptococci, *Neisseria* species, staphylococci, diph-

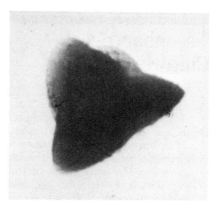

The absence of RBCs around this colony of group A beta-hemolytic streptococci characterizes the organism. Early identification of group A beta-hemolytic streptococci may avert the progression of pharyngitis to rheumatic heart disease or glomerulonephritis.

theroids, some hemophilus, pneumococci, yeasts, and enteric gram-negative rods.

Implications of results
Possible pathogens cultured include group A beta-hemolytic streptococci (*S. pyogenes*), which can cause scarlet fever or pharyngitis; *Candida albicans*, which can cause thrush; *Corynebacterium diphtheriae*, which can cause diphtheria; and *B. pertussis*, which can cause whooping cough. The laboratory report should indicate the prevalent organisms and the quantity of pathogens cultured.

Post-test care
None.

Interfering factors
☐ Failure to report recent or current antibiotic therapy on the laboratory slip may cause erroneous evaluation of bacterial growth.
☐ Failure to send the specimen to the laboratory within 15 minutes may permit bacteria to grow or deteriorate; failure to use the proper transport media may cause the specimen to dry out and the bacteria to die.

DEBORAH L. DALRYMPLE, RN, BSN

Nasopharyngeal Culture

This test evaluates nasopharyngeal se-cretions for the presence of pathogenic organisms. Direct microscopic inspec-tion of a gram-stained smear of the spec-imen provides preliminary identification of organisms that may guide clinical management, and determines the need for additional testing. Streaking a cul-ture plate with the swab and allowing any organisms present to grow permit isolation and identification of patho-gens. Cultured pathogens may then re-quire sensitivity testing to determine appropriate antibiotic therapy. Naso-pharyngeal cultures are often useful for identifying Bordetella pertussis and Neisseria meningitidis, especially in very young, elderly, or debilitated patients.

Nasopharyngeal culture can also be used to isolate viruses, especially to identify carriers of influenza virus A and B. However, the laboratory procedure re-quired for such testing is complex, time-consuming, and costly and so such a culture is performed infrequently.

Purpose
□ To identify pathogens causing upper respiratory tract symptoms
□ To identify proliferation of normal na-sopharyngeal flora, which may prove pathogenic in debilitated and other im-munologically vulnerable persons
□ To detect asymptomatic carriers of in-fectious organisms such as N. meningi-tidis and B. pertussis.

Patient preparation
Describe the procedure to the patient, and explain that this test isolates the cause of nasopharyngeal infection and allows identification of the organism and testing for antibiotic sensitivity. Tell him that secretions will be obtained from the back of the nose and the throat, using a cotton-tipped swab, and who will per-form this procedure. Warn him that he may experience slight discomfort and may gag, but reassure him that obtaining the specimen takes less than 15 seconds. Inform him that initial test results are generally available in 48 to 72 hours but that viral test results take longer to ob-tain.

Equipment
Penlight/sterile, flexible wire swab/ small, sterile, open-ended glass Pyrex tube or sterile nasal speculum/tongue depressor/culture tube/transport me-dium (broth).

Procedure

Ask the patient to cough be-fore you begin collection of the specimen. Then, position the patient with his head tilted back. Using a penlight and a tongue depressor, inspect the na-sopharyngeal area. Next, gently pass the swab through the nostril and into the nasopharynx, keeping the swab near the

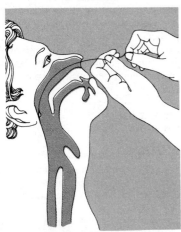

OBTAINING A NASOPHARYNGEAL SPECIMEN

When the swab passes into the nasophar-ynx, *gently* but quickly rotate the swab to collect a specimen. Then remove the swab, taking care not to injure the nasal mucous membrane.

septum and floor of the nose. Rotate the swab quickly, and remove it. Or, place the Pyrex tube in the patient's nostril, and carefully pass the swab through the tube into the nasopharynx. Rotate the swab for 5 seconds, and then place it in the culture tube with transport medium. Remove the Pyrex tube. Label the specimen appropriately, including the date and time of collection, and the origin of the material. Also indicate the suspected organism.

If the specimen is being collected for isolation of a virus, check with the laboratory for the recommended collection techniques.

Precautions
□ Maintain aseptic technique.
□ Make sure the swab doesn't touch the sides of the patient's nostril, or his tongue, to prevent any contamination of the specimen.
□ Note recent antibiotic therapy or chemotherapy on the laboratory slip.
□ Keep the container upright.
□ Since certain organisms, such as Corynebacterium diphtheriae and B. pertussis, require special growth media, inform the laboratory if they are suspected.
□ Refrigerate or freeze a viral specimen, according to your laboratory's procedure.

Findings
Flora commonly found in the nasopharynx include nonhemolytic streptococci, alpha-hemolytic streptococci, Neisseria species (except N. meningitidis and Neisseria gonorrhoeae), coagulase-negative staphylococci such as Staphylococcus epidermidis, and occasionally, the coagulase-positive Staphylococcus aureus.

Implications of results
Pathogens include group A beta-hemolytic streptococci; occasionally groups B, C, and G beta-hemolytic streptococci; B. pertussis; C. diphtheriae; S. aureus; and large amounts of H. influenzae, pneumococci, or C. albicans.

Post-test care
None.

Interfering factors
□ Recent antibiotic therapy decreases bacterial growth.
□ Improper collection technique may contaminate the specimen.
□ Failure to place the specimen in transport medium allows the specimen to dry out and the bacteria to deteriorate.
□ Failure to send the specimen to the laboratory immediately after collection permits proliferation of organisms.
□ Failure to keep a viral specimen cold allows the viruses to deteriorate.

DEBORAH L. DALRYMPLE, RN, BSN

Sputum Culture

Bacteriologic examination of sputum—material raised from the lungs and bronchi during deep coughing—is an important aid to the management of lung disease. During passage through the throat and oropharynx, sputum specimens are commonly contaminated with indigenous bacterial flora, such as alpha-hemolytic streptococci, Neisseria *species, diphtheroids, and some hemophili, pneumococci, staphylococci, and yeasts, such as* Candida. *Pathogenic organisms most often found in sputum include* Streptococcus pneumoniae, Mycobacterium tuberculosis, Klebsiella pneumoniae *(and other* Enterobacteriaceae), Hemophilus influenzae, Staphylococcus aureus, *and* Pseudomonas aeruginosa. *Other agents, such as* Pneumocystis carinii, *the* Legionellae, Mycoplasma pneumoniae, *and respiratory viruses may exist in the sputum and can cause lung disease, but they usually require serologic or histologic diagnosis rather than diagnosis by sputum culture.*

The usual method of specimen collection is expectoration (which may require ultrasonic nebulization, hydration, physiotherapy, or postural drainage);

ATTACHING AN IN-LINE TRAP TO A SUCTION CATHETER

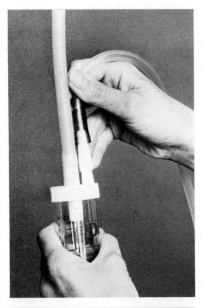

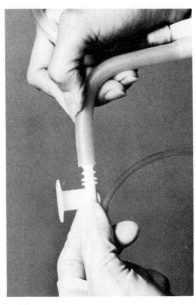

TOP LEFT:
Push the suction tubing onto the male adapter of the in-line trap.

TOP RIGHT:
Put on a sterile glove; with the gloved hand, insert the suction catheter into the rubber tubing of the trap.

LEFT:
After suctioning, disconnect the in-line trap from the suction tubing and catheter. To seal the container, connect the rubber tubing to the female adapter of the trap.

other methods include tracheal suctioning or bronchoscopy.

A Gram's stain of expectorated sputum must be examined to ensure that it's a representative specimen of secretions from the lower respiratory tract *(many WBCs, few epithelial cells) rather than one contaminated by oral flora (few WBCs, many epithelial cells). Careful examination of an acid-fast smear of sputum may provide presumptive evidence of a mycobacterial infection, such as tuberculosis.*

Purpose
□ To isolate and identify the cause of a pulmonary infection, thus aiding diagnosis of respiratory diseases (most frequently bronchitis, tuberculosis, lung abscess, and pneumonia).

Patient preparation
Explain to the patient that this test helps to identify the organism causing respiratory tract infection. Tell him the test requires a sputum specimen and who will perform the procedure. If the suspected organism is *M. tuberculosis*, tell the patient that at least three morning specimens may be required.

Test results are usually available in 48 to 72 hours. However, since cultures for tuberculosis take up to 2 months, diagnosis of this disorder generally depends on clinical symptoms, a smear for acid-fast bacilli, chest X-ray, and response to a purified protein derivative (PPD) skin test.

If the specimen is to be collected by expectoration, encourage fluid intake the night before collection, to help sputum production. Teach the patient how to expectorate by taking three deep breaths and forcing a deep cough. Emphasize that sputum isn't the same as saliva, which will be rejected for culturing. Tell him not to brush his teeth or use mouthwash before the specimen collection, although he may rinse his mouth with water.

If the specimen is to be collected by tracheal suctioning, tell the patient he'll experience discomfort as the catheter passes into the trachea.

If the specimen is to be collected by bronchoscopy, instruct the patient to fast for 6 hours before the procedure. Make sure he or a responsible member of the family has signed a consent form. Tell

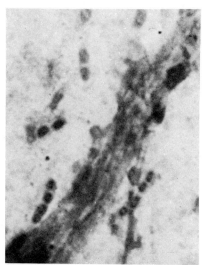

In this sputum smear, inflammatory cells and encapsulated gram-negative bacilli rods typify **Klebsiella pneumoniae.**

him he'll receive a local anesthetic just before the test, to minimize discomfort during passage of the tube.

Equipment
For expectoration: sterile, disposable, impermeable container with a tight-fitting cap/10% sodium chloride, acetylcysteine, propylene glycol, or sterile or distilled water aerosols, to induce cough, as ordered/leakproof bag.

For tracheal suctioning: size 16 or size 18 French suction catheter/water-soluble lubricant/sterile gloves/sterile specimen container or in-line specimen trap/normal saline solution.

For bronchoscopy: bronchoscope/local anesthetic/sterile needle and syringe/sterile specimen container/normal saline solution/bronchial brush/sterile gloves.

Procedure
Expectoration: Instruct the patient to cough deeply and expectorate into the container. If the cough is nonproductive, use chest physiotherapy, heated aerosol spray (nebulization), or intermittent positive pressure breathing with prescribed aerosol to induce sputum, as ordered. Using aseptic technique, close the

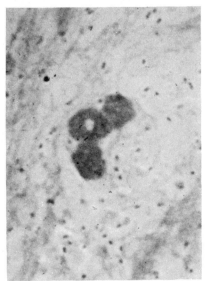

Many small, lightly stained, gram-negative coccoids appear in this sputum smear of Hemophilus influenzae.

container securely. Dispose of equipment properly; seal the container in a leakproof bag before sending it to the laboratory.

Tracheal suctioning: Administer oxygen to the patient before and after the procedure, if necessary. Attach the sputum trap to the suction catheter. Using sterile gloves, lubricate the catheter with normal saline solution, and pass the catheter through the patient's nostril, without suction. (The patient will cough when the catheter passes through the larynx.) Advance the catheter into the trachea. Apply suction for no longer than 15 seconds to obtain the specimen. Stop suction, and gently remove the catheter. Discard the catheter and gloves in the proper receptacle. Then, detach the inline sputum trap from the suction apparatus and cap the opening.

Bronchoscopy: After a local anesthetic is sprayed into the patient's throat or the patient gargles with a local anesthetic, the bronchoscope is inserted through the pharynx and trachea, into the bronchus. Secretions are then collected with a bronchial brush or aspirated through the inner channel of the scope, using an ir-

rigating solution, such as normal saline solution, if necessary. After the specimen is obtained, the bronchoscope is removed.

Label the container with the patient's name. Include on the test request form the nature and origin of the specimen, the date and time of collection, the initial diagnosis, and any current antibiotic therapy.

Precautions
□ Tracheal suctioning is contraindicated in patients with esophageal varices or cardiac disease.

□ In a patient with asthma or chronic bronchitis, watch for aggravated bronchospasms with use of more than 10% concentration of sodium chloride or acetylcysteine in an aerosol.

□ During tracheal suctioning, suction for only 5 to 10 seconds at a time. *Never* suction longer than 15 seconds. If the patient becomes hypoxic or cyanotic, remove the catheter immediately, and administer oxygen.

□ Since the patient may cough violently during suctioning, wear a mask to avoid exposure to respiratory pathogens.

□ *Don't* use more than 20% propylene glycol with water as an inducer for a specimen scheduled for tuberculosis culturing, since higher concentrations inhibit the growth of *M. tuberculosis.* (If propylene glycol isn't available, use 10% to 20% acetylcysteine with water or sodium chloride.)

□ Send the specimen to the laboratory immediately after collection.

Findings
Flora commonly found in the respiratory tract include alpha-hemolytic streptococci, *Neisseria* species, and diphtheroids. However, the presence of normal flora doesn't rule out infection.

Implications of results
Since sputum is invariably contaminated with normal oropharyngeal flora, interpretation of a culture isolate must relate

to the patient's overall clinical condition. Isolation of *M. tuberculosis* is always a significant finding.

Post-test care
☐ Provide good mouth care.
☐ After tracheal suctioning, offer the patient a drink of water.
☐ After bronchoscopy, observe the patient carefully for signs of hypoxemia (cyanosis), laryngospasm (laryngeal stridor), bronchospasm (paroxysms of coughing or wheezing), pneumothorax (dyspnea, cyanosis, pleural pain, tachycardia), perforation of the trachea or bronchus (subcutaneous crepitus), or trauma to respiratory structures (bleeding). Also, check for difficulty in breathing or swallowing. *Don't* give liquids until the gag reflex returns.

Interfering factors
☐ Improper collection or handling of the specimen may interfere with accurate determination of results.
☐ Failure to report current or recent antibiotic therapy doesn't allow the laboratory to correctly interpret decreased bacterial growth.
☐ Sputum collected over an extended period may allow pathogens to deteriorate or become overgrown by commensals and will not be accepted as a valid specimen by most laboratories.

SUSAN A. KAYES, BS, SM(ASCP)
DEBORAH L. DALRYMPLE, RN, BSN

Blood Culture

A blood culture is performed by inoculating a culture medium with a blood sample and incubating it for isolation and identification of the pathogens in bacteremia (bacterial invasion of the bloodstream) and septicemia (systemic spread of such infection). Blood culture can identify about 67% of pathogens within 24 hours and up to 90% within 72 hours.

Bacteria from local tissue infection usually invade the bloodstream through the lymphatic system by way of the thoracic duct. Occasionally, they enter the bloodstream directly through infusion lines, thrombophlebitis, or bacterial endocarditis from prosthetic heart valve replacements. Bacteremia may be transient, intermittent, or continuous. Timing of the specimens for blood cultures is somewhat debatable. Usually, it reflects the suspected type of bacteremia (intermittent or continuous) and the need to begin drug therapy.

Purpose
☐ To confirm bacteremia
☐ To identify the causative organism in bacteremia and septicemia.

Patient preparation
Explain to the patient that this procedure may identify the organism causing his symptoms. Inform him he needn't restrict food or fluids before the test. Tell him how many samples the test will require; who will perform the venipunctures and when; and that he may experience transient discomfort from the needle punctures and the pressure of the tourniquet. Reassure the patient that collecting each sample usually takes less than 5 minutes.

Equipment
Tourniquet/small adhesive bandages/alcohol swabs/povidone-iodine swabs/10- to 20-ml syringe for an adult; 6-ml syringe for a child/three or four sterile needles/two blood culture bottles, one vented (aerobic) and one unvented (anaerobic), with nutritionally enriched broths and sodium polyethanol sulfonate [SPS] added; or bottles with resin; or a lysis-centrifugation tube.

Procedure
After cleansing the venipuncture site with an alcohol swab, clean it again with an iodine swab, starting at the site and working outward, in a circular motion. Wait at least 1 minute for the skin to dry, and remove the residual iodine with an

THE LYMPHATIC SYSTEM

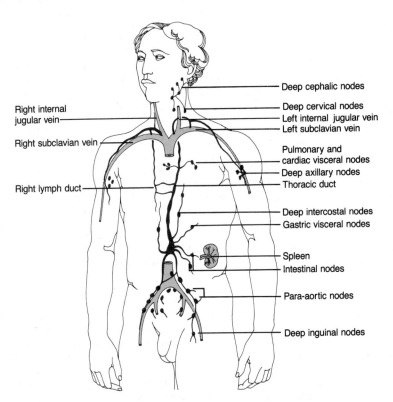

Deep cephalic nodes

Right internal jugular vein

Deep cervical nodes

Left internal jugular vein

Left subclavian vein

Right subclavian vein

Pulmonary and cardiac visceral nodes

Deep axillary nodes

Thoracic duct

Right lymph duct

Deep intercostal nodes

Gastric visceral nodes

Spleen

Intestinal nodes

Para-aortic nodes

Deep inguinal nodes

The lymphatic system—a network of capillary and venous channels—returns excess interstitial fluids and proteins to the blood. Materials flowing through these channels pass into the thoracic and right lymph ducts. The thoracic duct, the larger of the two, drains the lymphatic vessels from all but the upper right quadrant. This lymphatic drainage (commonly called lymph, the tissue fluid absorbed in the lymphatic vessels) then flows into the junction of the left internal jugular and the left subclavian veins. The right lymph duct drains interstitial fluid from the upper right quadrant into the right subclavian vein.

Bacteria from local tissue infection usually enter the bloodstream through this system. When functioning properly, however, the lymphatic system provides strong defense against bacteria and viruses. Before lymph reenters the bloodstream, afferent lymphatic vessels transport it to lymph nodes or glands—clusters of lymphatic tissues throughout the body—where numerous lymphocytes destroy microorganisms and foreign particles.

If the lymphatic system fails to destroy harmful particles before they enter the bloodstream, white cells in the spleen, liver, and bone marrow act as another defense mechanism. As blood circulates through the body, it flows into the spleen, where it's filtered. There, residing lymphocytes ingest abnormal or foreign cells while normal cells pass through. Bacteria that accompany digested food particles into the portal vein—which supplies the liver—are ingested by reticulum cells. Likewise, white cells formed in the bone marrow protect the body from invading bacteria.

Macrophages comprise still another defense system. These white cells in the tissues, lymph nodes, and red bone marrow are usually immobile. They migrate to inflamed areas, however, where they ingest and destroy infective particles.

alcohol swab. (Or you can remove the iodine after venipuncture.)

Perform a venipuncture; draw 10 to 20 ml of blood for an adult, and one syringe of 2 to 6 ml for a child. Clean the diaphragm tops of the culture bottles with alcohol or iodine, and change the needle on the syringe. If you're using broth, add blood to each bottle until you obtain a 1:5 or 1:10 dilution. For example, add 10 ml of blood to a 100-ml bottle. (Size of the bottle may vary depending on individual hospital protocol.) If you're using a special resin, such as Bactec resin medium or Antimicrobial Removal Device, add blood to the resin in the bottles and invert them gently to mix. Draw the blood directly into a special collection/processing tube, if you're using the lysis-centrifugation technique (Isolator). Indicate the tentative diagnosis on the laboratory slip, and note any current or recent antibiotic therapy.

Precautions

Send each sample to the laboratory immediately after collection.

Findings

Normally, blood cultures should be sterile.

Implications of results

Positive blood cultures do not necessarily confirm pathologic septicemia, since many organisms may temporarily invade the bloodstream during the early stages of infection. Mild, transient bacteremia may occur during the course of many infectious diseases or may complicate other disorders. Persistent, continuous, or recurrent bacteremia reliably confirms the presence of serious infection.

Isolation of most organisms takes about 72 hours; however, negative cultures are held for 1 week or more before being reported as negative. For example, cultures for suspected *Brucella* are generally held for 4 weeks before they are reported as negative.

Common blood pathogens include *Neisseria meningitidis*, *Streptococcus pneumoniae*, *Hemophilus influenzae*, other *Streptococcus* species, *Staphylococcus aureus*, *Pseudomonas aeruginosa*, Bacteroidaceae, *Brucella*, and Enterobacteriaceae. Although 2% to 3% of blood samples cultured are contaminated by skin bacteria, such as *Staphylococcus epidermidis*, diphtheroids, and *Propionibacterium*, these organisms may be clinically significant when isolated from multiple cultures.

Post-test care

If a hematoma develops at the venipuncture site, apply warm soaks.

Interfering factors

☐ Improper collection technique may contaminate the sample.

☐ Previous or current antimicrobial therapy may result in negative cultures or delayed growth.

☐ Removal of culture bottle caps at bedside may prevent anaerobic growth; use of incorrect bottle and media may prevent aerobic growth.

SUSAN A. KAYES, BS, SM(ASCP)

Wound Culture

A wound culture consists of microscopic analysis of a specimen from a lesion to confirm infection. Wound cultures may be aerobic (for detection of organisms that usually require oxygen to grow and usually appear in a superficial wound) or anaerobic (for organisms that need little or no oxygen and appear in areas of poor tissue perfusion, such as postoperative wounds, ulcers, or compound fractures). Indications for wound culture include fever, and inflammation and drainage in damaged tissue.

Purpose

☐ To identify an infectious microbe in a wound.

Patient preparation

Explain to the patient that this test iden-

ANAEROBIC SPECIMEN COLLECTOR

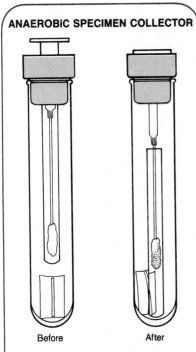

Before   After

Some anaerobes die when exposed to the slightest bit of oxygen. To facilitate anaerobic collection and culturing, tubes filled with carbon dioxide or nitrogen are used for oxygen-free transport.

The anaerobic specimen collector shown here consists of a rubber-stoppered tube filled with carbon dioxide, a small inner tube, and a swab attached to a plastic plunger. The drawing above (left) shows the tube before specimen collection. The small inner tube containing the swab is held in place by the rubber stopper.

After specimen collection (right), the swab is quickly replaced in the inner tube and the plunger depressed. This separates the inner tube from the stopper, forcing it into the larger tube, and thus exposes the specimen to the CO_2-rich environment.

tifies infectious microbes. Describe the procedure, advising him that a drainage specimen from the wound is withdrawn by a syringe or removed on cotton swabs. Tell him who will perform the procedure and when. Reassure him that collecting the drainage specimen takes less than 3 minutes.

Equipment

Sterile cotton swabs and sterile culture tube, or commercial sterile collection and transport system (for aerobic culture)/sterile cotton swabs or sterile 10-ml syringe with 21G needle, and special culture tube containing carbon dioxide or nitrogen (for anaerobic culture)/sterile gloves/alcohol sponges/sterile gauze and povidone-iodine solution.

Procedure

Prepare a sterile field and cleanse the area around the wound with antiseptic solution.

For *aerobic culture*, express the wound and swab as much exudate as possible, or insert the swab deeply into the wound and gently rotate. Immediately place the swab in the aerobic culture tube.

For *anaerobic culture*, insert the swab deeply into the wound, gently rotate, and immediately place the swab in the anaerobic culture tube; or insert the needle into the wound, aspirate 1 to 5 ml of exudate into the syringe, and immediately inject the exudate into the anaerobic culture tube. If the needle is covered with a rubber stopper, the aspirate may be sent to the laboratory in the syringe.

Record on the laboratory slip recent antibiotic therapy, the source of the specimen, and the suspected organism. Also, label the specimen container appropriately with the patient's name and room number, the doctor's name, and the wound site and the time of specimen collection.

Precautions

□ Cleanse the area around the wound thoroughly to limit contamination of the culture by normal skin flora, such as diphtheroids, *Staphylococcus epidermidis*, and alpha-hemolytic streptococcus. However, *don't* cleanse the area around a perineal wound.

□ Make sure no antiseptic enters the wound.

□ Obtain exudate from the entire wound, using more than one swab.

□ Since some anaerobes die in the presence of even a small amount of oxygen, place the specimen in the culture tube quickly, take care that no air enters into the tube, and check that double stoppers are secure.

□ Keep the specimen container upright, and send it to the laboratory within 15 minutes to prevent growth or deterioration of microbes.

□ Use aseptic technique during the procedure, and necessary isolation precautions when sending the specimen to the laboratory.

Findings
Normally, no pathogenic organisms are present in a clean wound.

Implications of results
The most common aerobic pathogens for wound infection include *Staphylococcus aureus*, Group A beta-hemolytic streptococci, *Escherichia coli* and other Enterobacteriaceae, Group D streptococci including enterococci and *Streptococcus bovis*, and some *Pseudomonas* species; the most common anaerobic pathogens include some *Clostridium*, *Proteus*, and *Bacteroides* species.

Post-test care
Dress the wound, as ordered.

Interfering factors
□ Failure to report recent or current antibiotic therapy may cause erroneous evaluation of bacterial growth.

□ Poor collection technique may contaminate or invalidate the specimen; failure to use the proper transport media may cause the specimen to dry up and the bacteria to die.

DEBORAH L. DALRYMPLE, RN, BSN

Gastric Culture

This test requires aspiration of gastric contents and cultivation of any microbes present to identify mycobacterial infection. It's performed in conjunction with a chest X-ray and a purified protein derivative (PPD) skin test, and is especially useful when a sputum sample can't be obtained by expectoration or nebulization. Gastric aspiration also provides a specimen for rapid presumptive identification of bacteria (by Gram's stain) in neonatal septicemia.

Purpose
□ To aid diagnosis of mycobacterial infections

□ To identify the infecting bacteria in neonatal septicemia.

Patient preparation
Explain to the patient (or to the parents if the patient is a child) that gastric culture helps diagnose tuberculosis. Instruct him to fast for 8 hours before the test. Tell him who will perform the procedure, and that the same procedure may be performed on three consecutive mornings. Instruct him to remain in bed each morning until specimen collection has been completed, to prevent premature emptying of stomach contents.

Describe the procedure to the patient. Tell him the nasogastric tube may make him gag but passes more easily if he relaxes and follows instructions about breathing and swallowing. Just before the procedure, obtain baseline heart rate and rhythm, and place the patient in high Fowler's position.

Advise the patient (or his parents) that test results may take 2 months, since acid-fast bacteria generally grow slowly. Check history for recent antibiotic therapy.

Equipment
Water-soluble lubricating jelly/sterile water/size 16 or 18 French, disposable, plastic nasogastric tube//50-ml sterile syringe/sterile specimen container/sterile gloves/emesis basin/stethoscope/clamp (if necessary).

Procedure
Perform nasogastric intubation when the patient awakens and obtain gastric washings. Clamp the tube before re-

moving quickly. Note recent antibiotic therapy on the laboratory slip, along with the site and time of collection. Label the specimens with the patient's name and room number (if applicable), and the doctor's name.

Precautions
□ Gastric intubation is contraindicated in conditions such as pregnancy, esophageal disorders (varices, stenosis, diverticula), malignant neoplasms, recent severe gastric hemorrhage, aortic aneurysm, congestive heart failure, and myocardial infarction.
□ If possible, obtain the specimens before the start of antibiotic therapy.
□ Watch for signs that the tube has entered the trachea—coughing, cyanosis, or gasping.
□ *Never* inject water into a nasogastric tube unless you're sure the tube is correctly placed in the patient's stomach. During lavage, use sterile, distilled water, to decrease risk of contamination with saprophytic myobacteria.
□ Since some patients develop arrhythmias during this procedure, check the pulse rate for irregularities.
□ Send the specimens to the laboratory immediately. Be sure the specimen container is tightly capped. Wipe the outside of the container with disinfectant, and send it to the laboratory, upright in a plastic bag.
□ Handle the nasogastric tube with gloved hands, and dispose of all equipment carefully in order to prevent staff contamination.

Findings
Normally, culture specimen is negative for pathogenic mycobacteria.

Implications of results
Isolation and identification of the organism *M. tuberculosis* indicates the presence of active tuberculosis; other species of *Mycobacterium*, such as *Mycobacterium bovis*, *Mycobacterium kansasii*, and *Mycobacterium avium-intracellulare* complex, may cause pulmonary disease that is clinically indistinguishable

from tuberculosis. Treatment of these mycobacterial diseases may be difficult and commonly requires sensitivity studies to determine effective antibiotic therapy. Pathogenic bacteria causing neonatal septicemia may also be identified through culture.

Post-test care
□ As ordered, resume administration of medications discontinued before the test.
□ Instruct the patient not to blow his nose for at least 4 to 6 hours, to prevent bleeding.
□ The patient may resume normal diet.

Interfering factors
□ Failure to observe an 8-hour fast before the test may decrease the amount of bacteria by diluting stomach contents or removing contents through digestion.
□ Drugs such as tetracycline and aminoglycosides can weaken bacilli, causing false-negative culture results.
□ The presence of saprophytic mycobacteria in gastric contents may cause false-positive acid-fast smears, since these bacteria can't be microscopically distinguished from pathogenic mycobacteria.

SUSAN A. KAYES, BS, SM(ASCP)

Duodenal Contents Culture

This test requires duodenal intubation, aspiration of duodenal contents, and cultivation of any microbes present to isolate and identify a duodenal or biliary pathogen. Occasionally, a specimen may be obtained during surgery, such as a cholecystectomy. Duodenal contents (pancreatic and duodenal enzymes and bile) are normally almost sterile, but are subject to infection by many pathogens, such as Escherichia coli, Staphylococcus aureus, *and* Salmonella. *Such microbial infection of the biliary tract and duo-*

denum can result in duodenitis, cholecystitis, or cholangitis.

Purpose
☐ To detect bacterial infection of the biliary tract and duodenum; to differentiate between such infection and gallstones

☐ To rule out bacterial infection as the cause of persistent gastrointestinal symptoms (epigastric pain, nausea, vomiting, and diarrhea).

Patient preparation
Explain to the patient that this test helps to determine the cause of his symptoms. Instruct him to restrict food and fluids for 12 hours before the test. Tell him who will perform the procedure and where it will be done.

Describe the intubation procedure to the patient. Assure him that although this procedure is uncomfortable, it isn't dangerous. Explain that passage of the tube may make him gag, but following the examiner's instructions about proper positioning, breathing, swallowing, and relaxing will minimize discomfort. Suggest to the patient that he empty his bladder before the procedure, to increase his general comfort.

Equipment
Double-lumen tube with olive tip/water-soluble jelly/30-ml sterile syringe/emesis basin/sterile specimen container/½" (1.2 cm) adhesive tape.

Procedure
After the nasoenteric tube is inserted, place the patient in a left lateral decubitus position, with his feet elevated, to allow peristalsis to move the tube into the duodenum. The pH of a small amount of aspirated fluid determines tube position: if the tube is in the stomach, pH is lower than 7.0; if the tube is in the duodenum, pH is higher than 7.0.

Correct position of the tube can also be confirmed by fluoroscopy. After it's confirmed, duodenal contents are aspirated.

Occasionally, a specimen for culture of duodenal contents is obtained during duodenoscopy (see ESOPHAGOGASTRODU-ODENOSCOPY in Chapter 27).

Transfer the specimen to a sterile container, and label with the patient's name and room number, doctor's name, date and time of collection.

Precautions
☐ Duodenal intubation is contraindicated in conditions such as pregnancy; acute pancreatitis; acute cholecystitis; esophageal varices, stenosis, diverticula or malignant neoplasms; recent severe gastric hemorrhage; aortic aneurysm; congestive heart failure; or myocardial infarction.

☐ Collect the specimen for culture before antibiotic therapy begins.

☐ Send the specimen to the laboratory immediately.

☐ Withdraw the tube slowly (6″ to 8″ [15 to 20 cm] every 10 minutes) until it reaches the esophagus; then clamp the tube and remove it quickly. Notify the doctor if the tube can't be withdrawn easily; *never* force the tube.

Findings
Normally, a duodenal contents culture contains small amounts of polymorphonuclear leukocytes and epithelial cells with no pathogens. The bacterial count is usually less than 100,000.

Implications of results
Generally, bacterial counts of 100,000 or more, or the presence of pathogens, such as *Salmonella,* in any number indicates infection. Sensitivity testing may be required. Numerous polymorphonuclear leukocytes, copious mucous debris, and bile-stained epithelial cells in the bile fluid suggest inflammation of the biliary tract; many segmented neutrophils and exfoliated epithelial cells suggest inflammation of the pancreas, the duodenum, or bile ducts. The presence of bile sand indicates cholelithiasis or calculi in the biliary tract. Differential diagnosis requires further testing, including oral or I.V. cholecystography; WBC count; cholangiography, measurement of serum bilirubin, alkaline phosphatase, serum

amylase, and urine urobilinogen; and culture of surgical material.

Post-test care
□ After duodenal intubation or duodenoscopy, observe the patient carefully for signs of perforation from tube passage, such as dysphagia, epigastric or shoulder pain, dyspnea, or fever.
□ After duodenoscopy, monitor vital signs until the patient is stable; keep the side rails up, and enforce bed rest until the patient is fully alert.
□ As ordered, resume diet discontinued before the test.

Interfering factors
□ Failure to observe a 12-hour fast can dilute the specimen, which decreases the bacterial count.
□ Improper collection technique can contaminate the specimen.

SUSAN A. KAYES, BS, SM(ASCP)

Culture for Gonorrhea

A stained smear of genital exudate can confirm gonorrhea in 90% of males with characteristic symptoms; nevertheless, a culture is often necessary, especially in asymptomatic females. Possible culture sites include the urethra (usual site in males), endocervix (usual site in females), anal canal, and oropharynx.

Gonorrhea, the most prevalent venereal disease, nearly exclusively results from sexual transmission of Neisseria gonorrhoeae. Its most common effect in females is a greenish-yellow cervical discharge; but in many females, it produces no symptoms at all—a factor that contributes to the epidemic prevalence of this infection. In males, gonorrhea generally causes painful urination and a mucopurulent urethral discharge, symptoms of acute anterior urethritis.

Purpose
□ To confirm gonorrhea.

Patient preparation
Describe the procedure to the patient, and explain that this test confirms gonorrhea. Inform the patient who will perform the test and when, and that results are usually available within 24 to 72 hours. Instruct the female patient not to douche for 24 hours before the test. Tell the male patient that he should not void during the hour preceding the test. Warn him that males sometimes experience nausea, sweating, weakness, and fainting from the emotional stress associated with fear or discomfort when the cotton swab or wire loop is introduced into the urethra.

Equipment
Sterile gloves/sterile cotton swabs/wire bacteriologic loop or thin urogenital alginate swabs (for male)/vaginal speculum/modified Thayer-Martin medium in plates (or Transgrow medium in specimen bottles if laboratory isn't readily available)/ring forceps/cotton balls.

Procedure
Endocervical culture: The patient is placed in the lithotomy position, draped, and instructed to take deep breaths. A vaginal speculum, lubricated only with warm water, is inserted. Mucus is cleaned from the cervix, using cotton balls in ring forceps. Then a dry, sterile cotton swab is inserted into the endocervical canal and rotated from side to side. The swab is left in place for several seconds for optimum absorption of organisms.

Urethral culture: Place the patient in supine position, and drape appropriately. Cleanse the urethral meatus with sterile gauze or a cotton swab, then insert a thin urogenital alginate swab or a wire bacteriologic loop $3/8''$ to $3/4''$ (1 to 2 cm) into the urethra, and rotate the swab or loop from side to side. Leave it in place for several seconds for optimum absorption of organisms. If permitted, the patient may milk the urethra, bringing urethral secretions to the meatus for collection on a cotton swab.

Rectal culture: After obtaining an en-

CULTURING FOR *NEISSERIA GONORRHOEAE*

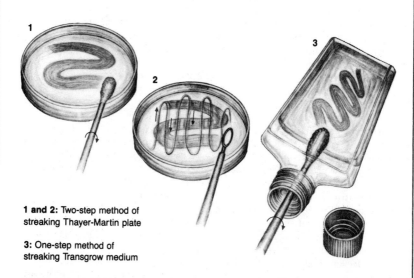

1 and 2: Two-step method of streaking Thayer-Martin plate

3: One-step method of streaking Transgrow medium

Modified Thayer-Martin (MTM) medium is a combination of hemoglobin, gonococcal growth-enhancing chemicals, and antimicrobial agents for culturing endocervical, urethral, or rectal specimens. To inoculate a culture plate treated with MTM medium and to spread organisms out of their associated mucus, roll the swab in a Z pattern (1). Using the swab or a sterile wire loop, immediately cross-streak the plate (2). To demonstrate *Neisseria gonorrhoeae*, incubate within 15 minutes of streaking.

Transgrow, a modification of MTM medium, is available in a screw-cap bottle containing air and carbon dioxide. Transgrow bottles are used to transport suspect cultures when laboratory facilities aren't available at the site of specimen collection. To prevent loss of carbon dioxide, inoculate the specimen bottle while it's in an upright position. After uncapping the bottle, immediately insert the swab and soak up all excess moisture. Then, starting at the bottom of the bottle, roll the swab from side to side across the medium (3). Recap the bottle, and send it to the laboratory immediately. Subculturing should begin within 24 to 48 hours.

docervical or urethral specimen (while the patient is still on the examining table), insert a sterile cotton swab into the anal canal about 1″ (2.5 cm), move the swab from side to side, and leave it in place for several seconds for optimum absorption. If the swab is contaminated with feces, discard it and repeat the procedure with a clean swab.

Throat culture: Position the patient with his head tilted back and his eyes closed. Check his throat for inflamed areas, using a tongue depressor. Rub a sterile swab from side to side over the tonsillar areas, including any inflamed

or purulent sites. Be careful not to touch the teeth, cheeks, or tongue with the swab.

After collecting any of these specimens: Roll the swab in a Z pattern in a plate containing modified Thayer-Martin medium. Then, cross-streak the medium with a sterile wire loop or the tip of the swab, and cover the plate. Label the specimen with the patient's name and room number (if applicable), the doctor's name, and the time and the date of collection.

If laboratory facilities aren't readily available: Uncap the Transgrow medium specimen bottle just before inserting the swab of test material into the bottle. Keep the bottle upright to minimize loss of carbon dioxide. With the swab, absorb the excess moisture within the bottle; then roll the swab across the Transgrow medium. Discard the swab, and place the lid on the bottle. Label the bottle appropriately.

Precautions
□ Place the male patient in supine position to prevent falling if vasovagal syncope occurs during introduction of the cotton swab or wire loop into the urethra. Observe for profound hypotension, bradycardia, pallor, and sweating.
□ Collect a urethral specimen at least 1 hour after the patient has voided, to prevent loss of urethral secretions.
□ After collecting the specimens, carefully dispose of gloves, swabs, and speculum, to prevent staff exposure to the organism.
□ Send the specimen to the laboratory immediately, or arrange for immediate transport of Transgrow bottle, since the specimen requires subculturing within 24 to 48 hours to obtain successful growths.

Findings
Normally, no *N. gonorrhoeae* appears in the culture.

Implications of results
A positive culture confirms gonorrhea.

Post-test care
□ Advise the patient to avoid intercourse and all sexual contact, until test results are available. Explain that treatment usually begins after confirmation of positive culture, except in a patient with symptoms of gonorrhea or in a person who has had intercourse with someone known to have gonorrhea.
□ Advise the patient that a repeat culture is required 1 week after completion of treatment to evaluate therapy.
□ Inform the patient that positive culture findings must be reported to the local health department.

Interfering factors
□ Improper collection technique may provide a nonrepresentative specimen or may contaminate the specimen.
□ Fecal material may contaminate an anal culture.
□ In males, voiding within 1 hour of specimen collection washes secretions out of the urethra, making fewer organisms available for culture.
□ In females, douching within 24 hours of specimen collection washes out cervical secretions, making fewer organisms available for culture.

KAREN DYER VANCE, RN, BSN

TESTS FOR OVA AND PARASITES

Examination of Stool for Ova and Parasites

Examination of a stool specimen can detect several types of intestinal parasites. Some of these parasites live in nonpathogenic symbiosis; others cause intestinal disease. In the United States, the most common parasites include the roundworms Ascaris lumbricoides and Necator americanus (commonly called hookworm); the tapeworms Diphyllobothrium latum, Taenia saginata, and rarely, Taenia solium; the ameba Entamoeba histolytica; and the flagellate Giardia lamblia.

Purpose
□ To confirm or rule out intestinal parasitic infection and disease.

Patient preparation
Explain to the patient that this test detects intestinal parasitic infection. Instruct him to avoid treatments with

castor or mineral oil, bismuth, magnesium or antidiarrheal compounds, barium enemas, and antibiotics for 7 to 10 days before the test. Tell him the test requires three stool specimens—one every other day or every third day. Up to six specimens may be required to confirm the presence of E. *histolytica*.

If the patient has diarrhea, record recent dietary and travel history. Check the patient's drug history for use of antiparasitic agents, such as carbarsone, tetracycline, paromomycin, metronidazole, and diiodohydroxyquin, within 2 weeks before the test.

Equipment
Waterproof container with tight-fitting lid/bedpan (if necessary)/tongue depressor.

Procedure
Collect a stool specimen directly into the container. If the patient is bedridden, collect the specimen into a clean, dry bedpan; then, using a tongue depressor, transfer it into a properly labeled container. Note on the laboratory form the date and time of collection, specimen consistency, any recent or current antibiotic therapy, and any pertinent travel or dietary history.

Precautions
☐ Do not contaminate the stool specimen with urine, which can destroy trophozoites.
☐ Don't collect stool from a toilet bowl, since water is toxic to trophozoites and may contain organisms that interfere with test results.
☐ Send the specimen to the laboratory immediately. If a liquid or soft stool specimen can't be examined within 30 minutes of passage, place some of it in a preservative; if a formed stool specimen can't be examined immediately, refrigerate it or place it in preservative.
☐ If the entire stool can't be sent to the laboratory, include macroscopic worms or worm segments, and bloody and mucoid portions of the specimen.
☐ Observe aseptic precautions when

COLLECTION PROCEDURE FOR PINWORMS

The ova of the pinworm *Enterobius vermicularis* seldom appear in feces, because the female migrates to the anus and deposits her ova there. To collect them, place a piece of cellophane tape, sticky side out, on the end of a tongue depressor, and press it firmly on the anal area. Then transfer the tape, sticky side down, to a slide (kits with tape and a slide or a sticky paddle are available). Since the female usually deposits her ova at night, collect the specimen early in the morning, before the patient bathes or defecates.

---

handling the specimen, disposing of equipment, sealing the container, and transporting it. Wash hands thoroughly after specimen collection.

Findings
Normally, no parasites or ova appear in stool.

Implications of results
The presence of E. *histolytica* confirms amebiasis; G. *lamblia*, giardiasis. However, the extent of infection depends on the degree of tissue invasion. If amebiasis is suspected but stool examinations are negative, specimen collection after saline cathartic using buffered sodium biphosphate or during sigmoidoscopy may be necessary. If giardiasis is suspected but stool examinations are negative, examination of duodenal contents may be necessary.

Since injury to the host is difficult to detect—even when helminth ova or larvae appear—the number of worms is usually correlated with the patient's clinical symptoms to distinguish between helminth infestation and helminth diseases. Eosinophilia may also indicate parasitic infection. Helminths may migrate from the intestinal tract, producing pathologic changes in other parts of the body. For example, the roundworm *Ascaris* may perforate the bowel wall, causing peritonitis, or may migrate to the lungs, causing pneumonitis. Hookworms can cause hypochromic microcytic anemia secondary to bloodsucking and hemorrhage, especially in patients with iron-deficient diets. The tapeworm *D. latum* may cause megaloblastic anemia by removing vitamin B_{12}.

Post-test care

As ordered, resume administration of medications discontinued before the test.

Interfering factors

☐ Improper collection technique or the presence of urine may cause false-negative results.

☐ Collection of too few specimens may cause failure to detect the organism.

☐ Failure to transport the specimen promptly or to refrigerate or preserve it if transport is delayed may influence test results.

☐ Excessive heat or excessive cold can destroy parasites.

☐ Failure to observe pretest restrictions of castor or mineral oil, bismuth, magnesium or antidiarrheal compounds, barium enemas, or antibiotics may interfere with microscopic analysis or reduce the number of parasites.

SUSAN A. KAYES, BS, SM(ASCP)

Examination of Urogenital Secretions for Trichomonads

Microscopic examination of urine or vaginal, urethral, or prostatic secretions can detect urogenital infection by Trichomonas vaginalis—*a parasitic, flagellate protozoan, usually transmitted sexually. This test is performed more often on females than on males, since females more often exhibit symptoms. Males with trichomoniasis may have symptoms of urethritis or prostatis.*

Purpose

☐ To confirm trichomoniasis.

Patient preparation

Explain to the patient that this test helps to determine the cause of urogenital infection. Tell the female patient the test requires a specimen of vaginal secretion or urethral discharge. Instruct her not to douche before the test. Tell the male patient the test requires a specimen of urethral or prostatic secretion. Inform the patient who will perform the procedure and when.

Equipment

Cotton swab/test tube containing small amount of normal saline solution (0.85% sodium chloride)/vaginal speculum/specimen cup, if a urine specimen.

Procedure

Vaginal secretion: With the patient in lithotomy position, an unlubricated vaginal speculum is inserted, and discharge is collected with a cotton swab. The swab is then placed in the tube containing normal saline solution, and the speculum is removed.

Prostatic material: After prostatic massage, collect secretions with a cotton swab, and place the swab in normal saline solution.

Urethral discharge: Collect the discharge with a cotton swab, and place the swab in normal saline solution.

Urine: Include the first portion of a voided random specimen (not midstream).

Label the specimen appropriately, including the date and time of collection.

Precautions

☐ If possible, obtain the urogenital specimen before treatment with a trichomonacide begins.

☐ Send the specimen to the laboratory immediately, since trichomonads can be identified only while still motile.

Findings

Trichomonads are normally absent from the urogenital tract. In approximately 25% of women and most infected males, trichomonads may be present without associated pathology.

Implications of results

Trichomonads confirm trichomoniasis.

Post-test care

Provide perineal care.

Interfering factors

□ Failure to send the specimen to the laboratory immediately causes trichomonads to lose their motility.
□ Improper collection technique may interfere with detection.
□ Collection of the specimen after trichomonacide therapy begins decreases the parasites in the specimen.

SUSAN A. KAYES, BS, SM(ASCP)

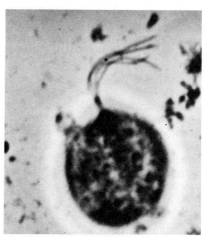

Identifying Trichomonas vaginalis, *an actively motile flagellate, in vaginal, urethral, or prostatic secretions strongly suggests trichomoniasis.*

Examination of Sputum for Ova and Parasites

This test evaluates a sputum specimen for parasites. Such infestation is rare in the United States but may result from exposure to Entamoeba histolytica, Ascaris lumbricoides, Echinococcus granulosus, Strongyloides stercoralis, Paragonimus westermani, *or* Necator americanus. *The specimen is obtained by expectoration or by tracheal suctioning.*

Purpose

□ To identify pulmonary parasites.

Patient preparation

Explain to the patient that this test helps identify parasitic pulmonary infection. Tell him the test requires a sputum specimen or, if necessary, tracheal suctioning. Inform him that early morning collection is preferred, because secretions accumulate overnight.

For expectoration, encourage fluid intake the night before collection, to help sputum production. Teach the patient how to expectorate by taking three deep breaths and forcing a deep cough. For tracheal suctioning, tell him he'll experience some discomfort from the catheter.

Equipment

For expectoration: Sterile, disposable, impermeable container with screw cap or tight-fitting cap/nebulizer, intermittent positive-pressure breathing ventilator, and 10% sodium chloride, acetylcysteine, or sterile or distilled water aerosols, to induce cough, as ordered.

For tracheal suctioning: size 16 or size 18 French suction catheter/sterile gloves/ sterile specimen container or sputum trap/sterile normal saline solution.

Procedure

Expectoration: Instruct the patient to breathe deeply a few times and then to "deep cough" and expectorate into the container. If cough is nonproductive, use chest physiotherapy, heated aerosol spray (nebulization), or intermittent positive pressure breathing with prescribed aerosol to induce sputum, as ordered. Close the container securely, and clean the outside of it. Dispose of equipment properly; take proper precautions in sending the specimen to the laboratory.

Tracheal suctioning: Administer oxygen before and after the procedure, if necessary. Attach a sputum trap to the suction catheter. While wearing a sterile glove, lubricate the tip of the catheter, and pass the catheter through the patient's nostril, without suction. (The patient will cough when the catheter passes into the larynx.) Advance the catheter into the trachea. Apply suction for no longer than 15 seconds, to obtain the specimen. Stop suction, and gently remove the catheter. Discard the catheter and glove in a proper receptacle. Then, detach the sputum trap from the suction apparatus and cap the opening.

Label all specimens carefully.

Precautions
□ Tracheal suctioning is contraindicated in patients with esophageal varices or cardiac disease.

□ In a patient with asthma or chronic bronchitis, watch for aggravated bronchospasms with use of more than 10% concentration of sodium chloride or acetylcysteine in an aerosol.

□ During tracheal suctioning, suction for only 5 to 10 seconds at a time. *Never* suction longer than 15 seconds. If the patient becomes hypoxic or cyanotic, remove the catheter immediately, and administer oxygen.

□ Send the specimen to the laboratory immediately, or place it in preservative.

Findings
Normally, no parasites or ova are present.

Implications of results
The parasite identified indicates the type of pulmonary infection and the presence of adult-stage intestinal infection.
□ *E. histolytica* trophozoites: pulmonary amebiasis
□ *A. lumbricoides* larvae and adults: pneumonitis
□ *E. granulosus* cysts of larval stage: hydatid disease
□ *P. westermani* ova: paragonimiasis
□ *S. stercoralis* larvae: strongyloidiasis
□ *N. americanus* larvae: hookworm disease.

Post-test care
□ Provide good mouth care.
□ After suctioning, offer water; monitor vital signs every hour until stable.

Interfering factors
□ Recent therapy with anthelmintics or amebicides may alter test results.
□ Improper collection may produce a nonrepresentative specimen.

SUSAN A. KAYES, BS, SM(ASCP)

Test for Duodenal Parasites

This test evaluates duodenal contents for the presence of parasites in a specimen obtained by duodenal intubation and aspiration or by the string test (Entero test). Such parasites include trophozoites of Giardia lamblia; *the ova and larvae of* Strongyloides stercoralis; *or the ova of* Necator americanus *or* Ancylostoma duodenale *in various stages of cleavage. This test can also detect ova of the liver flukes* Clonorchis sinensis *and* Fasciola hepatica *in the biliary tract. Liver fluke infestations are rare in the United States.*

Examination of duodenal contents for ova and parasites is performed only in a symptomatic patient with negative stool examinations.

Purpose
□ To detect parasitic infection when stool examinations are negative.

Patient preparation
Explain to the patient that this test detects parasitic infection of the gastrointestinal tract. Instruct him to restrict food and fluids for 12 hours before the test. Tell him who will perform the test and when. If the test will be done with a nasoenteric tube, warn him that he may gag during the tube's passage, but assure him that following the examiner's

instructions about positioning, breathing, and swallowing will minimize discomfort. Just before the procedure, instruct the patient to empty his bladder.

Equipment
Double-lumen tube with olive tip (or weighted gelatin capsule with string attached, for string test)/water-soluble jelly/30-ml sterile syringe/emesis basin/sterile specimen container/adhesive tape (½" [1.2 cm] wide).

Procedure
Using a nasoenteric tube: After the nasoenteric tube is inserted, place the patient in a left lateral decubitus position, with his feet elevated, to allow peristalsis to move the tube into the duodenum. The pH of a small amount of aspirated fluid determines tube position: if the tube is in the stomach, pH is lower than 7.0; if the tube is in the duodenum, pH is higher than 7.0. Correct positioning of the tube can also be determined by fluoroscopy. After position of the tube is confirmed, residual duodenal contents are aspirated. Transfer the entire specimen to a sterile container; label it appropriately.

Using an Entero Test capsule with string: Tape the free end of the string to the patient's cheek. Then, instruct him to swallow the capsule (on the other end of the string) with water. Leave the string in place for 4 hours; then pull it out gently and place it in a sterile container. Label the container appropriately.

Precautions
☐ Duodenal intubation is contraindicated during pregnancy or for patients with acute cholecystitis; acute pancreatitis; esophageal varices, stenosis, diverticula, or malignant neoplasms; recent severe gastric hemorrhage; aortic aneurysm; or congestive heart failure.
☐ When possible, obtain the specimen before the start of drug therapy.
☐ Send the specimen to the laboratory immediately, since detection may rest on observing the parasite's motility.
☐ Withdraw the tube slowly (6" to 8" [15 to 20 cm] every 10 minutes) to the esophagus; then clamp the tube and remove it quickly. *Never* force the tube.

Findings
Normally, no ova or parasites appear.

Implications of results
The presence of *G. lamblia* indicates giardiasis, possibly causing malabsorption syndrome; *S. stercoralis* suggests strongyloidiasis; and *A. duodenale* and *N. americanus* imply hookworm disease. The presence of *C. sinensis* and *F. hepatica* signifies histopathologic changes in the bile ducts.

Post-test care
☐ Dispose of equipment properly.
☐ Provide mouth care, and offer water.
☐ Observe carefully for signs of perforation, such as dysphagia or fever.
☐ As ordered, resume diet.

Interfering factors
☐ Failure of the patient to observe the 12-hour fast can dilute the specimen.
☐ Delay in sending the specimen may interfere with detection of parasites.
☐ Previous drug therapy may decrease the amount of parasites in the specimen.
SUSAN A. KAYES, BS, SM(ASCP)

Selected References
Finegold, Sidney M., and Martin, William J. *Bailey and Scott's Diagnostic Microbiology,* 6th ed. St. Louis: C.V. Mosby Co., 1982.
Henry, John Bernard, ed. *Todd-Sanford-Davidsohn Clinical Diagnosis and Management by Laboratory Methods,* 17th ed. Philadelphia: W.B. Saunders Co., 1984.
Lennette, E.H., et al, eds. *Manual of Clinical Microbiology,* 3rd ed. Washington, D.C.: American Society for Microbiology, 1980.
Volk, Wesley A. *Essentials of Medical Microbiology.* 2nd ed. Philadelphia: J.B. Lippincott Co., 1982.

20 Thyroid

LEARNING OBJECTIVES

After completing this chapter, the reader will be able to:
- describe the five categories of thyroid function tests.
- explain the anatomy and physiology of the thyroid.
- state the usual sequence of thyroid testing procedures.
- list common disorders caused by thyroid dysfunction.
- state the purpose of each test discussed in the chapter.
- prepare the patient physically and psychologically for each test.
- describe the procedure for performing each test.
- specify appropriate precautions for safe administration of each test.
- recognize signs of adverse reaction and respond appropriately.
- implement appropriate post-test care.
- identify the normal findings of each test.
- discuss the implications of abnormal test results.
- list factors that may interfere with accurate test results.

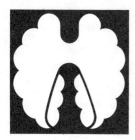

Thyroid

Introduction

A number of sensitive and specific laboratory tests are available to evaluate thyroid function and hormone use. These tests make diagnosis of thyroid dysfunction possible even in patients with marginal or obscure thyroid abnormalities. However, since no one test diagnoses all thyroid disorders and interpretation of test results may be complicated by many factors, a combination of laboratory tests is usually required to ensure accurate diagnosis.

Laboratory tests of thyroid function can be classified into the following categories:

☐ *direct tests of thyroid function* that measure thyroid hormone synthesis and excretion, such as the radioactive iodine uptake test

☐ *tests that measure concentration and binding of the thyroid hormones* and other iodinated materials in the blood, such as serum free thyroxine and T_3 resin uptake (see such tests in Chapter 5, Hormones), and protein-binding iodine

☐ *tests that assess the metabolic effects* of thyroid hormones on the tissues, such as serum cholesterol, basal metabolism rate (BMR), and Achilles reflex time; however, BMR and Achilles reflex time have largely been replaced by other tests

☐ *tests that evaluate hormonal regulating mechanisms,* such as the thyroid-stimulating hormone test, and thyroid suppression and stimulation tests (see such tests in Chapter 5, Hormones)

☐ *tests that evaluate anatomic detail* of the thyroid gland and aid in evaluation of thyroid masses, such as radionuclide thyroid imaging and thyroid ultrasonography.

Thyroid disorders

Thyroid dysfunction can cause several disorders, most commonly hyperthyroidism, hypothyroidism, thyroiditis, and goiter.

Simple goiter results from inadequate intake of iodine and tends to occur in certain geographic areas ("goiter belts"). Hyperthyroidism, which affects females four times more often than males, results from excessive secretion of thyroid hormone. Conversely, hypothyroidism results from inadequate production of thyroid hormone. Thyroiditis may occur as an acute inflammation, as a subacute viral inflammation that generally subsides spontaneously, or as a chronic disorder (Hashimoto's thyroiditis).

Benign adenomas and malignant tumors cause one third of all thyroid enlargements. Well-encapsulated and noninvasive, a benign adenoma usually causes no symptoms until it grows large enough to cause respiratory distress by compressing the trachea. Malignant thyroid tumors are rare, accounting for only 0.5% of cancer deaths. However, large doses of radiation to the head and neck

THYROID ANATOMY AND PHYSIOLOGY REVIEWED

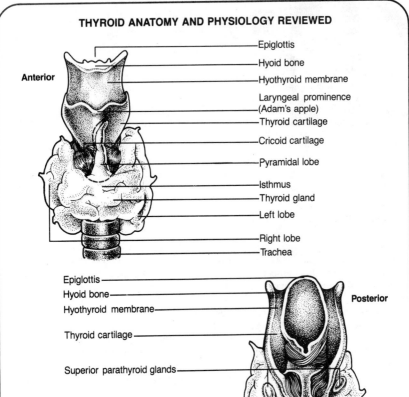

Anterior

- Epiglottis
- Hyoid bone
- Hyothyroid membrane
- Laryngeal prominence (Adam's apple)
- Thyroid cartilage
- Cricoid cartilage
- Pyramidal lobe
- Isthmus
- Thyroid gland
- Left lobe
- Right lobe
- Trachea

Epiglottis
Hyoid bone
Hyothyroid membrane

Thyroid cartilage

Superior parathyroid glands

Thyroid gland

Inferior parathyroid glands
Trachea

Posterior

The thyroid gland is located in the neck just below the cricoid cartilage. Its two lateral lobes straddle the trachea, usually but not always connected by an isthmus that crosses in front of the trachea. The right lobe is a bit larger and higher in the neck than the left. About 50% of normal persons have a third, pyramidal lobe (dotted line in illustration) rising from the isthmus. Occasionally, it's the site of a malignant tumor. Visualization of the thyroid can determine abnormalities in gland size and ability to absorb iodine, and the presence and quality of tumors and cysts. The parathyroid glands, two upper and two lower, sit behind the thyroid, so closely involved in its tissue that they're often inadvertently removed during thyroid surgery, causing hypoparathyroidism.

Thyroid tissue is composed of follicles filled with colloid, a substance consisting primarily of an iodine-containing protein known as *thyroglobulin*. Normally, the thyroid weighs about 20 g, but certain disorders, such as goiter, can grossly enlarge it to more than several hundred grams.

Primarily, the thyroid controls the body's metabolism through the secretion of two hormones, *thyroxine* (T_4) and *triiodothyronine* (T_3). T_4 regulates body metabolism and helps control physical and mental development, resistance to infection, and vitamin requirements. Its production is regulated by release of thyroid-stimulating hormone, a pituitary hormone, and the ingestion of iodine and protein. T_4 may also be converted to T_3, a more potent hormone, by deiodination. A third thyroid hormone, thyrocalcitonin, is a polypeptide whose function is limited to lowering plasma phosphate and calcium levels.

may predispose a person to later development of thyroid nodules and carcinoma, and prolonged thyroid-stimulating hormone production may lead to malignant transformation of benign adenomas.

Testing procedures

Thyroid evaluations usually begin with determinations of serum hormone levels; abnormal hormone levels indicate the need for visualization of the thyroid gland to assess function and detect anatomic abnormalities. Thyroid tests can determine glandular size, identify tumors or cysts, and measure the thyroid's ability to retain iodine, essential for thyroid hormone synthesis. Such tests, which often include the radioactive iodine uptake test, T_3 resin uptake study, radionuclide thyroid imaging, and thyroid ultrasonography, are commonly performed as part of a series to provide a complete analysis.

Radioactive iodine tests

Measuring thyroid uptake of radioactive iodine reflects the gland's ability to handle stable dietary iodine and allows direct evaluation of thyroid function. This measurement is especially significant in thyroid hyperfunction, assessment of thyrotoxicosis factitia, and subacute thyroiditis. In the radioactive iodine uptake test, the patient's thyroid is scanned at specific intervals after oral administration of a radioisotope of iodine (usually ^{131}I) to help determine the degree of iodine retention.

Three radioisotopes of iodine—^{123}I, ^{125}I, and ^{131}I—have been useful because they demonstrate differences in half-life and amount of radiation emitted. All are synthetic isotopes and are indistinguishable from the naturally occurring stable isotope, ^{127}I. All emit gamma radiation, which allows their external measurement in sites of concentration, such as the thyroid gland or aberrant thyroid tissue.

Radionuclide thyroid imaging

Thyroid imaging uses radionuclides to locate radioiodine accumulation sites. It's of great value in diagnosis or management of thyroid disease. In this test, the patient is given a radiopharmaceutical; then, a gamma camera is placed near the anterior portion of the patient's neck, where it assesses and processes the radioactivity of the radionuclide, producing a precise image of the thyroid gland.

Radionuclide thyroid imaging provides information on overall thyroid size and shape. More important, it can define areas of hyperfunction (hot spots) or hypofunction (cold spots), and is especially valuable in detecting cancer. Palpable nodules that can be shown to be nonfunctioning may be malignant. Conversely, functioning nodules, particularly if they are more active than surrounding tissue, are unlikely to be malignant. Accurate interpretation also requires careful correlation between the findings on palpation and thyroid imaging. Radionuclide thyroid imaging may also reveal substernal goiters or the location of ectopic thyroid tissue in the tongue, chest, or ovary, and can detect functioning metastases of thyroid carcinoma.

Rectilinear scintiscanning, an alternative thyroid imaging technique, is rarely used today. In this test, a mechanical device moves a highly focused scintillation detector across the area of study while a printing device simultaneously makes a visual record of the radioactivity. This produces a life-sized image of the thyroid gland in which landmarks and palpable nodules are clearly indicated.

Ultrasonography

Thyroid ultrasonography allows visualization of the thyroid gland through high-frequency sound waves converted to images on an oscilloscope screen. This is especially useful for distinguishing cystic from solid thyroid nodules. When used during pregnancy, thyroid ultrasonography doesn't expose the fetus to radioactive materials.

BONNIE L. ANDERSON, MD

SCANNING TESTS

Radioactive Iodine Uptake Test

The radioactive iodine uptake (RAIU) test evaluates thyroid function by measuring the amount of orally ingested ^{123}I or ^{131}I that accumulates in the thyroid gland after 6 and 24 hours. An external single counting probe measures the radioactivity in the thyroid as a percentage of the original dose, thus indicating the ability of the gland to trap and retain iodine. The test accurately diagnoses hyperthyroidism (about 90%) but is less accurate for hypothyroidism. When performed concurrently with radionuclide thyroid imaging and the T_3 resin uptake test, the RAIU test helps differentiate Graves' disease from hyperfunctioning toxic adenoma. Indications for this test include abnormal results of chemical tests used to evaluate thyroid function (see Chapter 5).

Purpose
□ To evaluate thyroid function
□ To aid diagnosis of hyper- or hypothyroidism
□ In combination with other tests, to help distinguish between primary and secondary thyroid disorders.

Patient preparation
Explain to the patient that the test assesses thyroid function. Instruct him to fast from midnight before the test. Tell him that after he receives the radioactive iodine capsule or liquid, he'll be scanned 6 and 24 hours later to determine the amount of radioactive substance present in the thyroid gland—an indicator of proper thyroid function. Assure him that the test is painless and that the small amount of radioactivity used for the procedure is harmless. Tell him that the test results will be available within 24 hours.

Check patient history for past or present iodine exposure, which may inter-

fere with test results. If the patient has previously undergone radiologic tests using contrast media or nuclear medicine procedures, or if he's currently receiving iodine preparations or thyroid medications, note this on the film request slip.

Since the amount of iodine used in this test is similar to the amount obtained through dietary intake, a history of iodine hypersensitivity is not considered a contraindication to the test.

Equipment
Oral dose of ^{123}I or ^{131}I (radiologist determines the exact dosage)/external single counting probe.

Procedure
At 6 and 24 hours after administration of an oral dose of radioactive iodine, the patient's thyroid is scanned by placing the anterior portion of his neck in front of an external single counting probe. The amount of radioactivity that the probe detects is compared to the amount in the original dose in order to determine the percentage of radioactive iodine retained by the thyroid.

Precautions
Radioactive iodine uptake testing is contraindicated during pregnancy and lactation because of possible teratogenic effects.

Values
After 6 hours, 3% to 16% of the radioactive iodine should have accumulated in the thyroid; after 24 hours, 8% to 29%. The remaining radioactive iodine is excreted in the urine.

Local variations in the normal range of iodine uptake may occur due to regional differences in dietary iodine intake and procedural differences among individual laboratories.

Implications of results
Below-normal percentages of iodine up-

take may indicate hypothyroidism, sub-acute thyroiditis, or iodine overload. Above-normal percentages may indicate hyperthyroidism, early Hashimoto's thy-roiditis, hypoalbuminemia, lithium in-gestion, or iodine-deficient goiter. How-ever, in hyperthyroidism, the rate of turnover may be so rapid that the 24-hour measurement appears falsely nor-mal.

Post-test care
□ As ordered, instruct the patient to re-sume a light diet 2 hours after taking the oral dose of ^{123}I or ^{131}I.
□ After the study is complete, tell the patient to resume a normal diet.

Interfering factors
□ Renal failure, diuresis, severe diar-rhea, X-ray contrast media studies, ingestion of iodine preparations (includ-ing iodized salt, cough syrups, and some multivitamins) or of other drugs (thyroid hormones, thyroid hormone antagonists, salicylates, penicillin, antihistamines, anticoagulants, corticosteroids, and phenylbutazone) can decrease iodine uptake, thereby interfering with accu-rate determination of iodine uptake test results.
□ Iodine-deficient diet or ingestion of phenothiazines can increase iodine up-take, interfering with accurate deter-mination of test results.

BONNIE L. ANDERSON, MD

Radionuclide Thyroid Imaging

Radionuclide thyroid imaging is the vi-sualization of the thyroid gland by a gamma camera after administration of a radioisotope—usually ^{123}I, ^{99m}Tc per-technetate, or ^{131}I. The first two radio-isotopes are used most often because of their short half-lives (which limit expo-sure to radiation) and because of their abilities to measure thyroid function.

Thyroid imaging is usually recom-mended after discovery of a palpable mass, enlarged gland, or asymmetric goiter. Generally, this test is performed concurrently with measurement of serum triiodothyronine (T_3) and serum thyrox-ine (T_4) levels, and thyroid uptake tests. Later, thyroid ultrasonography may be done.

Purpose
□ To assess the size, structure, and po-sition of the thyroid gland
□ To evaluate thyroid function, in con-junction with specific thyroid uptake studies.

Patient preparation
Explain to the patient that this test helps determine the cause of thyroid dysfunc-tion. If he's scheduled to receive an oral dose of ^{123}I or ^{131}I, instruct him to fast from midnight the night before the test; he needn't fast if he's to receive an I.V. injection of ^{99m}Tc pertechnetate. Tell the patient that after he receives the radio-pharmaceutical, his thyroid will be im-aged with a gamma camera. Assure him that neither the radiopharmaceutical medication nor the equipment will ex-pose him to dangerous radiation levels, and that the actual imaging takes only 30 minutes.

Check patient history for diet and medication. Ask the patient if he has un-dergone tests that used radiographic contrast media within the past 60 days. Note drugs or previous radiographic contrast media exposure that may inter-fere with iodine uptake on the X-ray re-quest slip.

As ordered, 2 to 3 weeks before the test, discontinue administration of thy-roid hormones, thyroid hormone antag-onists, and iodine preparations (Lugol's solution, some multivitamins, and cough syrups). One week before the test, dis-continue phenothiazines, corticoste-roids, salicylates, anticoagulants, and antihistamines, as ordered. Also, as or-dered, instruct the patient to avoid in-gesting iodized salt, iodinated salt

THYROID IMAGES: NORMAL AND ABNORMAL

NORMAL

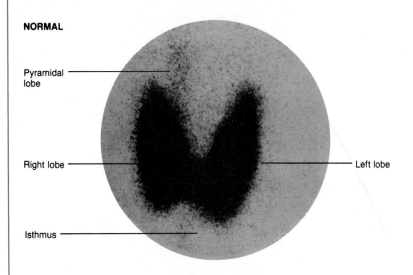

Pyramidal lobe

Right lobe

Left lobe

Isthmus

ABNORMAL

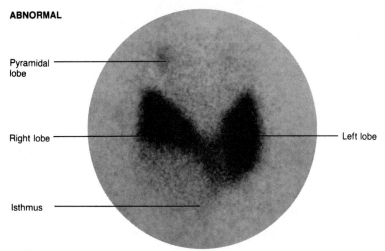

Pyramidal lobe

Right lobe

Left lobe

Isthmus

The top photograph shows an even distribution of black areas characteristic of a normal thyroid gland. The right and left lobes are clearly visible; the pyramidal lobe appears behind the right lobe. In the photograph at bottom, a hypofunctioning thyroid appears as a diminished gland with cold nodules (white or light gray areas) of decreased iodine concentration. Diagnostic evaluation of such nodules may be the most important function of radionuclide thyroid imaging. Malignant areas generally appear cold, while benign adenomas may be cold or hot. The patient with cold nodules requires subsequent thyroid ultrasonography to rule out cysts, possibly followed by fine needle aspiration and biopsy to rule out malignancy.

RESULTS OF THYROID IMAGING IN THYROID DISORDERS

CONDITION	FINDINGS	CAUSES
Hypothyroidism	• Glandular damage or absent gland	• Surgical removal of gland • Inflammation • Radiation • Neoplasm (rare)
Hypothyroid goiter	• Enlarged gland • Decreased uptake if glandular destruction is present • Increased uptake possible from congenital error in thyroxine synthesis	• Insufficient iodine intake • Hypersecretion of TSH caused by thyroid hormone deficiency
Myxedema (cretinism in children)	• Normal or slightly reduced gland size • Uniform pattern • Decreased uptake	• Defective embryonic development, resulting in congenital absence or underdevelopment of thyroid gland • Maternal iodine deficiency
Hyperthyroidism (Graves' disease)	• Enlarged gland • Uniform pattern • Increased uptake	• Unknown, but may be hereditary • Production of thyroid-stimulating immunoglobulins
Toxic nodular goiter	• Multiple hot spots	• Long-standing simple goiter
Hyperfunctioning adenomas	• Solitary hot spot	• Adenomatous production of T_3 and T_4, suppressing TSH secretion and producing atrophy of other thyroid tissue
Hypofunctioning adenomas	• Solitary cold spot	• Cyst or nonfunctioning nodule
Benign multinodular goiter	• Multiple nodules with variable or no function	• Local inflammation • Degeneration
Thyroid carcinoma	• Usually a solitary cold spot with occasional or no function	• Neoplasm

substitutes, and seafood during this period.

As ordered, give ^{123}I or ^{131}I orally. Alternatively, you or a laboratory technician may be asked to give ^{99m}Tc pertechnetate I.V., depending on your training and the hospital's protocol. Record the date and the time of administration. The patient receiving an oral dose should fast for another 2 hours after administration of the radioisotope.

Equipment

Radionuclide solutions—^{123}I or ^{131}I for oral administration; ^{99m}Tc pertechnetate solutions for I.V. administration/scanning equipment/gamma camera.

Procedure

The test follows P.O. administration of ^{123}I or ^{131}I by 24 hours; I.V. injection of ^{99m}Tc pertechnetate by 20 to 30 minutes. Just before the test, tell the patient to

---

T₃ THYROID SUPPRESSION TEST

The T₃ (Cytomel) thyroid suppression test helps determine whether areas of excessive iodine uptake in the thyroid (hot spots) are autonomous (as in some cases of Graves' disease) or reflect pituitary overcompensation (as in iodine-deficient goiter). Autonomous hot spots function independently of pituitary control. However, hot spots caused by iodine deficiency stem from reduced T₄ production, which decreases T₃ production and increases thyroid-stimulating hormone (TSH) production. Increased TSH production, in turn, overstimulates the thyroid and causes excessive iodine uptake.

After a baseline reading of thyroid function is obtained by a radioactive iodine uptake (RAIU) test, a dosage of 100 mcg of synthetic T₃ (Cytomel) is administered for 7 days. (Normally, T₃ acts through a negative feedback mechanism to suppress pituitary release of TSH; TSH suppression then suppresses thyroid function and iodine uptake.) During the last 2 days of Cytomel administration, RAIU tests are repeated to assess thyroid response. Suppression of RAIU to at least 50% of baseline indicates that the hot spot is under pituitary control and suggests iodine deficiency as the cause of increased iodine uptake. Failure to suppress RAIU by 50% suggests autonomous thyroid hyperfunction, resulting perhaps from Graves' disease or a toxic thyroid nodule.

---

remove his dentures and all jewelry that may interfere with visualization of the thyroid.

The patient's thyroid gland is palpated. Then, with the patient in a supine position with his neck extended, the gamma camera is placed over the anterior portion of his neck. The radioactive substance within the thyroid gland projects an image of the gland on an oscilloscope screen and X-ray film. Three views of the thyroid are obtained: one straight-on anterior view and two bilateral oblique views.

Precautions

Radionuclide thyroid imaging is contraindicated during pregnancy and lactation.

Findings

Normally, radionuclide thyroid imaging reveals a thyroid gland that is about 2″ (5 cm) long and 1″ (2.5 cm) wide, with a uniform uptake of the radioisotope and without tumors. The gland is butterfly-shaped, with the isthmus located at the midline. Occasionally, a third lobe called the pyramidal lobe may be present; this is a normal variant.

Implications of results

During radionuclide thyroid imaging, hyperfunctioning nodules (areas of excessive iodine uptake) appear as black regions called "hot spots." The presence of hot spots requires a follow-up T₃ (Cytomel) thyroid suppression test to determine if the hyperfunctioning areas are autonomous.

Hypofunctioning nodules (areas of little or no iodine uptake) appear as white or light gray regions called "cold spots." If a cold spot appears, subsequent thyroid ultrasonography may be performed to rule out cysts; in addition, fine needle aspiration and biopsy of such nodules may be performed to rule out malignancy.

Post-test care

□ As ordered, resume administration of any medications that were discontinued before the test.

□ Instruct the patient to resume his normal diet.

Interfering factors

□ Iodine-deficient diet and phenothiazines increase uptake of radioactive iodine.

□ Renal disease, ingestion of iodized salt, iodine preparations, iodinated salt substitutes, seafood, thyroid hormones, thyroid hormone antagonists, aminosalicyclic acid, corticosteroids, multivitamins, and cough syrups containing inorganic iodides decrease uptake of radioactive iodine. Severe diarrhea and vomiting can also decrease uptake by impairing gastrointestinal absorption of radioiodine.

BONNIE L. ANDERSON, MD

ULTRASONOGRAPHY

Thyroid Ultrasonography

In this safe, noninvasive procedure, ultrasonic pulses emitted from a piezoelectric crystal in a transducer and directed at the thyroid gland are reflected back to the transducer. These pulses are then converted electronically to produce structural visualization on an oscilloscope screen.

When a mass is located by palpation or by thyroid imaging, thyroid ultrasonography can differentiate between a cyst and a tumor larger than ⅜" (1 cm) with about 85% accuracy.

Thyroid ultrasonography is particularly useful in the evaluation of thyroid nodules during pregnancy, since it doesn't expose the fetus to the radioactive iodine used in other diagnostic procedures.

Purpose
□ To evaluate thyroid structure
□ To differentiate between a cyst and a solid tumor
□ To monitor the size of the thyroid gland during suppressive therapy.

Patient preparation
Describe the procedure to the patient, and explain that this test defines the size and shape of the thyroid gland. Inform him that he needn't restrict food or fluids before the test. Tell him who will perform the procedure and where, and that it only takes approximately 30 minutes. Reassure the patient that the procedure is painless and safe, and that test results are usually available within 24 hours.

Equipment
Sonographic equipment/camera and film, or videotape/water-soluble contact solution.

Procedure
The patient is placed in a supine position, with a pillow under his shoulder blades to hyperextend his neck. Next, his neck is coated with water-soluble gel. The transducer then scans the thyroid, projecting its echographic image on the oscilloscope screen. The image on the screen is photographed for subsequent examination. Accurate visualization of the anterior portion of the thyroid necessitates use of a short-focused transducer.

Precautions
None.

Findings
Normally, thyroid ultrasonography exhibits a uniform echo pattern throughout the gland.

Implications of results
Cysts appear as smooth-bordered, echo-free areas with enhanced sound transmission; adenomas and carcinomas appear either solid and well demarcated, with identical echo patterns, or less frequently, solid, with cystic areas. Carcinoma infiltrating the gland may not be well demarcated.

Identification of a tumor is generally followed up by fine needle aspiration or an excisional biopsy to determine malignancy.

PARATHYROID ULTRASONOGRAPHY

On ultrasonography, the parathyroid glands appear as solid masses, 5 mm or smaller in size, with an echo pattern of less amplitude than thyroid tissue. Glandular enlargement is usually characteristic of tumor growth or of hyperplasia. Normally, on a scan, the parathyroid glands are indistinguishable from the nearby neurovascular bundle.

HOW ULTRASONOGRAPHY WORKS

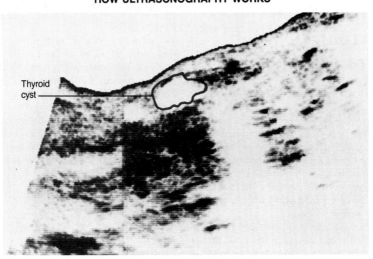

Thyroid
cyst

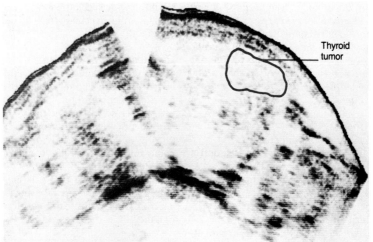

Thyroid
tumor

To understand how ultrasonography can differentiate between a thyroid cyst and tumor, you must first understand how ultrasonography works.

During ultrasonography, the technician guides a transducer over the pertinent area of the patient's body. The transducer sends an ultrasound beam, composed of sound waves, through the tissue. These sound waves travel at varying speeds, depending on the density of the tissue they're passing through. For example, sound waves travel through bone at 13,200' (4,000 m) per second; they travel through muscle at 5,230' (1,585 m) per second.

After passing through the tissue, the sound waves reflect to the transducer, where they're converted into electrical impulses. Then, these impulses are amplified and displayed on a screen.

Because the densities of the cyst and tumor differ, sound waves pass through them at different speeds. The image on the display screen reflects this difference. As these photographs show, the cyst (top photograph) is clearly defined, because it's filled with fluid and transmits sound waves very well. Conversely, the tumor (bottom photograph), which is a solid mass, is vaguely defined.

Post-test care
Thoroughly cleanse the patient's neck to remove the contact solution.

Interfering factors
None.

BONNIE L. ANDERSON, MD

Selected References

Conn, Howard F., and Conn, Rex B., eds. *Current Diagnosis,* 6th ed. Philadelphia: W.B. Saunders Co., 1980.

DeGroot, Leslie J., et al. *Endocrinology.* New York: Grune & Stratton, 1979.

Endocrine Disorders. Nurse's Clinical Library. Springhouse, Pa.: Springhouse Corp., 1984.

Ganga, Thomas S. *Laboratory Aids in Thyroid Problems,* Van Nuys, Calif.: Bio-Science Laboratories, 1981.

Grossman, Zachary D., et al. *The Clinician's Guide to Diagnostic Imaging.* New York: Raven Press Pubs., 1983.

Guyton, Arthur C. *Textbook of Medical Physiology,* 6th ed. Philadelphia: W.B. Saunders Co., 1981.

Harvey, A. McGehee, ed. *The Principles and Practice of Medicine,* 21st ed. East Norwalk, Conn.: Appleton-Century-Crofts, 1984.

Henry, John Bernard, ed. *Todd-Sanford-Davidson Clinical Diagnosis and Management by Laboratory Methods,* vol. 1, 17th ed.

Philadelphia: W.B. Saunders Co., 1984.

Lamb, Jane O. *Laboratory Tests for Clinical Nursing.* Bowie, Md.: Robert J. Brady Co., 1984.

Petersdorf, Robert G., and Adams, Raymond D., eds. *Harrison's Principles of Internal Medicine,* 10th ed. New York: McGraw-Hill Book Co., 1983.

Price, Sylvia, and Wilson, Lorraine. *Pathophysiology: Clinical Concepts of Disease Processes,* 2nd ed. New York: McGraw-Hill Book Co., 1982.

Ravel, Richard, *Clinical Laboratory Medicine,* 4th ed. Chicago: Year Book Medical Pubs., 1984.

Tilkian, Sarko M., et al. *Clinical Implications of Laboratory Tests,* 3rd ed. St. Louis: C.V. Mosby Co., 1983.

Widmann, Frances K. *Clinical Interpretation of Laboratory Tests,* 9th ed. Philadelphia: F.A. Davis Co., 1983.

Williams, Robert H. *Textbook of Endocrinology,* 6th ed. Philadelphia: W.B. Saunders Co., 1981.

21 Eye

LEARNING OBJECTIVES

After completing this chapter, the reader will be able to:
- explain the anatomy and physiology of the eye.
- discuss the nurse's role in the routine eye examination.
- define four common eye conditions related to age.
- identify common ophthalmic abbreviations.
- state the purpose of each test discussed in the chapter.
- prepare the patient physically and psychologically for each test.
- describe the procedure for performing each test.
- specify appropriate precautions for safe administration of each test.
- recognize signs of adverse reaction and respond appropriately.
- implement appropriate post-test care.
- identify the normal findings of each test.
- discuss the implications of abnormal test results.
- list factors that may interfere with accurate test results.

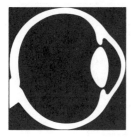

Eye

Introduction

Tests to diagnose eye disorders fall into three categories. *Subjective tests,* such as visual acuity tests and the tangent screen examination, require oral responses from the patient that must be interpreted by the examiner. These tests need to be correlated with *objective tests,* such as tonometry and ophthalmoscopy, in which the examiner obtains measurements or directly visualizes the interior of the eye. Finally, when severe abnormalities result from ocular disease or trauma, the ophthalmologist can resort to *special procedures,* like computed tomography. Understanding the diagnostic application and significance of these tests begins with review of the anatomical structure and physiology of the eye.

Outer layer

The cornea and sclera constitute the outermost portion of the eye's three layers. The *cornea* lies in the anterior portion of the eye. A transparent structure composed of avascular tissue, the cornea bends light rays that enter the eye and helps to focus the images on the retina. Adjoining the cornea is the *sclera,* an opaque, white, fibrous coat covering the posterior three fourths of the eye, through which nerves and blood vessels pass in order to penetrate the eye's interior.

Middle layer

The middle vascular layer, known as the uveal tract, consists of the iris, the ciliary body, and the choroid. The *iris,* the colored part of the eye, is composed of muscle fibers that regulate the amount of light admitted to the eye's interior through the pupil, the circular opening in its center. Behind the iris lies the *lens,* a biconvex, transparent structure that can change its shape to focus light rays precisely on the retina. The *ciliary body* produces aqueous humor and permits flexibility of the lens for clearer vision. The highly vascular and pigmented *choroid* supplies blood to the retina and conducts blood and nerve impulses to the eye's anterior structures.

Inner layer

The third layer of the eye, the *retina,* consists of a complicated network of rods, cones, and other nerve cells lined with pigment epithelium. In the posterior portion of the retina lies the *fovea;* composed entirely of cones, the fovea is the area of most acute vision.

Chambers and their fluids

The *anterior chamber* of the eye, which is situated behind the cornea and in front of the iris and lens, is filled with aqueous humor. Secreted by the ciliary body, aqueous humor nourishes the internal structures of the eye and maintains constant pressure within the eyeball. Defective drainage of this fluid can increase

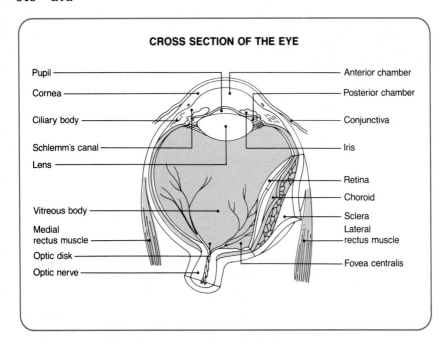

CROSS SECTION OF THE EYE

Pupil — Anterior chamber
Cornea — Posterior chamber
Ciliary body — Conjunctiva
Schlemm's canal — Iris
Lens —
— Retina
— Choroid
Vitreous body — Sclera
Medial rectus muscle — Lateral rectus muscle
Optic disk —
Optic nerve — Fovea centralis

intraocular pressure and eventually cause glaucoma. The iris forms a curtain that divides the space between the cornea and the lens into the anterior and posterior chambers of the eye. Aqueous humor secreted by the ciliary processes in the posterior chamber flows through the pupil, into the anterior chamber.

The vitreous cavity is surrounded by the retina and the optic nerve and constitutes four fifths of the back of the eye. It is filled with vitreous humor—a clear, avascular, gelatinous substance. Vitreous humor helps maintain the transparency and shape of the eye.

How the eye moves
The eye rests on a cushion of fat within its bony orbit, which also contains the eye's appendages—eyelids, lacrimal system, and conjunctiva. Six extraocular muscles attached to the sclera control the movements of the eyeball. Although each has at least one specific action, these muscles never act independently. Complex muscular interactions allow the eyes to move in different directions and make possible coordinated use of both eyes.

Progressive change
The eye is a dynamic organ that changes progressively throughout life. Because the elasticity of the lens greatly affects its ability to change its shape, changes in visual acuity from adolescence to adulthood are quite common, as the lens becomes increasingly less elastic.

Presbyopia, impaired near vision caused by loss of the natural elasticity of the lens, occurs commonly in middle age. This disorder often requires the use of reading glasses. In older persons, eye tissue may degenerate and seriously affect vision, especially in those patients with chronic diseases, such as diabetes. *Cataracts*—degenerative clouding of the lens—commonly afflict elderly patients.

Examination
A thorough eye examination begins with a patient history, including documentation of medical conditions and eye surgery. Identify the patient's chief complaint, such as discharge, pain or itching, blurred vision, vertigo, difficulty in distinguishing color, the presence of

blind spots, or poor visual acuity. Determine how long the symptom has been present and when it is most intense. Ask the patient about his occupation and what effect it has on his eyes. Also ask if he's had facial pain or headaches. Remember to consider the patient's age and understanding when phrasing your questions.

The next step in the examination is visual acuity testing, using standardized vision charts such as the Snellen chart and the Jaeger card. After assessing visual acuity, look for clinical features such as redness, excessive tearing or blinking, displacement of the eye within the orbit, and asymmetry of ocular and facial structures. External examination includes assessment of pupillary light reflexes, inspection of anterior segments, and evaluation of extraocular muscle function and ocular alignment. The interior structures of the eye are then inspected with an ophthalmoscope and a slit-lamp biomicroscope. Tonometry, which measures intraocular pressure, may be performed to help diagnose glaucoma.

Abnormalities detected by these routine procedures may indicate the need for more refined tests. For example, suspected pathologies and foreign bodies—although sometimes visible with an ophthalmoscope—can often be located more precisely with orbital radiography, orbital computerized tomography, ocular ultrasonography, or a combination of these tests.

Nursing considerations

In several routine tests, the doctor may request ophthalmic drugs. *Cycloplegics* cause paralysis of accommodation and are often required before refraction. *Mydriatics* cause pupillary dilation and are commonly used to inspect intraocular structures. Generally, two instillations are required to induce maximum mydriasis. To help prevent contamination, avoid touching the eye dropper to the eye or lids during instillation.

COMMON OPHTHALMIC ABBREVIATIONS	
When recording the patient's responses during eye examinations, use the following ophthalmic abbreviations:	
AC	anterior chamber
c̄c̄	with spectacles
CF	count fingers (visual acuity)
EOM	extraocular muscles
HM	hand motion (visual acuity)
IOP	intraocular pressure
LP	light perception
NLP	no light perception
NPC	near point of convergence
OD	right eye *(oculus dexter)*
OS	left eye *(oculus sinister)*
OU	both eyes (oculi uterque)
PERRLA	pupils equal, round, reactive to light, and accommodation
PH	pinhole
s̄c̄	without spectacles
VF	visual field
Δ	prism diopters
D	lens diopters
(+)	convex lens
(−)	concave lens

Never instill dilating drops in a patient who has or is suspected of having narrow-angle glaucoma. In such a patient, pupillary dilation may trigger an acute attack of angle closure.

To ensure the patient's cooperation during an eye examination, provide a thorough explanation of each test and reassure him that the procedures are painless. These measures are essential with those tests requiring subjective responses from the patient. The first section of this chapter deals with subjective tests; the second section focuses on objective tests. The final section covers definitive diagnostic procedures that are usually performed in a hospital or radiology department.

PATRICIA A. DOWEN, BA, COT, OT

SUBJECTIVE TESTS

Visual Acuity Tests

Part of a routine eye examination, a visual acuity test evaluates the patient's ability to distinguish the form and detail of an object. In this test, the patient is asked to read letters on a standardized visual chart, commonly called the Snellen chart, from a distance of 20' (6 m). Charts showing the letter E in various positions and sizes are used for young children and other persons who can't read. The smaller the symbol the patient can identify, the sharper his visual acuity. A patient's near, or reading, vision may be tested as well, using a standardized chart such as the Jaeger card. The Snellen test should be performed on all patients with eye complaints. It's also performed by doctors and by school or occupational health nurses on persons who have no complaints. Near-vision testing is routine for those complaining of eyestrain or reading difficulty, and for everyone over age 40. Results serve as a baseline for treatments, follow-up examinations, and referrals.

Purpose
☐ To test distance and near visual acuity
☐ To identify refractive errors in vision.

Patient preparation
Explain to the patient that these tests evaluate distant and near vision. Tell him the tests take only a few minutes. If he wears glasses, tell him to bring them to the examination.

Equipment
Standardized eye charts: to test distance visual acuity, the Snellen chart or the E chart; to test near visual acuity, the Jaeger card/occlusion supplies: hand-held occluder, disposable tissues for insertion between the patient's eyes and glasses (useful for some patients, particularly geriatric or pediatric patients who can't or won't use a hand-held occluder), or disposable eyepatches/standard 20' (6 m) room, or equipment to simulate correct distance (such as mirrors or chart with proportionately reduced letters)/illumination: 10 to 30 footcandles.

Procedure
Distance visual acuity: Have the patient sit 20' (6 m) away from the eye chart. If he's wearing glasses, tell him to remove them so his uncorrected vision can be tested first. Begin with the right eye, unless vision in the left eye is known to be more acute. Have the patient occlude the left eye, then ask him to read the smallest line of letters he can see on the chart. Encourage him to try to read lines he can't see clearly, because intelligent guesses usually indicate the patient can recognize some of the symbols' details.

Visual acuity is reported as a fraction: the numerator is the distance from the chart, and the denominator is the distance at which a normal eye can read this line.

Record the number of the smallest line the patient can read as the denominator. If he makes an error on a line, record the results with a minus number. For example, if the patient reads the 20/40 line but makes one error, record his vision as 20/40 − 1. If the patient reads the 20/40 line and one symbol on the following line, record his vision as 20/40 + 1.

Have the patient occlude the right eye, and repeat the test with the left eye. However, to minimize recall, use a different set of symbols or have the patient read the lines backward.

If the patient wears glasses, test his corrected vision, using the same procedure. If the patient normally wears glasses but doesn't have them with him, note this on the test results. In recording the patient's responses, indicate which eye was tested and whether it was tested with or without correction.

If the patient can't read the largest letter on the chart, further testing is necessary to determine what he can see. (See *Special Procedures for Testing Vision.*)

Near visual acuity: Have the patient remove his glasses and occlude the left eye. Ask him to read the Jaeger card (a card designed for this purpose, with print in graded sizes) at his customary reading distance. Both eyes are tested with and without corrective lenses. In reporting near visual acuity, specify both the size of the smallest print legible to the patient and the nearest distance at which reading is possible.

Precautions
None.

Findings
Most charts for distance visual acuity are read at 20' (6 m). If the patient's vision is normal, results are expressed as 20/20, which means that the smallest symbol he can identify at 20' (6 m) is the same symbol the normal eye can identify from the same distance.

The normal value for near visual acuity is 14/14, where 14 represents the distance in inches and /14 represents the correct identification of symbols that a person with normal vision can identify at 14".

Implications of results
Persons who can read the 20/20 line on the Snellen chart are considered to have normal distance visual acuity. If the denominator is more than 20, the patient's visual acuity is less than normal. For

---

SPECIAL PROCEDURES FOR TESTING VISION

Pinhole test: If the patient's visual acuity is less than 20/20, perform the pinhole test to determine whether reduced visual acuity is due to refractive error or organic disease. In this test, the patient is asked to look through a pinhole in the center of a disk at the visual acuity chart; the same effect can be achieved by punching a pinhole in a card. Looking through the tiny opening eliminates peripheral light rays and improves the patient's vision if impairment is due to refractive error. If impairment results from organic disease, the patient's vision fails to improve.

Changing the distance: If the patient can't identify the largest letter or symbol on the chart (line 20/200), tell him to walk toward the chart until he can correctly identify the largest symbol. Record the distance at which the patient can identify the symbol as the numerator. For example, 2/200 means the patient can identify at 2' (60 cm) a symbol that a person with normal vision can identify at 200' (60 m).

Counting fingers: If the patient can't identify the largest symbol at any distance, hold up your fingers at various distances in front of his eyes. When the patient correctly identifies the number of fingers in front of him, note the distance, for example, 4'/CF.

Hand movements: If the patient can't identify the number of fingers at any distance, wave your hand in front of his eyes at various distances. If he can detect hand movement, note the distance, for example, 2'/HM.

Light projection: If the patient can't identify hand movement at any distance, darken the room, and tell him to look straight ahead. Shine a penlight in each quadrant—nasal, temporal, superior, and inferior—of each eye. Note in which quadrants the patient can perceive light, for example, light projection/superior and nasal quadrants.

Light perception: If the patient can't perceive light projection at all, ask if he can tell whether the light is on or off. If the patient has no light perception, note NLP; otherwise, note that light perception exists.

---

example, 20/40 vision means the patient reads at 20' (6 m) what a person with normal vision can read at 40' (12 m). A patient with 20/200 visual acuity or less in the best corrected eye is considered legally blind.

If the denominator is less than 20, the patient's distance visual acuity is better than normal. For example, 20/15 vision means the patient reads at 20' (6 m) what a person with normal visual acuity can see at 15' (4.5 m).

Normal near visual acuity is usually recorded as 14/14, since standard testing charts, like the Jaeger card, are generally held 14" (35 cm) from the patient's eyes. Most charts aren't designed to measure better-than-normal near vision. Decreased near visual acuity is indicated by a larger denominator. For example, 14/20 near vision means the patient reads at 14" (35 cm) what a person with normal vision reads at 20" (50 cm).

Patients with less-than-normal visual acuity require further testing, including refraction and a complete ophthalmologic examination, to determine whether visual loss is due to injury, disease, or a need for corrective lenses.

Normal or better-than-normal visual acuity doesn't necessarily indicate normal vision, however. For example, a visual field defect may be present if the patient consistently misses the letters on one side of all the lines. A field defect is certainly present if the patient states that one or more of the letters disappears or becomes illegible when he is looking at a nearby letter. Such findings indicate the need for further visual field testing, such as the Amsler grid test and the tangent screen examination.

Post-test care
None.

Interfering factors
□ The patient's failure to cooperate or to bring his glasses to the examination interferes with accurate determination of test results.
□ If the patient wears glasses that were improperly prescribed or that are outdated in their degree of correction, he may have better visual acuity without his glasses.

PATRICIA A. DOWEN, BA, COT, OT

Amsler Grid Test

Composed of horizontal and vertical lines that form 5-mm squares, and a central black dot, the Amsler grid helps detect central scotomas—blind or partially blind spots in the macular area of the retina. The macula comprises the central visual field and has the greatest visual acuity of any retinal segment. This test can also detect microscopic areas of macular or perimacular edema that cause visual distortions. However, the Amsler grid test is only a screening procedure and must be supplemented with other tests, such as ophthalmoscopy, visual field testing, and fluorescein angiography, to determine the cause of abnormal vision.

Purpose
□ To detect central scotomas
□ To evaluate the stability or progression of macular disease.

Patient preparation
Explain to the patient that this test screens the central area of vision and takes about 5 to 10 minutes to perform. If he normally wears corrective lenses, instruct him to keep them on during the test.

Equipment
Amsler grid/occlusion supplies (hand-held occluder, disposable tissues for insertion between the patient's eyes and glasses, or disposable eyepatches).

Procedure
Occlude one of the patient's eyes. Hold the Amsler grid at his customary reading distance, approximately 11" to 12" (28 to 30 cm) in front of the unoccluded eye. Tell the patient to stare at the central dot on the Amsler grid, then ask these questions:
□ Can you see the black dot in the center?
□ When you look directly at the dot, can

you see all four sides of the grid? All the little squares?

□ Do all the lines appear ruler-straight?

□ Is there any blurring, distortion, or movement?

If the patient answers yes to any of these questions, ask him to elaborate on what he sees. Give him a pencil and paper, and encourage him to outline and describe the specific areas that appear distorted.

After recording the patient's observations, occlude the other eye and repeat the procedure.

Precautions

□ Remind the patient to keep his unoccluded eye fixed on the central black dot on the grid.

□ Perform this test on the patient with undilated pupils, before examining the fundus or conducting the refraction test.

Findings

The patient should be able to see the central black dot and, while staring at the dot, all four sides of the grid and all the little squares. All the lines should appear ruler-straight. He should not see any blurring, distortion, or missing squares.

Implications of results

Inability to see the black dot in the center of the grid suggests a central scotoma. If any of the lines do not appear ruler-straight to the patient, metamorphopsia (distorted perception of objects) may be indicated. Blurring, distortion, or movement may signal an imminent scotoma. Abnormal findings indicate the need for further evaluation by ophthalmoscopy, visual field testing, and fluorescein angiography.

Post-test care

None.

Interfering factors

□ The patient's inability to see the Amsler grid due to poor eyesight, or his failure to cooperate or to keep his unoccluded eye fixed on the central dot

---

NORMAL AND ABNORMAL VIEW OF AN AMSLER GRID

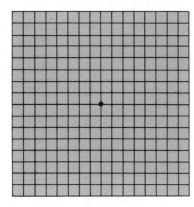

Normal view

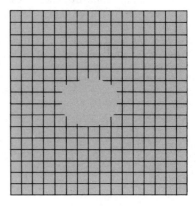

Abnormal view

On the left is a normal view of an Amsler grid. On the right is an Amsler grid as it might look to a patient with a central scotoma due to a macular hole. The center dot is entirely absent, as are the lines around it. The lines on the periphery of the scotoma appear bowed in an asymmetric pattern.

interferes with test results.
□ Bleaching of the retina with the bright light of a retinoscope or ophthalmoscope before the test impairs the patient's ability to see the Amsler grid.

PATRICIA A. DOWEN, BA, COT, OT

Tangent Screen Examination

The area within which objects can be seen as the eye fixates on a central point is called the visual field. It consists of a central field—a 25° area surrounding the fixation point—and a peripheral field— the remainder of the area within which objects can be visualized. The tangent screen examination evaluates a patient's central visual field through systematic movement of a test object across a tangent screen, usually a piece of black felt with concentric circles and lines radiating from a central fixation point, much like a spider web.

Monocular visual field examinations are important in detecting and following the progression of ocular diseases, such as glaucoma and optic neuritis. They are also indicated for detecting and evaluating neurologic disorders, such as brain tumors and cerebrovascular accidents. Localization of a specific visual field defect often points to the underlying pathology. The tangent screen examination provides only a general evaluation of the patient's visual field, however. Abnormal findings warrant further examination with a perimeter, to evalutate areas of the peripheral visual field. Perimeters are used almost exclusively by ophthalmologists.

Purpose
□ To detect central visual field loss and evaluate its progression or regression.

Patient preparation
Explain to the patient that this test evaluates his central field of vision. Tell him

the procedure takes about 30 minutes to perform. Reassure him that it causes no pain, but requires his full cooperation. If he normally wears corrective lenses, tell him to wear them during the test.

Equipment
Tangent screen/black-tipped straight pins/hand-held occluder, disposable tissues for insertion between the patient's eyes and glasses, or disposable eyepatches/test objects (usually 1- to 10-mm objects that can be inserted into a black wand)/visual field recording charts/stick or other object (to assist the patient in signaling).

Procedure
Have the patient sit comfortably about 3¼' (1 m) from the tangent screen, so the eye being tested is directly in line with the central fixation target on the screen. Occlude the patient's left eye, and tell him that while he fixates on the central target, you'll move a test object into his visual field. The test object is white on one side and black on the other; its diameter varies in size from 1 to 10 mm, depending on the patient's visual acuity (for example, if he has 20/20 vision, the test object should be 1 mm). Tell him not to look for the test object, but to wait for it to appear and then to signal when he sees it. Stand to the side of the eye being tested. Move the test object inward from the periphery of the screen at 30° intervals, as represented by the radiating lines on the screen. Using black-tipped straight pins, plot the points on the screen at which the patient can see the object. When connected, these points define areas of equal visual acuity. The boundaries of a visual field for a specific target size and distance is called an isopter.

To guarantee the adequacy of fixation, the blind spot (projection of optic nerve into the visual field) should be clearly identified.

After the boundaries of the patient's central visual field have been plotted, test how well he can see within his visual field. To do this, turn the test object to

CONFRONTATION TEST

If a tangent screen or perimeter isn't available, or if the patient is unable to cooperate for other tests, use this simple method to screen the visual field. Sit about 2' (60 cm) from the patient, directly in front of him. Test the patient's right eye first. Have the patient occlude his left eye and tell him to look at your right eye and maintain fixation during the test. Explain to the patient that you will hold up fingers or a fist in various positions. When he sees your hand, he should tell you what he can see—a fist or the number of fingers. Instruct him not to look for your hand, but to stare at your eye and signal when your hand appears.

Occlude your right eye. In each quadrant, hold up your hand midway between yourself and the patient. Move it from nonseeing to seeing areas. Alternate between presenting fingers and a fist. You and the patient should see your hand at the same time, and the patient should correctly identify what you're presenting.

If the patient responds correctly in all quadrants, present fingers on both sides of fixation to test horizontal, vertical, and oblique meridians. If the patient responds correctly, wiggle the index finger of each hand in the horizontal, vertical, and oblique meridians, and ask the patient if one finger is clearer than the other. If the patient reports that both fingers appear equally clear, occlude and fixate opposite eyes, and repeat the procedure to test the left visual field.

However, if the patient reports that one finger is clearer than the other, you'll need to pinpoint the questionable area. To do this, simultaneously hold fingers above and below the area, and ask the patient which finger he sees better. Then, proceed to test the other eye. If any areas of the visual field remain questionable, the patient should be tested with a tangent screen or a perimeter.

Although this confrontation test provides a simple means of screening a patient's visual field for gross abnormalities, it can't replace quantitative methods of evaluation. Also, the examiner's own visual field must be normal to produce valid test results.

the black side. Then turn it over within each 30° interval, and ask the patient to signal when he sees the test object. Plot suspicious areas—those in which the patient has failed to identify the test object—for size, shape, and density. Record the patient's visual field on the recording chart, marked in degrees, and note any abnormal areas within the field.

Since isopters vary with the patient's age, visual acuity, and pupil size; the size and color of the test object; and the distance between the patient and the screen, careful recording of all measurements is mandatory.

Occlude the patient's right eye, and repeat the test.

Precautions
Remind the patient that he must maintain fixation on the central target on the tangent screen; watch his eyes carefully to make sure he is following your instructions.

Findings
Normally, the central visual field forms a circle, extending 25° superiorly, nasally, inferiorly, and temporally. The physiologic blind spot lies 12° to 15° temporal to the central fixation point, approximately 1.5° below the horizontal meridian. It extends approximately 7.5° in height and 5.5° in width.

The test object should be visible throughout the patient's entire central visual field, except within the physiologic blind spot.

Implications of results
Visual field defects appear in a variety of forms and may arise from many causes. For example, inability to see the test object within the temporal half of the central visual field may indicate bitemporal hemianopia. Lesions of the optic chiasm, often caused by pituitary tumor; craniopharyngiomas in the young; and meningiomas or aneurysm of the circle of Willis in adults can cause bitemporal hemianopias. Hemianopia may also occur following a cerebrovascular accident. Although bilateral homonymous hemianopia is uncommon, it

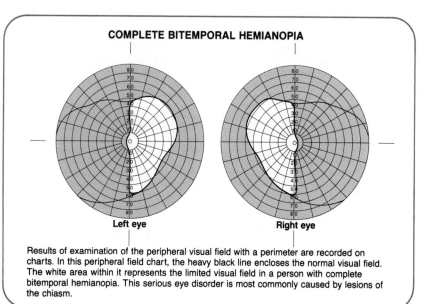

COMPLETE BITEMPORAL HEMIANOPIA

Left eye

Right eye

Results of examination of the peripheral visual field with a perimeter are recorded on charts. In this peripheral field chart, the heavy black line encloses the normal visual field. The white area within it represents the limited visual field in a person with complete bitemporal hemianopia. This serious eye disorder is most commonly caused by lesions of the chiasm.

may follow multiple thrombosis in the posterior cerebral circulation. Plotting visual fields following a cerebrovascular accident aids in locating cerebrovascular lesions.

When a disease, such as glaucoma, involves the optic nerve, an enlarged blind spot, a central scotoma, or a centrocecal scotoma may result. A ring scotoma (a scotoma 10° or more away from the fixation point) is characteristic of retinitis pigmentosa, a slowly progressive disease that leads to night blindness. The peripheral area beyond this ring is usually spared. Retinal detachments can be outlined as well.

Repeat tangent screen examinations can help evaluate progression or regression of a diagnosed disorder.

Post-test care
None.

Intefering factors
If the patient is uncooperative or has severe loss of vision that causes him to have difficulty in seeing even the largest test object, the test results will be invalid.

PATRICIA A. DOWEN, BA, COT, OT

Color Vision Tests

The human eye perceives color through the cones of the retina, which are also responsible for central visual acuity. The most widely accepted theories of color vision propose that these retinal cones contain three different photosensitive pigments, each of which absorbs light of different wavelengths. Specifically, these pigments are sensitive to red, green, and blue—the primary colors of light. Mixtures of these three pigments allow perception of other colors.

Color vision tests assess the ability to recognize differences in color. They may be performed routinely, and are often used to evaluate patients with suspected retinal disease or with family histories of color vision deficiency. A color vision deficiency may be inherited—a sex-linked recessive trait affecting approximately 8% to 10% of males and less than 1% of females—or acquired as a result of disease. These tests are also used to screen applicants for jobs in which ac-

curate color perception is vital, as in the military and electronics fields.

The most common color vision tests use pseudoisochromatic plates made up of dot patterns of the primary colors superimposed on backgrounds of randomly mixed colors. A patient with normal color vision can identify the dot pattern; a patient with a color deficiency can't distinguish between the pattern and the background. Basic color vision tests merely indicate the presence of a deficiency; more sophisticated tests can determine the degree of deficiency.

Purpose

☐ To detect color vision deficiency.

Patient preparation

Explain to the patient that this test evaluates color perception and takes only a few minutes to perform and causes no pain. If he normally wears glasses or contact lenses, tell him to wear them during the test.

Equipment

Color vision test kit (Hardy-Rand-Rittler [H-R-R] or Ishihara pseudoisochromatic plates)/occlusion supplies: hand-held occluder, disposable tissues for insertion between the patient's eyes and glasses, or disposable eyepatches/pointer (an artist's paintbrush is recommended, since secretions from the patient's fingertip may discolor the plates).

Procedure

After seating the patient comfortably, occlude one of his eyes. Hold the test book approximately 14″ (35 cm) in front of his unoccluded eye, and give him the pointer.

Explain to the patient what patterns or symbols he may see. Show him the sample plates—which can be deciphered by most patients—and tell him you'll ask him to identify the symbols and then to trace them with the pointer. Advise the patient that some symbols are more difficult to see than others.

Conduct the test, eliciting immediate responses from the patient. Record the responses according to the instructions included with the test kit. If the test must be repeated, or when testing the other eye, rotate the plates 90° to 180° to minimize recall.

Precautions

To prevent discoloration of the plates, keep the test book closed when it isn't being used and turn the pages by their edges.

Findings

A person with normal color vision—a trichromat—can identify all the patterns or symbols.

Implications of results

A patient with deficient color vision—an anomalous trichromat—can't identify all the patterns or symbols. This deficiency may be diagnosed more precisely by noting the combinations of colors that elicit incorrect responses. For example, protanopia is a deficiency of the retinal cone pigment that is sensitive to red. A patient with protanopia has difficulty discriminating between red/green and blue/green. A patient with deuteranopia, a deficiency of the retinal pigment sensitive to green, can't distinguish between green/purple and red/purple. Tritanopia, a deficiency of the pigment sensitive to blue, causes the patient to have difficulty discriminating between blue/green and yellow/green.

Achromatopia—true color blindness—is a rare disease inherited as a Mendelian autosomal dominant or autosomal recessive trait. Patients with achromatopia, called monochromats, see all colors as shades of gray. These patients may also have impaired visual acuity, nystagmus, and photophobia, due to reduced or absent cone function.

Inherited color deficiencies affect both eyes; acquired deficiencies may affect only one eye. Patients with acquired deficiencies may complain of inability to recognize colors that were formerly recognizable.

Abnormalities of the ocular media, retina, or optic nerve can cause deficient color vision. For this reason, a patient with an acquired color vision deficiency or an inherited deficiency accompanied by a loss of visual acuity should be referred for a complete ophthalmologic examination to determine the source of color deficiency.

Post-test care
None.

Interfering factors
□ Poor patient cooperation, the patient's inability to see the plates because of reduced visual acuity or failure to wear his glasses, or improper lighting interferes with test results.

□ Errors in the testing procedure, such as inaccurately recording the patient's responses or allowing too much time for response, interfere with accurate determination of test results.

PATRICIA A. DOWEN, BA, COT, OT

Refraction

Refraction—the bending of light rays by the cornea, aqueous, lens, and vitreous in the eye—enables images to focus on the retina and directly affects visual acuity. This test, done routinely during a complete eye examination or whenever a patient complains of a change in vision, defines the refractive error and determines the degree of correction required to improve visual acuity with glasses or contact lenses. The ophthalmologist generally performs a refraction both objectively, by using a retinoscope, and subjectively, by questioning the patient concerning his visual acuity while placing trial lenses before his eyes.

Purpose
□ To diagnose refractive error and prescribe corrective lenses, if necessary.

Patient preparation
Explain to the patient that this test helps determine whether he needs corrective lenses. Tell him eyedrops may be instilled to dilate the pupils and inhibit accommodation by the lens, and that the test takes about 10 to 20 minutes. Reassure him that the test is painless and safe.

Check the patient's history for narrow-angle glaucoma. Also check for previous use of and hypersensitivity to dilating eyedrops.

Equipment
Retinoscope/trial lens set/cycloplegic eyedrops//Snellen chart/occlusion supplies: hand-held occluder, disposable tissues for insertion between the patient's eyes and glasses, or disposable eyepatches.

Procedure
After cycloplegic eyedrops are administered (if ordered), the examiner directs the light of the retinoscope at the pupillary opening. Through the aperture at

---

PRESBYOPIA

Normally, the ability of the lens to change its shape or to accommodate to focus on objects closer than 20' (6 m) gradually decreases with age. This process, known as presbyopia, is so inexorable that determination of the convex lens strength needed for correction can usually be estimated on the basis of age. Even a patient with normal vision eventually needs the aid of lenses for close work. Onset of presbyopia usually begins between ages 42 and 47 and progresses steadily, so that a 75-year-old patient requires a stronger correction than a 45-year-old patient.

Since presbyopia is normally part of aging, failure to wear corrective lenses doesn't affect the progression of this condition. However, after correction, a patient should be reexamined every 1 to 2 years, since he'll probably need new lenses at such intervals.

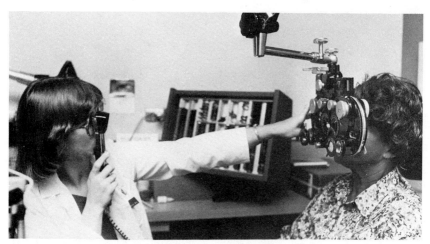

The ophthalmologist uses the retinoscope to project a beam of light into the eye of a patient wearing trial lens glasses. By manipulating the retinoscope beam, the ophthalmologist can illuminate retinal movement and test optic refraction.

the top of the instrument he looks for an orange glow—the retinoscopic, or red, reflex, which represents the reflection of light from the retinoscope—and notes its brightness, clarity, and uniformity. Moving the retinoscope's light across the pupil, he observes the reflex for any movement. The examiner then places trial lenses before the patient's eyes and adjusts the lens power to make the reflex clear, bright, and uniform, and to neutralize its motion. The lens power necessary to make this adjustment is recorded.

Objective findings can be refined by altering the trial lenses and having the patient read lines on a standardized visual chart. This step helps to determine which lens or combination of lenses provides the best correction of his visual acuity.

Precautions

Don't administer dilating eyedrops to any patient who has had a hypersensitivity reaction to such drops or to the patient who has narrow-angle glaucoma.

Findings

Refractive power, measured in diopters,

is greatest at the cornea (approximately 44 diopters) because of its curvature. The aqueous has the same refractive power as the cornea and is considered to be the same medium. The lens, normally a convex structure, has a refractive power of approximately 10 to 14 diopters but can alter this power by changing its shape. This phenomenon is known as accommodation and occurs when the eye views objects closer than 20′ (6 m).

The vitreous, a gelatinous medium, has little refractive power and mainly transmits light. In the absence of accommodation, the average refractive power of the human eye is 58 diopters.

Ideally, the eyes have no refractive error (emmetropia). Parallel light rays emanating from a point source can be focused directly on the retina to produce a clear image.

Implications of results

Most patients show some degree of refractive error, or ametropia. Three major types of ametropia exist. *Hyperopia*, commonly called farsightedness, occurs when the eyeball is too short, and parallel light rays focus behind the retina. Examination with the retinoscope shows a red reflex moving in the same direction as the retinoscope's light. A patient with

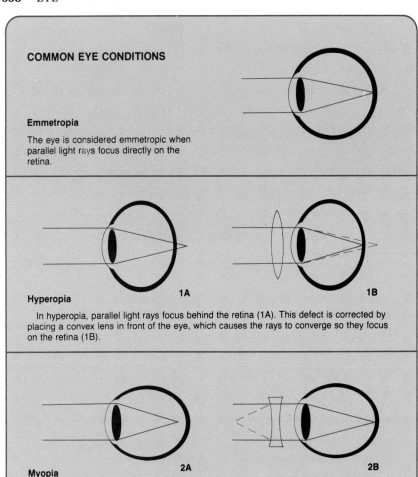

COMMON EYE CONDITIONS

Emmetropia

The eye is considered emmetropic when parallel light rays focus directly on the retina.

Hyperopia

1A 1B

In hyperopia, parallel light rays focus behind the retina (1A). This defect is corrected by placing a convex lens in front of the eye, which causes the rays to converge so they focus on the retina (1B).

Myopia

2A 2B

In myopia, parallel light rays focus in front of the retina (2A). A concave lens placed in front of the eye can correct this defect by diverging the rays so they focus on the retina (2B).

hyperopia sees clearly at a distance but experiences blurring of near objects.

Myopia, or nearsightedness, occurs when the eyeball is too long, and parallel light rays focus in front of the retina. Retinoscopic examination reveals reflex motion opposite to movement of the retinoscope's light. A patient with myopia sees near objects clearly but experiences blurring of distant images.

When light rays entering the eye are not refracted uniformly and a clear focal point on the retina is not attained, the patient has *astigmatism.* Usually caused by unequal curvature of the cornea, astigmatism is usually associated with some degree of hyperopia or myopia.

Post-test care

If corrective lenses are prescribed, advise the patient that images may appear blurred the first time he wears the lenses, but eventually his eyes will adjust to the prescription. If the patient has worn glasses or contact lenses previously, tell him to wear only his new prescription lenses, since changing back and forth from the old prescription to the new prescription doesn't permit the required adjustment to the new corrective lenses to take place.

Interfering factors
Inadequate paralysis of accommodation or pupil dilation, or poor patient cooperation interferes with test results.

PATRICIA A. DOWEN, BA, COT, OT

OBJECTIVE TESTS

Exophthalmometry

This test determines the relative forward protrusion of the eye from its orbit by using an exophthalmometer to measure the distance from the apex of the cornea to the lateral orbital margin. The exophthalmometer is a horizontal calibrated bar with movable carriers on both sides. These carriers hold mirrors inclined at 45° angles that reflect both the scale readings and the corneal apex in profile.

Exophthalmometry provides information useful in detecting and evaluating thyroid disease, tumors of the eye, and any condition that displaces the eye in the orbit.

Purpose
☐ To measure the amount of forward protrusion of the eye
☐ To evaluate the progression or regression of exophthalmos.

Patient preparation
Explain to the patient that this test de-termines the degree of eye protrusion, and that it takes less than 5 minutes to perform.

Equipment
Exophthalmometer.

Procedure
Ask the patient to sit upright facing you, with your eyes on the same level as his. Hold the horizontal bar of the exophthalmometer in front of the patient's eyes, parallel to the floor. Move the two small concave carriers of the exophthalmometer against the lateral orbital margins, and carefully record the calibrated bar reading. This baseline reading should be used during follow-up examinations. If the patient has already been measured with an exophthalmometer, set the calibrated bar at the baseline reading. Tighten the locking screws on the mirrors to keep them properly positioned.

Measure each eye separately. First, instruct the patient to fixate his right eye on your left eye. Using the inclined mirrors, superimpose the apex of the right cornea on the millimeter scale, and re-

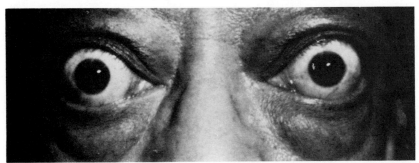

Bilateral bulging of the eyeballs and upper lid retraction characterize exophthalmos, which usually results from a thyroid disorder. Exophthalmometry evaluates the severity of exophthalmos.

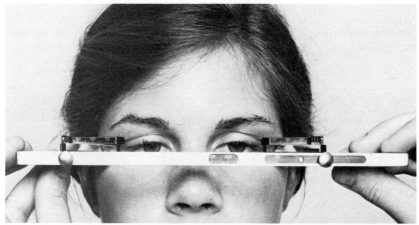

An exophthalmometer, shown properly positioned above, measures the degree that the center of the cornea protrudes beyond the lateral orbital rim. This forward displacement of the eye, exophthalmos, rarely exceeds 18 mm.

cord the reading, which represents the eye's relative forward displacement from its orbit. Then tell the patient to fixate his left eye on your right eye, and repeat the procedure.

Precautions
For follow-up examinations, be sure to set the calibrated bar at the baseline reading.

Findings
Normally, readings range from 12 to 20 mm. Measurements for each eye are similar, usually differing by 1.5 mm or less and rarely by more than 3 mm.

Implications of results
A difference between the eyes of more than 3 mm may indicate exophthalmos or enophthalmos. A single reading that exceeds 20 mm may indicate exophthalmos; readings under 12 mm may indicate enophthalmos.

A patient with exophthalmos should receive a thorough ophthalmologic examination, since the underlying cause may be local in origin. Any mass in the orbital cavity, edematous or hemorrhagic conditions, inflammatory diseases such as periostitis or cellulitis, hyperostosis of the orbit, or other conditions causing reduction in the normal size of the orbit will result in exophthalmos. However, it may also result from a systemic disorder, notably thyroid disease, as well as xanthomatosis and blood dyscrasia, in which case a complete medical examination is indicated. In such a case, exophthalmos is usually bilateral. Enophthalmos may arise following trauma, such as a fractured orbital floor. Less commonly, enophthalmos is congenital or is associated with inflammation.

Post-test care
The patient should be referred to an appropriate specialist, as needed.

Interfering factors
Failure to set the calibrated bar of the exophthalmometer at the baseline distance interferes with test results.

PATRICIA A. DOWEN, BA, COT, OT

Slit-lamp Examination

The slit lamp, an instrument equipped with a special lighting system and a bin-

ocular microscope, allows an ophthalmologist to visualize in detail the anterior segment of the eye, which includes the eyelids, eyelashes, conjunctiva, sclera, cornea, tear film, anterior chamber, iris, crystalline lens, and vitreous face. To evaluate normally transparent or near-transparent ocular fluids and tissues, the size, shape, intensity, and depth of the light source as well as the magnification of the microscope may be altered. If any abnormalities are noted, special devices may be attached to the slit lamp to allow more detailed investigation.

Purpose

☐ To detect and evaluate abnormalities and pathologies of anterior segment tissues and structures.

Patient preparation

Explain to the patient that this examination evaluates the front portion of the eyes. Tell him that the test takes about 5 to 10 minutes and requires that he remain still. Reassure him that the examination is painless.

Contact lenses are removed before the test, unless the test is being performed to evaluate the fit of the contact lens. If dilating eyedrops have been ordered, check the patient's history for adverse reactions to mydriatics or for the presence of narrow-angle glaucoma before administering. For a routine eye examination, dilating drops aren't used, because the slit lamp's bright light would hurt the dilated eyes. However, some diseases require pupillary dilation before a slit-lamp examination. Iritis, for

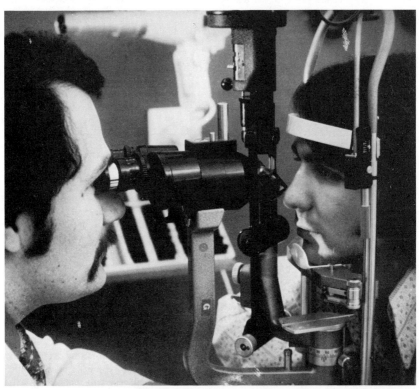

The patient shown at right is undergoing a slit-lamp biomicroscopy examination. The slit lamp directs an intense, narrow beam of light on optic tissue, allowing the ophthalmologist to see the patient's cornea and lens as layers of different optical densities, not transparent structures. This method permits accurate detection of pathologic conditions in the eye's anterior segment.

OTHER SLIT-LAMP PROCEDURES

Fluorescein staining: When a patient complains of a scratching sensation or when corneal or conjunctival abnormalities are suspected, fluorescein staining provides a better view of the anterior portion of the eye than the basic slit-lamp examination. Since the corneal layers and conjunctiva are transparent, the slit lamp can't detect minute scratches or breaks in tissue. By staining the eye's surface with a sodium fluorescein dye and observing the resulting fluorescence through a cobalt blue filter (a special attachment to the slit lamp) corneal and conjunctival injuries—such as abrasions, foreign bodies, damage from ultraviolet light, and drying due to exposure—can be visualized, as well as their area, depth, and pattern. Such injuries have specific staining patterns that aid diagnosis.

To stain the eye's surface, the tip of a sterile fluorescein strip is moistened with sterile normal saline solution, and the strip is touched to the patient's lower conjunctival sac. The patient is asked to close his eyes gently, and a film of fluorescein dye spreads over the corneal and conjunctival surfaces. Surface defects absorb more dye than normal areas. When the corneal epithelium is broken or scratched, for example, the underlying Bowman's membrane stains bright green. Injuries or chemical insults to the conjunc-

tiva or cornea also fluoresce green.

Hruby lens: A −55 diopter lens placed in front of—not on—the eye permits binocular, magnified examination of the posterior vitreous and retina, when used with the slit lamp. The pupils must be widely dilated for this examination. Following mydriasis and placement of the lens, a pencil of light from the slit lamp is directed through the center of the lens toward the posterior portion of the eye. Pathologies can be further studied by direct or indirect ophthalmoscopy.

Gonioscopy: The angle of the anterior chamber may be evaluated by using focal illumination, a microscope, and a special contact lens. This special lens (goniolens) eliminates the corneal curvature, allowing light to be reflected from the angle so its structures can be seen in detail. Before the lens is placed on the eye, the cornea is anesthetized and a thin layer of fluid (usually 2% methylcellulose solution) is applied to the contact surface of the lens, to separate the lens from the cornea. The goniolens deflects the beam of light from the slit lamp into the opposite angle of the anterior chamber, revealing the image of the angle structure. Gonioscopy is essential in evaluating glaucoma, especially when caused by angle closure, since prompt action is needed to prevent further rise in pressure.

example, a painful condition aggravated by pupillary constriction, mandates pupillary dilation to alleviate pain and allow the ophthalmologist to examine the eyes with adequate illumination.

Equipment
Slit lamp/mydriatics, as ordered.

Procedure
After seating the patient in the examining chair, with both his feet on the floor, ask him to place his chin on the rest and his forehead against the bar. Dim the lights in the room. The ophthalmologist examines the patient's eyes—starting with the lids and lashes, and progressing to the vitreous face—altering light and magnification, as necessary. In some cases, a special camera can be attached to the slit lamp to pho-

tograph portions of the eye.

Precautions

Don't instill mydriatic drops into the eyes of a patient who has had a hypersensitive reaction to them or who has narrow-angle glaucoma.

Findings
Slit-lamp examination should reveal no abnormalities or pathologies of anterior segment tissues and structures.

Implications of results
Slit-lamp examination may detect pathologic conditions—such as corneal abrasions and ulcers, lens opacities, iritis, and conjunctivitis—and irregular corneal shapes—such as in keratoconus. A parchmentlike consistency of the lid skin,

with redness, minor swelling, and moderate itching, may indicate a hypersensitive reaction. If a corneal abrasion or ulcer is detected, a fluorescein stain may be applied to enable better viewing of the area. If a tearing deficiency is suspected, the ophthalmologist may examine the eye after applying a fluorescein or rose bengal stain; he may also perform the Schirmer tearing test. Some abnormal findings may indicate impending disorders. For example, early-stage lens opacities may signal the development of cataracts.

Post-test care

If dilating drops were instilled, tell the patient that his near vision will be blurred for 40 minutes to 2 hours.

Interfering factors

Poor patient cooperation interferes with test results.

PATRICIA A. DOWEN, BA, COT, OT

Schirmer Tearing Test

The Schirmer test assesses the function of the major lacrimal glands, which are responsible for reflex tearing in response to stressful situations, such as the presence of a foreign body. Reflex tearing is stimulated by the insertion of a strip of filter paper into the lower conjunctival sac, followed by measurement of the amount of moisture absorbed by the paper. Both eyes are tested simultaneously. A variation of this test evaluates the function of the accessory lacrimal glands of Krause and Wolfring, by instillation of a topical anesthetic before insertion of the filter papers. The anesthetic inhibits reflex tearing by the major lacrimal glands, assuring measurement of only the basic tear film that is normally produced by the accessory glands. This tear film usually maintains

adequate corneal moisture under normal circumstances.

Purpose

☐ To measure tear secretion in persons with suspected tearing deficiency.

Patient preparation

Explain to the patient that this test measures secretion of tears. Tell him the test requires that a strip of filter paper be placed in the lower part of each eye for 5 minutes. Reassure him that the procedure isn't painful.

If the patient wears contact lenses, ask him to remove them before the test. If an anesthetic is instilled, he will not be able to reinsert the lenses for 2 hours after the test.

Equipment

Schirmer test kit (standardized sterile strips of individually wrapped filter paper in millimeter-ruled envelopes)/topical anesthetic (such as proparacaine) for evaluation of accessory lacrimal glands.

Procedure

Seat the patient in the examining chair, with his head against the headrest. To remove the test strip from the wrapper, bend the rounded wick end at the indentation, and cut open the envelope at the other end. Tell the patient to look up,

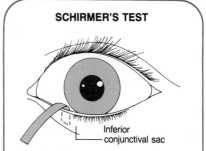

SCHIRMER'S TEST

Inferior
conjunctival sac

This illustration shows the proper placement of the filter paper for the Schirmer test. The filter paper should be inserted into the inferior conjunctival sac of each eye.

then gently lower the inferior eyelid. Hook the bent end of the strip over the inferior eyelid, at the junction of the medial and nasal segments. Insert one strip in each eye, and note the time of insertion. Tell the patient not to squeeze or rub his eyes, but to blink normally or to keep his eyes closed lightly.

After 5 minutes, remove the strips from the patient's eyes, and measure the length of the moistened area from the indentation, using the millimeter scale on the envelope. Report the results as a fraction: the numerator is the length of the moistened area; the denominator is the time the strips were left in place. Also note which eye was tested. Thus, if a strip inserted in the right conjunctival sac for 5 minutes shows 8 mm of moisture, the correct notation is OD (*oculus dexter,* or right eye), 8 mm/ 5 minutes.

To measure the function of the accessory lacrimal glands of Krause and Wolfring, instill one drop of topical anesthetic into each conjunctival sac before inserting the Schirmer strips.

Precautions
To prevent patient discomfort, be careful not to touch the cornea while inserting the test strip.

Findings
Normally, a Schirmer test strip shows at least 15 mm of moisture after 5 minutes. However, since tear production decreases with age, normal test results in patients over age 40 may range from 10 to 15 mm after 5 minutes. Both eyes usually secrete the same amount of tears.

Implications of results
While the Schirmer tearing test is a simple and usually efficient method for measuring the rate of tear secretion, as many as 15% of the patients tested have false-positive or false-negative results. Since the test is rapid and simple, it may be repeated and findings compared. Additional testing, such as a slit-lamp examination with fluorescein or rose bengal stain, is necessary to corroborate results.

A positive result confirmed by additional testing indicates a definite tearing deficiency, which may result from aging or, more seriously, from Sjögren's syndrome, a systemic disease of unknown origin that is most common among postmenopausal women. Tearing deficiency may also arise secondarily to systemic diseases such as lymphoma, leukemia, and rheumatoid arthritis. Regardless of cause, tearing deficiency is a matter of clinical concern, since it can lead to corneal erosions, scarring, and secondary infection.

Post-test care
If a topical anesthetic was instilled, advise the patient not to rub his eyes for at least 30 minutes after instillation, since this can cause a corneal abrasion. Patients who wear contact lenses should not reinsert them for at least 2 hours.

Interfering factors
□ If the patient closes his eyes too tightly during the test, tearing will increase.
□ Reflex tearing due to contact of the test strip with the cornea affects test results.
PATRICIA A. DOWEN, BA, COT, OT

Tonometry

Tonometry allows indirect measurement of intraocular pressure and serves as an effective screen for early detection of glaucoma, a common cause of blindness. Intraocular pressure rises when the rate of production of aqueous humor—the clear fluid secreted continuously by the ciliary processes in the eye's posterior chamber—exceeds the rate of drainage. This rise in pressure causes the eyeball to harden and become more resistant to extraocular pressure. Indentation tonometry tests this resistance by measuring how deeply a known weight depresses the cornea; applanation tonometry provides the same information by measuring the amount of force re-

APPLANATION TONOMETRY

The most precise test of intraocular pressure, applanation tonometry measures the force required to flatten a certain area of the cornea. The applanation tonometer (the most popular is the Goldmann tonometer) is mounted on a slit-lamp biomicroscope.

This test is performed with minimal corneal trauma and may be done after a routine slit-lamp examination. However, since the slit-lamp biomicroscope is used only by an ophthalmologist, applanation tonometry is less available than indentation tonometry for large-scale screening of the general population.

In applanation tonometry, a topical anesthetic is instilled, and the tear film is stained with fluorescein drops or a moistened fluorescein paper strip inserted into the lower conjunctival sac. The patient is seated as for a slit-lamp examination and is instructed to look straight ahead. The examiner moves the slit lamp forward until the tonometer comes in contact with the cornea. Through the eyepiece of the slit lamp, the examiner sees two fluorescein semicircles. He adjusts the tension dial on the tonometer until the inner, straight-edged margins of the semi-

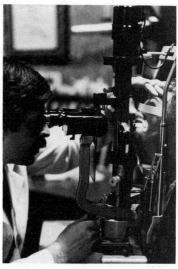

circles touch.

The reading on the tension dial provides a direct indication of the patient's intraocular pressure.

quired to flatten a known area of the cornia. Both procedures necessitate corneal anesthetization and careful examination technique. Tonometry should never be performed on a patient with a corneal ulcer or infection except by a skilled examiner, and then only under extreme circumstances, as in suspected acute narrow-angle glaucoma.

The diagnostic significance of tonometry is readily apparent, because glaucoma—which can be treated if detected early enough—accounts for 12% to 15% of blindness in the United States. This test should be performed routinely on persons over age 40, since glaucoma strikes 2% of persons past this critical age. Nurses may perform tonometry in emergency or occupational health settings. Findings must be confirmed by visual field testing and ophthalmoscopy.

Purpose
□ To measure intraocular pressure

□ To aid diagnosis and follow-up evaluation of glaucoma.

Patient preparation
Explain to the patient that this test measures the pressure within his eyes. Tell him the test requires that his eyes be anesthetized and that the test takes only a few minutes. Reassure him that the procedure is painless. If the patient wears contact lenses, instruct him to remove them before the procedure. Inform him that he shouldn't reinsert them for 2 hours after the test, or until the anesthetic wears off completely.

Ask the patient to assume a supine position. Make sure he's relaxed, since anxiety may raise intraocular pressure. Have him loosen or remove restrictive clothing around his neck, which can also raise intraocular pressure. Instruct him not to cough or squeeze his eyelids together. Explain that his cooperation will ensure accurate test results.

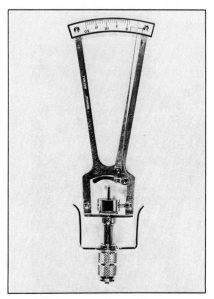

The Schiøtz tonometer consists of a concave footplate that rests on the cornea, a plunger to apply pressure to the cornea, and a calibrated scale to measure the amount of pressure applied by the plunger.

Equipment
Indentation tonometer (the Schiøtz tonometer is the most popular), sterilized or used with disposable sterile tonofilms/topical anesthetic.

Procedure
Ask the patient to look down. Raise his superior eyelid with your thumb, and place one drop of the topical anesthetic at the top of the sclera. The solution spreads over the entire sclera when the patient blinks.

Check the tonometer for a zero reading on the steel test block that comes with the instrument. Make sure the plunger moves freely. The first measurement on each eye is obtained with the 5.5 g weight.

Have the patient look up and stare at a spot on the ceiling. Then ask him to open his mouth, take a deep breath, and exhale slowly. This distracts the patient, preventing forceful closure of the lids. After this initial breath, instruct the patient to breathe normally during the procedure. With the thumb and forefinger of one hand, hold the lids of his right eye open, against the orbital rim. Hold the tonometer vertically with the thumb and forefinger of the other hand, and rest the footplate on the apex of the cornea. Be especially careful to avoid resting your fingers on the cornea or pressing on the cornea, since this increases intraocular pressure. With the footplate in place, check the indicator needle for a rhythmic transmission caused by the ocular pulse. Then record the calibrated scale reading that converts to a measurement of intraocular pressure. If the reading doesn't exceed 4, add an additional weight (7.5, 10, or 15 g) to obtain a reliable result.

Repeat the procedure on the left eye, and record the time when the test was performed.

Precautions

To avoid corneal abrasion, hold the tonometer still. Don't touch the lashes; this could trigger a blink response or Bell's phenomenon (upward movement of the eyes with forced closure of the lids), which can cause the footplate to move and scratch the cornea.

Findings
Intraocular pressure normally ranges from 12 to 20 mmHg, with diurnal variations. The highest point is reached at the time of waking; the lowest point, in the evening.

Implications of results
Elevated intraocular pressure requires further testing for glaucoma. Since intraocular pressure varies diurnally, findings must be supplemented with serial measurements obtained at different times on different days.

Indentation tonometry by itself can't diagnose glaucoma; applanation tonometry, visual field testing, and ophthalmoscopy must confirm the diagnosis.

Post-test care
☐ Because an anesthetic was instilled, tell the patient not to rub his eyes for at

least 20 minutes after the test, to prevent corneal abrasion. If the patient wears contact lenses, tell him not to reinsert them for at least 2 hours.

□ If the tonometer moved across the cornea during the test, tell the patient he may feel a slight scratching sensation in the eye when the anesthetic wears off. This sensation should disappear within 24 hours, since most corneal abrasions resulting from tonometry affect only the corneal epithelium, which regenerates within 24 hours, without scarring.

Interfering factors

□ Deformed corneal curvature prohibits proper placement of the footplate.

□ Corneoscleral rigidity or flaccidity, as determined by an ophthalmologist, may cause falsely elevated or depressed readings, since the Schiøtz tonometer measures the pressure required for corneal indentation.

□ Poor patient cooperation or careless examination technique interferes with test results.

PATRICIA A. DOWEN, BA, COT, OT

Ophthalmoscopy

Ophthalmoscopy—an important part of routine physical examinations and eye evaluations—allows magnified examination of living vascular and nerve tissue of the fundus, including the optic disk, retinal vessels, macula, and retina. The instrument used in this test—either the direct or the indirect ophthalmoscope—is considered one of the most important diagnostic tools in ophthalmology. Generally, examiners use the direct ophthalmoscope—a small, hand-held instrument consisting of a light source, viewing device, reflecting device to channel light into the patient's eyes, and spherical lenses to correct refractive error of the patient or examiner. This direct model is easier to use than the indirect model. If a slit lamp is not available, the examiner may also use the ophthalmoscope to examine the patient's cornea, iris, and lens.

Purpose

To detect and evaluate eye disorders as well as ocular manifestations of systemic disease.

Patient preparation

Explain to the patient that this test permits examination of the back of the eye. Tell him who will perform the test and where, and that the procedure takes less than 5 minutes. Advise him that eyedrops may be instilled to dilate the pupils for a clearer examination, but reassure him that he'll feel no discomfort during the test.

Check the patient's history for previous use of dilating eyedrops, possible hypersensitivity to the eyedrops, and narrow-angle glaucoma.

Equipment

Direct ophthalmoscope/mydriatic eyedrops/disposable tissues.

Procedure

Routine examination of the ocular media and fundus is usually possible without dilation of the pupil if there is sufficient light in the ophthalmoscope and room lighting is subdued. However, if indicated, mydriatic eyedrops may be ordered; usually two instillations are necessary to achieve maximum mydriasis.

Have the patient sit upright in the examination chair. Darken the room to keep irregular reflections from interfering with the examination. Sit about 2' (60 cm) away from the patient, at his eye level. Examine the patient's right eye first, holding the ophthalmoscope in your right hand and in front of your right eye. Position your right index finger on the lens selection dial to facilitate rapid lens changes, and sit slightly to the patient's right. Set the illuminated dial to zero, and tell the patient to look straight ahead at a specific object 20' (6 m) away—a large symbol on a standardized vision chart, for example. Tell him to maintain

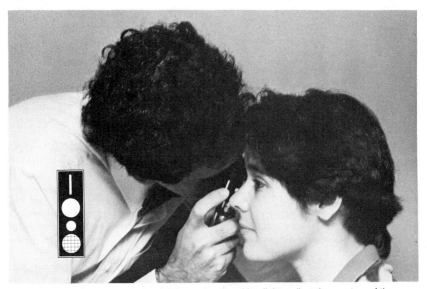

The ophthalmologist in this photograph is rotating the white dial to adjust the aperture of the ophthalmoscope, to obtain the best possible visualization of the patient's eye. The aperture controls the amount of light directed onto the patient's retina. Usually, the large aperture allows the best visualization of the fundus, but only when the pupils are dilated. The small aperture allows visualization of the fundus when the pupils are small, undilated, or miotic from glaucoma medications and unable to be dilated beyond 3 to 4 mm.

The grid permits an estimate of the size of fundal lesions. The slit helps determine the levels of such lesions as tumors or swollen disks. The red free filter (not shown), a special attachment, excludes red rays from the field to make minute retinal changes more pronounced and easier to evaluate.

fixation throughout the examination. Remaining on the patient's right side, move forward slightly, until you're about 6" (15 cm) from him.

Direct the light beam into the pupil; select the proper lens aperture on the ophthalmoscope, and look through it for the red reflex. This can be seen without magnification and represents a red reflection from the fundus. Keeping this reflection in view and reminding the patient to maintain fixation, move slowly toward the patient until you're 1½" to 2" (3.8 to 5 cm) from him. Rotate the lenses on the scope to focus on the optic disk, and note its size, shape, and color.

Next, look for a white, central depression in the disk—the physiologic cup. Observe the retinal vessels that emerge from the optic disk. They normally bifurcate and extend toward all quadrants of the retina. Follow each vessel as far as possible to the periphery.

Examine the macula—a yellowish depression lying approximately two disk diameters away from and slightly below the center of the optic disk—and its center, the fovea. To examine the extreme periphery, tell the patient to look up, down, and to each side. Examine the superior, inferior, temporal, and nasal portions of the retina, respectively.

Repeat the procedure to examine the patient's left eye, moving slightly to the patient's left side and holding the ophthalmoscope in your left hand and in front of your left eye. Adjust the lens selection dial to account for a different refractive state, if necessary.

Precautions

NURSING ALERT

Don't administer dilating eyedrops to a patient who has a history of hypersensitive reaction to them or who has narrow-angle glaucoma.

□ Make sure the patient maintains fixation throughout the procedure.

Findings

With the beam of light from the ophthalmoscope directed into the patient's pupil, the red reflex should be visible through the aperture. The slightly oval optic disk, measuring approximately 1.5 mm vertically, lies to the nasal side of the fundus center. Although its color varies widely, it's usually pink, with darker edges at its nasal border. The physiologic cup, a pale depression in the center of the disk, varies widely in size; it tends to be larger in patients with myopia and smaller in those with hyperopia.

The semitransparent retina surrounds the optic disk. Branching out from the disk are the retinal vessels, including venules and the slightly smaller arterioles. Vessel diameter progressively decreases with distance from the optic disk. Retinal arterioles generally have a medium red color; venules appear dark red or blue.

The macula, a small avascular area that appears darker than the surrounding retina, is located approximately 2½ disk diameters temporal from the optic disk and slightly beneath the horizontal meridian. In its center lies a small, even darker spot—the fovea. A tiny light reflex can be seen at the center of the fovea, caused by reflection of the ophthalmoscopic light from the concave inner surface of the area.

Implications of results

Absent or diminished red reflex may be due to gross corneal lesions, dense opacities of the aqueous or vitreous (such as from blood following hemorrhage), cataracts, or detached retina. Cloudy vitreous that obscures the fundus may be caused by inflammatory disease of the optic disk, retina, or uvea. Fundal lesions should be sketched or photographed for further study.

Optic neuritis causes the optic disk to become elevated and more vascular; small hemorrhages may also occur. Optic nerve atrophy causes the disk to appear white. Papilledema, which may result from increased intracranial pressure, causes abnormal elevation of the disk, blurring of disk margins, engorged vessels, and hemorrhages. In glaucoma, the physiologic cup may appear enlarged and gray, with white edges. A milky-white retina characterizes the acute phase of a central retinal artery occlusion; the fovea, in contrast to the ischemic macula, appears as a bright red spot. Central retinal vein occlusion is marked by widespread retinal hemorrhaging, patches of white exudate, and disk elevation. Retinal detachments ap-

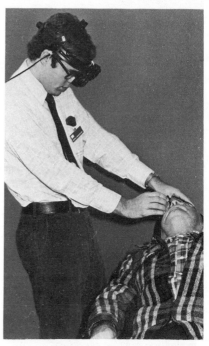

A more expensive and more sophisticated instrument than the direct ophthalmoscope, the indirect ophthalmoscope is used with convex lens, which the ophthalmologist holds a few inches from the patient's eye, and a headlamp, which provides a strong source of illumination. The lens focuses light reflected from the retina, producing an image that is rotated 180° but is unaffected by refractive errors or opacities in the media. Since the indirect ophthalmoscope provides a wide-angle, stereoscopic view of the peripheral retina, many surgeons depend on it for preoperative diagnosis and during retinal detachment surgery.

COMPARISON OF DIRECT AND INDIRECT OPHTHALMOSCOPES

CHARACTERISTICS	DIRECT OPHTHALMOSCOPE	INDIRECT OPHTHALMOSCOPE
Image	True	Rotated 180°
Intensity of illumination	Medium to high	Dazzling
Magnification	15×	2× to 4×
Field of vision (disk diameters)	2	8
Affected by major refractive errors	Yes	No
Good view despite opacities in the media	No	Yes
Stereopsis	No (monocular)	Yes (binocular)
Easy to use	Yes	No

pear as gray, elevated areas, possibly with areas of red vascular choroid exposed by retinal tears. A choroidal tumor appears as a dark lesion.

The integrity of retinal vessels is commonly evaluated to aid diagnosis of systemic disease. Hypertension, for example, causes vasospasm, sclerosis, and eventual occlusion of retinal arterioles, leading to retinal edema and hemorrhage, and papilledema. Diabetes mellitus may be complicated by retinal fibroses, patches of white exudate, and microaneurysms. Other systemic disorders present similar findings.

Interpretation of ophthalmoscopy findings depends largely on the examiner's knowledge and experience, since an abnormality can arise from several sources. After an ophthalmologic evaluation, referral for complete medical evaluation may be necessary.

Post-test care
None.

Interfering factors
□ Poor patient cooperation or conditions that prohibit a good view of the fundus, such as insufficient dilation, dense cataracts, cloudy media, or gross nystagmus, may affect test results.

□ Proper examination conditions (darkened room, adequate light source on ophthalmoscope) are essential to accurate diagnosis.

PATRICIA A. DOWEN, BA, COT, OT

Fluorescein Angiography

In this test, rapid-sequence photographs of the fundus are taken with a special camera, following I.V. injection of sodium fluorescein, a contrast medium. The fluorescein dye and the use of sophisticated photographic equipment enhance the visibility of microvascular structures of the retina and choroid, allowing evaluation of the entire retinal vascular bed, including retinal circulation. Thus, fluorescein angiography records the appearance of blood vessels inside the eye.

Purpose
□ To document retinal circulation as an aid in evaluating intraocular abnormalities, such as retinopathy, tumors, and

circulatory or inflammatory disorders.

Patient preparation

Explain to the patient that this test evaluates the small blood vessels in the eyes. Tell him that the procedure takes about 30 minutes.

Make sure the patient or a responsible family member has signed a consent form, if required. Check the patient's history for glaucoma and hypersensitive reactions, especially reactions to contrast media and dilating eyedrops. If ordered, tell a patient with glaucoma not to use miotic eyedrops on the day of the test.

Explain to the patient that eyedrops will be instilled to dilate his pupils and that a dye will be injected into his arm. Tell him that his eyes will be photographed with a special camera before and after the injection. Stress that these are photographs, *not* X-rays. Warn him that his skin and urine may appear yellow, but these effects disappear within 24 to 48 hours.

Equipment

Fundus camera and film/mydriatic eyedrops/alcohol swabs/tourniquet/21-G scalp-vein needle/5- to 10-ml syringe/2-ml of 25% or 5 ml of 10% sodium fluorescein/small sterile dressing/emesis basin/emergency resuscitation kit.

Procedure

Administer mydriatic eyedrops, as ordered. Usually, two instillations are necessary to achieve maximum mydriasis within 15 to 40 minutes. Following mydriasis, seat the patient comfortably in the examining chair, facing the camera. Have him loosen or remove any restrictive clothing around his neck. Ask the patient to place his chin in the chin rest and his forehead against the bar. Instruct him to keep his teeth together, to open his eyes as widely as possible, to stare straight ahead, and to breathe and blink normally.

The antecubital vein is prepared and punctured, but the dye isn't injected yet. A few preinjection photographs may be taken at this time. Tell the patient to keep his arm extended; if necessary, use an arm board.

 When ordered, the dye is injected rapidly into the vein. Remind the patient to maintain his position and fixation. The patient may briefly experience nausea and a feeling of warmth. Reassure him, as necessary, and observe for hypersensitivity reactions, such as vomiting, dry mouth, metallic taste, sudden increased salivation, sneezing, lightheadedness, fainting, and hives. Rarely, anaphylactic shock may result.

As the dye is injected, 25 to 30 photographs are taken in rapid sequence (1 second apart). The needle and syringe are removed carefully; pressure and a dressing are applied to the injection site. If late-phase photographs have been requested, tell the patient to sit comfortably and relax for 20 minutes. After 20 minutes, reposition the patient for 5 to 10 late-phase photographs. If ordered, photographs may be taken up to 1 hour after the injection.

Precautions

☐ Don't leave the patient unattended while waiting to take late-phase photographs.

☐ Be sure to check for proper placement of the needle in the patient's vein, since extravasation of the dye around the injection site is very painful.

Findings

After rapid injection into the antecubital vein, sodium fluorescein normally reaches the retina in 12 to 15 seconds. This *filling phase* varies with cardiac output, blood viscosity, and blood vessel caliber. As the choroidal vessels and choriocapillaries fill, the background of the retina fluoresces, taking on an evenly mottled appearance. Known as the *choroidal flush*, this usually occurs just before the *arterial phase*, the point at which the dye appears and fills the arteries. The *arteriovenous phase* occurs next, extending from the complete filling of the arteries and capillaries to the earliest evidence of dye in the veins. From the time

ANGIOGRAMS REVEAL RETINAL CIRCULATION

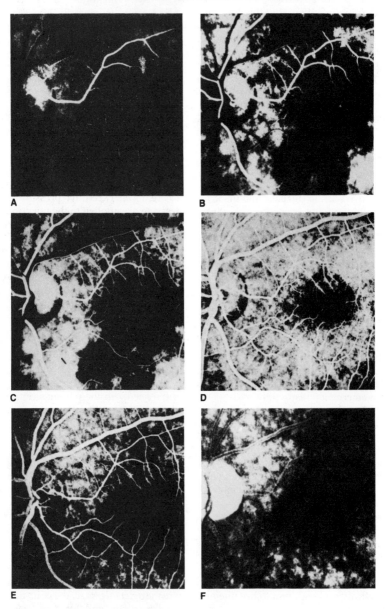

These six angiograms chronicle the phases of retinal circulation in the right eye: (A) filling phase, (B) early arterial phase, (C) laminar venous filling phase, (D) full venous phase, (E) late venous phase, and (F) recirculation phase. By examining and interpreting these angiograms, the doctor can evaluate the circulatory status within the eye.

the arteries begin to empty to the time the veins fill and empty is known as the *venous phase*. Finally, the *recirculation phase* occurs 30 to 60 minutes after the injection, when the fluorescein—if at all present—is barely detectable in the retinal vessels. Normally, there is no leakage from the retinal vessels.

Implications of results
The varying and complex findings after fluorescein angiography require interpretation by a highly skilled ophthalmologist with extensive experience in the diagnosis of retinal disorders. Abnormalities in the early filling phase may include microaneurysms, arteriovenous shunts, and neovascularization. The test may identify arterial occlusion by showing delayed or absent flow of the dye through the arteries, stenosis, and prolonged venous drainage. Venous occlusion may be associated with dilation of the vessels and fluorescein leakage. Chronic obstruction may produce recanalization and collateral circulation. In hypertensive retinopathy, abnormalities may include areas of increased vascular tortuosity, microaneurysms around zones of capillary nonperfusion, and generalized suffusion of the dye in the retina. Aneurysms and capillary hemangiomas may leak fluorescence and are often surrounded by hard, yellow exudate. Tumors exhibit variable fluorescein patterns, depending on histologic type. Retinal edema, or inflammation and fibrous tissue may show variable degrees of fluorescence. Papilledema produces vascular leakage in the disk area.

Post-test care
□ Remind the patient that his skin and urine will be slightly discolored for 24 to 48 hours after the test.
□ Tell the patient that his near vision will be blurred for up to 12 hours.

Interfering factors
Inadequate view of the fundus, resulting from insufficient pupillary dilation, a cataract, media opacity, or inability of the patient to keep his eyes open and to maintain fixation interferes with accuracy of test results.

PATRICIA A. DOWEN, BA, COT, OT

SPECIAL PROCEDURES

Orbital Radiography

The orbit is a deep-set cavity that houses the eye, lacrimal gland, blood vessels, nerves, muscles, and fat. It is enclosed anteriorly by the eyeball and the eyelids. Since portions of the orbit are composed of thin bone that is easily fractured, radiographs of these structures are commonly taken following facial trauma. Radiographs are also useful in diagnosing ocular and orbital pathology. Special radiographic techniques can visualize foreign bodies in the orbit or in the eye that can't be seen with an ophthalmoscope. To further define abnormalities, tomograms may be taken concurrently with standard radiographs. Comput-erized tomography and ultrasonography can provide further information.

Purpose
□ To aid in diagnosis of orbital fractures and pathology
□ To help locate intraorbital or intraocular foreign bodies.

Patient preparation
Explain to the patient that this test assesses the condition of the bones around the eye. Tell him that several X-ray films will be taken of his eye, who will perform the test and where, and that the procedure takes about 15 minutes. Reassure him that this procedure is usually painless unless he's suffered facial trauma, in which case positioning may cause some discomfort.

RADIOGRAPHY EVALUATES ORBITAL STRUCTURES

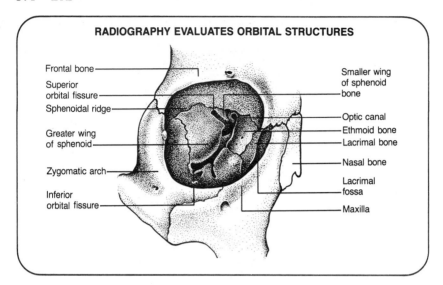

Frontal bone
Superior orbital fissure
Sphenoidal ridge
Greater wing of sphenoid
Zygomatic arch
Inferior orbital fissure

Smaller wing of sphenoid bone
Optic canal
Ethmoid bone
Lacrimal bone
Nasal bone
Lacrimal fossa
Maxilla

Tell the patient he'll be asked to turn his head from side to side and to flex or extend his neck, to achieve correct positioning. Instruct him to remove all metal and jewelry in the X-ray field.

Procedure

The patient is placed in a supine position on the radiographic table, or is seated in a chair, and is instructed to remain still while the radiographs are taken. A standard series of orbital radiographs usually includes a lateral view, posteroanterior view, submento-vertical (base) view, stereo Waters' views (views from both sides), Towne's (half-axial) projection, and optic canal projections. If enlargement of the superior orbital fissure is suspected, apical views are also obtained. Before the patient leaves the radiography department, the films are developed and checked for quality.

Precautions

None.

Findings

Each orbit is composed of a roof, a floor, and medial and lateral walls. The bones that form the roof and floor are very thin; the thickness of the floor may be only 1 mm or less. The medial wall is slightly thicker than the roof and floor, except for the portion formed by the ethmoidal bone. The medial walls of both orbits parallel each other. The lateral wall—the thickest part of the orbit—is strongest at the orbital rim. The lateral walls of both orbits project toward each other; if they were straight and extended farther into the head, they would meet at a 90° angle.

The superior orbital fissure lies in the back of the orbit, between the lateral wall and the roof, and is actually a gap between the greater and the lesser wings of the sphenoidal bone. The optic canal, found at the apex of the orbit, is an opening in the lesser wing of the sphenoidal bone, through which the optic nerve and the ophthalmic artery pass.

Implications of results

Orbital fractures resulting from facial trauma usually occur in the floor and in the ethmoidal bone, since these structures are extremely thin.

To detect abnormalities, the size and shape of the orbital structures on the affected side are compared with those on the other side. Enlargement of an orbit, for example, generally indicates the presence of a lesion that has caused proptosis from increased intraorbital pressure.

Any growing tumor can produce these changes. Specifically, superior orbital fissure enlargement can result from orbital meningioma, from intracranial conditions such as pituitary tumors, or more characteristically, from vascular anomalies. Optic canal enlargement may result from extraocular extension of a retinoblastoma or, in children, it may be due to optic nerve glioma. In adults, only prolonged pathology can increase orbital size. In children, however, even a rapidly growing lesion can cause orbital enlargement due to incomplete development of the orbital bones. A decrease in the size of the orbit may follow childhood enucleation of the eye or conditions such as congenital microphthalmia.

Destruction of the orbital walls may indicate a malignant neoplasm or infection. A benign tumor or cyst produces a clear-cut local indentation of the orbital wall. Lesions of adjacent structures may also produce radiographic changes due to enlargement and erosion of the orbit.

Increased bone density may be seen in conditions such as osteoblastic metastasis, sphenoid ridge meningioma, or Paget's disease. To confirm orbital pathology, however, radiographic findings must be supplemented with results from other appropriate tests and procedures.

Post-test care
None.

Interfering factors
None.

PATRICIA A. DOWEN, BA, COT, OT

Orbital Computed Tomography

Orbital computed tomography (CT) allows visualization of abnormalities not readily seen on standard radiographs, delineating their size, position, and relationship to adjoining structures. The orbital CT scan—a series of tomograms reconstructed by a computer and displayed as anatomic slices on an oscilloscope screen—identifies space-occupying lesions earlier and more accurately than other radiographic techniques; it also provides three-dimensional images of orbital structures, especially the ocular muscles and the optic nerve.

Contrast enhancement may be used in CT to define ocular tissues and evaluate a patient with such conditions as suspected circulatory disorder, hemangioma, or subdural hematoma. Application of CT to ophthalmology extends beyond the evaluation of the orbital and adjoining structures; it also permits precise diagnosis of many intracranial lesions that affect vision.

Purpose
□ To evaluate pathologies of the orbit and eye—especially expanding lesions and bone destruction
□ To evaluate fractures of the orbit and adjoining structures
□ To determine the cause of unilateral exophthalmos.

Patient preparation
Describe the procedure to the patient, and explain that this test visualizes the anatomy of the eye and its surrounding structures. Unless contrast enhancement is scheduled, inform him he needn't restrict food or fluids. If contrast enhancement is scheduled, withhold food and fluids from the patient for 4 hours before the test.

Tell the patient that a series of X-ray films will be taken of his eye, and who will perform the test and where. Reassure him that the test will cause him no discomfort and will take 15 to 30 minutes to perform.

Tell the patient he'll be positioned on an X-ray table, and that the head of the table will be moved into the scanner, which will rotate around his head and make loud, clacking sounds. If a contrast agent will be used for the procedure, tell the patient he may feel flushed and warm, and experience a transient headache, a salty taste, and nausea or vomiting after the dye is injected. Reassure him that these reactions to the contrast medium are typical.

Make sure the patient or a responsible member of the family has signed a consent form. Check the patient's history for hypersensitivity reactions to iodine, shellfish, or radiographic dyes. Instruct the patient to remove jewelry, hairpins, or other metal objects in the X-ray field to allow for precise imaging of the orbital structures.

Procedure

The patient is placed in a supine position on the radiographic table, with his head immobilized by straps, and is asked to lie still. The head of the table is then moved into the scanner, which rotates around the patient's head, taking radiographs.

The information obtained is stored on magnetic tapes, and the images are displayed on an oscilloscope screen, which may be photographed if a permanent record is desired.

When this series of radiographs has been taken, contrast enhancement is performed, if ordered. The contrast agent is injected and a second series of scans is recorded.

Precautions

Use of contrast enhancement, if ordered, is contraindicated in those patients with known hypersensitivity reactions to iodine, shellfish, or radiographic dyes used in other tests.

Findings

Orbital structures are evaluated for size, shape, and position. Dense orbital bone provides a marked contrast to less dense periocular fat. The optic nerve and the medial and lateral rectus muscles are clearly defined. The rectus muscles appear as thin dense bands on each side, behind the eye. The optic canals should be equal in size.

Implications of results

Orbital CT can identify intra- and ex-traorbital space-occupying lesions that obscure the normal structures or cause orbital enlargement, indentation of the orbital walls, or bone destruction. This test can also help determine the type of lesion. For example, infiltrative lesions, such as lymphomas and metastatic carcinomas, appear as irregular areas of density. However, encapsulated tumors, such as benign hemangiomas and meningiomas, appear as clearly defined masses of consistent density. CT can also visualize intracranial tumors that invade the orbit, thickening of the optic nerve that may occur with gliomas, meningiomas, and secondary tumors that may cause enlargement of the optic canal.

In evaluating fractures, CT allows a complete three-dimensional view of the affected structures. In determining the cause of unilateral exophthalmos, CT can show early erosion or expansion of the medial orbital wall that may arise from lesions in the ethmoidal cells. It can also detect space-occupying lesions in the orbit or paranasal sinuses that cause exophthalmos. CT can also show thickening of the medial and lateral rectus muscles in proptosis, resulting from Graves' disease.

Enhancement with a contrast agent can yield important information on the circulation through abnormal ocular tissues.

Post-test care

None, if test was performed without contrast enhancement. If a contrast agent was used, watch for its residual side effects, including headache, nausea, or vomiting. Advise the patient he may resume his usual diet withheld before the test, if he is not experiencing such reactions.

Interfering factors

Movement of the head during scanning or failure to remove radiopaque objects from the X-ray field may cause unclear images, interfering with accurate determination of test results.

PATRICIA A. DOWEN, BA, COT, OT

Ocular Ultrasonography

Ocular ultrasonography involves the transmission of high-frequency sound waves through the eye and the measurement of their reflection from ocular structures. An A-scan converts the resulting echoes into waveforms whose crests represent the positions of different structures, giving a linear dimensional picture. The B-scan converts the echoes into patterns of dots that form a two-dimensional, cross-sectional image of the ocular structure.

Because the B-scan is easier to interpret than the A-scan, it is used more often to evaluate the structures of the eye and to diagnose abnormalities. However, the A-scan is of much greater value in measuring the axial length of the eye and characterizing the tissue texture of abnormal lesions. Thus, the combination of A- and B-scans produces the most useful test results.

Illustrating the eyes' structures through ultrasound is especially helpful in evaluating a fundus clouded by an opaque medium, such as a cataract. In such a patient, this test can identify pathologies that are normally undetectable through ophthalmoscopy.

Ophthalmologists may also perform this test before surgery—for example, cataract removal—to ensure the integrity of the retina. If an intraocular lens is to be implanted, ultrasound may be used preoperatively to measure the length of the eye and the curvature of the cornea, as a guide for the surgeon. Unlike computed tomography, ocular ultrasonography is readily available and has the advantage of providing information immediately.

Purpose
□ To aid in evaluating the fundus in an eye with an opaque medium, such as a cataract

□ To aid diagnosis of vitreous disorders and retinal detachment
□ To diagnose and differentiate between intraocular and orbital lesions, and to follow their progression through serial examinations
□ To help locate intraocular foreign bodies.

Patient preparation
Describe the procedure to the patient, and explain that this test evaluates the eye's structures. Inform him that he needn't restrict food or fluids before the test.

Tell the patient who will perform the test and where. Reassure him that the procedure is safe and painless, and takes about 5 minutes to perform.

Tell the patient that a small transducer will be placed on his closed eyelid, and that the transducer transmits high-frequency sound waves that are reflected by the structures in the eye. Inform him that he may be asked to move his eyes or change his gaze during the procedure, and that his cooperation is required to ensure accurate determination of test results.

Equipment
Ultrasound transducer/water-soluble jelly/eye cup (for A-scan)/oscilloscope and photographic equipment.

Procedure
Place the patient in a supine position on a radiographic table. For the B-scan, the patient is asked to close his eyes, and water-soluble jelly (such as Goniosol) is applied to his eyelid. The transducer is then placed on the eyelid. For the A-scan, the patient's eye is numbed with anesthetizing drops, and a clear plastic eye cup is placed directly on the eyeball. Water-soluble jelly is then applied to the eye cup, and the transducer positioned on this medium. The transducer then transmits high-frequency sound waves into the patient's eye, and the resulting echoes are transformed into images or waveforms on the oscilloscope screen, which may be photographed.

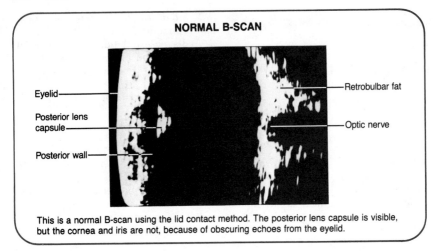

NORMAL B-SCAN

Eyelid

Posterior lens capsule

Posterior wall

Retrobulbar fat

Optic nerve

This is a normal B-scan using the lid contact method. The posterior lens capsule is visible, but the cornea and iris are not, because of obscuring echoes from the eyelid.

Precautions
None.

Findings
The optic nerve and posterior lens capsule produce echoes that take on characteristic forms on A- and B-scan images. The posterior wall of the eye appears as a smooth, concave curve; retrobulbar fat can also be identified. The lens and vitreous, which don't produce echoes, can also be identified. Normal orbital echo patterns depend on the position of the transducer and the position of the patient's gaze throughout the ultrasonography procedure.

Implications of results
In eyes that are clouded by a vitreous hemorrhage, the organization of the hemorrhage can be identified according to the degree of density that appears on the image. In some instances, the cause of the hemorrhage, the prognosis, and associated abnormalities can also be determined.

Other vitreous abnormalities, such as massive vitreous organization and vitreous bands, may also be detected by ultrasonography. Retinal detachment, commonly found in a patient with an opaque medium, characteristically produces a dense sheetlike echo on a B-scan. The extent of retinal detachment or choroidal detachment can be defined by transmitting ultrasound waves through the quadrants of the patient's eye.

Ocular ultrasonography can be used to diagnose and differentiate intraocular tumors according to size, shape, location, and texture. The most common tumors identified are melanomas, metastatic tumors, and hemangiomas. This test can also identify retinoblastomas and can measure the dimensions of other tumors detectable by ophthalmoscopy.

Orbital lesions, such as hemangiomas and cystic lesions, produce characteristic ultrasound patterns. Other orbital lesions detectable by ultrasound testing include meningiomas, neurofibromas, gliomas, neurilemomas, and the inflammatory changes associated with Graves' disease.

In addition to its diagnostic capabilities, ocular ultrasonography can also identify intraocular foreign bodies and determine their position in relation to ocular structures, and can assess the severity of resulting ocular damage.

Post-test care
□ Be sure the water-soluble jelly has been removed from the patient's eyelid.

Interfering factors
None.

PATRICIA A. DOWEN, BA, COT, OT

Selected References

Anderson, Douglas R. *Testing the Field of Vision*. St. Louis: C.V. Mosby Co., 1982.

Assessment. Nurse's Reference Library. Springhouse, Pa.: Springhouse Corp., 1984.

Brunner, Lillian S., and Suddarth, Doris. *Textbook of Medical-Surgical Nursing*, 5th ed. Philadelphia: J.B. Lippincott Co., 1984.

Bredemeyer, Hans G., and Bullock, Kathleen. *Orthoptics: Theory and Practice*. St. Louis: C.V. Mosby Co., 1968.

Coleman, J.D., and Dallow, R.L. *Introduction to Ophthalmic Ultrasonography: Clinical Ophthalmology*, vol. 2. New York: Harper & Row Pubs., 1978.

Diseases, 2nd ed. Nurse's Reference Library. Springhouse, Pa.: Springhouse Corp., 1986.

Duane, Thomas D., ed. *Clinical Ophthalmology*, vols. 2 and 3. New York: Harper & Row Pubs., 1978.

Emergencies. Nurse's Reference Library. Springhouse, Pa.: Springhouse Corp., 1985.

Harrington, David O. *The Visual Fields: A Textbook and Atlas of Clinical Perimetry*, 5th ed. St. Louis: C.V. Mosby Co., 1981.

Havener, William H., and Goeckner, Sallie L. *Introductory Atlas of Perimetry*. St. Louis: C.V. Mosby Co., 1972.

Leibowitz, Howard M., et al. "The Framingham Eye Study Monograph," *Survey of Ophthalmology Supplement*, May/June 1980.

Leitman, M., et al. *Manual for Eye Examination and Diagnosis*. New York: Van Nostrand Reinhold Co., 1975.

Moses, Robert A. *Adler's Physiology of the Eye: Clinical Application*. 7th ed. St. Louis: C.V. Mosby Co., 1981.

Procedures. Nurse's Reference Library. Springhouse, Pa.: Springhouse Corp., 1983.

Scheie, Harold G., and Albert, Daniel M. *Textbook of Ophthalmology*, 9th ed. Philadelphia: W.B. Saunders Co., 1977.

Sloane, Albert E., and Garcia, George E. *Manual of Refraction*, 3rd ed. Boston: Little, Brown & Co., 1979.

22 Ear

LEARNING OBJECTIVES

After completing this chapter, the reader will be able to:
- explain the anatomy and physiology of the ear.
- distinguish a sensorineural from a conductive hearing loss.
- identify screening programs used to detect hearing impairment in children.
- list categories of job-related hearing loss.
- explain how to use an audiometer.
- state guidelines for communicating effectively with the hearing impaired.
- describe common abnormalities of the tympanic membrane.
- evaluate eustachian tube function.
- state the purpose of each test discussed in the chapter.
- prepare the patient physically and psychologically for each test.
- describe the procedure for performing each test.
- specify appropriate precautions for safe administration of each test.
- recognize signs of adverse reaction and respond appropriately.
- implement appropriate post-test care.
- identify the normal findings of each test.
- discuss the implications of abnormal test results.
- list factors that may interfere with accurate test results.

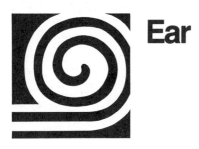

Ear

Introduction

Auditory tests serve a dual purpose; they can detect hearing impairment and can reveal the presence of lesions or disorders requiring treatment. Vestibular tests, which are concerned primarily with the complex function of labyrinthine structures of the inner ear, help detect a vestibular lesion and determine its location. However, no single auditory or vestibular test provides full diagnostic information; only a complete otologic and neurologic workup can do so.

Anatomy and physiology

The ear is conveniently divided into three parts: external, middle, and inner. The external ear consists of the auricle, or pinna (the visible flap), and the external ear canal. These structures direct and transmit sound waves toward the tympanic membrane (eardrum). The external ear canal also serves as a resonating tube, amplifying sound frequencies between 2,000 and 6,000 hertz (Hz). These frequencies are critical for perceiving consonants, which have both phonemic and morphologic importance.

The middle ear, which lies directly behind the tympanic membrane, is a small air space in the tympanic region of the temporal bone. Three small bones—the malleus (hammer), the incus (anvil), and the stapes (stirrup)—make up the auditory ossicles. These bones' vibrations transmit sound waves from the tympanic membrane toward the inner ear through a membrane known as the oval window.

The inner ear contains the sensory end organs for hearing and balance. These interconnected, fluid-filled, membranous structures are surrounded and protected by the temporal bone. The auditory end organ, or cochlea, is a coiled tube divided along its length into three compartments; vibration of the ossicles sets the fluid in these compartments into motion. The middle compartment, or cochlear duct, contains the organ of Corti, in which an array of sensitive hair cells convert fluid disturbance into neural impulses. These impulses travel along the eighth cranial nerve to the brain stem and to the auditory cortex.

The vestibular organs include the utricle, saccule, and semicircular canals. Changes in body orientation disturb the fluid in the canals and stimulate vestibular hair cells—called cristae in the semicircular canals, and maculae in the saccule and utricle. These hair cells dispatch messages to the cerebellum and other portions of the brain, enabling coordination of muscles of the eyes, head, neck, and other parts of the body to respond to changes in position.

Types of hearing loss

Hearing loss can result from injury to or disease of any part of the auditory

AUDITORY TESTS EVALUATE EAR STRUCTURES

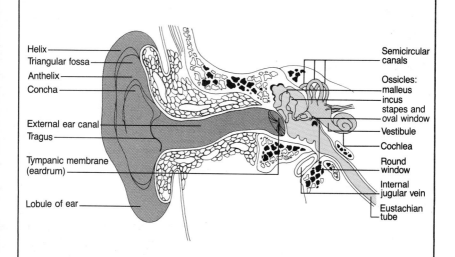

Helix
Triangular fossa
Anthelix
Concha

External ear canal
Tragus

Tympanic membrane
(eardrum)

Lobule of ear

Semicircular
canals

Ossicles:
malleus
incus
stapes and
oval window

Vestibule

Cochlea

Round
window

Internal
jugular vein

Eustachian
tube

The ear is divided into three anatomic parts—the external ear, the middle ear, and the internal ear—as illustrated by the shading above. Because the ear is so complex, thorough examination of all its structures requires a battery of diagnostic tests. For example, otoscopy provides direct visualization of the external ear canal and tympanic membrane; acoustic immittance tests evaluate middle ear and eustachian tube function; and electronystagmography, and falling and past-pointing tests evaluate the vestibular system. The ear has two functional parts—conductive, which includes the external ear canal, tympanic membrane, and ossicles; and sensorineural, which includes the vestibular system, the cochlea, and associated neural pathways. Pure tone audiometry and tuning fork tests evaluate conductive and sensorineural function and help determine the cause and extent of hearing loss.

system. For example, foreign objects, impacted cerumen, or growths can obstruct the external ear canal; perforation may damage the tympanic membrane; and various diseases may affect the delicate parts of the middle and inner ear. In a strict sense, the type of hearing loss refers to the site of the lesion or to the pathology.

A conductive hearing loss results from impairment of sound transmission through the external or middle ear since these parts conduct mechanical vibrations to the inner ear or sensorineural system. Such loss may result from impacted cerumen, a perforated tympanic membrane, accumulation of pus or serous fluid in the middle ear (as in otitis media), or impaired ossicular mobility (as in otosclerosis). In audiometric testing, a conductive loss is associated with better conduction thresholds in bone than in air, since bone-conducted sound, or skull vibration, doesn't pass through the external or middle ear, whereas air-conducted sound does; a lesion in the conductive system thus depresses only air-conduction thresholds.

A sensorineural hearing loss indicates a lesion in the inner ear (cochlear lesion), or the eighth cranial nerve or higher neural pathways (retrocochlear lesion). It's important to distinguish cochlear from retrocochlear lesions, since the latter may prove life threatening. Cochlear hearing loss may result from Ménière's disease, ototoxic agents, and viral labyrinthitis; retrocochlear loss, from tumors and multiple sclerosis.

A mixed hearing loss results from a combined sensorineural-conductive dysfunction. A central hearing loss results from damage to the brain's auditory receptors.

Audiologic tests

A thorough otoscopic examination of the external ear, the ear canal, and the tympanic membrane should precede any auditory or vestibular test. After otoscopy, basic audiologic examination consists of the following tests: pure tone audiometry to measure thresholds for air- and bone-conducted sound; spondee threshold; word discrimination; and acoustic immittance measurements, such as tympanometry, acoustic reflexes, and eustachian tube function. Tuning fork tests may be omitted, because the preceding tests prove more accurate.

Audiologic examination reveals the degree and type of hearing loss. When this examination or the patient's history suggests the presence of a lesion, site of lesion, vestibular, and radiographic tests may be ordered. Site of lesion tests distinguish cochlear from retrocochlear lesions; vestibular tests, such as electronystagmography and falling and past-pointing, help detect and locate vestibular lesions; numerous radiographic techniques, such as standard radiography, computerized tomography, and pneumoencephalography, may detect a lesion and determine its type. Standard radiographs can reveal congenital malformations of the middle and inner ears, mastoid inflammation, cholesteatoma, or acoustic tumors. Computerized tomography also provides radiographic evidence of tumors, as does pneumoencephalography, and helps detect neural degeneration, hydrocephalus, brain abscesses, and central tumors that disrupt auditory and vestibular function.

Neonatal screening

Early identification of high-risk infants to detect hearing impairment is essential to promote learning potential and minimize the effects of hearing loss. High-risk infants include those with family histories of hearing impairment, congenital anomalies of the face and skull, low birth weight, hyperbilirubinemia, or those with mothers who had intrauterine infections.

To promote early detection of hearing impairment, neonatal screening programs have been instituted in hospitals and well-baby clinics. Such neonatal screening may include the auditory brain stem response (ABR) and behavioral tests. The ABR objectively measures the integrity of the auditory system through the brain stem with mid- and high-frequency stimuli, while subjective behavioral tests check for reflexes, such as Moro's, in response to intense sound. An audiologist usually oversees these programs, although a nurse may perform some testing and provide follow-up care and parent training.

Screening school children

Screening programs in nursery and elementary schools aim to identify children with hearing losses that interfere with language development and general learning. These screening tests, performed by a nurse or audiologist and graded pass-fail, simply identify the need for more precise testing. Their overall effectiveness depends on the quality of follow-up services. The school screening program can be successful only if it provides audiologic or medical referral, or both; if it involves consultation with parents; and if it dispenses information to teachers and others responsible for the child's educational program.

Annual screening for hearing impairment for all children from nursery school to grade 3 is recommended by the American Speech-Language-Hearing Association (ASHA), since this age group has a high incidence of hearing loss. The association also recommends screening for children with:

☐ speech or language problems

☐ learning difficulties or special education needs

☐ classroom behavior problems, such as inattention to auditory signals, unusual visual alertness, or giving wrong answers to simple questions

☐ patient histories of allergies, or repeated colds or earaches

☐ recent placement in a new school.

Screening should take place early in the school year, to allow enough time for follow-up testing and referral. If comprehensive screening isn't possible, testing of at-risk groups should take priority.

If you're performing hearing screening tests, present pure tones—at levels established by state public health regulations—to each child individually. Failure to respond to any single tone constitutes failure of the test. If a child fails the initial screening, retest him later that day or within 1 week. Remember that many children who fail the first screening pass the second one after reinstruction. If a child fails the second screening, refer him to an audiologist for a complete workup. When notifying parents of screening test results, remember to explain that screening doesn't confirm a hearing loss but only suggests the need for further evaluation. Provide them with adequate information for obtaining audiologic and medical services. If a doctor or audiologist confirms hearing loss, you can help parents, teachers, and the child understand its implications.

Although pure tone screening is a valuable tool, many children with active middle ear pathology pass this test. To identify such pathology, the ASHA Committee on Audiological Evaluation recommends otologic examination; pure-tone bone conduction screening; or acoustic immittance tests, which are easily and quickly administered.

Preventing industrial hearing impairment

Noise affects people in an industrial environment in various ways. High noise levels result in changes in heart rate and blood pressure, and cause annoyance, decreased productivity, and distress, as well as hearing impairment. Workmen's Compensation claims for hearing-related disability, passage of the Occupational Safety and Health Act (OSHA) in 1970, and other legislation have stimulated development of industrial programs for hearing conservation.

Job-related hearing loss has been divided into two general categories of severity: temporary threshold shift (TTS) and permanent threshold shift (PTS). In the latter, hearing loss is permanent and generally results from years of exposure to noise. It may also result from acoustic trauma, in which one or more very intense sounds damage the tympanic membrane, ossicles, or organ of Corti. TTS may result from any sound intense enough to cause ringing in the ears, a sensation of fullness in the ears, or difficulty in one-to-one conversation. It causes temporary deafness lasting for hours to weeks; however, repeated, intermittent exposure to such noise may cause permanent hearing impairment. Consider TTS when evaluating any employees for permanent hearing loss,

---

MEASURES OF SOUND

Frequency and intensity are the two measures of sound. Frequency, measured in Hertz (Hz), is the number of sound vibrations per second. Although the ear can detect frequencies of 20 to 20,000 Hz, those between 500 and 2,000 Hz are the most important for speech recognition in a quiet environment.

Intensity is measured in decibels (dB). One decibel is roughly the smallest difference in intensity that the human ear can detect. Decibels express a logarithmic, not a linear, relationship: a 10-dB sound is 10 times the intensity of a 0-dB sound; a 20-dB sound, 100 times the intensity of a 0-dB sound; and a 30-dB sound, 1,000 times the intensity of a 0-dB sound. Decibel units require specification of a reference sound pressure level; for audiometric purposes, this level is dB HL (hearing level). A faint whisper registers 10 to 15 dB HL; average conversation registers 50 to 60 dB HL, and a shout registers 70 to 80 dB HL.

since both TTS and PTS produce a similar audiometric pattern. Accurate audiograms can be obtained only after a minimum of 16 hours have elapsed since exposure to intense noise.

Noise hazard includes not just loudness but frequency and duration of noise. Since noise levels may fluctuate considerably during the work day and some persons are more susceptible to it than others, official guidelines for hazardous noise in the workplace necessarily represent a compromise between complete protection and agreed-on thresholds of hearing loss.

Some industries require their employees to wear protective devices, such as earplugs or earmuffs. As part of the hearing conservation program, nurses should encourage such use of ear protection devices and promote routine screening for hearing loss to monitor their effectiveness.

Audiometer specifications

The audiometer, the instrument for hearing evaluation, should meet specifications established by the American National Standards Institute (ANSI) in 1969 and should deliver precisely calibrated tones at octave frequencies between 250 and 8,000 Hz. Such tones can be delivered by air or bone conduction. Pure tone and speech levels should each be calibrated in dB HL (hearing level). If the audiometer has a masking noise generator, noise levels should be calibrated in dB EL (effective level) or EM (effective masking); EL or EM designates the amount of threshold shift or masking caused by a noise.

Accurate testing requires a calibrated audiometer in good working order and a quiet test environment. A properly functioning audiometer should emit signals of the correct frequency and intensity, deliver those signals only to the selected transducer (for example, earphone or bone vibrator), and produce signals free of extraneous noise.

The test environment should have low ambient noise, since noise may mask test signals and falsely depress thresholds.

PSEUDOHYPACUSIS: NONORGANIC HEARING LOSS

Some patients, both children and adults, may not understand test procedures or may be malingering to gain some psychological or financial advantage. Often, you can identify such a patient by watching for behavioral cues.

• Watch the patient in the waiting room; he may converse normally with the receptionist but not with you or the examiner.

• During pure tone testing, the patient may never signal when a stimulus is absent. Most patients, if they are listening as well as expected, occasionally respond falsely, thinking they've heard a tone. Repeated threshold measurements may vary by 15 dB or more. If the patient reports a unilateral hearing loss, he may not respond on the side with diminished hearing by air or bone conduction, even at levels where crossover responses are anticipated. His bone conduction thresholds may be significantly poorer than the corresponding air conduction thresholds, and masked thresholds may prove better than unmasked ones.

• Abnormal behavior on speech tests often suggests malingering. The patient may refuse to guess, take long pauses before responding, or provide only half-word responses to spondee (easily understood, bisyllabic, equally stressed) words. The pure tone average and spondee threshold should agree; if they differ by 12 dB or more, malingering is possible. The patient may have excellent speech discrimination at or slightly above his voluntary spondee threshold or pure tone average.

If test results are questionable, instruct him again. Emphasize that he should respond to the softest tone he can detect. Give the equipment a quick listening check. If the problem persists, reschedule the test. Don't confront the patient with your suspicions of malingering, but give him a chance to yield gracefully. If these maneuvers fail, refer him to an audiologist.

(No factor can correct for the presence of noise.)

Each component of the audiometer—stimulus selection, frequency selection, attenuator, and transducers—must be checked. You can set up the equipment to listen through earphones while sitting at the control panel, or you may have a colleague with normal hearing listen in the test booth. Begin by selecting a pure tone stimulus (typically 1,000 Hz) and an earphone output (right or left ear). Except as indicated, set the tone at a comfortable listening level (for example, 50 dB HL), so you can detect changes in tonal quality and loudness.

□ *Attenuator linearity and scratchiness:* Starting at zero dB HL, decrease attenuation in 10-dB steps to maximum output. Listen for corresponding increases in loudness (which should double with each step). If you hear a scratchy sound as the attenuator is moved, the contacts are dusty; rotate the dial rapidly to clean them.

□ *Signal rise time, extraneous noise, and distortion:* At each signal presentation, listen for clicks; they indicate noise in the presentation switch or that the signal rises to maximum amplitude too fast. If the latter is the case, electronic adjustment is required. At high output levels, listen for excessive distortion in the signal. Gently flex the earphone cords at the phone connections and listen for interruptions; this indicates a poor connection or a frayed cord.

□ *Hum:* Extraneous noise produced by the audiometer may mask test signals. Set the attenuator to 90 dB, 60 dB, and 0 dB. At each setting, turn the signal on and off, and listen for noise. You may hear noise at 90 dB but not at 60 dB.

□ *Frequency selectivity:* To make sure each test tone can be generated, you can set the attenuator to 50 dB HL and listen to the output at each frequency.

□ *Auxiliary channels:* Perform each of the above steps with each attenuator. In addition, check frequency selectivity for narrow-band noises.

□ *Earphone balance and simultaneity of output:* Send a pure tone stimulus to one earphone and the corresponding narrow-band noise to the other at 50 dB HL and EL. Verify that the signal and noise go to the appropriate outputs. Reverse the stimuli, and verify that the sounds are equally loud in each earphone.

□ *Crosstalk:* Crosstalk occurs when the signal in one channel of the audiometer leaks across to the other channel, so it may be heard in the ear not being tested. Select the right earphone on the control panel, and unplug the corresponding earphone jack. Listen to the left earphone, which should be silent. Repeat for the opposite earphone.

□ *Bone vibrator:* Remove the earphones, and place the bone vibrator on your mastoid. You don't need to check attenuator linearity again, since the same attenuator is used for both air and bone conduction testing. However, listen to the output of each test frequency at 50 dB HL. Also listen for excessive distortion at the machine's output limit.

□ *Visual inspection:* Examine all cords, especially near the transducer connections. Earphone and vibrator headbands should be springy enough to provide a snug fit. When hung freely, the earphones should collapse together. Check for physical damage to the vibrator and for cracked or hard earphone cushions. (Worn-out headbands and cushions fit the ears poorly and interfere with reliability of the test.) You can wipe the cushions with a moist cloth; don't use alcohol to moisten the cloth, since it causes the cushions to harden and crack.

Keep the earphone itself dry.

Any suspected change in calibration should be confirmed by electronic and acoustic measurements. Calibration should be checked every 6 months by a qualified electronics technician.

CHERYL LONGINOTTI, PhD
CYNTHIA G. FOWLER, PhD

AUDIOLOGIC TESTS

Otoscopy

Otoscopy is the direct visualization of the external auditory canal and the tympanic membrane through an otoscope. It's the basic element of any physical examination of the ear and should be performed before other auditory or vestibular tests. Otoscopy indirectly provides information about the eustachian tube and the middle ear cavity.

Purpose
☐ To detect foreign bodies, cerumen or stenosis in the external canal
☐ To detect external or middle ear pathology, such as infection or tympanic membrane perforation.

Patient preparation
Describe the procedure to the patient, and explain that this test permits visualization of the ear canal and eardrum. Reassure him that the examination is usually painless and takes less than 5 minutes to perform. Inform him the ear will be pulled upward and backward to straighten the canal, to facilitate insertion of the otoscope.

Procedure
When assembling the otoscope, test the

COMMON ABNORMALITIES OF THE TYMPANIC MEMBRANE	
ABNORMAL FINDINGS	**USUAL CAUSE**
Bright red	Inflammation (otitis media)
Yellowish	Pus or serum behind the tympanic membrane (acute or chronic otitis media)
Bubble behind tympanic membrane	Serous fluid in middle ear (serous otitis media)
Absent light reflection	Bulging tympanic membrane (acute otitis media)
Absent or diminishing landmarks	Thickened tympanic membrane (chronic otitis media, otitis externa, or tympanosclerosis)
Oval dark areas	Perforated or scarred tympanic membrane (otitis media or trauma)
Very prominent malleus	Retracted tympanic membrane (nonfunctional eustachian tube)
Reduced mobility	Stiffened middle ear system (serous otitis media or, more rarely, middle ear adhesions)

lamp and be sure to attach the largest speculum that fits comfortably into the patient's ear; the speculum straightens and dilates the ear canal. With the patient seated, tilt his head slightly away from you, so the ear to be examined is pointed upward. (If the patient is restless or unable to sit up during the procedure, he may lie down, as long as the ear is positioned upward. However, in conditions such as serous otitis media, recumbency may displace the accumulated fluid in the middle ear, making the condition harder to detect.)

Pull the auricle upward and backward (pull downward if the patient is under age 3); insert the otoscope gently into the ear canal, with a downward and forward motion. If insertion is difficult, the speculum may be too large; replace it with a smaller one. If the ear canal resists the smaller speculum, withdraw the otoscope and notify the doctor. When the otoscope is placed comfortably, look through the lens, and gently advance the speculum until the eardrum becomes visible. Obtain as full a view as possible, and note redness, swelling, lesions, or scaling in the canal. Check the eardrum for a cone of light that appears at the 5-o'clock position in the right ear, and at the 7-o'clock position in the left; this

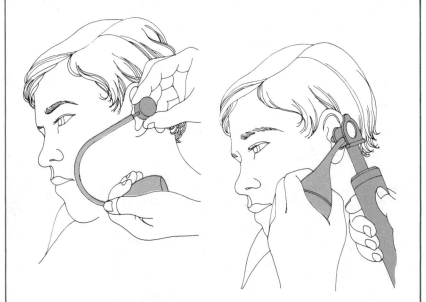

PNEUMATIC OTOSCOPY

This technique demonstrates the tympanic membrane's capacity to adjust to changes in air pressure in the middle ear. The otoscope may be fitted with a pneumatic bulb (at right) but, if not, a separate device for performing this test is available (at left). Once a tight seal is achieved on insertion of the speculum, air pressure from the bulb forces the tympanic membrane to flex inward or outward. Suction reveals pinhole perforations in the tympanic membrane when middle ear secretions issue from them. A perforated tympanic membrane is unable to move, since suction can't be maintained; adhesions or fluid in the middle ear may also prevent normal movement. A tympanic membrane previously perforated, but now healed, may appear abnormally flaccid.

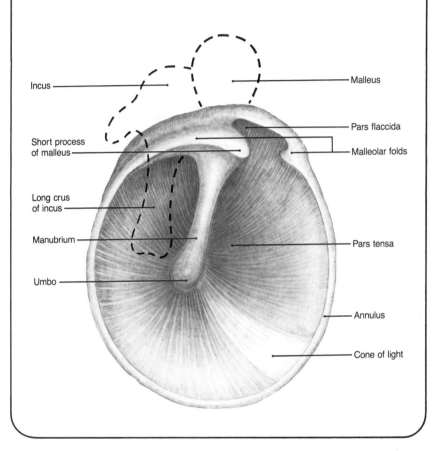

OTOSCOPIC VIEW OF TYMPANIC MEMBRANE

The normal tympanic membrane is shiny and pearl-gray or pale pink in color. It reflects the light of the otoscope as a "cone of light."

Incus

Short process of malleus

Long crus of incus

Manubrium

Umbo

Malleus

Pars flaccida

Malleolar folds

Pars tensa

Annulus

Cone of light

is a reflection of the otoscope lamp. Locate the *malleus,* which should be partially visible through the translucent tympanic membrane. The malleus—comprised of the short process, manubrium mallei, and umbo—extends downward to the center of the tympanic membrane. Examine the membrane itself and the surrounding fibrous rim (annulus).

Precautions
□ The otoscope should be advanced slowly and gently through the medial portion of the ear canal to avoid irritation of the canal lining, especially if an infection is suspected.
□ Continuing to insert an otoscope against resistance may cause a perforation or damage.

Findings
The normal tympanic membrane is thin, translucent, shiny, and slightly concave. It appears as a pearl-gray or pale pink disk that reflects light in its inferior por-

tion. The short process, manubrium mallei, and umbo should be visible but not prominent.

Implications of results
Scarring, discoloration, or retraction or bulging of the tympanic membrane indicates pathology (see chart on page 587). Movement of the tympanic membrane in tandem with respiration suggests abnormal patency of the eustachian tube.

Post-test care
None.

Interfering factors
□ Obstruction of the ear canal by cerumen or foreign matter obscures the tympanic membrane.
□ Recumbent positioning of a patient during otoscopy can mask serous otitis media.

CHERYL LONGINOTTI, PhD
CYNTHIA G. FOWLER, PhD

Tuning Fork Tests
[Weber, Rinne, and Schwabach tests]

Despite their limitations, the Weber, Rinne, and Schwabach tuning fork tests are quick, valuable screening tools for detecting hearing loss and providing preliminary information as to its type. The Weber test determines whether a patient lateralizes the tone of the tuning fork to one ear. The Rinne test compares air and bone conduction in both ears. The Schwabach test compares the patient's bone conduction response with that of the examiner, who is assumed to have normal hearing. Although the results of these tests are most reliable when a low-frequency tuning fork is used, they're not definitive since they depend on subjective factors, such as the examiner's ability to strike the fork with

equal force each time and the patient's ability to report audible tones correctly. Also, the Weber test results may be misleading, and the Rinne test frequently doesn't detect a mild conductive loss (10 to 35 dB). Thus, abnormal test results require confirmation by pure tone audiometry.

Purpose
□ To screen for or confirm hearing loss
□ To help distinguish conductive from sensorineural hearing loss.

Patient preparation
Describe the procedure to the patient, and explain that these tests help detect hearing loss and give information on the type of loss. Tell him who will perform the tests, and reassure him that the tests are painless and take only a few minutes.

Advise the patient that his concentration and prompt responses are essential to accurate testing. Have the patient use hand signals to indicate whether a tone is louder in his right ear or left ear, and also when he stops hearing the tone.

Inform him that tuning fork tests are not definitive and that further testing may be necessary to confirm abnormal results.

Procedure
Using a low-frequency tuning fork (256 or 512 hertz), practice achieving a consistent tone. You can vibrate the tuning fork by gently striking one prong against your elbow or the heel of your hand, by stroking the prongs upward, or by pinching them together.

Weber test: Vibrate the fork and place its base on the midline of the skull at the forehead. Ask the patient if he hears the tone in his left ear, right ear, or equally in both. Record the results as *Weber left, Weber right,* or *Weber midline,* respectively.

Rinne test: To test bone conduction, hold the tuning fork between your thumb and index finger and place the base of the vibrating fork against the patient's mastoid process. Then, to test air conduction, move the still-vibrating prongs next to but not touching the external ear. Ask the patient which location has the louder or longer sound. Repeat the procedure for the other ear. Record the results as *Rinne positive,* if the air-conducted sound is heard louder or longer, and *Rinne negative,* if the bone-conducted sound is heard louder or longer.

Schwabach test: Hold the tuning fork between your thumb and index finger, and place the base of the vibrating tuning fork against his left mastoid process, and ask him if he hears the tone. If he does, immediately place the tuning fork on *your* left mastoid process, and listen for the tone. Alternate the tuning fork between the patient's left mastoid process and your own until one of you stops hearing the sound; record the length of time the other continues to hear it. Then, repeat the procedure on the right mastoid process.

Precautions

Strike the tuning fork with equal force each time. Hold the fork at its base to allow the prongs to vibrate freely. Record the name of the test, the result, and the vibrating frequency of the tuning fork.

Findings

In the Weber test, a patient with normal hearing hears the same tone equally loud in both ears—a Weber-midline result. In the Rinne test, a patient hears the air-conducted tone louder or longer than the bone-conducted tone—a Rinne-positive result. In the Schwabach test, both the patient and the examiner hear the tone equally long.

Implications of results

In the Weber test, lateralization of the tone to one ear suggests a conductive loss on that side or a sensorineural loss on the other side. Physiologically, lateralization results from the tone being louder in one ear (Stenger effect) or from the tone reaching one ear sooner than the other (phase effect). If one ear has a sensorineural loss, the Stenger effect causes lateralization to the unaffected ear; if one ear has a conductive loss, either the Sten-

ger or phase effect produces lateralization to that ear. If a patient's hearing loss is unilateral, the Weber test may suggest the type of loss. When a patient's hearing loss is bilateral, this test may help to identify the ear with the better bone conduction.

In the Rinne test, hearing of the bone-conducted tone louder or for a longer duration than the air-conducted tone indicates a conductive loss. In a unilateral hearing loss, the tone may be heard louder when conducted by bone, but in the opposite ear. This is a false-negative Rinne. A sensorineural loss is indicated when the sound is heard louder by air conduction.

In the Schwabach test, prolonged duration of the tone, compared with that of the examiner, suggests a conductive loss; conversely, shortened duration indicates a sensorineural loss. A conductive loss attenuates (decreases the energy of) air-conducted sound in a room with ambient noise, enabling patients with this type of loss to hear bone-conducted sound longer than the examiner can hear such sound.

A patient with abnormal results on any or all tuning fork tests should be retested. Similar results on retesting require pure tone audiometry to confirm the hearing loss and determine its type and severity.

Post-test care

Refer the patient for further audiologic testing if tuning fork tests suggest a hearing loss.

Interfering factors

□ Failure to strike the tuning fork with equal force or to hold it correctly during the procedure interferes with accurate testing.

□ Undetected hearing loss in the examiner invalidates results of the Schwabach test.

□ Inaccurate patient response due to poor understanding of his task interferes with accurate testing.

CHERYL LONGINOTTI, PhD
CYNTHIA G. FOWLER, PhD

HOW TO USE THE TUNING FORK

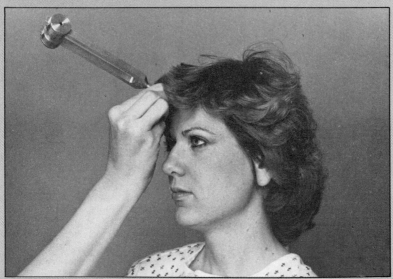

Weber test (above): Place the vibrating tuning fork on the midline of the patient's skull. Ask her if she hears the tone in her left ear, right ear, or equally in both. Record the results as Weber left, Weber right, or Weber midline, respectively.

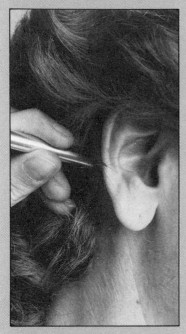

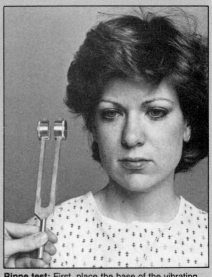

Rinne test: First, place the base of the vibrating tuning fork on the patient's mastoid process to test bone conduction (at left), then hold the prongs ½" (1 cm) from the ear canal to test air conduction (above).

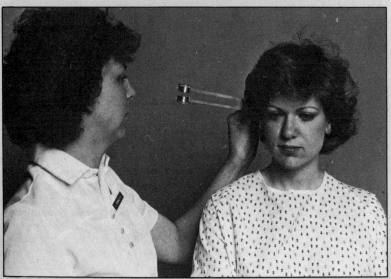

Schwabach test: First, place the vibrating tuning fork on the patient's right mastoid process (top), then on your own (bottom). Continue alternating the fork until one of you stops hearing the sound, and record how long the sound is heard. Repeat the procedure on the left mastoid process.

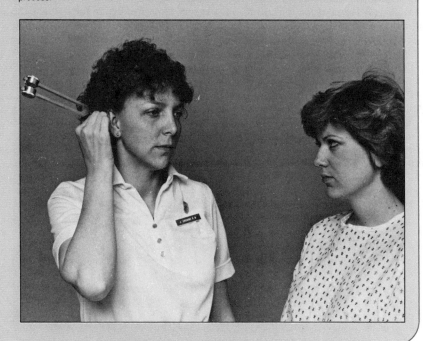

Pure Tone Audiometry

This test, performed with an audiometer, provides a record of the thresholds—the lowest intensity levels—at which a patient can hear a set of test tones introduced through earphones or bone conduction (sound) vibrator. These tones, called pure tones, have their energy concentrated at discrete frequencies. The octave frequencies between 125 and 8,000 Hz are used to obtain air conduction thresholds; frequencies between 250 and 4,000 Hz, to obtain bone conduction thresholds.

Comparison of air and bone conduction thresholds can suggest a conductive, sensorineural, or mixed hearing loss, but does not indicate the cause of the loss; further audiologic and vestibular tests and radiographs may provide the etiology. Pure tone audiometry results may also suggest the need for referral to an audiologist for evaluation of communication difficulties and planning of appropriate rehabilitation.

Pure tone audiometry is indicated in any child or adult who needs quantitative hearing assessment. Although this test has no contraindications, results depend on the cooperation of the patient. Acoustic immittance may provide additional information.

Purpose
□ To determine the presence, type, and degree of hearing loss
□ To assess communication abilities and rehabilitation needs.

Patient preparation
Describe the procedure to the patient, and explain that this test determines the presence and degree of hearing loss. Tell him who will perform the test and where, and that the test takes about 20 minutes.

Inform him that each ear will be tested separately, starting with the ear with the better hearing acuity. Advise him that he will hear tones at various intensities, and that he will be instructed to give a signal (or press the response button) each time he hears the tone. Emphasize that he should respond even if the tone is very faint. Just before the test, ask the patient to remove all obstructions to proper earphone placement. If he has been exposed to loud noises (loud enough to cause tinnitus or make face-to-face

RELATING PURE TONE AVERAGE TO HEARING LOSS AND SPEECH AUDIBILITY		
PURE TONE AVERAGE	**DEGREE OF HEARING LOSS**	**SPEECH AUDIBILITY**
0 to 25 dB	Normal limits	No significant difficulty
26 to 40 dB	Mild	Difficulty with faint or distant speech
41 to 55 dB	Moderate	Difficulty with conversational speech
56 to 70 dB	Moderately severe	Speech must be loud; difficulty with group conversation
71 to 90 dB	Severe	Difficulty with loud speech; understands only shouted or amplified speech
91 + dB	Profound	May not understand amplified speech

communication difficult) within the past 16 hours, postpone the test.

Equipment

Otoscope/calibrated audiometer with earphones and bone conduction vibrator/quiet test environment (sound-treated room).

Procedure

The patient's ear canal is checked with the otoscope for impacted cerumen. Then, the examiner presses a finger first on the auricle, then on the tragus, to rule out possible closure of the canal under pressure from the earphones. If the canal tends to close, a stiff-walled plastic tube is carefully inserted into the canal, and this modification is recorded on the audiogram; children and the elderly are most likely to require this modification.

The earphones are positioned so they are lined up opposite the ear canals, and the headband is tightened. The patient is familiarized with the test tone by presenting it to his better ear for less than 1 second at a level 15 to 25 dB above the expected threshold. If he responds to the tone, *air conduction* testing is begun at 1,000 Hz, by decreasing intensity in 10-dB steps until the patient fails to respond. Then, intensity is increased in 5-dB steps until he hears the tone again. After he responds to the ascending run, intensity is decreased in 10-dB steps. Sequences of 10-dB decrements and 5-dB increments are repeated until the patient responds to at least two of three presentations at a single level. The threshold level is the lowest decibel level at which the response rate is at least 50%.

Using this procedure, tones are presented to the better ear in this order: 1,000 Hz, 2,000 Hz, 4,000 Hz, 8,000 Hz, 1,000 Hz, 500 Hz, and 250 Hz. After testing the better ear, the worse ear is tested. In each ear, test/retest differences may be ± 5 dB. If the difference between the first and second threshold at 1,000 Hz is greater than 10 dB, test results are unreliable; equipment is checked for malfunction, and the patient is reinstructed and retested.

CROSSOVER

A sufficiently intense test tone presented to one ear causes the skull to vibrate. The tone then passes by bone conduction to the opposite ear (crossover). For air conduction testing, this crossover generally occurs when the test tone exceeds 40 dB HL (125 to 750 Hz) or 50 dB HL (1,000 to 8,000 Hz). During bone conduction, crossover occurs at all levels.

Crossover can be prevented by masking the ear not being tested with narrow-band noise from the audiometer. If crossover isn't prevented, test results will underestimate the degree of hearing loss.

Because of the difficulty involved, masking is generally performed by an audiologist.

For *bone conduction* testing, the earphones are removed and the vibrator is placed on the mastoid process of the better ear (the auricle shouldn't touch the vibrator). Ascending and descending tones are used as in air conduction testing, using 250 Hz, 500 Hz, 1,000 Hz, 2,000 Hz, and 4,000 Hz.

Precautions

Record on the audiogram any modifications to the standard testing procedure, such as insertion of a plastic tube into the ear canal to avoid ear canal collapse.

Findings

The normal range of hearing sensitivity is 0 to 25 dB HL for adults and 0 to 15 dB HL for children. However, normal test results do not rule out pathology; a mild middle ear infection or other pathology may exist but not interfere with auditory function.

Implications of results

The pure tone average (PTA)—the average of pure tone air conduction thresholds obtained at 500 Hz, 1,000 Hz, and 2,000 Hz—quantifies the degree of hearing loss. When these three thresholds vary widely, the mean of the best two—the Fletcher average—indicates the degree of hearing loss.

The relationship between threshold

PURE TONE AUDIOGRAMS

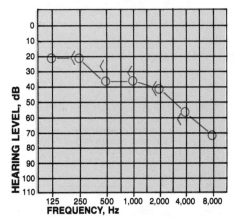

Sensorineural hearing loss depresses both air (circles) and bone (arrows) conduction thresholds to about the same degree. No matter how sound vibrations reach the inner ear, they must be transmitted to higher neural centers through the sensorineural system.

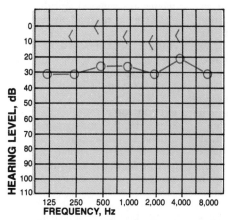

Conductive hearing loss, produced by interference with the conductive mechanism, depresses air conduction thresholds but generally doesn't affect bone thresholds.

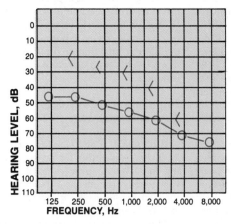

Mixed hearing loss involves abnormal air and bone conduction thresholds. Air conduction thresholds demonstrate a greater loss due to a conductive lesion.

responses for air and bone conduction tones determines the type of hearing loss. In *sensorineural* loss, both thresholds are depressed; in *conductive* loss, air thresholds are depressed, but bone thresholds are unchanged; and in *mixed* hearing loss, both thresholds are abnormal, with air conduction being more depressed than bone conduction.

The chart on page 594 shows the relationship among PTA, the degree of hearing loss, and the audibility of speech in a quiet environment.

Post-test care

If test results aren't reliable or if they are confounded by possible crossover, refer the patient to an audiologist.

Interfering factors

☐ Impacted cerumen or a closed ear canal can cause a 35- to 40-dB artifactual conductive hearing loss.

☐ A patient who confuses vibrotactile with auditory sensation or tinnitus with the signal will give invalid responses.

☐ Cracked or poorly-fitting earphones result in low-frequency leakage and falsely elevated thresholds.

☐ An uncalibrated audiometer or background noise can invalidate test results.

☐ Presentation of extraneous cues to the patient, such as a rhythmic pattern of test tones or hand movement near the attenuator dial, can invalidate results.

☐ An uncooperative or inattentive patient may give invalid responses.

CHERYL LONGINOTTI, PhD
CYNTHIA G. FOWLER, PhD

Acoustic Immittance Tests

[Admittance testing: tympanometry, acoustic reflexes]

Immittance tests evaluate middle ear function by measuring the flow of sound energy into the ear (admittance) and the opposition to that flow (impedance). Not all sound energy that impinges on the tympanic membrane reaches the inner ear; some reflects into the external ear canal. The relationship of incident to reflected sound energy determines the admittance, which depends on the resistance, stiffness, and mass of the auditory system. Normally, stiffness is the predominant factor in the middle ear.

Admittance is commonly measured by two tests—tympanometry and acoustic reflexes. Each test employs an electronic tone generator, an air pressure manometer, and a tone probe that delivers both sound and air pressure stimuli to the ear canal and tympanic membrane through an airtight seal. Tympanometry measures middle ear admittance in response to changes in air pressure in the ear canal; the acoustic reflexes test measures the change in admittance produced by contraction of the stapedius muscle as it responds to an intense sound. Stapedial contraction stiffens the tympanic membrane and ossicular chain, causing a measurable change in middle ear admittance. Reflex decay, part of the acoustic reflexes test, is a function of eighth nerve adaptation or fatigue in response to a reflex-eliciting stimulus.

Admittance tests help diagnose middle ear pathology, lesions in the seventh (facial) or eighth cranial nerve, and eustachian tube dysfunction. They can also help verify the presence of a labyrinthine fistula and identify pseudohypacusis (nonorganic hearing loss). Because admittance tests require little patient cooperation, they can reliably test very young children, or mentally or physically handicapped patients.

Purpose

Tympanometry:
☐ To assess the continuity and admittance of the middle ear
☐ To evaluate status of the tympanic membrane
Acoustic reflexes and reflex decay:
☐ To distinguish cochlear from retrocochlear lesions

INTERPRETING TYMPANOGRAMS:
SAMPLE RESULTS AND DESCRIPTIVE TERMS

Tympanograms can be classified according to pressure, amplitude, and shape. This chart depicts a series of tympanograms and describes these related features.

TYMPANOGRAM	SHAPE	AMPLITUDE	PRESSURE
	Normal	Normal	Normal
	Peaked	Flaccid	Normal
	Normal	Stiff	Normal
	Flat	Stiff	Absent-Negative
	Flat	Stiff	Absent-Negative
	Normal	Stiff	−125 daPa
	Normal	Normal	+90 daPa
	Notched	Flaccid	Normal
	Deep, broad notching	Flaccid	Normal
	Normal	Flaccid	−200 daPa
	Deep, broad notching	Flaccid	−200 daPa
	Vascular perturbation	Stiff	Normal

−300   0   +300
PRESSURE in daPa
(.983 daPa = 1 mm H_2O)

Adapted with permission from A. Feldman, "Tympanometry: Applications and Interpretation," *Annals of Otology, Rhinology, and Laryngology,* Supp. 24, 85, 1976.

☐ To discern eighth nerve-peripheral brain stem lesions from intra-axial brain stem lesions
☐ To locate seventh nerve lesions relative to stapedius muscle innervation
☐ To confirm conductive hearing loss
☐ To help confirm pseudohypacusis.

Patient preparation

Describe the procedure to the patient, and explain that these tests evaluate the condition of the middle ear. Inform him who will perform the tests and where, and that each test takes approximately 2 or 3 minutes.

Instruct the patient not to move, speak, or swallow while admittance is being recorded, and caution him not to startle during the loud tone reflex-eliciting measurement. Advise him that changes in ear

TYMPANOGRAMS: CORRELATION WITH SELECTED DISORDERS

Shape	Altered smoothness	• Eardrum abnormality • Ossicular discontinuity • Vascular tumor
	Flat	• Serous otitis • Perforated tympanic membrane • Canal wall or cerumen artifact • Middle ear tumor
	Peaked	• Eardrum abnormality • Ossicular discontinuity
Amplitude	Increased	• Eardrum abnormality • Ossicular discontinuity
	Normal	• Blocked eustachian tube • Early acute otitis media
	Reduced	• Ossicular fixation • Serous otitis media • Cholesteatoma, polyps, granuloma • Glomangioma
Pressure	Positive	• Early acute otitis media
	Normal	• Ossicular fixation or adhesive fixation • Ossicular discontinuity • Middle ear tumor • Eardrum abnormality
	Negative	• Blocked eustachian tube • Early serous otitis media

canal pressure rarely may cause transient vertigo, but tell him to report any discomfort or dizziness. Reassure him that while the probe, which forms an airtight seal in the ear canal, may cause discomfort, it will not harm the ear.

Equipment

Admittance meter/calibrated probe cavity to calibrate the meter (supplied by manufacturer)/strip chart recorder (optional)/probe tips and cuffs (to seal probe in ear canal)/silicone putty (for difficult seal)/otoscope with speculum/wire (to clean bores of probe)/pure tone audiometer (to provide stimulus for acoustic reflex [optional]).

Procedure

A quick otoscopic examination is performed to verify that no impacted cerumen or other obstruction is present in the ear canal. The size and shape of the canal is checked in order to select the appropriate size probe cuff, which is then attached to the probe. The probe tip is inserted into the ear canal while pulling upward and backward on the auricle; a proper seal can maintain a negative pressure of −200 daPa. If necessary, silicone putty is used to ensure a snug, leakproof seal; care must be taken to avoid clogging the probe tip with putty.

Tympanometry: After a seal is obtained, the admittance meter sensitivity and probe tone level is set, if it's not automatic. The patient is informed when the test is about to begin. Air pressure is then changed, and the admittance is recorded. If recording is manual, at least six measurements between −200 and +200 daPa are taken. Additional measurements are taken if there are large admittance changes. Although the direction of air pressure change (positive to negative, or vice versa) is arbitrary, the direction is kept consistent throughout the test.

If a flat tympanogram is obtained (no change in admittance), the possibility that the probe tip may have rested against the canal wall or that it was clogged with cerumen must be ruled out with ear canal volume measurements. The probe is moved very slightly and the tympanogram is observed for a large admittance change. The probe tip is removed, cleaned, and reinserted, and the test is repeated.

Acoustic reflexes: A broad-band noise or a pure tone (500 to 4,000 Hz) is presented monaurally; a monaural stimulus causes bilateral reflex activation. Depending on the equipment available, the change in admittance in the stimulated ear (ipsilateral measurement) or in the opposite ear (contralateral or trans–brain stem measurement) is monitored. The results for the stimulated ear are recorded, regardless of whether monitoring is ipsilateral or contralateral.

The patient is told that stimuli will be presented. Reflex threshold is determined by presenting stimuli in ascending steps of 10 dB; when the first reflex occurs, decrease the level by 10 dB and start an ascending run in 5-dB steps. The lowest level stimulus that elicits a reflex is recorded. Then, reflex decay is measured contralaterally at 500 and 1,000 Hz by presenting the stimulus at 10 dB above the reflex threshold for 10 seconds; the magnitude of the reflex during the first second of stimulation is the baseline. Reflex magnitude at 5 or 10 seconds is compared with baseline at 1 second; significant reflex decay occurs when reflex magnitude declines to less than half of baseline.

Precautions

☐ Admittance tests should be performed cautiously in patients with recent middle ear surgery, head trauma, or possible labyrinthine fistula; in such patients, medical clearance should be obtained before testing.

☐ Check equipment carefully. If the probe tip is clogged with cerumen or debris, the measured admittance will not change, even when the probe isn't coupled to the ear. Clean the probe by carefully inserting a wire through each bore, wiping the wire, and then withdrawing it.

☐ If you can't obtain a seal even though the probe seems well seated, look for leakage elsewhere in the air system. Check the system by putting your finger over the probe tip and cuff and determine if nonzero pressure can be maintained. If it can't, seal the air outlet behind the meter with your finger, and check admittance. Then check each subsequent link in the system for possible leakage.

☐ Although the capability for monitoring acoustic reflexes both ipsilateral and contralateral to the stimulated ear is diagnostically useful, ipsilateral measurement is subject to equipment artifact. To check for this, put the probe tip in a calibrated cavity supplied by the manufacturer. Presentation of the reflex stimulus in this cavity should not change the measured admittance.

ACOUSTIC IMMITTANCE TESTING

With the probe tip sealed in the external meatus, the examiner can deliver both sound and air pressure stimuli to the ear canal and tympanic membrane.

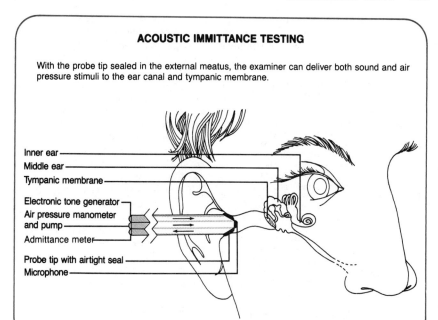

Inner ear
Middle ear
Tympanic membrane
Electronic tone generator
Air pressure manometer and pump
Admittance meter
Probe tip with airtight seal
Microphone

Findings

In tympanometry, the normal middle ear air pressure range is ± 100 daPa. The overall shape of the tympanogram is smooth and symmetric.

In acoustic reflexes, the normal trans–brain stem reflex threshold levels for pure tones range from 70 to 100 dB HL; ipsilateral thresholds are 3 to 12 dB lower. Reflex decay is normally slight—not more than one half of baseline over 10 seconds.

Implications of results

A flat tympanogram indicates no change in admittance with changing air pressure and can result from fluid in the middle ear, a perforated eardrum, or impacted cerumen. Large changes in admittance can reflect tympanic membrane scarring or disarticulated ossicular chain. If the eustachian tube is patent, admittance may change with the patient's respiration, resulting in periodic fluctuations on the tympanogram. Fluctuations synchronous with the patient's pulse suggest the presence of a gloman-

gioma in the middle ear space. The accompanying chart relates variations in tympanograms to selected underlying disorders; however, actual diagnosis of these disorders requires additional tests.

Absence of acoustic reflexes may indicate poor residual sensitivity in the stimulated ear (hearing loss greater than 70 dB HL); a conductive loss of sufficient magnitude (greater than 25 dB) to prevent adequate stimulus levels from reaching the inner ear; damage to the eighth nerve in the stimulated ear and/or lower brain stem; absence of the stapedius muscle in the probe ear; a conductive loss greater than 5 dB in the probe ear; or damage to the seventh nerve of the probe ear central to the innervation of the stapedius muscle. Reflexes can't be monitored if middle ear reconstructive surgery has removed the stapedius muscle or if the muscle is congenitally absent. A suprastapedial lesion of the seventh nerve paralyzes the stapedius. Thus, the presence of the reflex in a patient with seventh nerve pathology suggests that the lesion is inferior or peripheral to stapedial innervation.

Ipsilateral stimulation and monitoring doesn't require transmission of stimulus information across the brain stem. Comparison of ipsilateral and trans–brain stem findings may help distinguish eighth nerve and peripheral brain stem lesions from intra-axial brain stem lesions.

A change in reflex magnitude in response to a sustained stimulus suggests an eighth nerve and/or brain stem lesion. Using the first second of stimulation as the baseline magnitude, reflex decay to less than one half baseline in 5 or 10 seconds is a significant sign of a retro-cochlear lesion.

If cochlear sensitivity is poor, reflexes are absent; therefore, if reflex thresholds are better than voluntary thresholds, suspect malingering. In such a case, reemphasize the importance of this test to the patient, inform him that the admittance meter reveals actual ability to hear, and ask for his complete cooperation.

Post-test care

None.

Interfering factors

□ Clogged tone probe, poor air seal, or movement of probe tip during measurement interferes with accurate testing.

□ The patient's talking, swallowing, or startling during measurement interferes with the accurate determination of test results.

CHERYL LONGINOTTI, PhD
CYNTHIA G. FOWLER, PhD

> ### EVALUATING EUSTACHIAN TUBE FUNCTION
>
> An oxygen-absorbing mucosal lining covers the middle ear cavity and mastoid air cells. The eustachian tube periodically opens to ensure the middle ear's oxygen supply. If this tube is blocked, negative air pressure in the middle ear results, causing edema and a buildup of effusions.
>
> Testing eustachian tube function in an ear with an intact tympanic membrane generally involves three steps: inducing negative (preferable) or positive pressure in the middle ear cavity (verified tympano-metrically); having the patient swallow or yawn to open the tube; and recording another tympanogram to determine if this maneuver altered middle ear pressure. However, since it's difficult to artificially induce sufficient negative pressure, this test doesn't duplicate the most critical conditions for eustachian tube function. The test also can't be performed if the tympano-gram is abnormally shaped and middle ear pressure isn't known.
>
> However, if the patient has a tympano-gram with a well-defined peak, peak admittance pressure is a useful indicator of eustachian tube function. If pressure is normal (± 100 daPa), it usually means that the middle ear is properly ventilated and the eustachian tube is functioning adequately; if it's abnormal, the examiner asks the patient to swallow or yawn several times, and repeats the tympanogram to verify that negative pressure isn't transient.
>
> If the patient has a perforated tympanic membrane or a ventilatory tube in place, the ear canal and middle ear form a single cavity; pressure within this cavity can be varied directly with the admittance meter air system. The examiner creates a negative pressure of − 100 daPa in the cavity, asks the patient to swallow four to six times, and watches the manometer for changes in air pressure. If pressure doesn't return to within ±50 daPa, the procedure is repeated with + 100 daPa and again with + 200 daPa. Although positive pressure isn't as accurate as negative pressure, it does suggest the degree of eustachian tube dysfunction.
>
> Tympanometry can also verify abnormal patency or opening of the eustachian tube. If the eustachian tube is open, air pressure in the middle ear cavity fluctuates with respiration, and this can be recorded with the admittance meter.

Spondee Threshold

[Speech reception threshold, spondaic word threshold]

This simple, reliable and widely used test determines the faintest level at which a patient correctly repeats 50% of a live or recorded set of spondee words presented to him through earphones in a quiet environment. Spondees are two-syllable words—such as baseball, airplane, or birthday—with equal stress placed on each syllable. The spondees selected for the test are familiar words, uniformly audible, and dissimilar in phonetic construction. The spondee threshold test is commonly performed after pure tone audiometry to check the validity of audiometric hearing thresholds; the pure tone (Fletcher) average should agree with the spondee threshold within 10 dB.

Purpose
☐ To measure the degree of hearing loss for speech recognition
☐ To discern true hearing loss from nonorganic hearing loss (pseudohypacusis)
☐ To confirm the results of pure tone audiometry for frequencies most important for speech recognition.

Patient preparation
Describe the procedure to the patient, and explain that this test evaluates his ability to hear conversational speech. Tell him the test is performed by an audiologist, and that the procedure takes approximately 5 minutes. Tell the patient that he'll hear a series of two-syllable words transmitted to him through earphones while he is in a soundproof booth, to repeat each word after he hears it, and to guess if he isn't sure of a word. Advise him that the volume of each word spoken becomes progressively softer as the test continues, and each ear will be tested separately.

If the patient has difficulty understanding English, provide him with a printed list of words before the test and, if necessary, help him learn them. Advise him that he won't be able to refer to the list during the test.

Equipment
Calibrated speech audiometer/earphones/recorded spondee list/sound treated room.

Procedure
The patient is instructed to enter the soundproof booth, and the audiologist places the earphones securely over the patient's ears. The ear with better hearing acuity is tested first, with the sound

level set about 20 dB above the patient's pure tone threshold. After familiarizing the patient with the spondees, the spondee threshold is determined in a fashion similar to the pure tone threshold. The intensity is decreased and then raised until it reaches the faintest level at which the patient gives a 50% correct response rate.

After determining the spondee threshold of the better ear, the procedure is repeated for the other ear.

Precautions
Although the spondee threshold provides a direct and reliable measure of hearing loss for speech in most adults, it cannot measure it reliably in very young children or in persons with language difficulties.

Findings
Normally, the spondee threshold should fall within ± 10 dB of the pure tone threshold. However, this relationship may vary in patients with precipitous sloping hearing losses or in those whose tests demonstrate irregular audiometric configuration.

Implications of results
If the spondee threshold differs by more than 10 dB from the pure tone threshold, the patient may be unable to respond to the lowest audible levels, or may be malingering. In such cases, the instructions are repeated to the patient and the test is performed again.

Any patient with abnormal test results should be referred to an audiologist for tests of malingering or pseudohypoacusis.

Post-test care
None.

Interfering factors
Very young children or persons unfamiliar with the English language or terminology used in the test may give inaccurate responses.

CHERYL LONGINOTTI, PhD
CYNTHIA G. FOWLER, PhD

Word Recognition Tests

Word recognition tests measure the ability to recognize and repeat a series of monosyllabic words presented by a live or recorded voice at suprathreshold levels (about 40 dB above the spondee threshold) in a quiet environment. The phonetically balanced test words represent the relative frequency of occurrence of sounds in English. Commonly used word recognition tests include the PAL PB-50 (Psychoacoustics Laboratories, Harvard University, Cambridge, Mass.), the CID W-22 (Central Institute for the Deaf, St. Louis), and the NU auditory test # 4 or # 6 (Northwestern University, Evanston, Ill.).

Most speech energy is contained in vowel sounds and concentrated in low frequencies; less energy, in consonantal sounds and high frequencies. Since consonants distinguish most words (such as pin, thin, and bin), a patient with high-frequency hearing loss misses consonantal cues and commonly complains that he hears speech but doesn't understand it.

Word recognition is tested because patients with similar audiograms may have markedly different word recognition abilities. Poor word recognition is the result of the distortion imposed by hearing loss. In real-life situations, nonauditory factors such as the ability to speech read or use contextual information are important for understanding speech.

Purpose
□ To evaluate the clarity of speech reception at suprathreshold levels
□ To determine the need for and potential benefits from a hearing aid or speech reading instruction
□ To help locate auditory tract and CNS lesions.

Patient preparation
Describe the procedure to the patient, and explain that these tests assess his ability to hear and understand speech presented at above-normal tones and to determine if he would benefit from a hearing aid. Tell him the test will be performed by an audiologist, and that each ear will be tested separately. Tell the patient that he'll hear a series of short

---

CLASSIFYING WORD RECOGNITION ABILITY

Word recognition tests evaluate a patient's hearing by measuring the percentage of test words he recognizes and repeats correctly. This illustration provides general guidelines for classifying a patient's word recognition ability according to the percentage of correct responses.

Classification	Percentage
Excellent	90% to 100% correct
Good	75% to 90% correct
Fair	60% to 75% correct
Poor	40% to 60% correct
Very poor	less than 40% correct

words transmitted to him through earphones while he is in a soundproof booth, to repeat each word after he hears it, and to guess when unsure.

If the patient is wearing a hearing aid, ask him to remove it.

Equipment
Calibrated speech audiometer and earphones/standardized word list.

Procedure
After the patient is seated in a soundproof booth, earphones are placed on his ears. The live voice or recorded word list is presented at a sensation level of approximately 40 dB greater than the patient's spondee threshold or at a level considered comfortable by the patient. The number of correct responses is recorded and converted to a percentage score.

Precautions
None.

Findings
A person with normal hearing can correctly repeat 90% to 100% of the test words.

Implications of results
The chart to the left provides general guidelines for classifying word recognition ability. Test scores may differ by as much as 12%—the result of sampling error or normal test-retest differences. However, if the score for one ear differs from that of the other ear by more than 12%, or if the scores are significantly poorer than expected (in comparison with the pure tone audiogram), a retrocochlear lesion may be present.

Conductive hearing loss can permit excellent word recognition, if speech is loud enough. Sensorineural loss may distort neural representation of sound and cause poor recognition. Amplification allows hearing-impaired individuals to hear speech at conversational levels. A hearing aid may improve understanding by amplifying frequencies important for distinguishing speech sounds. Individuals may also benefit from increased awareness of environmental sounds.

If test scores suggest (or the patient reports) difficulty hearing or understanding speech, refer the patient for aural rehabilitation; if scores suggest a retrocochlear lesion, refer the patient for neuro-otologic examination.

Post-test care
None.

Interfering factors
☐ The characteristics of the test equipment (particularly the earphones) or changes in the presentation level of the word list may affect test scores.
☐ Scores obtained using earphones at a particular presentation level may not agree with those obtained using a hearing aid at the same level.

CHERYL LONGINOTTI, PhD
CYNTHIA G. FOWLER, PhD

Site of Lesion Tests

When patient history or pure tone audiogram suggests the presence of a lesion, site of lesion tests can be performed to locate it. Indications from patient history include difficulty in understanding speech that's disproportionate to the degree of pure tone loss; dizziness, tinnitus, or sudden or fluctuating hearing loss; or other neural symptoms. The primary indication from the pure tone audiogram is a difference between ears in the sensorineural components. However, not all lesions impair pure tone sensitivity. Since the auditory system contains many different neural pathways in the brain stem and cortex, a pure tone signal can bypass a lesion and be carried by relatively few neural fibers. More difficult stimuli, presented in the site of lesion test battery, are required to test auditory system function and to reveal the effects of lesions.

Site of lesion tests help distinguish

BÉKÉSY AUDIOMETRY

Békésy audiometry: In this test, pure tone frequencies are presented in a sweep of 100 to 10,000 Hz, changing at a rate of one octave per minute. They are first presented as pulsed tones (broken tracings), then as continuous tones (solid tracings). The patient controls tone intensity by pushing a response button whenever he

Figure A: Type I Békésy audiogram, typically obtained from normal patients or from those suffering conductive hearing losses. The tracings overlap closely. The broken tracing is the pulsed tone; the solid tracing, the continuous tone.

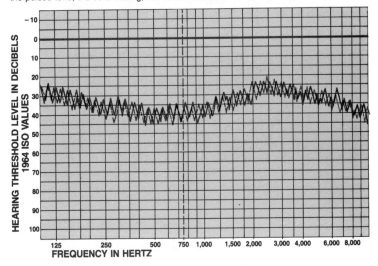

Figure B: Type II tracing that shows characteristic 10 to 20 dB separation of curves; seen in patients with cochlear hearing losses.

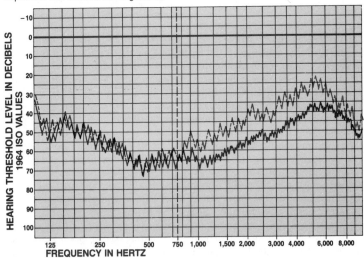

hears a tone. Except in cases of functional hearing loss, the pulsed tone always has a better pure tone threshold than the continuous tone. Audiometric tracings show excursions above and below the patient's actual threshold. Test results fall into one of five categories, four of which are illustrated here (see chart for explanations).

Figure C: Type III tracings similar to this one may appear with retrocochlear pathology. This tracing, conducted at three discrete frequencies, shows rapid decline in threshold only for the continuous tone.

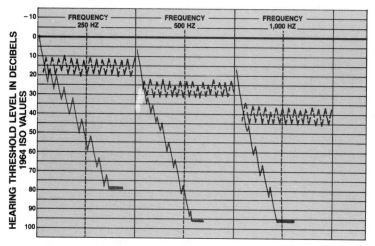

Figure D: Type IV tracing that shows marked curve separation with the continuous tone tracing reaching a plateau more than 20 dB below that for the pulsed tone. This pattern may be seen in patients with neural or severe cochlear lesions.

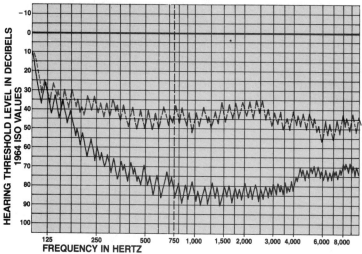

Adapted with permission from Jack Katz, *The Handbook of Clinical Audiology* (2nd ed.; Baltimore: Williams & Wilkins Co., 1978).

cochlear from retrocochlear lesions, and often can localize lesions in the retrocochlear system at the eighth nerve, extra-axial (peripheral) or intra-axial brain stem, and in the cortex. Some commonly used site of lesion tests include alternate binaural loudness balance (ABLB), simultaneous binaural midplane localization (SBMPL), tone decay, Békésy audiometry, masking level differences (MLD), difficult speech discrimination tasks, auditory brain stem electrical response measures (ABR), and competing message (CM) tasks.

When performing site of lesion tests, the intensity of the test signal is distinguished from the sensation level. Intensity is the hearing level (HL) shown on the audiometer dial, and sensation level (SL) is the number of decibels above the patient's threshold for that signal. For example, a patient with a threshold of zero dB HL hears a 60 dB HL tone at 60 dB SL; a patient with a 40 dB HL threshold (or a 40 dB hearing loss) hears the same tone at 20 dB SL. The distinction between HL and SL is diagnostically important because, in many tests, a person with a cochlear hearing loss performs as well as a person with normal hearing if intensity levels are held constant; sensation levels, however, may be quite different.

By itself, the site of lesion test battery cannot diagnose a disorder, but it can suggest the location and extent of damage to the auditory system. However, air and bone conduction thresholds and aural immittance tests must rule out or measure the extent of conductive hearing before site of lesion tests can be performed.

Purpose

☐ To distinguish cochlear from retrocochlear hearing loss
☐ To localize lesions in the retrocochlear component of the auditory system.

Patient preparation

Explain to the patient that this group of tests helps locate the probable cause of hearing impairment. Inform him that the tests are performed by an audiologist who thoroughly explains each procedure before it is done, and that the test battery takes approximately 90 minutes.

Procedure

Earphones are used for each test.

ABLB: A tone is alternately presented to one ear and then the other. The tone in one ear is held at a constant intensity of 90 dB HL, whereas the other tone is varied. The patient indicates when the tones sound equally loud to both ears.

SBMPL: A 90 dB HL tone is presented to one ear and tones of varying intensity are simultaneously presented to the other ear. The patient indicates when he perceives a single tone in the center of his head.

Tone decay: A tone is presented at or near threshold and the patient indicates how long he can hear it. If the tone becomes inaudible or changes to a buzzing or hissing sound, the tone is raised 5 dB, which produces a tone that the patient should again be able to hear. The process is repeated until the patient hears the tone continuously for 60 seconds.

Békésy audiometry: In this test, the patient controls the tone intensity by depressing a response button whenever he hears a tone. When the tone softens and disappears, he releases the button; the tone then becomes louder. The patient repeats this procedure for several minutes, and the resulting audiometric tracing shows excursions above and below the actual threshold. The audiometer is set to sweep across frequencies or to record at one frequency. When the test is being used for site of lesion studies, the threshold for a pulsing tone is determined; then the threshold for a continuous tone is determined. Test results conform to one of five types of curves (see accompanying illustration for more information).

MLD: A 500-Hz tone and a narrow-band masking noise are presented to both ears at once. The noise is held at a constant intensity, and the patient's threshold for the tonal stimulus in that noise is determined. Then, the phase of the tone to one ear is changed by 180°.

AUDITORY BRAIN STEM ELECTRIC RESPONSE
(4,000 Hz TONE PIP AT 75 dB nHL)

Auditory brain stem response: In this test, auditory neural activity is recorded as it passes from the peripheral or cochlear end organ through the brain stem to the cortex. Wave I is associated with the acoustic nerve response, while Wave V is associated with an upper brain stem response.

Waves I and V are considered to be the most clinically useful. The test is repeated for accuracy; thus each graph below shows two sets of wave forms. Both wave forms follow the same pattern, confirming test results.

Normal tracing

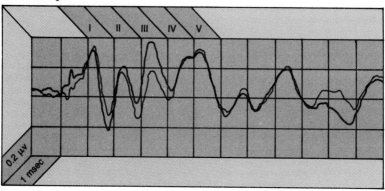

Tracing in cochlear hearing loss

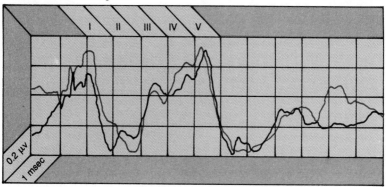

INTERPRETING SITE OF LESION TEST RESULTS

TEST	FINDINGS	IMPLICATIONS
Alternate binaural loudness balance	Patient interprets two sounds of equal intensity as being equally loud	• *Cochlear lesion:* tones sound equally loud at 90 dB HL; recruitment, a sudden growth in loudness in the recruiting ear, occurs • *Retrocochlear lesion:* no recruitment; difference between ears at 90 dB HL equals or exceeds the difference between ears at threshold levels
Simultaneous binaural midplane localization	Single tone heard in center of head when both tone intensities are equal	• *Cohlear lesion:* response same as normal • *Retrocochlear lesion:* tones never sound centered; or, both ears may require significantly different intensities for midline perception; may indicate nerve or intra-axial brain stem lesion
Tone decay	Patient may require 0 to 10 dB above threshold to perceive tone for 60 seconds	• *Cochlear lesion:* may require a tone up to 30 dB above threshold • *Retrocochlear lesion:* may require a tone greater than 30 dB above threshold
Békésy audiometry	*Type I audiogram:* tracings generally overlap in both pulsed and continuous mode	• *Type I:* same as normal with conductive hearing loss (see p. 606) • *Type II:* continuous trace falls 10 to 20 dB below pulsed trace (see p. 606); may indicate cochlear loss • *Type III:* pulsed trace continues at threshold level; continuous trace drops to equipment limits (see p. 607); may indicate auditory fatigue, possible neural lesion, such as acoustic neuroma • *Type IV:* pulsed trace continues at threshold level; continuous trace drops more than 20 dB and plateaus (see p. 607); may occur with neural or severe cochlear lesions • *Type V:* pulsed trace drops below continuous trace; suggests uncooperative patient; no physiological explanation

INTERPRETING SITE OF LESION TEST RESULTS

TEST	FINDINGS	IMPLICATIONS
Masking level differences	Tone heard subjectively louder in antiphasic mode; threshold difference between homophasic and antiphasic conditions is about 12 dB	• Little or no difference between conditions may suggest eighth nerve or intra-axial brain stem lesion
Difficult speech discrimination tasks (in white noise)	Scores in quiet and in noise differ by 40% or less	• Difference of more than 40% between scores may indicate a lesion anywhere in the auditory system
Auditory brainstem electrical response	Series of 5 potentials: wave I appears 2 milliseconds after stimulus; other waves follow at 1-millisecond intervals. Waves diminish as stimulus level is lowered; wave V, occurring within 10 dB of behavioral threshold, disappears last (see normal tracing, p. 609)	• *Cochlear lesion:* normal response at high intensities; depending on the degree and configuration of cochlear loss, wave V may occur slightly later than normal and earlier waves may be distorted (see p. 609) • *Retrocochlear lesion:* possible absent or late waves at high intensities; possible increased interval between waves I and V; possible decreased amplitude of wave V to less than half that of wave I
Gross competing message tasks (Northwestern University test #20)	Same score with and without competing message	• *Cortical damage:* poor scores from ear opposite the damage
Precise competing message tasks (dichotic nonsense syllables test)	About 80% in right ear; about 65% in left ear	• *Cortical damage:* poor scores from ear opposite the damage; better than normal scores from other ear • *Lesions of left hemisphere:* possible low scores from both ears • *Lesions of the corpus callosum:* possible lower scores from left ear

This minimal change, which cannot be heard by either ear individually, makes the tone subjectively louder for the binaural system. A new threshold is then obtained at this level. Although MLD is quite sensitive to small neural lesions, it must be used cautiously, because peripheral losses can affect the results. The test can also employ spondaic words in noise instead of a tone in noise.

Difficult speech discrimination tasks: An example of this type of test is speech discrimination in white noise. A speech stimulus is presented to one ear and the result is scored, then white noise and speech stimulus are simultaneously presented to the same ear and the result is scored. The two scores are compared; then the task is repeated for the other ear and its scores compared. Finally, each ear's score is compared with the other's and with normal range.

ABR: Electrodes are placed at the vertex of the patient's scalp (active), the mastoid process or earlobe of the stimulated ear (reference), and the mastoid process, or earlobe of the opposite ear (ground). Stimuli, in the form of clicks or rapid rise time (1 millisecond) tone pips, are presented at 10/second until 2,000 time-locked responses are collected and averaged.

The origins of the peaks are complex, but primary contributors may be the eighth nerve (Wave I), cochlear nucleus (Wave II), superior olive (Wave III), and lateral lemniscus and inferior colliculus (Waves IV and V). To estimate thresholds, responses to stimuli are collected at decreasing intensities until Wave V disappears from the trace. Cochlear and retrocochlear lesions are differentiated by presenting click stimuli at high intensities and comparing the absolute latencies of waves I, III, and V, and the interwave latency differences between ears and to normal data.

CM tasks: In these tests, a different message is presented to each ear and the patient is asked to discriminate between the messages. In a gross measure test, such as the Northwestern University test #20, speech discrimination words are presented to one ear and the patient is asked to repeat them. Then, speech discrimination words are presented to the same ear and short sentences are simultaneously presented to the other ear, and the patient is asked to repeat the words and ignore the sentences. The patient's scores at each task are then compared.

Dichotic nonsense syllables test: In a precise measure test such as this, carefully aligned nonsense syllables are presented to both ears at once, and the patient is asked to repeat or write both syllables. The number of syllables correctly identified during the testing of each ear are compared with each other and with a normal range.

Precautions

Patient cooperation is essential for adequate test results.

Findings

Basing the choice of site of lesion tests on the patient's history and other medical information, the audiologist selects the appropriate test battery. The charts on pages 607 and 609 list normal responses to different site of lesion tests.

Implications of results

Site of lesion tests can rule out cochlear and retrocochlear lesions. If a lesion is present, these tests help distinguish its type. The chart on pages 610 and 611 gives specific implications of each test in a typical site of lesion battery.

Post-test care

None.

Interfering factors

□ Severe hearing loss can interfere with accurate testing.
□ Poor electrode placement or equipment failure can interfere with the ABR test.
□ A tense or uncooperative patient may cause unreliable test results.
□ Cochlear or brain stem lesions interfere with competing message tests.

CHERYL LONGINOTTI, PhD
CYNTHIA G. FOWLER, PhD

VESTIBULAR TESTS

Falling and Past-pointing Tests

Falling and past-pointing tests, performed as part of a neuro-otologic examination, screen for vestibular or cerebellar dysfunction in a patient who complains of dizziness, dysequilibrium, or nystagmus. These tests evaluate balance and coordination as the patient performs various maneuvers with eyes open and closed. Abnormal results suggest the need for further evaluation.

Purpose
□ To help identify vestibular or cerebellar disorders affecting the entire body (falling test)
□ To help identify vestibular or cerebellar disorders affecting the arms (past-pointing test).

Patient preparation
Describe the tests to the patient, and explain that these tests help identify neurologic dysfunction. Tell him some tests are performed to evaluate sense of balance. Reassure him that he will not fall and that someone will stand next to him.

Assess the patient's general physical condition, since it influences his ability to perform the maneuvers. Check the patient's history for ingestion of drugs that affect the CNS and for recent alcohol consumption.

Procedure
Falling test: Instruct the patient to perform as many of the following maneuvers as possible, and observe for marked swaying or falling. First, ask him to stand with feet together, arms at his sides, and eyes open for 20 seconds; then tell him to maintain this position for another 20 seconds with eyes closed (Romberg test). Next, have the patient stand on one foot for 5 seconds, then on

the other foot for 5 seconds; instruct him to repeat the procedure with eyes closed. Then tell him to stand heel to toe for 20 seconds with eyes opened, then to maintain the same position with eyes closed for another 20 seconds. Finally, instruct him to walk forward and backward in a straight line, heel to toe, first with eyes open, then with eyes closed.

Past-pointing test: With the patient seated and facing you, hold out your index finger at his shoulder level. Instruct him to touch your finger with his right index finger. Then tell him to lower his arm, close his eyes, and touch your finger again. Have the patient repeat the entire maneuver using his left index finger. Observe the degree and direction of past-pointing.

Precautions
□ The falling and past-pointing tests, or parts of them, are contraindicated in patients physically unable to perform all or some of the maneuvers.
□ During the falling test, the examiner should stand close to the patient to catch him if he falls. If the patient is tall or heavy, someone should assist the examiner.

Findings
In the falling test, a healthy person maintains his balance with eyes open and closed. In the past-pointing test, a healthy person touches the examiner's finger with eyes open and closed.

Implications of results
A peripheral vestibular lesion can cause swaying or falling in the direction opposite to the nystagmus when the patient's eyes are closed; a cerebellar lesion causes swaying or falling when eyes are open or closed. A labyrinthine disorder can lead to past-pointing in the opposite direction to the nystagmus when the patient's eyes are closed; a cerebellar lesion can lead to past-pointing when eyes are

open or closed; and a lateralized lesion, past-pointing only with the arm on the affected side.

Post-test care
None.

Interfering factors
Drugs that affect the CNS—such as stimulants, anti-anxiety agents, sedatives, and medications to relieve vertigo—and alcohol interfere with accurate testing.

CHERYL LONGINOTTI, PhD
CYNTHIA G. FOWLER, PhD

Electronystagmography

In *electronystagmography, eye movements in response to specific stimuli are permanently recorded and used to evaluate the interactions of the vestibular system and the muscles controlling eye movement, in what is known as the vestibulo-ocular reflex. Nystagmus, the involuntary back-and-forth eye movement caused by this reflex, results from the vestibular system's attempts to maintain visual fixation during head movements. When the head turns in one direction, the eyes deviate slowly in the opposite direction; on reaching their deviation limit, they quickly return to the center. If the head continues to turn, the pattern of eye movements continues.*

The nystagmus cycle has two parts: slow deviation against the direction of the turn, or the slow phase, is controlled by the vestibular system; rapid return to center, or the fast phase, is controlled by the CNS. Nystagmus is described as "beating" in the direction of the fast phase. Thus, a head turn to the right yields a right-beating nystagmus, with its slow phase to the left and its fast phase to the right.

Nystagmus accompanying a head turn is normal; prolonged nystagmus following a head turn is abnormal. Because of the interaction of the vestibular and

ocular systems, abnormal nystagmus can result from lesions of either system; such lesions can be peripheral (end organ or vestibular nerve involvement) or central (CNS—cerebellar or brain stem involvement). Abnormal nystagmus is the primary sign of vestibular disturbances, such as dizziness or vertigo. Electronystagmography is the technique for monitoring nystagmus; the battery of tests used to elicit the nystagmus includes calibration, gaze, pendulum tracking, optokinetics, positional methods, and caloric tests. Electronystagmography relies on the corneoretinal potential—the difference of 1 millivolt between the positive charge of the cornea and the negative charge of the retina—to record nystagmus through electrodes placed near the eyes. As the eyes move horizontally or vertically, the electrodes pick up the corneoretinal potential and feed it to a recorder, which amplifies the signal and charts it. This method permits recording of the nystagmus in dimly lit surroundings, with the patient's eyes open or closed.

Purpose
□ To help identify the cause of dizziness, vertigo, or tinnitus
□ To help diagnose unilateral hearing loss of unknown origin
□ To confirm the presence of a lesion, and to determine its location (central, peripheral, or both).

Patient preparation
Describe the tests to the patient, and explain that this battery of tests evaluates visual and balance control mechanisms. Instruct him to observe the following pretest restrictions: if ordered, to abstain from stimulants, antianxiety agents, sedatives, antivertigo drugs, and alcohol for 24 to 48 hours before the test; to abstain from tobacco and beverages containing caffeine the day of the test; and not to eat a heavy meal immediately before electronystagmography, since caloric testing may cause transient nausea. Tell him who will perform the tests, that he will receive instructions before each

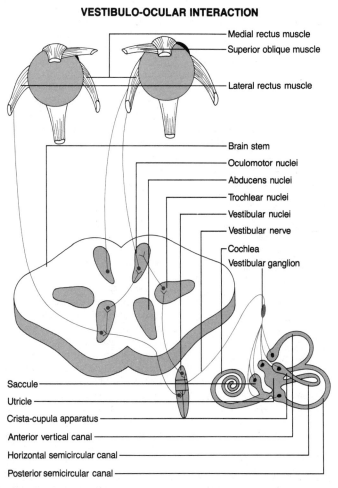

VESTIBULO-OCULAR INTERACTION

Medial rectus muscle
Superior oblique muscle
Lateral rectus muscle

Brain stem
Oculomotor nuclei
Abducens nuclei
Trochlear nuclei
Vestibular nuclei
Vestibular nerve
Cochlea
Vestibular ganglion

Saccule
Utricle
Crista-cupula apparatus
Anterior vertical canal
Horizontal semicircular canal
Posterior semicircular canal

Head movement causes the fluid in the vestibular apparatus to move against receptor cells in the semicircular canals (cristae and cupulae) and in the saccule and utricle. This simplified innervation scheme shows the brain stem nuclei that control the extrinsic eye muscles with their connections to the sensory receptors in the horizontal semicircular canal. In the right labyrinth, note the main connections to the medial rectus muscle of the right eye and the lateral rectus of the left eye.

Adapted with permission from T.J. Glattke, "Electronystagmography," in J. Katz, ed., *Handbook of Clinical Audiology* (Baltimore: Williams & Wilkins Co., 1978.)

test, and that the battery of tests takes 60 to 90 minutes to perform. Reassure him that someone will be nearby during all tests and won't permit him to fall.

If the patient wears glasses, tell him to bring them with him. Emphasize the importance of fully documenting his ex-

perience to ensure an accurate diagnosis. Provide emotional support, since the test can be very uncomfortable at times. Keep in mind that the patient must cooperate fully to achieve accurate test results.

Obtain a complete patient history, including general emotional and physical

GLOSSARY

Conjugate deviation: drawing of the eyes to one side in unison.

Directional preponderance: a difference in beat intensity in one direction versus the other direction.

Nystagmus: the involuntary, rhythmic, back-and-forth movement of the eyes, usually composed of a slow deviation in one direction and a rapid return in the other; *fast phase of nystagmus:* the quick jerky component of nystagmus controlled by the CNS; *horizontal nystagmus:* nystagmus in the horizontal plane, either left- or right-beating; *inverted nystagmus:* nystagmus that beats in the direction opposite to that anticipated; *positional nystagmus:* a persistent nystagmus that appears on assumption of a particular head position; *positioning nystagmus:* a transient nystagmus occurring immediately after a change in head position; *rotary nystagmus:* a nystagmus that rotates about the axis of the eye; *slow phase of nystagmus:* the vestibular phase of nystagmus or the slow deviation of the eyes from the midline; *spontaneous nystagmus:* a nystagmus occurring in the absence of stimuli; *vertical nystagmus:* occurring in the vertical plane, either up- or down-beating.

Saccades: the rapid, involuntary jerky movements that occur simultaneously in both eyes when they change their fixation to a new point.

Unilateral weakness: a decreased intensity of nystagmus after one ear stimulus as compared to the other.

condition, recent medication history, and a description of symptoms, such as the nature of the sensation and its frequency, severity, duration, and first occurrence. Also include data on related problems, such as hearing loss, tinnitus, fullness in the ears, ear infection or surgery, or headaches; visual disorders or head trauma; weakness, numbness, slurred speech, difficulty in swallowing, or confusion; and neck or back conditions that limit the patient's ability to assume the positions required for the positional test portion of electronystagmography.

Just before electronystagmography, perform an otoscopic examination. If the patient's ear canals are filled with cerumen, they should be cleaned.

Equipment

Two-channel differential amplifier with high- and low-frequency filters/strip-chart recorder/electrodes (one for ground; two for horizontal and two for vertical recordings)/electrode paste/adhesive tape/cotton and 70% alcohol/examining table with headrest and adjustable back.

For *water caloric tests:* two water pans/water pump and hose, with foot switch control/two thermostatically controlled heaters: one set at 86° F. (30° C.), the other set at 111.2° F. (44° C.)/timer/emesis basin/fingercot (for protecting middle ear if the patient has a perforated eardrum).

For *air caloric tests:* air pump and hose, with foot switch control/timer/air heater with thermostat.

For *ice water caloric tests:* 20 ml of ice water/irrigating syringe.

Procedure

The electronystagmography battery and test sequence discussed here is representative. Although test sequence may vary, caloric tests are usually done last. When performing the tests, indicate the name of the test, and note if the recording stylus has been recentered or if any unusual event occurs during the test. Tell the patient to follow all instructions. For the ocular tests, allow adequate opportunity for him to learn the tasks. For the positional tests, do *not* permit him to practice the positions before the recording, since this movement may fatigue the nystagmus and give inaccurate results.

Because the corneoretinal potential is labile, calibrate the equipment at the start of the battery and before each caloric test. Don't touch the gain knob on the amplifier except for calibration, but the balance knob may be adjusted, as needed, without affecting calibration. If the stylus becomes pinned to one side of the graph and cannot be centered, the electrodes may need to be repositioned.

Calibration test: Have the patient sit upright on the examining table, with his head against the headrest and his eyes directed toward a light bar 6' to 10' (180 to 300 cm) away. Tell him to hold

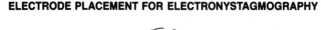

ELECTRODE PLACEMENT FOR ELECTRONYSTAGMOGRAPHY

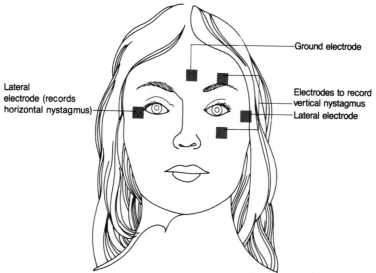

Ground electrode

Lateral electrode (records horizontal nystagmus)

Electrodes to record vertical nystagmus

Lateral electrode

To insure accurate electronystagmography results, test electrodes must be positioned properly. However, before placing the electrodes, the patient's skin must be prepared as follows. First, the contact points of each electrode are scrubbed with a cotton pad saturated with alcohol, and they are air dried. A small amount of electrode paste is then rubbed into the patient's skin at each contact point. Just before placement, an adhesive collar is placed on the electrode and the electrode cup is filled with paste. Next, the backing is peeled from the adhesive collar and the electrode is pressed firmly against the patient's skin.

The ground electrode, which minimizes line noise interference, is positioned in the neutral position in the center of the patient's forehead, midway between the eyes. If horizontal nystagmus is being recorded, two lateral electrodes are placed as close to the outer canthus of each eye as possible without interfering with eye closure. If vertical nystagmus is being recorded, two additional electrodes are positioned directly above and below the center of one eye. (Generally, only one eye is monitored for vertical nystagmus.) It is important that the eye isn't artificial or paralyzed, and that there is no disconjugate movement between the eyes.

After the electrodes are positioned, the impedance in each pair is determined; if impedance exceeds 10,000 ohms, the electrode is reapplied. The electrode paste must be allowed to stablize for 5 minutes before starting the test.

his head still and to follow the light only with his eyes. Center the stylus, set the paper speed to 5 mm/second, and start the recorder. Move the light so that the patient's eyes deviate 10° to the right of center. By adjusting gain and balance, fix the stylus sensitivity so the 10° deviation of the eyes corresponds to a 10-mm deflection of the stylus on the chart. Move the light back to the center, then to the left, and readjust the stylus

position until its deflection again matches eye deviation.

To detect ocular dysmetria, move the light in this sequence: center, 10° right, center, and 10° left, stopping in each position for about 2 seconds. Repeat this sequence until you get two cycle tracings that represent the patient's best tracking ability.

Gaze nystagmus test: Remove the visual target from the previous test. Place the patient in a comfortable seated or supine position, and have him close his eyes. To keep his mind off the eye motion itself, give him a mental arithmetic task to do, while you record spontaneous eye motion for 30 seconds.

To record center gaze nystagmus, have the patient look straight ahead, with his eyes fixed on the center light. Record for 30 seconds. Then, tell him to close his eyes without changing their position; record for another 30 seconds. On the chart, mark the transition point from open to closed eyes.

EDITING ELECTRONYSTAGMOGRAPHY FINDINGS

Only a small part of the charts produced during electronystagmography is diagnostically useful. It's important to edit these charts carefully, because the doctor generally uses only the edited version to prepare his report, and the patient's permanent records contain only the edited charts and report. Before editing the charts, however, be sure to check with the doctor. He may prefer to see the unedited version and, should there be legal action, the edited version wouldn't stand up in court. When editing the charts, clearly mark any factors affecting the test procedure such as poor eyesight, drowsiness, neck or back conditions that caused some tests to be eliminated, medications, or the patient's refusal to undergo certain tests. Then, for each test, select the most representative portions, as follows:

- *Calibration:* two or three cycles
- *Spontaneous nystagmus:* 20 seconds
- *Gaze:* 20 seconds of eyes opened and closed for each condition
- *Optokinetics:* 20 seconds each of eyes opened and closed following tracking
- *Pendulum tracking:* 20 seconds each of eyes opened and closed following tracking
- *Positional tests:* 3 seconds baseline and 20 seconds following assumption of the posture.

If nystagmus lasted longer than 20 seconds, indicate the duration. If a posture was repeated, save this tracing, and label it clearly. Report any of the patient's sensations.

- *Calorics:* 20 seconds of the most intense nystagmus; include the part used for velocity measurements, as well as 10 seconds of tracing made with the eyes open. Report any of the patient's sensations.

Calculating slow-phase velocity (SPV)

In caloric tests, nystagmus strength is measured in terms of total duration, frequency of beats, and highest velocity of the slow phase. SPV, the most reliable measurement, is expressed as the highest average velocity over a 5-second period. A unilateral weakness (more than 20% difference in maximum SPV for the two ears) or a directional preponderance (more than 20% to 30% difference in the maximum SPV for right- and left-beating nystagmus) can be determined by the following formulas:

$$\text{unilateral weakness} = \frac{(LC+LW) - (RC+RW)}{(LC+LW+RC+RW)} \times 100\%$$

$$\text{directional preponderance} = \frac{(LC+RW) - (RC+LW)}{(LC+LW+RC+RW)} \times 100\%$$

in which: LC = maximum SPV for the left ear, cold stimulus
RC = maximum SPV for the right ear, cold stimulus
LW = maximum SPV for the left ear, warm stimulus
RW = maximum SPV for the right ear, warm stimulus

You can read the SPV directly from the velocity channel, if one is available, or you can obtain them from the nystagmus channel in the following way: On the chart, draw 10 lines that parallel the slow-phase segments of the nystagmus trace so they intersect the vertical chart lines spanning 1 second. These lines form 10 small triangles; each triangle has as its baseline the time interval of 1 second, and as its hypotenuse the sloped line parallel to the slow phase segment of the nystagmus trace. Count the number of millimeters along the vertical side of each triangle. Because the initial calibration established a relation of 1 mm to 1°/second, you obtain 10 readings of eye speed in degrees per second. Average these to obtain SPV.

To read SPV from the velocity trace (assuming the same calibration), count the vertical difference in millimeters from the peaks to the baselines of 10 representative intervals and take the average. Both methods should yield similar results.

To record right-gaze nystagmus, tell the patient to look at the center light, and start the stylus near the right margin of the chart. Instruct him to move his eyes to the right, on cue, and to fix them on a light 25° to the right of center; record for 30 seconds. Then tell the patient to close his eyes but to maintain eye position; record for 30 seconds. Mark the transition from open to closed eyes. To record left-gaze nystagmus, proceed as above, but have the patient look at a light set at 20° and then at 30° to the left of center. Start the stylus near the left margin of the chart.

Pendulum tracking test: Have the patient look straight ahead. Activate the pendulum movement or a light that mimics this movement, and ask the patient to follow the target with his eyes. Record until you obtain 20 seconds of tracings that reflect the patient's best tracking ability. Then tell the patient to close his eyes while looking straight ahead, and record for 30 seconds.

Optokinetics test: Tell the patient to look straight ahead. If there is a velocity channel, set it to read *left*-beating nystagmus. Adjust the stimulus to travel across the patient's visual field, from left to right, at about 20°/second. Instruct the patient to follow the target across his visual field until it disappears, then to snap his eyes back to meet the next target and follow it across, and so on. Continue recording until you've obtained 20 seconds of the patient's best responses. Then instruct him to look straight ahead with his eyes closed, and record for another 30 seconds.

Repeat the procedure, setting the velocity channel to read *right*-beating nystagmus and adjusting the stimulus to move from right to left. Mark the transition from right to left on the chart.

Positional tests: Obtain a baseline recording for about 5 seconds before having the patient assume each of the nine test positions and identify each transition on the chart.

□ Erect to head right: Instruct the patient to sit erect, with eyes forward and closed. On cue, have him turn his head quickly to the right as far as he can. Instruct him to maintain this posture; record for 30 seconds or until nystagmus subsides (if it doesn't, stop recording after 90 seconds). Then have him slowly turn his head back to center. If nystagmus occurs, repeat the maneuver. If dizziness occurs, note this on the chart.

□ Erect to head left: Repeat the above maneuver, with the patient's head turned to the left.

□ Erect to supine: Lower the back of the examining table to the horizontal position. Instruct the patient to sit erect at one end, with his eyes closed and centered. On cue, have him quickly lie flat on his back; record for 30 seconds or until nystagmus subsides, or stop recording after 90 seconds if nystagmus continues. If nystagmus occurs, repeat the maneuver.

□ Supine to erect: Repeat as above, but have the patient quickly sit erect from a supine position.

□ Supine to lateral right: Have the patient lie supine, with eyes closed and head supported by a pillow. Instruct him to turn his body and head quickly to the right; record for 30 seconds or until nystagmus subsides, or stop recording after 90 seconds if nystagmus continues. Instruct the patient to return slowly to the supine position; repeat the maneuver if nystagmus occurred.

□ Supine to lateral left: Repeat the procedure above, with the patient quickly turning his body and head to the left.

□ Erect to head hanging: Remove the headrest from the examining table. Instruct the patient to sit erect, with eyes forward and closed. Position him so his head will clear the other end of the table when he lies down. On cue, instruct him to lie back quickly, letting his head hang over the edge; record for 30 seconds or until nystagmus subsides, or stop recording after 90 seconds if nystagmus continues. Repeat the maneuver if nystagmus occurred. Record on the chart any sensation reported by the patient.

□ Head hanging to erect: Repeat as above, but have the patient move from the head-hanging position to an erect position.

RESULTS OF ELECTRONYSTAGMOGRAPHY

TEST AND NORMAL FINDINGS	ABNORMAL FINDINGS	USUAL INDICATIONS
Calibration Square wave pattern indicates accurate, repeatable eye movement (1)	*Ocular dysmetria:* results from inability of the ocular system to exert fine control over eye movements; results in "overshoots" or "undershoots" in pattern (2)	Lesion in cerebellum or cerebellar brain stem pathways
Spontaneous nystagmus (No external stimulus) Eyes open: no nystagmus; eyes closed: some weak horizontal (less than 7°/second) or vertical (less than 10°/second) nystagmus (4)	*Ocular nystagmus:* diminishes at a particular angle of gaze and with convergence of eyes; with upward gaze, it's horizontal	Most prevalent as a congenital, nonlesional disorder; some forms caused by poor vision
	Vestibular nystagmus: horizontal direction; suppressed with visual fixation; unidirectional beats; fast and slow components (3)	Peripheral or central (brain stem or cerebellar) lesion
	Central nystagmus: unclassified as above	Central lesion
Positional (head in position) **Positioning** (head in movement to the position usually taken together)	*Type I—persistent, direction-changing nystagmus:* duration, more than 1 minute; beats in different directions, depending on head position	Nonlocalized lesion
	Type II—persistent, direction-fixed nystagmus: duration, more than 1 minute; beats in same direction regardless of head position; intensity may vary	Nonlocalized lesion
Eyes open: no nystagmus; eyes closed: weak nystagmus (less than 7°/second) in one or more positions (5)	*Type III—transitory, fixed, or changeable direction nystagmus:* duration, less than 1 minute; benign paroxysmal nystagmus is the most common form, marked by a latent period, a transient burst of nystagmus, severe vertigo, and fatigue upon repeating the position (6A and 6B)	Peripheral lesion (usually); occurs in the elderly, after head trauma, with middle ear pathology. Nystagmus that changes direction during a position may indicate cerebellar or brain stem pathology. (Drug effects must be ruled out.)
Pendulum tracking Sinusoidal waveform for stimuli with excursions of 40° and eye speeds of 40° to 50°/second (7)	Sinusoidal tracking with superimposed *saccades* or nystagmus	End organ or brain stem pathology
	Disrupted (ataxic) sinusoidal tracking (8)	Brain stem pathology (If spontaneous nystagmus wasn't present before the test, there should be none following it when eyes are closed. Its presence, a form of provoked nystagmus, is a nonlocalizing sign.)

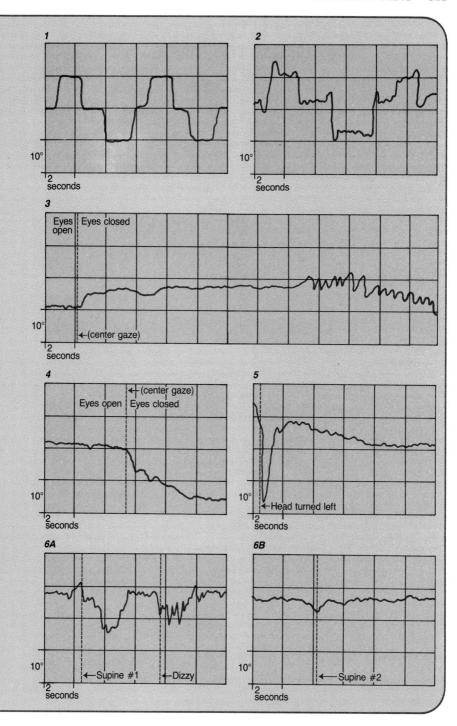

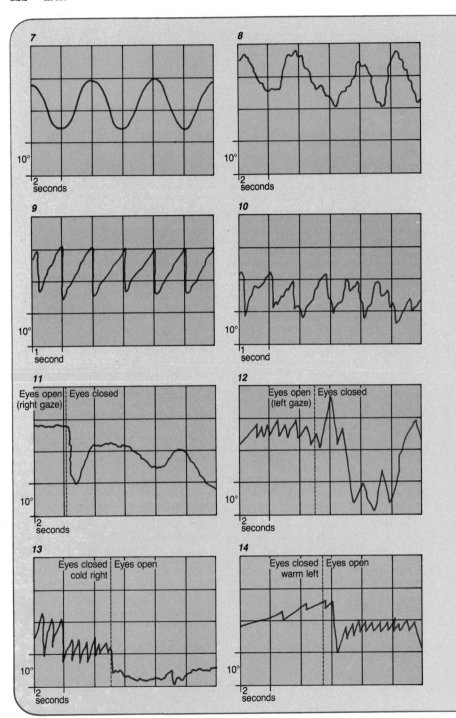

RESULTS OF ELECTRONYSTAGMOGRAPHY

TEST AND NORMAL FINDINGS	ABNORMAL FINDINGS	USUAL INDICATIONS
Optokinetics Stimulus followed up to 30°/second; clear triangular wave pattern; similar pattern for stimuli travelling in both directions (9)	Difference in slow-phase velocities of the nystagmus resulting from stimuli to left and right greater than 20°/second	Nonlocalized lesion
	Disconjugate eye movements or reduced velocity in both directions (10)	Cerebellar or brain stem pathology
	Asymmetry in velocities in the direction of spontaneous nystagmus	Peripheral lesion producing strong spontaneous vestibular nystagmus; may also result from drug use, inattention, and advancing age. (When the eyes are closed, nystagmus should cease; its persistence is a sign of nonlocalized pathology.)
Gaze nystagmus (eyes deviated from center) Eyes closed: weak nystagmus (less than 7°/second). End point nystagmus may occur when eyes are deviated to their limit (11)	*Peripheral gaze nystagmus:* horizontal or horizontal-rotatory; inhibited by visual fixation; beats strongest with gaze in direction of fast phase	Peripheral lesion
	Central gaze nystagmus: bilateral nystagmus that beats in different directions, depending on direction of gaze; suppressed with eyes closed; nystagmus may change direction even though gaze remains constant, or it may move in a horizontal, vertical, oblique, and rotary direction (12)	Central lesion (Drug effects must be ruled out.)
Water calorics Eyes closed: nystagmus occurs in all conditions; suppressed by visual fixation (13). With cold stimuli, nystagmus beats to the opposite ear; with warm stimuli, it beats to the same ear. (The acronym COWS—cold opposite, warm same—helps to recall this phenomenon.)	*Unilateral weakness:* more than 20% difference in maximum slow-phase velocities	Peripheral lesion of weaker side
	Bilateral weakness: slow-phase velocity less than 7°/second	Bilateral peripheral lesion (usually); possibly a brain stem lesion
	Hyperexcitability of vestibular system: slow-phase velocity more than 50°/second	Possible CNS lesion or anxious patient
	Directional preponderance: more than 20% to 30% difference in slow-phase velocities for right and left beating nystagmus	Pathologic but may indicate peripheral or cerebellar/brain stem lesions
	Failure to suppress fixation: visual fixation fails to reduce nystagmus by at least 20% (14)	Cerebellar or brain stem pathology
	Inverted or distorted nystagmus	Cerebellar or brain stem pathology

□ Erect to head hanging right/left: Repeat as above, but as the patient moves from the erect to the head-hanging position, tell him to turn his head to the right. Then ask him to repeat the movement, but to turn his head to the left.

Water caloric test: Have the patient lie supine with his head elevated 30°, so his lateral semicircular canals are perpendicular to the floor. Place a towel and emesis basin under his ear to collect the water as it drains from the ear. Except as noted below, instruct the patient to close his eyes during and after stimulation. Inform him when stimulation is about to begin, so he isn't startled by the sudden rush of water in his ear. Introduce water into the ear canal so it hits the tympanic membrane directly, and continue the stimulation for 30 seconds. Then begin the recording immediately; give the patient some mental tasks to keep him alert. After about 60 seconds, tell the patient to open his eyes and fix them on a target, such as his raised thumb. After 10 seconds, tell him to close his eyes; continue recording until the nystagmus subsides, or for a total of 3 minutes. Record on the chart any sensation reported by the patient, as well as the transition from open to closed eyes. Wait 5 minutes before starting the next caloric stimulation. Repeat the test if the stimulation seems inadequate; recalibrate before starting the next test.

Repeat the above procedure with each of these stimuli: 86° F. (30° C.) to the right ear (set velocity channel for left-beating nystagmus), 86° F. (30° C.) to the left ear (set velocity channel for right-beating nystagmus), 111.2° F. (44° C.) to the right ear (set velocity channel for right-beating nystagmus), and 111.2° F. (44° C.) to the left ear (set velocity channel for left-beating nystagmus). Be sure to recalibrate each time.

If the patient has a punctured eardrum, insert a fingercot into the canal to protect the middle ear, and change temperatures to 87° F. (25° C.) for the cool stimulus and to 120.2° F. (49° C.) for the warm stimulus. Alternatively, use air calorics to obtain the same information. Deliver 8 liters of air at 85.2° F. (24° C.) and at 122° F. (50° C.) to each ear separately over 60 seconds.

If the patient fails to respond to standard caloric stimulation, use ice water calorics. Use a blunt syringe to irrigate the ear with 20 ml of ice water. Then, record as you would with standard calorics. After completing caloric testing, carefully lift the electrodes from the patient's face. To avoid spreading the electrode paste, tell him not to rub his eyes. Wipe the paste from his skin.

Precautions

□ Electronystagmography is contraindicated in patients with pacemakers, since the equipment may interfere with pacemaker function.

□ If the patient has a back or neck condition that may be aggravated by rapid changes in position, check with the doctor to determine if any of the positional tests should be omitted.

□ Don't use the usual water caloric tests if the patient has a perforated eardrum. If there is any question about the condition of the eardrum, make sure a doctor has examined the patient and authorized the test. Modified air or water caloric tests, with fingercots in place, may also be substituted. When fingercots are used in such tests, be certain one is placed in each ear equidistant from the tympanic membrane, so both labyrinths are stimulated equally.

Findings

The chart on page 620 shows normal responses to the electronystagmography test battery.

Implications of results

Electronystagmography results are reported as normal, borderline, or abnormal. If results are abnormal, they're further described as indicating a peripheral, central, or undetermined (nonlocalized) lesion. (See the chart on page 620.) A peripheral lesion may involve the end organ or the vestibular branch of the eighth cranial nerve, and may result from conditions such as ototoxicity and eighth nerve tumors. A central lesion may involve the brain stem, cerebellum, cerebrum, or any of the connecting structures, and may result from demyelinating diseases, tumors, and circulatory disorders.

Post-test care

Observe for signs of weakness, dizziness, or nausea. Assist the patient to an area where he can sit comfortably or lie down until he recovers.

Interfering factors

□ CNS stimulants, depressants, and antivertigo agents may suppress nystagmus, cause gaze or positional nystagmus, or reduce the patient's ability to concentrate on the test tasks.

□ Poor eyesight may reduce the patient's ability to perform ocular tests and to suppress nystagmus visually.

□ Drowsiness may suppress any nystagmus that might otherwise occur, and may produce wide, pendular eye movements and alter test results.

□ Blinking the eyes may mimic nystagmus, and thus alter test results.

□ Loose or poorly applied electrodes invalidate test findings.

□ Poor patient cooperation influences test results.

CHERYL LONGINOTTI, PhD
CYNTHIA G. FOWLER, PhD

Selected References

Assessing Your Patients. Nursing Photobook series. Springhouse, Pa.: Springhouse Corp., 1982.

Barber, Hugh O., and Stockwell, Charles W. *Manual of Electronystagmography,* 2nd ed. St. Louis: C.V. Mosby Co., 1980.

Feldman, Alan S., and Wilber, Laura A. *Acoustic Impedance and Admittance: Measurement of Middle Ear Function.* Baltimore: Williams & Wilkins Co., 1976.

Goodhill, Victor. *Ear Disease, Deafness, and Dizziness.* Philadelphia: J.B. Lippincott Co., 1979.

House, W.F., and Luetje, C.M. *Acoustic Tumors: Diagnosis and Management.* Baltimore: University Park Press, 1979.

Jerger, J., and Northern, J., eds. *Clinical Impedance Audiometry,* 2nd ed. Acton, Mass.: American Electromedics, 1980.

Katz, Jack. *The Handbook of Clinical Audiology,* 2nd ed. Baltimore: Williams & Wilkins Co., 1978.

Keith, R.W., ed. *Audiology for the Physician.* Baltimore: Williams & Wilkins Co., 1980.

Lipscomb, D.M. "Anatomy and Physiology of the Hearing Mechanism," in Lass, N.J., et al., eds. *Speech, Language and Hearing.* Philadelphia: W.B. Saunders Co., 1982.

Margolis, R. "Fundamentals of Acoustic Immittance," in Popelka, G.R., ed. *Hearing Assessment with the Acoustic Reflex.* New York: Grune & Stratton, 1981.

Martin, Frederick N., ed. *Introduction to Audiology,* 2nd ed. Englewood Cliffs, N.J.: Prentice-Hall, 1981.

Martin, Frederick N., ed. *Pediatric Audiology.* Englewood Cliffs, N.J.: Prentice-Hall, 1978.

Newby, Hayes A. *Audiology* 4th ed. Englewood Cliffs, N.J.: Prentic Hall, 1979.

Northern, J., ed. *Hearing Disorders,* 2nd ed. Boston: Little, Brown & Co., 1984.

Northern, J., and Downs, M.P. *Hearing in Children,* 3rd ed. Baltimore: Williams & Wilkins Co., 1984.

Rintelmann, W. *Hearing Assessment.* Baltimore: University Park Press, 1979.

Rosenblum, Estelle. *Fundamentals of Hearing for Health Professionals.* Boston: Little, Brown & Co., 1979.

Simmons, F.B., et al. *An Atlas of Electronystagmography.* New York: Grune & Stratton, 1979.

Singh, Roderick P. *Anatomy of Hearing and Speech.* New York: Oxford University Press, 1980.

23 Respiratory System

LEARNING OBJECTIVES

After completing this chapter, the reader will be able to:
- explain the physiology of respiration and list its control mechanisms.
- describe the procedures for evaluating pulmonary dysfunction.
- state the characteristics of pulmonary transudate and exudate.
- explain the staging system for lung cancer.
- describe six common radiographic views of the chest and list anatomic landmarks.
- state the purpose of each test discussed in the chapter.
- prepare the patient physically and psychologically for each test.
- describe the procedure for performing each test.
- specify appropriate precautions for safe administration of each test.
- recognize signs of adverse reaction and respond appropriately.
- implement appropriate post-test care.
- identify the normal findings of each test.
- discuss the implications of abnormal test results.
- list factors that may interfere with accurate test results.

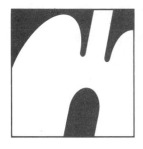

Respiratory System

Introduction

The pulmonary and circulatory systems are designed to provide the body with a continuous supply of oxygen and a quick, efficient removal of carbon dioxide. The pulmonary system controls the exchange of gases between the atmosphere and blood, while the circulatory system transports these gases between the lungs and cells. A dysfunction in either system disrupts homeostasis and causes anoxia and even cell death. Tests described in this chapter are designed to identify and assess such dysfunction.

Pulmonary physiology reviewed

The organs involved in the exchange of gases between the atmosphere and blood are the nose, pharynx, larynx, trachea, bronchi, and lungs. The trachea branches into primary bronchi, secondary bronchi, bronchioles, terminal bronchioles, and finally, alveolar sacs. The walls of the alveolar sacs are called alveoli and are covered by a capillary network of arterioles and venules. The alveoli are the functional units of the lungs responsible for the exchange of gases between the air and blood.

Three concurrent processes permit gas exchange during respiration:

□ *Ventilation* is the movement of air between the atmosphere and the alveoli. This process is the result of the contraction and relaxation of the respiratory muscles (primarily the diaphragm), which compress and distend the lungs and cause the rise or fall of pressure in the alveoli. Inspiration occurs when the pressure in the alveoli is less than atmospheric pressure, and expiration occurs when the pressure in the alveoli is greater than atmospheric pressure.

□ *Diffusion* is the process by which oxygen and carbon dioxide cross the alveolar capillary membrane. Oxygen (at a higher concentration in alveolar air than in blood) and carbon dioxide (at a higher concentration in blood than in alveolar air) move from their respective region of higher concentration to one of lower concentration.

□ *Perfusion* is the injection of blood into an artery that supplies blood to an organ or tissue.

Primary controls

The following mechanisms are the primary controls of respiration:

□ The *nervous system* adjusts the rate of respiration to satisfy physiologic demands. The respiratory center in the brain, which consists of the medulla oblongata and the pons, directs the contraction and relaxation of respiratory muscles.

□ The *Hering-Breuer reflex* controls the depth and rhythm of respiration and prevents overinflation of the lungs. This reflex occurs in response to nerve impulses transmitted from stretch receptors in the bronchi and bronchioles to the respiratory center in the brain.

□ *Carbon dioxide, oxygen, and hydrogen ion concentrations* determine the rate of respiration by acting directly on the respiratory center in the brain or on chemoreceptors located in the carotid arteries and the aorta.

Together, these control mechanisms keep blood oxygen and carbon dioxide levels remarkably stable.

Pulmonary assessment

Clinical evaluation of a patient suspected of pulmonary dysfunction begins with a physical examination and a thorough patient history. A *chest X-ray* usually follows initial assessment and, depending on its results, may be followed by collection of a *sputum specimen,* to deter-

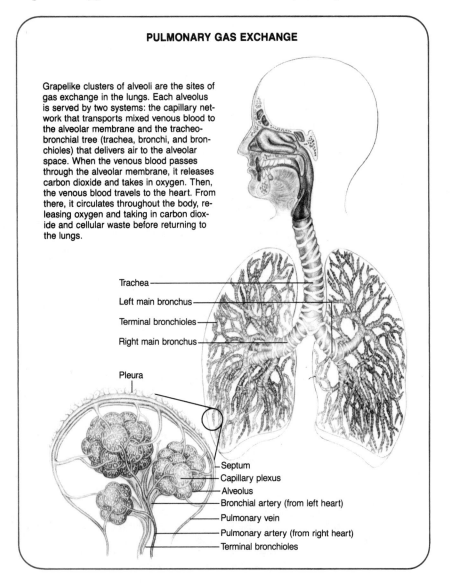

PULMONARY GAS EXCHANGE

Grapelike clusters of alveoli are the sites of gas exchange in the lungs. Each alveolus is served by two systems: the capillary network that transports mixed venous blood to the alveolar membrane and the tracheobronchial tree (trachea, bronchi, and bronchioles) that delivers air to the alveolar space. When the venous blood passes through the alveolar membrane, it releases carbon dioxide and takes in oxygen. Then, the venous blood travels to the heart. From there, it circulates throughout the body, releasing oxygen and taking in carbon dioxide and cellular waste before returning to the lungs.

Trachea

Left main bronchus

Terminal bronchioles

Right main bronchus

Pleura

Septum

Capillary plexus

Alveolus

Bronchial artery (from left heart)

Pulmonary vein

Pulmonary artery (from right heart)

Terminal bronchioles

EVALUATING PULMONARY FUNCTION AND STRUCTURE

TEST	PURPOSE
Volumetric tests	**Assess function**
Lung capacity *Vital capacity* *Inspiratory capacity* *Functional residual capacity* *Total lung capacity* *Forced vital capacity* *Flow-volume curve* *Forced expiratory volume* *Peak expiratory flow* *Maximal midexpiratory flow* *Maximal voluntary ventilation*	• Evaluates ventilatory function of lungs and chest wall; screens for pulmonary disorders • Helps classify pulmonary disorders as restrictive or obstructive • Evaluates severity of any pulmonary disorders
Lung volume *Tidal volume* *Minute volume* *CO_2 response* *Inspiratory reserve volume* *Expiratory reserve volume* *Residual volume* *Thoracic gas volume*	• Evaluates ventilatory function of lungs and chest wall; screens for pulmonary disorders • Helps classify pulmonary disorders as restrictive or obstructive • Evaluates severity of any pulmonary disorders
Endoscopic tests	**Assess structure**
Bronchoscopy	• Directly examines larger airways of tracheobronchial tree
Mediastinoscopy	• Directly examines mediastinum for biopsy (usually supplements bronchoscopy)
Radiographic and scanning tests	**Assess structure, function, and vascular status**
Chest radiography	• Visualizes appearance and status of respiratory system
Paranasal sinus radiography	• Visualizes appearance and status of paranasal sinuses
Fluoroscopy	• Visualizes thoracic organs in motion
Tomography	• Supplements radiographs; visualizes target areas in a series of planes to reveal occult pathology
Bronchography	• Visualizes size and appearance of tracheobronchial tree
Pulmonary angiography	• Visualizes pulmonary vascular system
Lung perfusion scan	• Visualizes distribution of blood flow patterns in lungs
Ventilation scan	• Evaluates ventilatory function
Thoracic computed tomography	• Locates suspected neoplasms, mediastinal nodes, and pleural involvement

mine if dysfunction results from cancer cells, bacteria, or parasites. *Arterial blood gas determinations* can evaluate the patient's ability to exchange a sufficient amount of carbon dioxide for oxygen.

As indicated, *pulmonary function tests* may then identify obstructive or restrictive ventilatory defects. Such tests measure lung capacity and volume, and are useful in screening patients preoperatively to evaluate surgical risk.

Endoscopic examinations permit direct observation of the larger airways.

Such examinations may serve both diagnostic and therapeutic purposes. For example, they allow removal of foreign bodies (with a rigid bronchoscope), secretions, and blood.

Finally, *radiographic and scanning tests* serve a variety of purposes, from screening for asymptomatic cancer to determining perfusion and ventilation abnormalities. These tests visualize the entire pulmonary system or can provide a three-dimensional view of a specific area.

SR. EILEEN MARIE HOLLEN, RN, BSN, CCRN

FUNCTION TESTS

Pulmonary Function Tests

Pulmonary function tests (volume and capacity tests) are a series of measurements that evaluate ventilatory function through spirometric measurements, and are performed on patients with suspected pulmonary dysfunction. Of the seven tests to determine volume, tidal volume (V_T) and expiratory reserve volume (ERV) are direct spirographic measurements; minute volume (V_E), CO_2 response, inspiratory reserve volume (IRV), and residual volume (RV) are calculated from the results of other pulmonary function tests; and thoracic gas volume (TGV) is calculated from body plethysmography. Of the pulmonary capacity tests, vital capacity (VC), inspiratory capacity (IC), functional residual capacity (FRC), total lung capacity (TLC), and maximal midexpiratory flow (MMEF) may be measured directly or calculated from the results of other tests. Forced vital capacity (FVC), flow-volume curve, forced expiratory volume (FEV), peak expiratory flow rate (PEFR), and maximal voluntary ventilation (MVV) are direct spirographic measurements. The diffusing capacity for carbon mon-

oxide (DL_{CO}) is calculated from the amount of carbon monoxide exhaled.

Purpose
☐ To determine the cause of dyspnea
☐ To assess the effectiveness of specific therapeutic regimen
☐ To determine whether a functional abnormality is obstructive or restrictive
☐ To estimate the degree of pulmonary dysfunction.

Patient preparation
Explain to the patient that these tests evaluate pulmonary function. Instruct him not to eat a heavy meal before the tests and not to smoke for 4 to 6 hours before the tests. Tell him who will perform these tests and where, and explain the operation of a spirometer. Advise him that the accuracy of the tests depends on his cooperation. Assure him that the procedure is painless and that he will be able to rest between tests.

Inform the laboratory if the patient is taking an analgesic that depresses respiration. As ordered, withhold bronchodilators and intermittent positive-pressure breathing therapy.

Just before the test, tell the patient to void and to loosen tight clothing. If he wears dentures, tell him to wear them during the test to help form a seal around the mouthpiece. Advise him to put on the nose clip, to adjust to it before the test.

Equipment

For direct spirography: spirometer/recording paper/nose clip/mouthpiece. *For body plethysmography:* body plethysmograph/mouthpiece/transducer.

Procedure

Tidal volume: The patient is told to breathe normally into the mouthpiece 10 times.

Expiratory reserve volume: The patient is told to breathe into the mouthpiece 10 times and to exhale as completely as possible after each breath.

Vital capacity: The patient is told to inhale as deeply as possible and to exhale into the mouthpiece as completely as possible. This procedure is repeated three times, and the test result showing the largest volume is used.

Inspiratory capacity: The patient is instructed to inhale fully, to exhale normally into the mouthpiece, and then to breathe normally 10 times, inhaling as deeply as possible after the 10th breath.

Functional residual capacity: The patient is told to breathe normally into a spirometer that contains a known concentration of an insoluble gas (usually helium or nitrogen) in a known volume of air. After a few breaths, the concentrations of gas in the spirometer and in the lungs reach equilibrium. The point of equilibrium and the concentration of gas in the spirometer is recorded.

Alternatively, the patient is placed in an airtight box called a body plethysmograph and told to breathe air through a tube connected to a transducer. At end-expiration the tube is occluded, the patient is told to pant, and changes in

---

READING A SPIROGRAM

The plotting of a spirogram, or lung signature, is based on the following: the patient's tidal volume (V_T), and his maximum inspiration (A) and expiration (B) capabilities, which constitute forced vital capacity (FVC). After these are plotted, a spirogram can be used to calculate inspiratory reserve volume (IRV); expiratory reserve volume (ERV); residual volume (RV); inspiration capacity (IC); functional residual capacity (FRC): and total lung capacity (TLC).

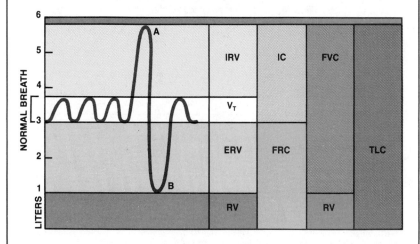

Adapted with permission from R.F. Wilson, ed., *Critical Care Manual: Principles and Techniques of Critical Care*, (Vol. 1; Kalamazoo, Mich.: Upjohn Co., 1976).

INTERPRETING PULMONARY FUNCTION TESTS

MEASUREMENT OF PULMONARY FUNCTION	METHOD OF CALCULATION	IMPLICATIONS
Tidal volume V_T: amount of air inhaled or exhaled during normal breathing	Determine the spirographic measurement for 10 breaths, and then divide by 10.	Decreased V_T may indicate restrictive disease and requires further testing, such as full pulmonary function studies or chest radiography.
Minute volume V_E: total amount of air breathed per minute	Multiply V_T by the respiration rate.	Normal V_E can occur in emphysema; decreased V_E may indicate other diseases, such as pulmonary edema. Increased V_E can occur with acidosis, increased CO_2, decreased PO_2, exercise, and low compliance states.
CO_2 response: increase or decrease in V_E after breathing various CO_2 concentrations	Calculated by plotting changes in V_E against increasing inspired CO_2 concentrations	Reduced CO_2 response may indicate chronic bronchitis or other obstructive disease.
Inspiratory reserve volume (IRV): amount of air inspired over above-normal inspiration	Subtract V_T from inspiratory capacity (IC).	Abnormal IRV alone doesn't indicate respiratory dysfunction; IRV decreases during normal exercise.
Expiratory reserve volume (ERV): amount of air exhaled after normal expiration	Direct spirographic measurement	ERV varies, even in healthy persons, but usually decreases in the obese.
Residual volume (RV): amount of air remaining in the lungs after forced expiration	Subtract ERV from functional residual capacity (FRC).	RV greater than 35% of TLC after maximal expiratory effort may indicate obstructive disease.
Vital capacity (VC): total volume of air that can be exhaled after maximum inspiration	Direct spirographic measurement, or add V_T, IRV, and ERV	Normal or increased VC with decreased flow rates may indicate any condition that causes a reduction in functional pulmonary tissue, such as pulmonary edema. Decreased VC with normal or increased flow rates may indicate decreased respiratory effort resulting from neuromuscular disease, drug overdose, or head injury; decreased thoracic expansion; or limited movement of diaphragm.
Inspiratory capacity (IC): amount of air that can be inhaled after normal expiration	Direct spirographic measurement, or add IRV and V_T.	Decreased IC indicates restrictive disease.
Thoracic gas volume (TGV): total volume of gas in lungs from both ventilated and non-ventilated airways	Body plethysmography	Increased TGV indicates air trapping, which may result from obstructive disease.
Functional residual capacity (FRC): amount of air remaining in lungs after normal expiration	Body plethysmography, helium dilution technique, or add ERV and RV	Increased FRC indicates overdistention of lungs, which may result from obstructive pulmonary disease.

INTERPRETING PULMONARY FUNCTION TESTS

MEASUREMENT OF PULMONARY FUNCTION	METHOD OF CALCULATION	IMPLICATIONS
Total lung capacity (TLC): total volume of the lungs when maximally inflated	Add V_T, IRV, ERV, and RV; or FRC and IC; or VC and RV.	Low TLC indicates restrictive disease; high TLC indicates overdistended lungs caused by obstructive disease.
Forced vital capacity (FVC): measurement of the amount of air exhaled forcefully and quickly after maximum inspiration	Direct spirographic measurement; expressed as a percentage of the total volume of gas exhaled	Decreased FVC indicates flow resistance in respiratory system from obstructive disease, such as chronic bronchitis, or from restrictive disease, such as pulmonary fibrosis.
Flow-volume curve [also called flow-volume loop]: greatest rate of flow (Vmax) during FVC maneuvers versus lung volume change	Direct spirographic measurement at 1-second intervals; calculated from flow rates (expressed in liters/second) and lung volume changes (expressed in liters) during maximal inspiratory and expiratory maneuvers	Decreased flow rates at all volumes during expiration indicate obstructive disease of the small airways, such as emphysema. A plateau of expiratory flow near TLC, a plateau of inspiratory flow at mid-VC, and a square wave pattern through most of VC indicate obstructive disease of large airways. Normal or increased PEF, decreased flow with decreasing lung volumes, and markedly decreased VC indicate restrictive disease.
Forced expiratory volume (FEV): volume of air expired in the 1st, 2nd, or 3rd second of FVC maneuver	Direct spirographic measurement; expressed as percentage of FVC	Decreased FEV_1, and increased FEV_2 and FEV_3 may indicate obstructive disease; decreased or normal FEV_1 may indicate restrictive disease.
Maximal midexpiratory flow (MMEF) [also called forced expiratory flow (FEF) or FEF 25%-75%]: average rate of flow during middle half of FVC	Calculated from the flow rate and the time needed for expiration of middle 50% of FVC	Low MMEF indicates obstructive disease of the small airways.
Peak expiratory flow (PEF): Vmax during forced expiration	Calculated from flow-volume curve, or by direct spirographic measurement, using a pneumotachometer or electronic tachometer with a transducer to convert flow to electrical output display	Decreased PEF may indicate a mechanical problem, such as upper airway obstruction, or obstructive disease. PEF is usually normal in restrictive disease but decreases in severe cases. Because PEF is effort-dependent, it's also low in a person who has poor expiratory effort or doesn't understand the procedure.
Maximal voluntary ventilation (MVV) [also called maximum breathing capacity (MBC)]: greatest volume of air breathed per unit of time	Direct spirographic measurement	Decreased MVV may indicate obstructive disease; normal or decreased MVV may indicate restrictive disease, such as myasthenia gravis.
Diffusing capacity for carbon monoxide (DL_{CO}): milliliters of carbon monoxide diffused per minute across the alveolar-capillary membrane	Calculated from analysis of amount of carbon monoxide exhaled compared with amount inhaled	Decreased DL_{CO} in the presence of thickened alveolar-capillary membrane indicates interstitial pulmonary disease, such as pulmonary fibrosis and emphysema.

RESTRICTIVE AND OBSTRUCTIVE LUNG DISEASE

A spirogram helps determine if a patient's lung disorder is restrictive or obstructive. As these graphs of forced vital capacity (FVC) maneuvers show, in restrictive disease, FVC and forced expiratory volume (FEV) are reduced. But FEV is reduced less in restrictive disease, which doesn't change airway resistance. In obstructive disease, all the parameters are reduced because the patient takes a longer time per unit to exhale.

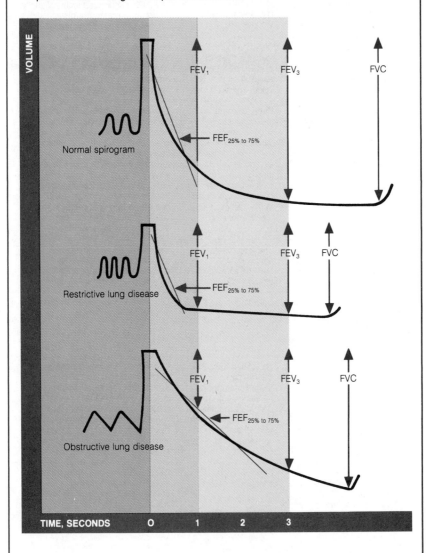

Adapted with permission from N.B. Slonim and L.H. Hamilton, *Respiratory Physiology* (3rd ed.; St. Louis: C.V. Mosby Co., 1976).

intrathoracic and plethysmographic pressures are measured. The results are used to calculate total TGV and FRC.

Forced vital capacity and *forced expiratory volume:* The patient is instructed to inhale as slowly and deeply as possible and then asked to exhale into the mouthpiece as quickly and completely as possible. This procedure is repeated three times, and the largest volume is recorded. The volume of air expired at 1 second (FEV_1), at 2 seconds (FEV_2), and at 3 seconds (FEV_3) during all three repetitions is also recorded.

Maximal voluntary ventilation: The patient is told to breathe into the mouthpiece as quickly and deeply as possible for 15 seconds.

Diffusing capacity for carbon monoxide: The patient is told to inhale a gas mixture with a low concentration of carbon monoxide, and then to hold his breath for 10 seconds before exhaling.

Precautions

 □ Pulmonary function tests are contraindicated in patients with acute coronary insufficiency, angina, or recent MI. During such tests, watch for respiratory distress, changes in pulse rate and blood pressure, coughing or bronchospasm.

Values

Normal values are predicted for each patient based on age, height, weight, and sex, and are expressed as a percentage. Usually, results are considered abnormal if they're less than 80% of these values.

Values such as the following can be calculated at bedside with a portable spirometer: V_T: 5 to 7 ml/kg of body weight; ERV: 25% of VC; IC: 75% of VC; FEV_1: 83% of VC (after 1 second); FEV_2: 94% of VC (after 2 seconds); and FEV_3: 97% of VC (after 3 seconds).

Post-test care

□ As ordered, resume medications, diet, and activities.

Interfering factors

□ Lack of patient cooperation, hypoxia, or metabolic disturbances can make testing difficult or impossible.

□ Pregnancy or gastric distention may displace lung volume.

□ Poor seal around the mouthpiece or the tube can decrease volumes.

□ A narcotic analgesic or sedative administered before the test can decrease inspiratory and expiratory forces.

□ Bronchodilators may temporarily improve pulmonary function, thereby producing misleading results.

SR. EILEEN MARIE HOLLEN, RN, BSN, CCRN

FLUID ANALYSIS TESTS

Pleural Fluid Analysis
[Thoracentesis]

The pleura, a two-layer membrane covering the lungs and lining the thoracic cavity, maintains a small amount of lubricating fluid between its layers to minimize friction during respiration. Increased fluid in this space—the result of diseases such as cancer or tuberculosis, or of blood or lymphatic disorders—can cause respiratory difficulty.

In pleural fluid aspiration (thoracen-

tesis), the thoracic wall is punctured to obtain a specimen of pleural fluid for analysis; or to relieve pulmonary compression and resultant respiratory distress. The specimen is examined for color, consistency, glucose and protein content, cellular composition, and the enzymes lactic dehydrogenase (LDH) and amylase; it's also examined cytologically for malignant cells and cultured for pathogens. Preceding thoracentesis with physical examination and chest radiograph or ultrasound study, to locate the fluid, lessens the risk of puncturing the lung, liver, or spleen.

POSITIONING THE PATIENT FOR THORACENTESIS

To prepare the patient for thoracentesis, place him in one of the three positions shown below: (1) sitting on the edge of the bed with arms on overbed table; (2) sitting up in bed with arms on overbed table; (3) lying partially on the side, partially on the back with arms over the head. These positions serve to widen the intercostal spaces and permit easy access to the pleural cavity. Using pillows as shown will make the patient more comfortable.

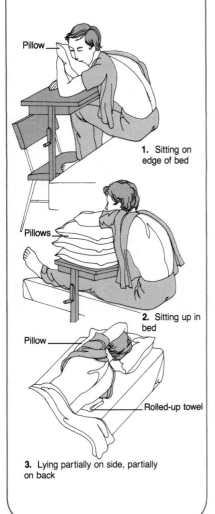

Pillow

1. Sitting on edge of bed

Pillows

2. Sitting up in bed

Pillow

Rolled-up towel

3. Lying partially on side, partially on back

Purpose

☐ To provide a fluid specimen to determine the cause and nature of pleural effusion.

Patient preparation

Explain to the patient that the test assesses the space around the lungs for fluid. Inform him that he needn't restrict food or fluids. Tell him who will perform the test and where.

Inform the patient that chest radiography or ultrasound study may precede the test, to help locate the fluid. Check the patient's history for hypersensitivity to local anesthetics. Warn the patient that he may feel a stinging sensation on injection of the anesthetic and some pressure during withdrawal of the fluid. Advise him not to cough, breathe deeply, or move during the test, to minimize the risk of injury to the lung.

Equipment

Sterile collection bottles/sterile gloves/adhesive tape/sterile thoracentesis tray (a prepackaged, disposable tray with the following: 70% alcohol or povidone-iodine solution/drapes/local anesthetic [usually 1% lidocaine]/5-ml sterile syringe for local anesthetic/25G needle/50-ml syringe for removing fluid/17G aspiration needle/sterile specimen bottle or tube/three-way stopcock or sterile tubing to prevent air from entering the pleural cavity/small sterile dressing).

Procedure

Record baseline vital signs. Shave the area around the needle insertion site, if necessary. Position the patient properly to widen intercostal spaces and to allow easier access to the pleural cavity; make sure he's well-supported and comfortable. Preferably, seat him at the edge of the bed, with a chair or stool supporting his feet, and his head and arms resting on a padded overbed table. If he can't sit up, position him on his unaffected side, with the arm on the affected side elevated above his head. Remind him not to cough, breathe deeply, or move suddenly during the procedure.

After the patient is properly positioned, the doctor disinfects the skin, drapes the area, injects local anesthetic into the subcutaneous tissue, and inserts the thoracentesis needle above the rib, to avoid lacerating intercostal vessels. When the needle reaches the pocket of fluid, he attaches the 50-ml syringe and the stopcock, and opens the clamps on the tubing to aspirate fluid into the container. During aspiration, check the patient for signs of respiratory distress, such as weakness, dyspnea, pallor, cyanosis, changes in heart rate, tachypnea, diaphoresis, blood-tinged frothy mucus, and hypotension.

After the needle is withdrawn, apply slight pressure and a small adhesive bandage to the puncture site.

Label the specimen, and record the date and time of the test, and the amount, color, and character of the fluid (clear, frothy, purulent, bloody) on the request slip. Note any signs of distress the patient exhibited during the procedure. Document the exact location where fluid was removed, since this information may aid diagnosis.

Precautions

□ Thoracentesis is contraindicated in patients who have histories of bleeding disorders.

□ Use strict aseptic technique.

□ Note the patient's temperature and antibiotic therapy, if applicable, on the laboratory slip.

□ Add a small amount (about 0.5 ml) of sterile heparin to the container to prevent coagulation of the fluid.

□ Send the specimen to the laboratory immediately.

Values

Normally, the pleural cavity maintains negative pressure and contains less than 20 ml of serous fluid.

Implications of results

Pleural effusion results from the abnormal formation or reabsorption of pleural fluid. Certain characteristics classify pleural fluid as either a transudate (a low-protein fluid that has leaked from normal blood vessels) or an exudate (a protein-rich fluid that has leaked from blood vessels with increased permeability). Pleural fluid may contain blood (hemothorax), chyle (chylothorax), or pus and necrotic tissue. Blood-tinged fluid may indicate a traumatic tap; if so, the fluid should clear as aspiration progresses.

Transudative effusion generally results from diminished colloidal pressure, increased negative pressure within the pleural cavity, ascites, systemic and pulmonary venous hypertension, congestive heart failure, hepatic cirrhosis, and nephritis.

Exudative effusion results from disorders that increase pleural capillary permeability (possibly with changes in hydrostatic or colloid osmotic pressures), lymphatic drainage interference, infections, pulmonary infarctions, and neoplasms. Exudative effusion associated with depressed glucose levels, elevated LDH, rheumatoid arthritis cells, and negative smears, cultures, and cytologic examination may indicate pleurisy associated with rheumatoid arthritis.

The most common pathogens that ap-

RECOGNIZING COMPLICATIONS OF THORACENTESIS

Identify the following possible complications of thoracentesis by watching for their characteristic signs and symptoms:

• *pneumothorax:* apprehension, increased restlessness, cyanosis, sudden breathlessness, tachycardia, chest pain
• *tension pneumothorax:* dyspnea, chest pain, tachycardia, hypotension, absent or diminished breath sounds on the affected side
• *fluid reaccumulation:* increasing and persistent cough, respiratory distress, hemoptysis, subcutaneous emphysema
• *mediastinal shift:* labored breathing, cardiac arrhythmias, cardiac distress, pulmonary edema (pink frothy sputum, paradoxical pulse).

CHARACTERISTICS OF PULMONARY TRANSUDATE AND EXUDATE		
CHARACTERISTIC	**TRANSUDATE**	**EXUDATE**
Appearance	Clear	Cloudy, turbid
Specific gravity	< 1.016	> 1.016
Clot (fibrinogen)	Absent	Present
Protein	< 3 g/dl	> 3 g/dl
WBCs	Few lymphocytes	Many; may be purulent
RBCs	Few	Variable
Glucose	Equal to serum level	May be less than serum level
LDH	Low	High

pear in culture studies of pleural fluid include *Mycobacterium tuberculosis, Staphylococcus aureus, Streptococcus pneumoniae* and other streptococci, *Hemophilus influenzae,* and in the case of a ruptured pulmonary abscess, anaerobes, such as bacteroides. Generally, cultures are positive during the early stages of infection; however, antibiotic therapy may produce a negative culture despite a positive Gram's stain and grossly purulent fluid. Empyema may result from complications of pneumonia, pulmonary abscess, perforation of the esophagus, or penetration from mediastinitis. A high percentage of neutrophils suggests septic inflammation; predominating lymphocytes suggest tuberculosis, or fungal or viral effusions.

Serosanguineous fluid may indicate pleural extension of a malignant tumor. Elevated LDH in a nonpurulent, nonhemolyzed, nonbloody effusion may also suggest malignancy. Pleural fluid glucose levels that are 30 to 40 mg/dl lower than blood glucose levels may indicate malignancy, bacterial infection, nonseptic inflammation, or metastases. Increased amylase levels occur with pleural effusions associated with pancreatitis.

Post-test care
☐ Reposition the patient comfortably on the affected side or as ordered by the doctor. Tell the patient to remain on this side for at least 1 hour to seal the puncture site. Elevate the head of the bed to facilitate breathing.
☐ Monitor vital signs every 30 minutes for 2 hours, then every 4 hours until they are stable.
☐ Tell the patient to call a nurse immediately if he experiences difficulty breathing.
☐ Watch for signs of pneumothorax, tension pneumothorax, fluid reaccumulation, and if a large amount of fluid was withdrawn, pulmonary edema or cardiac distress due to mediastinal shift. Usually, a post-test radiograph is ordered to detect these complications before clinical symptoms appear.
☐ Check the puncture site for any fluid leakage. A large amount of leakage is abnormal.

Interfering factors
☐ Failure to use aseptic technique may contaminate the specimen.
☐ Antibiotic therapy before aspiration of fluid for culture may decrease the number of bacteria, making isolation of the infecting organism difficult.
☐ Failure to send the specimen to the laboratory immediately or to add heparin to the container may alter test results.

DEBORAH L. DALRYMPLE, RN, BSN
SUSAN A. KAYES, BS, SM(ASCP)

Sweat Test

The sweat test quantitatively measures electrolyte concentrations (primarily sodium and chloride) in sweat, usually through pilocarpine iontophoresis (pilocarpine is a sweat inducer). This test is used almost exclusively in children to confirm cystic fibrosis, a congenital condition that raises the sodium and chloride electrolyte levels in sweat.

Sweat glands are found over most body surfaces. When stimulated by the sympathetic nerves, these glands secrete a watery solution that contains sodium chloride, most plasma components (except proteins), urea, and lactate ions in greater amounts than in plasma. Elevated sodium and chloride sweat concentrations may also occur in persons predisposed to cystic fibrosis, such as those with family histories of the disease, or in those suspected of the disease because of malabsorption syndrome or failure to thrive.

Purpose
☐ To confirm cystic fibrosis.

Patient preparation
Since the patient is generally a child, explain the test to him as simply as possible (if he is old enough to understand). Inform the patient and his parents that there are no restrictions of diet, medication, or activity before the test. Tell the patient who will perform the test and where, and that it takes 20 to 45 minutes (depending on the equipment used).

Tell the child he may feel a slight tickling sensation during the procedure but won't feel any pain. If he becomes nervous or frightened during the test, try to distract him with a book, television, or other appropriate diversion.

Encourage the parents to assist with preparations and to stay with their child during the test. Their presence will minimize the child's anxiety.

Equipment
Analyzer/two skin chloride electrodes (positive and negative)/distilled water/two standardizing solutions (chloride concentrations)/2″ x 2″ sterile gauze pads (kept in airtight container)/pilocarpine pads/forceps (for handling pads)/straps (for securing electrodes)/gram scale/normal saline solution.

Procedure
With distilled water, wash the area to be iontophoresed, and dry it. (The flexor surface of the right forearm is commonly used, or when the patient's arm is too small to secure electrodes, as with an infant, the right thigh.) Place a gauze pad saturated with premeasured pilocarpine solution on the positive electrode; place the pad saturated with normal saline solution on the negative electrode. Apply both electrodes to the area to be iontophoresed, and secure them with straps.

Lead wires to the analyzer—which are attached in a manner similar to that used for EKG electrodes—are given a current of 4 milliamperes in 15 to 20 seconds. This process (iontophoresis) is continued at 15- to 20-second intervals for 5 minutes. After iontophoresis, remove both electrodes. Discard the pads, cleanse the skin with distilled water, then dry it.

Using forceps, place a dry gauze pad or filter paper (previously weighed on a gram scale) on the area where the pilocarpine was iontophoresed. Cover the pad or filter paper with a slightly larger piece of plastic, and seal the edges of the plastic with waterproof adhesive tape. Leave the gauze pad or filter paper in place for about 30 to 40 minutes. (The appearance of droplets on the plastic usually indicates induction of an adequate amount of sweat.)

Remove the pad or filter paper with the forceps, and place it immediately in the weighing bottle, and insert the stopper in the bottle. (The difference between the first and second weights indicates the weight of the sweat specimen collected.)

Precautions

 □ Always perform iontophoresis on the right arm (or right thigh) rather than on the left. *Never* perform iontophoresis on the chest, especially in a child, since the current can induce cardiac arrest.

□ To prevent electric shock, use battery-powered equipment, if possible.

 □ Stop the test immediately if the patient complains of a burning sensation, which usually indicates that the positive electrode is exposed or positioned improperly. Adjust the electrode, and continue the test.

□ Make sure at least 100 mg of sweat is collected for analysis.

□ Carefully seal the gauze pad or filter paper in the weighing bottle, and send the bottle to the laboratory immediately.

Values

Normal sodium values in sweat range from 10 to 30 mEq/liter. Normal chloride values range from 10 to 35 mEq/liter.

Implications of results

Abnormal sodium values range from 50 to 130 mEq/liter. Abnormal chloride values range from 50 to 110 mEq/liter. Sodium and chloride concentrations of 50 to 60 mEq/liter strongly suggest cystic fibrosis. Concentrations greater than 60 mEq/liter, with typical clinical features, confirm the diagnosis. Only a few conditions other than cystic fibrosis cause elevated sweat electrolyte levels—most notably, untreated adrenal insufficiency, as well as type I glycogen storage disease, vasopressin-resistant diabetes insipidus, meconium ileus, and renal failure. However, cystic fibrosis is the only condition that raises sweat electrolyte levels above 80 mEq/liter.

In females, sweat electrolyte levels fluctuate cyclically: chloride concentrations usually peak 5 to 10 days before onset of menses, and most women retain fluid before menses. Males also show fluctuations (up to 70 mEq/liter).

Post-test care

□ Wash the iontophoresed area with soap and water, and dry it thoroughly.

□ If the iontophoresed area looks red, reassure the patient that this is normal and will disappear within a few hours.

□ Tell the patient he may resume his usual activities.

Interfering factors

□ Failure to obtain an adequate amount of sweat (common in newborns) prevents proper testing.

□ Presence of pure salt depletion (common during hot weather) may cause false-normal test results.

□ Failure to cleanse the skin thoroughly or to use sterile gauze pads may cause false elevations.

□ Failure to seal the gauze pad or filter paper carefully may falsely elevate electrolyte levels, due to evaporation.

□ Unstable clinical conditions allow erroneous interpretation of test results.

MARILEE J. WARNER, RN, BSN, BSPA

ENDOSCOPY

Direct Laryngoscopy

Direct laryngoscopy, the visualization of the larynx by the use of a fiberoptic endoscope or laryngoscope passed through the mouth and pharynx to the larynx, usually follows indirect laryngoscopy, the more common procedure. Direct laryngoscopy permits visualization of areas that are inaccessible through indirect laryngoscopy, and is indicated for children; for patients with strong gag reflexes due to anatomic abnormalities; for those with symptoms of pharyngeal or laryngeal disease, such as stridor or hemoptysis; or for those who have had no response to short-term symptomatic therapy. The procedure may include the collection of secretions or tissue for further study and the removal of foreign bodies. Normally, the test is contraindicated for patients with epiglottitis, since trauma can quickly cause edema and airway obstruction; however, when this test is absolutely necessary in such patients, it may be performed in the operating room, with resuscitative equipment available.

Purpose
□ To detect lesions, strictures, or foreign bodies in the larynx
□ To aid diagnosis of laryngeal cancer
□ To remove benign lesions or foreign bodies from the larynx
□ To examine the larynx when the view provided by indirect laryngoscopy is inadequate.

Patient preparation
Explain to the patient that this test determines laryngeal abnormalities. Instruct him to fast for 6 to 8 hours before the test. Tell him who will perform the laryngoscopy and that it will be performed in a dark operating room.

Inform the patient that he'll receive a sedative to help him relax, atropine to reduce secretions, and during the procedure, a general or local anesthetic. Also, reassure him that this procedure won't obstruct the airway.

Make sure the patient or a responsible member of his family has signed a consent form. Check the patient's history for hypersensitivity to the anesthetic. Obtain baseline vital signs. Administer the sedative and atropine to the patient, as ordered (usually 30 minutes to 1 hour before the test). Just before the test, instruct the patient to remove dentures, contact lenses, and jewelry, and tell him to void.

Equipment
Laryngoscope / sedative / atropine / local anesthetic (spray or jelly, as ordered) or general anesthetic/sterile container for microbiology specimen/sterile gloves/

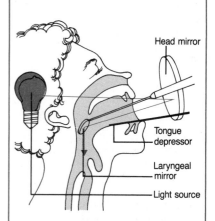

INDIRECT LARYNGOSCOPY

Head mirror — Tongue depressor — Laryngeal mirror — Light source

Indirect laryngoscopy, normally an office procedure, allows visualization of the larynx, using a warm laryngeal mirror positioned at the back of the throat, a head mirror held in front of the mouth, and a light source.

The patient sits erect in a chair and sticks his tongue out as far as possible. The tongue is grasped with a piece of gauze and held in place with a tongue depressor. If the patient's gag reflex is sensitive, a local anesthetic may be sprayed on the pharyngeal wall. Then, the larynx is observed at rest and during phonation. A simple excision of polyps may also be performed during this procedure.

Coplin jar with 95% ethyl alcohol for cytology smears/container with 10% formaldehyde solution for histology specimen/forceps for biopsy/emesis basin/resuscitative equipment.

Procedure
Place the patient in a supine position. Encourage him to relax with his arms at his sides and to breathe through his nose. A general anesthetic is administered or the patient's mouth and throat are sprayed with local anesthetic. The patient's head is positioned and held, while the doctor introduces the laryn-

goscope through the patient's mouth. The larynx is examined for abnormalities and a specimen or secretions may be removed for further study. Minor surgery, such as removal of polyps or nodules, may be performed at this time. Place specimens for histology, cytology, and microbiology in their respective containers.

Precautions
Send the specimens to the laboratory immediately.

Findings
A normal larynx shows no evidence of inflammation, lesions, strictures, or foreign bodies.

Implications of results
The combined results of direct laryngoscopy, biopsy, and radiography may indicate laryngeal carcinoma. Direct laryngoscopy may show benign lesions, strictures, or foreign bodies, and with a biopsy, may distinguish laryngeal edema from radiation reaction or tumor.

Post-test care
□ As ordered, place the conscious patient in semi-Fowler's position; place the unconscious patient on his side with his head slightly elevated to prevent aspiration.
□ Check vital signs every 15 minutes until stable, then every 30 minutes for 4 hours, every hour for the next 4 hours, and then every 4 hours for 24 hours. Immediately report any adverse reaction to anesthetic or sedative (tachycardia, palpitations, hypertension, euphoria, excitation, and rapid, deep respirations).
□ Apply an ice collar to prevent or minimize laryngeal edema.
□ Provide an emesis basin, and instruct the patient to spit out saliva rather than swallow it. Observe sputum for blood, and notify the doctor immediately if excessive bleeding occurs.
□ Instruct the patient to refrain from clearing his throat and coughing, which may dislodge the clot at the biopsy site

and cause hemorrhaging. Also, advise the patient to avoid smoking until vital signs are stable and there is no evidence of complications.
□ Immediately report any subcutaneous crepitus around the patient's face and neck—a possible indication of tracheal perforation.

 □ Observe the patient with epiglottitis for signs of airway obstruction. Immediately report signs of respiratory difficulty, such as laryngeal stridor and dyspnea, resulting from laryngeal edema or laryngospasm. Keep emergency resuscitative equipment available; keep a tracheotomy tray nearby for 24 hours.
□ Restrict food and fluids until the gag reflex returns (usually 2 hours). Then the patient may resume his usual diet, beginning with sips of water.
□ Reassure the patient that voice loss, hoarseness, and sore throat are temporary. Provide throat lozenges or a soothing liquid gargle when his gag reflex returns.

Interfering factors
Failure to place the specimens in the appropriate containers and to send the specimens to the laboratory immediately may interfere with the accurate determination of test results and diagnosis.

MARCIA S. SLAUGHTER, RRT

Bronchoscopy

Bronchoscopy is the direct visualization of the trachea and tracheobronchial tree through a standard metal bronchoscope or a fiberoptic bronchoscope, a slender flexible tube with mirrors and a light at its distal end. A brush, biopsy forceps, or a catheter may be passed through the bronchoscope to obtain specimens for cytologic examination.

A flexible fiberoptic bronchoscope is

used most often since it's smaller, allows a greater range of view of the segmental and subsegmental bronchi, and carries less risk of trauma than the rigid bronchoscope. However, a large rigid bronchoscope is necessary to remove foreign objects, excise endobronchial lesions, and control massive hemoptysis.

Complications resulting from bronchoscopy may include bleeding, infection, and pneumothorax.

Purpose

□ To visually examine possible tumor, obstruction, secretion, or foreign body in the tracheobronchial tree, as demonstrated on radiograph

□ To help diagnose bronchogenic carcinoma, tuberculosis, interstitial pulmonary disease, or fungal or parasitic pulmonary infection, by obtaining a specimen for bacteriologic and cytologic examination

□ To locate a bleeding site in the tracheobronchial tree

□ To remove foreign bodies, malignant or benign tumors, mucous plugs, or excessive secretions from the tracheobronchial tree.

Patient preparation

Describe the procedure to the patient, and explain that this test determines the nature of pulmonary dysfunction. Instruct him to fast for 6 to 12 hours before the test. Tell him who will perform the test and where; that the room will be darkened; and that the procedure takes 45 to 60 minutes. Advise him that test results are usually available in 1 day— except the tuberculosis report, which may take up to 6 weeks.

Tell the patient that chest X-ray studies and blood studies (prothrombin time, activated partial thromboplastin time, platelet count, and possibly arterial blood gases) will be performed before the bronchoscopy. Advise him that he may receive a sedative I.V. to help him relax. If the procedure is not being performed under a general anesthetic, inform the patient that a local anesthetic will be sprayed into his nose and mouth to sup-

press the gag reflex. Warn him that the spray has an unpleasant taste and that he may experience some discomfort during the procedure. Reassure him that his airway won't be blocked during the procedure, and that oxygen will be administered through the bronchoscope.

Make sure the patient or a responsible member of the family has signed the consent form. Check the patient's history for hypersensitivity to anesthetic. Obtain baseline vital signs. Administer the preoperative sedative, as ordered. If the patient is wearing dentures, instruct him to remove them just before the test.

Equipment

Flexible fiberoptic bronchoscope/sedative/local anesthetic (spray, jelly, or liquid, as ordered)/sterile gloves/sterile container for microbiology specimen/container with 10% formalin solution for histology specimen/Coplin jar with 95% ethyl alcohol for cytology smears/six glass slides (all frosted, if possible, or with frosted tips)/emesis basin/AMBU bag with face mask/oral and endotracheal airways/laryngoscope/oxygen set-up/ventilating bronchoscope for a patient requiring controlled mechanical ventilation.

Procedure

Place the patient in a supine position on a table or bed, or have him sit upright in a chair. Tell him to remain relaxed, with his arms at his sides, and to breathe through his nose. After the local anesthetic is sprayed into the patient's throat and takes effect (usually 1 or 2 minutes), the doctor introduces the bronchoscope (possibly tipped with lidocaine jelly) through the patient's mouth or nose. When the bronchoscope is just above the vocal cords, approximately 3 to 4 ml of 2% to 4% lidocaine is flushed through the inner channel of the scope to the vocal cords, to anesthetize deeper areas. The doctor inspects the anatomic structure of the trachea and bronchi, observes the color of the mucosal lining, and notes unusual masses or inflamed areas. Then, biopsy forceps may be used to remove a tissue specimen from a

PERFORMING BRONCHOSCOPY

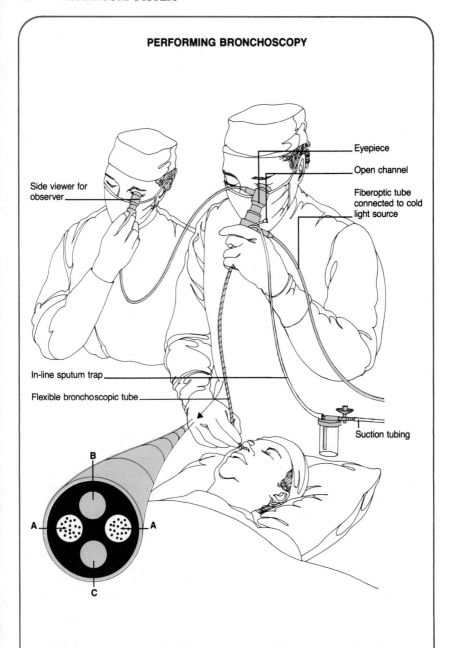

The bronchoscopic tube, inserted through the nostril into the bronchi, has four channels (see inset). Two light channels (A) provide a light source: one visualizing channel (B) to see through, and one open channel (C) that accommodates biopsy forceps, cytology brush, suctioning, lavage, anesthetic, or oxygen.

suspect area, a bronchial brush to obtain cells from the surface of a lesion, or suction apparatus to remove foreign bodies or mucous plugs. Place the resulting specimens for microbiology, histology, and cytology in their respective, properly labeled containers.

Bronchoscopy requires fluoroscopic guidance for distal evaluation of lesions or for a transbronchial biopsy in alveolar areas.

Precautions

 □ A patient with severe respiratory failure who can't breathe adequately by himself should be placed on a ventilator before bronchoscopy.

□ Send the specimens to the laboratory immediately.

Findings

The trachea, a 4½″ (11.3 cm) tube extending from the larynx to the bronchi, normally consists of smooth muscle containing C-shaped rings of cartilage at regular intervals, and is lined with ciliated mucosa. The bronchi appear structurally similar to the trachea; the right bronchus is slightly larger and more vertical than the left. Smaller secondary bronchi, bronchioles, alveolar ducts, and eventually alveolar sacs and alveoli branch off from the main bronchi. The walls of the microscopic end structures consist of a single layer of squamous epithelial tissue.

Implications of results

Abnormalities of the bronchial wall include inflammation, swelling, protruding cartilage, ulceration, tumors, enlargement of the mucous gland orifices, or submucosal lymph nodes. Abnormalities of endotracheal origin include stenosis, compression, ectasia (dilation of tubular vessel), anomalous (irregular) bronchial branching, and abnormal bifurcation due to diverticulum. Abnormal substances in the bronchial lumen include blood, secretions, calculi, and foreign bodies.

Results of tissue and cell studies may indicate interstitial pulmonary disease, bronchogenic carcinoma, tuberculosis, or other pulmonary infections. Bronchogenic carcinomas include epidermoid or squamous cell carcinoma, small cell (oat cell) carcinoma, adenocarcinoma, and large cell (undifferentiated) carcinoma. Correlation of radiographic, bronchoscopic, and cytologic findings with clinical signs and symptoms is essential.

Post-test care

□ Monitor vital signs. Notify the doctor immediately of any adverse reaction to anesthetic or sedative.

□ As ordered, place the conscious patient in semi-Fowler's position; place the unconscious patient on his side with the head of the bed slightly elevated to prevent aspiration.

□ Provide an emesis basin, and instruct the patient to spit out saliva rather than swallow it. Observe sputum for blood, and notify the doctor immediately if excessive bleeding occurs.

□ Collect all sputum for 24 hours after bronchoscopy for cytologic examination, since irritation produced during bronchial brushing often results in delayed shedding of malignant cells.

□ Tell the patient who had a biopsy to refrain from clearing his throat and coughing, which may dislodge the clot at the biopsy site and cause hemorrhaging.

□ Immediately report any subcutaneous crepitus around the patient's face and neck—a possible indication of tracheal or bronchial perforation.

 □ Watch for and immediately report symptoms of respiratory difficulty, such as laryngeal stridor and dyspnea, resulting from laryngeal edema or laryngospasm. Observe for signs of hypoxemia (cyanosis), pneumothorax (dyspnea, cyanosis, diminished breath sounds on affected side), bronchospasm (dyspnea, wheezing), or bleeding (hemoptysis). Keep resuscitative equipment and tracheotomy tray available for 24 hours after the test.

□ Restrict food and fluids until the gag

reflex returns (usually in 2 hours). Then the patient may resume his usual diet, beginning with sips of clear liquid or ice chips.

□ Reassure the patient that hoarseness, loss of voice, and sore throat after this procedure are only temporary. Provide lozenges or a soothing liquid gargle to ease discomfort when his gag reflex returns.

Interfering factors
Failure to place the specimens in the appropriate containers and to send the specimens to the laboratory immediately may interfere with accurate determination of test results and diagnosis.

SR. EILEEN MARIE HOLLEN, RN, BSN, CCRN
SHIRLEY GIVEN, HT(ASCP)

Mediastinoscopy

Mediastinoscopy allows direct visualization of mediastinal structures—through an exploring speculum with built-in fiber light and side slit—and palpation and biopsy of paratracheal and carinal lymph nodes. The mediastinum is the mass of tissues and organs behind the sternum, separating the lungs. Its major contents include the heart and its vessels, the trachea, esophagus, thymus, and lymph nodes. Examination of the nodes, which receive lymphatic drainage from the lungs, can detect lymphoma (including Hodgkin's disease) and sarcoidosis, and aids in staging lung cancer. A surgical procedure, mediastinoscopy is indicated when tests such as sputum cytology, lung scans, radiography, and bronchoscopic biopsy, fail to confirm diagnosis.

The right side of the mediastinum allows easy exploration, and since mediastinoscopy can diagnose bronchogenic carcinoma at an early stage, this procedure is now replacing the scalene fat pad biopsy. Exploring the left side, however, is less satisfactory and more haz-

ardous, due to the close proximity of the aorta. Although rare, complications of the test may include pneumothorax, perforation of the esophagus, infection, hemorrhage, and left recurrent laryngeal nerve damage. Scarring of the area as a result of a previous mediastinoscopy contraindicates this test.

Purpose
□ To detect bronchogenic carcinoma, lymphoma, and sarcoidosis
□ To determine staging of lung cancer.

Patient preparation
Describe the procedure to the patient and answer any questions he may have. Explain that this test evaluates the lymph nodes and other structures in the chest. Instruct the patient to fast after midnight before the test. Tell him who will perform the procedure and where; that a general anesthestic will be administered; and that the procedure will take approximately 1 hour.

Tell him he may temporarily experience chest pain, tenderness at the incision site, or a sore throat (from intubation). Reassure him that although complications are possible with this procedure, they rarely occur.

Make sure the patient or a responsible member of the family has signed a consent form. Check the patient's history for hypersensitivity to the anesthetic. As ordered, administer a sedative the night before the test and before the procedure is performed.

Equipment
Mediastinoscope/light carriers/suction tubes/long aspiration needle/cup biopsy forceps/laryngeal scissors/spreader.

Procedure
After the patient has an endotracheal tube in place, the surgeon makes a small transverse suprasternal incision. Using finger dissection, a channel is formed and the lymph nodes are palpated. A mediastinoscope is inserted into the mediastinum, and tissue specimens are collected and sent to the laboratory for

STAGING OF LUNG CANCER

This staging system was developed by the American Joint Committee on Cancer (formerly the American Joint Committee for Cancer Staging and End Results Reporting) in 1979.

CLASSIFICATION	DEFINITION
Primary Tumor (T)	
TX	Tumor proven by the presence of malignant cells in bronchopulmonary secretions but not visualized roentgenographically or bronchoscopically; or any tumor that cannot be assessed
T0	No evidence of primary tumor
TIS	Carcinoma in situ
T1	Tumor 1¼″ (3 cm) or less in greatest diameter, surrounded by lung or visceral pleura, and without evidence of invasion proximal to a lobar bronchus at bronchoscopy
T2	Tumor more than 1¼″ (3 cm) in greatest diameter, or a tumor of any size that either invades the visceral pleura or has associated atelectasis or obstructive pneumonitis extending to the hilar region. At bronchoscopy, the proximal extent of demonstrable tumor must be within a lobar bronchus or at least ¾″ (2 cm) distal to the carina. Any associated atelectasis or obstructive pneumonitis must involve less than an entire lung, and there must be no pleural effusion.
T3	Tumor of any size with direct extension into an adjacent structure, such as the parietal pleura or the chest wall, the diaphragm, or the mediastinum and its contents; or a tumor demonstrated bronchoscopically to involve a main bronchus less than ¾″ (2 cm) distal to the carina; or any tumor associated with atelectasis or obstructive pneumonitis of an entire lung or pleural effusion
Nodal Involvement (N)	
N0	No demonstrable metastasis to regional lymph nodes
N1	Metastasis to lymph nodes in the peribronchial or the ipsilateral hilar region, or both, including direct extension
N2	Metastasis to lymph nodes in the mediastinum
Distant Metastasis (M)	
MX	Not assessed
M0	No (known) distant metastasis
M1	Distant metastasis present

STAGE GROUPING

Occult Carcinoma			Stage 1			Stage 2			Stage 3
TX	N0	M0	TIS	N0	M0	T2	N1	M0	T3; any N or M
			T1	N0	M0				N2; any T or M
			T1	N1	M0				M1; any T or N
			T2	N0	M0				

Reprinted with permission from *Staging of Lung Cancer* (Chicago: American Joint Committee for Cancer Staging and End Results Reporting, 1979).

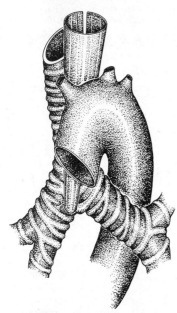

POSITIONING THE MEDIASTINOSCOPE

The mediastinoscope shown here has been inserted suprasternally to inspect the paratracheal and carinal lymph nodes. The path of the mediastinoscope is cleared digitally before the scope is introduced. If the scope meets resistance while it's being advanced, a blunt dissection may be performed to clear the path.

frozen section examination. If analysis confirms malignancy of a resectable tu-mor, a thoracotomy and pneumonectomy may follow immediately.

Precautions
None.

Findings
Normally, lymph nodes appear as small, smooth, flat oval bodies of lymphoid tissue.

Implications of results
Malignant lymph nodes usually indicate inoperable—but not always untreatable—lung or esophageal cancer, or lymphomas (such as Hodgkin's disease). Staging of lung cancer helps determine therapeutic regimen. Multiple nodular involvement, for example, can contraindicate surgery.

Post-test care
□ Monitor vital signs, and check the dressing for bleeding or fluid drainage.
□ Observe for signs of the following complications: fever (mediastinitis); crepitus (subcutaneous emphysema); dyspnea, cyanosis, and diminished breath sounds on the affected side (pneumothorax); tachycardia and hypotension (hemorrhage).
□ Administer the prescribed analgesic, as needed.

Interfering factors
None.
SR. EILEEN MARIE HOLLEN, RN, BSN, CCRN

RADIOGRAPHY

Chest Radiography
[Chest roentgenography]

In a chest radiograph, X-rays or gamma rays penetrate the chest and react on specially sensitized film. Since normal pulmonary tissue is radiolucent, foreign bodies, infiltrates, fluids, tumors, and other abnormalities appear as densities on the chest film. A chest radiograph is most useful when compared with the patient's previous films, allowing the radiologist to detect changes.

Although chest radiography was once routinely performed as a cancer screening test, the associated expense and exposure to radiation has caused many authorities to question its usefulness. The American Cancer Society recom-

mends sputum cultures rather than chest radiography—even in patients at high-risk —and the Food and Drug Administration has convened a panel for the development of guidelines concerning the use of chest radiography.

Purpose
□ To detect pulmonary disorders, such as pneumonia, atelectasis, pneumothorax, pulmonary bullae, and tumors
□ To detect mediastinal abnormalities, such as tumors, and cardiac disease
□ To determine the location and size of a lesion
□ To help assess pulmonary status.

Patient preparation
Describe the procedure to the patient, and explain that this test assesses his respiratory status. Inform him that he needn't restrict food or fluids. Tell him who will perform the test, and where and when the X-ray film will be taken.

Provide a gown without snaps, and instruct the patient to remove all jewelry

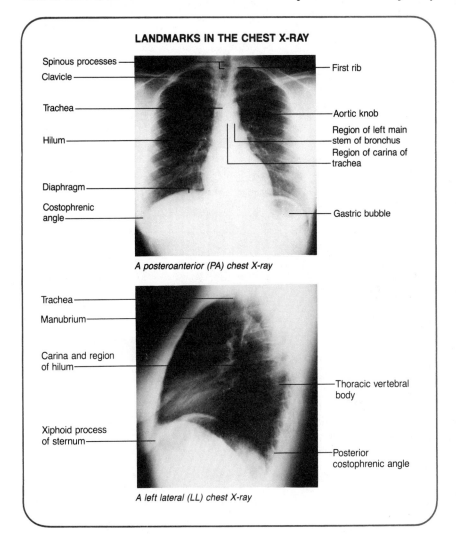

LANDMARKS IN THE CHEST X-RAY

Spinous processes
Clavicle
Trachea
Hilum
Diaphragm
Costophrenic angle

First rib
Aortic knob
Region of left main stem of bronchus
Region of carina of trachea
Gastric bubble

A posteroanterior (PA) chest X-ray

Trachea
Manubrium
Carina and region of hilum
Xiphoid process of sternum

Thoracic vertebral body
Posterior costophrenic angle

A left lateral (LL) chest X-ray

SOME CLINICAL IMPLICATIONS OF CHEST X-RAY FILMS

NORMAL ANATOMIC LOCATION AND APPEARANCE	POSSIBLE ABNORMALITY	IMPLICATIONS
Trachea Visible midline in the anterior mediastinal cavity; translucent tubelike appearance	• Deviation from midline	• Tension pneumothorax, atelectasis, pleural effusion, consolidation, mediastinal nodes, or in children, enlarged thymus
	• Narrowing, with hourglass appearance and deviation to one side	• Substernal thyroid
Heart Visible in the anterior left mediastinal cavity; solid appearance due to blood contents; edges may be clear in contrast with surrounding air density of the lung.	• Shift • Hypertrophy of right heart • Cardiac borders obscured by stringy densities ("shaggy heart")	• Atelectasis • Cor pulmonale, congestive heart failure • Cystic fibrosis
Aortic knob Visible as water density; formed by the arch of the aorta	• Solid densities, possibly indicating calcifications • Tortuous shape	• Atherosclerosis • Atherosclerosis
Mediastinum (mediastinal shadow) Visible as the space between the lungs; shadowy appearance that widens at the hilum of the lungs	• Deviation to nondiseased side; deviation to diseased side by traction • Gross widening	• Pleural effusion or tumor, fibrosis or collapsed lung • Neoplasms of esophagus, bronchi, lungs, thyroid, thymus, peripheral nerves, lymphoid tissue; aortic aneurysm; mediastinitis; cor pulmonale
Ribs Visible as thoracic cavity encasement	• Break or misalignment • Widening of intercostal spaces	• Fractured sternum or ribs • Emphysema
Spine Visible midline in the posterior chest; straight bony structure	• Spinal curvature • Break or misalignment	• Scoliosis, kyphosis • Fractures

SOME CLINICAL IMPLICATIONS OF CHEST X-RAY FILMS

NORMAL ANATOMIC LOCATION AND APPEARANCE	POSSIBLE ABNORMALITY	IMPLICATIONS
Clavicles Visible in upper thorax; intact and equidistant in properly centered X-ray films	• Break or misalignment	• Fractures
Hila (lung roots) Visible above the heart where pulmonary vessels, bronchi, and lymph nodes join the lungs; appear as small, white, bilateral densities	• Shift to one side • Accentuated shadows	• Atelectasis • Emphysema, pulmonary abscess, tumor, enlarged lymph nodes
Mainstem bronchus Visible, part of the hila with translucent tubelike appearance	• Spherical or oval density	• Bronchogenic cyst
Bronchi Usually not visible	• Visible	• Bronchial pneumonia
Lung fields Usually not visible throughout, except for the blood vessels	• Visible • Irregular, patchy densities	• Atelectasis • Resolving pneumonia, silicosis, fibrosis, metastatic neoplasm
Hemidiaphragm Rounded, visible; right side ⅜″ to ¾″ (1 to 2 cm) higher than left	• Elevation of diaphragm (difference in elevation can be measured on inspiration and expiration to detect movement) • Flattening of diaphragm • Unilateral elevation of either side • Unilateral elevation of left side only	• Active tuberculosis, pneumonia, pleurisy, acute bronchitis, active disease of the abdominal viscera, bilateral phrenic nerve involvement, atelectasis • Asthma, emphysema • Possible unilateral phrenic nerve paresis • Perforated ulcer (rare), gas distention of stomach or splenic flexure of colon, free air in abdomen

COMMON RADIOGRAPHIC VIEWS

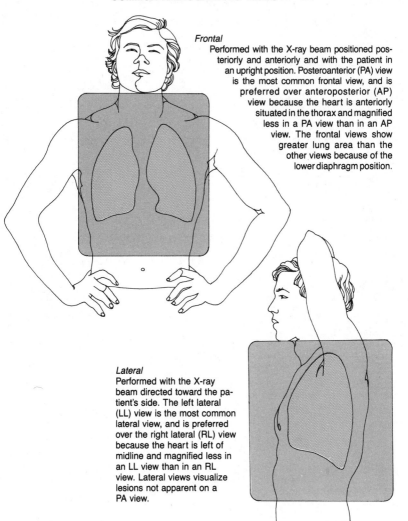

Frontal
Performed with the X-ray beam positioned posteriorly and anteriorly and with the patient in an upright position. Posteroanterior (PA) view is the most common frontal view, and is preferred over anteroposterior (AP) view because the heart is anteriorly situated in the thorax and magnified less in a PA view than in an AP view. The frontal views show greater lung area than the other views because of the lower diaphragm position.

Lateral
Performed with the X-ray beam directed toward the patient's side. The left lateral (LL) view is the most common lateral view, and is preferred over the right lateral (RL) view because the heart is left of midline and magnified less in an LL view than in an RL view. Lateral views visualize lesions not apparent on a PA view.

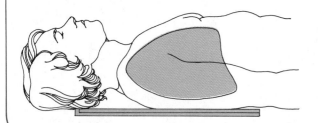

Recumbent
Performed with the X-ray beam overhead and with the patient supine. This view helps distinguish free fluid from encapsulated fluid and from an elevated diaphragm.

Oblique

Performed with the X-ray beam angled between the frontal and lateral views. This view helps evaluate intrathoracic disorders, pleural disease, esophageal abnormalities, hilar masses, and mediastinal masses (rarely, it is also used to localize lesions within the chest).

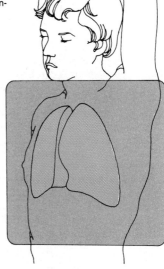

Lordotic

Performed with the X-ray beam directed through the axis of the middle thoracic lobe and with the patient leaning back against the film plate. This view evaluates the apices of the lungs (usually obscured by bony structures) and helps localize sites of tuberculosis.

Decubitus

Performed with the X-ray beam parallel to the floor and with the patient in one of several horizontal positions (supine, prone, or side). This view demonstrates the extent of pulmonary abscess or cavity, the presence of free pleural fluid or pneumothorax, and the mobility of mediastinal mass when the patient changes positions.

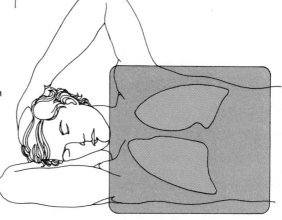

in the X-ray field. Tell him he'll be asked to take a deep breath and to hold it momentarily while the film is being taken, to provide a clearer view of pulmonary structures.

Equipment
X-ray machine (stationary or portable).

Procedure
If a *stationary X-ray machine* is being used, the patient stands or sits in front of the machine, so films can be taken of the posteroanterior and left lateral views.

When the radiograph is taken by the *portable X-ray machine,* at the patient's bedside, assist with the positioning of the patient. Since an upright chest radiograph is preferable, move the patient to the top of the bed, if he can tolerate it. Elevate the head of the bed for maximum upright positioning. Move cardiac monitoring cables, I.V. tubing from subclavian lines, pulmonary artery catheter lines, and safety pins as far from the X-ray field as possible.

Precautions
□ Chest radiography is usually contraindicated during the first trimester of pregnancy; however, when radiography is absolutely necessary, a lead apron placed over the patient's abdomen can shield the fetus.
□ If the patient is intubated, check that no tubes have been dislodged during positioning.
□ To avoid exposure to radiation, leave the room or the immediate area while the films are being taken. If you must stay in the area, wear a lead-lined apron or protective clothing.

Findings
For normal chest radiography findings, see chart on pages 650 and 651.

Implications of results
For an accurate diagnosis, radiography findings require correlation with additional radiologic and pulmonary tests. Pulmonary hyperinflation with low diaphragm and generalized increased radiolucency may suggest emphysema but

may also occur in radiographs of healthy persons. (For common radiography findings, see chart on pages 650 and 651.)

Post-test care
None.

Interfering factors
□ Portable chest radiographs taken in the anteroposterior position may show larger cardiac shadowing than other radiographs, because the distance of the anterior structures from the beam is shorter. Portable chest radiographs— primarily those taken to detect atelectasis, pneumonia, pneumothorax, and mediastinal shift, or to evaluate treatment—may be less reliable than stationary radiographs.
□ Films taken with the patient in a supine position will not show fluid levels.
□ Since chest radiographs vary with the patient's age, sex, and habitus, these factors should be considered when the films are evaluated.
□ Underexposure or overexposure of the film may result in radiographs of poor quality.

SR. EILEEN MARIE HOLLEN, RN, BSN, CCRN

Paranasal Sinus Radiography

The paranasal sinuses—air-filled cavities lined with mucous membrane—lie within the maxillary, ethmoid, sphenoid, and frontal bones. Sinus abnormalities, resulting from inflammation, trauma, cysts, mucoceles, granulomatosis, and other conditions, may include distorted bony sinus walls, altered mucous membranes, and fluid or masses within the cavities.

In paranasal sinus radiography, X-rays or gamma rays penetrate the paranasal sinuses and react on specially sensitized film, forming an image of sinus structures. The air that normally fills the paranasal sinuses appears black on film, but fluid in a sinus appears as a clouded to opaque density and may reveal an air-fluid level. A bone fracture is visible as a linear, radiolucent defect; cysts, polyps, and tumors are visible as soft-tissue masses projecting into the sinus.

When surrounding facial structures—superimposed on the paranasal sinuses—interfere with visualization of relevant areas, tomography may be done to provide further information. Tomography is especially useful in evaluating facial trauma and neoplastic disease.

Purpose
□ To detect unilateral or bilateral abnormalities, possibly indicating trauma or disease

□ To confirm diagnosis of neoplastic or inflammatory paranasal sinus disease

□ To determine the location and size of a malignant neoplasm.

Patient preparation
Describe the procedure to the patient, and explain that this test helps evaluate abnormalities of the paranasal sinuses. Tell him who will perform the test, where and when it will be performed, and that it usually takes 10 or 15 minutes to complete.

Tell the patient that his head may be immobilized in a foam vise during the test to help him maintain the correct position, but that the vise doesn't hurt. Explain that he'll be asked to sit upright and avoid moving while the X-rays are being taken, to prevent blurring of the image and to allow visualization of air-fluid levels, if present. Emphasize the importance of his cooperation. Instruct him to remove dentures, all jewelry, or metal in the X-ray field.

Equipment
Franklin radiographic head unit.

Procedure
The patient sits upright (possibly with his head in a foam vise), between the X-ray tube and a film cassette. During the test, the X-ray tube is positioned at

PARANASAL SINUS TOMOGRAPHY

Tomography of the paranasal sinuses is performed by moving an X-ray beam and X-ray film simultaneously and in opposite directions around a pivot point during film exposure. The resulting image produces a sharply focused selected section, with blurred areas above and below it. This test supplements radiography when surrounding facial structures obscure relevant areas. Because tomography visualizes the paranasal sinuses in very thin sections, one section at a time, it's especially useful in detecting involvement of bone by tumor and locating fractures of bony sinus walls and foreign bodies.

To prepare a patient for paranasal sinus tomography, describe the procedure to him and advise him to remain motionless while the tomograms are being taken; patient movement during filming interferes with test results. A normal paranasal sinus tomogram shows structures equivalent to a normal X-ray film of this area without superimposition of other structures.

specific angles and the patient's head is placed in various standard positions, while his paranasal sinuses are filmed from different angles. If necessary, assist with positioning the patient.

Precautions
□ Paranasal sinus radiography is usually contraindicated during pregnancy; however, when it's absolutely necessary, a lead-lined apron placed over the patient's abdomen can shield the fetus.

□ To avoid exposure to radiation, leave the room or the immediate area during the test; if you must stay in the area, wear a lead-lined apron.

Findings
Normal paranasal sinuses are radiolucent and filled with air, which appears black on paranasal sinus films.

Implications of results
See the chart on page 656 for common implications of abnormal radiographic findings.

Post-test care
None.

IMPLICATIONS OF ABNORMAL FINDINGS

DISORDER	ABNORMAL FINDINGS
Paranasal sinus trauma or fracture	• Edema or hemorrhage in mucous membrane lining or sinus cavity • Clouded sinus air cells • Air-fluid level • Radiolucent, linear bone defects • Irregular, overriding bone edges • Depression or displacement of bone fragments • Foreign bodies
Acute sinusitis	• Swollen, inflamed mucous membrane • Inflammatory exudate • Hazy to opaque sinus air cells • Air-fluid level
Chronic sinusitis	• Thickened mucous membrane • Hazy to opaque sinus air cells • Air-fluid level • Thickening or sclerosis of bony wall of affected sinus
Wegener's granulomatosis	• Clouded to opaque sinus air cells • Destruction of bony sinus wall
Malignant neoplasm	• Rounded or lobulated soft-tissue mass, projecting into sinus • Destruction of bony sinus wall
Benign bone tumor	• Distortion of bony sinus wall in specific patterns
Cyst, polyp, or benign tumor	• Rounded or lobulated soft-tissue mass, projecting into sinus
Mucocele	• Clouded sinus air cells • Destruction of bony sinus wall resulting in various degrees of radiolucency

Interfering factors

□ Failure to remove dentures, jewelry, and metal within the X-ray field, or the presence of numerous metallic foreign bodies in or around the paranasal sinuses may interfere with accurate determination of test results.

□ Patient movement during filming may necessitate additional X-ray films.

□ The patient's inability to sit upright during filming may necessitate performing the test on an X-ray table. This impairs visualization and diminishes the diagnostic values of the test.

□ The superimposition of surrounding facial structures on the film may impair visualization of paranasal sinuses.

BONNIE L. ANDERSON, MD

Fluoroscopy

In fluoroscopy, a continuous stream of X-rays passes through the patient, casting shadows of the heart, lungs, and diaphragm on a fluorescent screen. Since fluoroscopy reveals less detail than standard chest radiography, it's indicated only when diagnosis requires visualization of physiologic or pathologic motion of thoracic contents, such as to rule out paralysis in patients with diaphragmatic elevation.

Purpose
□ To assess lung expansion and contraction during quiet breathing, deep breathing, and coughing
□ To assess movement and paralysis of the diaphragm
□ To detect bronchiolar obstructions and pulmonary disease.

Patient preparation
Describe the procedure to the patient, and explain that this test assesses respiratory structures and their motion. Tell him who will perform the test and where, and that the test usually takes 5 minutes.

Tell the patient he'll be asked to follow specific instructions, such as to breathe deeply and to cough, while X-ray images depict his breathing. Instruct him to remove all jewelry in X-ray field.

Equipment
X-ray machine (X-ray transformer, X-ray tube and special fluorescent screen)/videotape recorder (optional).

Procedure
If necessary, assist with positioning the patient. Move cardiac monitoring cables, I.V. tubing from subclavian lines, pulmonary artery catheter lines, and safety pins as far from the X-ray field as possible. During the test, the patient's cardiopulmonary motion is observed on a screen. Special equipment may be used to intensify the images, or a videotape recording of the fluoroscopy may be made, for later study.

Precautions
□ Fluoroscopy is contraindicated during pregnancy.
□ If the patient is intubated, check that no tubes have been dislodged during positioning.
□ To avoid exposure to radiation, leave the room or the immediate area during the test; if you must stay in the area, wear a lead-lined apron.

Findings
Normal diaphragmatic movement is synchronous and symmetric. Normal diaphragmatic excursion ranges from ¾" to 1⅝" (2 to 4 cm).

Implications of results
Diminished diaphragm movement may indicate pulmonary disease. Increased lung translucency may indicate loss of elasticity or bronchiolar obstruction. In elderly persons, the lowest part of the trachea may be displaced to the right by an elongated aorta. Diminished or paradoxical diaphragm movement may indicate diaphragmatic paralysis; however, fluoroscopy may not detect such paralysis in patients who compensate for diminished diaphragm function by using forceful contraction of their abdominal muscles to aid expiration.

Post-test care
None.

Interfering factors
Failure to remove jewelry and metal within the X-ray field may interfere with accurate determination of test results.
SR. EILEEN MARIE HOLLEN, RN, BSN, CCRN

Chest Tomography
[Laminagraphy, planigraphy, stratigraphy, body-section roentgenography]

Tomography provides clearly focused radiographic images of selected body sections otherwise obscured by shadows of overlying or underlying structures. In this procedure, the X-ray tube and film move around the patient (the linear tube sweep) in opposite directions, producing exposures in which a selected body plane appears sharply defined and the areas above and below it are blurred.

Since tomography emits high radiation levels, it's used only for further evaluation of a chest lesion.

Purpose

□ To demonstrate pulmonary densities (for cavitation, calcification, and presence of fat), tumors (especially those obstructing the bronchial lumen), or lesions (especially those located deep within the mediastinum, such as lymph nodes at the hilum).

Patient preparation

Describe the procedure to the patient, and explain that this test helps evaluate structures within the chest. Inform him that he needn't restrict food or fluids before the test. Tell him who will perform the test and where, and that it takes 30 to 60 minutes.

Warn the patient that the equipment is noisy, due to rapidly moving metal-on-metal parts, and that the X-ray tube swings overhead. Advise him to breathe normally during the test but to remain immobile; tell him that foam wedges will be used to help him maintain a comfortable, motionless position. Suggest he close his eyes to prevent involuntary movement. Instruct him to remove all jewelry within the X-ray field.

Equipment

Tomograph.

Procedure

The patient is placed in a supine position or in different degrees of lateral rotation on the X-ray table. The X-ray tube then swings over the patient, taking numerous films from different angles.

For lung tomography, the X-ray tube is usually moved in a linear direction but may be moved in a hypocycloid, or in a circular, elliptic, trispiral, or figure-eight pattern. Pluridirectional films aid diagnosis of mediastinal lesions or tumors.

Precautions

□ Tomography is contraindicated during pregnancy.
□ To avoid exposure to radiation, leave the room or the immediate area during the test; if you must stay in the area, wear a lead-lined apron.

Findings

A normal chest tomogram shows structures equivalent to a normal chest X-ray film.

Implications of results

Central calcification in a nodule suggests a benign lesion; an irregularly bordered tumor suggests malignancy; a sharply defined tumor suggests granuloma or nonmalignancy. Evaluation of the hilum can help differentiate blood vessels from nodes; identify bronchial dilation, stenosis, and endobronchial lesions; and detect tumor extension into the hilar lung area. Tomography can also identify extension of a mediastinal lesion to the ribs or spine.

Post-test care

None.

Interfering factors

□ Failure to remove jewelry and metal within the X-ray field may interfere with accurate determination of test results.
□ The patient's inability to lie still may interfere with test results and necessitate additional X-ray films, with greater exposure to radiation.

SR. EILEEN MARIE HOLLEN, RN, BSN, CCRN

Bronchography

Bronchography is X-ray examination of the tracheobronchial tree after instillation of a radiopaque iodine contrast agent through a catheter into the lumens of the trachea and bronchi. The contrast agent coats the bronchial tree, permitting visualization of any anatomic deviations. Bronchography has been performed infrequently since the development of tomography and the flexible bronchoscope. Currently, it is used primarily for guidance during a bronchoscopy or to provide permanent films of pathologic findings.

Bronchography may be performed us-

ing a local anesthetic instilled through the catheter or bronchoscope, although a general anesthetic may be necessary for children or during a concurrent bronchoscopy (see BRONCHOSCOPY).

Purpose

☐ To help detect bronchiectasis, bronchial obstruction, pulmonary tumors, cysts, and cavities, and indirectly, to pinpoint the cause of hemoptysis

☐ To provide permanent films of pathologic findings

☐ To provide guidance while performing a bronchoscopy.

Patient preparation

Explain to the patient that this test helps evaluate abnormalities of the bronchial structures. Instruct him to fast for 12 hours before the test, and to perform good oral hygiene the night before and the morning of the test. Tell him who will perform the test, and where and when it will be performed.

Make sure the patient or a responsible member of the family has signed a consent form. Check the patient's history for hypersensitivity to anesthetics, iodine, or X-ray dyes. If the patient has a productive cough, administer an expectorant and perform postural drainage 1 to 3 days before the test is performed, as ordered.

If the procedure is to be performed under a local anesthetic, tell the patient he'll receive a sedative to help him relax and to suppress the gag reflex. Prepare him for the unpleasant taste of the anesthetic spray. Warn him that he may experience some difficulty breathing during the procedure, but reassure him that his airway won't be blocked and that he'll receive enough oxygen. Tell him the catheter or bronchoscope will pass more easily if he relaxes. Just before the test, instruct the patient to remove his dentures and to void.

If bronchography is to be performed under a general anesthetic, at the time of bronchoscopy, inform the patient that he'll receive a sedative before the test, to help him relax.

Equipment

X-ray machine/tilting table/sedative/anesthetic/catheter or bronchoscope/radiopaque oils or water-soluble dye solution for contrast agent/emergency resuscitation equipment.

Procedure

After a local anesthetic is sprayed into the patient's mouth and throat, a bronchoscope or catheter is passed into the trachea, and the anesthetic and contrast agent are instilled. The patient is placed in various positions during the test, to promote movement of the contrast agent into different areas of the bronchial tree. After radiographs are taken, the dye is removed through postural drainage or nebulization.

Precautions

☐ Bronchography is contraindicated during pregnancy, in persons with hypersensitivity to iodine or X-ray dyes, and usually in persons with respiratory insufficiency.

☐ Observe the patient with asthma for laryngeal spasm secondary to the instillation of the contrast agent.

☐ Observe the patient with chronic obstructive pulmonary disease for airway occlusion secondary to the instillation of the contrast agent.

Findings

Right main stem bronchus is shorter, wider, and more vertical than the left bronchus. Successive branches of the bronchi become smaller in diameter and are free of obstruction or lesions.

Implications of results

Bronchography may demonstrate bronchiectasis or bronchial obstruction due to tumors, cysts, cavities, or foreign objects. Findings require correlation with physical examination, patient history, and possibly other pulmonary diagnostic studies.

Post-test care

☐ Watch for signs of laryngeal spasms

(dyspnea) or edema (hoarseness, dyspnea, laryngeal stridor) secondary to traumatic intubation.

☐ Immediately report signs of allergic reaction to contrast agent or anesthetic—itching, dyspnea, tachycardia, palpitations, excitation, hypo- or hypertension, or euphoria.

☐ Withhold food, fluid, and oral medications until gag reflex returns (usually 2 hours). Fluid intake before the gag reflex returns may cause aspiration.

☐ Watch for signs of chemical or secondary bacterial pneumonia—fever, dyspnea, rales, or rhonchi—the result of incomplete expectoration of the contrast agent.

☐ If the patient has a sore throat, reassure him it is only temporary, and provide throat lozenges or a liquid gargle when his gag reflex returns.

☐ Advise the outpatient to postpone resuming his usual activities until the following day.

Interfering factors

The presence of secretions or failure to position the patient properly may inhibit the contrast agent from adequately filling the bronchial tree.

SR. EILEEN MARIE HOLLEN, RN, BSN, CCRN

Pulmonary Angiography

[Pulmonary arteriography]

Pulmonary angiography is the radiographic examination of the pulmonary circulation following injection of a radiopaque iodine contrast agent into the pulmonary artery or one of its branches. Most commonly, it's used to confirm symptomatic pulmonary emboli when scans prove nondiagnostic, especially before anticoagulant therapy or in patients in whom it's contraindicated. It also provides accurate preoperative evaluation of

patients with congenital heart disease.

Possible complications include arterial occlusion, myocardial perforation or rupture, ventricular arrhythmias from myocardial irritation, and acute renal failure from hypersensitivity to the contrast agent.

Purpose

☐ To detect pulmonary embolism in a patient who is symptomatic but whose lung scan is indeterminate or normal

☐ To evaluate pulmonary circulation preoperatively in the patient with congenital heart disease.

Patient preparation

Describe the procedure to the patient, and explain that this test permits evaluation of the blood vessels, to help identify the cause of his symptoms. Instruct him to fast for 8 hours before the test, or as ordered. Tell him who will perform the test and where, and that the test takes approximately 1 hour.

Tell the patient a small incision will be made in the right arm where blood samples are usually drawn, or in the right groin, and that a local anesthetic is used to numb the area. Inform him that a small catheter is then inserted into the blood vessel and passed into the right side of the heart, to the pulmonary artery. Tell him the contrast agent is then injected into this artery, to allow visualization of blood flow to the lungs on the X-ray film. Warn him that he may experience an urge to cough, a flushed feeling, nausea, or a salty taste for approximately 5 minutes after the injection. Inform him that his heart rate will be monitored continuously during the procedure.

Make sure the patient or a responsible member of the family has signed a consent form. Check the patient's history for hypersensitivity to anesthetics, iodine, seafood, or radiographic contrast agents.

Equipment

50 ml of 60% meglumine diatrizoate or of 45% diatrizoate/60 ml thimerosal/ 60 ml of 70% alcohol/500 ml physiologic

saline solution/epinephrine for emergency administration/30 ml of 2% procaine/3-ml, 6-ml, and 20-ml syringes/ two 2½" 18G needles/polyethylene catheter/extension tubing (Venotube) with stopcock/two sterile graduated cups/ knife blade and handle/mechanical contrast agent injector/radiographic equipment.

Procedure

After the patient is placed in a supine position, the local anesthetic is injected and the cardiac monitor is attached to the patient. An incision is made, and a catheter is introduced into the antecubital or femoral vein. As the catheter passes through the right atrium, the right ventricle, and the pulmonary artery, pressures are measured and blood samples are drawn from various regions of the pulmonary circulatory system. The contrast agent is then injected, and circulates through the pulmonary artery and lung capillaries while X-ray films are taken.

Precautions

□ Pulmonary angiography is contraindicated during pregnancy and in patients who are hypersensitive to iodine, seafood, or radiographic contrast agents.
□ Monitor for ventricular arrhythmias, due to myocardial irritation from passage of the catheter through the heart chambers.
□ Observe for signs of hypersensitivity to the contrast agent, such as dyspnea, nausea, vomiting, sweating, increased heart rate, and numbness of extremities.
□ Keep emergency equipment available in case of hypersensitivity reaction to the contrast agent.

Findings

Normally, the contrast agent flows symmetrically and without interruption through the pulmonary circulatory system.

Implications of results

Interruption of blood flow may result from emboli, vascular filling defects, or stenosis.

Post-test care

□ Apply a pressure dressing over the catheter insertion site, and note any bleeding.
□ Observe for signs of myocardial per-

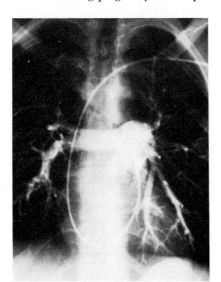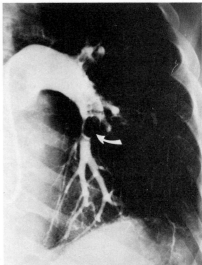

Shown at left is a normal pulmonary angiogram, taken during the arterial phase. At right is a close-up of an abnormal angiogram, showing a blood clot in the left pulmonary artery (indicated by arrow).

foration or rupture by monitoring vital signs, as ordered.

□ Be alert for signs of acute renal failure, such as sudden onset of oliguria, nausea, and vomiting.

□ Check the catheter insertion site for inflammation or hematoma formation and report symptoms of a delayed hypersensitive response to the contrast agent or to the local anesthetic (dyspnea, itching, tachycardia, palpitations, hypo- or hypertension, excitation, or euphoria).

□ Advise the patient about any restriction of activity. He may resume his usual diet after the test.

Interfering factors

None.

SR. EILEEN MARIE HOLLEN, RN, BSN, CCRN

SCANNING TESTS

Lung Scan

[Lung perfusion scan, lung scintiscan]

The lung scan produces a visual image of pulmonary blood flow after I.V. injection of a radiopharmaceutical—human serum albumin microspheres (particles) or macroaggregated albumin, both of which are bonded to technetium. This test is useful in confirming pulmonary vascular obstruction, such as pulmonary emboli. The lung scan, performed with a ventilation scan, assesses ventilation-perfusion patterns.

Purpose

□ To assess arterial perfusion of the lungs

□ To detect pulmonary emboli

□ To evaluate, preoperatively, the pulmonary function of a patient with marginal lung reserves.

Patient preparation

Explain to the patient that this test helps evaluate respiratory function. Inform him he needn't restrict food or fluids before the test. Tell him who will perform the test and where, and that it takes 15 to 30 minutes.

Inform the patient that the radiopharmaceutical will be injected into a vein in the arm and that the amount of radioactivity is minimal. Tell him he'll ei-

ther sit in front of the camera or lie under it, and that neither the camera nor the uptake probe emits any radiation. Assure him that he'll be comfortable during the test and that he doesn't have to remain perfectly still.

On the test request slip, note conditions such as chronic obstructive pulmonary disease (COPD), vasculitis, pulmonary edema, tumor, sickle cell disease, or parasitic disease.

Equipment

Scintiscanner/radiopharmaceutical.

Procedure

Half the total amount of radiopharmaceutical is injected I.V. while the patient is in a supine position, and half is injected while the patient is in a prone position. After the uptake of the radiopharmaceutical, the gamma camera takes a series of single stationary images in the anterior, posterior, oblique, and both lateral chest views. Images projected on an oscilloscope screen show the distribution of radioactive particles.

Precautions

A lung scan is contraindicated in patients hypersensitive to the radiopharmaceutical.

Findings

Hot spots—areas with normal blood perfusion—show a high uptake of the radioactive substance; a normal lung shows a uniform uptake pattern.

Implications of results

Cold spots—areas of low radioactive uptake—indicate poor perfusion, suggesting an embolism; however, a ventilation scan is necessary to confirm diagnosis. Decreased regional blood flow that occurs without vessel obstruction may indicate pneumonitis.

Post-test care

If a hematoma develops at the injection site, apply warm soaks.

Interfering factors

□ Scheduling the patient for more than one radionuclide test a day (especially if different trace substances are used) can

NORMAL AND ABNORMAL LUNG SCANS

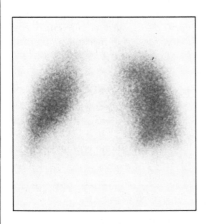 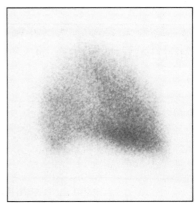

In the normal posteroanterior and lateral lung scan views (top), note the smooth outlines and the uniform, complete visualizations of both fields. Compare them with the abnormal views (bottom). Note the uneven densities, particularly in the right lung field of the abnormal posteroanterior view. This indicates impaired blood flow, resulting from a pulmonary embolus.

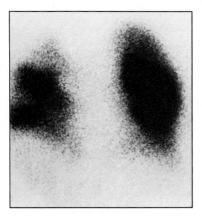 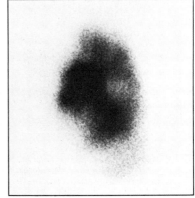

inhibit adequate diffusion of the radioactive substance in the second test.

□ I.V. injection of the radiopharmaceutical while the patient is sitting can produce abnormal images, since a large proportion of the particles settle to the lung bases.

□ Conditions such as COPD, vasculitis, pulmonary edema, tumor, sickle cell disease, or parasitic disease may cause abnormal perfusion, interfering with accurate determination of test results.

SR. EILEEN MARIE HOLLEN, RN, BSN, CCRN

Ventilation Scan

Ventilation scan—a nuclear scan performed after inhalation of air mixed with radioactive gas—delineates areas of the lung ventilated during respiration.

The scan consists of recording the distribution of the gas during three phases: during the buildup of radioactive gas (wash-in phase), after the patient rebreathes from a bag and the radioactivity reaches a steady level (equilibrium phase), and after removal of the radioactive gas from the lungs (wash-out phase). Performed with a perfusion scan (see LUNG SCAN), a ventilation scan helps distinguish between parenchymal disease, such as emphysema, sarcoidosis, bronchogenic carcinoma, and tuberculosis, and conditions due to vascular abnormalities, such as pulmonary emboli.

In a patient on mechanical ventilation, krypton gas must be substituted for xenon gas during the test.

Purpose
□ To help diagnose pulmonary emboli
□ To identify areas of the lung capable of ventilation
□ To help evaluate regional respiratory function

NORMAL AND ABNORMAL VENTILATION SCANS

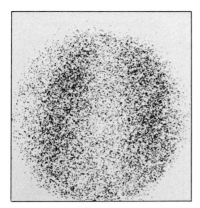 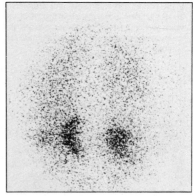

Ventilation scans record the distribution of radioactive gas during three phases: buildup of radioactive gas (wash-in phase), after the patient rebreathes from a bag and the radioactivity reaches a steady level (equilibrium phase), and after removal of the radioactive gas from the lungs (wash-out phase). The normal ventilation scan (at left), taken 30 minutes to 1 hour after wash-out phase, shows equal gas distribution. The abnormal scan (at right), taken 1½ to 2 hours after the start of the wash-out phase, shows unequal gas distribution represented by the area of poor wash-out on both the left and right sides.

□ To locate regional hypoventilation, which usually results from excessive smoking or chronic obstructive pulmonary disease.

Patient preparation

Describe the procedure to the patient, and explain that this test helps evaluate respiratory function. Inform him he needn't restrict food or fluids. Tell him who will perform the test and where, and that the test takes 15 to 30 minutes.

Instruct the patient to remove all jewelry or metal in the X-ray field. Tell him he'll be asked to hold his breath for a short time after inhaling gas, and that a machine will scan his chest, at which time he must remain still. Reassure the patient that the amount of radioactive gas used is kept to a minimum.

Equipment

Breathing mask that fits tightly over the nose and mouth/radioactive gas (xenon 133 or krypton 85)/nuclear scanner.

Procedure

After the patient inhales air mixed with a small amount of radioactive gas through a mask, its distribution in the lungs is monitored on a nuclear scanner. The patient's chest is scanned as he exhales.

Precautions

Watch for leaks in the closed system of radioactive gas, such as through the mask, which can contaminate the surrounding atmosphere.

Findings

Normal findings include an equal distribution of gas in both lungs, and normal wash-in and wash-out phases.

Implications of results

Unequal gas distribution in both lungs indicates poor ventilation or airway obstruction in areas with low radioactivity. When compared with a lung scan (perfusion scan), in vascular obstruc-

tions—such as pulmonary embolism—the perfusion to the embolized area is decreased, but the ventilation to this area is maintained; in parenchymal disease—such as pneumonia—ventilation is abnormal within the areas of consolidation.

Post-test care

None.

Interfering factors

Failure to remove jewelry and metal in the X-ray field during scanning may interfere with accurate determination of test results.

SR. EILEEN MARIE HOLLEN, RN, BSN, CCRN

Thoracic Computed Tomography

Thoracic computed tomography (CT) provides cross-sectional views of the chest by passing an X-ray beam from a computerized scanner through the body at different angles. CT scanning may be done with or without an injected radioiodine contrast agent, which is primarily used to highlight blood vessels and to allow greater visual discrimination.

This test is especially useful in detecting small differences in tissue density. With nuclear medicine scanning, thoracic CT is one of the most accurate and informative diagnostic tests, and may replace mediastinoscopy in diagnosis of mediastinal masses and Hodgkin's disease; its clinical application in the evaluation of pulmonary pathology is proven.

Purpose

□ To locate suspected neoplasms (such as in Hodgkin's disease), especially with mediastinal involvement

□ To differentiate coin-sized calcified lesions (indicating tuberculosis) from tumors

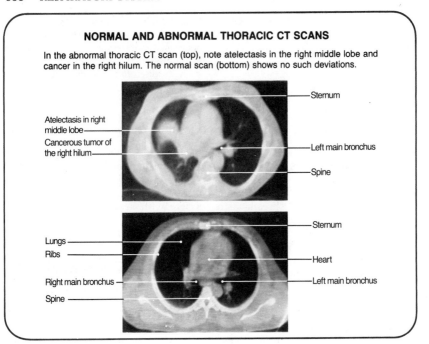

NORMAL AND ABNORMAL THORACIC CT SCANS

In the abnormal thoracic CT scan (top), note atelectasis in the right middle lobe and cancer in the right hilum. The normal scan (bottom) shows no such deviations.

Top scan labels: Atelectasis in right middle lobe — Cancerous tumor of the right hilum — Sternum — Left main bronchus — Spine

Bottom scan labels: Lungs — Ribs — Right main bronchus — Spine — Sternum — Heart — Left main bronchus

☐ To distinguish tumors adjacent to the aorta from aortic aneurysms

☐ To detect the invasion of a neck mass in the thorax

☐ To evaluate primary malignancy that may metastasize to the lungs, especially in patients with primary bone tumors, soft-tissue sarcomas, and melanomas

☐ To evaluate the mediastinal lymph nodes.

Patient preparation

Explain to the patient that this test provides cross-sectional views of the chest and distinguishes small differences in tissue density. If a contrast agent will not be used, inform him that he needn't restrict food or fluids. If the test is to be performed with contrast enhancement, instruct the patient to fast for 4 hours before the test. Tell him who will perform the test and where, and that the procedure usually takes 1½ hours and will not cause him any discomfort.

Tell the patient he'll be positioned on an X-ray table that moves into the center of a large ring-shaped piece of X-ray equipment, and that the equipment may be noisy. Inform him that a radiographic contrast agent may be injected into a vein in his arm. If so, he may experience nausea, warmth, flushing of the face, or a salty taste. Reassure him that the amount of radiation exposure is minimal. Tell him not to move during the test, but to breathe normally. Instruct him to remove all jewelry and metal in the X-ray field.

Make sure the patient or a responsible member of the family has signed a consent form. Check the history for hypersensitivity to iodine or radiographic contrast agents.

Equipment

CT scanner/oscilloscope/Polaroid film/ contrast agent for injection, if ordered.

Procedure

After the patient is placed in a supine position on the radiographic table and the contrast agent has been injected, the machine scans the patient at different angles, while the computer calculates small differences in the densities of various tissues, water, fat, bone, and air. This information is displayed as a printout of numerical values and as a projection on an oscilloscope screen. Images may be recorded for further study.

Precautions

Thoracic CT is contraindicated during pregnancy and, if a contrast agent is used, in persons who have a history of hypersensitivity reactions to iodine, shellfish, or radiographic contrast agents.

Findings

Black and white areas on a thoracic CT scan refer, respectively, to air and bone densities. Shades of gray correspond to water, fat, and soft-tissue densities.

Implications of results

Abnormal thoracic CT findings include tumors, nodules, cysts, aortic aneurysm, enlarged lymph nodes, pleural effusion, and accumulations of blood, fluid, or fat.

Post-test care

Watch for signs of delayed hypersensitivity to the contrast agent. These signs include itching, hypo- or hypertension, and respiratory distress.

Interfering factors

☐ Failure to remove jewelry or metal from the X-ray field may interfere with an accurate diagnosis.

☐ The patient's inability to lie still during scanning may interfere with accurate diagnosis or may require repetition of the test, which increases his exposure to radiation.

☐ Obese patients may not fit on the X-ray table.

SR. EILEEN MARIE HOLLEN, RN, BSN, CCRN

Selected References

Bordow, Richard A., et al. *Manual of Clinical Problems in Pulmonary Medicine*. Boston: Little, Brown & Co., 1980.

Brunner, Lillian S., and Suddarth, Doris S. *The Lippincott Manual of Nursing Practice*, 3rd ed. Philadelphia: J.B. Lippincott Co., 1982.

Brunner, Lillian S., and Suddarth, Doris S. *Textbook of Medical-Surgical Nursing*, 5th ed. Philadelphia: J.B. Lippincott Co., 1984.

French, Ruth M. *Guide to Diagnostic Procedures*, 5th ed. New York: McGraw-Hill Book Co., 1980.

Glauser, Frederick L., ed. *Signs and Symptoms in Pulmonary Medicine*. Philadelphia: J.B. Lippincott Co., 1983.

Grossman, Zachary D., et al. *The Clinician's Guide to Diagnostic Imaging*. New York: Raven Press Pubs., 1983.

Henry, John Bernard, ed. *Todd-Sanford-Davidsohn Clinical Diagnosis and Management by Laboratory Methods*, 17th ed. Philadelphia: W.B. Saunders Co., 1984.

Holloway, Nancy M. *Nursing the Critically Ill Adult*. Reading, Mass.: Addison-Wesley Publishing Co., 1978.

Luckmann, Joan, and Sorensen, Karen C. *Medical-Surgical Nursing: A Psychophysiologic Approach*, 2nd ed. Philadelphia: W.B. Saunders Co., 1980.

Nursing85 Drug Handbook. Springhouse, Pa.: Springhouse Corp., 1985.

Petersdorf, Robert G., and Adams, Raymond D. eds. *Harrison's Principles of Internal Medicine*, 10th ed. New York: McGraw-Hill Book Co., 1983.

Proto, A.V., et al. "The Chest Radiologic Workup—Special Studies," *Basics of RD* 9:1-6, September 1980.

Respiratory Disorders. Nurse's Clinical Library. Springhouse, Pa.: Springhouse Corp., 1984.

Swett, Henry A. "Thoracic CT: When X-rays Are Not Enough," *Journal of Respiratory Diseases* 1(8):48-64, July/August 1980.

Wallach, Jacques B. *Interpretation of Diagnostic Tests: A Handbook Synopsis of Laboratory Medicine*, 3rd ed. Boston: Little, Brown & Co., 1978.

24 Skeletal System

LEARNING OBJECTIVES

After completing this chapter, the reader will be able to:
- explain the anatomy and physiology of the skeletal system.
- describe the procedure for evaluating skeletal disorders.
- list the puncture sites for joint aspiration.
- identify the types of tests used to evaluate the skeletal system.
- state the purpose of each test discussed in the chapter.
- prepare the patient physically and psychologically for each test.
- describe the procedure for performing each test.
- specify appropriate precautions for safe administration of each test.
- recognize signs of adverse reaction and respond appropriately.
- implement appropriate post-test care.
- identify the normal findings of each test.
- discuss the implications of abnormal test results.
- list factors that may interfere with accurate test results.

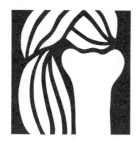

Skeletal System

Introduction

Diagnostic tests of the skeletal system efficiently evaluate bones and their inner structures, as well as the joints and lubricating fluids within them. These tests commonly utilize a wide range of techniques—radiography, nuclear medicine, endoscopy, joint aspiration, and biopsy.

Several skeletal tests combine diagnosis and treatment. For example, arthroscopy permits direct visualization of a joint as well as removal of loose bodies within the joint, menisectomy, meniscal repair, abrasion arthroplasty, and release of the vastus lateralis muscle. Arthrocentesis provides a fluid sample for laboratory analysis as well as an avenue for local drug therapy.

Structure of bone

Bones are complex structures composed of living cells and nonliving intercellular substance. The intercellular matrix consists of inorganic salts—mostly calcium and phosphate—embedded in collagen fibers. All bones have some basic structures in common. They are covered by the periosteum—a dense layer of connective tissue that contains osteoblasts, blood vessels, nerves, and lymphatics—and have an inner generative membrane called the marrow (medullary) cavity.

Histologically, bone is of two basic types. *Cancellous* (spongy) bone contains many open spaces between thin strands of bone called *trabeculae,* which are oriented along lines of stress or pressure and give the bone extra structural strength. *Compact* bone is strong and dense, with many networks of interconnecting canals, each of which is known as a *haversian system.* A haversian canal runs centrally through each system, parallel to the bone's long axis, and contains one or two blood vessels, which provide much of the bone's blood supply. The haversian canals are surrounded by concentric cylindric layers *(lamellae),* which are closely spaced in compact bone. Small cavities *(lacunae)* appear between the lamellae; each lacuna contains *osteocytes,* mature bone-forming cells, suspended in tissue fluid. The lacunae are joined by a network of tiny canals called *canaliculi,* each of which contains one or more capillaries and provides an additional route for tissue fluids.

Red marrow, which produces blood cells, occupies the spaces of cancellous bone. In adults, red marrow appears mainly in the spongy part of cranial bones, in the ribs and sternum, in the vertebrae, and in portions of the femur, humerus, and other long bones. In newborns and children, it appears in many other bones. *Yellow marrow* is present in the shafts of long bones and extends into the haversian system. It is composed of adipose cells and can change to red marrow, if necessary.

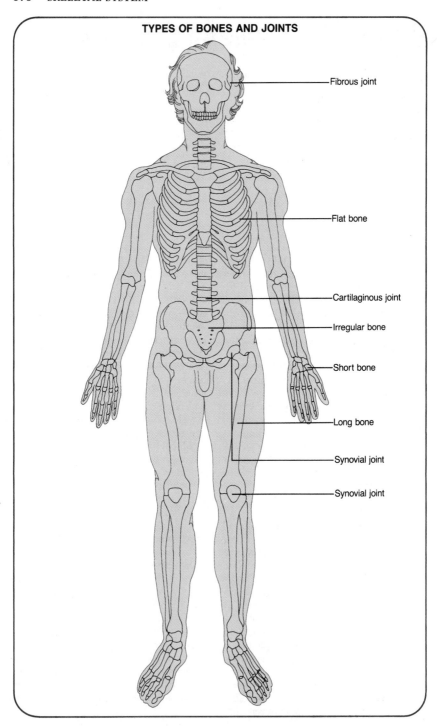

TYPES OF BONES AND JOINTS

Fibrous joint

Flat bone

Cartilaginous joint

Irregular bone

Short bone

Long bone

Synovial joint

Synovial joint

Types of bones
Bones are classified by shape.

□ *Long bones* are found in the extremities and consist of a shaft, or *diaphysis,* and two bulbous ends called *epiphyses.* The parts of the shaft that flare to join the epiphyses are called *metaphyses;* these contain the bone's growth zones and become continuous with the epiphyses at maturity. Long bones are composed primarily of compact bone, and include the humerus, radius, ulna, femur, tibia, fibula, phalanges, and metatarsals.

□ *Short bones* consist mainly of cancellous bone with a thin compact bone shell, and include the tarsal and carpal bones.

□ *Flat bones* have a large surface area and provide protection for soft body parts. They comprise an inner layer of cancellous bone, surrounded by compact bone. Examples are the frontal and parietal bones of the cranium, and the ribs, sternum, scapulae, ilium, and pubis.

□ *Irregular bones* are of various shapes and composition, and include the spine (vertebrae, sacrum, coccyx) and certain skull bones—sphenoid, ethmoid, and mandible.

Bones not classified by shape include the sesamoid (free-floating) bones—such as the patella—and wormian bones—small clusters of bones found between some cranial bones. All bones are covered with a fibrous layer called the *periosteum*—except at joints, where they're covered by articular cartilage.

Types of joints
Joints consist of two bones joined in various ways and, like bones, have varying forms.

□ *Fibrous joints* (synarthroses) have only minute motion and provide stability when tight union is necessary, as in the sutures joining the cranial bones.

□ *Cartilaginous joints* (amphiarthroses) allow limited movement, as between vertebrae.

□ *Synovial joints* (diarthroses), the most common type, allow angular and circular movement. To achieve freedom of movement, synovial joints have special characteristics: the bones' two articulating surfaces have a smooth hyaline covering (articular cartilage) that is resilient to pressure; their opposing surfaces are congruous, and glide smoothly on each other; a fibrous capsule holds them together. Lining the joint cavity is the synovial membrane, which secretes a clear viscous fluid called synovial fluid. This fluid lubricates the two opposing surfaces during motion and nourishes the articular cartilage. Surrounding a synovial joint are ligaments, muscles, and tendons, which strengthen and stabilize the joint but allow free movement.

In some synovial joints, the synovial membrane forms two additional structures—bursae and tendon sheaths—which reduce friction. *Bursae* are small cushionlike sacs lined with synovial membranes and filled with synovial fluid; most are located between tendons and bones, as in the shoulders, knees, or elbows, but others can be found between muscles and bones, ligaments and bones, or skin and bone. *Tendon sheaths* are modified bursae that wrap around a tendon to cushion it as it stretches across a joint.

Evaluating skeletal disorders
When a patient's chief complaint involves the skeletal system, be sure to obtain an accurate medical and personal history. Ask the patient about general activity that may be altered by skeletal disease or trauma. Inquire about his job, diet, recreation, sexual activity, and elimination habits. Does he have difficulty getting around or performing normal daily activities?

Ask the patient to describe his symptoms. When did they begin? Have they lessened or worsened? Has he previously sought treatment for the problem? If so, what was the result? Did he comply with the prescribed treatment? Ask if he is in pain at the moment. Has he been able to get relief from the pain? Does he require medication? If so, ask what it is and how much he takes.

Since joint or bone pain symptoms

usually indicate a systemic disease, a complete physical examination is essential. Observe the patient's general appearance; check for localized edema, reddening of pressure points, point tenderness, and other deformities. Check the range of motion of the joint; this may be restricted or painful. Palpate swollen joints to determine the nature of the swelling, which may result from synovial thickening, bone enlargement, or simple fluid effusion.

Pain thought to originate in a major joint may actually come from a minor one. Check the patient's neurovascular status, including motion sensation and circulation. Measure and record any dissimilarities in muscle circumference or limb length. Compare the size and shape of the affected joint with its unaffected opposite.

Diagnostic tests

Radiography is probably the most widely used skeletal test. Because osseous tissue is quite dense, radiography readily demonstrates the skeletal system. A plain X-ray film doesn't require any special patient preparation or restrictions, but does require patient cooperation in assuming various positions during the procedure. Radiographs are usually taken with the patient in the anteroposterior, lateral, or oblique position, or a combination of these. Although the basic views provide valuable diagnostic information, radiography doesn't allow visualization of certain areas.

Bone scan is the examination of bone after I.V. injection of radioiostopes, which accumulate in abnormal bone. Bone scan permits detection of primary and metastatic tumors 3 to 6 months ear-

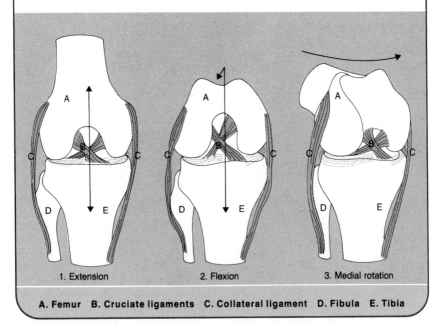

MOVEMENTS OF THE SYNOVIAL KNEE JOINT

The three major movements of the synovial knee joint are extension, flexion, and medial rotation. During extension, both collateral ligaments and cruciate liagments are tensed. During flexion, the collateral ligaments are relaxed and the cruciate ligaments are tensed. During medial rotation, the collateral and cruciate ligaments are twisted.

1. Extension   2. Flexion   3. Medial rotation

A. Femur   B. Cruciate ligaments   C. Collateral ligament   D. Fibula   E. Tibia

lier than X-ray films alone, and helps detect infection and trauma.

Arthrography is the radiographic examination of a joint after injection of air, a radiopaque dye, or both into the joint space. It can detect a torn meniscus or the presence of loose bodies, capsular leaks, and other joint abnormalities.

Arthrocentesis is the aspiration of synovial fluid from a joint space (usually the knee) for diagnosis or to relieve pain caused by fluid accumulation.

Arthroscopy, the direct visualization of joint structures (usually the knee) using a fiberoptic endoscope, is particularly useful for detecting knee disorders—such as arthritis, a torn meniscus, cysts, or loose bodies—that aren't readily revealed by radiography or arthrography.

For a discussion of bone and synovial membrane biopsies commonly performed on patients with skeletal disorders, see chapter 18, HISTOLOGY.

JANE FARRELL, RN, BS

RADIOGRAPHY & NUCLEAR MEDICINE

Vertebral Radiography

Vertebral radiography visualizes all or part of the vertebral column. A commonly performed test, it is used to evaluate the vertebrae for deformities, fractures, dislocations, tumors, and other abnormalities.

In a newborn, the vertebral column normally consists of 33 interlocked vertebrae, most of which are separate and moveable. Anatomically, the vertebral column is divided in descending order into five segments: cervical, thoracic, lumbar, sacral, and coccygeal. The cervical segment, the most flexible part of the column, includes the 7 vertebrae that form the bony framework of the neck. The thoracic segment, with 12 vertebrae, lies behind the thorax and supports the 12 pairs of ribs. The lumbar segment, with 5 vertebrae, supports the small of the back. The sacral segment, originally 5 separate vertebrae, fuses into a single bone by adulthood. The coccygeal segment begins as 4 or 5 small vertebrae and eventually fuses to form the coccyx. The fusion of the vertebrae in these last two segments reduces the number of vertebrae from 33 at birth, to 26 in the adult spine.

All vertebrae are similar in structure,

but vary in size, shape, and articular surface, according to their location in the vertebral column. Fibrocartilaginous intervertebral disks allow some movement between the individual vertebrae.

The type and extent of vertebral radiography depends on the patient's clinical condition. For example, a patient with suspected scoliosis usually requires radiographic study of the entire vertebral column; one with lower back pain requires only study of the lumbar and sacral segments.

Purpose
□ To detect vertebral fractures, dislocations, subluxations, and deformities
□ To detect vertebral degeneration, infection, and congenital disorders
□ To detect disorders of the intervertebral disks
□ To determine the vertebral effects of arthritic and metabolic disorders.

Patient preparation
Explain to the patient that this test permits examination of the spine. Inform him he needn't restrict food or fluids. Tell him that the test requires X-ray films; who will perform the test and where; and that the procedure usually takes 15 to 30 minutes. Advise him that he'll be placed in various positions for the X-ray films, and that, although some positions may produce slight discomfort, he should cooperate to ensure accurate results.

Procedure
Initially, the patient is placed in a supine position on the radiograph table for an anteroposterior view. He may then be repositioned for lateral or right and left oblique views. However, specific positioning depends on the vertebral segment or adjacent structure of interest. For example, to obtain a lateral view of C_7 (and possibly T_1 and T_2), the patient's shoulders should be depressed or pulled down and rotated.

Precautions
□ Vertebral radiography is contraindicated during the first trimester of pregnancy, except when the value of this test outweighs the risk of fetal radiation exposure.

□ Exercise extreme caution when handling trauma patients with suspected spinal injuries, particularly of the cervical area. Such patients should be filmed while on the stretcher to avoid further injury during transfer to the radiographic table.

Findings
Normal vertebrae show no fractures, subluxations, dislocations, curvatures, or other abnormalities. Specific positions and spacing of the vertebrae vary with the patient's age. In the lateral view, adult vertebrae are aligned to form four alternately concave and convex curves. The cervical and lumbar curves are convex anteriorly; the thoracic and sacral curves are concave anteriorly. Although the structure of the coccyx varies, it usually points forward and downward. Neonatal vertebrae form only one curve, which is concave anteriorly.

Implications of results
The vertebral radiograph readily shows spondylolisthesis, fractures, subluxations, dislocations, wedging, and such deformities as kyphosis, scoliosis, and lordosis. However, to confirm other disorders, spinal structures and their spatial relationships on the radiograph must be examined, and the patient's history and clinical status must be considered. These disorders include congenital abnormalities, such as torticollis (wryneck), absence of sacral or lumbar vertebrae, hemivertebrae, and Klippel-Feil syndrome; degenerative processes, such as hypertrophic spurs, osteoarthritis, and narrowed disk spaces; tuberculosis (Pott's disease); benign or malignant intraspinal tumors; ruptured disk and cervical disk syndrome; and systemic disorders, such as rheumatoid arthritis, Charcot's disease, ankylosing spondylitis, osteoporosis, and Paget's disease.

Depending on radiographic results, definitive diagnosis may also require additional tests, such as myelography or computerized tomography.

Post-test care
None.

Interfering factors
Improper positioning of the patient or movement during radiography may produce inaccurate films.

KATHY A. HAUSMAN, RN, MS

Arthrography

Arthrography is the radiographic examination of a joint—usually the knee or shoulder—following the injection of air (pneumoarthrography), a radiopaque contrast medium, or both into the joint space. Arthrography outlines soft tissue not usually visualized by standard radiographs such as the meniscus, cartilage, or ligaments of the knee, and structures of the joint capsule, rotator cuff, and subacromial bursa.

Arthrography, performed as an outpatient procedure under a local anesthetic, is indicated in a patient with persistent unexplained knee or shoulder discomfort. Complications may include occasional infection at the puncture site or in the joint or, rarely, allergic reac-

tions to the contrast medium.

Purpose

□ To detect abnormalities of the menisci, cartilage, and ligaments of the knee

□ To detect shoulder abnormalities, such as a torn rotator cuff and anterior capsule derangement.

Patient preparation

Describe the procedure to the patient, and answer any questions he may have. Explain that this test permits examination of a joint. Inform him he needn't restrict food or fluids. Tell him who will perform the procedure and where. Explain that the fluoroscope is different than an ordinary X-ray machine, and that it allows the doctor to track the contrast medium as it fills the joint space. Inform him that standard X-ray films will also be taken after diffusion of the contrast medium.

Tell the patient that, while the joint area will be anesthetized, he may experience a tingling sensation or pressure in the joint on injection of the contrast medium. Instruct him to remain as still as possible during the procedure, except when following instructions to change position. Stress the importance of his cooperation in assuming various positions, since films must be taken as quickly as possible to ensure optimum quality.

Check the patient's history for hypersensitivity to local anesthetics, iodine, seafood, or the dyes used for other diagnostic tests, such as intravenous pyelography.

Equipment

Fluoroscope/povidone-iodine solution/local anesthetic/two 2″ 20G needles/two 24G needles/three 3-ml syringes/short lumbar puncture needle (3″ 22G for arthrography of the shoulder)/water-soluble radiopaque dye (5 to 15 ml), to be used alone or with air/four sterile sponges/elastic knee bandage/sterile towels/sterile specimen container for fluid/culture tube/sterile adhesive bandage/collodion (optional)/shave preparation kit.

Procedure

Knee arthrography: The knee is cleansed with an antiseptic solution, and the area around the puncture site anesthetized. (It's not usually necessary to anesthetize the joint space itself.) A 2″ needle is then inserted into the joint space between the patella and femoral condyle, and fluid is aspirated. While the needle is still in place, the aspirating syringe is removed and replaced with one containing dye. If fluoroscopic examination demonstrates correct placement of the needle, the dye is injected into the joint space. The aspirated fluid is usually sent to the laboratory for analysis. (See SYNOVIAL FLUID ANALYSIS in this chapter.) After the needle is removed, the site is rubbed with a sterile sponge to prevent air from escaping, and the wound may be sealed with collodion. The patient is asked to walk a few steps or to move his knee through range of motion, as directed, to distribute the dye in the joint space. A film series is quickly taken—before the contrast medium can be absorbed by the joint tissue—with the knee held in various positions. If the films are clean and demonstrate proper dye placement, the knee is bandaged.

Shoulder arthrography: The skin is prepared, and a local anesthetic is injected subcutaneously, just in front of the acromioclavicular joint. Additional anesthetic is injected directly onto the head of the humerus. The short lumbar puncture needle is then inserted until the point is embedded in the joint cartilage. The stylet is removed, a syringe of contrast medium attached, and using fluoroscopic guidance, about 1 ml of dye is injected into the joint space, as the needle is withdrawn slightly. If fluoroscopic examination demonstrates correct placement of the needle, the remainder of the dye is injected, while the needle is withdrawn slowly, and the site is wiped with a sterile sponge. A film series is then taken quickly to achieve maximum contrast.

Precautions

This procedure is contraindicated dur-

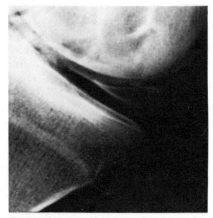
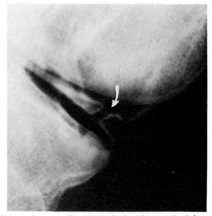

These arthrograms of the knee show a normal medial meniscus, as it appears in the view on the left, and a torn medial meniscus, as indicated by the arrow in the view on the right.

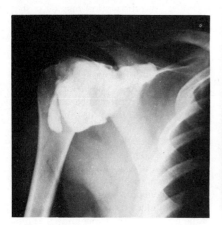
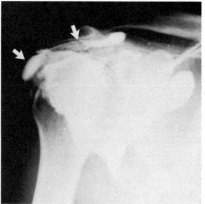

The arthrogram on the left is of a normal shoulder. The arthrogram on the right shows a shoulder with a ruptured rotator cuff. Contrast medium has collected in the subacromial bursa (indicated by arrows).

ing pregnancy or for patients with active arthritis, joint infection, or previous sensitivity to radiopaque media.

Findings

A normal knee arthrogram shows a characteristic wedge-shaped shadow, pointed toward the interior of the joint, that indicates a normal medial meniscus. A normal shoulder arthrogram shows the bicipital tendon sheath, redundant inferior joint capsule, and subscapular bursa intact.

Implications of results

Arthrography accurately detects medial meniscal tears and lacerations in 90% to 95% of cases. Since the entire joint lining is opacified, arthrography can demonstrate extrameniscal lesions, such as osteochondritis dissecans, chondromalacia patellae, osteochondral fractures, cartilaginous abnormalities, synovial abnormalities, tears of the cruciate ligaments, and disruption of the joint capsule and collateral ligaments.

Arthrography can demonstrate shoulder abnormalities, such as adhesive capsulitis, bicipital tenosynovitis or rupture, and rotator cuff tears. It can also evaluate the extent of damage from recurrent dislocations.

Post-test care

□ Tell the patient to rest the joint for at least 12 hours. If knee arthrography was performed, wrap the knee in an elastic bandage, if ordered. Tell the patient to keep the bandage in place for several days, and teach him how to rewrap it.

□ Inform the patient that he may experience some swelling or discomfort, or may hear crepitant noises in the joint after the test, but that these symptoms usually disappear after 1 or 2 days; tell him to contact the doctor if symptoms persist. Advise him to apply ice to the joint if swelling occurs, and to take a mild analgesic for pain.

Interfering factors

□ Incomplete aspiration of the joint fluid dilutes the contrast medium, diminishing quality of the film.

□ Improper injection technique may cause misplacement of contrast medium.

JANE FARRELL, RN, BS

Bone Scan

Bone scan is a test that permits imaging of the skeleton by a scanning camera after I.V. injection of a radioactive tracer compound. The tracer of choice, radioactive technetium diphosphonate, collects in bone tissue in increased concentrations at sites of abnormal metabolism. When scanned, these sites appear as "hot spots" that are often detectable months before a radiograph can reveal any lesion.

This test is primarily indicated in patients with symptoms of metastatic bone disease, with bone trauma, or with a known degenerative disorder that requires monitoring for signs of progres-

NORMAL AND ABNORMAL BONE SCANS

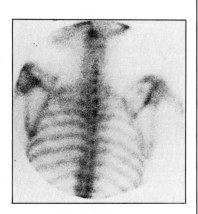

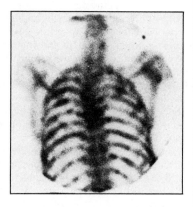

The bone scan of the thorax shown in top photo above is normal. The isotope ^{99m}Tc diphosphonate is distributed evenly throughout the skeletal tissue; darker areas indicate the density of bone masses, as in the vertebrae. However, the scan depicted below reveals isotope accumulation in multiple metastases in the ribs and spine. Although bone scans can detect metastatic and primary bone tumors as early as 3 to 6 months before they appear on plain films, radiographs are usually taken after a scan, for comparison. Using such isotopes, whole-body scans of the entire skeletal system expose the patient to much less radiation than comparable procedures using X-rays. Bone scanning can also monitor the progress of bone grafts and can detect infection after total hip arthroplasty.

sion. It may be performed with a gallium scan to promote early detection of lesions.

Purpose
□ To detect or rule out malignant bone lesions when radiographic findings are normal but cancer is confirmed or suspected
□ To detect occult bone trauma due to pathologic fractures
□ To monitor degenerative bone disorders
□ To detect infection.

Patient preparation
Describe the procedure to the patient, and answer any questions he may have. Explain that this test often detects abnormal skeletal pathology sooner than is possible with ordinary X-ray films. Since the patient is required to drink several glasses of water or tea in the interval between injection of the tracer and the actual scanning (about 1 to 3 hours), advise him not to drink large amounts of fluids before the test. Tell him who will perform the test and where, and that he may have to assume various positions on a scanner table.

Assure the patient that the scan itself, which takes about 1 hour, is painless and that the isotope, although radioactive, emits less radiation than a standard X-ray machine.

Make sure the patient or a family member has signed a consent form. If a bone scan is ordered to diagnose cancer, evaluate the patient's emotional state and offer supportive care, as needed. Administer an analgesic, as ordered.

Equipment
Bone mineral tracer/3-ml syringe/21G needle/70% alcohol or povidone-iodine solution/sterile sponge/tourniquet/scanning camera.

Procedure
After the patient receives an I.V. injection of the tracer and imaging agent, encourage him to increase his intake of fluids for the next 1 to 3 hours, to facil-

itate renal clearance of the circulating free tracer (not being picked up by the bone). Instruct him to void immediately before the procedure; then position him on the scanner table.

As the scanner head moves back and forth over the patient's body, it detects low-level radiation emitted by the skeleton and translates this into a film or paper chart, or both, to produce two-dimensional pictures of the area scanned. The scanner takes as many views as needed to cover the specified area; the patient may have to be repositioned several times during the test to obtain adequate views.

Precautions
To avoid exposing the fetus or infant to radiation, a bone scan is contraindicated during pregnancy or lactation.

Findings
The tracer concentrates in bone tissue at sites of new bone formation or increased metabolism. The epiphyses of growing bone are normal sites of high concentration, or hot spots.

Implications of results
Although a bone scan demonstrates hot spots that identify sites of bone formation, it doesn't distinguish between normal and abnormal bone formation. However, scan results can identify all types of bone malignancy, infection, fracture, and other disorders, when interpreted in light of the patient's medical and surgical history, radiographs, and other laboratory tests.

Post-test care
Check the injection site for redness or swelling. If a hematoma develops, ease discomfort by applying warm soaks.

Interfering factors
□ A distended bladder may obscure pelvic detail.
□ Improper injection technique allows the tracer to seep into muscle tissue, producing erroneous hot spots.

JANE FARRELL, RN, BS

ENDOSCOPY & JOINT ASPIRATION
Arthroscopy

Arthroscopy is the visual examination of the interior of a joint with a specially designed fiberoptic endoscope. It is most commonly used to examine the knee. In evaluating a patient with suspected or confirmed joint disease, arthroscopy is usually considered a secondary tool; the initial diagnostic approach consists of a complete history and physical examination, plain X-ray films, and arthrography. However, the diagnostic accuracy of arthroscopy (about 98%) surpasses that of arthrography and radiographs, and it may prove to be the definitive diagnostic procedure.

Unlike radiographic studies, arthroscopy permits concurrent surgery or biopsy using a technique called triangulation, in which instruments are passed through a separate cannula. Thus, arthroscopy provides a safe, convenient alternative to open surgery (arthrotomy) or separate biopsy. Although arthroscopy is commonly performed under a local anesthetic, it may also be performed under a spinal or general anesthetic, particularly when surgery is anticipated. When the joint is properly anesthetized, a cannula is positioned in the joint cavity, and the arthroscope inserted through it. Visual findings may be recorded by attaching a camera to the arthroscope and photographing specific areas for later study.

Complications associated with arthroscopy rarely occur but may include infection, hemarthrosis, swelling, synovial rupture, thrombophlebitis, infrapatellar anesthesia, and joint injury.

Purpose
☐ To detect and diagnose meniscal, patellar, condylar, extrasynovial, and synovial diseases
☐ To monitor the progression of disease
☐ To perform joint surgery
☐ To monitor effectiveness of therapy.

Patient preparation
Describe the procedure to the patient, and answer any questions he may have. Explain that this test permits examination of the interior of the joint and evaluation of joint disease. If appropriate, tell the patient this test monitors his response to therapy. (If surgery or other treatment is anticipated, explain that in many cases this may be safely and conveniently accomplished through the arthroscope.) Instruct the patient to fast after midnight before the procedure. Tell him who will perform this procedure and where.

If local anesthesia is to be used, tell the patient he may experience transient discomfort from the injection of the local anesthetic and the pressure of the tourniquet on his leg.

Make sure the patient or a responsible member of the family has signed a consent form. Check the patient's history for hypersensitivity to the anesthetic. Just before the procedure, shave the area 5″ (12.5 cm) above and below the joint, then administer a sedative, as ordered.

Equipment
Skin antiseptic (povidone-iodine solution)/arthroscope and accessory equipment/pointed scalpel/sterile gloves/local anesthetic/sterile needle/12-ml and 60-ml syringes/waterproof stockinette/elastic bandages/pneumatic tourniquet/epinephrine (1:100,000 in 1% lidocaine solution)/500 ml sterile normal saline solution/continuous drainage system/sponges/2″ x 2″ sterile gauze pads/sterile drapes/small adhesive bandages.

Procedure
Although arthroscopic techniques vary, depending on the surgeon and the type of arthroscope used, the following knee arthroscopy procedure is typical.

After the patient is placed in a supine position on the operating table, a pneu-

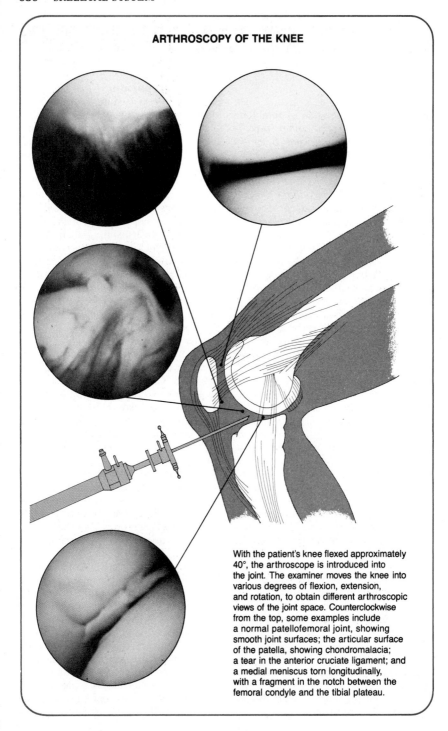

ARTHROSCOPY OF THE KNEE

With the patient's knee flexed approximately 40°, the arthroscope is introduced into the joint. The examiner moves the knee into various degrees of flexion, extension, and rotation, to obtain different arthroscopic views of the joint space. Counterclockwise from the top, some examples include a normal patellofemoral joint, showing smooth joint surfaces; the articular surface of the patella, showing chondromalacia; a tear in the anterior cruciate ligament; and a medial meniscus torn longitudinally, with a fragment in the notch between the femoral condyle and the tibial plateau.

matic tourniquet may be placed around his leg but not tightened. The patient's leg is scrubbed according to standard surgical procedure, and a waterproof stockinette is applied. The patient's leg is elevated and wrapped with an elastic bandage—from toes to lower thigh—to drain as much blood from the leg as possible. Then, the tourniquet is inflated and the elastic bandage removed; the tourniquet may be used at 300 mmHg and may remain in place during the procedure, depending on the surgeon's preference and the patient's comfort. (For techniques that don't require a tourniquet, 10 ml of 1% lidocaine with epinephrine 1:100,000 is mixed with 500 ml of sterile normal saline solution. Then 50 ml of this solution is instilled into the patient's knee immediately before insertion of the arthroscope; this instillation distends the knee and helps reduce bleeding.)

After the foot of the table is lowered so the patient's knee is bent at about 45°, the stockinette is opened, and the local anesthetic is administered. Infiltration of the capsule at many sites blocks impulses from the infrapatellar branch of the saphenous nerve as far back as possible. A pointed scalpel is used to make a 3- to 5-mm incision in either the anteromedial or the anterolateral aspect of the knee, above the tibial plateau. (When a posteromedial tear is suspected, the knee is entered posteromedially.) If the procedure is being performed under a local anesthetic, warn the patient that he will feel a thumping sensation as the cannula with sharp trocar is inserted into the capsule at a point medial to the patellar tendon, just lateral to the anterior cruciate and immediately above the meniscus. Next, the trocar is removed and replaced with a blunt obturator, which penetrates the synovia, causing transient pain. The arthroscope is then inserted through the cannula. To provide a viewing medium, normal saline and epinephrine solutions are introduced into the joint through the arthroscope, which also provides drainage from the joint into a container on the floor.

The arthroscope is inserted in and out of various joint spaces, or is held steady as the knee is bent, extended, and turned to aid visualization. Generally, examination of the tibial plateaus, the back recesses of the joint, the menisci, the posterior two thirds of the femoral condyles, the cruciate structures, and the under surface of the patella takes about 10 minutes. Although the entire joint can be viewed from one puncture site, an obstruction may necessitate additional punctures. After visual examination, a synovial biopsy or appropriate surgery may be performed, or treatment applied, as indicated.

When the examination is completed, the arthroscope is removed, the joint irrigated by way of the cannula, the cannula removed, and gentle manual pressure applied to the knee to help remove the saline solution. An adhesive strip and compression dressing are then applied over the incision site.

Precautions
Arthroscopy is contraindicated in a patient with fibrous ankylosis with flexion of less than 50°. It is also contraindicated in a patient with local skin or wound infections, because of the risk of subsequent joint involvement.

Findings
The knee is a typical diarthrodial joint surrounded by muscles, ligaments, cartilage, and tendons, and is lined with synovial membrane. In children, the menisci are smooth and opaque, with their thick outer edges attached to the joint capsule and their inner edges lying snugly against the condylar surfaces, unattached. Articular cartilage appears smooth and white; ligaments and tendons appear cable-like and silvery. The synovium is smooth and marked by a fine vascular network. Degenerative changes begin during adolescence.

Implications of results
Arthroscopic examination can reveal meniscal disease, such as torn medial or lateral meniscus or other meniscus in-

juries; patellar disease, such as chon-dromalacia, dislocation, subluxation, fracture, and parapatellar synovitis; condylar disease, such as degenerative articular cartilage, osteochondritis dis-secans, and loose bodies; extrasynovial disease, such as torn anterior cruciate or tibial collateral ligaments, Baker's cyst, and ganglion cyst; and synovial disease, such as synovitis, rheumatoid and de-generative arthritis, and foreign bodies associated with gout, pseudogout, and osteochondromatosis.

Depending on test findings, appropri-ate treatment or surgery can follow ar-throscopy. If arthroscopic surgery can't be performed, arthrotomy is the proce-dure of choice.

Post-test care

□ Watch for fever, and for swelling, in-creased pain, and localized inflamma-tion at the incision site. If the patient reports discomfort, administer aspirin, as ordered.

□ Tell the patient that he may walk as soon as he's fully awake but should avoid excessive use of the joint for a few days.

□ Advise the patient that he may resume his usual diet that was discontinued be-fore the test.

Interfering factors

Failure to use the arthroscope properly can result in an incomplete examination of the joint.

JANE FARRELL, RN, BS

Synovial Fluid Analysis

Synovial fluid is normally a viscid, colorless-to-pale-yellow liquid found in small amounts in the diarthrodial (sy-novial) joints, bursae, and tendon sheaths. It's thought to be produced by the dialysis of plasma across the sy-novial membrane and by the secretion of hyaluronic acid, a mucopolysacchar-ide. Although its functions aren't clearly understood, synovial fluid probably lu-bricates the joint space, nourishes the articular cartilage, and protects the car-tilage from mechanical damage while stabilizing the joint.

In synovial fluid aspiration, or ar-throcentesis, a sterile needle is inserted into a joint space—most commonly the knee—under strict aseptic conditions, to obtain a fluid specimen for analysis. This procedure is indicated in patients with undiagnosed articular disease and symptomatic joint effusion—the exces-sive accumulation of synovial fluid.

Although rare, complications associ-ated with synovial fluid aspiration in-clude joint infection and hemorrhage leading to hemarthrosis (accumulation of blood within the joint).

Purpose

□ To aid differential diagnosis of ar-thritis, particularly septic or crystal-induced arthritis

□ To identify the cause and nature of joint effusion

□ To relieve the pain and distention re-sulting from accumulation of fluid within the joint

□ To administer local drug therapy, usu-ally corticosteroids.

Patient preparation

Describe the procedure to the patient, and answer any questions he may have. Explain that this test helps determine the cause of joint inflammation and swell-ing, and also helps relieve the associated pain. If glucose testing of synovial fluid is ordered, instruct him to fast for 6 to 12 hours before the test; otherwise, in-form him he needn't restrict food or fluids before the test. Tell him who will perform the test and where. Warn him that while he'll receive a local anesthetic, he may still feel transient pain when the needle penetrates the joint capsule.

Make sure the patient or a responsible member of the family has signed a con-sent form. Check the patient's history for hypersensitivity to iodine compounds (such as povidone-iodine), procaine, lidocaine, or other local anesthetics. Administer a sedative as ordered.

Equipment

Surgical detergent/skin antiseptic (usually tincture of povidone-iodine)/alcohol sponges/local anesthetic (procaine or lidocaine, 1% or 2%)/sterile, disposable 1½″, 25G needle/sterile, disposable 1½″ to 2″, 20G needle/sterile 5-ml syringe for injecting anesthetic/sterile 20-ml syringe for aspiration/3-ml syringe for administering sedative/2″ x 2″ sterile gauze pads/sterile dressings/sterile drapes/elastic bandage/tubes for culture, cytologic, clot, and glucose analysis/anticoagulants—heparin, EDTA, and potassium oxalate/venipuncture equipment, if ordered.

For corticosteroid administration: corticosteroid suspension, such as hydrocortisone/2-ml and 5-ml syringes (or one 10-ml syringe if procaine and steroid are to be injected simultaneously).

Procedure

Position the patient, as ordered. Explain that he will need to maintain this position throughout the procedure. Tell him that although he'll receive a local anesthetic to minimize pain, he will probably feel some discomfort when the needle is inserted. (A sedative is sometimes ordered for a young child.) Clean the skin over the puncture site with surgical detergent and alcohol. Paint the site with tincture of povidone-iodine, and allow it to air-dry for 2 minutes. After the local anesthetic is administered, the aspirating needle is quickly inserted through the skin, subcutaneous tissue, and synovial membrane, into the joint space. As much fluid as possible is aspirated into the syringe; a minimum of 10 to 15 ml should be obtained, although a lesser amount is usually adequate for analysis. The joint (except for the area around the puncture site) may be wrapped with an elastic bandage to compress the free fluid into this portion of the sac, ensuring maximal collection of fluid.

If a corticosteroid is being injected,

prepare the dosage, as ordered. For instillation, the syringe is detached, leaving the needle in the joint, and the syringe

NORMAL FINDINGS IN SYNOVIAL FLUID

ANALYSIS	RESULTS
Gross	
Color	Colorless to pale yellow
Clarity	Clear
Quantity (in knee)	0.3 to 3.5 ml
Viscosity	5.7 to 1,160
pH	7.2 to 7.4
Mucin clot	Good
Microscopic	
WBC count	0 to 200/µl
WBC differential	
• Lymphocytes	0 to 78/µl
• Monocytes	0 to 71/µl
• Clasmatocytes	0 to 26/µl
• Polymorphonuclears	0 to 25/µl
• Other phagocytes	0 to 21/µl
• Synovial lining cells	0 to 12/µl
Microbiologic	
Formed elements	Absence of cartilage debris and crystals
Bacteria	None
Serologic	
Complement	
• for 10 mg protein/dl	3.7 to 33.7 u/ml
• for 20 mg protein/dl	7.7 to 37.7 u/ml
Rheumatoid arthritis cells	None
Lupus erythematosus cells	None
Chemical	
Total protein	10.7 to 21.3 mg/dl
Fibrinogen	None
Glucose	70 to 100 mg/dl
Uric acid	2 to 8 mg/dl (men) 2 to 6 mg/dl (women)
Hyaluronate	0.3 to 0.4 g/dl
PaCO₂	40 to 60 mmHg
PaO₂	40 to 80 mmHg

SYNOVIAL FLUID ANALYSIS IN ARTHRITIS

	DISEASE	COLOR	CLARITY	VISCOSITY
Group I noninflammatory	Traumatic arthritis	Straw to bloody to yellow	Transparent to cloudy	Variable
	Osteoarthritis	Yellow	Transparent	Variable
Group II inflammatory	Systemic lupus erythematosus	Straw	Clear to slightly cloudy	Variable
	Rheumatic fever	Yellow	Slightly cloudy	Variable
	Pseudogout	Yellow	Slightly cloudy (if acute)	Low (if acute)
	Gout	Yellow to milky	Cloudy	Low
	Rheumatoid arthritis	Yellow to green	Cloudy	Low
Group III septic	Tuberculous arthritis	Yellow	Cloudy	Low
	Septic arthritis	Gray or bloody	Turbid, purulent	Low

MUCIN CLOT	WBC COUNT/ % NEUTRO- PHILS	CARTILAGE DEBRIS	CRYSTALS	RA CELLS	BACTERIA
Good to fair	1,000; 25%	None	None	None	None
Good to fair	700; 15%	Usually present	None	None	None
Good to fair	2,000; 30%	None	None	LE cells	None
Good to fair	14,000; 50%	None	None	LE cells may be present	None
Fair to poor	15,000; 70%	Usually present	Calcium pyrophosphate	None	None
Fair to poor	20,000; 70%	None	Urate	None	None
Fair to poor	20,000; 70%	None	Occasionally, cholesterol	Usually present	None
Poor	20,000; 60%	None	None	None	Usually present
Poor	90,000; 90%	None	None	None	Usually present

Adapted with permission from R. Jessar, "Synovianalysis in Arthritis," in Donald J. McCarty, *Arthritis and Allied Conditions: A Textbook of Rheumatology* (8th ed.; Philadelphia: Lea & Febiger, 1972).

PUNCTURE SITES FOR JOINT ASPIRATIONS

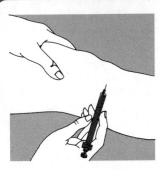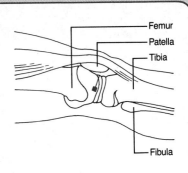

Femur
Patella
Tibia

Fibula

Knee: The needle is introduced with a single thrust in the slight depression under the patella and is kept parallel with the underside of the patella.

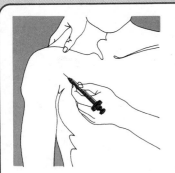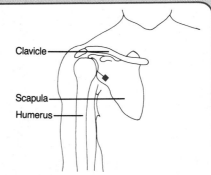

Clavicle

Scapula
Humerus

Shoulder: The needle is introduced just below the coracoid process (on the upper anterior surface of the scapula) and is aimed laterally.

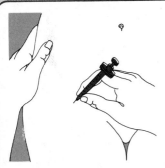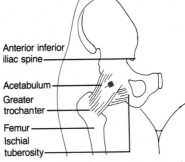

Anterior inferior
iliac spine

Acetabulum

Greater
trochanter

Femur
Ischial
tuberosity

Hip: The needle is introduced just above or anterior to the trochanter and parallel to the femoral neck and is aimed at the acetabulum.

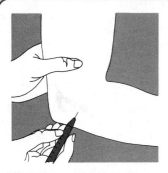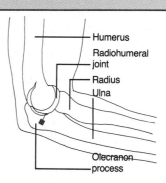

Elbow: The needle is introduced into the radiohumeral joint area just above the olecranon of the ulna, while the elbow is held at 90°.

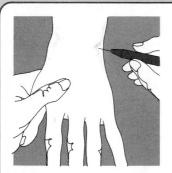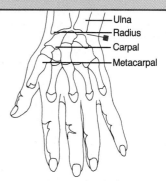

Wrist: The needle is introduced perpendicular to the skin just distal to the radius until the needle touches the carpal bone.

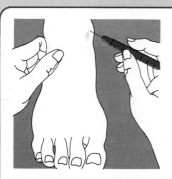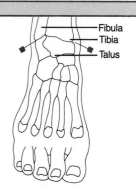

Ankle: The needle is introduced laterally just inside the fibula or medially just inside the tibal malleolus at the depression, with the foot fully flexed.

containing the steroid attached to the needle instead. After the steroid is injected and the needle withdrawn, wipe the puncture site with alcohol. Apply pressure to the puncture site for about 2 minutes to prevent bleeding, then apply a sterile dressing.

If synovial fluid glucose is being measured, perform venipuncture to obtain a specimen for blood glucose analysis.

Precautions

□ Adhere to strict aseptic technique throughout aspiration to prevent contamination of joint space or the synovial fluid specimen.

□ Add anticoagulants to the specimen, according to the laboratory tests requested. Gently invert the tube several times to mix the specimen and anticoagulant adequately. *For cultures,* obtain 2 to 5 ml of synovial fluid and, if possible, inoculate the medium immediately. Otherwise, add 1 or 2 drops of heparin to the specimen. *For cytologic analysis,* add 5 mg of EDTA or 1 or 2 drops of heparin to 2 to 5 ml of synovial fluid. *For glucose analysis,* add potassium oxalate, as specified by the laboratory, to 3 to 5 ml of fluid. *For crystal examination,* add heparin, if specified by the laboratory. *For other studies,* such as general appearance and clot evaluation, obtain 2 to 5 ml of synovial fluid, but don't add an anticoagulant.

□ Send the properly labeled specimens to the laboratory immediately—gonococci are particularly labile. If a WBC count is being performed, clearly label the specimen "Synovial Fluid" and "Caution—Don't use acid diluents."

Values

Examination of synovial fluid in the laboratory can take many forms. Routine examination includes gross analysis for color, clarity, quantity, viscosity, pH, and the presence of a mucin clot, as well as microscopic analysis for WBC count and differential. Special examination includes microbiologic analysis for formed elements (including crystals) and bacteria, serologic analysis, and chemical

analysis for such components as glucose, protein, and enzymes. (See the chart on page 683 for representative values.)

Implications of results

Examination of synovial fluid may reveal various joint diseases, including noninflammatory disease (traumatic arthritis and osteoarthritis), inflammatory disease (systemic lupus erythematosus, rheumatic fever, pseudogout, gout, and rheumatoid arthritis), and septic disease (tuberculous and septic arthritis). The chart on pages 684-685 shows findings that implicate these diseases.

Post-test care

□ Apply ice or cold packs to the affected joint for 24 to 36 hours after aspiration, to decrease pain and swelling. Use pillows for support. If a large quantity of fluid was aspirated, apply an elastic bandage to stabilize the joint.

□ If the patient's condition permits, tell him he may resume normal activity immediately after the procedure. However, warn him to avoid excessive use of the joint for a few days after the test, even though pain and swelling may have subsided. Excessive use may cause transient pain, swelling, and stiffness.

□ Watch for increased pain or fever, which may indicate joint infection.

□ Carefully handle the dressings and linens of patients with drainage from the joint space, especially if septic arthritis is confirmed or suspected.

□ Advise the patient that he may resume his usual diet.

Interfering factors

□ Acid diluents added to the specimen for WBC count precipitate the mucin and alter the cell count.

□ Failure to mix the specimen and the anticoagulant adequately or to send the specimens to the laboratory immediately may cause inaccurate test results.

□ Patient failure to adhere to dietary restrictions can affect glucose levels.

□ Contamination of the specimen can invalidate test results.

DEBORAH M. BERKOWITZ, RN, MSN

Selected References

Birkner, R. *Normal Radiologic Patterns and Variances of the Human Skeleton: An X-ray Atlas of Adults and Children.* Baltimore: Urban & Schwarzenberg, 1978.

Brunner, Lillian S., and Suddarth, Doris S. *Textbook of Medical-Surgical Nursing,* 5th ed. Philadelphia: J.B. Lippincott Co., 1984.

Diseases, 2nd ed. Nurse's Reference Library. Springhouse, Pa.: Springhouse Corp., 1986.

Farrell, Jane. *Illustrated Guide to Orthopedic Nursing,* 2nd ed. Philadelphia: J.B. Lippincott Co., 1982.

Feldman, Frieda. *Radiology, Pathology and Immunology of Bones and Joints.* East Norwalk, Conn.: Appleton-Century-Crofts, 1979.

Fischbach, Frances. *A Manual of Laboratory Diagnostic Tests,* 2nd ed. Philadelphia: J.B. Lippincott Co., 1984.

Grossman, Zachary D., et al. *The Clinician's Guide to Diagnostic Imaging.* New York: Raven Press Pubs., 1983.

Guyton, Arthur C. *Textbook of Medical Physiology,* 6th ed. Philadelphia: W.B. Saunders Co., 1981.

Harvey, A. McGehee, ed. *The Principles and Practice of Medicine,* 21st ed. East Norwalk, Conn.: Appleton-Century-Crofts, 1984.

Henry, John Bernard, ed. *Todd-Sanford-Davidsohn Clinical Diagnosis and Management by Laboratory Methods,* vol. 1, 17th ed. Philadelphia: W.B. Saunders Co., 1984.

Hilt, Nancy E., and Cogburn, Shirley B. *Manual of Orthopedics.* St. Louis: C.V. Mosby Co., 1979.

Luckmann, Joan, and Sorensen, Karen C. *Medical-Surgical Nursing: A Psychophysiologic Approach,* 2nd ed. Philadelphia: W.B. Saunders Co., 1980.

Nursing85 Drug Handbook. Springhouse, Pa.: Springhouse Corp., 1985.

Petersdorf, Robert G., and Adams, Raymond D., eds. *Harrison's Principles of Internal Medicine,* 10th ed. New York: McGraw-Hill Book Co., 1983.

Price, Sylvia, and Wilson, Lorraine. *Pathophysiology: Clinical Concepts of Disease Processes,* 2nd ed. New York: McGraw-Hill Book Co., 1984.

Ravel, Richard. *Clinical Laboratory Medicine,* 4th ed. Chicago: Year Book Medical Pubs., 1984.

Tilkian, Sarko M., et al. *Clinical Implications of Laboratory Tests,* 3rd ed. St. Louis: C.V. Mosby Co., 1983.

Widmann, Frances K. *Clinical Interpretation of Laboratory Tests,* 9th ed. Philadelphia: F.A. Davis Co., 1983.

Wyngaarden, James, and Smith, Lloyd. *Cecil Textbook of Medicine,* 16th ed. Philadelphia: W.B. Saunders Co., 1982.

25 Reproductive System

LEARNING OBJECTIVES

After completing this chapter, the reader will be able to:
- explain the anatomy and physiology of the reproductive system.
- describe normal fetal development and the three stages of labor.
- identify the sequence of tests used to evaluate the reproductive system.
- describe the technique for performing testicular self-examination.
- explain how DNA and RNA influence protein synthesis.
- discuss how cell division occurs.
- discuss chromosomal analysis and its clinical implications.
- list the major sex chromosome anomalies.
- explain how to use the Doppler stethoscope correctly.
- state the purpose of each test discussed in the chapter.
- prepare the patient physically and psychologically for each test.
- describe the procedure for performing each test.
- specify appropriate precautions for safe administration of each test.
- recognize signs of adverse reaction and respond appropriately.
- implement appropriate post-test care.
- identify the normal findings and values for each test.
- discuss the implications of abnormal test results.
- list factors that may interfere with accurate test results.

Reproductive System

Introduction

Diagnostic testing of the reproductive system may be performed to assess the organs and associated structures for abnormalities, to detect malignancies, or to determine the cause of infertility or sexual dysfunction. Some diagnostic tests are especially useful during pregnancy: first, to confirm pregnancy and, later, to detect genetic defects and monitor fetal well-being.

Reproductive organs

The reproductive system comprises essential and accessory organs for procreation. Essential organs are the gonads—the testes and the ovaries. The testes produce the germ cells known as spermatozoa and the hormone testosterone, which induces and maintains secondary sexual characteristics; the ovaries produce ova and the hormones estrogen and progesterone, which also promote and maintain secondary sexual characteristics.

Male accessory organs consist of the scrotum and a transport system of ducts and glands, including the urethra, epididymis, vas deferens, ejaculatory duct, seminal vesicles, the prostate and the bulbourethral glands, and the penis.

Female accessory organs include the fallopian tubes, the uterus, and the vagina. External structures of female genitalia, collectively called the vulva, are the mons pubis, labia majora, labia mi-

nora, clitoris, vestibule, urethral meatus, hymen, Bartholin's glands, Skene's glands, fourchette, and perineum. The mammary glands, whose primary function is lactation, are also generally considered part of the reproductive system.

Fetal development

Normally, the spermatozoon fertilizes the ovum in the upper to middle third of the fallopian tube. At fertilization, the sperm, which contains 22 autosomes and either an X or a Y chromosome, fuses with the ovum, which contains 22 autosomes and an X chromosome, to form a zygote made up of 44 autosomes and 2 sex chromosomes. The 44 autosomes determine genetic characteristics; the sex chromosomes determine sex. Two X chromosomes produce a female zygote; the combination of an X and a Y, a male zygote.

After fertilization, the fertilized ovum develops in two stages over a 40-week gestation period:
□ During the *embryonic* stage, which begins at conception and lasts 8 weeks, the blastocyst develops and is implanted, and primitive chorionic villi start to form. The amnion begins to ensheath the body stalk, which will become the umbilical cord. Embryonic heart chambers develop, and a primitive cardiovascular system begins to function. By the end of this stage, the eyes, ears, nose, and mouth

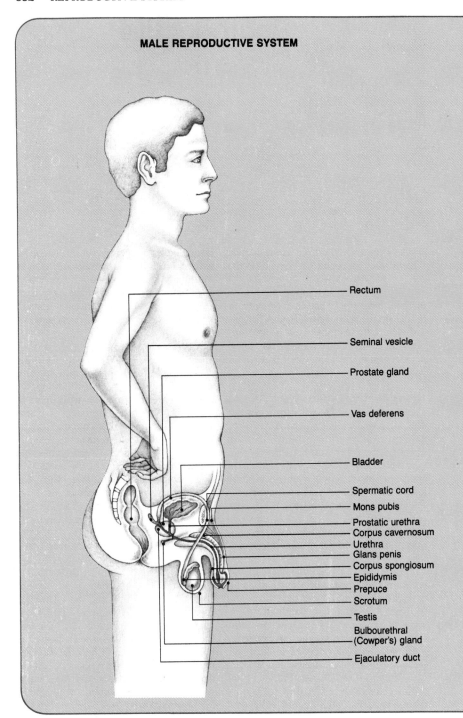

MALE REPRODUCTIVE SYSTEM

Rectum

Seminal vesicle

Prostate gland

Vas deferens

Bladder

Spermatic cord

Mons pubis

Prostatic urethra

Corpus cavernosum

Urethra

Glans penis

Corpus spongiosum

Epididymis

Prepuce

Scrotum

Testis

Bulbourethral (Cowper's) gland

Ejaculatory duct

FEMALE REPRODUCTIVE SYSTEM

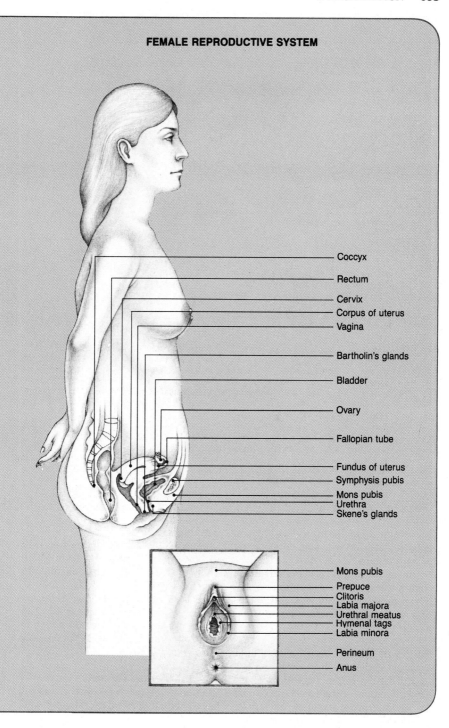

Coccyx

Rectum

Cervix
Corpus of uterus
Vagina

Bartholin's glands

Bladder

Ovary

Fallopian tube

Fundus of uterus
Symphysis pubis
Mons pubis
Urethra
Skene's glands

Mons pubis

Prepuce
Clitoris
Labia majora
Urethral meatus
Hymenal tags
Labia minora

Perineum

Anus

FETAL GROWTH AND DEVELOPMENT

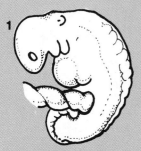

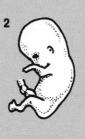

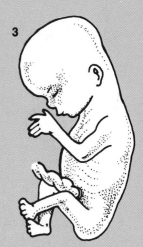

1 month (10 times actual size)

2 months
(actual size)

3 months (actual size)

1. At the end of 1 month, the embryo has a definite form. The head and trunk are apparent, and the tiny buds that will become the arms and legs are discernible. The cardiovascular system has begun to function, and the umbilical cord is visible in its most primitive form.

2. In the next month, the embryo—called a fetus from the seventh week on—grows to 1″ in length and weighs ⅓₀ oz. The head and facial features develop as the eyes, ears, nose, lips, tongue, and tooth buds form. The arms and legs also take shape, with the elbows, forearms, hands, fingers, thighs, knees, ankles, and toes becoming visible. Although the gender of the fetus is not yet discernible, all external genitalia are present. Cardiovascular function is complete, and the umbilical cord has a definite form. At the end of 2 months, the fetus resembles a full-term baby except for size.

3. During the third month, the fetus grows to 3″ in length and weighs 1 oz (28 g). Teeth and bones begin to appear, and the kidneys start to function. Although the mother can't yet feel its activity, the fetus is moving. It opens its mouth to swallow, grasps with its fully developed hands, and—even though its lungs are not functioning—it prepares for breathing by inhaling and exhaling. At the end of the first trimester, its gender is distinguishable.

are recognizable; the arms, legs, fingers, and toes are formed; and development of most organs has begun.

□ During the *fetal* stage, a period lasting from 8 weeks after conception until delivery, the major structures and organs that are already developed grow and mature.

Stages of labor
□ *Stage I* is the time between the beginning of regular contractions and full cervical dilatation—usually, about 12 hours for a primigravida and about 6 hours for a multigravida.

□ *Stage II,* the period lasting from full dilatation until delivery, lasts about 1½ hours for a primigravida, 30 minutes for a multigravida.

□ *Stage III* lasts from delivery to the expulsion of the placenta—normally, 3 to 4 minutes for a primigravida and 4 to 5 minutes for a multigravida but possibly as long as 1 hour.

Special diagnostic tests
Evaluation of the reproductive system begins with a physical examination and

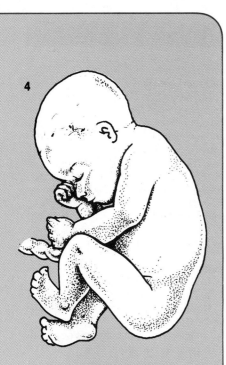

9 months (⅓ actual size)

4. In the remaining 6 months, fetal growth continues as internal and external structures develop at a rapid rate. In the third trimester, the fetus stores fats and minerals it will need to live outside the womb. At birth, the average full-term fetus measures 20″ (51 cm) and weighs 7 to 7½ lbs (3 to 3.5 kg).

a detailed history to detect abnormalities that may require further testing. Special tests using various techniques include the following:

□ *Pap test,* the cytologic examination of cervical scrapings, allows early detection of cervical cancer.

□ *Semen analysis* evaluates male fertility, validates the effectiveness of a vasectomy, and detects the presence of semen for medicolegal investigations.

□ *Sex chromatin tests* screen for abnormalities of the sex chromosomes.

□ *Chromosomal analysis* can evaluate genetic defects in the fetus, thus aiding genetic counseling.

□ *Amniotic fluid analysis, chorionic villi biopsy,* and *pelvic ultrasonography* can facilitate early diagnosis of fetal abnormalities, some of which may be successfully treated in utero. (For instance, amniotic fluid analysis can identify Rh isoimmunization before birth, allowing treatment with intrauterine transfusions to prevent stillbirth.)

□ *Colposcopy* provides direct visualization of cervical and vaginal abnormalities, such as benign lesions and invasive carcinoma.

□ *Laparoscopy* can determine if female infertility results from anatomic defects. Laparoscopy also detects pathology of the ovaries, fallopian tubes, and uterus, through direct visualization, thus allowing early treatment of life-threatening conditions, such as malignancies or severe hemorrhage.

□ *Internal* and *external fetal monitoring,* and *Doppler stethoscope testing* can rapidly assess fetal distress during pregnancy, labor, and delivery.

□ *Mammography* and *thermography* can aid assessment of breast lumps.

□ *Hysterosalpingography* provides visualization of malformations, adhesions, and occlusions of the uterus and fallopian tubes through fluoroscopic examination.

Emotional support significant

For many patients scheduled for diagnostic tests of the reproductive system, emotional support has special significance. Fertility or ability to deliver a child may be closely related to self-image. Also, the tests themselves may cause anxiety. For example, if amniocentesis is recommended, the patient may fear having a deformed or retarded infant. A patient scheduled for mammography is likely to fear cancer and mastectomy. Therefore, make sure you assess a patient's psychological state before the test so you can deal with it appropriately.

RONALD J. WAPNER, MD
MARTIN WEISBERG, MD

TISSUE ANALYSES

Papanicolaou Test

The Papanicolaou (Pap) test, a cytologic test, is widely known for its use in early detection of cervical cancer. To perform this test, a doctor or a specially trained nurse scrapes secretions from the patient's cervix and spreads these secretions on a slide. After the slide is immersed in a fixative, it is sent to the laboratory for cytologic analysis. This test relies on the ready exfoliation of malignant cells from the cervix. Although cervical scrapings are the most common test specimen, this test also permits cytologic evaluation of the vaginal pool, prostatic secretions, urine, gastric secretions, cavity fluids, bronchial aspirations, sputum, and solid tumor cells obtained by fine needle aspiration. It also shows cell maturity, metabolic activity, and morphology variations.

The American Cancer Society recommends a Pap test every 3 years for women between ages 20 and 40 who are not in a high-risk category and who have had negative results from two previous Pap tests. Yearly tests (or at intervals dictated by the patient's doctor) are advisable for women over age 40, for those in a high-risk category, and for those who have had a positive test. If a Pap test is positive or suggests malignancy, cervical biopsy can confirm diagnosis.

Purpose
☐ To detect malignant cells
☐ To detect inflammatory tissue changes
☐ To assess response to chemotherapy and radiation therapy
☐ To detect viral, fungal, and occasionally, parasitic invasion.

Patient preparation
Explain to the patient that the test allows the study of cervical cells. Stress its importance as an aid for detection of cancer at a stage when the disease is often asymptomatic and still curable. The test should not be scheduled during the menstrual period: the best time is mid-cycle. Instruct the patient not to douche or insert vaginal medications for 24 hours before the test, since doing so can wash away cellular deposits and change the vaginal pH. Tell her the test requires that the cervix be scraped, who will perform the procedure and when, and that she may experience slight discomfort but no pain from the speculum. Reassure her that the procedure takes only 5 to 10 minutes to perform—slightly longer if the vagina, pelvic cavity, and rectum are examined bimanually.

Obtain an accurate patient history, and ask the following questions: When did you last have a Pap test? Have you ever had an abnormal Pap test? When was your last menstrual period? Are your

---

HISTORY OF THE PAP TEST

The Pap test derives its name from George N. Papanicolaou, the father of modern cytology. Although Dr. Papanicolaou began his research in 1910 and developed the test by 1928, he did not see the test gain popular acceptance until the early 1950s. Once the importance of the test was recognized, the American Cancer Society instituted a sophisticated advertising campaign to popularize the Pap test. Because of early detection made possible by this test, mortality from cervical cancer has greatly decreased.

The Pap test evolved from Dr. Papanicolaou's study of vaginal contents as a key to understanding the exact timing of ovulation. He used specimens taken from his wife to help establish the normal cyclic changes in women, from onset of menses (puberty) to menopause. Later, he was able to test patients admitted to the gynecologic service at New York Hospital. In 1954, his research enabled him to complete *An Atlas of Exfoliative Cytology*, which classifies specimens into five diagnostic categories and is still in use in some institutions today.

PERFORMING A PAP TEST

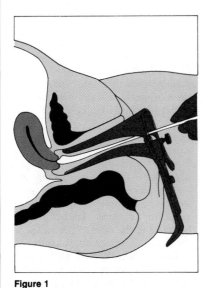

Figure 1

An unlubricated speculum is inserted into the vagina. To make insertion easier and more comfortable, the speculum is held under warm running water before insertion.

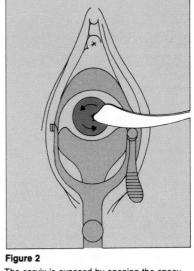

Figure 2

The cervix is exposed by opening the speculum blades. A saline-moistened Pap stick is inserted through the speculum and secretions are scraped from the cervical canal.

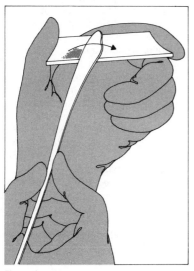

Figure 3

The specimen is spread on a slide.

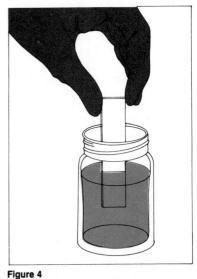

Figure 4

Immediately, the slide is placed in a fixative solution, or sprayed with a commercial fixative.

VAGINAL SMEARS

Although the Pap test was not developed to detect vaginitis, a cytologist can usually identify cells associated with vaginitis while examining the stained cells for cancer. The most reliably detected cells are *Trichomonas vaginalis, Candida,* and herpes progenitalis. If such cells are present, the Pap test indicates Class II findings—atypical cells, but no evidence of malignancy.

The most conventional way to detect vaginitis is the vaginal smear. Using a cotton-tipped applicator or wooden spatula, the examiner collects vaginal secretions and places them at opposite ends of a slide. After adding a drop of normal saline solution to one end of the slide and a drop of 10% to 20% potassium hydroxide (KOH) to the other end (wet mount preparation), he examines the slide immediately. Trichomonads, white cells, epithelial cells, "clue" cells, and bacteria readily appear at the saline-treated end; *Candida,* at the KOH-treated end.

In the vaginal pool smear, secretions are aspirated through a pipette that's attached to a bulb for suction. Part of the secretion is smeared on a slide and fixed. Vaginal pool smears are more sensitive to uterine cancer than cervical smears. However, the latter are better detectors of cervical cancer.

Scrapings for cytohormonal evaluation can also be taken from the vaginal pool. In this procedure, the lateral vaginal wall is gently scraped, and the scrapings spread on a glass slide and fixed. Using the pyknotic index, the estrogenic effect is assessed by determining the percentage of superficial and intermediate squamous cells with a fatty pyknotic nucleus.

periods regular? How many days do they last? Is bleeding heavy or light? Have you taken or are you presently taking hormones or oral contraceptives? Do you use an intrauterine device? Do you have any vaginal discharge, pain, or itching? What, if any, gynecologic disorders have occurred in your family? Have you ever had gynecologic surgery, chemotherapy, or radiation therapy? If so, describe it fully. Note any pertinent patient history on the laboratory slip. If the patient is anxious, be supportive and tell her that test results should be available within a few days.

Just before the test, ask the patient to empty her bladder.

Equipment

Drape/vaginal speculum/collection device, such as a Pap stick (wooden spatula), cotton-tipped swab, or clean, dry glass pipette with rubber bulb/saline/glass microscopic slides/fixative (commercial spray or 95% ethyl alcohol solution in a jar) for slides.

Procedure

After instructing the patient to disrobe from the waist down and to drape herself, ask her to lie on the examining table and to place her heels in the stirrups. (She may be more comfortable if she keeps on her shoes.) Tell her to slide her buttocks to the edge of the table. Adjust the drape to minimize exposure.

To avoid startling the patient, tell her when the examiner will begin the examination. First, an unlubricated speculum is inserted into the vagina. To make insertion easier, the speculum may be moistened with saline or warm water.

After the examiner locates the cervix, he will collect secretions from the cervix and material from the endocervical canal with a saline-moistened cotton-tipped swab or wooden spatula. Then the specimen is spread on the slide, according to laboratory recommendation, and the slide is immediately immersed in a fixative or is sprayed. Alternatively, posterior vaginal pool secretions and pancervical material may be collected and smeared on a single slide, which must be fixed immediately according to laboratory instructions.

Label the specimen appropriately, including the date; the patient's name, age, and date of her last menstrual period; and the collection site and method.

A bimanual examination may follow removal of the speculum. When the examination is completed, assist the patient to an upright position and instruct her to dress.

Precautions

☐ Be sure the cervical specimen is aspirated and scraped from the cervix. Aspiration of the posterior fornix of the vagina can supplement a cervical specimen but should not replace it.

□ If vaginal or vulval lesions are present, scrapings taken directly from the lesion are preferred.

□ In a patient whose uterus is involuting or atrophying from age, use a small pipette, if necessary, to aspirate cells from the squamocolumnar junction and the cervical canal.

□ Preserve the slides *immediately.*

Findings
Normally, no malignant cells or abnormalities are present.

Implications of results
Usually, malignant cells have relatively large nuclei and only small amounts of cytoplasm. They show abnormal nuclear chromatin patterns and marked variation in size, shape, and staining properties, and may have prominent nucleoli.

A Pap smear may be graded in different ways, so check your laboratory's reporting format. The following system is the traditional classification method:

□ *Class I*: Normal pattern; absence of atypical or abnormal cells

□ *Class II*: Benign abnormality; atypical, but nonmalignant, cells present

□ *Class III*: Atypical cells consistent with dysplasia

□ *Class IV*: Suggestive of, but inconclusive for, malignancy

□ *Class V*: Conclusive for malignancy.

To confirm a suggestive or positive cytology report, the test may be repeated and/or followed by a biopsy.

Post-test care
□ If cervical bleeding occurs, supply the patient with a sanitary napkin.

□ Tell the patient when to return for her next Pap test.

Interfering factors
□ Delay in fixing a specimen allows the cells to dry, destroys effectiveness of the nuclear stain, and makes cytologic interpretation difficult.

□ Excessive use of lubricating jelly on the speculum can alter the specimen.

□ Douching within 24 hours of a Pap test can wash away cellular deposits.

□ Exclusive use of a specimen collected from the vaginal fornix may yield false-negative test results.

□ Collection of the specimen during menstruation may interfere with accurate determination of test results.

SUSAN A. KAYES, BS, SM(ASCP)

Semen Analysis

Inexpensive, technically simple, and reasonably definitive, semen analysis is usually the first test performed on the male to evaluate fertility. The procedure for analyzing semen for infertility usually includes measuring the volume of seminal fluid, assessing sperm counts, and microscopic examination. Sperm are counted in much the same way that WBCs, RBCs, and platelets are counted on an anticoagulated blood sample. Staining and microscopic examination of a drop of semen permits the motility and morphology of the spermatozoa to be evaluated.

Abnormal semen may require further testing (such as liver, thyroid, pituitary, and adrenal function tests) to identify its underlying cause and screening for metabolic abnormalities (such as diabetes mellitus). Significantly abnormal semen—such as greatly decreased sperm count or motility, or marked increase in morphologically abnormal forms—may require testicular biopsy.

Semen analysis can also be used to detect semen on a rape victim, to identify the blood group of an alleged rapist, or to prove sterility in a paternity suit. Some laboratories offer specialized semen tests, such as screening for antibodies to spermatozoa.

Purpose
□ To evaluate male fertility in an infer-

tile marriage (most common use)
□ To substantiate the effectiveness of vasectomy
For medicolegal purposes:
□ To detect semen on the body or clothing of a suspected rape victim, or elsewhere at the crime scene
□ To identify blood group substances to exonerate or incriminate a criminal suspect (rare)
□ To rule out paternity on grounds of complete sterility (rare).

Patient preparation

For evaluation of fertility: Provide written instructions, and inform the patient that the most desirable specimen requires masturbation, ideally in a doctor's office or a laboratory. Instruct him to follow the doctor's orders regarding the period of continence before the test, since it may increase his sperm count. Some doctors specify a fixed number of days, usually between 2 and 5; others advise a period of continence equal to the usual interval between episodes of sexual intercourse.

If the patient prefers to collect the specimen at home, emphasize the importance of delivering the specimen to the laboratory within 3 hours after collection. Warn him not to expose the specimen to extreme temperatures or to direct sunlight (which can also increase its temperature). Ideally, the specimen should remain at body temperature until liquefaction is complete (about 20 minutes). To deliver a semen specimen to the laboratory during cold weather, suggest the patient protect the specimen from exposure to cold by keeping the specimen container in a coat pocket on the way to the laboratory.

Alternatives to collection by masturbation include coitus interruptus or the use of a condom. For collection by coitus interruptus, instruct the patient to withdraw immediately before ejaculation during intercourse and to deposit the ejaculate in a suitable specimen container. For collection by condom, tell the patient to wash the condom with soap and water, rinse it thoroughly, and allow it to dry completely. (Powders or lubricants applied to the condom may be spermicidal.) After collection, instruct him to tie the condom, place it in a glass jar, and promptly deliver it to the laboratory.

Fertility may also be determined by collecting semen postcoitally from the female, to assess the ability of the spermatozoa to penetrate the cervical mucus and remain active. For the postcoital cervical mucus test, instruct the patient to report for examination during the ovulatory phase of her menstrual cycle, as determined by basal temperature records, and as soon as possible after sexual intercourse (within 8 hours). Explain to the patient scheduled for this test that the procedure takes only a few minutes. Tell her she'll be placed in lithotomy position, and that the doctor will insert a speculum in the vagina to collect the specimen. She may feel some pressure but no pain during this procedure.

Semen collection from rape victim: Explain to the patient that the doctor will try to obtain a semen specimen from her vagina. Prepare her for insertion of the speculum as you would the patient scheduled for postcoital examination. Handle the victim's clothes as little as possible. If her clothes are moist, put them in a paper bag—not a plastic bag (which causes seminal stains and secretions to mold). Label the bag properly, and send it to the laboratory immediately. Provide emotional support by speaking to the patient calmly and reassuringly. Encourage her to express her fears and anxieties. Listen sympathetically. If the rape victim is scheduled for vaginal lavage, tell her to expect a cold sensation when saline solution is instilled to wash out the specimen. To help her relax during this procedure, instruct her to breathe deeply and slowly through her mouth. Just before the test, instruct the victim to urinate, but warn her not to wipe the vulva afterward, because this may remove semen.

Equipment

For semen collection by masturbation, coitus interruptus, or with a condom:

clean plastic specimen container (for example, disposable urine or sputum container, with lid).

For semen collection from rape victim: clean plastic specimen container/vaginal speculum/rubber gloves/cotton applicator sticks/glass microscopic slides with frosted ends/physiologic (0.85%) saline solution/Pap sticks/Coplin jars containing 95% ethanol/large syringe, rubber bulb, or other device suitable for vaginal lavage.

For a postcoital specimen collection: clean plastic specimen container/vaginal speculum/rubber gloves/cotton applicator sticks/glass microscopic slides with frosted ends/1-ml tuberculin syringe, without a cannula or needle.

Procedure

To obtain a semen specimen for a fertility study, ask the patient to collect semen in a clean, plastic specimen container.

The doctor obtains a specimen from the vagina of a rape victim by direct aspiration, saline lavage, or a direct smear of vaginal contents, using a Pap stick or, less desirably, a cotton applicator stick. Dried smears are usually collected from the suspected rape victim's skin by gently washing the skin with a small piece of gauze, moistened with physiologic saline solution. Prepare direct smears on glass microscopic slides after labeling the frosted end. Immediately place smeared slides in Coplin jars containing 95% ethanol.

Before postcoital examination, the examiner wipes any excess mucus from the external cervix and collects the specimen by direct aspiration of the cervical canal, using a 1-ml tuberculin syringe, without a cannula or needle.

Precautions

☐ Instruct the male patient who wants to collect the specimen during coitus interruptus to prevent any loss of semen during ejaculation.

☐ Deliver all specimens, regardless of source or method of collection, to the laboratory promptly.

☐ Protect semen specimens for fertility

SEMEN IDENTIFICATION FOR MEDICOLEGAL PURPOSES

Spermatozoa (or their fragments) persist in the vagina for more than 72 hours after sexual intercourse. This allows detection and positive identification of semen from vaginal aspirates or smears, or from stains on clothing, other fabrics, skin, or hair, which is often necessary for medicolegal purposes, usually in connection with rape or homicide investigations. Spermatozoa taken from the vagina of an exhumed body that has been properly embalmed and remains reasonably intact can also be identified.

To determine which stains or fluids require further investigation, clothing or other fabrics can be scanned with ultraviolet light to detect the typical green-white fluorescence of semen. Soaking appropriate samples of clothing, fabric, or hair in physiologic saline solution elutes the semen and spermatozoa. Suspect deposits of dried semen can be gently sponged from the victim's skin.

The two most common tests to identify semen are the determination of *acid phosphatase concentration* (the more sensitive test) and *microscopic examination* for the presence of spermatozoa. Acid phosphatase appears in semen in significantly greater concentrations than in any other body fluid. In microscopic examination, spermatozoa or head fragments can be identified on stained smears prepared directly from vaginal scrapings or aspirates, or from the concentrated sediment of eluates or lavages.

Like other body fluids, semen contains the soluble A, B, and H blood group substances in the approximately 80% of males who are genetically determined secretors (males who have the dominant secretor gene in a homozygous or heterozygous state). Thus, the male who is group A blood and is a secretor has soluble blood group A substance in his seminal fluid and group A substance on the surface of his RBCs. This fact may be of considerable medicolegal importance. Semen analysis can demonstrate that the semen of a suspect in a rape or homicide investigation is different from or consistent with semen found in or on the victim's body.

studies from extremes of temperature and direct sunlight during delivery to the laboratory.

□ *Don't* lubricate the vaginal speculum. Oil or grease hinders examination of spermatozoa by interfering with smear preparation and staining, and by inhibiting sperm motility through toxic ingredients. Instead, moisten the speculum with water or physiologic saline.

□ Use extreme caution in securing, labeling, and delivering all specimens to be used for medicolegal purposes. You may be asked to testify as to when, where, and from whom the specimen was obtained; the specimen's general appearance and identifying features; steps taken to ensure the specimen's integrity; and when, where, and to whom the specimen was delivered for analysis. If your hospital or clinic uses routing slips for such specimens, fill them out carefully, and submit them to the permanent *medicolegal* file.

Findings

Normal semen volume ranges from 0.7 to 6.5 ml. Paradoxically, the semen volume of males in infertile marriages is frequently increased. Continence for 1 week or more results in progressively increased semen volume (sperm counts increase with abstinence up to 10 days; sperm motility progressively decreases; and sperm morphology stays the same). Liquefied semen is generally highly viscid, translucent, and gray-white, with a musty or acrid odor. After liquefaction, specimens of normal viscosity can be poured in drops. Normally, semen is slightly alkaline, with a pH of 7.3 to 7.9.

Other normal characteristics of semen: it coagulates immediately and liquefies within 20 minutes; normal spermatozoa count ranges from 20 to 150 million/ml; at least 40% of sper-

---

MORPHOLOGY OF NORMAL AND ABNORMAL SPERMATOZOA

Normal spermatozoon

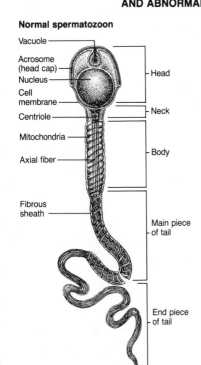

The mature spermatozoon consists of three principal parts: the head, midpiece or body, and the tail. Covered with a tightly fitting acrosome, or cap, the ovoid head has a large nucleus, which contains the paternal chromosomes. The body is attached to the neck and holds the mitochondria, the energy source necessary for spermatic movement. Contracting protein fibers comprise the tail, the longest part of the spermatozoon, and drive the spermatozoon forward.

Abnormal spermatozoa

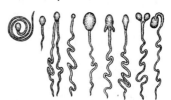

Morphologic abnormalities of spermatozoa include enlarged, undersized, or deformed heads; double heads or tails; and immaturity due to the retention of cytoplasmic remnants from the parent germ cells in the testicular tubules. Such morphologic abnormalities may be associated with decreased fertility.

matozoa have normal morphology; at least 20% of spermatozoa show progressive motility within 4 hours of collection.

The normal postcoital cervical mucus test shows at least ten motile spermatozoa per microscopic high-power field; spinnbarkeit (a measurement of the tenacity of the mucus) of at least 4″ (10 cm). These findings indicate adequate spermatozoa and receptivity of the cervical mucus.

Implications of results

Abnormal semen is *not* synonymous with infertility. Only one viable spermatozoon is needed to fertilize an ovum. Although a normal sperm count is more than 20 million/ml, many males with sperm counts below 1 million/ml have fathered normal children. Only males who can't deliver *any* viable spermatozoa in their ejaculates during sexual intercourse are absolutely sterile. Nevertheless, subnormal sperm counts, decreased sperm motility, and abnormal morphology are usually associated with decreased fertility. Other tests may be necessary to evaluate the patient's general health, metabolic status, or the function of specific endocrine systems (pituitary, thyroid, adrenal, or gonadal).

Post-test care

☐ Inform a patient who is undergoing infertility studies that test results should be available in 24 hours.

☐ Refer the suspected rape victim to an appropriate specialist for counseling—a gynecologist, psychiatrist, clinical psychologist, nursing specialist, member of the clergy, or representative of a community support group, such as Women Organized Against Rape (WOAR).

Interfering factors

☐ Delayed delivery of specimen, exposure of specimen to extremes of temperature or direct sunlight, or the presence of toxic chemicals in the specimen container or the condom can decrease the number of viable sperm.

☐ An incomplete specimen—from faulty

TESTICULAR SELF-EXAMINATION

Experts believe that the death rate from testicular cancer could be notably reduced if all males aged 15 years and older realized the importance of early detection and treatment. Besides a regular physical checkup that includes examination of the testes, the American Cancer Society recommends monthly testicular self-examination according to the following procedure:

After a warm bath or shower, when the scrotal skin is relaxed, each testis should be examined with both hands. Placing the index and middle fingers below one testis and the thumbs on top, the testis should be rolled gently between the fingers and thumbs to discover any lump, thickening, or change in consistency. (Most lumps are pea-sized and are found on either side or at the front of the testes. It's important not to confuse the epididymis, located at the lower rear portion of the testis, with a lump.) If any such abnormalities are discovered, the doctor should be notified. Early discovery and *immediate* treatment of testicular cancer greatly increase the chance of cure.

---

collection by coitus interruptus, for example—diminishes the volume of the specimen.

DONALD C. CANNON, MD, PhD

Sex Chromatin Tests

Although sex chromatin tests can screen for abnormalities in the number of sex chromosomes, they've been largely replaced by the full karyotype (chromosome analysis) test, which is faster, simpler, and more accurate. Sex chromatin tests are usually indicated for abnormal sexual development, ambiguous genitalia, amenorrhea, and suspected chromosomal abnormalities.

Fluorescent-staining techniques have identified the Y chromosome as the most fluorescent chromosome in a karyotype. Such fluorescence is confined to the long arm of the Y chromosome, which is tightly condensed in cells during interphase. When these cells are stained with quinacrine, a bright dot—known as the Y chromatin mass—appears in the nuclei of cells containing a Y chromosome. The number of such masses is identical to the number of Y chromosomes in the cell. Barr bodies (the X chromatin mass) can be stained with any nuclear stain, usually carbolfuchsin, to reveal the number of X chromatin bodies.

Purpose
□ To quickly screen for abnormal sexual development (both X and Y chromatin tests)
□ To aid assessment of an infant with ambiguous genitalia (X chromatin test only)
□ To determine the number of Y chromosomes in an individual (Y chromatin test only).

Patient preparation
Explain to the patient or to his parents, if appropriate, why the test is being performed. Tell him the test requires that the inside of his cheek be scraped to obtain a specimen and who will perform the test. Assure the patient the test takes only a few minutes but may require a follow-up chromosome analysis. Inform him that the laboratory generally requires as long as 4 weeks to complete the analysis.

Equipment
Wooden or metal spatula/clean glass slide/cell fixative.

Procedure
Scrape the buccal mucosa firmly with a wooden or metal spatula at least twice to obtain a specimen of healthy cells (vaginal mucosa is occasionally used in young women). Rub the spatula over the glass slide, making sure the cells are evenly distributed. Spray the slide with cell fixative, and send the slide to the laboratory with a brief patient history and indications for the test.

Precautions
Make sure the buccal mucosa is scraped firmly to ensure a sufficient number of cells. Check that the specimen isn't saliva, which contains no cells.

CYTOGENETICS

Modern cytogenetics began with the discovery of a small mass of chromatin in the nuclei of somatic cells in female mammals. This mass—called the chromatin mass, or Barr body—has been identified as a highly condensed X chromosome. It appears as a dark oval body at or near the nuclear membrane.

Research also indicates the X chromosome is inactivated during embryonic implantation in the uterus. Regardless of the number of X chromosomes in a cell, only one is biologically active; the rest condense and appear as Barr bodies. Consequently, the number of Barr bodies is one less than the total number of X chromosomes (active and inactive) in a cell.

Another fundamental discovery in cytogenetics is that mammalian eggs fertilized by X-bearing sperm become females (XX), while those fertilized by Y-bearing sperm become males (XY). The presence of the Y chromosome induces the indifferent gonad to organize testes; the testes then secrete testosterone, inducing the male body type. In the absence of the Y chromosome and testosterone secretion, ovaries form, and the embryo becomes a female.

Occasionally, XX embryos develop testes and become males, or XY embryos develop ovaries and become females. Moreover, either type of embryo may exhibit a combination of testicular and ovarian tissue (true hermaphroditism). It's believed that only a small portion of the Y chromosome—probably that portion clustered near the centromere—determines the male sex. This male-determining portion produces a substance called H-Y antigen, which is associated with testicular formation. Therefore, XX persons with testicular differentiation have probably conserved this critical portion of the Y chromosome, which remains active.

SEX CHROMOSOME ANOMALIES

DISORDER AND CHROMOSOMAL ANEUPLOIDY	CAUSE AND INCIDENCE	PHENOTYPIC FEATURES
Klinefelter's syndrome • 47,XXY • 48,XXXY • 49,XXXXY • 48,XX,YY • 49,XXX,YY • Mosaics: XXY, XXXY, or XXXXY/XX or XY	Nondisjunction or improper chromatid separation during anaphase I or II of oogenesis or spermatogenesis results in abnormal gamete 1/500 to 600 male births	• Syndrome usually inapparent until puberty • Small penis and testes • Sparse facial and abdominal hair; feminine distribution of pubic hair • Somewhat enlarged breasts (gynecomastia) • Sexual dysfunction • Sterility • Possible mental retardation (greater incidence with increased X chromosomes)
Polysomy Y • 47,XYY	Nondisjunction during anaphase II of spermatogenesis causes both Y chromosomes to pass to the same pole and results in a YY sperm 1/1,000 male births	• Above average stature (often over 72″ [1.8 m]) • May display aggressive, psychopathic, or criminal behavior • Normal fertility
Turner's syndrome (ovarian dysgenesis) • 45,XO • Mosaics: XO/XX or XO/XXX • Aberrations of X chromosomes, including deletion of short arm of one X chromosome, presence of a ring chromosome, or presence of an isochromosome on the long arm of an X chromosome	Nondisjunction during anaphase I or II of spermatogenesis results in sperm without any sex chromosomes 1/3,500 female births (most common chromosome complement in first trimester abortions)	• Short stature (usually under 57″ [130 cm]) • Webbed neck • Low hairline • Broad chest with widely spaced nipples • Underdeveloped breasts • Juvenile external genitalia • Primary amenorrhea common • Sterility due to underdeveloped internal reproductive organs (ovaries are merely strands of connective tissue) • No mental retardation, but possible problems with space perception and orientation
Other X Polysomes	Nondisjunction at anaphase I or II of oogenesis	
• 47,XXX	1/1,400 female births	• Often, no obvious anatomical abnormalities • Normal fertility
• 48,XXXX	Rare	• Mental retardation • Ocular hypertelorism • Reduced fertility
• 49,XXXXX	Rare	• Severe mental retardation • Ocular hypertelorism, with uncoordinated eye movement • Abnormal development of sexual organs • Various skeletal anomalies

Findings

A normal female (XX) has only one X chromatin mass (the number of X chromatin masses discernible is one less than the number of X chromosomes in the cells examined). For various reasons, an X chromatin mass is ordinarily discernible in only 20% to 50% of the buccal mucosal cells of a normal female.

A normal male (XY) has only one Y chromatin mass (the number of Y chromatin masses equals number of Y chromosomes in the cells examined).

Implications of results

In most laboratories, if less than 20% of the cells in a buccal smear contain an X chromatin mass, some cells are presumed to contain only one X chromosome, necessitating full karyotyping. Persons with female phenotypes and positive Y chromatin masses run a high risk of developing malignancies in their intra-abdominal gonads. In such persons, removal of these gonads is indicated, and should generally be performed before age 5.

Post-test care

After the cause of chromosomal abnormal sexual development has been identified, the patient or his parents require genetic counseling. If a child is phenotypically of one sex and genotypically of the other, a medical team comprised of knowledgeable doctors, psychologists, psychiatrists, and possibly, educators, must decide the child's sex. This careful evaluation should be made early to prevent developmental problems related to incorrect gender identification.

Interfering factors

□ Obtaining saliva instead of buccal cells provides a false specimen.
□ Failure to apply cell fixative to the slide allows cells to deteriorate.
□ Laboratory artifacts, such as the presence of bacteria or wrinkles in the cell membrane, analysis of degenerating cells, or use of outdated stain, can cause misleading results.

RONALD J. WAPNER, MD

DNA, RNA, AND PROTEIN SYNTHESIS

The chromosomes in every body cell are composed of genes, individual units of deoxyribonucleic acid (DNA) that carry genetic information. DNA also synthesizes the proteins which comprise the enzymes fundamental to cellular growth and function.

Located primarily in the nucleus, the DNA molecule consists of two tightly coiled helical chains. The backbone of each chain consists of alternating units of deoxyribose (a 5-carbon sugar) and phosphate. A mixture of four nitrogenous bases—adenine (A); guanine (G); cytosine (C); and thymine (T)—form the links of each chain. (The sequential arrangement of these four bases represents the inherited genetic code of a particular trait.) From chain to chain, adenine (A) is always paired with thymine (T), and cytosine (C) with guanine (G).

Ribonucleic acid (RNA) transmits genetic messages from DNA to the cytoplasmic ribosomes, site of protein formation. Single-stranded, RNA consists of alternating ribose-phosphate units and a mixture of four bases, three of which comprise DNA. The fourth base, uracil (U) replaces thymine. Various types of RNA are distinguished by the number of their components and the arrangement of their bases.

When a cell needs a specific protein enzyme to carry out a chemical reaction, the cell alerts the appropriate DNA molecule and protein synthesis begins. The double-stranded DNA helix unwinds, and separates into individual chains. The bases of each chain are arranged in sequential triplets or codons that eventually determine the arrangement of amino acids in the final protein molecule. (The human body has only 20 types of amino acids available for protein construction. The total number and sequential combinations of these amino acids determine the many protein molecules in the body and their various biological properties.)

Next, the DNA code is transcribed onto a single strand of RNA. Before transcription can occur, however, the individual strands of

Chromosome Analysis

Chromosomes—threadlike bodies in the cellular nucleus—each contain thousands of genes with biochemical programs for cell function that are stored in deoxyribonucleic acid (DNA), the ba-

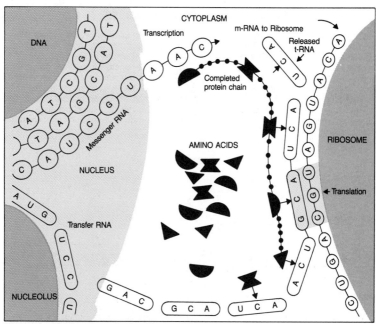

KEY: A = adenine, **G** = guanine, **C** = cytosine
T = thymine, **U** = uracil (which replaces thymine)

DNA become a template or blueprint for a matching RNA molecule. The bases of DNA and RNA pair off according to the A-T, C-G pattern previously described. (However, in RNA uracil replaces thymine; therefore, the adenine in DNA takes on a new partner.) When base pairing is complete, the RNA and DNA strands separate.

Carrying a specific DNA code or message for amino acid formation, the newly-formed RNA [messenger RNA (mRNA)] leaves the nucleus and enters the cytoplasm. There, mRNA attaches itself to one or more ribosomes, spherical bodies of protein and ribosomal RNA (rRNA) running through the cytoplasm. Attached, the ribosome travels the length of the mRNA, reading the genetic message in a process called translation.

As the ribosome translates the message, it calls for the insertion of the proper amino acids into the growing protein chain. To facilitate its entry into the protein chain, each amino acid binds with a complementary molecule of RNA [transfer RNA (tRNA)]. While one end of the tRNA molecule is firmly attached to its complementary amino acid, the other end (specific triplet arrangement of bases) joins corresponding triplet bases of mRNA. After alignment of tRNA and mRNA bases, the newly-formed protein frees itself of the ribosome to produce the enzyme needed for chemical reaction.

sic genetic material. Chromosome analysis, an integral facet of cytogenetics, studies the relationship between the microscopic appearance of chromosomes and the person's phenotype—the expression of the genes in physical, biochemical, or physiologic traits.

Light microscopy can visualize the chromosomes but is not yet capable of showing individual genes. Ideally, chromosomes require study during meta-phase, the middle phase of mitosis, when new cell poles appear. Only rapidly dividing cell lines, such as bone marrow or neoplastic cells, permit direct, immediate study. Most other cell types require stimulation of mitosis by addition of phytohemagglutinin to the culture. Subsequently, the addition of colchicine (a cell poison) arrests the cell division in metaphase. Harvested, stained, and viewed under a microscope, the cells are

CELL DIVISION: MITOSIS AND MEIOSIS

All living cells arise from existing living cells. During an uninterrupted process of nuclear division known as mitosis (see illustrations 1A to 6A on this and the following page), newly formed daughter nuclei receive the same diploid number (2n) of chromosomes as the parent cell.

Meiosis (see illustrations 1B to 10B on pages 710 and 711)—another kind of cell division, which takes place in two sequences—occurs in the gonads and produces ova or spermatozoa. During meiosis, the chromosomes in each sex cell or gamete are reduced to one half the number (haploid or n) found in somatic cells. Despite this reduction, the diploid number is restored when an ovum and spermatozoon unite to form a new cell, or zygote. Without this reduction in each sex cell, the union of gametes would result in a zygote with twice the number of chromosomes as the parent cells.

MITOSIS

1A:

INTERPHASE

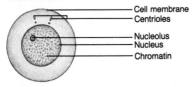

— Cell membrane
— Centrioles
— Nucleolus
— Nucleus
— Chromatin

During interphase and before mitosis, the nondividing cell must duplicate its genetic material before distributing it to daughter cells. Although the nucleus and one or more nucleoli are visible, the chromosomes are seen only as a chromatinic mass. In this preliminary phase, the cylindrical centrioles migrate from their right angular position and equip themselves for cellular division.

2A:

LATE PROPHASE

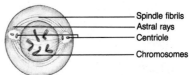

— Spindle fibrils
— Astral rays
— Centriole
— Chromosomes

Throughout prophase, the first stage of mitosis, both the nucleus and nucleoli become less distinct and finally disappear. Conversely, the chromosomes take shape and eventually appear as short, rodlike, mobile structures. As the centrioles continue to migrate toward opposite sides of the nucleus, they align thin, projecting fibrils or spindles. (Astral fibrils radiate from each centriole; spindle fibrils link them.) At the end of prophase, each chromosome has moved to the midpoint of one of the spindle fibrils comprising the biconical spindle.

---

finally photographed to provide a karyotype, the systematic arrangement of chromosomes in groupings according to size and shape. Indications for the test determine the specimen required (blood, bone marrow, amniotic fluid, skin, or placental tissue) and the procedure.

Purpose
□ To identify chromosomal abnormalities, such as hypoploidy or hyperploidy, as the underlying cause of malformation, maldevelopment, or disease.

Patient preparation
Explain to the patient or to his parents,

if appropriate, that this test identifies the underlying cause of malformation, maldevelopment, or disease. Tell him who will perform the test and what kind of specimen will be required. Inform him when results will be available, according to the specimen required. For example, test results on a blood sample are generally available 72 to 96 hours after stimulation; analysis of skin biopsy specimens or amniotic fluid cells may take several weeks.

Procedure
Collect a blood sample (in a 5 to 10 ml *green-top* [heparinized] tube), a tissue

3A:
METAPHASE

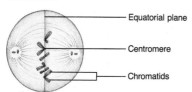

- Equatorial plane
- Centromere
- Chromatids

When metaphase begins, the chromosomes are double-stranded structures consisting of two chromatids united by a single body called a centromere. Each chromosome is attached by its centromere to a fibril in the equatorial plane of the spindle. This brief phase ends when each centromere divides and each chromatid becomes a single-stranded chromosome.

4A:
LATE ANAPHASE

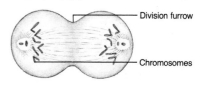

- Division furrow
- Chromosomes

Anaphase marks the migratory separation of each set of single-stranded chromosomes. By late anaphase, the chromosomes have neared their respective poles and cytokinesis—division of the cytoplasm—has begun.

5A:
TELOPHASE

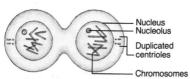

- Nucleus
- Nucleolus
- Duplicated centrioles
- Chromosomes

Telophase, the last stage of mitosis, reverses the processes of prophase. Having reached their respective poles, the two sets of chromosomes become encapsulated in newly developing nuclei that evolve as the spindles disappear. Likewise, the nucleoli slowly reappear as the chromosomes become less visible, resembling the thin, intertwined filaments of early prophase. By late telophase, the centriole of each nucleus has replicated and cytokinesis has ended.

6A:
LATE TELOPHASE
(Interphase)

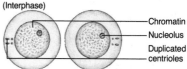

- Chromatin
- Nucleolus
- Duplicated centrioles

When telophase, and hence mitosis, is complete, the newly formed nuclei typify interphase. Furthermore, each new daughter cell has the same number (46) and types of chromosomes (23) as its parent cell, and can thus function characteristically.

specimen, 1 ml of bone marrow, or at least 20 ml of amniotic fluid. (For additional information, see SKIN BIOPSY and BONE MARROW ASPIRATION AND BIOPSY in Chapter 18, and also AMNIOTIC FLUID ANALYSIS in this chapter.)

Precautions
□ Keep all specimens sterile, especially those requiring a tissue culture.
□ To facilitate interpretation of test results, send the specimen to the laboratory immediately, with a brief patient history and indication for the test. If transport must be delayed, refrigerate the specimen but *never* freeze it.

□ Before skin biopsy, make sure the povidone-iodine solution is thoroughly removed with alcohol. This solution may prevent cell growth in tissue culture.

NURSING ALERT

Findings
The normal cell contains 46 chromosomes: 22 pairs of nonsex chromosomes (autosomes) and 1 pair of sex chromosomes (Y for the male-determining chromosome, X for the female-determining chromosome). On a karyotype, chromosomes are arranged according to size and the location of their primary con-

CELL DIVISION (continued): MEIOSIS

1B:

LATE PROPHASE I

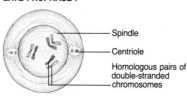

— Spindle

— Centriole

Homologous pairs of double-stranded chromosomes

Usually, first meiotic prophase resembles mitotic prophase. Individual chromosomes become more apparent as the nucleoli and nuclear membrane fade, spindles form and centrioles polarize. In meiotic prophase I, paired homologous chromosomes—from the male and female pronuclei—move together toward the spindles' equator.

2B:

METAPHASE I

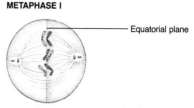

— Equatorial plane

Since these double-stranded, homologous chromosomes are traveling side by side, each pair occupies a single fibral spindle during first metaphase. (In mitosis, each chromosome travels alone and thus occupies a separate fibral spindle.)

3B:

ANAPHASE I

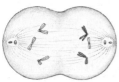

During mitosis, metaphase ends and anaphase begins when the centromeres linking the double-stranded chromosomes divide, leaving single-stranded chromosomes. In meiosis, however, such division does not occur. During anaphase I, therefore, double-stranded chromosomes comprising each homologous pair separate and polarize. Consequently, when cytokinesis occurs, the two daughter nuclei will have one of each type of chromosome or one half the number of chromosomes as each parent cell.

4B:

TELOPHASE I

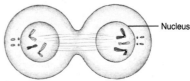

— Nucleus

Meiotic and mitotic telophase are essentially alike. As cytokinesis ends, two new nuclei are formed and the spindles disappear. The difference, however, lies in the number of chromosomes per newly formed nuclei. When mitosis is complete, each daughter cell has the same number of chromosomes as the parent cell and is therefore diploid. Following meiosis, each new nucleus has only one of each type of chromosome or one half the number of each parent cell, and is therefore haploid.

strictions, or centromeres. The centromere may be medial (metacentric), slightly to one end of the chromosome (submetacentric), or entirely to one end (acrocentric). The largest chromosomes are displayed first; the others are arranged in order of decreasing size, with the two sex chromosomes traditionally placed last. By convention, the centromere is always placed at the top in a karyotype. Thus, if the two pairs of chromosomal arms are of unequal length, the arm above the centromere will be shorter. The letter "p" designates the short arm;

the letter "q," the long arm.

Special stains identify individual chromosomes, and locate and enumerate particular portions of chromosomes. Trypsin, alkali, heat denaturization, and Giemsa's stain are used for visible light microscopy; quinacrine stain, for ultraviolet microscopy. These staining techniques produce nonuniform staining of each chromosome in a repetitive, banded pattern. The mechanism of chromosome banding is unknown, but seems related to primary DNA sequence and protein composition of the chromosome.

5B:

INTERKINESIS

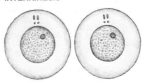

Interkinesis, the brief period following first telophase and preceding the second sequence of meiosis, resembles mitotic interphase. Since the chromosomes are already double-stranded, however, there is no replication of genetic material and no new chromatid formation.

6B:

PROPHASE II

Second prophase triggers the final series of meiotic divisions. Since the two newly formed daughter cells are haploid, their chromosomes are not homologous and therefore move independently, as in mitosis.

7B:

METAPHASE II

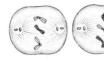

Each double-stranded chromosome is attached by its centromere to a separate spindle. At the end of metaphase II, the centromeres divide, leaving single-stranded chromosomes that polarize during anaphase II.

8B:

ANAPHASE II

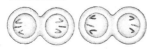

Single-stranded chromosomes

9B:

TELOPHASE II

The two additional newly formed nuclei of telophase II are haploid, but unlike the two daughter cells of telophase I, their chromosomes are single-stranded.

10B:

LATE TELOPHASE II

Nucleus

At the end of meiosis, four new haploid cells contain single-stranded chromosomes.

Implications of results

Chromosome abnormalities may be numerical or structural. Numerical deviation from the norm of 46 chromosomes is called aneuploidy. Less than 46 chromosomes is called hypoploidy; more than 46, hyperploidy. Special designations exist for whole multiples of the haploid number 23: diploidy for the normal somatic number of 46, triploidy for 69, tetraploidy for 92, and so forth. When the deviation occurs within a single pair of chromosomes, the suffix -somy is used, as in trisomy for the presence of three chromosomes instead of the usual pair, or monosomy for the presence of only one chromosome.

Aneuploidy most commonly follows failure of the chromosomal pair to separate (nondisjunction) during anaphase, the mitotic stage that follows metaphase. It may also result from anaphase lag, in which one of the normally separated chromosomes fails to move to a pole and is left out of the daughter cells. If nondisjunction or anaphase lag occurs during meiosis, the cells of the zygote will all be the same. Errors in mitotic

CHROMOSOME ANALYSIS FINDINGS

SPECIMEN AND INDICATION	RESULT	IMPLICATION
Blood • To evaluate abnormal appearance or development suggesting chromosomal irregularity	• Abnormal chromosome number (aneuploidy) or arrangement	• Identifies specific chromosomal abnormality
• To evaluate couple with history of miscarriages, or to identify balanced translocation carriers having unbalanced offspring	• Normal chromosomes	• Miscarriage unrelated to parental chromosomal abnormality
	• Parental balanced translocation carrier	• Increased risk of repeated abortion or unbalanced offspring indicates need for amniocentesis in future pregnancies
• To detect chromosomal rearrangements in rare genetic diseases predisposing patient to malignant neoplasms	• Chromosomal rearrangements, gaps, and breaks	• Occurs in Bloom's syndrome, Fanconi's syndrome, telangiectasia; patient predisposed to malignant neoplasms
Blood or bone marrow • To identify Philadelphia chromosome and confirm chronic myelogenous leukemia	• Translocation of chromosome 22q (long arm) to another chromosome (often chromosome 9)	• Aids diagnosis of chronic myelogenous leukemia
	• Aneuploidy (usually due to abnormalities in chromosomes 8 and 12)	• Occurs in acute myelogenous leukemia
	• Trisomy 21	• Occasionally occurs in chronic lymphocytic leukemia cells
Skin • To evaluate abnormal appearance or development suggesting chromosomal irregularity	• All chromosomal abnormalities possible	• Same as chromosomal abnormality in blood; rarely, mosaic individual has normal blood but abnormal skin chromosomes
Amniotic fluid • To evaluate developing fetus with possible chromosomal abnormality	• All chromosomal abnormalities possible	• Same as chromosomal abnormality in blood or fetus
Placental tissue • To evaluate products of conception after a miscarriage to determine if abnormality is fetal or placental in origin	• All chromosomal abnormalities possible	• Over 50% of aborted tissue is chromosomally abnormal
Tumor tissue • For research purposes only	• Many chromosomal abnormalities possible	• Although malignant tumors are not associated with specific chromosomal aberrations, most are aneuploid, usually hyperploid.

division after the formation of the zygote will produce more than one cell line (mosaicism).

Structural chromosome abnormalities result from chromosome breakage. Intrachromosomal rearrangement occurs within a single chromosome in various forms:

□ *Deletion:* loss of an end (terminal) or middle (interstitial) portion of a chromosome·

□ *Inversion:* end-to-end reversal of a chromosome segment, which may be pericentric inversion (including the centromere) or paracentric inversion (occurring in only one arm of the chromosome)

□ *Ring chromosome formation:* breakage of both ends of a chromosome and reunion of the ends

□ *Isochromosome formation:* abnormal splitting of the centromere in a transverse rather than a longitudinal plane.

Interchromosomal rearrangements (of more than one chromosome, usually two) also occur. The most common rearrangement is translocation, or exchange, of genetic material between two chromosomes. Translocations may be balanced, in which the cell neither loses nor gains genetic material; unbalanced, in which a piece of genetic material is gained or lost from each cell; reciprocal (in chil-

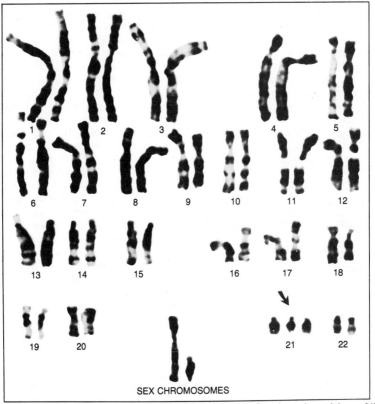

DOWN'S SYNDROME KARYOTYPE

This karyotype, obtained from the amniotic fluid of a fetus with Down's syndrome (trisomy 21), reveals a third chromosome instead of the usual pair (see arrow).

dren), in which two chromosomes exchange material; or Robertsonian, in which two chromosomes join to form one combined chromosome, with little or no loss of material.

Implications of chromosome analysis results depend on the specimen and indications for the test (see chart on page 712).

Post-test care
☐ Provide appropriate post-test care, depending on the procedure used to collect the specimen.
☐ Explain the test results and their implications to the patient or to the parents of a child with a chromosomal abnormality.
☐ If necessary, recommend appropriate genetic or other counseling and follow-up care, such as an infant stimulation program for Down's syndrome.

Interfering factors
☐ Chemotherapy may cause abnormal results, such as chromosome breaks.
☐ Contamination of tissue with bacteria, fungus, or a virus may inhibit growth of the culture.
☐ Inclusion of maternal cells in a specimen obtained by amniocentesis, with subsequent culturing, may cause false results.

RONALD J. WAPNER, MD

Amniotic Fluid Analysis

Amniocentesis is the transabdominal needle aspiration of 10 to 20 ml of amniotic fluid for laboratory analysis. Such analysis can detect several birth defects (especially Down's syndrome and spina bifida), determine fetal maturity, detect hemolytic disease of the newborn, and, through karyotyping, detect gender and chromosomal abnormalities. This test can be performed only when the amniotic
fluid level reaches 150 ml, usually after the 16th week of pregnancy.

Amniotic fluid reflects important metabolic changes in the fetus, the placenta, or the mother. It protects the fetus from external trauma, allows fetal movement, and provides an even body temperature and limited source of protein (10% to 15%) for the fetus. Although the origin of amniotic fluid is uncertain, it may arise as a water-permeable transudate from fetal skin, or as a dialysate from the maternal serum through the fetal membranes into the amniotic cavity. Its original composition is essentially the same as that of interstitial fluid. As the fetus matures, however, the amniotic fluid becomes progressively more diluted with hypotonic fetal urine.

One of the chief differences between amniotic fluid and maternal plasma during intrauterine development is the amniotic fluid's relatively high levels of uric acid, urea, and creatinine. The volume of amniotic fluid steadily rises from 50 ml at the end of the first trimester to an average of 1,000 ml near term; at 40 weeks' gestation, the volume decreases to 700 to 800 ml.

Amniocentesis is indicated during pregnancy associated with advanced maternal age (over 35); family history of genetic, chromosomal, or neural tube defects; or previous miscarriage. Adverse effects from this test are rare; potential risks include spontaneous abortion, trauma to the fetus or placenta, bleeding, premature labor, infection, and Rh sensitization from fetal bleeding into the maternal circulation. However, because such complications are possible, amniocentesis is contraindicated as a general screening test. Abnormal test results or failure of the tissue cultures to grow may necessitate repetition of the test.

Purpose
☐ To detect fetal abnormalities, particularly chromosomal and neural tube defects
☐ To detect hemolytic disease of the newborn

ANALYSIS OF AMNIOTIC FLUID

TEST	NORMAL FINDINGS	FETAL IMPLICATIONS OF ABNORMAL FINDINGS
Color	Clear, with white flecks of vernix caseosa in a mature fetus	Blood of maternal origin is usually harmless. "Port wine" fluid may indicate abruptio placentae. Fetal blood may indicate damage to the fetal, placental, or umbilical cord vessels.
Bilirubin	Absent at term	High levels indicate hemolytic disease of the newborn in isoimmunized pregnancy
Meconium	Absent (except in breech presentation)	Presence indicates fetal hypotension or distress.
Creatinine	More than 2 mg/100 ml in a mature fetus	Decrease may indicate immature fetus (less than 37 weeks).
L/S ratio	More than 2 generally indicates fetal pulmonary maturity	Less than 2 indicates pulmonary immaturity and subsequent respiratory distress syndrome.
Phosphatidylglycerol	Present	Absence indicates pulmonary immaturity.
Glucose	Less than 45 mg/100 ml	Excessive increases at term or near term indicates hypertrophied fetal pancreas and subsequent neonatal hypoglycemia.
Alpha-fetoprotein	Variable, depending on gestational age and laboratory technique. Highest concentration (about 18.5 mcg/ml) occurs at 13 to 14 weeks	Inappropriate increases indicate neural tube defects, such as spina bifida or anencephaly, impending fetal death, congenital nephrosis, or contamination by fetal blood.
Bacteria	Absent	Presence indicates chorioamnionitis.
Chromosome	Normal karyotype	Abnormal karyotype may indicate fetal sex and chromosome disorders.
Acetycholinesterase	Absent	Presence may indicate neural tube defects, exomphalos, or other serious malformations.

□ To diagnose metabolic disorders, amino acid disorders, and mucopolysaccharidoses

□ To determine fetal age and maturity, especially pulmonary maturity

□ To assess fetal health by detecting the presence of meconium or blood, or measuring amniotic levels of estriol and fetal thyroid hormone

□ To identify fetal gender when one or both parents are carriers of a sex-linked disorder.

Patient preparation

Describe the procedure to the patient, and explain that this test detects fetal abnormalities. Assess her understanding of the test, and answer any questions she may have. Inform her that she needn't restrict food or fluids. Tell her the test requires a specimen of amniotic fluid and who will perform the test. Advise her that normal test results can't guarantee a normal fetus, since some fetal disorders are undetectable.

Make sure the patient has signed a consent form. Explain that she'll feel a stinging sensation when the local anesthetic is injected. Provide emotional support before and during the test and reassure her that adverse effects are rare.

Just before the test, ask her to void to minimize the risk of puncturing the bladder and aspirating urine instead of amniotic fluid.

Equipment

70% alcohol or povidone-iodine solution/sponge forceps/2″ x 2″ gauze pads/local anesthetic (1% lidocaine)/25G sterile needle/3-ml syringe/20G sterile spinal needle with stylet/10-ml syringe/amber or foil-covered sterile 10-ml test tube.

Procedure

After determining fetal and placental position, usually through palpation and ultrasonic visualization, the doctor locates a pool of amniotic fluid. Following skin preparation with an antiseptic and alcohol, 1 ml of 1% lidocaine is injected with a 25G needle, first intradermally and then subcutaneously. Then the 20G spinal needle, with a stylet, is inserted into the amniotic cavity and the stylet is withdrawn. After a 10-ml syringe is attached to the needle, the fluid is aspirated and placed in an amber or foil-covered test tube. After the needle is withdrawn, an adhesive bandage is

---

SHAKE TEST OR FOAM STABILITY TEST

Positive foam test

Amniotic fluid from mature fetal lungs contains surface-active material (surfactants). In this test, bubbles should appear on the surface of a test tube of amniotic fluid that is shaken vigorously if adequate amounts of surfactants are present.

Numerically label five clean, dry test tubes and add 1 ml, 0.75 ml, 0.50 ml, 0.25 ml, and 0.20 ml of amniotic fluid to test tubes 1, 2, 3, 4, and 5 respectively. Add normal saline: 0.25 ml, 0.50 ml, 0.75 ml, and 0.80 ml to tubes 2, 3, 4, and 5. Then add 1 ml of 95% ethanol to each test tube. Cap each test tube with a clean rubber stopper (don't use your finger since it contains surface-active material). Shake each test tube for 15 seconds and place upright in rack (undisturbed) for 15 minutes.

A complete ring of bubbles is a positive result. Negative results in tube 1 (the 1:1 dilution) indicates a high risk of respiratory distress syndrome (RDS). A positive result in tube 3 (1:2 dilution) indicates pulmonary maturity. Negative results in the other tubes indicate varying degrees of RDS risks (62% develop mild to severe respiratory problems). Blood or meconium in the fluid invalidates the test.

placed over the needle insertion site.

Precautions

☐ Instruct the patient to fold her hands behind her head to prevent her from accidently touching the sterile field and causing contamination.
☐ Send the specimen to the laboratory immediately.

Findings

Normal amniotic fluid is clear but may contain white flecks of vernix caseosa when the fetus is near term. For detailed analysis of the appearance and components of amniotic fluid, see the chart on page 715.

Implications of results

Blood in amniotic fluid is usually of maternal origin and doesn't indicate abnormality. However, it does inhibit cell growth and changes the level of other amniotic fluid constituents.

Large amounts of *bilirubin,* a breakdown product of RBCs, may indicate hemolytic disease of the newborn. Normally, the bilirubin level increases from the 14th to the 24th week of pregnancy, then declines as the fetus matures, essentially reaching zero at term. Testing for bilirubin usually isn't performed until the 26th week, since that's the earliest time successful therapy for Rh sensitization can begin. Bilirubin level is determined by spectrophotometric measurement of the optic density of the amniotic fluid. The deviation of the scan at 450 mμ from a straight line drawn between 375 and 525 mμ represents the bilirubin peak.

Meconium, a semisolid viscous material found in the fetal gastrointestinal tract, consists of mucopolysaccharides, desquamated cells, vernix, hair, and cholesterol. Meconium passes into the amniotic fluid when hypoxia causes fetal distress and relaxation of the anal sphincter. Meconium is a normal finding in breech presentation. Meconium in the amniotic fluid produces a peak of 410 mμ on the spectrophotometric analysis. However, serial amniocentesis may show

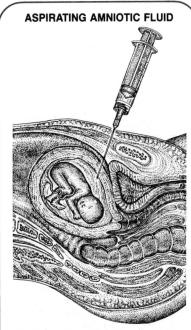

ASPIRATING AMNIOTIC FLUID

After the position of the placenta and fetus are determined, the aspirating needle is inserted through the abdominal wall at a right angle. To avoid penetrating the placenta or puncturing the fetus, the needle is inserted by the back of the neck or the small body parts of the fetus.

a clearing of meconium over a 2- to 3-week period. If meconium is present during labor, the newborn's nose and throat require thorough cleaning to prevent meconium aspiration.

Creatinine, a product of fetal urine, increases in the amniotic fluid as the fetal kidneys mature. Generally, the creatinine value exceeds 2 mg/100 ml in a mature fetus.

Alpha-fetoprotein is a fetal alpha globulin produced first in the yolk sac and, later, in the parenchymal cells of the liver and gastrointestinal tract. Fetal serum levels of alpha-fetoprotein are about 150 times more than amniotic fluid levels; maternal serum levels are far less than amniotic fluid levels. High amniotic fluid levels indicate neural tube defects, but the alpha-fetoprotein level may remain normal if the defect is small and closed. Elevated alpha-fetoprotein level may occur in multiple pregnancy; in disorders such as omphalocele, congenital nephrosis, esophageal or duodenal atresia, cystic fibrosis, exomphalos, Turner's syndrome, and fetal bladder neck obstruction with hydronephrosis; and in impending fetal death.

The amount of *uric acid* in the amniotic fluid increases as the fetus matures, but these levels fluctuate widely and can't accurately predict maturity. Laboratory studies indicate that severe erythroblastosis fetalis, familial hyperuricemia, and Lesch-Nyhan syndrome tend to increase the level of uric acid.

Estrone, estradiol, estriol, and *estriol conjugates* appear in amniotic fluid in varying amounts. Estriol, the most prevalent estrogen, increases from 25.7 ng/ml during the 16th to 20th weeks to almost 1,000 ng/ml at term. Severe erythroblastosis fetalis decreases the estriol level.

Blood in the amniotic fluid occurs in about 10% of amniocenteses and results from a faulty tap. If the origin is maternal, the blood generally has no special significance; however, "port wine" fluid may be a sign of abruptio placentae, while blood of fetal origin may indicate damage to the fetal, placental, or umbilical cord vessels by the amniocentesis needle.

THE APT TEST

Blood in the amniotic fluid can be of maternal or fetal origin. The Apt test, based on the premise that fetal hemoglobin is alkali-resistant and adult hemoglobin changes to alkaline hematin after the addition of alkali, can differentiate the two. This test may be performed on all bloody amniotic fluid samples.

Dilute 1 ml of amniotic fluid with water until it turns pink. Centrifuge for 10 minutes, and decant the supernatant. Add five parts supernatant to one part 0.25 N (1%) sodium hydroxide, and observe for 1 or 2 minutes. Fetal blood appears red; maternal blood, yellow-brown. To confirm results, repeat the test with known maternal blood.

The Type II cells lining the fetal lung alveoli produce *lecithin* slowly in early pregnancy, and then markedly increase production around the 35th week.

The *sphingomyelin* level parallels that of lecithin until the 35th week, when it gradually decreases. Measuring the ratio of lecithin to sphingomyelin (L/S ratio) confirms fetal pulmonary maturity (L/S ratio>2) or suggests a risk of respiratory distress (L/S ratio<2). However, fetal respiratory distress may develop in the fetus of a patient with diabetes, even though the L/S ratio is greater than 2, a level usually indicative of pulmonary maturity.

Phosphatidylglycerol levels are present with pulmonary maturity; *phosphatidylinositol* levels decrease. Measuring *glucose* levels in the fluid can aid in assessing glucose control in the patient with diabetes, but this isn't done routinely. A level greater than 45 mg/100 ml indicates poor maternal and fetal control. *Insulin* levels normally increase slightly from the 27th to the 40th week but increase sharply (up to 27 times normal) in a poorly controlled patient with diabetes.

Laboratory analysis can identify at least 25 different *enzymes* (usually in low concentrations) in amniotic fluid. The enzymes have few known clinical implications, although elevated acetylcholinesterase levels may occur with neural tube defects, exomphalos, and other serious malformations.

When the mother carries an *X-linked disorder*, determination of fetal sex is important. If chromosome karyotyping identifies a male fetus, there's a 50% chance he'll be affected; a female fetus won't be affected but has a 50% chance of being a carrier. (See CHROMOSOME ANALYSIS for more information.)

Post-test care

☐ Monitor fetal heart rate and maternal vital signs every 15 minutes for at least 30 minutes.

☐ If the patient feels faint or nauseated, or sweats profusely, position her on the left side to counteract uterine pressure

CHORIONIC VILLI SAMPLING

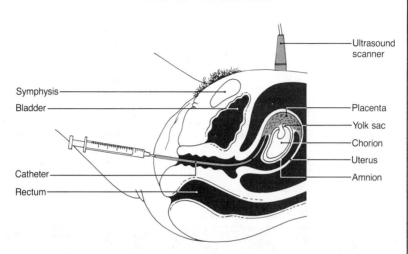

- Ultrasound scanner
- Symphysis
- Bladder
- Placenta
- Yolk sac
- Chorion
- Uterus
- Catheter
- Amnion
- Rectum

Chorionic villi sampling, or biopsy, is an experimental prenatal test that may someday replace amniocentesis for quick, safe detection of fetal chromosomal and biochemical disorders. Developed in Europe and now being tested in the United States, the procedure is performed during the first trimester of pregnancy. Preliminary results may be available within hours; complete results within a few days. In contrast, amniocentesis cannot be performed before the 16th week of pregnancy, and the results aren't available for at least 2 weeks. Thus, chorionic villi sampling offers the advantage of earlier detection of fetal abnormalities.

The chorionic villi are finger-like projections that surround the embryonic membrane and eventually give rise to the placenta. Cells obtained from an appropriate sample are of fetal, rather than maternal, origin and thus can be analyzed for fetal abnormalities. Samples are best obtained between the 8th and 10th weeks of pregnancy. Before 7 weeks, the villi cover the embryo and make selective sampling difficult. After 10 weeks, maternal cells begin to grow over the villi and the amniotic sac begins to fill the uterine cavity, making the procedure difficult and potentially dangerous.

To collect a chorionic villi sample, place the patient in the lithotomy position. The doctor checks the placement of the patient's uterus bimanually, and then inserts a Graves speculum and swabs the cervix with an antiseptic solution. If necessary, he may use a tenaculum to straighten an acutely flexed uterus, permitting cannula insertion. Guided by ultrasound and, possibly, endoscopy, he directs the catheter through the cannula to the villi. Suction is applied to the catheter to remove about 30 mg of tissue from the villi. The sample is withdrawn, placed in a Petri dish, and examined with a dissecting microscope. Part of the specimen is then cultured for further testing.

Results of a chorionic villi testing can be used to detect about 200 diseases prenatally. For example, direct analysis of rapidly dividing fetal cells can detect chromosome disorders; DNA analysis can detect hemoglobinopathies; and lysosomal enzyme assays can screen for lysosomal storage disorders, such as Tay-Sachs disease.

The test appears to provide reliable results except when the sample contains too few cells or the cells fail to grow in culture. Patient risks for this procedure are considered similar to those for amniocentesis—a small chance of spontaneous abortion, cramps, infection, and bleeding.

Unlike amniocentesis, chorionic villi sampling can't detect complications in cases of Rh sensitization, uncover neural tube defects, or determine pulmonary maturity. However, it may prove to be the best way to detect other serious fetal abnormalities early in pregnancy.

on the vena cava.

□ Before the patient is discharged, instruct her to notify the doctor immediately if she experiences abdominal pain or cramping, chills, fever, vaginal bleeding or leakage of serous vaginal fluid, or fetal hyperactivity or unusual fetal lethargy.

Interfering factors

□ Failure to place the fluid specimen in an appropriate amber or foil-covered tube may result in abnormally low bilirubin levels.

□ Blood or meconium in the fluid adversely affects the L/S ratio.

□ Maternal blood in the fluid may lower creatinine levels.

□ Fetal blood in the fluid specimen invalidates the alpha-fetoprotein results, since even small amounts of fetal blood (50 μl/10 ml) can double alpha-fetoprotein concentrations.

□ Several disorders that are not associated with pregnancy (including infectious mononucleosis, cirrhosis, hepatic cancer, teratoma, endodermal sinus tumor, gastric carcinoma, pancreatic carcinoma, and subacute hereditary tyrosinemia) can cause increased alpha-fetoprotein levels.

□ Plastic disposable syringes can be toxic to amniotic fluid cells.

FRANK C. RIGGALL, MD

ENDOSCOPY

Colposcopy

In colposcopy, the cervix and vagina are visually examined by means of an instrument containing a magnifying lens and a light (colposcope). Although originally used as a screening test for cancer, colposcopy is now used primarily to evaluate abnormal cytology or grossly suspicious lesions, and to examine the cervix and vagina after a positive Papanicolaou (Pap) test. During the examination, a biopsy may be performed and photographs taken of suspicious lesions with the colposcope and its attachments. Risks of biopsy include bleeding (especially during pregnancy) and infection.

Purpose

□ To help confirm cervical intraepithelial neoplasia or invasive carcinoma after a positive Pap test

□ To evaluate vaginal or cervical lesions

□ To monitor conservatively treated cervical intraepithelial neoplasia

□ To monitor patients whose mothers received diethylstilbestrol during pregnancy.

Patient preparation

Explain to the patient that this test permits magnified visualization of the vagina and cervix, and thus provides more information than a routine vaginal examination. Inform her that she needn't restrict food or fluids. Tell her who will perform the examination and where, that it's safe and painless, and takes 10 to 15 minutes.

Tell the patient a biopsy may be performed at the time of examination, and that this may cause minimal but easily controlled bleeding.

Equipment

Colposcopy: colposcope/vaginal speculum/3% acetic acid solution/ swabs.

Biopsy: biopsy forceps/endocervical curette/forceps for uterine dressing/tenaculum/ring forceps/Monsel's (ferric subsulfate) solution/biopsy bottle and preservative/sterile cotton balls/Pap test equipment (glass slide, wooden spatula, swabs, and fixative).

Procedure

With the patient in lithotomy position, the examiner inserts the speculum and, if indicated, performs a Pap test. (Help the patient relax during insertion by telling her to breathe through her mouth and to concentrate on relaxing her abdominal muscles.) Then the cervix is swabbed with acetic acid solution, to remove mucus. After the cervix and vagina are examined, biopsy is performed on areas that appear abnormal (in blood vessel pattern or tissue color, for example). Finally, the bleeding is stopped by applying pressure or hemostatic solutions, or by cautery.

Precautions
None.

Findings
Normally, cervical vessels show a network and hairpin capillary pattern, with about 100 microns between them. Surface contour is smooth and pink; columnar epithelium appears grapelike. Different tissue types are sharply demarcated.

Implications of results
Abnormal colposcopy findings include white epithelium or punctation and mosaic patterns, which may indicate underlying cervical intraepithelial neoplasia; keratinization in the transformation zone, which may indicate cervical intraepithelial neoplasia or invasive carcinoma; and atypical vessels, which may indicate invasive carcinoma. Other abnormalities visible on colposcopic examination include inflammatory changes (usually from infection), atrophic changes (usually from aging or, less often, the use of oral contraceptives), erosion (probably from increased pathogenicity of vaginal flora, due to changes in vaginal pH), and papilloma and condyloma (possibly from viruses).

Histologic study of the biopsy specimen confirms colposcopic findings. However, if the results of the examination and biopsy are inconsistent with the results of the Pap test and biopsy of the squamocolumnar junction, conization of the cervix for biopsy may be indicated.

Post-test care
After biopsy, instruct the patient to abstain from intercourse, and tell her not to insert anything in her vagina (except a tampon) until healing of the biopsy site is confirmed.

Interfering factors
Failure to cleanse the cervix of foreign materials, such as creams and medications, may impair visualization.

RONALD J. WAPNER, MD
MARTIN WEISBERG, MD

Laparoscopy

Laparoscopy permits visualization of the peritoneal cavity by the insertion of a small fiberoptic telescope (laparoscope) through the anterior abdominal wall. This surgical technique may be used diagnostically to detect abnormalities, such as cysts, adhesions, fibroids, and infection; it can be used therapeutically as well to perform procedures such as lysis of adhesions, ovarian biopsy, tubal sterilization, removal of foreign bodies, and fulguration of endometriotic implants. Since laparoscopy requires a smaller incision, it can be completed in less time, causes less physiologic stress and therefore allows faster recovery, reduces the risk of postoperative adhesions, and is less costly. For all these reasons, it has often replaced laparotomy; nevertheless laparotomy is usually preferred when extensive surgery is indicated. Potential risks of laparoscopy include a punctured visceral organ, causing bleeding or spilling of intestinal contents into the peritoneum.

Purpose
☐ To identify the cause of pelvic pain
☐ To help detect endometriosis, ectopic pregnancy, or pelvic inflammatory disease (PID)
☐ To evaluate pelvic masses or the fallopian tubes of infertile patients
☐ To stage carcinoma.

Patient preparation

Explain the procedure to the patient and tell her the test helps detect abnormalities of the uterus, fallopian tubes, and ovaries. Instruct her to fast after midnight before the test or at least 8 hours before surgery. Tell her who will perform the procedure and that it takes only 15 to 30 minutes.

Assure the patient she'll receive a local or general anesthetic, and tell her whether the procedure will require an outpatient visit or overnight hospitalization. Warn her she may experience pain at the puncture site and in the shoulder.

Make sure the patient or responsible member of the family has signed a consent form. Check the patient's history for hypersensitivity to the anesthetic. Be sure all laboratory work is completed and results reported before the test.

Equipment

Foley or straight catheter/sterile tray with scalpel, hemostats, needle holder, suture, and suture scissors/Verees needle/gas insufflator/laparoscope/fiberoptic light source and cable/laparoscope sheath and trocar/electrosurgical generator/tenaculum and intrauterine manipulator/probes, scissors, or forceps/adhesive bandages.

Procedure

The patient is anesthesized and is placed in lithotomy position. The examiner catheterizes the bladder, and then performs a bimanual examination of the pelvic area to detect abnormalities that may contraindicate the test and to ensure that the bladder is empty. After the tenaculum is placed on the cervix and a uterine manipulator is inserted, an incision is made at the inferior rim of the umbilicus. The Verees needle is inserted into the peritoneal cavity, and approximately 2 to 3 liters of carbon dioxide or nitrous oxide are insufflated to distend the abdominal wall and provide an organ-free space for insertion of the trocar. Next, the needle is removed and a trocar and sheath are inserted into the peritoneal cavity. After removal of the trocar, the laparoscope is inserted through the sheath, to examine the pelvis and abdomen. To evaluate tubal patency, the examiner infuses a dye through the cervix and observes the fimbria of the tubes for spillage.

Following the examination, minor surgical procedures, such as ovarian biopsy, may be performed. A second trocar may be inserted at the pubic hairline to provide a channel for the insertion of other instruments.

Precautions

□ Laparoscopy is contraindicated in patients with advanced abdominal wall malignancy, advanced respiratory or cardiovascular disease, intestinal obstruction, palpable abdominal mass, large abdominal hernia, chronic tuberculosis, or history of peritonitis.

□ During the procedure, check for proper drainage of the catheter.

Findings

The uterus and fallopian tubes are of normal size and shape, free of adhesions, and mobile. The ovaries are of normal size and shape; cysts and endometriosis are absent. Dye injected through the cervix flows freely from the fimbria.

Implications of results

An ovarian cyst appears as a bubble on the surface of the ovary. The cyst may be clear; filled with follicular fluid, or serous or mucous material; or red, blue, or brown if filled with blood. Adhesions appear as sheets or strands of tissue that are almost transparent, or thick and fibrous. Endometriosis resembles small, blue powder burns on the peritoneum or the serosa of any pelvic or abdominal structure. Fibroids appear as lumps on the uterus; hydrosalpinx, as an enlarged fallopian tube; ectopic pregnancy, as an enlarged or ruptured fallopian tube. In PID, infection or abscess is evident.

Post-test care

□ Monitor vital signs and urinary output. Report sudden changes immediately; they may indicate complications.

☐ After administration of a general anesthetic, check for allergies; monitor electrolyte balance and hemoglobin and hematocrit levels, as ordered. Ambulate the patient, as ordered, after recovery.
☐ Resume diet, as ordered.
☐ Instruct the patient to restrict activity for 2 to 7 days, as ordered.
☐ Reassure the patient that some abdominal and shoulder pain is normal and should disappear within 24 to 36 hours. Provide aspirin, as ordered.

Interfering factors
Adhesions or marked obesity may obstruct the field of vision.

RONALD J. WAPNER, MD
MARTIN WEISBERG, MD

DIRECT GRAPHIC RECORDING

External Fetal Monitoring

In external fetal monitoring, a noninvasive test, an electronic transducer and cardiotachymeter amplify and record fetal heart rate (FHR), while a pressure-sensitive transducer, the tokodynamometer, simultaneously records uterine contractions. This procedure records the baseline FHR (average FHR over two contraction cycles or 10 minutes), periodic fluctuations in the baseline FHR, and beat-to-beat heart rate variability. Fluctuations in FHR can occur as baseline changes (unrelated to uterine contractions) or as periodic changes (in response to uterine contractions). Such fluctuations are described in terms of amplitude (difference in beats per minute [bpm] between baseline readings and maximum or minimum fluctuation), lag time (difference between the peak of the contraction and the lowest point of deceleration), and recovery time (difference between the end of the contraction and the return to the baseline FHR).

External fetal monitoring is also used for other tests of fetal health—the non-stress test and the contraction stress test (CST). The relationship between FHR and the uterine contraction pattern is described by acceleration (transient rise in FHR lasting longer than 15 seconds and associated with a uterine contraction) and deceleration (transient fall in FHR related to a uterine contraction).

Purpose
☐ To measure FHR and the frequency of uterine contractions
☐ To evaluate antepartum and intrapartum fetal health during stress and nonstress situations
☐ To detect fetal distress
☐ To determine the necessity for internal fetal monitoring.

Patient preparation
Describe the procedure to the patient and answer any questions she may have. Explain that the test assesses fetal health. If monitoring is to be performed antepartum, instruct the patient to eat a meal just before the test, to increase fetal ac-

---

USING THE DOPPLER STETHOSCOPE

The Doppler stethoscope is used antepartum and intrapartum to confirm fetal life by monitoring the fetal heart rate (FHR) through continuous ultrasonic vibration electronically converted to audible sound. Testing for fetal life takes only a few seconds; evaluating fetal health may take several hours. No risks or side effects are associated with this procedure.

To perform this test, mineral oil or water-soluble jelly is rubbed on the patient's abdomen, and the transducer attached to the Doppler stethoscope is moved over the abdomen until fetal heart tones are heard. For continuous FHR monitoring, the transducer is strapped to the mother's abdomen.

Obesity or hydramnios may cause difficulty in obtaining results, by absorbing sound waves.

COMPARISON OF DECELERATED FETAL HEART RATES AND UTERINE CONTRACTIONS

Unlike variable decelerations, early and late decelerations in the fetal heart rate correspond to uterine contractions.

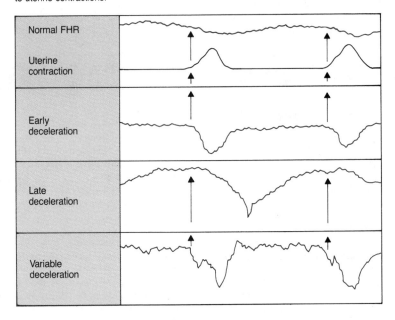

Decelerations in fetal heart rate (FHR) may be affected by uterine contractions. The three types of FHR decelerations—early, late, and variable—occur at different points in the contraction phase.

Early FHR decelerations occur at onset of uterine contraction and reach their lowest point at the peak of the contraction. In early deceleration, FHR returns to the average baseline by the end of the contraction. FHR produces a smooth wave pattern that mirrors the uterine contraction. There is a consistent relationship between the fall in fetal heart rate and the uterine contractions. Early deceleration is usually benign and is most commonly caused by compression of the fetal head.

Late decelerations begin about 20 seconds after onset of a contraction and reach their lowest point well after the contraction has peaked. In late deceleration, FHR recovery occurs later than 15 seconds following the contraction. Although the FHR tracing in late deceleration resembles the smooth wave of early deceleration, its implications are far more serious. Late decelerations usually result from uteroplacental insufficiency and may lead to fetal death. When associated with increased variability or with tachycardia and no variability, late decelerations indicate fetal CNS depression and myocardial hypoxia.

Variable decelerations—sudden drops in the FHR—may occur at any time during a contraction. Following the decline, baseline FHR recovery may be rapid or prolonged. Since the fall in FHR is unrelated to uterine contractions, wave patterns also vary. Variable decelerations are common, occurring in about 50% of all labors, and are usually associated with transitory umbilical cord compression. However, a severe drop (to less than 70 beats per minute for more than 60 seconds) may indicate fetal acidosis, hypoxia, and low Apgar scores.

tivity, which decreases the test time. Assure her that external fetal monitoring is painless and noninvasive, and that it won't hurt the fetus or interfere with the normal progress of labor. Tell her she may have to restrict movement during baseline readings, but that she may change position between the readings.

Make sure the patient has signed a consent form.

Equipment

Tokodynamometer—pressure transducer (to measure uterine contractions)/ ultrasonic transducer (to amplify FHR)/ cardiotachymeter (to record FHR)/mineral oil or ultrasound transmission jelly/ elastic band, stockinette, or abdominal strap.

Procedure

Place the patient in semi-Fowler's or left lateral position, with her abdomen exposed. Cover the ultrasonic transducer receiver crystal with ultrasound transmission jelly. After palpating the abdomen to identify the fetal chest area, locate the most distinct fetal heart sounds, and secure the ultrasound transducer over this area with the elastic band, stockinette, or abdominal strap. Check the recordings to assure an adequate printout, and verify the fetal monitor's alarm boundaries. During monitoring, periodically check the elastic band, stockinette, or abdominal strap securing the transducer to ensure the fit is tight enough to produce good tracing but loose enough to be comfortable. As labor progresses, reposition the pressure transducer, as necessary, so that it remains on the fundal portion of the uterus. You may have to reposition the ultrasonic transducer as fetal position changes.

Antepartum monitoring with nonstress tests: Tell the patient to hold the pressure transducer in her hand and to push it each time she feels the fetus move. Within a 20-minute period, monitor the baseline FHR until you record two fetal movements that last longer than 15 seconds each and cause heart rate accelerations of more than 15 bpm from the baseline. If you can't obtain two FHR accelerations, wait 30 minutes, shake the patient's abdomen to stimulate the fetus, and repeat the test.

Antepartum monitoring with CST: Induce contractions by oxytocin infusion or nipple stimulation (endogenous oxytocin). If you administer oxytocin, infuse a dilute solution at a rate of 1 mU/minute, and increase the oxytocin rate until the patient experiences three contractions within 10 minutes, each lasting longer than 45 seconds. If nipple stimulation is used, tell the patient to stimulate one nipple by hand until contractions begin. If a second contraction doesn't occur in 2 minutes, have her restimulate the nipple. Stimulate both nipples if contractions don't occur in 15 minutes. Continue the test until 3 contractions occur in 10 minutes. If no decelerations occur during three contractions, the patient may be discharged. Late decelerations during any of the contractions require notification of the doctor and additional testing.

Intrapartum monitoring: Secure the pressure transducer with an elastic band, stockinette, or abdominal strap over the area of greatest uterine electrical activity during contractions (usually the fundus). Adjust the machine to record 0

CONTRACTION STRESS TEST

The contraction stress test (CST) measures fetal ability to withstand the stress of contractions induced before actual labor begins. Late decelerations in the fetal heart rate in response to uterine contractions during this test may indicate that the placenta can't deliver enough oxygen to the fetus. Placental insufficiency may result from maternal vascular disease, associated with diabetes mellitus, preeclampsia, or chronic hypertension. Intrauterine growth retardation, postmaturity syndrome, and Rh isoimmunization may also cause fetal compromise.

Since CST mimics labor, it's contraindicated in patients with placenta previa or when premature labor is likely, as in premature rupture of the membrane, multiple pregnancy, or incompetent cervix.

to 10 mmHg pressure between palpable contractions. (Readings during contractions vary, depending on the tightness of the bands, the amount of adipose tissue, and the placement of the pressure transducer.) Reposition the ultrasound and pressure transducers, as necessary, to assure continuous accurate readings. Review the tracings frequently for baseline abnormalities, periodic changes, variability changes, and uterine contraction abnormalities. Record maternal movement, administration of drugs, and procedures performed directly on the tracing, so changes in the tracing can be evaluated in view of these activities. Report any abnormalities immediately.

Precautions
During CST, watch for fetal distress with oxytocin infusion or nipple stimulation.

Values
Normally, FHR baseline ranges from 120 to 160 bpm, with 5 to 25 bpm variability.

Antepartum nonstress test: If two fetal movements associated with more than 15 bpm heart rate acceleration from baseline FHR occur within 20 minutes, the fetus is considered healthy and should remain so for another week.

Contraction stress test: If three contractions occur during a 10-minute period, with no late decelerations, fetal health is assumed and should continue for another week.

Implications of results
Bradycardia—an FHR of less than 120 bpm—may indicate fetal heart block, malposition, or hypoxia. Fetal bradycardia may also be drug-induced.

Tachycardia—an FHR of more than 160 bpm—may result from vagolytic drugs; maternal fever, tachycardia, or hyperthyroidism; early fetal hypoxia; or fetal infection or arrhythmia. Decreased variability—a fluctuation of less than 5 bpm in the FHR—may be caused by fetal cardiac arrhythmia or heart block; by fetal hypoxia, CNS malformation, or infections; or by vagolytic drugs. When

FHR patterns indicate fetal distress, fetal oxygenation can often be improved by turning the mother on her side (preferably the left) to alleviate supine hypoxia; by giving oxygen to the mother; or by loading maternal fluids to increase placental perfusion. If the fetal heart rate returns to normal, labor may continue. If abnormal FHR patterns persist, cesarean birth may be required.

Accelerations in FHR may result from early hypoxia. They may precede or follow variable decelerations and may indicate a breech position.

Antepartum nonstress tests: A positive nonstress test result (less than two accelerations of FHR that last longer than 15 seconds each, with a heart rate acceleration over 15 bpm) indicates an exaggerated risk of perinatal morbidity and mortality, and usually necessitates performance of the CST. But CST produces a high rate of false-positive results.

CST: Persistent late decelerations during two or more contractions may indicate increased risk of fetal morbidity or mortality. Hyperstimulation (long or frequent uterine contractions) or suspicious results require repetition of the test on the following day. If results are still positive, internal fetal monitoring or cesarean birth may be necessary.

Post-test care
Repeat antepartum monitoring weekly as long as indications, such as pregnancy over 42 weeks' gestation or fetal growth retardation, persist.

Interfering factors
☐ Drugs that affect the sympathetic and the parasympathetic nervous systems may depress FHR.
☐ Maternal position, particularly if the patient is lying supine, may cause artifactual fetal distress.
☐ Maternal obesity, or excessive maternal or fetal activity may inhibit recording of uterine contractions or of FHR.
☐ Loose or dirty leads or transducer connections may cause artifacts.

RONALD J. WAPNER, MD
MARTIN WEISBERG, MD

Internal Fetal Monitoring

In internal fetal monitoring, an invasive procedure, an electrode attached directly to the fetal scalp measures the fetal heart rate (FHR)—especially its beat-to-beat variability—and a fluid-filled catheter that has been introduced into the uterine cavity measures the frequency and pressure of uterine contractions. This procedure is performed exclusively during labor, after the membranes have ruptured and the cervix has dilated 1¼" (3 cm), with the fetal head lower than the −2 station. Internal monitoring is indicated when external monitoring pro-vides inadequate or suspicious data. Since internal monitoring records FHR directly, it supplies more accurate information about fetal health than external monitoring; measuring the pressure of uterine contractions allows better assessment of the progress of labor. Consequently, internal monitoring is especially useful in determining if cesarean birth is necessary. Risks to the mother (perforated uterus or intrauterine infection) or to the fetus (scalp abscess or hematoma) are small, and the benefit is more accurate information about fetal health.

Purpose
□ To monitor FHR, especially beat-to-beat variability
□ To measure the frequency and pressure of uterine contractions
□ To evaluate intrapartum fetal health

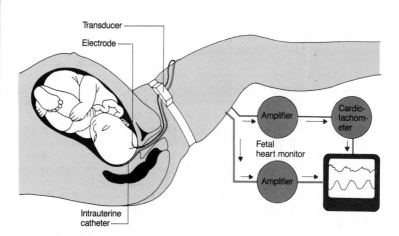

INTERNAL FETAL MONITORING

Transducer
Electrode
Amplifier
Cardio-tachom-eter
Fetal heart monitor
Amplifier
Intrauterine catheter

In internal fetal monitoring, an electrode is attached to the fetal scalp. The resultant fetal electrocardiograms (FECGs) are transmitted to an amplifier. Subsequently, a cardiotachometer measures the interval between FECGs and plots a continuous fetal heart rate (FHR) graph, which is displayed on a two-channel oscilloscope screen. Intrauterine catheters attached to a transducer in the leg plate measure the frequency and pressure of uterine contractions, which are plotted below the FHR graph.

Adapted with permission from an original figure by Carol Donner, in Edward H. Hon, "Direct Monitoring of the Fetal Heart," *Hospital Practice*, Vol. 5, No. 9, September 1970.

□ To supplement or replace external fetal monitoring.

Patient preparation

Describe the procedure to the patient, and answer any questions she may have. Explain that this test provides an accurate assessment of fetal health and doesn't necessarily indicate a problem. Warn her that she may feel mild discomfort when the uterine catheter and scalp electrode are inserted, but reassure her that this part of the procedure takes only a few minutes.

Make sure the patient has signed a consent form.

Equipment

Sterile fetal scalp electrode and guide tube/intrauterine pressure catheter/catheter guide/pressure transducer/fetal heart monitor.

Procedure

Measuring FHR: Place the patient in dorsal lithotomy position, and prepare her perineal area for a vaginal examination, explaining each step of the procedure as it's performed. As the procedure begins, ask the patient to breathe through her mouth and to concentrate on relaxing her abdominal muscles. After the vaginal examination, the fetal scalp is palpated, and an area not over a fontanelle is identified. Then the plastic guide tube surrounding the small corkscrew-type electrode is introduced into the cervix, pressed firmly against the fetal scalp, and rotated 180° clockwise to insert the electrode into the scalp. After the electrode wire is tugged slightly to make sure it's attached properly, the tube is withdrawn, leaving the electrode in place.

Next, after a conduction medium is applied to a leg plate, the leg plate is strapped to the mother's thigh. The electrode wires are attached to the leg plate, and a cable from the leg plate is plugged into the fetal monitor. To check proper placement of the scalp electrode, the monitor is turned on and the EKG button is pressed; an FHR signal indicates proper electrode attachment.

Measuring uterine contractions: Before inserting the uterine catheter, fill it with sterile normal saline solution, to prevent air emboli. Explain each step of the procedure to the patient, and ask her to breathe deeply through her mouth and to concentrate on relaxing her abdominal muscles. After the vagina has been examined and the presenting part of the fetus has been palpated, the fluid-filled catheter and catheter guide are inserted ⅜" to ¾" (1 to 2 cm) into the cervix, usually between the fetal head and the posterior cervix. The catheter is then gently inserted into the uterus until the black mark on the catheter is flush with the vulva (the catheter guide should *never* be passed deeply into the uterus). Next, the guide is removed and the catheter is connected to a transducer that converts the intrauterine pressure, as measured by the fluid in the catheter, to an electrical signal. To standardize pressure readings, the transducer is exposed to air (it should measure zero pressure). The system is then closed to the air and intrauterine pressure readings are checked.

Precautions

□ Internal fetal monitoring is contraindicated in the presence of uncertainty as to the fetal presenting part, technical inability to attach the lead, or cervical or vaginal herpes lesions.

□ Prevent artifactual pressure readings by flushing the pressure transducer with normal saline solution; to relieve catheter obstruction (by vernix caseosa, for example), inject a small amount of sterile normal saline solution into the catheter (while the transducer is isolated from the system).

□ Be sure a low heart rate is actually the FHR (the fetal tachymeter may be recording a maternal heart rate).

□ Check that the fetal scalp electrode and the uterine catheter are removed before cesarean birth.

Values

Normally, FHR ranges from 120 to 160 beats per minute (bpm), with a variability of 5 to 25 bpm from FHR baseline (for normal uterine contractions, see chart on this page).

Implications of results

Bradycardia—a FHR of less than 120 bpm—may indicate fetal heart block, malposition, or hypoxia. Fetal bradycardia may result from maternal ingestion of certain drugs, such as propanolol or from administration of narcotic analgesics.

Tachycardia—a FHR greater than 160 bpm—may result from vagolytic drugs; maternal fever, tachycardia, or hyperthyroidism; early fetal hypoxia; fetal infection or arrhythmia; or prematurity.

Decreased variability—fluctuation of less than 5 bpm from FHR baseline—may result from vagolytic drugs; fetal cardiac arrhythmia or heart block; fetal hypoxia, CNS malformation, or infections.

Early decelerations (slowing of FHR at onset of the contraction, with recovery to baseline no greater than 15 seconds after completion of the uterine contraction) is related to fetal head compression and usually assures fetal health. Late decelerations (slowing of FHR, with onset after the start of the contraction, a lag time greater than 20 seconds, and a recovery time greater than 15 seconds) may be related to uteroplacental insufficiency, fetal hypoxia, or acidosis. Recurrent and

persistent late decelerations with decreased variability usually indicate serious fetal distress; they may result from conduction (spinal, caudal, or epidural) anesthesia or fetal depression. Variable decelerations (sudden precipitous drops in FHR unrelated to uterine contractions) are commonly related to cord compression. A severe drop in fetal heart rate (to less than 70 bpm for longer than 60 seconds) with decreased variability indicates fetal distress and may result in a depressed neonate.

When FHR patterns indicate fetal distress, fetal oxygenation often can be improved by loading maternal fluids to increase placental perfusion, turning the mother on her side (preferably the left) to alleviate supine hypotension, and administering oxygen to the mother. If these measures return heart rate patterns to normal, labor may continue. If abnormal patterns persist, cesarean birth may be necessary. Poor beat-to-beat variability without periodic patterns may indicate fetal stress, requiring further evaluation, such as analysis of fetal blood gases.

Decreased intrauterine pressure during labor that's not progressing normally may require oxytocin stimulation. Elevated intrauterine pressure readings may indicate abruptio placentae or overstimulation from oxytocin, possibly resulting in fetal distress due to decreased placental perfusion.

NORMAL INTRAUTERINE PRESSURE READINGS DURING LABOR			
STAGE OF LABOR	FREQUENCY (Number of contractions per 10 minutes)	BASELINE PRESSURE (mmHg)	PRESSURE DURING CONTRACTION (mmHg)
Prelabor	1 to 2	—	25 to 40
First stage	3 to 5	8 to 12	30 to 40 (or more)
Second stage	5	10 to 20	50 to 80

Post-test care

☐ After removal of the fetal scalp electrode, apply antiseptic or antibiotic solution to the site of attachment.

☐ Watch for signs of fetal scalp abscess or maternal intrauterine infection.

Interfering factors

Drugs that affect the parasympathetic and the sympathetic nervous systems may influence FHR.

RONALD J. WAPNER, MD
MARTIN WEISBERG, MD

RADIOGRAPHY AND THERMOGRAPHY

Mammography

Mammography is a radiographic technique used to detect breast cysts or tumors, especially those not palpable on physical examination. In xeromammography, an electrostatically charged plate records the X-ray images and transfers them to a special paper. Biopsy of suspicious areas may be required to confirm malignancy. Mammography may follow screening procedures such as ultrasonography or thermography. Although 90% to 95% of breast malignancies can be detected by mammography, this test carries a 75% false-positive result rate. The American College of Radiologists and the American Cancer Society have established separate guidelines for the use and potential risks of mammography; both agree that despite low radiation levels (0.1 to 0.3 rads), the test

USING LIGHT AND SOUND TO FIND BREAST CANCERS

Two noninvasive tests that do not require radiographs are being developed for safe, early detection of cancer and other breast diseases. In most cases, their diagnostic accuracy isn't as high as that of conventional mammography, but they can be repeated as often as needed without risk to the patient.

In *diaphanography*, also known as transillumination of the breast, infrared light is directed through the breast with a fiberoptic device, and the transmitted light is photographed with infrared film. The denser the tissues, the darker they appear on the film, which allows a trained examiner to distinguish them. Healthy breast tissue is reddish-yellow and translucent; fluid-filled cysts and fatty tissue appear as bright spots; benign tumors are red; blood vessels are dark red to black, and malignant tumors are dark brown or black. The technique can also be used to guide a needle for biopsy or cyst drainage.

Currently, diaphanography is used by only a few specialists in the United States. Although the method has a detection rate of 98% with modified equipment, it is less reliable than mammography and can't accurately distinguish cancer from benign mastitis, which causes lumps

and inflammation, or from hemorrhage, which resembles malignant tissue in transmitted light.

Ultrasonography is a test that's especially useful for diagnosing tumors less than ¼" in diameter and in distinguishing cysts from solid tumors in dense breast tissue. As in other diagnostic ultrasound techniques, a transducer is used to focus a beam of high-frequency sound waves through the patient's skin and into the breast. The sound waves bounce back to the transducer as an echo that varies in strength with the density of the underlying tissues. A computer processes these echoes and displays them on a screen, for interpretation.

Ultrasound can show all areas of a breast, including the difficult area close to the chest wall, which is hard to study with radiographs. When used as an adjunct to mammography, the technique increases diagnostic accuracy, and when used alone it's more accurate than mammography in examining the denser breast tissue of young patients. While still largely experimental, ultrasonography is being studied as a possible replacement for mammography in breast cancer screening programs.

is contraindicated during pregnancy.

Purpose
□ To screen for breast malignancy
□ To investigate palpable and unpalp-
able breast masses, breast pain, or nipple
discharge
□ To help differentiate between benign
breast disease and breast malignancy.

Patient preparation
Assess the patient's understanding of the
test, answer her questions, and correct
any misconceptions. Tell her who will
perform the test and where, and that the
procedure is painless. Inform her that
although the test takes only about 15 to
30 minutes to perform, she may be asked
to wait while the films are checked to
make sure they're readable. Advise her
that this test has a high rate of false-
positive results.

Just before the test, give her a gown
to wear that opens in the front, and ask
her to remove all jewelry and clothing
above the waist.

Equipment
Mammograph/X-ray film/plastic compressor.

Procedure
The patient is seated on a chair and is
asked to rest one of her breasts on a table
above an X-ray cassette. The compressor
is placed on the breast, and the patient
is told to hold her breath. Then a radiograph is taken of the craniocaudal view.
The machine is rotated, the breast is
compressed again, and a radiograph of
the lateral view is taken. The procedure
is then repeated on the other breast.
After the films are developed, they are
checked to make sure they're readable.

Findings
A normal mammogram reveals normal
duct, glandular tissue, and fat architecture. No abnormal masses or calcifications should be seen.

Implications of results
Well-outlined, regular, and clear spots

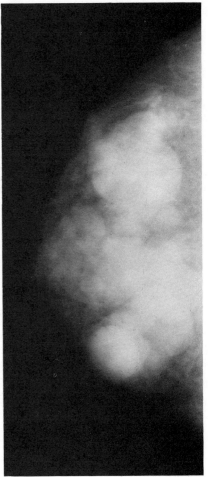

Mammogram showing multiple benign cysts

suggest benign cysts; irregular, poorly
outlined, and opaque areas suggest malignancy. Benign cysts tend to be bilateral, while malignant tumors are generally
solitary and unilateral. Findings that
suggest cancer require further tests, such
as biopsy, for confirmation.

Post-test care
□ None.

Interfering factors
□ Very glandular breasts (common under age 30) and previous breast surgery
can impair readability of the films.

☐ Powders and salves on the breast may cause false-positive results.
☐ Failure to remove jewelry and clothing from the X-ray field may cause false-positive results or unsatisfactory films.

RONALD J. WAPNER, MD
MARTIN WEISBERG, MD

Breast Thermography

Breast thermography is an infrared photographic procedure that measures and records heat patterns within breast tissue. Since body changes that increase the breast's metabolic rate raise the breast's surface temperature, thermography can aid detection of breast cancer. However, because of a high rate of false-positive results with this test (possibly 25%), thermography is being replaced by ultrasonography and low-dose mammography.

Purpose
☐ To screen for breast cancer
☐ To predict the risk of breast cancer
☐ To detect breast cancer, fibrocystic disease of the breast (Schimmelbusch's disease), and breast abscesses
☐ To evaluate the prognosis of breast cancer.

Patient preparation
Assess the patient's understanding of the test, and correct any misconceptions. Instruct her to avoid excessive exposure to sunlight before the test, since a recent sunburn invalidates results, and not to put ointment or powder on her breasts the day of the test. Tell her who will perform the test and where, that it takes about 15 minutes, and is painless. Inform her that test results are usually available in 1 or 2 days.

Just before the test, provide a gown for her to wear that opens in the front, and ask her to remove all clothing and jewelry above the waist.

Tell the patient that the temperature in the room where the test is performed may be a little cool, and that she may be asked to wait a few minutes after the test while the thermograms are checked for readability.

Equipment
Infrared camera and film.

Procedure
After the patient has been in the room where the test is to be performed for about 10 minutes, to lower the skin temperature of the breasts, photographs of the breasts are taken from three different angles, usually with the patient holding her hands above her head or on her hips. After the procedure, the patient may be asked to wait while the films are checked for readability.

Precautions
None.

Findings
Normally, breasts appear symmetric on the thermogram.

Implications of results
Asymmetric appearance of the breasts may indicate malignancy, fibrocystic disease, or abscesses. Inflammatory or

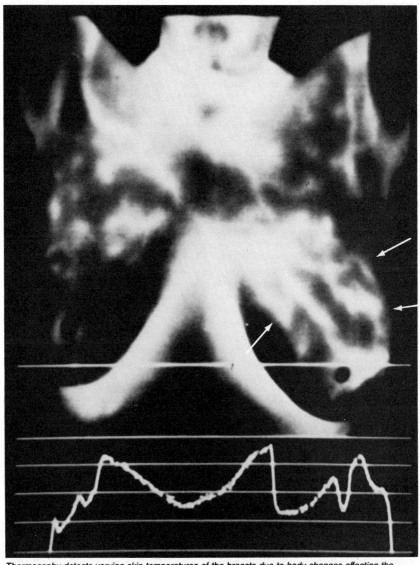

Thermogaphy detects varying skin temperatures of the breasts due to body changes affecting the breasts' metabolic rate and surface temperature and displays them in both pictorial and graphic forms. Since inflammatory or malignant lesions have greater vascularity than normal tissue, white hot spots may indicate the site of tumors. This thermogram reveals a hot spot (see arrows) in the enlarged left breast. Such abnormal results require additional tests to confirm malignancy.

malignant lesions have a greater vascularity than normal tissue, which increases venous drainage and raises the surface temperature of the skin. Such abnormalities in the breast are represented on thermograms as white areas, or "hot spots." Additional tests, such as mammography and biopsy, are necessary to confirm breast cancer.

Post-test care

Remind the patient to keep her follow-up appointment with the doctor, who'll inform her of the test results.

Interfering factors
Insufficient cooling of the breasts, recent sunburn, skin lesions, or ointment on the breasts can cause false-positive results by altering skin temperature.

RONALD J. WAPNER, MD
MARTIN WEISBERG, MD

Hysterosalpingography

Hysterosalpingography is a radiologic examination for visualizing the uterine cavity, the fallopian tubes, and the peritubal area. The procedure consists of taking fluoroscopic X-ray films as contrast medium flows through the uterus and the fallopian tubes. Generally performed as part of an infertility study, this test also helps evaluate repeated fetal loss and may be utilized as a follow-up to surgery, especially uterine unification procedures and tubal reanastomosis.

Although ultrasonography has virtually replaced hysterosalpingography in the detection of foreign bodies, such as a dislodged intrauterine device, it can't evaluate tubal patency, which is the main purpose of hysterosalpingography. Risks of this test include uterine perforation, intravascular injection of the contrast medium, and exposure to potentially harmful radiation.

Purpose
□ To confirm tubal abnormalities, such as adhesions and occlusion
□ To confirm uterine abnormalities, such as the presence of foreign bodies, congenital malformations, and traumatic injuries
□ To confirm the presence of fistulas or peritubal adhesions.

Patient preparation
Explain to the patient that this test con-

firms uterine and fallopian tube abnormalities. Tell her who will perform the test and where, and that it takes about 15 minutes.

Advise the patient that she may experience moderate cramping from the procedure; however, she may receive a mild sedative, such as diazepam.

Equipment
Povidone-iodine solution/sterile needle/contrast medium (oil- or water-based)/vaginal speculum/tenaculum/cannula, with acorn tip on one end and Luer-Lok on the other/X-ray machine with fluoroscopic capabilities.

Procedure
With the patient in lithotomy position, a scout film is taken. Then a speculum is inserted in the vagina, the tenaculum is placed on the cervix, and the cervix is cleansed. Next, the cannula is inserted into the cervix and anchored to the tenaculum. After the contrast medium is injected through the cannula, the uterus and the fallopian tubes are viewed fluoroscopically, and radiographs are taken. To take oblique views, the radiographic table may be tilted or the patient asked to change position. Films may also be taken later, to evaluate spillage of contrast medium into the peritoneal cavity.

Precautions
□ Hysterosalpingography is contraindicated in patients with menses, undiagnosed vaginal bleeding, or pelvic inflammatory disease.
□ Watch for an allergic reaction to the contrast medium, such as hives, itching, or hypotension.

Findings
Normally, radiographs reveal a symmetric uterine cavity; the contrast medium courses through fallopian tubes of normal caliber, spills freely into the peritoneal cavity, and doesn't leak from the uterus.

Implications of results
An asymmetric uterus suggests intra-

uterine adhesions or masses, such as fibroids or foreign bodies; impaired contrast flow through the fallopian tubes suggests partial or complete blockage, resulting from intraluminal agglutination, extrinsic compression by adhesions, or perifimbrial adhesions; leakage of contrast through uterine wall suggests fistulas. Laparoscopy with contrast instillation confirms positive or equivocal findings.

Post-test care
□ Watch for signs of infection, such as fever, pain, increased pulse rate, malaise, and muscle ache.
□ Assure the patient that cramps and vagal reaction (slow pulse rate, nausea, and dizziness) are transient.

Interfering factors
□ Tubal spasm or excessive traction may cause the appearance of a stricture in normal fallopian tubes.
□ Excessive traction can displace adhesions, making tubes appear normal.

RONALD J. WAPNER, MD
MARTIN WEISBERG, MD

ULTRASONOGRAPHY

Pelvic Ultrasonography

In pelvic ultrasonography, a piezoelectric crystal generates high-frequency sound waves that are reflected to a transducer, which in turn converts sound energy into electrical energy and forms images of the interior pelvic area on an oscilloscope screen. Techniques of sound imaging include A-mode (amplitude modulation), a one-dimensional system that records only distances between interfaces (recorded as spikes); B-mode (brightness modulation), a two-dimensional or cross-sectional image that reflects the intensity of the returning sound wave by the brightness of the dot; gray scale, a representation of organ texture in shades of gray on a television screen; and real-time imaging, instantaneous images of the tissues in motion, similar to fluoroscopic examination. Selected views may be photographed for later examination and a permanent record of the test.

The most common uses of pelvic ultrasonography include evaluation of symptoms that suggest pelvic disease, confirmation of tentative diagnosis, and determination of fetal growth during pregnancy. It's often required during pregnancy for women with histories or signs of fetal anomalies or multiple pregnancies, histories of bleeding, inconsistency of fetal size and conception date, or indications for amniocentesis.

Purpose
□ To detect foreign bodies and distinguish between cystic and solid masses (tumors)
□ To measure organ size
□ To evaluate fetal viability, position, gestational age, and growth rate
□ To detect multiple pregnancy
□ To confirm fetal abnormalities (such as molar pregnancy, and abnormalities of the arms and legs, spine, heart, head, kidneys, and abdomen) and maternal abnormalities (such as posterior placenta and placenta previa)
□ To guide amniocentesis by determining placental location and fetal position.

Patient preparation
Describe the test to the patient, and tell her the reason it is being performed. Assure her this procedure is safe, noninvasive, and painless. Since pelvic ultrasonography requires a full bladder as a landmark to define pelvic organs, instruct the patient to drink liquids and not to void before the test. Tell her who will perform the procedure and where,

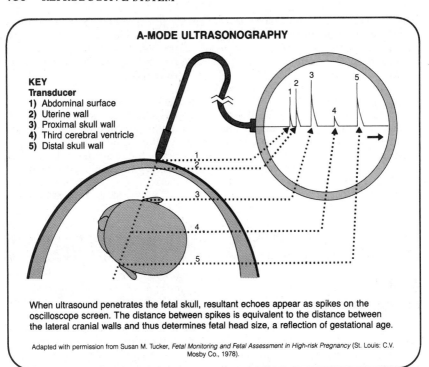

A-MODE ULTRASONOGRAPHY

KEY
Transducer
1) Abdominal surface
2) Uterine wall
3) Proximal skull wall
4) Third cerebral ventricle
5) Distal skull wall

When ultrasound penetrates the fetal skull, resultant echoes appear as spikes on the oscilloscope screen. The distance between spikes is equivalent to the distance between the lateral cranial walls and thus determines fetal head size, a reflection of gestational age.

Adapted with permission from Susan M. Tucker, *Fetal Monitoring and Fetal Assessment in High-risk Pregnancy* (St. Louis: C.V. Mosby Co., 1978).

and that it can vary in length from a few minutes to several hours.

Explain to the patient that a water enema may be necessary to produce a better outline of the large intestine. Reassure her that the test won't harm the fetus. Provide emotional support during the test.

Equipment
Mineral oil or water-soluble jelly/ultrasound machine and transducer/camera and film, or videotape/oscilloscope.

Procedure
With the patient in supine position, the pelvic area is coated with mineral oil or water-soluble jelly to increase sound wave conduction. Then the transducer crystal is guided over the area, images observed on the oscilloscope screen, and a good image is photographed.

Precautions
None.

Findings
The uterus is normal in size and shape. The ovaries are normal in size, shape, and sonographic density. No other masses are visible. If the patient is pregnant, the gestational sac and fetus are of normal size for date.

Implications of results
Although both cystic and solid masses have homogeneous densities, solid masses (such as fibroids) appear more dense on ultrasonography. Inappropriate fetal size may indicate miscalculation of conception or delivery date, or a dead fetus. Abnormal echo patterns may indicate foreign bodies (such as an intrauterine device), multiple pregnancy, maternal abnormalities (such as placenta previa or abruptio placentae), or fetal abnormalities (such as molar pregnancy, or abnormalities of the arms and legs, spine, heart, head, kidneys, and abdomen). Ultrasonography can also delineate fetal malpresentation (such as breech [at term]

or shoulder presentation), and cephalo-pelvic disproportion.

Post-test care

Allow the patient to empty her bladder immediately after the test.

Interfering factors

Failure to fill the bladder, obesity, or fetal head positioned deep in the pelvis can render the image uninterpretable.

RONALD J. WAPNER, MD
MARTIN WEISBERG, MD

Selected References

Danforth, David N., ed. *Obstetrics and Gynecology*, 4th ed. Philadelphia: J.B. Lippincott Co., 1982.

Diseases, 2nd ed. Nurse's Reference Library. Springhouse, Pa.: Springhouse Corp., 1986.

Glass, Robert H. *Office Gynecology*. 2nd ed. Baltimore: Williams & Wilkins Co., 1981.

Grossman, Zachary D., et al. *The Clinician's Guide to Diagnostic Imaging*. New York: Raven Press Pubs., 1983.

Haughey, Cynthia W. "Understanding Ultrasonography," *Nursing81* 11:100-04, April 1981.

Henry, John Bernard, ed. *Todd-Sanford-Davidsohn Clinical Diagnosis and Management by Laboratory Methods*, vol. 1, 17th ed. Philadelphia: W.B. Saunders Co., 1984.

Jensen, Margaret, et al. *Maternity Care: The Nurse and the Family*, 2nd ed. St. Louis: C.V. Mosby Co., 1981.

Kolstad, O., and Stafl, A. *Atlas of Colposcopy*, 3rd ed. Baltimore: University Park Press, 1982.

Lamb, Jane O. *Laboratory Tests in Clinical Nursing*. Bowie, Md.: Robert J. Brady Co., 1984.

Nursing85 Drug Handbook. Springhouse, Pa.: Springhouse Corp., 1985.

Pritchard, Jack A., and MacDonald Paul C. eds. *Williams Obstetrics*, 16th ed. East Norwalk, Conn.: Appleton-Century-Crofts, 1980.

Ravel, Richard. *Clinical Laboratory Medicine*, 4th ed. Chicago: Year Book Medical Pubs., 1984.

Sanders, R., and James, A.E., Jr., eds. *Principles and Practice of Ultrasonography in Obstetrics and Gynecology*, 2nd ed. East Norwalk, Conn.: Appleton-Century-Crofts, 1980.

Thompson, James S., and Thompson, Margaret W. *Genetics in Medicine*, 3rd ed. Philadelphia: W.B. Saunders Co., 1980.

Tucker, Susan M., and Bryant, Sandra. *Fetal Monitoring and Fetal Assessment in High Risk Pregnancy*. St. Louis: C.V. Mosby Co., 1978.

Wallach, Jacques B. *Interpretation of Diagnostic Tests: A Handbook Synopsis of Laboratory Medicine*, 3rd ed. Boston: Little, Brown, & Co., 1978.

Widmann, Frances K. *Clinical Interpretation of Laboratory Tests*, 9th ed. Philadelphia: F.A. Davis Co., 1983.

26 Nervous System

LEARNING OBJECTIVES

After completing this chapter, the reader will be able to:
- explain the anatomy and physiology of the nervous system.
- describe how to position the patient for a routine skull X-ray series.
- discuss the diagnostic applications of magnetic resonance imaging.
- explain why computed tomography typically yields better diagnostic information than conventional X-rays.
- state the purpose of each test discussed in the chapter.
- prepare the patient physically and psychologically for each test.
- describe the procedure for performing each test.
- specify appropriate precautions for safe administration of each test.
- recognize signs of adverse reaction and respond appropriately.
- implement appropriate post-test care.
- identify the normal findings of each test.
- discuss the implications of abnormal test results.
- list factors that may interfere with accurate test results.

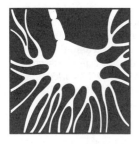

Nervous System

Introduction

The human nervous system is the final frontier of modern medicine, and its study—neurology—draws closer than any other discipline to examining the fundamental mystery of life. It seeks to understand how we come to feel, to think, to be aware of who and what we are.

The field of neurodiagnostics faces an equally difficult challenge: to devise safe, effective methods of detecting the diseases and disorders that affect what is one of the most powerful body systems and yet contains (or is made up of) some of the most fragile tissues. Sophisticated procedures such as computed tomography help to meet this challenge. The tests discussed in this chapter allow diagnosis of the major disorders of the brain and its cavities, vasculature, and coverings; the brain stem and cranial nerves; the spinal cord and spinal roots; as well as the peripheral nerves and the major skeletal muscle groups they innervate. These disorders comprise the substance of clinical neurology, a clear understanding of which is essential to modern nursing practice.

Neurons and synapses
The nervous system has three major divisions: *central (CNS)*, *peripheral*, and *autonomic*. The CNS consists of the brain, the brain stem, and the spinal cord. The peripheral system comprises the cranial and spinal nerves; the autonomic system—a mainly involuntary division that is actually part of the peripheral nervous system—consists of sympathetic and parasympathetic divisions, which influence the function of glands, blood vessels, smooth muscle, and internal organs.

The basic structural unit of the nervous system is the *neuron*, or nerve cell. Neurons carry electrical impulses along their axons (or major processes) and transmit them electrochemically across junctions called *synapses*; these impulses are received by the branching dendrites of other nerve cells.

Synaptic transmission is the basis for all cellular transactions within the CNS and in certain parts of the peripheral and autonomic systems. The typical central synapse is 200 angstroms across (1 angstrom = 10^{-8} cm) and serves as the arena for electrical and chemical events that excite (depolarize) or inhibit (hyperpolarize) cells, depending on the neurotransmitters they receive from other cells across the synaptic cleft.

Original data processing
The processes (axons or fibers) of nerve cells join in bundles like cables in a communications system. These cables or nerves contain afferent nerve fibers that carry impulses from the periphery to the nervous system (sensory nerves), or ef-

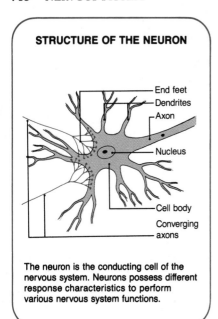

STRUCTURE OF THE NEURON

End feet
Dendrites
Axon
Nucleus
Cell body
Converging axons

The neuron is the conducting cell of the nervous system. Neurons possess different response characteristics to perform various nervous system functions.

hypothesis exists as to precisely how the human brain functions, it is generally considered to function in a manner analogous to a probability computer. Thus, when confronted with a problem or situation about which it has incomplete information, the brain quickly makes a "best guess," based on experience and learning, as to what this new state of affairs might be. To some extent, learning depends on memory, and memory depends on the number of functioning cellular elements. In the human brain, which contains approximately one trillion neurons, a rich cellular substratum exists for learning and memory.

Normal brain function depends on the integrity of cerebral circulation and the metabolism of brain substance. Blood flows to the brain through the two internal carotid arteries and the two vertebral arteries. The latter two vessels unite posteriorly to form the basilar artery. The *circle of Willis* is situated at the base of the brain and is the origin of six large vessels supplying the cortex. Venous drainage occurs by way of deep veins and dural sinuses emptying into the internal jugular veins.

Many vessels in the brain are amply supplied by various kinds of nerve fibers. When a major cerebral artery is occluded, cerebral ischemia occurs distal to the occlusion. Collateral circulation may develop in the presence of gradual occlusion or reduced blood flow through certain areas of the brain, particularly in aging individuals. However, sudden occlusion of a carotid artery, especially in older persons, may cause serious symptoms of cerebral ischemia.

ferent fibers that carry impulses from the nervous system to the periphery (motor nerves). Mixed nerves are composed of both afferent and efferent fibers. Several types and sizes of nerve fiber may exist in a single sensory or motor nerve; each fiber type and size has a different conduction velocity. Moreover, different peripheral sensations may be carried by specific fiber types within nerves.

During development, the growth of nerve cells and the sprouting of processes appear to be partially regulated by various factors of great interest to biochemists and neurobiologists. Within the CNS, for example, cells known as *glia* (from the Greek word for glue) support and help nourish nerve tissue. Glia may also be involved in the biosynthesis of myelin, the insulating material that surrounds certain portions of central and peripheral axons and that assists the conduction of nerve impulses. Pathologically, glia may undergo malignant metamorphosis, forming glial tumors.

Making the "best guess"
While no completely accepted or unified

Blood-brain barrier
A complex combination of factors and structural elements exists to form a functional blood-brain barrier. This barrier consists partly of tight endothelial junctions that prohibit passage of many substances; through the capillary beds and cellular membranes that must also be traversed by substances leaving the circulation and entering the brain. The blood-brain barrier helps maintain a

constant environment for brain cells. Because a breakdown in the blood-brain barrier commonly occurs at the site of tumor growth, it can be identified by substances that rapidly penetrate the tumor tissue (such as radioiodine-labeled albumin), allowing it to stand out photographically.

Protective fluid

Cerebrospinal fluid (CSF) is formed mainly by the choroid plexuses within the brain's four ventricles; it's also formed around the cerebral vessels and along ventricular walls. The composition of CSF depends on filtration and diffusion from the blood, and it's very similar to the brain's extracellular fluid. Both fluids flow out through the foramina of Magendie and Luschka, and are absorbed thereafter through the arachnoid villi into the cerebral venous sinuses.

Few conditions cause CSF pressure to fall below normal (dehydration might be one), but many conditions can cause large amounts of fluid to accumulate— sometimes under pressure. This may lead to communicating hydrocephalus, or to noncommunicating hydrocephalus, in which the flow of CSF from one or more ventricles is blocked.

Along with the meninges, CSF protects and supports the brain, as evidenced by the pain generated by the withdrawal of spinal fluid. Without this cushion of fluid, the brain settles, and its weight—combined with traction on pain-sensitive vessels—causes a severe headache.

Neurologic tests

Brain diseases or disorders related to the diagnostic tests in this chapter include congenital defects and anomalies, perinatal defects, ventricular abnormalities, the epilepsies, the so-called degenerative diseases, and space-occupying lesions. This last finding includes solid tumors and other neoplasms originating in the brain or metastasizing to it.

These tests can also diagnose infectious diseases, including those caused by bacteria (such as meningitis), viruses (such as encephalitis or polioencephalo-

myelitis), spirochetes (such as neurosyphilis), parasitic infestations of various kinds (rare in North America), and fungal and related infections. Demyelinating diseases (such as multiple sclerosis), cerebrovascular disorders (including stroke, transient ischemic attacks, aneurysms of the blood vessels, and subdural and subarachnoid hemorrhages or hematomas), and disorders of the skull, vertebral column, and other non-neural tissues may also be diagnosed using the tests in this chapter.

Disorders of the brain stem and cranial nerves that can be detected by these tests include vascular insufficiency, resulting from obstruction to specific regions of the brain stem; cranial nerve syndromes (such as trigeminal neuralgia); headache disorders; and congenital disorders that occur as distortions of normal relationships between the skull and vertebral column, or as abnormal formations of the base of the skull.

The spinal cord may be affected by metastasis from non-nervous primary tumors that spread to the vertebrae and meninges, producing extradural tumors that distort the spinal cord or interrupt CSF flow in the spinal subarachnoid spaces. This causes a block in CSF circulation, accompanied by spinal cord dysfunction. Both the brain stem and the spinal cord may be affected by Guillain-Barré syndrome, which is typically a myeloradiculopathy.

Because disorders of the peripheral nervous system are often toxic or metabolic in origin, the tests covered in this chapter are generally not as useful as investigation for exposure to toxins or as a systemic metabolic workup. In addition, diagnosis of peripheral neuropathies often depends on nerve biopsy, which allows identification of specific pathologic change in the nerve fibers. This applies also to the identification of myopathies or muscle disorders, which commonly depends on muscle biopsy.

Noninvasive tests

Skull radiography is an X-ray evaluation of the skull taken at various planes and

NORMAL CIRCULATION OF CSF

CSF is produced from blood in the capillary networks called the choroid plexus. Choroid plexuses are complex structures of vascular folds in the pia mater in the brain's lateral, third, and fourth ventricles. From these sites of origin, CSF passes into the lateral ventricles. It flows through the foramen of Monro, into the third ventricle; through the aqueduct of Sylvius, into the fourth ventricle; and through the foramina of Luschka and Magendie, to the cisterna of the subarachnoid space. The cisterna is continuous with the subarachnoid space, surrounding the entire brain and spinal cord. Then, the fluid passes under the base of the brain, upward over the brain's upper surface, and down around the spinal cord. When CSF reaches the arachnoid villi, it's absorbed into venous blood at the venous sinuses. Normally, the amount of CSF produced (500 to 800 ml/day) equals the amount absorbed. The average amount circulating at one time is 125 to 175 ml.

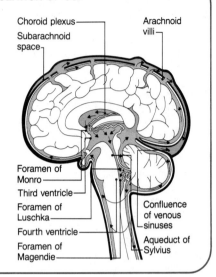

from different angles that allows examination of almost all intracranial structures.

Computed tomography (CT) provides a computerized image that reproduces a section of the brain or spinal column as if sliced from front to back, in the horizontal plane. Recent advances permit reconstruction in other planes as well. Although generally considered a noninvasive test, CT has an invasive variation in the form of the contrasted or enhanced scan, which allows for uptake—by an intracranial or spinal lesion—of a radiopaque medium injected into a peripheral vein.

The revolutionary *magnetic resonance imaging* (MRI) relies on the magnetic properties of the body's atoms. It uses radiofrequency energy and a powerful magnetic field to produce computerized multiplanar images of startling detail and resolution.

Echoencephalography, less commonly used now than before CT scanning, involves the reflection of ultrasound waves from structures within the skull. This procedure determines the position of the cerebral midline structures and, from this information, the existence or nonexistence of a midline shift.

Electroencephalography (EEG) detects, records, and amplifies electrical potentials on the scalp that are generated by the brain's neurons, using a noninvasive technique that requires small electrodes to be applied in carefully defined patterns on the scalp. The findings depict the electrical activity of the brain's surface. This surface activity reflects, and can be used to interpret, changes in electrical activity of deeper structures.

Evoked potential studies directly evaluate sensory and somatosensory neurologic pathways by recording the brain's electrical response to external stimuli.

Lumbar, thoracic, and *cervical thermography* may graphically demonstrate abnormal heat patterns caused by nerve root irritation.

Oculoplethysmography indirectly measures ocular artery pressure and reflects the adequacy of cerebrovascular blood flow.

Invasive tests

The *radionuclide scan of the brain* gives an overall picture of the integrity of the blood-brain barrier. If a defect in this barrier exists, an injected radionuclide *may* penetrate the area, producing a localized increase in the concentration of the radioisotopic tracer, as shown on a scintillation camera.

Cerebral angiography allows visualization of blood vessels through injection of a substance that is opaque to X-rays and therefore stands out as a white contrast. *Digital subtraction angiography* (DSA) uses computers and sophisticated video equipment to eliminate interfering images of bone and soft tissue and further reveal details of the opacified vessels. In addition to detecting disorders of the blood vessels themselves, angiography may also help detect displacement of blood vessels by other lesions, such as tumors.

Electromyography assesses the electrical potential across the muscle membrane through a needle electrode. This procedure yields information on the conduction of the nerve impulse to the muscle, as well as the muscle's response to the nerve impulse. The *nerve conduction* part of this test determines whether the velocity of propagation of the nerve impulse along a particular sensory, motor, or combined sensory-motor nerve is normal. This test also provides general information concerning the possibility of neuropathy.

Cerebrospinal fluid analysis provides a general profile of the cellular and chemical composition of CSF at a particular time. Since CSF is secreted and represents a highly refined distillate of the blood, concentrations of certain substances are different in CSF than in serum. The pressure under which CSF is circulating can be determined during lumbar puncture, before the CSF specimen is obtained.

Myelography involves injection of a radiopaque contrast medium into the subarachnoid space. CSF is removed for analysis at the time of myelography—thereby accomplishing two tests with one procedure—and is replaced by the heavier contrast medium, which gravitates toward the head or elsewhere within the spinal canal when the radiographic table is tilted.

In the *Tensilon test,* a short-acting potent anticholinesterase drug is administered intravenously, for the diagnosis of myasthenia gravis.

New techniques

Knowledge gained through research and technology makes possible the advancement of new techniques for the investigation of clinical neurologic disorders. A number of these techniques have been used by laboratories for many years to conduct fundamental research on the nervous system. One such technique is *positron emission tomography* (PET), which creates an image of a slice of the

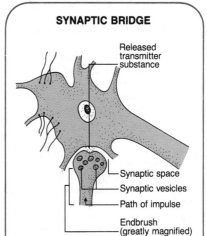

SYNAPTIC BRIDGE

Released transmitter substance

Synaptic space
Synaptic vesicles
Path of impulse

Endbrush
(greatly magnified)

A synapse is the junction place between neurons across which nervous impulses travel. The impulses cross the minute synaptic space by an electrochemical process. The terminal portion of the neuron capable of transmission is called an endbrush, and contains vesicles filled with transmitter substances. When the nerve impulse reaches the endbrush, the vesicles release the transmitter substance, bridging the space to the adjacent neuron. The substance depolarizes the adjacent neuron's dendrites. This generates an action potential capable of carrying the impulse forward.

Adapted with permission from James Chaplin, *Primer of Neurology and Neurophysiology* (New York: John Wiley & Sons, 1978).

brain similar to a CT image but is based on different biophysical and radiochemical techniques. Many advanced mathematical models of EEG are being used and developed to widen and extend its application. A new clinical application of EEG is *somnography,* the scientific evaluation of sleep and its disorders. These promising new techniques are still essentially investigational and have limited clinical application.

ROGER MORRELL, MD, PhD

NONINVASIVE TESTS

Skull Radiography

Skull radiography is the oldest noninvasive neurologic test and is frequently the second step—after routine neurologic examination—in a complete neurologic workup. In patients with head injuries, X-ray films of the skull offer limited information about skull fractures. However, this test is extremely valuable for studying increased intracranial pressure (ICP), abnormalities of the base of the skull and the cranial vault, congenital and perinatal anomalies, and many systemic diseases that produce bone defects of the skull.

Skull radiography evaluates the three groups of bones that comprise the skull— the calvaria or vault, the mandible or jaw bone, and the facial bones. The calvaria and the facial bones are closely connected by immovable joints with irregular serrated edges, called sutures. The bones of the skull form an anatomic structure so complex that several radiologic views of each area are required for a complete skull examination.

Purpose
☐ To detect fractures in patients with head trauma
☐ To help detect and assess increased ICP, tumors, bleeding, and infections
☐ To aid diagnosis of pituitary tumors
☐ To detect congenital anomalies.

Patient preparation
Explain to the patient that this test helps establish a diagnosis. Inform him that he needn't restrict food or fluids. Tell him that several X-ray films of his skull will be taken from various angles, and who will perform the test and where. Reassure him that the procedure will cause him no discomfort, and that it takes about 15 minutes. Instruct him to remove glasses, dentures, jewelry, and metal objects in the X-ray field.

Equipment
X-ray machine and film.

Procedure
The patient is placed in a supine position on a radiographic table, or is seated in a chair, and is instructed to remain still while the radiographs are taken. A head band, foam pads, or sandbags may be used to immobilize the patient's head and increase his comfort. Routinely, five views of the skull are taken: left and right lateral, anteroposterior Townes, posteroanterior Caldwell, and axial (or base). Films are developed and checked for quality before the patient leaves the radiography department.

Precautions
None.

Findings
A radiologist interprets the radiographs, evaluating the size, shape, thickness, and position of cranial bones, as well as the vascular markings, sinuses, and sutures; all should be normal for the patient's age.

Implications of results
Skull radiography is often diagnostic for fractures of the vault or base, although basilar fractures may not show on the

ROUTINE SKULL SERIES

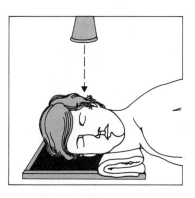

Right lateral and left lateral

The sagittal plane is parallel to the tabletop and the film. A support, such as the patient's clenched fist, or a folded towel, is placed under the chin. (Adequate film shows both halves of the mandible directly superimposed.)

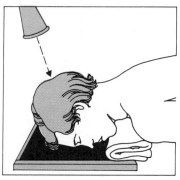

Posteroanterior (PA) Caldwell

The patient lies prone (his chin may be supported with his fist or a folded towel). The sagittal plane and the canthomeatal line are perpendicular to the tabletop and the film. The X-ray beam is angled 15° toward the feet.

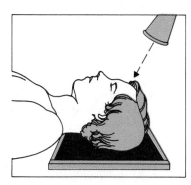

Anteroposterior (AP) Towne's

The patient lies supine, with his chin flexed toward the neck, the canthomeatal line is perpendicular to the tabletop and the film. The X-ray beam is angled 30° toward the feet.

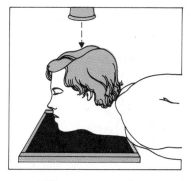

Axial (base)

The patient lies prone, with chin fully extended; his head rests in such a way that the line of the face is perpendicular and the canthomeatal line is parallel to the tabletop and the film.

film if the bone is dense. This test may confirm congenital anomalies and may show erosion, enlargement, or decalcification of the sella turcica that result from increased ICP. A marked rise in pressure may cause the brain to expand and press against the inner bony table of the skull, leaving marks or impressions that have been compared in appearance to beaten silver.

X-ray films of the skull may also show abnormal areas of calcification in conditions such as osteomyelitis (with possible calcification of the skull itself) and chronic subdural hematomas. They can detect neoplasms within the brain substance that contain calcium, such as oligodendrogliomas or meningiomas, or the midline shifting of a calcified pineal gland caused by a space-occupying lesion. Skull radiography may also detect other changes in bone structure, for example, those that arise from metabolic disorders like acromegaly or Paget's disease.

Post-test care
None.

Interfering factors
Improper positioning of the patient, excessive head movement by the patient, or failure to remove radiopaque objects from the X-ray field produces films that are inadequate for radiologic interpretation.

KATHY A. HAUSMAN, RN, MS

Intracranial Computed Tomography

Intracranial computed tomography (CT) provides a series of tomograms, translated by a computer and displayed on an oscilloscope screen, representing cross-sectional images of various layers (or slices) of the brain. This technique can reconstruct cross-sectional, horizontal, sagittal, and coronal plane images. Hundreds of thousands of readings of radiation levels absorbed by brain tissues may be combined to depict anatomic slices of varying thickness. Specificity and accuracy are enhanced by the degree of resolution, which depends on the number of radiation density calculations made by the computer. This, in turn, depends on the number of collimated (parallel) radiographs taken. Newer versions of the scanner take more radiographs than earlier models, producing more detailed images. These images identify intracranial tumors and other brain lesions as areas of altered density.

The increasing availability of CT scanners allows faster and safer diagnosis than in the past. Often, intracranial CT scanning eliminates the need for painful and hazardous invasive procedures, such as pneumoencephalography and cerebral angiography. CT, which often uses contrast enhancement, is especially valuable in assessing a patient with focal neurologic abnormalities and other clinical features that suggest an intracranial mass. In a patient with suspected head injury, intracranial CT may allow diagnosis of subdural hematoma before it causes characteristic symptoms. In short, indications for this test are legion, and their number is growing with new technologic refinements of the scanner.

Purpose
□ To diagnose intracranial lesions and abnormalities
□ To monitor the effects of surgery, radiotherapy, or chemotherapy on intracranial tumors.

Patient preparation
Explain to the patient that this test permits assessment of the brain. Unless contrast enhancement is scheduled, inform him he needn't restrict food or fluids. If contrast enhancement is scheduled, instruct him to fast for 4 hours before the test. Tell him a series of X-ray films will be taken of his brain, and who will perform the test and where. Reassure him that the test will cause him no discomfort and takes 15 to 30 minutes.

Tell the patient he'll be positioned on an X-ray table, with his head immobilized and his face uncovered. The head of the table is moved into the scanner,

NORMAL AND ABNORMAL CT SCANS

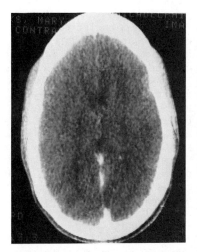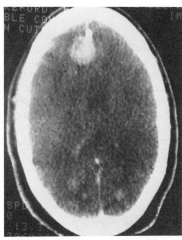

Shown here are two intracranial CT scans. The scan on the left is normal. The scan on the right shows a large meningioma in the frontal region, represented by the white area.

which rotates around his head and makes clacking sounds. If a contrast agent is used, tell the patient he may feel flushed and warm, and experience a transient headache, a salty taste, or nausea and vomiting after injection of the dye.

Instruct the patient to wear a hospital gown (outpatients may wear any comfortable clothing) and to remove all metal objects and jewelry in the X-ray field. If the patient is restless or apprehensive, notify the doctor, and administer a sedative, if ordered.

Make sure the patient or responsible family member has signed a consent form. Check the patient's history for hypersensitivity to shellfish, iodine, or other contrast media. Inform the doctor of any sensitivities, since he may order prophylactic medications or may choose not to perform contrast enhancement.

Equipment
CT scanner/oscilloscope/contrast medium, as ordered (meglumine iothalamate or sodium diatrizoate)/60-ml syringe/19G to 21G needle/tourniquet.

Procedure
The patient is placed in a supine position on a radiographic table, with his head immobilized by straps, and is asked to lie still. The head of the table is moved into the scanner, which rotates around the patient's head, taking radiographs at 1° intervals in a 180° arc.

When this series of radiographs is complete, contrast enhancement is performed, if ordered. Usually, 50 to 100 ml of contrast medium are injected I.V. or by drip method over 1 to 2 minutes, and the patient is observed for hypersensitive reactions, such as urticaria, respiratory difficulty, and a rash. Such reactions usually develop within 30 minutes.

After injection of the contrast medium, another series of scans is taken. Information from the scans is stored on magnetic tapes, fed into a computer, and converted into images on an oscilloscope screen. Photographs of selected views are taken for further study.

Precautions
Intracranial CT with contrast enhance-

ment is contraindicated in persons who are hypersensitive to iodine or contrast medium.

Findings

The density of tissue determines the amount of radiation that will pass through it. Tissue densities appear as black, white, or shades of gray on the computerized image obtained by intracranial CT scanning. Bone, the densest tissue, appears white; brain matter appears in shades of gray; ventricular and subarachnoid CSF—the least dense—appears black. Structures are evaluated according to their density, size, shape, and position.

Implications of results

Areas of altered density (they may be lighter or darker) or displaced vasculature or other structures may indicate intracranial tumor, hematoma, cerebral atrophy, infarction, edema, or congenital anomalies, such as hydrocephalus.

Intracranial tumors vary significantly in appearance and characteristics. *Metastatic tumors* generally cause extensive edema in early stages, and can usually be defined by contrast enhancement. *Primary tumors* vary in density and in their capacity to cause edema, displace ventricles, and absorb dye in contrast enhancement. Astrocytomas, for example, usually have low densities; meningiomas have higher densities and can generally be defined with contrast enhancement; glioblastomas, usually ill-defined, are also enhanced after injection of a contrast medium.

Both subdural and epidural hematomas, and other acute hemorrhages are normally easy to detect, because the high density of blood contrasts markedly with low-density brain tissue. Contrast enhancement usually helps locate subdural hematomas.

Cerebral atrophy customarily appears as enlarged ventricles with large sulci. Cerebral infarction may appear as low-density areas at the obstruction site or may not be apparent if the infarction is small or doesn't cause edema. With con-

trast enhancement, the infarcted area may not show in the acute phase, but will show clearly after resolution of the lesion. Cerebral edema usually appears as an area of marked generalized lucency. In children, enlargement of the fourth ventricle generally indicates hydrocephalus.

Normally, the cerebral vessels don't appear on computerized tomogram images. However, in patients with arteriovenous malformation, cerebral vessels may appear with slightly increased density. Contrast enhancement allows a better view of the abnormal area. Definitive diagnosis requires correlation of intracranial CT results with patient history and clinical status.

Post-test care

None, if the test was performed without contrast enhancement. If a contrast agent was used, watch for residual side effects (headache, nausea, and vomiting), and inform the patient he may resume his usual diet.

Interfering factors

☐ Artifact caused by the patient moving his head makes CT scan images difficult to interpret.
☐ Failure to remove radiopaque objects from X-ray field may produce unclear images.

KATHY A. HAUSMAN, RN, MS

Magnetic Resonance Imaging

Although its full range of clinical applications has yet to be established, magnetic resonance imaging (MRI) is already recognized as a safe, valuable tool for neurologic diagnosis. Like computed tomography (CT), MRI produces cross-sectional images of the brain and spine in multiple planes. However, unlike CT, MRI produces images without use of ion-

POSITRON EMISSION TOMOGRAPHY

Like computed tomography (CT) scanning and magnetic resonance imaging (MRI), positron emission tomography (PET) provides images of the brain through sophisticated computer reconstruction algorithms. However, PET images detail brain function as well as structure and thus differ significantly from the images provided by these other advanced techniques.

Positron emission tomography combines elements of both CT scanning and conventional radionuclide imaging. For example, PET measures the emissions of injected radioisotopes and converts these to a tomographic image of the brain. But, unlike conventional radionuclide imaging, PET uses radioisotopes of biologically important elements—oxygen, nitrogen, carbon, and fluorine—that emit particles called *positrons*.

During positron emission, pairs of gamma rays are emitted; the PET scanner detects these and relays the information to a computer for reconstruction as an image. Positron-emitters can be chemically "tagged" to biologically active molecules such as carbon monoxide, neurotransmitters, hormones, and metabolites (particularly glucose), enabling study of their uptake and distribution in brain tissue. For example, blood tagged with ^{11}C-carbon monoxide allows study of hemodynamic patterns in brain tissue, whereas tagged neurotransmitters, hormones, and drugs allow mapping of receptor distribution. Isotope-tagged glucose (which penetrates the blood-brain barrier rapidly) allows dynamic study of brain function, since PET can pinpoint the sites of glucose metabolism in the brain under various conditions. This last application is particularly promising—researchers expect it to prove useful in the diagnosis of psychiatric disorders, transient ischemic attacks, amyotrophic lateral sclerosis, Parkinson's disease, Wilson's disease, multiple sclerosis, seizure disorders, cerebrovascular disease, and Alzheimer's disease. The reason: All of these disorders may alter the location and patterns of cerebral glucose metabolism.

Positron emission tomography is a costly test because the radioisotopes used have very short half-lives and must be produced at an on-site cyclotron and attached quickly to the desired tracer molecules. So far, this prohibitive cost has limited PET's use, except as a research tool. However, PET has already provided significant information about the brain and may someday have widespread clinical applications.

izing radiation or injected contrast solutions.

MRI's greatest advantages are its ability to "see through" bone and to delineate fluid-filled soft tissue in great detail. Thus far, it's proved useful in the diagnosis of cerebral infarction, tumors, abscesses, edema, hemorrhage, nerve fiber demyelination (as in multiple sclerosis), and other disorders that increase the fluid content of affected tissues. It can also show irregularities of the spinal cord with a resolution and detail previously unobtainable. And it holds promise for producing images of organs in motion.

MRI relies on the magnetic properties of the atom. (Hydrogen, the most abundant and magnetically sensitive of the body's atoms, is most commonly selected for MRI studies.) The scanner uses a powerful magnetic field and radio-frequency (RF) energy to produce images based on the hydrogen (primarily water) content of body tissues. Exposed to an external magnetic field, positively charged atomic nuclei and their negatively charged electrons align uniformly in the field. RF energy is then directed at the atoms, knocking them out of this magnetic alignment and causing them to precess, or spin. When the RF pulse is discontinued, the atoms realign themselves with the magnetic field, emitting RF energy as a tissue-specific signal based on the relative density of nuclei and the realignment time. These signals are monitored by the MRI computer, which processes them and displays the information on a video monitor as a high-resolution image.

The magnetic fields and RF energy used

for MRI are imperceptible by the patient; no harmful effects have been documented. Research is continuing on the optimal magnetic fields and RF waves for each type of tissue.

Purpose
□ To aid diagnosis of intracranial and spinal lesions and soft-tissue abnormalities.

Patient preparation
Explain to the patient that this test assesses his brain or spinal cord. Tell him who will perform the test and where. Stress that the test is painless and involves no exposure to radiation. Tell him that the procedure may take up to 90 minutes.

Explain to the patient that he'll be positioned on a narrow bed and slid into a large cylinder that houses the MRI magnets. Have him change to a loose-fitting hospital gown (outpatients may wear any comfortable clothing). Since watches and jewelry can be damaged by the strong magnetic field, ask the patient to remove all metal objects before the test begins.

Equipment
MRI scanner and computer/display screen/recorder (film or magnetic tape).

Procedure
The patient is placed in a supine position on a narrow bed and told to lie still. The bed then slides him to the desired position inside the scanner, where RF energy is directed at his head or spine. The resulting images are displayed on a monitor and recorded on film or magnetic tape for permanent storage. The radiologist may vary RF waves and use the computer to manipulate and enhance the images.

Precautions
Because MRI works through a powerful magnetic field, it can't be performed on patients with pacemakers, intracranial aneurysm clips, or other ferrous metal implants.

Findings
Magnetic resonance imaging can show normal anatomic details of the central nervous system in any plane, without bone interference. Brain and spinal cord structures should appear distinct and sharply defined. Tissue color and shading will vary, depending on the RF energy, magnetic strength, and degree of computer enhancement.

Implications of results
Because the MRI signal represents proton density (water content) of tissue, MRI clearly shows structural changes resulting from disorders that increase tissue water content, such as cerebral edema, demyelinating disease, and pontine and cerebellar tumors. Edematous fluid, for example, generally appears cloudy or gray, whereas blood generally appears dark. Lesions of multiple sclerosis appear as areas of demyelination (curdlike, gray or gray-white areas) around the edges of ventricles. Tumors show as changes in normal anatomy, which computer enhancement may further delineate.

Post-test care
None.

Interfering factors
Excessive movement can blur images.
ROGER M. MORRELL, MD, PhD

Echoencephalography

In echoencephalography, an ultrasonic beam is transmitted through the skull by a transducer. The time required for midline cerebral structures to reflect the beam back to the transducer is converted to an electrical impulse, and is then displayed on an oscilloscope screen and measured to determine the position of the brain's midline structures, particularly the third ventricle. Echoencephalography has largely been replaced by computerized tomography.

CAROTID IMAGING FACTS

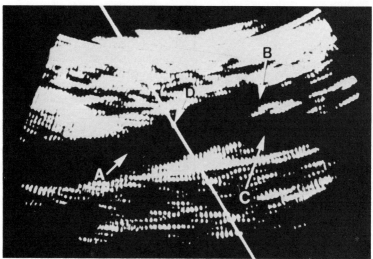

Normal real-time image, taken by echo technique, shows the common carotid artery (A), external carotid artery (B), internal carotid artery (C), and Doppler beam (D).

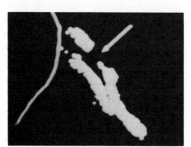 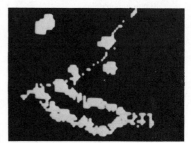

Abnormal pulsed Doppler image (at left) shows total occlusion (arrow) of the internal carotid artery. Compare this to the normal pulsed Doppler image (at right).

What is it? Carotid imaging is a diagnostic test that assesses the carotid arteries for occlusive disease. In this test, a pulsed Doppler ultrasonic flow transducer or a real-time imager permits imaging and recording of the carotid artery.
• *Real-time imaging* (top photo) uses the echo technique, which also permits visualization of the carotid artery. In this technique, a Doppler signal can be directed to specific points along the vessel. The audio signal is then evaluated.
• *Pulsed Doppler technique* (bottom photos) uses a transducer with a range-gating system that allows alternate transmission and reception of ultrasonic signals. The sound reflected from moving RBCs within the lumen is then collected and stored in a computer, for subsequent intraluminal image reconstruction.
How is it done? The patient is placed in a supine position, and the probe is placed on his neck and is moved slowly from the vicinity of the common carotid artery to that of the bifurcation, then to the site of the internal and external carotids.
What are its advantages? Carotid imaging detects ulcerating plaques that can't be detected by other methods; it can also differentiate between total and near-total arterial occlusion.
What are its disadvantages? Intramural calcification prevents sound penetration and may lead to false-positive results.

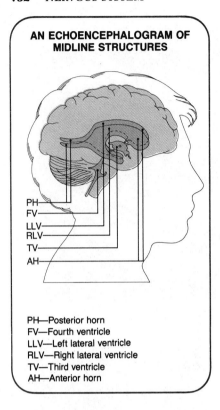

AN ECHOENCEPHALOGRAM OF MIDLINE STRUCTURES

PH—Posterior horn
FV—Fourth ventricle
LLV—Left lateral ventricle
RLV—Right lateral ventricle
TV—Third ventricle
AH—Anterior horn

Purpose
□ To determine the position and size of midline cerebral structures.

Patient preparation
Describe the procedure to the patient, and explain that this test determines the position and size of several brain structures. Inform him he needn't restrict food or fluids. Tell him who will perform the test and where. Reassure him that the procedure is safe and painless, and takes approximately 1 hour.

Tell the patient a small transducer will be placed on the side of his head, just above the ear, and that this transducer will send an ultrasonic beam into the brain. As the cerebral structures reflect the beam, he may hear an echo that sounds like repetitive humming or a musical note. Instruct the patient to remove jewelry or other metal objects from his head and neck.

Equipment
Echoencephalograph / transducer / oscilloscope / water-soluble jelly.

Procedure
Place the patient in a supine position on a radiographic table. Water-soluble jelly is applied to the transducer, which is then placed on the temporoparietal region of the patient's head. The transducer transmits an ultrasonic beam to the underlying structures. The time required for cerebral structures to reflect the beam to the transducer is converted to an electrical impulse, and is visualized on an oscilloscope screen. This image is photographed for later study and a permanent record.

Precautions
None.

Findings
Normally, an echoencephalogram shows the third ventricle centered in the skull, no more than 2 to 3 mm from the midline. Other midline structures, such as the right and the left lateral ventricles, also appear in their normal anatomic positions.

Implications of results
A shift in midline structures of more than 3 mm indicates an abnormality. If the third ventricle is enlarged by 10 mm or more (7 mm or more in children), further investigation for a possible space-occupying lesion is necessary. However, two sets of identical impulses are required to confirm abnormal results. Echoencephalography may also reveal structural shifts due to cerebral edema or to subdural and extradural hemorrhage.

Post-test care
None.

Interfering factors
Failure to remove jewelry or metal objects from the patient's head and neck interferes with test results.

KATHY A. HAUSMAN, RN, MS

Electroencephalography

In electroencephalography, electrodes attached to standard areas of the patient's scalp record a portion of the brain's electrical activity. These electrical impulses are transmitted to an electroencephalograph, which magnifies them 1 million times and records them as brain waves on moving strips of paper. Especially valuable in assessing patients with seizure disorders, electroencephalography is also used to evaluate patients with symptoms of brain tumors, abscesses, and cerebral damage due to other causes. The procedure is usually performed in a room designed to eliminate electrical interference and minimize distractions. Portable units are available, however, to perform electroencephalography at bedside, which is commonly done to confirm brain death.

Purpose
□ To determine the presence and type of epilepsy
□ To aid diagnosis of intracranial lesions, such as abscesses and tumors
□ To evaluate the brain's electrical activity in metabolic disease, head injury, meningitis, encephalitis, mental retardation, and psychological disorders
□ To confirm brain death.

Patient preparation
Describe the procedure to the patient, and explain that this test records the brain's electrical activity. Inform him that, except for fluids containing caffeine, he needn't restrict food or fluids before the test (in fact, skipping the meal before the test can cause relative hypoglycemia and alter brain wave patterns). Thoroughly wash and dry the patient's hair to remove hair sprays, creams, or oils.

Tell the patient he'll be asked to relax in a reclining chair or lie on a bed, and that electrodes will be attached to his scalp. Assure him that the electrodes won't shock him. If needle electrodes are used, he'll feel pricking sensations when they're inserted; however, flat electrodes are more commonly used. Do your best to allay the patient's fears, since mental tension can affect brain wave patterns.

Check the patient's medication history for drugs that may interfere with test results. As ordered, withhold anticonvulsants, tranquilizers, barbiturates, and other sedatives for 24 to 48 hours before the test. Infants and very young children occasionally require sedation to prevent crying and restlessness during the test.

To evaluate a patient with a seizure disorder, a "sleep electroencephalogram" (EEG) may be ordered. In this case, keep the patient awake the night before the test, and as ordered, administer a sedative (such as chloral hydrate) to help him sleep during the test.

Equipment
Electroencephalograph and recorder/electrodes with leads/electrode paste.

Procedure
The patient is positioned comfortably on a bed or a reclining chair, and electrodes are attached to his scalp. Before the recording procedure begins, the patient is instructed to close his eyes, relax, and remain still. During the recording, the patient is carefully observed through a window in an adjoining room, and blinking, swallowing, talking, or other movements that may cause artifacts on the tracing are noted. The recording may be stopped periodically to allow the patient to reposition himself and get comfortable. This is important, since restlessness and fatigue can alter brain wave patterns.

After an initial baseline recording, the patient may be tested in various stress situations to elicit abnormal patterns not obvious in the resting state. For example, the patient may be asked to breathe deeply and rapidly for 3 minutes (hyperventilation), which may elicit brain wave patterns typical of seizure disorders or other abnormalities. This technique is commonly used to detect petit mal epilepsy. Photic stimulation—another technique—tests central cerebral activity in response to bright light, accentuating abnormal activity in petit mal or myoclonic seizures. A strobe light placed in front of the patient is flashed 1 to 20 times/second. Recordings are made with the patient's eyes opened and closed.

Precautions
Observe the patient carefully for seizure activity. Record seizure patterns, and be prepared to provide assistance in the rare event of a severe seizure. Have suction equipment and diazepam for I.V. injection readily available.

Findings
Electroencephalography records a portion of the brain's electrical activity as waves; some are irregular, while others demonstrate frequent patterns. Among the basic waveforms are the alpha, beta, theta, and delta rhythms. *Alpha waves* occur at frequencies of 8 to 12 cycles/second in a regular rhythm. They're present only in the waking state when the patient's eyes are closed but he's mentally alert; usually, they disappear with visual

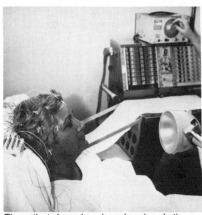

The patient shown here is undergoing photic stimulation during electroencephelography. The flashing light can cause myoclonic seizures in the patient with central cerebral damage.

activity or mental concentration. *Beta waves* (13 to 30 cycles/second)—generally associated with anxiety, depression, or sedative drugs—are seen most readily in the frontal and central regions of the brain. *Theta waves* (4 to 7 cycles/second) are most common in children and young adults, and appear in the frontal and temporal regions. *Delta waves* (0.5 to 3.5 cycles/second) normally occur only in young children and during sleep.

Implications of results
Usually, 100′ to 200′ (30 to 60 m) of the recording are evaluated, with particular attention paid to basic waveforms, symmetry of cerebral activity, transient discharges, and responses to stimulation. A specific diagnosis depends on the patient's clinical status.

In patients with epilepsy, EEG patterns may identify the specific disorder. In patients with *petit mal epilepsy,* for example, the EEG shows spikes and waves at a frequency of 3 cycles/second. In grand mal epilepsy, it generally shows multiple, high-voltage, spiked waves in both hemispheres. In temporal lobe epilepsy, the EEG usually shows spiked waves in the affected temporal region. And in patients with focal seizures, it usually shows localized, spiked discharges.

In patients with intracranial lesions, such as tumors or abscesses, the EEG may show slow waves (usually delta waves, but possibly unilateral beta waves). Vascular lesions, such as cerebral infarcts and intracranial hemorrhages, generally produce focal abnormalities in the injured area.

Generally, any condition that causes a diminishing level of consciousness alters the EEG pattern in proportion to the degree of consciousness lost. For example, in a patient with a metabolic disorder, an inflammatory process (such as meningitis or encephalitis), or increased intracranial pressure, the EEG recording shows brain waves that are generalized, diffuse, and slow. The most pathologic finding of all, of course, is absence of an EEG pattern, or a "flat" tracing (except

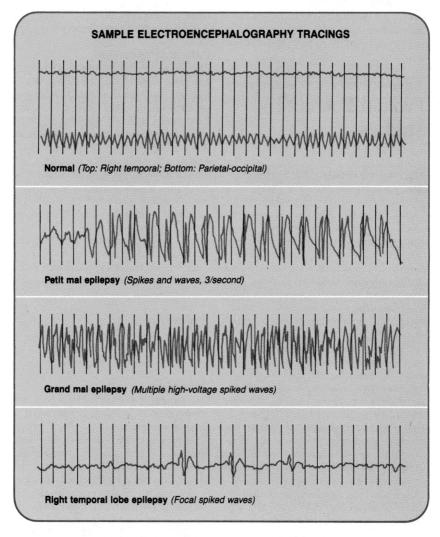

SAMPLE ELECTROENCEPHALOGRAPHY TRACINGS

Normal *(Top: Right temporal; Bottom: Parietal-occipital)*

Petit mal epilepsy *(Spikes and waves, 3/second)*

Grand mal epilepsy *(Multiple high-voltage spiked waves)*

Right temporal lobe epilepsy *(Focal spiked waves)*

for artifacts) which may indicate brain death.

Post-test care

☐ Review with the doctor the reinstatement of anticonvulsant medication or other drugs that were withheld before the test.

☐ Carefully observe the patient for seizure activity.

☐ Help the patient remove electrode paste from his hair with acetone.

☐ If the patient received a sedative be-

fore the test, take safety precautions, such as raising the side rails.

Interfering factors

☐ Excessive artifacts may be caused by extraneous electrical activity; head, body, eye, or tongue movement; and muscular contractions.

☐ Anticonvulsants, tranquilizers, barbiturates, and other sedatives interfere with the accurate determination of test results.

☐ Acute drug intoxication or severe hypothermia resulting in loss of consciousness causes a flat EEG.

KATHY A. HAUSMAN, RN, MS

Evoked Potential Studies

These tests evaluate the integrity of visual, somatosensory, and auditory nerve pathways by measuring evoked potentials—the brain's electrical response to stimulation of the sense organs or peripheral nerves. Evoked potentials are recorded as electronic impulses by surface electrodes attached to the scalp and to the skin over various peripheral sensory nerves. A computer extracts these low-amplitude impulses from background brainwave activity and averages the signals from repeated stimuli.

Three types of responses are measured. Visual evoked potentials, *produced by exposing the eye to a rapidly reversing checkerboard pattern, help evaluate demyelinating disease, traumatic injury, and puzzling visual complaints.* Somatosensory evoked potentials, *produced by electrically stimulating a peripheral sensory nerve, help diagnose peripheral nerve disease and locate brain and spinal cord lesions.* Auditory brain stem evoked potentials, *produced by delivering clicks to the ear, help locate auditory lesions and evaluate brain stem integrity. (For a complete discussion of auditory brain stem evoked potentials, see* SITE OF LESION TESTS, *page 605.)*

Evoked potential studies are also useful for monitoring comatose patients and patients under anesthesia, monitoring spinal cord function during spinal cord surgery, and evaluating neurologic function in infants whose sensory systems normally can't be adequately assessed.

Purpose
□ To aid diagnosis of nervous system le-

sions and abnormalities
□ To assess neurologic function.

Patient preparation
Explain to the patient that this group of tests measures the electrical activity of his nervous system. Explain who will perform the procedure and where, and that it takes 45 to 60 minutes.

Tell the patient that he'll be positioned in a reclining chair or on a bed. If visual evoked potentials will be measured, tell him that electrodes will be attached to his scalp; if somatosensory evoked potentials will be measured, electrodes will be placed on his scalp, neck, lower back, wrist, knee, and ankle.

Assure the patient that the electrodes won't hurt him; encourage him to relax, since tension can affect neurologic function and interfere with test results. Have him remove all jewelry.

Equipment
Evoked potential unit/auditory, visual, or tactile stimuli/amplifier/oscilloscope tube face/magnetic tape.

Procedure
The patient is positioned in a reclining chair or on a bed and is instructed to relax and remain still.

To measure *visual evoked potentials,* electrodes are attached to the patient's scalp at occipital, parietal, and vertex locations; a reference electrode is placed on the midfrontal area or on the ear. The patient is positioned 1 meter from the pattern-shift stimulator—either an electronic stimulator, which displays the pattern on a television screen or uses an array of light-emitting diodes; or a mechanical stimulator, which projects the pattern from a slide projector onto a translucent screen. One eye is occluded, and the patient is instructed to fix his gaze on a dot in the center of the screen. A checkerboard pattern is projected and then rapidly reversed or shifted 100 times, once or twice per second. A computer amplifies and averages the brain's response to each stimulus, and the results are plotted as a waveform. The procedure is repeated for the other eye.

To measure *somatosensory evoked potentials,* electrodes are attached to the patient's skin over somatosensory pathways to stimulate peripheral nerves. Electrode sites usually include the wrist, knee, and ankle. Recording electrodes are placed on the scalp over the sensory cortex of the hemisphere opposite the limb to be stimulated. Additional electrodes may be placed at Erb's point (above the clavicle overlying the brachial plexus) and at the second cervical vertebra for upper-limb stimulation; and over the lower lumbar vertebrae for lower-limb stimulation. Midfrontal or noncephalic electrodes are placed for reference.

A painless electrical shock is delivered to the peripheral nerve through the stimulating electrode. The intensity of the shock is adjusted to produce a minor muscle response, such as a thumb twitch upon median nerve stimulation at the wrist. The shock is delivered at least 500 times, at a rate of five per second. A computer measures and averages the time it takes for the electrical current to reach the cortex; the results, expressed in milliseconds (msec), are recorded as waveforms. The test is repeated once to verify results; then the electrodes are repositioned and the entire procedure is repeated for the other side.

Findings

Visual evoked potentials: On the waveform, the most significant wave is P100, a positive wave appearing about 100 msec after the pattern-shift stimulus is applied. The most clinically significant measurements are absolute P100 latency (the time between stimulus application and peaking of the P100 wave) and the difference between the P100 latencies of each eye. Because many physical and technical factors affect P100 latency, normal results vary greatly between laboratories and patients. The chart on page 758 shows a typical response.

Somatosensory evoked potentials: The waveforms obtained vary, depending on locations of the stimulating and recording electrodes. The positive and negative peaks are labeled in sequence, based on normal time of appearance. For example, N19 is a negative peak normally recorded 19 msec after application of the stimulus. Each wave peak arises from a discrete location: N19 is generated mainly from the thalamus, P22 from the parietal sensory cortex, and so on. Interwave latencies (time between waves), rather than absolute latencies, are used as a basis for clinical interpretation. Latency differences between sides are significant. Normal waveforms for upper and lower limbs appear in the chart on page 758.

Implications of results

Visual evoked potentials: Generally, abnormal (extended) P100 latencies confined to one eye indicate a visual pathway lesion anterior to the optic chiasm. A lesion posterior to the optic chiasm usually doesn't produce abnormal P100 latencies: because each eye projects to both occipital lobes, the unaffected pathway transmits sufficient impulses to produce a normal latency response.

Bilateral abnormal P100 latencies have been found in patients with multiple sclerosis (see the waveform on page 758), optic neuritis, retinopathies, amblyopias (although abnormal latencies don't correlate well with impaired visual acuity), spinocerebellar degeneration, adrenoleukodystrophy, sarcoidosis, Parkinson's disease, and Huntington's chorea.

Somatosensory evoked potentials: Because somatosensory evoked potential components are assumed to be linked in series, an abnormal interwave latency indicates a conduction defect between the generators of the two peaks involved. This often enables precise location of a neurologic lesion.

Abnormal upper-limb interwave latencies may indicate cervical spondylosis, intracerebral lesions, or sensorimotor neuropathies. Abnormalities in the lower limb demonstrate peripheral nerve and root lesions, such as those in Guillain-Barré syndrome, compressive myelopathies, multiple sclerosis (see the

VISUAL AND SOMATOSENSORY EVOKED POTENTIALS

Pattern-shift evoked potentials: In this test, visual neural impulses are recorded as they travel along the pathway from the eye to the occipital cortex. Wave P100 is the most significant component of the resultant waveform—normal P100 latency is approximately 100 msec after the application of visual stimulus, as shown in the top diagram. Increased P100 latency, shown in the bottom diagram, is an abnormal finding indicating a lesion along the visual pathway.

Normal tracing

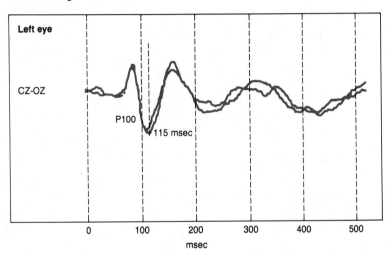

Tracing in multiple sclerosis

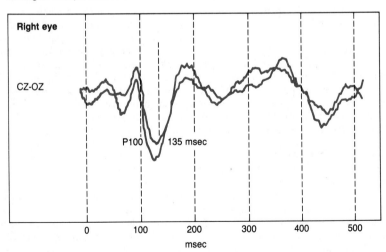

CZ = vertex   OZ = midocciput

Somatosensory evoked potentials: These tests measure the conduction time of an electrical impulse traveling along a somatosensory pathway to the cortex. Interwave latency is the most significant component of the resultant waveform. On the set of upper- and lower-limb tracings shown below, the top tracings represent normal interwave latencies; the bottom tracings, typical abnormal latencies found in a patient with multiple sclerosis. Because of the close correlation between waveforms and the anatomy of somatosensory pathways, such tracings allow precise localization of lesions that produce conduction defects.

Upper limb

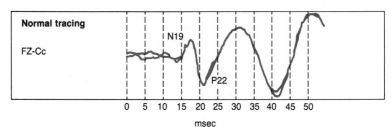

FZ = midfrontal   Cc = sensoparietal cortex contralateral to stimulated limb

Lower limb

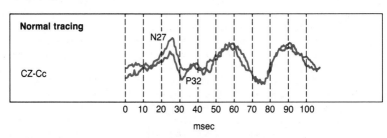

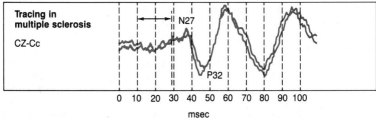

CZ = vertex   Cc = sensoparietal cortex contralateral to stimulated limb

chart on pages 758 and 759), transverse myelitis, and traumatic spinal cord injury.

Information from evoked potential studies is useful but insufficient to confirm a specific diagnosis. Test data must be interpreted in light of clinical information.

Post-test care
None.

Interfering factors
□ Incorrect placement of electrodes or equipment failure can alter test results.
□ Patient tension or failure to cooperate can impair the accuracy of test results.
□ Extremely poor visual acuity can hinder accurate determination of visual evoked potentials.

ROGER M. MORRELL, MD, PhD

Computed Tomography of the Spine

Much more versatile than conventional radiography, computed tomography (CT) of the spine provides detailed high-resolution images in the cross-sectional, longitudinal, sagittal, and lateral planes. Multiple X-ray beams from a computerized body scanner are directed at the spine from different angles; these pass through the body and strike radiation detectors, producing electrical impulses. A computer then converts these impulses into digital information, which is displayed as a three-dimensional image on a video monitor. Storage of the digital information allows electronic recreation and manipulation of the image, creating a permanent record of the images to enable reexamination without repeating the procedure.

Two variations of spinal CT further expand the procedure's diagnostic capabilities. Contrast-enhanced CT accen-tuates spinal vasculature and highlights even subtle differences in tissue density. Air CT, which involves removing a small amount of cerebrospinal fluid (CSF) and injecting air via lumbar puncture, intensifies the contrast between the subarachnoid space and surrounding tissue.

Purpose
□ To diagnose spinal lesions and abnormalities
□ To monitor the effects of spinal surgery or therapy.

Patient preparation
Explain to the patient that this procedure allows visualization of his spine. Unless contrast enhancement is ordered, tell him that he needn't restrict food or fluids. (If contrast enhancement is ordered, instruct him to fast for 4 hours before the test.) Tell him that a series of X-rays will be taken of his spine. Explain who will perform the procedure and where and that the test takes 30 to 60 minutes. Reassure him that the procedure is painless.

Explain to the patient that he'll be positioned on an X-ray table inside a CT body scanning unit and asked to lie still; the computer-controlled scanner will revolve around him taking multiple X-ray exposures. Stress that he should lie as still as possible when asked to do so because movement during the procedure may cause distorted images. If contrast dye is used, tell him that he may feel flushed and warm and may experience a transient headache, a salty taste, and nausea or vomiting after injection of the contrast dye. Reassure him that these effects are normal.

Instruct the patient to wear a radiologic examining gown and to remove all metal objects and jewelry that may appear in the X-ray field. Make sure the patient or a responsible family member has signed an appropriate consent form. Check the patient's history for hypersensitivity reactions to iodine, shellfish, or contrast media. If such reactions have occurred, notify the doctor, who may order prophylactic medications or choose not to use contrast enhancement.

If the patient appears restless or apprehensive about the procedure, notify the doctor, who may prescribe a mild sedative.

Equipment
Computerized body scanner/oscilloscope/recording equipment/contrast medium, as ordered (meglumine iothalamate or sodium diatrizoate)/60-ml syringe/19G to 20G needle/tourniquet.

Procedure
The patient is placed in a supine position on a radiographic table and is told to lie as still as possible. The table is then slid into the circular opening of the body CT scanner. The scanner revolves around the patient, taking radiographs at preselected intervals.

After the first set of radiographs is taken, the patient is removed from the scanner and contrast medium is administered, if ordered. Usually, 50 to 100 ml of contrast dye is injected. Observe the patient for signs and symptoms of a hypersensitivity reaction—pruritus, rash, and respiratory difficulty—for 30 minutes after the contrast dye has been injected.

After dye injection, the patient is moved back into the scanner, and another series of radiographs is taken. The images obtained from the scan are displayed on a video monitor during the procedure and stored on magnetic tape to create a permanent record for subsequent study.

Precautions
☐ Body CT scanning with contrast enhancement is contraindicated in patients who are hypersensitive to iodine, shellfish, or contrast media used in radiographic studies.
☐ Some patients may experience strong feelings of claustrophobia or anxiety when inside the body CT scanner. For such patients, the doctor may order administration of a mild sedative to help reduce anxiety.

Findings
In the CT image, spinal tissue appears black, white, or gray, depending on its density. Vertebrae, the densest tissues, are white; soft tissues appear in shades of gray; CSF is black.

Implications of results
By highlighting areas of altered density and depicting structural malformation, CT scanning can reveal all types of spinal lesions and abnormalities. It's particularly useful in detecting and localizing tumors, which appear as masses varying in density. Measuring this density and noting the configuration and location relative to the spinal cord can often identify the type of tumor. For example, a neurinoma (Schwannoma) appears as a spherical mass dorsal to the cord. A darker, wider mass lying more laterally or ventrally to the cord may be a meningioma.

CT also reveals degenerative processes and structural changes in detail. Herniated nucleus pulposus shows as an obvious herniation of disk material with unilateral or bilateral nerve root compression; if the herniation is midline, spinal cord compression will be evident. Cervical spondylosis shows as cervical cord compression due to bony hypertrophy of the cervical spine; lumbar stenosis as hypertrophy of the lumbar vertebrae, causing cord compression by decreasing space within the spinal column. Facet disorders show as soft-tissue changes, bony overgrowth, and spurring of the vertebrae, which result in nerve root compression. Fluid-filled arachnoidal and other paraspinal cysts show as dark masses displacing the spinal cord. Vascular malformations, evident after contrast enhancement, show as masses or clusters, usually on the dorsal aspect of the spinal cord.

Congenital spinal malformations such as meningocele, myelocele, and spina bifida show as abnormally large, dark gaps between the white vertebrae.

Post-test care
None, if the procedure was done without

contrast enhancement. After testing with contrast enhancement, observe the patient for residual effects, such as headache, nausea, and vomiting; inform the patient that he may resume his usual diet withheld before administration of contrast dye.

Interfering factors
☐ Excessive movement by the patient during the scanning procedure may create artifact, making the images difficult to interpret.
☐ Radiopaque objects not removed from the X-ray field may produce unclear images.

ROGER M. MORRELL, MD, PhD

Lumbar, Thoracic, and Cervical Thermography

Using infrared sensors, thermography measures and compares the heat emitted from two adjacent areas of skin surface. Irritation of a nerve root may produce an abnormal heat pattern along the course of its dermatome, the area of skin supplied with afferent fibers by the nerve root; thermography can often graphically demonstrate such changes. Lumbar, thoracic, and cervical thermography, specifically, can thus be helpful in evaluating sensory nerve irritation or significant soft tissue injury. The usual clinical indication for this test is back pain—often severe and possibly chronic—such as chronic lumbar pain. Thermography complements tests such as electromyography, myelography, and CT scans.

Purpose
To evaluate sensory nerve irritation or significant soft tissue injury.

Patient preparation
Explain to the patient that this test helps determine the cause of his back pain. Instruct him not to smoke for several hours before the test. Tell him who will perform the test and where, and that the procedure takes about 1½ hours. Reassure the patient that thermography is painless and doesn't expose him to radiation.

The patient should not undergo physical therapy or electromyography on the same day that thermography is to be performed.

Equipment
Electronic or liquid crystal thermography apparatus/hair dryer/spray bottle containing alcohol (if electronic apparatus is used)/oscilloscope/Polaroid camera/temperature reference.

Procedure
After the patient undresses, his back is cooled with room-temperature water (68° F.) [20° C.], and is blown dry with cool air from the hair dryer. The patient may then relax for 10 to 15 minutes before the procedure begins.

A lumbar examination includes scans of the low back, the buttocks, and both legs. For thoracic examination, only the posterior chest is scanned. For cervical examination, thermograms of the back of the neck, the back of the shoulders, and both arms are taken.

Findings
Normal thermograms show diffused heat patterns with relative left-right symmetry.

Implications of results
A difference of 1° C. between 25% of the surface area on one side of the spine and the other side is abnormal. If the abnormality follows the course of a specific dermatome, sensory nerve irritation may exist at this level. Soft tissue injuries appear as local abnormalities.

To verify test results, thermography is repeated three times at 20-minute intervals. An abnormality due to organic disease should be reproducible on the thermogram at any given time.

LUMBAR THERMOGRAMS

The thermograms below are pre- and postoperative studies of a patient with a herniated intervertebral lumbar disk which is pressing on the right fifth lumbar nerve root. The black areas represent heat. In the preoperative study of the lower back (A), the arrows point to increased heat emission from the lower portion of the lumbar stripe. In the postoperative study (three months after surgery) of the same view (B), this increase in heat emission is diffused.

In the preoperative study of the back of the thighs (C), a cold stripe—white blush along the outer back aspect of the right thigh—represents absence of heat emission. The cold stripe results from constriction of the very fine skin capillary blood vessels that accompany the nerve endings. The postoperative study of the same view (D) shows that the blush is gone and that the heat emission of both thighs is relatively symmetrical.

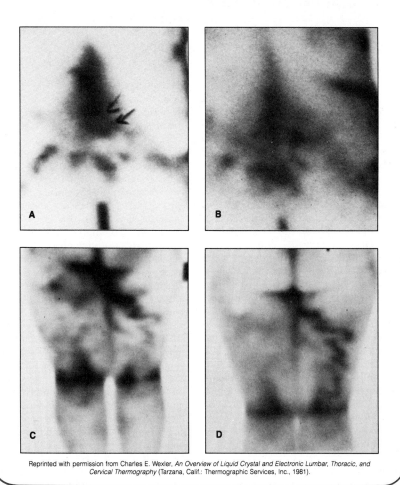

Reprinted with permission from Charles E. Wexler, *An Overview of Liquid Crystal and Electronic Lumbar, Thoracic, and Cervical Thermography* (Tarzana, Calif.: Thermographic Services, Inc., 1981).

Post-test care

Patient may resume smoking and therapies withheld before thermography.

Interfering factors

□ Smoking affects vascular distribution, producing abnormalities that reflect impaired circulation and do not follow the course of sensory dermatomes.

☐ Patient history of fractures, surgery, or grossly asymmetrical varicose veins may cause abnormal test results.

☐ Direct or indirect drafts on the patient interfere with test results.

CHARLES E. WEXLER, MD

Oculoplethysmography

An important cerebrovascular test, oculoplethysmography (OPG) is a noninvasive procedure that indirectly measures blood flow in the ophthalmic artery. Since the ophthalmic artery is the first major branch of the internal carotid artery, its blood flow accurately reflects carotid blood flow and ultimately that of cerebral circulation. Two techniques are used for this test. In OPG, pulse arrival times in the eyes and ears are measured and compared to detect carotid occlusive disease. In ocular pneumoplethysmography (OPG-Gee), ophthalmic artery pressures are indirectly measured and compared with the higher brachial pressure and with each other.

Indications for both oculoplethysmographic techniques include symptoms of transient ischemic attacks, asymptomatic carotid bruits, and nonhemispheric neurologic symptoms, such as dizziness, ataxia, or syncope. This test may also be performed as a follow-up procedure after carotid endarterectomy or with carotid phonoangiography or carotid imaging. If indicated, it may be followed by cerebral angiography.

Purpose

☐ To aid detection and evaluation of carotid occlusive disease.

Patient preparation

Explain to the patient that this test evaluates carotid artery function. Inform him he needn't restrict food or fluids. Tell him who will perform the test and where, and that the procedure takes only a few minutes.

Warn the patient that his eyes may burn slightly after the eyedrops are instilled. If OPG-Gee is scheduled, warn him that he may experience transient loss of vision when suction is applied to the eyes. Instruct him not to blink or move during the procedure. Obviously, if he wears contact lenses, tell him to remove them before the test. Patients with glaucoma may take their usual medications and eyedrops.

Equipment

Oculoplethysmograph or oculopneumoplethysmograph/anesthetic eyedrops (such as proparacaine 0.5%)/tissues.

Procedure

OPG: Anesthetic eyedrops are instilled to minimize patient discomfort during the test. Small photoelectric cells are attached to the earlobes; these cells can detect blood flow to the ear through the *external* carotid artery. Tracings for both ears are taken and compared, but only right ear tracings are compared with the eyes. (Tracings for the ears should be the same; if they're not, this is considered during interpretation of test results.)

Eyecups resembling contact lenses are applied to the corneas and are held in place with light suction (40 to 50 mm Hg). Tracings of the pulsations within each eye are compared with each other and with tracings for the right ear.

OPG-Gee: Anesthetic eyedrops are instilled, as for OPG, and eyecups like those used in OPG are attached to the *scleras* of the eyes. A vacuum of 300 mm Hg is applied to each eye, corresponding to a mean pressure of 100 mm Hg in the ophthalmic artery, and gradually released. With the application of suction, the pulse in both eyes disappears; with the gradual release of suction, both pulses should return simultaneously. Pulse arrival times are converted to ophthalmic artery pressures, and then compared. Both brachial pressures are taken. The higher systolic pressure is then compared with the ophthalmic artery pressures.

CAROTID PHONOANGIOGRAPHY

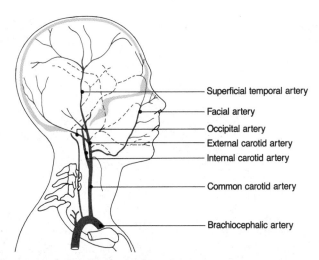

- Superficial temporal artery
- Facial artery
- Occipital artery
- External carotid artery
- Internal carotid artery
- Common carotid artery
- Brachiocephalic artery

An often valuable complement to oculoplethysmography, carotid phonoangiography graphically records the intensity of carotid bruits during systolic and diastolic phases. It thus helps identify the presence, site, and severity of carotid artery occlusive disease.

For this test, the patient assumes a supine position and holds his breath while a transducer is placed at several sites along the carotid artery. Soundings are made directly over the clavicle (common carotid artery), midway up the neck (carotid bifurcation), and directly below the mandible (internal carotid artery). Oscillographic recordings are obtained and stored on both Polaroid film and magnetic tape for later study.

Absence of bruits generally indicates an absence of significant carotid artery disease. However, bruits may also be absent when stenosis approaches total occlusion. Bruits heard at all three sites, but loudest over the clavicle, usually originate in the aortic arch or within the heart. Blood flow in the carotid artery itself is unobstructed. Bruits heard over the carotid bifurcation and internal carotid sites, but louder over the latter, indicate turbulent blood flow within the internal carotid artery and the likely presence of a lesion of greater than 40% occlusion.

Carotid phonoangiography is a quick test and relatively simple to perform, but it's less sensitive and less specific than other noninvasive techniques, such as carotid imaging with Doppler ultrasound. Nevertheless, this test is approximately 85% accurate in detecting a stenosis of the carotid artery of more than 40%.

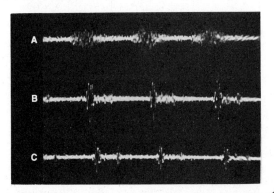

This is a phonoangiogram of a patient with an internal carotid artery bruit. Bruit is loudest directly below the mandible (A), present midway up the neck (B), and absent directly over the clavicle (C).

OPG EXAMINATION AND TRACINGS

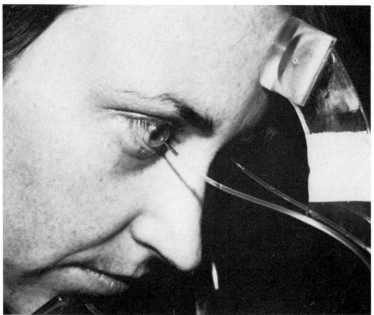

The patient shown here is undergoing OPG. The eyecups on her corneas detect ocular pulsations, which are compared with each other and with the blood flow in the ear. Blood flow in the ear is detected by a small photoelectric cell (not shown).

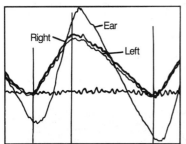 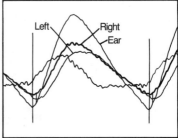

The OPG tracing on the left is normal, showing simultaneous pulsations in the right and left eyes and in the right ear. The differential waveform of ocular pulses (horizontal waveform), which amplifies pulse differences, and the vertical lines drawn on valleys and peaks of pulses to indicate pulse delays, confirm simultaneous pulsation. The OPG tracing on the right is abnormal; the left-eye pulsation (see vertical lines) arrives later than the other two pulsations, indicating a left internal carotid artery stenosis. Note the elevation of the differential waveform.

Precautions

☐ Oculoplethysmography is contraindicated in patients who have had recent eye surgery (within 2 to 6 months), enucleation, or a history of retinal detachment or lens implantation, or who are hypersensitive to the local anesthetic. Because of the risk of scleral hematoma or erythema, OPG-Gee is contraindicated in patients receiving anticoagulant therapy.

□ To limit the risk of corneal abrasions, both techniques must be performed only by specially trained personnel.

Findings

OPG: All pulses should occur simultaneously.

OPG-Gee: The difference between ophthalmic artery pressures should be less than 5 mm Hg. Ophthalmic artery pressure divided by the higher brachial systolic pressure should be more than 0.67.

Implications of results

OPG: Carotid occlusive disease reduces the rate of blood flow during systole and delays the arrival of a pulse in the ipsilateral eye or ear. When all pulses are compared, any delay can be measured and the degree of carotid artery stenosis estimated as mild, moderate, or severe. Although the length of the delay is related to the degree of stenosis, this test only estimates the extent of stenosis and can't give an exact percentage.

OPG-Gee: A difference between ophthalmic artery pressures of more than 5 mm Hg suggests the presence of carotid occlusive disease on the side with the lower pressure. A ratio between the ophthalmic artery pressure and the higher brachial systolic pressure of less than 0.67 reinforces this finding. In other words, the ratio is related to the degree of stenosis. The lower the ratio, the more severe the stenosis. As in OPG, OPG-Gee only estimates the degree of stenosis present, and angiography may be necessary for precise evaluation.

Post-test care

□ To prevent corneal abrasions, instruct the patient not to rub his eyes for 2 hours after the test. Observe for symptoms of corneal abrasion, such as pain or photophobia, and report them to the doctor.

□ Mild burning as the eyedrops wear off is normal. Report severe burning.

□ If the patient wears contact lenses, instruct him not to reinsert them for about 2 hours after OPG, to allow the effect of the anesthetic drops to wear off.

Interfering factors

□ In patients with hypertension, OPG-Gee test results may be more difficult to interpret due to elevated ophthalmic artery pressures.

□ Constant blinking or nystagmus may cause an artifact, making the tracings difficult to interpret.

□ Severe cardiac dysrhythmias may alter test results.

DONNA R. BLACKBURN, RN
LINDA K. PETERSON, RN

INVASIVE TESTS

Radionuclide Scan of the Brain

This test uses a gamma scintillation camera or rectilinear scanner to provide images of the brain after an I.V. injection of a radionuclide. The scintillation camera or scanner detects rays emitted by the radionuclide—usually technetium-99m pertechnetate (^{99m}Tc)—and converts them into images, which are then displayed on an oscilloscope screen. Normally, the radionuclide can't permeate the blood-brain barrier. However, if pathologic changes have destroyed the barrier, the radionuclide may concentrate in the abnormal area. Immediately after injection of the radionuclide, cerebral blood flow can also be evaluated. Radionuclide scan of the brain is valuable in the early detection of cerebritis and subdural hematomas; however, the test has largely been replaced by the more versatile and precise computed tomography.

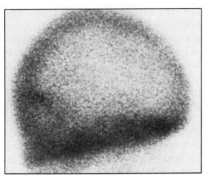

This lateral view of a normal radionuclide scan shows characteristic uptake of 99 ^{m}Tc around the brain. An intact blood-brain barrier prevents uptake by normal brain tissue.

Purpose

□ To detect an intracranial mass or vascular lesion

□ To locate areas of ischemia, cerebral infarction, and intracerebral hemorrhage

□ To evaluate the course of certain lesions postoperatively and during chemotherapy.

Patient preparation

Explain to the patient that this test helps detect abnormalities in the brain. Inform him he needn't restrict food or fluids. Tell him he'll receive an injection of a radioactive drug and that films will be taken of his brain at various intervals. Advise him who will perform the test and where, and that 1 to 1½ hours are required for each series of films.

Tell the patient he may feel a slight burning sensation at the injection site. Describe the scanning machine, and explain that it will move back and forth close to his head and may make some noise. Reassure him that the procedure is painless, and that the radiation poses no danger to him or his visitors and should be cleared from his body within 6 hours. Instruct the patient to remove all metal or jewelry in the X-ray field.

Equipment

Gamma scintillation camera or rectilinear scanner/oscilloscope/radiopharma-ceutical/tourniquet/70% alcohol, or povidone-iodine solution/19G or 21G sterile needle/20-ml syringe.

Procedure

If a cerebral blood flow study has been ordered, a bolus of ^{99m}Tc is injected into the antecubital fossa vein while the patient lies supine on a radiographic table. Rapid-sequence images are taken immediately to follow passage of the radionuclide through the carotid arteries and cerebral hemispheres. Although the images displayed on the oscilloscope screen are inferior by arteriographic standards, they usually show normal blood flow. Later, static scans can identify pathologic tissue, if the blood-brain barrier has been broken. The radionuclide may be allowed to circulate for at least 1 hour before static imaging is performed; the scanner moves back and forth, taking anteroposterior and lateral views at specific intervals. For a clearer picture of radionuclide accumulation, additional imaging is performed 3 or 4 hours after injection.

Findings

A negative, or normal, radionuclide scan reveals a barrier between the bloodstream and brain substance. Certain regions of bone and areas with increased blood supply may exhibit increased uptake of the radionuclide, which must be carefully evaluated. Minimal background uptake occurs in each cerebral hemisphere. Again, the amount signifying an abnormality must be carefully interpreted by an experienced examiner.

Implications of results

Results are interpreted by the doctor, radiologist, or hospital specialist in nuclear medicine, and must be correlated with the patient's clinical condition. For example, a negative scan, in the presence of clinical features indicating an abnormality, necessitates further testing. Usually, the scan can detect lesions, such as malignant gliomas, meningiomas, metastases, and abscesses, since the radionuclide readily accumulates in the presence of such abnormalities. However, the scan is less accurate for certain benign or low-grade malignant tumors, since the radionuclide doesn't accumulate as readily. The scan can detect cerebral infarctions and arteriovenous malformations with variable accuracy, depending on the extent of the lesion and the interim after onset.

Post-test care
If a hematoma develops at the injection site, warm soaks may ease discomfort and aid resolution.

Interfering factors
□ Significant head movement by the patient distorts the image.
□ Failure to remove radiopaque objects from the X-ray field may produce unclear images.

KATHY A. HAUSMAN, RN, MS

Cerebral Angiography

Cerebral angiography allows radiographic examination of the cerebral vasculature after injection of a contrast medium. Possible injection sites include the femoral, carotid, or brachial arteries; the femoral artery is used most often, because it allows visualization of four vessels (the carotid and the vertebral arteries). The usual clinical indication for this test is a suspected abnormality of the cerebral vasculature, often as suggested by intracranial computed tomography or a radionuclide scan of the brain.

Purpose
□ To detect cerebrovascular abnormalities, such as aneurysm or arteriovenous malformation, thrombosis, narrowing, or occlusion
□ To study vascular displacement caused by tumor, hematoma, edema, herniation, arterial spasm, increased intracranial pressure (ICP), or hydrocephalus

□ To locate clips applied to blood vessels during surgery and to evaluate the postoperative status of such vessels.

Patient preparation
Explain to the patient that this test shows blood circulation in the brain. Instruct him to fast for 8 to 10 hours before the test is scheduled to begin. Tell him who will perform the test and where, and that it takes about 2 hours.

Instruct the patient to wear a hospital gown and to remove jewelry, dentures, hairpins, and other radiopaque objects in the X-ray field. If ordered, administer a sedative and anticholinergic 30 to 45 minutes before the test. Make sure the patient voids before leaving his room.

Tell the patient he'll be positioned on an X-ray table, with his head immobilized, and will be asked to lie still. Tell him a local anesthetic will be administered. (Some patients—especially children—may receive a general anesthetic.) Explain that he'll probably feel a transient burning sensation as the contrast medium is injected, and that he may feel flushed and warm, and experience a transient headache, a salty taste, or nausea and vomiting after injection of the "dye."

Make sure the patient or responsible member of the family has signed a consent form. Check the patient's history for hypersensitivity to iodine, iodine-containing substances (such as shellfish), or other contrast media. Notify the doctor of any hypersensitivities; he may order prophylactic medications or may choose not to perform the test.

Equipment
Contrast medium/automatic contrast injector/X-ray machine, with rapid biplane cassette changer/arterial needles: 18G or 19G, 2½" needle for adults; 20G, 1½" needle for children/femoral arterial catheters for femoral injection.

Procedure
The patient is placed in a supine position on a radiographic table, and the injection site (femoral, carotid, or brachial

artery) is shaved. The patient is then instructed to lie still, with his arms at his sides. The skin is cleansed with alcohol and povidone-iodine, and the local anesthetic is injected. The artery is then punctured with the appropriate needle and catheterized. If the *femoral approach* is used, a catheter is threaded up to the aortic arch. If the *carotid artery* is to be used as the injection site, the patient's neck is hyperextended, and a rolled-up towel or sandbag is placed under his shoulders. His head is then immobilized with a restraint or tape. If the *brachial artery* (least common) is to be used, a blood pressure cuff is placed distal to the puncture site and inflated before injection, to prevent the contrast medium from flowing into the forearm and hand.

After placement of the needle (or catheter) is verified by radiography or fluoroscopy, the contrast medium is injected. The patient is observed for a reaction, such as hives, flushing, and laryngeal stridor. A first series of lateral and anteroposterior radiographs is taken, developed, and reviewed. Depending on the results of this initial series, more contrast medium may be injected and another series of radiographs taken. Arterial catheter patency is maintained by continuous or periodic flushing with normal saline or heparin solution. Vital and neurologic signs are monitored throughout the test.

When an acceptable series of radiographs have been obtained, the needle (or catheter) is withdrawn, and firm pressure is applied to the puncture site for 15 minutes. The patient is observed for bleeding, distal pulses are checked, and a pressure bandage applied.

Precautions

Cerebral angiography is contraindicated in patients with hepatic, renal, or thyroid disease, or with hypersensitivity to iodine or contrast media.

Findings

During the arterial phase of perfusion, the contrast medium fills and opacifies superficial and deep arteries and arterioles; it opacifies superficial and deep veins during the venous phase. The finding of apparently normal (symmetrical) cerebral vasculature, however, must be correlated with the patient's history and clinical status.

Implications of results

Changes in the caliber of vessel lumina suggest vascular disease, possibly due to spasms, plaques, fistulas, arteriovenous malformation, or arteriosclerosis. Diminished blood flow to vessels may be related to increased ICP.

Vessel displacement may reflect the presence and size of a tumor, areas of edema, or obstruction of the CSF pathway. Cerebral angiography may also show circulation within a tumor, often giving precise information on the tumor's position and nature. Meningeal blood supply originating in the external carotid artery may indicate an extracerebral tumor but usually designates a meningioma. Although such a tumor may arise outside the brain substance, it may still be within the cerebral hemisphere.

Post-test care

☐ Enforce bed rest for 12 to 24 hours, and provide pain medication, as ordered. Monitor vital signs and neurologic status for 24 hours—every hour for the first 4 hours, then every 4 hours.

☐ Check the puncture site for signs of extravasation, such as redness and swelling. To ease the patient's discomfort and minimize swelling, apply an ice bag to the site. If bleeding occurs, apply firm pressure to the puncture site.

☐ If the *femoral approach* was used, keep the affected leg straight for at least 12 hours, and routinely check pulses distal to the site (dorsalis pedis and popliteal). Check the temperature, color, and tactile sensations of the affected leg, since thrombosis or hematoma can occlude blood flow. Extravasation can also block blood flow by exerting pressure on the artery.

NORMAL AND ABNORMAL ANGIOGRAMS

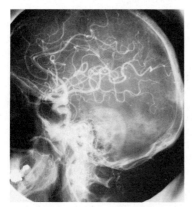 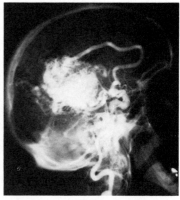

The cerebral angiogram on the left is a normal view. The cerebral angiogram on the right shows occluded vasculature caused by a large arterovenous malformation.

□ If a *carotid artery* was used as the injection site, watch for dysphagia or respiratory distress, which can result from extravasation. Also, watch for disorientation and weakness or numbness in the extremities (signs of thrombosis or hematoma), and for arterial spasms that produce symptoms of transient ischemic attacks. Notify the doctor if abnormal signs develop.

□ If the *brachial approach* was used, immobilize the arm for at least 12 hours, and routinely check the radial pulse. Place a sign above the patient's bed warning personnel against taking blood pressure readings from the affected arm. Observe the arm and hand, noting any change in color, temperature, or tactile sensations. If it becomes pale, cool, or numb, notify the doctor.

□ The patient may resume usual diet.

Interfering factors

□ Head movement during the test affects the clarity of the radiographs and interferes with accurate interpretation.

□ Radiopaque objects in the X-ray field may produce unclear images.

KATHY A. HAUSMAN, RN, MS

Digital Subtraction Angiography

Digital subtraction angiography (DSA) is a sophisticated radiographic technique that uses video equipment and computer-assisted image enhancement to examine the vascular systems. As in conventional angiography, X-ray images are obtained after injection of a contrast medium. However, unlike conventional angiography, in which images of bone and soft tissue often obscure vascular detail, DSA provides a better, high-contrast view of blood vessels, without interfering images or shadows.

This unique view is made possible by digital subtraction, in which fluoroscopic images are taken both before and after injection of a contrast medium. A computer converts these images into digital information, and then "subtracts" the first image from the second, eliminating most information (mainly bone and soft tissue) common to both images.

The result is a better image of the contrast-enhanced vasculature.

In addition to superior image quality, DSA has other important advantages over conventional angiography. Because the digital subtraction process allows intravenous, rather than intraarterial, injection of the contrast medium, DSA avoids one risk of conventional angiography—stroke—and reduces the pain and the discomfort associated with arterial catheterization.

Although DSA has been used to study peripheral and renal vascular disease, it's probably most useful in diagnosing cerebrovascular disorders such as carotid stenosis and occlusion, arteriovenous malformation, aneurysms, and vascular tumors. It's also useful in visualizing displacement of vasculature by other intracranial pathology or trauma and in detecting lesions often missed by CT scans, such as thrombosis of the superior sagittal sinus.

Purpose
□ To visualize extracranial and intracranial cerebral blood flow
□ To detect and evaluate cerebrovascular abnormalities
□ To aid postoperative evaluation of cerebrovascular surgery such as arterial grafts and endarterectomies.

Patient preparation
Explain to the patient that this test visualizes the blood vessels in his head. Instruct him to fast for 4 hours before the test, but inform him that he needn't restrict fluids. Explain that he'll receive an injection of a contrast medium, either by needle or through a venous catheter inserted in his arm, and that a series of X-rays will be taken of his head. Tell him who will perform the test and where, and that it takes 30 to 45 minutes.

Inform the patient that he'll be positioned on an X-ray table, with his head immobilized, and will be asked to lie still. (Some patients—especially children—may be given a sedative to prevent movement during the procedure.) Instruct him to remove all jewelry, dentures, and other radiopaque objects from the X-ray field. Tell him that he'll probably feel some transient pain from insertion of the needle or catheter, and that he may experience mild symptoms from injection of the contrast medium, such as a feeling of warmth, a headache, a metallic taste, and nausea or vomiting.

Make sure the patient or a responsible family member has signed a consent form. Check the patient's history for hypersensitivity to iodine, iodine-containing substances such as shellfish, and radiographic contrast media. Report any hypersensitivities to the doctor, who may order prophylactic medications or choose not to perform the test.

Equipment
I.V. equipment and 250 ml normal saline/contrast medium/automatic contrast medium injector/X-ray machine with biplane cassette changer/computer and video monitor/video recorder.

Procedure
The patient is placed in a supine position on an X-ray table and is told to lie still with his arms at his sides. After an initial series of fluoroscopic pictures *(mask images)* of his head is taken, the injection site—most commonly the antecubital basilic or cephalic vein—is shaved and cleansed with an antiseptic solution.

If catheterization is ordered, a local anesthetic is administered, a venipuncture is performed, and a catheter is inserted and advanced to the superior vena cava. After placement is verified by X-ray, I.V. lines from a bottle of normal saline solution and from an automatic contrast medium injector are connected. While the saline is administered, the injector delivers the contrast medium at a rate of about 14 ml/second.

If simple injection of the contrast medium is ordered, a bolus of 40 to 60 ml is administered intravenously by needle.

The patient's vital signs and neurologic status are monitored, and he's observed for signs of a hypersensitivity reaction, such as hives, flushing, and respiratory distress. After allowing time for the contrast medium to clear the pulmonary circulation and enter the cerebral vasculature, a second series of fluoroscopic images *(contrast images)* is taken. The computer digitizes the information received from both series and compares mask and contrast images, subtracting the information (images of bone and soft tissue) common to both. A detailed image of the contrast medium-filled vessels is displayed on a video monitor; the image may be stored on videotape or a videodisc for future reference.

Precautions

DSA may be contraindicated in patients with iodine or contrast media hypersensitivity or in those who have poor cardiac function; renal, hepatic, or thyroid disease; diabetes; or multiple myeloma.

Findings

The contrast medium should fill and opacify all superficial and deep arteries, arterioles, and veins, allowing visualization of normal cerebral vasculature. The digitized subtraction process may intensify areas that receive only contrast medium. However, conventional angiography provides a more detailed image of the carotids than DSA.

Implications of results

Vascular filling defects, seen as areas of increased vascular opacity, may indicate arteriovenous occlusion or stenosis, possibly due to vasospasm, vascular malformation or angiomas, arteriosclerosis, or cerebral embolism or thrombosis. Out-pouchings in vessel lumina may reflect cerebral aneurysms; such aneurysms frequently rupture, causing subarachnoid hemorrhage. Vessel displacement or vascular masses may indicate an intracranial tumor. DSA can clearly depict the vascular supply of some tumors, reflecting the tumor's position, size, and nature.

Post-test care

□ Because the contrast medium acts as a diuretic, encourage the patient to increase his fluid intake over the 24 hours after this test. Advise him that extra fluid intake will also speed excretion of the contrast medium. Monitor intake and output, as ordered.

□ Check the venipuncture site for signs of extravasation, such as redness or swelling. If bleeding occurs, apply firm pressure to the puncture site. If a hematoma develops, elevate the arm and apply warm soaks.

□ Observe the patient for a delayed hypersensitivity reaction to the contrast medium. Delayed reaction is rare but can occur up to 18 hours after the procedure.

□ Resume normal diet.

Interfering factors

□ Patient movement during the procedure may cause blurred images.

□ Radiopaque objects in the fluroscopic field may impair image clarity.

ROGER M. MORRELL, MD, PhD, FACP

Electromyography

Electromyography is the recording of the electrical activity of selected skeletal muscle groups at rest and during voluntary contraction. In this test, a needle electrode is inserted percutaneously into a muscle. The electrical discharge (or motor unit potential) of the muscle is then displayed and measured on an oscilloscope screen. Nerve conduction time—a separate procedure—is often measured simultaneously. Electromyography is a useful diagnostic technique for evaluating muscle disorders.

Purpose

□ To aid differentiation between primary muscle disorders, such as the muscular dystrophies, and those that are secondary

□ To help determine diseases characterized by central neuronal degeneration, such as amyotrophic lateral sclerosis

□ To aid diagnosis of neuromuscular disorders, such as myasthenia gravis.

NERVE CONDUCTION STUDIES

Nerve conduction studies aid diagnosis of peripheral nerve injuries and diseases affecting the peripheral nervous system, such as peripheral neuropathies. To measure nerve conduction time, a nerve is stimulated electrically through the skin and underlying tissues. The patient experiences mild electrical shock discomfort with each stimulation. At a known distance from the point of stimulation, a recording electrode detects the response from the stimulated nerve. The time between stimulation of the nerve and the detected response is measured on an oscilloscope. The speed of conduction along the nerve is then calculated by dividing the distance between the point of stimulation and the recording electrode by the time between stimulus and response. In peripheral nerve injuries and diseases such as peripheral neuropathies, nerve conduction time is abnormal.

Patient preparation

Explain to the patient that this test measures the electrical activity of his muscles. Normally, foods and fluids aren't withheld before this test, but some doctors may order restrictions on cigarettes, coffee, tea, or cola for 2 or 3 hours before the test. Tell the patient who will perform the test and where, and that it takes at least 1 hour.

The patient may wear a hospital gown for the test or any comfortable clothing that permits access to the muscles to be tested. Advise the patient that a needle will be inserted into selected muscles, and that he may experience some discomfort. Reassure him that side effects or complications rarely result from this test.

Make sure the patient or responsible member of the family has signed a consent form. Check the patient's history for medications that may interfere with test results. If the patient is receiving such medications, note this on the chart, and if ordered, withhold the medications.

Equipment

Electromyograph and recorder/needle electrodes/oscilloscope.

Procedure

The patient lies on a stretcher or bed, or sits on a chair, depending on the muscles to be tested. The arm or leg is positioned so the muscle to be tested is at rest. The needle electrodes are then quickly inserted into the selected muscle, and a metal plate is placed under the patient to serve as a reference electrode. The muscle's resulting electrical signal or motor unit potential, recorded during rest and contraction, is amplified 1,000,000 times and displayed on an oscilloscope screen. Photographs are taken of the display for a permanent record. Frequently, the lead wires of the recorder are attached to an audio-amplifier, so the fluctuation of voltage within the muscle can be heard.

Precautions

Electromyography is contraindicated in patients with bleeding disorders.

Findings

At rest, a normal muscle exhibits minimal electrical activity. During voluntary contraction, however, electrical activity increases markedly. A sustained contraction or one of increasing strength causes a rapid "train" of motor unit potentials that can be heard as a crescendo of sounds—similar to the sound of an outboard motor, over the audio-amplifier. At the same time, the oscilloscope screen displays a sequence of wave forms that vary in amplitude (height) and frequency. Wave forms that are close together indicate a high frequency; those that are far apart, a low frequency.

Implications of results

In primary muscle disease, such as the muscular dystrophies, motor unit potentials are short (low amplitude), with frequent, irregular discharges. In disorders such as amyotrophic lateral sclerosis (as well as in peripheral nerve disorders), motor unit potentials are isolated and irregular but show increased amplitude and duration. In myasthenia gravis, motor unit potentials initially may be normal but progressively diminish in amplitude with continuing contractions. The interpreter makes a distinction between wave forms that indicate a muscle disorder and those that indicate denervation. Findings must be correlated with the patient's history, clinical features, and results of other neurodiagnostic tests.

Post-test care
☐ If the patient experiences residual pain, apply warm compresses and administer analgesics, as ordered.
☐ Substances withheld before the test may be resumed, as ordered.

Interfering factors
☐ The patient's inability to comply with instructions during the test may invalidate results.
☐ Drugs that affect myoneural junctions, such as cholinergics, anticholinergics, and skeletal muscle relaxants, interfere with test results.

KATHY A. HAUSMAN, RN, MS

TESTING FOR QUECKENSTEDT'S SIGN

If an obstruction in the spinal subarachnoid space is suspected, you may be asked to assist with testing for Queckenstedt's sign. After inserting the spinal needle, the doctor takes an initial CSF pressure reading and then asks you to compress one or both of the patient's jugular veins with your fingers for 10 seconds. This obstructs blood flow from the cranium, increasing intracranial pressure and, in the absence of a subarachnoid block, causing CSF pressure to rise also. A partial subarachnoid block may cause CSF pressure to rise sluggishly; a complete block prevents it from rising at all.

Normally, the fluid column in the manometer should rise after 10 seconds of compression, then fall to the patient's initial pressure within 30 seconds. CSF pressure is recorded every 5 seconds from the time you begin compression until the pressure returns to baseline.

Because of the obvious danger of cerebellar tonsillar herniation and medullary compression, testing for Queckenstedt's sign is contraindicated in a patient with increased intracranial pressure.

Cerebrospinal Fluid Analysis

Cerebrospinal fluid (CSF), a clear substance that circulates in the subarachnoid space, has many vital functions. It protects the brain and spinal cord from injury and transports products of neurosecretion, cellular biosynthesis, and cellular metabolism through the CNS. For qualitative analysis, CSF is most commonly obtained by lumbar puncture (usually between the third and fourth lumbar vertebrae) and, occasionally, by cisternal or ventricular puncture. A sample of CSF for laboratory analysis is frequently obtained during other neurologic tests, including myelography and pneumoencephalography.

Purpose
☐ To measure CSF pressure as an aid in detecting obstruction of CSF circulation
☐ To aid diagnosis of viral or bacterial meningitis, and subarachnoid or intracranial hemorrhage, tumors, and brain abscesses
☐ To aid diagnosis of neurosyphilis and chronic CNS infections.

Patient preparation
Describe the procedure to the patient, and explain that this test analyzes the fluid within the spinal cord. Inform him he needn't restrict food or fluids. Tell him who will perform the procedure and where, and that it usually takes at least 15 minutes.

Advise the patient that a headache is the most common side effect of a lumbar puncture, but reassure him that his cooperation during the test minimizes such an effect. Make sure the patient or responsible member of the family has signed a consent form. If the patient is unusually anxious, assess his vital signs and notify the doctor.

CSF FINDINGS

TEST	NORMAL	ABNORMAL	IMPLICATIONS
Pressure	50 to 180 mm H_2O	Increase	Increased intracranial pressure due to hemorrhage, tumor, or edema caused by trauma
		Decrease	Spinal subarachnoid obstruction above puncture site
Appearance	Clear, colorless	Cloudy	Infection (elevated WBC count and protein, or many microorganisms)
		Xanthochromic or bloody	Subarachnoid, intracerebral, or intraventricular hemorrhage; spinal cord obstruction; traumatic tap (usually noted only in initial specimen)
		Brown, orange, or yellow	Elevated protein, RBC breakdown (blood present for at least 3 days)
Protein	15 to 45 mg/100 ml	Marked increase	Tumors, trauma, hemorrhage, diabetes mellitus, polyneuritis, blood in CSF
		Marked decrease	Rapid CSF production
Gamma globulin	3% to 12% of total protein	Increase	Demyelinating disease (such as multiple sclerosis), neurosyphilis, Guillain-Barré syndrome
Glucose	50 to 80 mg/100 ml (⅔ of blood glucose)	Increase	Systemic hyperglycemia
		Decrease	Systemic hypoglycemia, bacterial or fungal infection, meningitis, mumps, postsubarachnoid hemorrhage
Cell count	0 to 5 WBCs	Increase	Active disease: meningitis, acute infection, onset of chronic illness, tumor, abscess, infarction, demyelinating disease (such as multiple sclerosis)
	No RBCs	RBCs	Hemorrhage or traumatic tap
VDRL and other serologic tests	Nonreactive	Positive	Neurosyphilis
Chloride	118 to 130 mEq/liter	Decrease	Infected meninges (as in tuberculosis or meningitis)
Gram stain	No organisms	Gram-positive or gram-negative organisms	Bacterial meningitis

Equipment

Lumbar puncture tray/sterile gloves/local anesthetic (usually 1% lidocaine)/povidone-iodine/small adhesive bandage.

Procedure

Position the patient on his side at the edge of the bed, with his knees drawn up to his abdomen and his chin on his chest. Provide pillows to support the spine on a horizontal plane. With the patient in this position, full flexion of the spine and easy access to the lumbar subarachnoid space are possible. Help the patient maintain this position by placing one arm around his knees and the other arm around his neck. If a sitting position is preferred, have the patient sit up and bend his chest and head toward his knees. Help him maintain this position throughout the procedure.

After the skin is prepared for injection, the area is draped. Warn the patient that he'll probably experience a transient burning sensation when the local anesthetic is injected. Tell him that when the spinal needle is inserted, he may feel some local, transient pain as the needle transverses the dura mater. Ask him to report any pain or sensations that differ from or continue after this expected discomfort, as these may indicate irritation

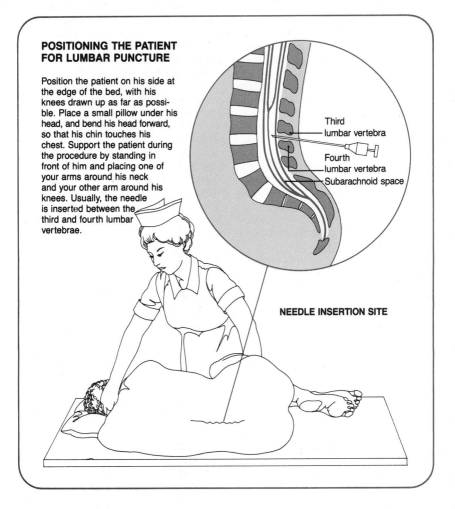

POSITIONING THE PATIENT FOR LUMBAR PUNCTURE

Position the patient on his side at the edge of the bed, with his knees drawn up as far as possible. Place a small pillow under his head, and bend his head forward, so that his chin touches his chest. Support the patient during the procedure by standing in front of him and placing one of your arms around his neck and your other arm around his knees. Usually, the needle is inserted between the third and fourth lumbar vertebrae.

Third lumbar vertebra

Fourth lumbar vertebra

Subarachnoid space

NEEDLE INSERTION SITE

or puncture of a nerve root, requiring repositioning of the needle. Instruct the patient to remain still and breathe normally; movement and hyperventilation can alter pressure readings or cause injury.

The anesthetic is injected, and the spinal needle is inserted in the midline, between the spinous processes of the vertebrae (usually between the third and fourth lumbar verbebrae). When the stylet is removed from the needle, CSF will drip from it if the needle is properly positioned. A stopcock and manometer are attached to the needle to measure initial (or opening) CSF pressure. After the specimen is collected, label the containers in the order in which they were filled, and ask the doctor if he has any specific instructions for the laboratory. A final pressure reading is taken, and the needle is removed. Clean the puncture site with a local antiseptic, such as povidone-iodine solution, and apply a small adhesive bandage.

Precautions
□ Infection at the puncture site contraindicates removal of CSF; in a patient with increased intracranial pressure, CSF should be removed with extreme caution, since the rapid reduction in pressure that follows withdrawal of fluid can cause cerebellar tonsillar herniation and medullary compression.

□ During the procedure, observe closely for signs of adverse reaction, such as elevated pulse rate, pallor, or clammy skin. Alert the doctor immediately to any significant changes.
□ Record the collection time on the test request form. Send it, and labeled specimens, to the laboratory immediately.

Findings
Normally, the doctor records CSF pressure and checks the appearance of the specimen. Three tubes are collected routinely and are sent to the laboratory for analysis of protein, sugar, and cells, as well as for serologic testing, such as the VDRL (Venereal Disease Research Lab-

oratory) test for neurosyphilis. A separate specimen is also sent to the laboratory for culture and sensitivity testing. Electrolyte analysis and Gram stain may be ordered as supplementary tests. CSF electrolyte levels are of special interest in patients with abnormal serum electrolyte levels or CSF infection, or in those receiving hyperosmolar agents. See the chart on page 776 for a summary of normal and abnormal findings in CSF analysis.

Post-test care
□ Check if the patient must lie flat or if the head of his bed may be slightly elevated. In most cases, you will be instructed to *keep the patient lying flat for 8 hours after lumbar puncture.* Some doctors, however, allow a 30° elevation at the head of the bed. Remind the patient that, although he must not raise his head, he can turn from side to side.
□ Encourage the patient to drink fluids. Provide a flexible straw.
□ Check the puncture site for redness, swelling, and drainage every hour for the first 4 hours, then every 4 hours for the first 24 hours.
□ If CSF pressure is elevated, assess neurologic status every 15 minutes for 4 hours. If the patient is stable, assess every hour for 2 hours, then every 4 hours or according to pretest schedule.

□ Watch for complications of lumbar puncture, such as reaction to the anesthetic, meningitis, bleeding into the spinal canal, and cerebellar tonsillar herniation and medullary compression. Signs of meningitis include fever, neck rigidity, and irritability; signs of herniation include decreased level of consciousness, changes in pupil size and equality, altered vital signs (including widened pulse pressure, decreased pulse rate, and irregular respirations), or respiratory failure.

Interfering factors
□ The patient's position and activity can alter CSF pressure. Crying, coughing, or straining may increase pressure.

ALTERNATE METHODS FOR OBTAINING CSF

Cisternal puncture

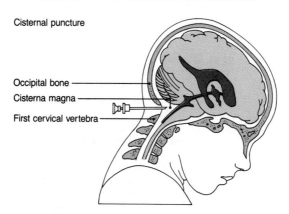

Occipital bone
Cisterna magna
First cervical vertebra

CISTERNAL PUNCTURE

When lumbar puncture is contraindicated by infection at the puncture site, lumbar deformity, or some other problem, the doctor may perform a cisternal puncture to obtain CSF. A short-beveled, hollow needle is inserted into the cisterna cerebellomedullaris, below the occipital bone, between the first cervical vertebra and rim of the foramen magnum. Side effects are minimal; the severe headaches that often occur after lumbar puncture are uncommon with this procedure. Cisternal puncture is hazardous, however, because the needle is positioned close to the brain stem. Contraindications are the same as for lumbar puncture—infection or deformity at the puncture site, or increased intracranial pressure.

Prepare the patient as for lumbar puncture; a cisternal puncture tray contains the necessary equipment. The patient's neck should be flexed forward, so his chin touches his chest. Hold his head firmly in place to bring the brain stem and spinal cord forward and allow more space for the cisternal needle to enter. (If the doctor prefers, the patient may assume a sitting position, with his neck flexed forward.)

Post-test care is the same as for lumbar puncture. If the procedure was performed on an outpatient, instruct a family member to check the puncture site for redness, swelling, and drainage, and to observe the patient for signs of complications, such as neck rigidity, irritability, and decreased level of consciousness.

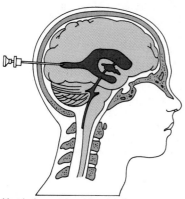

Ventricular puncture into posterior horn of right lateral ventricle

VENTRICULAR PUNCTURE

Although rarely performed, ventricular puncture is the procedure of choice when a spinal puncture may cause brain stem herniation or other complications. Ventricular puncture is usually done in the operating room. The doctor makes a small incision in the parieto-occipital region of the scalp, then drills a hole in the skull. A short-beveled, hollow needle is inserted through the hole and into a lateral ventricle, and CSF is withdrawn. Complications —such as ventriculitis and hemorrhage from ruptured blood vessels—are rare. Post-test care is the same as for lumbar puncture, but don't elevate the head of the patient's bed more than 15° to 20°. Bed rest is usually prescribed for 24 hours.

☐ Delay between collection time and laboratory testing can invalidate results, especially cell counts.

JOAN C. MCMANUS, RN, MA
KATHY A. HAUSMAN, RN, MS

Myelography

Myelography combines fluoroscopy and radiography to evaluate the spinal subarachnoid space after injection of a contrast medium. Because the contrast medium is heavier than CSF, it will flow through the subarachnoid space to the dependent area when the patient, lying prone on a fluoroscopic table, is tilted up or down. The fluoroscope allows visualization of the flow of the contrast medium and the outline of the subarachnoid space. Radiographs are taken for a permanent record.

Sometimes, myelography is performed to confirm the need for surgery; in such cases, a neurosurgeon may stand by. If this test confirms a spinal tumor, the patient may be taken directly to the operating room. Immediate surgery may also be necessary when the contrast medium causes a total block of the subarachnoid space.

Purpose
☐ To demonstrate lesions, such as tumors and herniated intervertebral disks, that partially or totally block the flow of CSF in the subarachnoid space
☐ To aid detection of arachnoiditis, spinal nerve root injury, or tumors in the posterior fossa of the skull.

Patient preparation
Explain to the patient that this test reveals obstructions in the spinal cord. Instruct him to restrict food and fluids for 8 hours before the test. However, if the test is scheduled for late in the day and hospital policy permits, the patient may have clear liquids before the test. Tell him who will perform the test and where,

and that the procedure takes 1 hour or more.

Explain to the patient that he'll probably feel a transient burning sensation as the contrast medium is injected, that he may feel flushed and warm, and experience a headache, a salty taste, or nausea and vomiting after injection of the contrast. Warn him that he may feel some pain during the procedure from the positions he'll assume, insertion of the needle, and in some cases, from removal of the contrast medium.

Make sure the patient or responsible member of the family has signed a consent form. Check the patient's history for hypersensitivity to iodine and iodine-containing substances (such as shellfish), radiographic contrast medium, and other medications associated with the procedure. If metrizamide is used as the contrast medium, discontinue phenothiazines 48 hours before the test is scheduled to begin. Notify the radiologist if the patient has a history of epilepsy or phenothiazine use.

Instruct the patient to remove jewelry and metal objects in the X-ray field. Administer pretest medications and perform pretest procedures, as ordered. In the lumbar region, a cleansing enema may be ordered to prevent gas shadows on the film. A sedative and anticholinergic (such as atropine sulfate) may be ordered to calm the patient and keep his mouth dry, to reduce swallowing during the procedure.

Equipment
Alcohol/1% lidocaine solution/lumbar puncture tray/contrast medium (iophendylate or metrizamide sodium/two 10-ml syringes/spinal needle—18G for iophendylate and 11G for metrizamide/X-ray machine capable of fluoroscopy/povidone-iodine solution/sterile gloves/small adhesive bandage.

Procedure
The patient is positioned on his side at the edge of the table, with his knees drawn up to his abdomen and his chin on his chest. (If the patient has lumbar

deformity or infection at the puncture site, cisternal puncture may be done.) A lumbar puncture is performed, and the fluoroscope is used to verify proper needle position in the subarachnoid space. Some CSF may be removed for routine laboratory analysis. The patient is then turned to the prone position and is secured with straps across his upper back, under his arms, and across his ankles. His chin is hyperextended to prevent the flow of contrast medium into the cranium; a towel or sponge is placed under his chin for comfort. In this position, the patient may complain of a headache, have trouble swallowing, or feel he's not inhaling enough oxygen. If so, reassure him that he'll have opportunities during the procedure to rest from this uncomfortable position.

With the spinal needle in place, the contrast medium is injected and the table tilted so that the contrast flows through the subarachnoid space. (Occasionally, air may be injected as a contrast agent [negative contrast], but this is rarely done except in patients with suspected congenital abnormalities, such as syringomyelia.) The flow of the contrast is studied on the fluoroscope, and radiographs are taken. If an obstruction in the subarachnoid space blocks the upward flow of the contrast, a cisternal puncture may be performed. When required radiographs have been obtained the contrast is withdrawn, if necessary, and the needle is removed. The puncture site is cleaned with povidone-iodine solution, and a small adhesive bandage applied.

Precautions
Generally, myelography is contraindicated in patients with increased intracranial pressure, hypersensitivity to iodine or contrast media, or infection at the puncture site.

Findings
Normally, the contrast medium flows freely through the subarachnoid space, showing no obstruction or structural abnormalities.

REMOVING CONTRAST MEDIA AFTER MYELOGRAPHY

Managing removal of the contrast medium after the test differs, depending on which contrast is used—iophendylate or metrizamide.

If *iophendylate* is injected as the contrast medium, it must be removed after the procedure, because it's not water-soluble and won't be excreted. Left in the body, it may cause inflammation or adhesive arachnoiditis.

One of two methods may be used to remove iophendylate: with the patient in the prone position, the contrast pools in the lumbar lordosis and can then be aspirated; or with the patient on his side, in the usual position for lumbar puncture, the contrast may be aspirated or allowed to drip from the needle. Removal of iophendylate may produce pain in the buttocks or legs, from nerve root irritation. The patient must return to his room on a stretcher and lie flat for 24 hours after myelography.

Metrizamide is water-soluble and doesn't have to be removed. After it's absorbed into the bloodstream, the kidneys excrete it. However, the patient who receives metrizamide sodium must return to his room in a wheelchair, or on a stretcher with the head elevated at least 60°. In his room, he must sit in a chair, or lie in bed with his head elevated at least 60°. He must *not* lie flat for at least 8 hours, because this contrast medium can irritate cervical nerve roots and cranial structures.

Implications of results
This test can identify and localize lesions within or surrounding the spinal cord or subarachnoid space. For example, common extradural lesions include herniated intervertebral disks and metastatic tumors. Common lesions within the subarachnoid space include neurofibromas and meningiomas; lesions within the spinal cord, ependymomas and astrocytomas. This test may also detect syringomyelia, a congenital abnormality marked by fluid-filled cavities within the spinal cord and widening of the cord itself. Myelography may also detect arachnoiditis, spinal nerve root injury, and tumors in the posterior fossa of the skull. Test results must be corre-

lated with the patient's history and clinical status.

Post-test care

☐ Find out which contrast medium was used for the test, and position the patient accordingly.

☐ Monitor vital signs and neurologic status at least every 30 minutes for the first 4 hours, then every 4 hours for 24 hours.

☐ Encourage the patient to drink extra fluids. He should void within 8 hours after returning to his room.

☐ If no complications or side effects occur, the patient may resume usual diet and activities the day after the test. If radicular pain, fever, back pain, or signs of meningeal irritation (headache, irritability, or neck stiffness) develop, keep the room quiet and dark, and provide an analgesic or an antipyretic, as ordered.

Interfering factors

Incorrect needle placement or patient failure to cooperate may alter results.

KATHY A. HAUSMAN, RN, MS

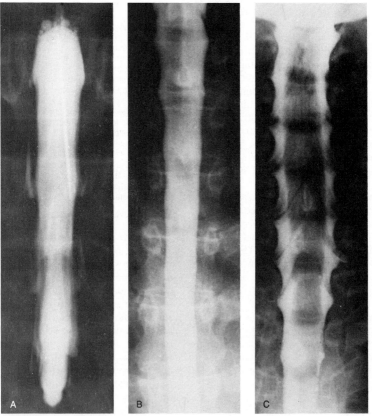

SPINAL MYELOGRAPHY SERIES

A   B   C

These myelograms of the spinal canal were taken in this order: lumbar region (A), thoracic region (B), and cervical region (C). Together, they reveal a normal-sized spinal cord, free of external compression.

Tensilon Test

This test involves careful observation of the patient following I.V. administration of Tensilon (edrophonium chloride), a rapid, short-acting anticholinesterase that improves muscle strength by increasing muscular response to nerve impulses. It is especially useful in diagnosing myasthenia gravis, an abnormality of the myoneural junction in which nerve impulses fail to induce normal muscular responses. Patients with myasthenia gravis experience extreme fatigue at the end of the day or after repetitive activity or stress. Results of other procedures, including electromyography, may supplement Tensilon test findings in diagnosing this disease.

Purpose
□ To aid diagnosis of myasthenia gravis
□ To aid in differentiation between myasthenic and cholinergic crises
□ To monitor oral anticholinesterase therapy.

Patient preparation
Explain to the patient that this test helps determine the cause of muscle weakness. Inform him he needn't restrict food or fluids. Tell him who will perform the test and where, and that it takes 15 to 30 minutes.

Don't describe the exact response that will be evaluated, since this knowledge may interfere with the test's objectivity. Simply tell the patient that a small tube will be inserted into a vein in his arm and that a drug will be administered periodically. He will then be closely observed as he is asked to make repetitive muscular movements. Advise him that Tensilon may produce some unpleasant side effects, but reassure him that someone will be with him at all times, and that any reactions will quickly disappear. To ensure accurate results, the test may be repeated several times.

Check the patient's history for medications that affect muscle function, and for anticholinesterase therapy, drug hypersensitivities, and respiratory disease. Withhold medication, as ordered. If the patient is receiving anticholinesterase therapy, note this on the requisition slip, with the last dose he received and the time it was administered. Patients with respiratory ailments, such as asthma, should receive atropine during the test, to minimize Tensilon side effects.

Equipment
Standard: 10 mg Tensilon/0.4 mg atropine (as ordered, for patients with respiratory distress)/one tuberculin and one 3-ml syringe/I.V. infusion set/50-ml bag of I.V. solution (5% dextrose in water or normal saline solution)/tape, tourniquet, alcohol swabs.

Emergency: 0.5 to 1 mg atropine I.V., for cholinergic crisis/0.5 to 2 mg neostigmine methylsulfate I.V., for myasthenic crisis (may be repeated up to 5 mg)/extra tuberculin and 3-ml syringes (for atropine or neostigmine injections)/resuscitation equipment, including a tracheotomy tray.

Procedure
Begin I.V. infusion of 5% dextrose in water or normal saline solution. To perform the Tensilon test on an adult patient suspected of having *myasthenia gravis,* 2 mg of Tensilon are administered initially. (Dosage must be adjusted for an infant or child.) Before the rest of the dosage is administered, the doctor may want to fatigue the muscles by asking the patient to perform various exercises, such as looking up until ptosis develops, counting to 100 until his voice diminishes, or holding his arms above his shoulders until they drop. When the muscles are fatigued, the remaining 8 mg of Tensilon are administered over 30 seconds.

Some doctors prefer to begin this test with a placebo injection to evaluate the patient's muscular response more accurately. If so, the placebo is administered and the patient observed. This placebo isn't necessary when cranial muscles are being tested, since cranial strength can't be simulated voluntarily.

After administration of Tensilon, the patient is asked to perform repetitive muscular movements, such as opening and closing his eyes and crossing and uncrossing his legs. Assist the doctor by closely observing the patient for improved muscle strength. If muscle strength doesn't improve within 3 to 5 minutes, the test may be repeated.

To differentiate between *myasthenic crisis* and *cholinergic crisis*, 1 to 2 mg of Tensilon is infused. After infusion, continually monitor the patient's vital signs. Watch closely for respiratory distress, and be prepared to provide respiratory assistance. If muscle strength doesn't improve, more Tensilon is infused cautiously—1 mg at a time up to a maximum of 5 mg—and the patient is observed for distress. Neostigmine is administered immediately if the test demonstrates myasthenic crisis; atropine is administered for cholinergic crisis.

To evaluate oral *anticholinesterase therapy*, 2 mg of Tensilon is infused 1 hour after the patient's last dose of the anticholinesterase. The patient is observed carefully for side effects and muscular response. After administration of

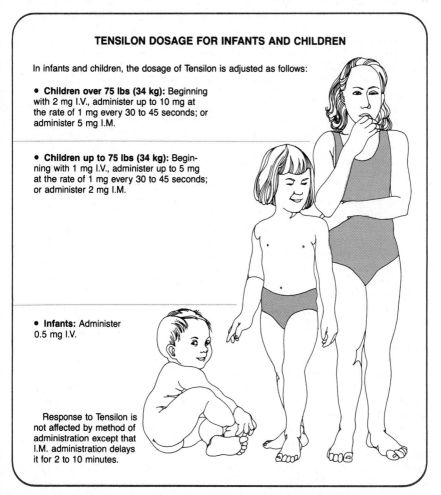

TENSILON DOSAGE FOR INFANTS AND CHILDREN

In infants and children, the dosage of Tensilon is adjusted as follows:

• **Children over 75 lbs (34 kg):** Beginning with 2 mg I.V., administer up to 10 mg at the rate of 1 mg every 30 to 45 seconds; or administer 5 mg I.M.

• **Children up to 75 lbs (34 kg):** Beginning with 1 mg I.V., administer up to 5 mg at the rate of 1 mg every 30 to 45 seconds; or administer 2 mg I.M.

• **Infants:** Administer 0.5 mg I.V.

Response to Tensilon is not affected by method of administration except that I.M. administration delays it for 2 to 10 minutes.

Tensilon, the I.V. line is kept open at a rate of 20 ml/hour until all the patient's responses have been evaluated. When the test is complete, discontinue the I.V., as ordered, and check the patient's vital signs. Check the puncture site for hematoma, excessive bleeding, and swelling.

Precautions

☐ Because of the systemic side effects Tensilon may produce, this test may be contraindicated in patients with hypotension, bradycardia, apnea, and mechanical obstruction of the intestine or urinary tract.

☐ Stay with the patient during the test, and observe him closely for side effects.

☐ Keep resuscitation equipment handy in case of respiratory failure.

Findings

Persons who don't have myasthenia gravis usually develop fasciculations in response to Tensilon. The doctor must interpret the responses carefully to distinguish a normal person from one with myasthenia gravis.

Implications of results

If the patient has *myasthenia gravis*, following administration of Tensilon, muscle strength should improve promptly. The degree of improvement depends on the muscle group being tested. Improvement usually becomes obvious within 30 seconds; although the maximum benefit lasts only several minutes, lingering effects may persist—up to 2 hours in a patient receiving prednisone, for example. Although all patients with *myasthenia gravis* show improved muscle strength in this test, some respond only slightly, and the test may need to be re-peated to confirm diagnosis. This test gives inconsistent results when *myasthenia gravis* affects only ocular muscles, as in mild or early forms of the disorder. It may produce a positive response in motor neuron disease and in some neuropathies and myopathies. However, the response is usually less dramatic and less consistent than in *myasthenia gravis*.

Patients in *myasthenic crisis* (exacerbation of the disease requiring increased anticholinesterase therapy) show brief improvement in muscle strength after Tensilon administration. In patients in *cholinergic crisis* (anticholinesterase overdose), Tensilon promptly exaggerates muscle weakness. If Tensilon increases the patient's muscle strength without increasing side effects, *oral anticholinesterase therapy* can be increased. If Tensilon decreases muscle strength in a person with prominent side effects, therapy should be reduced. If the test shows no change in muscle strength and only mild side effects occur, therapy should remain the same.

Post-test care

As ordered, resume medications.

Interfering factors

☐ In patients receiving prednisone, the effect of Tensilon on muscle strength may be delayed.

☐ Quinidine and anticholinergics interfere with test results by inhibiting the action of Tensilon.

☐ Procainamide and muscle relaxants interfere with test results by inhibiting normal muscular responses.

PAULA STEPHENS OKUN, RN, MSN
JOSEPH B. WARREN, RN, BSN

Selected References

Berkow, Robert, ed. *The Merck Manual of Diagnosis and Therapy*, 14th ed. Rahway, N.J.: Merck, Sharp & Dohme, 1982.

Chaplin, James P., and Demers, Aline. *Primer of Neurology and Neurophysiology*.

New York: John Wiley & Sons, 1978.

Petersdorf, Robert G., and Adams, Raymond D., eds. *Harrison's Principles of Internal Medicine*, 10th ed. New York: McGraw-Hill Book Co., 1983.

27 Gastrointestinal System

LEARNING OBJECTIVES

After completing this chapter, the reader will be able to:
- explain the anatomy and physiology of the digestive system.
- identify seven investigative techniques used in gastroenterology.
- state the purpose of each test discussed in the chapter.
- prepare the patient physically and psychologically for each test.
- describe the procedure for performing each test.
- specify appropriate precautions for safe administration of each test.
- recognize signs of adverse reaction and respond appropriately.
- implement appropriate post-test care.
- identify the normal values and findings for each test.
- discuss the implications of abnormal test results.
- list factors that may interfere with accurate test results.

Gastrointestinal System

Introduction

The gastrointestinal (GI) tract and the adjoining liver, gallbladder, and pancreas are responsible for the proper digestion and absorption of food and for the elimination of metabolic waste products. Numerous diagnostic tests evaluate this system to detect diseases, functional disorders, and abnormalities resulting from emotional stress. They range from laboratory analysis of stool and esophageal, gastric, and peritoneal contents, to specialized invasive and noninvasive procedures, such as endoscopy, contrast radiography, nuclear imaging, ultrasonography, and computerized tomography (CT). Specialized laboratory procedures are considered the most valuable, since they produce results that are usually specific for a particular disease. However, choice of an appropriate test or test battery always depends on the patient's signs and symptoms, and the results of a physical examination.

Anatomy and physiology
The GI tract includes the mouth, pharynx, esophagus, stomach (fundus, body, antrum), small intestine (duodenum, jejunum, ileum), and large intestine (cecum, colon, rectum, anal canal). Throughout the GI tract, peristalsis propels the ingested material along; sphincters prevent its reflux.

Digestion begins in the mouth through chewing and the action of the enzyme amylase—secreted in saliva—which breaks down starches. Food is lubricated by the glycoprotein mucin, then swallowed as a bolus. While the food is passing through the esophagus, it's also lubricated by mucous secretions. Digestion continues in the stomach through the action of glandular secretions, such as mucus, pepsinogen, hydrochloric acid, gastrin, and intrinsic factor, a glycoprotein essential in vitamin B_{12} absorption. The hormone gastrin, the most potent stimulus of gastric secretion, enhances the release of hydrochloric acid. In turn, hydrochloric acid lowers the pH of gastric contents, promoting the conversion of pepsinogen to pepsin, a proteolytic enzyme. Pepsin begins protein catabolism, breaking down dietary protein into products ranging from large polypeptides to amino acids. Through a churning motion, the stomach breaks food into tiny particles, mixes them with gastric juices, and pushes the mass toward the pylorus. The liquid portion (chyme) enters the duodenum in small amounts; solid material remains in the stomach until it liquefies (usually from 1 to 6 hours). Although limited amounts of water, alcohol, and certain drugs are absorbed in the stomach, chyme passes unabsorbed into the duodenum.

Digestion and absorption occur primarily in the small intestine, where millions of villi increase the surface area.

HOW TO INSERT A NASOGASTRIC TUBE

First, gather the following equipment: appropriate size nasogastric tube, water-soluble lubricant, glass of water with straw (or ice chips), towel, tissues, emesis basin, bulb or 50-ml catheter-tip syringe, hypoallergenic tape, safety pin, stethoscope, and clamp.

Place the patient in a sitting or high Fowler's position. Drape a towel across his chest. Then, determine how far to insert the tube by using the tube to measure the distance from the patient's earlobe to the tip of his nose (1). Then, measure the distance from his earlobe to the base of his xiphoid process (2). Total these measurements, and use adhesive tape to mark this length on the tube.

Lubricate 6" to 8" (15 to 20 cm) of the tube, and pass the tube down and back into the posterior nasopharynx (3). When the tube reaches the pharynx, the patient may gag. If so, have him lower his head and sip water (4) or suck ice chips. As he swallows, advance the tube. If you can't advance the tube, don't use force. Instead, rotate the tube gently and try advancing it. If this is unsuccessful, remove the tube and insert it in the other nostril. If the patient starts gasping, coughing, or develops cyanosis, remove the tube immediately and notify the doctor.

For digestion, the small intestine relies on the many enzymes produced by the pancreas or by the intestinal lining. Pancreatic enzymes empty into the duodenum through the ampulla of Vater. These enzymes include trypsin, which digests protein to amino acids; lipase, which digests fat to fatty acids and glycerol; and amylase, which digests starches to sugars. Intestinal enzymes include peptidases, which convert protein to amino acids; lactase, maltase, and sucrase, which digest complex sugars like glucose, fructose, and galactose; and enterokinase, which activates trypsin.

Bile also participates in digestion and absorption. After formation in the liver, bile is stored and concentrated in the gallbladder. It's released in response to cholecystokinin, a hormone secreted by the duodenum, and is then emptied into the duodenum through the ampulla of Vater. Bile helps neutralize stomach acid, and promotes the emulsification of fats and the absorption of the fat-soluble vitamins A, D, E, and K.

When food reaches the ileocecal valve and enters the large intestine (3 to 10 hours after ingestion), all its nutritional value has been absorbed. The first half of the large intestine absorbs water, sodium, and chloride, reducing bulk; the second half stores and further dehydrates the digestive material until defecation. The second half of the large intestine may also excrete water, potassium, and bicarbonate. Bacterial action in the colon putrefies undigested foods; synthesizes vitamins K, B_{12}, B_2 (riboflavin), and B_1 (thiamine); and produces gas, which helps propel feces toward the anus. Intestinal gas may also result from swallowed air or diffusion of blood gases. Rectal distention by feces stimulates the defecation reflex, which is assisted by voluntary sphincter relaxation. Normal passage of feces through the large intestine takes 24 to 40 hours.

HOW TO CHECK FOR PLACEMENT OF A NASOGASTRIC TUBE

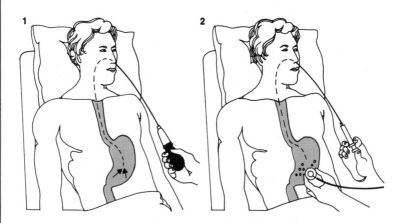

To check for proper tube placement, connect a syringe to the tube and try aspirating stomach contents (1). If you're successful, the tube's correctly placed in the stomach. In addition, place a stethoscope over the epigastrium (2). Then, inject 15 ml of air into the nasogastric tube. If the tube is correctly positioned, you'll hear a swooshing sound as the air enters the stomach.

When you're sure the tube's correctly placed, secure the tube to the patient's nose with hypoallergenic tape and to his gown. Finally, clamp the tube when not in use.

INVESTIGATIVE TECHNIQUES IN GASTROENTEROLOGY

PROCEDURE	DEFINITION AND TEST METHOD	TYPICAL CLINICAL OBJECTIVES
Endoscopy	*Direct visualization of the lining of a hollow viscus using an endoscope:* A cablelike cluster of glass fibers within the endoscope transmits light into the viscus, then returns an image to the scope's optical head.	• To diagnose inflammatory, ulcerative, and infectious diseases; benign and malignant neoplasms; and other lesions of the esophageal, gastric, and intestinal mucosa
Radiography	*Passage of X-radiation through the patient to create a radiograph:* X-ray films depict body structures and air in shades of gray, which reflect their density—air appears black, fat appears dark gray, soft tissue appears light gray, and bone appears white. Use of contrast media accentuates these densities.	• To detect obstruction, strictures, and deviations in the biliary tract • To detect inflammatory disease, tumors, ulcers, and other lesions • To diagnose hiatal hernia and other structural changes in the GI tract
Cineradiography	*Rapid-sequence X-ray examination that films motion:* Replay of this film at slow speeds allows close observation of such motion.	• To detect vascular abnormalities by recording the stages of perfusion • To evaluate the condition of the pharynx by recording its muscular contraction
Fluoroscopy	*Projection of X-ray films onto a fluoroscope, or specialized screen, to permit continuous observation of motion:* Spot films record significant findings.	• To detect obstruction, strictures, and deviations in the biliary tract • To detect inflammatory disease, tumors, ulcers, and other lesions • To diagnose hiatal hernia and other structural changes in the GI tract • To check catheter placement in angiography by observing small injections of dye

Esophageal, gastric, and peritoneal contents

Examination of esophageal and gastric contents reveals the secretory function of the mucosa in each organ; excessive or deficient mucosal secretions, or the presence of blood often aids diagnosis. Peritoneal fluid analysis provides a broader assessment of abdominal integrity, since this fluid lubricates all organs within the peritoneum.

Esophageal contents consist entirely of mucus, whereas gastric contents—(after a 12-hour fast)—include water, hydrochloric acid, mucus, electrolytes, and pepsin. The fasting interval normally clears food particles from the stomach into the duodenum, but a small amount of food residue may be present.

Gastric contents may vary too. For example, if excessive gagging accompanies nasogastric intubation, gastric juice may contain bile that gives it a lemon-yellow to cloudy green color. It may contain mucus that may arise from stomach glandular secretions or from swallowed saliva and nasorespiratory secretions. Although gastric content may normally contain flecks or streaks of bright red blood after minor trauma during intu-

INVESTIGATIVE TECHNIQUES IN GASTROENTEROLOGY *(continued)*

PROCEDURE	DEFINITION AND TEST METHOD	TYPICAL CLINICAL OBJECTIVES
Nuclear medicine imaging	*Use of a gamma camera or rectilinear scanner:* Distribution of a decaying radiopharmaceutical is recorded after I.V. injection.	• To screen for hepatocellular disease and for focal disease in the liver and spleen • To detect hepatomegaly and splenomegaly • To diagnose liver or spleen hematoma after abdominal trauma • To detect site of GI bleeding • To evaluate acute cholecystitis
Ultrasonography	*Focused beam of high-frequency sound waves:* The sound waves pass through the patient, creating echoes that vary with tissue density. These echoes are converted into electrical energy, are amplified by a transducer, and appear on an oscilloscope screen in shades of gray as spikes or dots.	• To detect splenomegaly • To differentiate neoplasms, cysts, and abscesses in the liver, spleen, and pancreas • To detect metastases in the liver • To diagnose liver or spleen hematoma after abdominal trauma • To differentiate obstructive and nonobstructive jaundice • To diagnose cholelithiasis
Computed tomography (CT scan)	*Multiple X-ray beams pass through the patient, detectors record tissue attenuation, and a computer then reconstructs this information as a three-dimensional image on an oscilloscope screen:* Attenuation varies with tissue density and appears in shades of gray on the oscilloscope screen. Use of contrast media accentuates density.	• To differentiate neoplasms, abscesses, and cysts in the liver, spleen, and pancreas • To detect liver metastases • To diagnose liver or spleen hematoma after abdominal trauma • To evaluate, diagnose, or confirm pancreatitis • To distinguish obstructive from nonobstructive jaundice • To evaluate retroperitoneal disease

bation, a large amount of blood is abnormal. Partially digested blood appears as dark, coffee-colored particles and indicates chronic bleeding, such as from ulceration or carcinoma.

Peritoneal fluid, which normally is clear and pale yellow, is removed from the abdominal cavity by needle aspiration. Less than 50 ml of this fluid normally lubricates the peritoneal surfaces; excessive volumes indicate pathology.

Nasogastric intubation

Aspiration of gastric contents through a nasogastric tube can evaluate both the secretory activity of the gastric mucosa and the efficiency of gastric emptying into the duodenum, aiding diagnosis of GI disorders. Such intubation is somewhat un-pleasant for the patient but can be accomplished quickly, safely, and with minimal discomfort. Diagnostic intubation is contraindicated in pregnant patients and those with aortic aneurysms, myocardial infarction, diverticula, or stenosis. However, it may be done with caution in an emergency.

Fecal contents

The GI tract processes about 10 liters of chyme daily, of which 100 to 300 g are eventually expelled as feces. Normal defecation patterns—influenced by food and fluid intake, medications, exercise, and rate of digestion—vary from two or three times daily to two or three times weekly. Fecal analysis can evaluate digestive efficiency and the integrity of

PATIENT TEACHING AID

Collecting a Stool Specimen at Home

Dear Patient:
Here's what you should know about collecting a stool specimen at home. To make sure you obtain a suitable specimen, follow these instructions carefully:
• Use a bedpan—if you have one—to collect the stool. Be sure the bedpan is clean. If you don't have a bedpan, use a large glass jar that you've carefully cleaned and then boiled.
• Collect a specimen of *every* stool passed within the period designated by your doctor. Consider your first stool as the starting time of the collection period. If you accidentally discard a specimen, call the doctor. Sometimes the doctor will ask you to save only a small portion of each stool or collect only one stool specimen for analysis.
• Don't contaminate the specimen by urinating or placing toilet tissue in the bedpan or jar.
• The doctor will give you a container— made of plastic, cardboard, or glass, with a tight lid to minimize odor—in which to collect the specimen. Use a tongue blade or piece of cardboard to transfer the stool from the bedpan or jar to the specimen container. When doing so, be careful not to contaminate the outside of the container with the stool.
• Don't overfill the container. Keep it in a cool place during the collection period. Carefully loosen the lid occasionally, to allow gas to escape.
• If you have difficulty defecating, call the doctor.

the stomach and intestines.

Feces normally consist of 75% water and 25% solids, such as cellulose and other indigestible fiber, bacteria, unabsorbed minerals, fat and fat derivatives, desquamated epithelial cells, mucus, and small amounts of digestive enzymes and secretions. Fecal analysis begins with gross examination of color, consistency, odor, and other characteristics, and concludes with microscopic, chemical, or bacterial analysis. Feces are usually light to dark brown, soft, and slightly acidic. Their color depends on diet, drugs, absorption efficiency, and bilirubin concentration; their normal brown color, on metabolism of bile pigments to stercobilin. Fecal pH depends on dietary influences: acidic pH results from a high carbohydrate intake, alkaline pH results from high protein intake. Fecal odor results from the presence of indole and skatole, end products of protein catabolism by bacterial action in the large intestine.

Stool is usually about 1″ (2.5 cm) in diameter and has the tubular shape of the colon, but may be larger or smaller, depending on the condition of the colon.

If the colon is partially obstructed or loses its elasticity, the passage of stool often traumatizes the colon and may cause bleeding; blood in the stool may also result from hemorrhoids. A black, tarry stool can result from bleeding high in the intestinal tract. A large, bulky, foul-smelling stool that floats on water may indicate malabsorption of fat (steatorrhea) or a large quantity of air or other gases in the stool. Diarrhea results from too rapid passage of food through the GI tract, often spurred by viral infection. Mucus-containing stool can indicate colitis or a mucus-producing tumor. Pus, detected in microscopic analysis, can result from rectal abscess or ulcerative colitis.

Stool specimen collection

Stool specimen collection is often required for diagnosis of infectious diseases, GI bleeding, and other GI tract disorders. Since stool specimens can't be obtained on demand, close cooperation between nurse and patient is necessary to secure a suitable specimen. Stool specimens may be collected randomly or for a specified period; for example, a random specimen is required for urobilinogen, and a 72-hour specimen, for lipids. Three specimens are usually required in testing for occult blood.

Before starting stool specimen collection, have ready a clean (preferably sterile), dry bedpan; a specimen container; and tongue blades. Then, instruct the patient how to collect a random or timed stool specimen. Tell him to notify you when he feels the urge to defecate.

To collect a random specimen: Provide the patient with a bedpan, and instruct him to avoid contaminating the stool with urine or toilet tissue, since urine will inhibit bacterial growth and toilet tissue contains bismuth which interferes with test results. Using a tongue blade, carefully transfer the stool from the bedpan to the specimen container. Then tightly secure the lid of the container. If the patient passes blood or mucus with the stool, be sure to include these with the specimen. Carefully label the container, and send it to the laboratory immediately, since a fresh specimen produces the most accurate results. If the specimen can't be transported immediately, keep it under refrigeration.

To collect a timed specimen: Consider the first stool passed by the patient as the start of the collection period. Prepare this specimen and all other stools passed during the collection period in the same manner as for a random specimen. As ordered, send each specimen to the laboratory immediately, or refrigerate the specimens collected during the test period and send them when collection is completed.

Endoscopy, radiography, and ultrasonography

Although the chart on pages 790 and 791 lists specialized tests and their indications, the accurate diagnosis of GI tract, hepatic, biliary, and pancreatic disorders often requires more than one test. Such tests often proceed in the following logical order:

□ *Fecal occult blood test* generally detects GI bleeding.

□ *Barium studies* (upper GI and small

bowel series, and barium enema) visualize GI structures. Barium studies may reveal inflammation or ulcers, tumors, strictures, or other lesions.

□ *Endoscopies* (esophagogastroduodenoscopy, colonoscopy, and proctosigmoidoscopy) directly visualize an abnormality, locate sources of bleeding, and, if necessary, provide a channel for biopsy.

The selection of a diagnostic test or test battery may depend on hospital resources. If they are available, noninvasive procedures, such as ultrasonography and CT, take precedence over invasive procedures, such as endoscopic retrograde cholangiopancreatography, in evaluating pancreatic disorders. Similarly, oral cholecystography and ultrasonography frequently replace percutaneous transhepatic cholangiography in evaluation of gallbladder and biliary tract disorders.

Other useful tests

Breath hydrogen analysis, a simple method of detecting lactose intolerance, measures the hydrogen content of breath samples in the fasting state before and after ingestion of lactose. Lactose, a disaccharide composed of glucose and galactose, normally breaks down in the small intestine and is then absorbed. When lactase, the enzyme that breaks down lactose, is deficient, lactose passes unabsorbed into the large intestine. Bacteria then ferment and split lactose, producing hydrogen and other gases that the lungs exhale. To produce a sample for this test, the patient exhales into an anesthesia balloon. The hydrogen content of the sample is then determined by gas chromatography and a thermistor detector. Increased hydrogen content after lactose ingestion indicates lactose intolerance.

The *HIDA scan* (technetium-labeled iminodiacetic acid, ^{99m}Tc HIDA) is a new, simple procedure for evaluating hepatobiliary function. Since the scan requires only a 2-hour fast before the test, it permits quicker diagnosis than oral cholecystography, particularly in a

NONPATHOLOGIC CAUSES OF VARIANT STOOL COLOR

STOOL COLOR	FOOD OR FLUID	DRUG
Red	Carrots, beets, tomatoes, red peppers	Pyrvinium
Black	Licorice, grape juice	Iron salts, phenylbutazone
Brown	Cocoa, high intake of meat protein (dark brown)	Anthraquinone
Green-blue or black	Spinach	Bismuth preparations
Yellow	Rhubarb; high intake of milk (yellow-brown)	Senna
White discoloration or speckling		Antacids (aluminum hydroxide types)

patient with severe abdominal pain that suggests acute gallbladder disease.

The injected radioisotope (HIDA) is taken up by the liver and excreted into the biliary tree. Serial imaging with a gamma camera then depicts radioactivity in the liver, bile ducts, gallbladder, and duodenum. Adequate visualization of the gallbladder requires normal gallbladder and liver function, as well as patency of the biliary tree. Failure to visualize the gallbladder can result from hepatocellular disease, which impairs the uptake of HIDA, and from biliary obstruction, which prevents the release of HIDA into the gallbladder. Abnormally diminished radioactivity in the liver characterizes hepatocellular disease; absence of radioactivity in both gallbladder and duodenum suggests biliary obstruction.

The *saline-load test,* a rarely used measure of gastric retention during fasting, requires aspiration of stomach contents before and after instillation of 750 ml of normal saline solution through a nasogastric tube. The amount of saline solution remaining in the stomach 30 minutes after instillation provides an index of intrinsic gastric motility. Excessive retention of saline solution (more than 300 ml) may indicate gastric outlet

obstruction stemming from edema, tumor, or stenosis.

The *secretin test* assesses pancreatic exocrine function. It involves insertion of a double-lumen oral tube into the duodenum and aspiration of gastric and duodenal contents before and after I.V. injection of secretin, an intestinal hormone that stimulates liver and pancreatic secretions. After such injection, an abnormal volume of secretions or of bicarbonate or enzymes may indicate pancreatic carcinoma, ductal obstruction, chronic pancreatitis, or advanced pancreatic insufficiency.

The rarely used *biliary drainage test* examines bile composition. This test requires insertion of a single-lumen oral tube into the duodenum of a fasting patient and aspiration of duodenal contents before and after instillation of 30 ml of 25% magnesium sulfate. Such instillation relaxes the sphincter of Oddi and allows bile to flow into the duodenum. (I.V. injection of sincalide, an acceptable substitute for magnesium sulfate, can also stimulate gallbladder contraction and release bile.) Aspirated duodenal contents are then examined for the presence of white cells, cholesterol, crystals, and parasites.

MAE E. PAULFREY, RN, MN

ESOPHAGEAL, GASTRIC, AND PERITONEAL CONTENTS

Esophageal Acidity Test

In contrast with the high acidity of the stomach (pH 1.1 to 2.4), the esophagus normally maintains a pH over 5.0. Although some reflux of gastric juices into the lower esophagus is common, a sharp increase in such backflow may acidify the intraesophageal pH to as low as 1.5. When repeated reflux occurs, esophageal mucosa becomes inflamed by the acidic gastric juices, resulting in pyrosis (heartburn).

The esophageal acidity test evaluates the competency of the lower esophageal sphincter—the major barrier to reflux—by measuring intraesophageal pH with an electrode attached to a manometric catheter. This test, the most sensitive indicator of gastric reflux, is indicated in patients who complain of persistent heartburn, with or without regurgitation.

Purpose
□ To evaluate competency of the lower esophageal sphincter.

Patient preparation
Explain to the patient that this test evaluates the function of the sphincter between the esophagus and stomach. Instruct him to fast and avoid smoking after midnight before the test. Tell the patient who will perform the test and where, and that it usually takes about 45 minutes.

Inform the patient that a tube will be passed through his mouth into the stomach, and that he may experience slight discomfort and may cough or gag. Just before the test, check the patient's pulse rate and blood pressure, and instruct him to void.

Withhold antacids, anticholinergics, cholinergics, adrenergic blockers, alcohol, corticosteroids, cimetidine, and reserpine for 24 hours before the test, as ordered. If these medications must be continued, note this on the laboratory slip.

Procedure
After placing the patient in high Fowler's position, introduce the catheter with pH electrode into his mouth, and instruct him to swallow when the electrode reaches the back of his throat. Locate the lower esophageal sphincter manometrically, then raise the catheter ¾″ (2 cm). Instruct the patient to perform Valsalva's maneuver or lift his legs, to stimulate reflux. After he does so, determine the intraesophageal pH.

If the pH remains normal, pass the catheter into the patient's stomach. Instill 300 ml of 0.1% N HCl over 3 minutes (100 ml/minute), then raise the catheter ¾″ (2 cm) above the sphincter. Again, to stimulate reflux, ask the patient to perform Valsalva's maneuver or lift his legs; after he does so, again determine the intraesophageal pH.

Precautions
□ During insertion, the electrode may enter the trachea instead of the esophagus. If the patient develops cyanosis or paroxysms of coughing, move the electrode immediately.
□ Observe the patient closely during intubation, since arrhythmias may develop.
□ Clamp the catheter before removing it, to prevent aspiration of fluid into the lungs.

Values
Normally, the pH of the esophagus is over 5.0.

ESOPHAGEAL MANOMETRY

Esophageal manometry measures esophageal sphincter pressure, and records the duration and sequence of peristaltic contractions to detect motility disorders, such as achalasia, diffuse esophageal spasm, and scleroderma. In this test, the patient is asked to swallow a manometric catheter that contains a small pressure transducer along its length. With the catheter placed at various levels in the esophagus, baseline measurements of pressures are made, followed by measurement of pressures in the lower esophageal sphincter immediately before and after swallowing, and then peristaltic contractions are recorded. It may be necessary to ask the patient to take wet swallows, as well as swallows with ice water, to obtain more specific information. Cholinergic and anticholinergic drugs are withheld and the patient is told to avoid tobacco and alcohol for 24 hours before the test; he's instructed to fast for 4 hours. These restrictions help prevent esophageal sphincter pressures from increasing or decreasing, which would interfere with test results. Normally, baseline sphincter pressure is about 20 mmHg; relaxation pressure (the pressure immediately before swallowing) is at least 18 mmHg. Peristalsis usually appears as a series of high-pressure peaks, representing sequential contractions of the esophagus.

In **achalasia,** baseline sphincter pressure commonly reaches 50 mmHg; relaxation pressure, less than 25 mmHg. Peristalsis is usually weak and nonpropulsive. Food and fluids accumulate in the esophagus until their weight can overcome sphincter resistance.

In **diffuse spasm of the esophagus,** sphincter pressure is generally normal, but peristalsis is disordered. Instead of sequential, orderly contractions, different segments of the esophagus contract simultaneously—and often with abnormal force—after swallowing. Contractions may also occur without the stimulus of swallowing, or more than one contraction may follow a single swallow.

In **esophageal scleroderma,** impaired sphincter function and peristalsis result from replacement of smooth muscle by fibrous tissue in the lower two thirds of the esophagus. Both baseline and relaxation pressures are depressed. Peristalsis is normal in the upper third of the esophagus, where striated muscle predominates, but it's weak or absent in the lower two thirds.

Implications of results
An intraesophageal pH of 1.5 to 2.0 indicates gastric acid reflux resulting from incompetency of the lower esophageal sphincter. Persistent reflux leads to chronic reflux esophagitis. Additional studies, such as barium swallow and esophagogastroduodenoscopy, are necessary to diagnose and determine the extent of esophagitis.

Post-test care
☐ As ordered, resume administration of medications withheld before the test, and tell the patient he may resume his usual diet.
☐ If the patient complains of a sore throat, provide soothing lozenges.

Interfering factors
☐ Failure to adhere to pretest restrictions interferes with accurate testing.
☐ Antacids, anticholinergics, and cimetidine may depress intraesophageal pH by decreasing gastric secretion or reducing its acidity; cholinergics, reserpine, alcohol, adrenergic blockers, and corticosteroids may elevate intraesophageal pH by increasing gastric secretion or by promoting reflux by relaxing the lower esophageal sphincter.

LOLITA M. ADRIEN, RN, BA, BSN
CLAIRE B. MAILHOT, RN, MS

Acid Perfusion Test
[Bernstein test]

The lower esophageal sphincter normally prevents gastric reflux. However, if this sphincter is incompetent, the recurrent backflow of such acidic juices (and of bile salts, if the pyloric sphincter is also incompetent) into the esophagus inflames the esophageal mucosa. This inflammation (esophagitis) is manifested by burning epigastric or retrosternal pain that radiates to the back or arms. To distinguish such pain from that caused by angina pectoris or other disorders, normal saline and acidic solutions are perfused separately into the esophagus through a nasogastric tube.

Purpose
□ To distinguish chest pains caused by esophagitis from those caused by cardiac disorders.

Patient preparation
Explain to the patient that this test helps determine the cause of chest pain. Instruct him to observe the following pretest restrictions: no antacids for 24 hours, as ordered; no food for 12 hours; and no fluids or smoking for 8 hours before the test. Tell him who will perform the test and where, and that it takes about 1 hour.

Inform the patient that the test requires passage of a tube through his nose into the esophagus, and that he may experience some discomfort and may cough or gag during tube passage. Tell him that liquid is slowly perfused through the tube into the esophagus; instruct him to report immediately pain or burning during perfusion.

Just before the test, check the patient's pulse rate and blood pressure. Ask him if he's experiencing any chest pain and, if so, to describe it.

Procedure
After seating the patient, insert a nasogastric tube that has been marked 12″ (30 cm) from the tip into his stomach. Attach a 20-ml syringe to the tube, and aspirate the stomach contents. Then, withdraw the tube into esophagus (to the 12″ [30-cm] mark).

Hang labeled containers of 0.9% normal saline solution and of 0.1 N HCl solution on an I.V. pole behind the patient, then connect the nasogastric tube to I.V. tubing. Open the line from the normal saline solution, and begin a drip at a rate of 60 to 120 drops/minute. Continue to perfuse this solution for 5 to 10 minutes. Then, ask the patient if he's experiencing any discomfort, and record his response. Without the patient's knowledge, close the line from the saline solution and open the line from the acidic solution. Begin a drip into the esophagus at the same rate as for the saline solution, but continue the perfusion for 30 minutes. Ask the patient if he's experiencing any discomfort, and record his response. If he experiences discomfort, immediately close the line from the acidic solution and open the line from the saline solution. Continue to perfuse saline solution until the discomfort subsides.

If ordered, repeat perfusion of the acidic solution to verify the patient's response. If this is not required, or if the patient experiences no discomfort after perfusion of the acidic solution for 30 minutes, withdraw the nasogastric tube.

Precautions
□ The acid perfusion test is contraindicated in patients with esophageal varices, congestive heart failure, acute myocardial infarction, or other cardiac disorders.
□ During intubation, make sure the tube enters the esophagus, and not the trachea. Withdraw the tube immediately if the patient develops cyanosis or paroxysms of coughing.
□ Observe the patient closely, because arrhythmias may develop.
□ Clamp the tube before removing it, to prevent aspiration of fluid into the lungs.

Findings
Absence of pain or burning during perfusion of either solution indicates a healthy esophageal mucosa.

Implications of results
In patients with esophagitis, acidic solution causes pain or burning; normal saline solution should produce no adverse effects. Occasionally, both solutions cause pain in patients with esophagitis; they may cause no pain in patients with asymptomatic esophagitis.

Post-test care
□ If the patient continues to experience pain or burning, administer an antacid, as ordered. If he complains of a sore

throat, provide soothing lozenges or obtain an order for an ice collar.

□ As ordered, the patient may resume his usual diet and medications withheld before the test.

Interfering factors
Failure to adhere to pretest restrictions may interfere with accurate determination of test results.

LOLITA M. ADRIEN, RN, BA, BSN
CLAIRE B. MAILHOT, RN, MS

Basal Gastric Secretion Test

Although gastric secretion peaks after ingestion of food, small amounts of gastric juice are also secreted between meals. This secretion, known as basal secretion, results from psychoneurogenic influences mediated by the vagus nerves and by hormones, such as gastrin.

This test measures basal secretion under fasting conditions by aspirating stomach contents through a nasogastric tube, and is indicated in patients with obscure epigastric pain, anorexia, and weight loss. Since external factors—such as the sight or odor of food—and psychological stress stimulate gastric secretion, accurate testing requires that the patient be relaxed and isolated from all sources of sensory stimulation. Although abnormal basal secretion can suggest various gastric and duodenal disorders, complete evaluation of secretion requires the gastric acid stimulation test.

Purpose
□ To determine gastric output in the fasting state.

Patient preparation
Explain to the patient that this test measures the stomach's secretion of acid. Instruct him to restrict food for 12 hours, and fluids and smoking for 8 hours before the test. Tell him who will perform the test, and that the procedure takes approximately 1½ hours (or 2½ hours, if followed by the gastric acid stimulation test).

Inform the patient that the test requires insertion of a tube through the nose and into the stomach, and that he may initially experience discomfort and may cough or gag.

Withhold antacids, anticholinergics, cholinergics, alcohol, cimetidine, reserpine, adrenergic blockers, and adrenocorticosteroids for 24 hours before the test, as ordered. If these medications must be continued, note this on the laboratory slip.

Just before the test, check the patient's pulse rate and blood pressure. Then, encourage him to relax.

Procedure
After seating the patient comfortably, insert the nasogastric tube. Then, attach a 20-ml syringe to it, and aspirate the stomach contents. To ensure complete emptying of the stomach, ask the patient to assume three positions in sequence—supine, and right and left lateral decubitus—while the stomach contents are aspirated. Label the specimen container "Residual Contents."

Then, connect the nasogastric tube to the suction machine. Aspirate gastric contents by continuous low suction for 1½ hours. (Aspiration can also be performed manually, with a syringe.) Collect a specimen every 15 minutes, but discard the first two; this eliminates the specimen that could be influenced by the stress of the intubation. Record the color and odor of each specimen, and note the presence of food, mucus, bile, or blood. Label these specimens "Basal Contents," and number them 1 through 4.

If the nasogastric tube is to be left in place, clamp it or attach it to low intermittent suction, as ordered.

Precautions
□ The basal gastric secretion test is contraindicated in patients with conditions that prohibit nasogastric intubation.

THE HOLLANDER TEST

I.V. injection of insulin in a patient with a normal blood sugar level causes hypoglycemia by promoting cellular absorption of glucose. In turn, hypoglycemia affects the vagus nerve, which stimulates acid secretion by the parietal and chief cells. A vagotomy—surgical transection of the vagus nerves—eliminates this neural stimulus for gastric acid secretion.

The Hollander test (insulin gastric analysis) evaluates the effectiveness of vagotomy, and is best performed 3 to 6 months after surgery. In this test, gastric contents are aspirated under fasting conditions through a nasogastric tube, before and after a dose of insulin, and then compared; simultaneously, blood glucose levels are determined before and after the insulin

injection. If the acid output after the insulin injection exceeds the preinjection acid output, the vagotomy is likely to be incomplete; if acid output fails to rise after the insulin injection, the vagotomy is considered complete. However, failure to increase acid output is significant only if achlorhydria persists after blood glucose falls below 50 mg/dl.

The Hollander test is contraindicated in patients with coronary artery or cerebrovascular disease, a predisposition to hypoglycemia, or other conditions that prohibit nasogastric intubation. It's not useful in patients with achlorhydria, as demonstrated by the gastric acid stimulation test, since such patients fail to respond to insulin injection.

□ During insertion, make sure the nasogastric tube enters the esophagus, and not the trachea; remove it immediately if the patient develops cyanosis or paroxysms of coughing.

□ Monitor vital signs during intubation, and observe carefully for arrhythmias.

□ To prevent contamination of the specimens with saliva, instruct the patient to expectorate excess saliva.

□ When collection is completed, send the specimens to the laboratory immediately.

Values

Normally, basal secretion ranges from 0.2 to 3.8 mEq/hour in females and from 1 to 5 mEq/hour in males.

Implications of results

Abnormal basal secretion findings are nonspecific and must be considered with the results of the gastric acid stimulation test. Elevated secretion may suggest duodenal or jejunal ulcer (after partial gastrectomy) or, when markedly elevated, Zollinger-Ellison syndrome. Depressed secretion may indicate gastric carcinoma or benign gastric ulcer. Absence of secretion may indicate pernicious anemia.

Post-test care

□ Watch for complications—such as

nausea, vomiting, and abdominal distention or pain—following removal of the nasogastric tube.

□ If the patient complains of a sore throat, provide soothing lozenges.

□ As ordered, the patient may resume his usual diet and medications withheld before the test unless the gastric acid stimulation test will also be performed.

Interfering factors

□ Failure to adhere to pretest restrictions increases basal secretion.

□ Psychological stress can stimulate excessive basal secretion.

□ Cholinergics, reserpine, alcohol, adrenergic blockers, and adrenocorticosteroids may increase basal secretion; antacids, anticholinergics, and cimetidine may depress it.

LOLITA M. ADRIEN, RN, BA, BSN
CLAIRE B. MAILHOT, RN, MS

Gastric Acid Stimulation Test

The gastric acid stimulation test measures the secretion of gastric acid for 1 hour after subcutaneous injection of pentagastrin or a similar drug that stimulates gastric acid output. It's indicated and usually follows the basal secretion test immediately, when the latter suggests abnormal gastric secretion.

Pentagastrin stimulates the parietal cells to secrete hydrochloric acid. If these cells are damaged or destroyed, acid secretion decreases or is absent; if the cells are hyperactive, acid secretion increases. Although this test detects abnormal gastric secretion, radiographic studies and endoscopy are necessary to determine the cause.

Purpose
□ To aid diagnosis of duodenal ulcer, Zollinger-Ellison syndrome, pernicious anemia, and gastric carcinoma.

Patient preparation
Explain to the patient that this test determines if the stomach is secreting acid properly. Instruct him to refrain from eating, drinking, and smoking from midnight before the test. Tell him who will perform the test, and that it takes 1 hour.

Tell the patient that the test requires passing a tube through the nose and into the stomach, and a subcutaneous injection of pentagastrin. Describe the possible side effects—abdominal pain, nausea, vomiting, flushing, transitory dizziness, faintness, and numbness of extremities—and instruct him to report such symptoms immediately.

Check the patient's history for hypersensitivity to pentagastrin. As ordered, withhold antacids, anticholinergics, adrenergic blockers, cimetidine, and reserpine. If these drugs must be continued, note this on the laboratory slip. Record baseline vital signs before beginning the procedure.

Procedure
After basal gastric secretions have been collected, keep the nasogastric tube in place. Pentagastrin is then injected subcutaneously. Wait 15 minutes, and then collect a specimen every 15 minutes for 1 hour. Record the color and odor of each specimen, and note the presence of food, mucus, bile, or blood. Label all specimens "Stimulated Contents," and number them 1 through 4.

If the nasogastric tube is to be left in place, clamp it or attach it to low intermittent suction, as ordered.

Precautions
□ The gastric acid stimulation test is contraindicated in patients with hypersensitivity to pentagastrin or with conditions that prohibit nasogastric intubation.
□ Observe for adverse effects of pentagastrin.
□ To prevent contamination of the specimens with saliva, instruct the patient to expectorate excess saliva.
□ When collection is completed, send the specimens to the laboratory immediately.

Values
Normally, gastric secretion following stimulation ranges from 11 to 21 mEq/hour for females and from 18 to 28 mEq/hour for males.

Implications of results
Elevated gastric secretion may indicate duodenal ulcer; markedly elevated secretion suggests Zollinger-Ellison syndrome. Depressed secretion may indicate gastric carcinoma; achlorhydria may indicate pernicious anemia.

Post-test care
□ Watch for nausea, vomiting, and abdominal distention and pain after removal of the nasogastric tube.
□ If the patient complains of a sore throat, provide soothing lozenges.
□ As ordered, the patient may resume his usual diet and medications withheld before the basal secretion test.

Interfering factors
□ Failure to adhere to pretest restrictions may interfere with the accuracy of test results.
□ Gastric acid levels are elevated by cholinergics, adrenergic blockers, and re-

serpine; such levels are depressed by antacids, anticholinergics, and cimetidine.

LOLITA M. ADRIEN, RN, BA, BSN
CLAIRE B. MAILHOT, RN, MS

Peritoneal Fluid Analysis

The peritoneum is a tough, semipermeable membrane that lines the abdominal and visceral cavities, and encloses, supports, and lubricates the organs within these cavities. It also serves an important osmoregulatory function; passive diffusion of water and solute particles (up to a certain size) occurs across this membrane, to maintain osmotic and chemical equilibrium with associated blood and lymphatic systems.

Accumulation of fluid in the peritoneal space—ascites—can be caused by conditions such as hepatic, renal, or cardiovascular disorders; inflammation; infection; or neoplasm.

Peritoneal fluid analysis includes examination of gross appearance, erythrocyte and leukocyte counts, cytologic studies, microbiologic studies for bacteria and fungi, and determinations of protein, glucose, amylase, ammonia, and alkaline phosphatase levels.

This test assesses a sample of peritoneal fluid obtained by paracentesis, a procedure which entails inserting a trocar and cannula through the abdominal wall with the patient under a local anesthetic. If the sample of fluid is being removed for therapeutic purposes, the trocar can be connected to a drainage system. If only a small amount of fluid is being removed for diagnostic purposes, an 18G needle can be substituted for the trocar and cannula. In a four-quadrant tap, fluid is aspirated from each quadrant of the abdomen, to verify abdominal trauma and confirm the need for surgery.

Complications associated with this test include shock and hypovolemia, perforation of abdominal organs, hemorrhage, and hepatic coma.

Purpose
□ To determine the cause of ascites
□ To detect abdominal trauma.

Patient preparation
Explain to the patient that this procedure helps determine the cause of ascites or detects abdominal trauma. Inform him he needn't restrict food or fluids before the test. Tell him that the test requires a peritoneal fluid sample, that he will receive a local anesthetic to minimize discomfort, and that the procedure takes 5 to 45 minutes to perform.

Provide psychological support to decrease the patient's anxiety, and assure him that complications are rare. If the patient has severe ascites, inform him that the procedure will relieve his discomfort and allow him to breathe more easily.

Make sure the patient or responsible family member has signed a consent form. Record baseline vital signs and weight for comparison with post-test readings; abdominal girth measurements may also be ordered. Tell the patient a blood sample may be taken for laboratory analysis (hemoglobin, hematocrit, prothrombin time, activated partial prothrombin time, and platelet count).

Just before the test, tell the patient to void. This helps prevent accidental bladder injury during needle insertion.

Procedure
Position the patient, as ordered. Seat the patient on a bed or in a chair, with his feet flat on the floor and his back well supported. If he can't tolerate being out of bed, place him in high Fowler's position. Make him as comfortable as you can. Except for the puncture site, keep him covered to prevent chilling. Provide a plastic sheet or absorbent pad to collect spillage and to protect the patient and bed linens.

PERITONEAL FLUID ANALYSIS

ELEMENT	NORMAL VALUE OR FINDING
Gross appearance	Sterile, odorless, clear to pale yellow color; scant amount (< 50 ml)
RBCs	None
WBCs	< 300/µl
Protein	0.3 to 4.1 g/dl (albumin, 50% to 70%; globulin, 30% to 45%; fibrinogen, 0.3% to 4.5%)
Glucose	70 to 100 mg/dl
Amylase	138 to 404 amylase units/liter
Ammonia	< 50 µg/dl
Alkaline phosphatase	Male: > age 18—90 to 239 units/liter Female: < age 45—76 to 196 units/liter Female: > age 45—87 to 250 units/liter
LDH	Equal to serum level
Cytology	No malignant cells present
Bacteria	None
Fungi	None

The puncture site is then shaved, the skin prepared, and the area draped. A local anesthetic is injected, and the needle or trocar and cannula are usually inserted 1″ to 2″ (2.5 to 5 cm) below the umbilicus. However, insertion may also be through the flank, the iliac fossa, the border of the rectus, or at each quadrant of the abdomen. If a trocar and cannula are used, a small incision is made to facilitate insertion. When the needle pierces the peritoneum, it "gives" with an audible sound. The trocar is removed, and a sample of fluid is aspirated with a 50-ml Luer-Lok syringe.

The paracentesis tray contains specimen tubes for the various tests. If additional fluid is to be drained, assist in attaching one end of an I.V. tube to the cannula and the other end to a collection bag. The fluid is then aspirated (no more than 1,500 ml). If fluid aspiration is difficult, reposition the patient, as ordered. After aspiration, the trocar or needle is removed, and a pressure dressing is applied. Occasionally, the wound may be sutured first. Label the samples in the order they were drawn. If the patient has received antibiotic therapy, note this on the laboratory slip. Carefully dispose of needles and contaminated articles if the patient has a history of hepatitis; incinerate disposable items and return reusable ones to the central supply area.

Precautions
□ Peritoneal fluid analysis should be used cautiously in patients who are pregnant and in those with bleeding tendencies or unstable vital signs.

□ Check vital signs every 15 minutes during the procedure. Watch for deviations from baseline findings. Observe for dizziness, pallor, perspiration, and increased anxiety.
□ If rapid fluid aspiration induces hypovolemia and shock, reduce the vertical

distance between the trocar and the collection bag, to slow the drainage rate. If necessary, stop drainage by turning the stopcock off or by clamping the tubing.
□ Avoid contamination of specimens, which alters their bacterial content. Send them to the laboratory immediately.

Values
The chart on opposite page gives normal values for peritoneal fluid.

Implications of results
Milk-colored peritoneal fluid may result from chyle escaping from a thoracic duct that is damaged or blocked by carcinoma, lymphoma, tuberculosis, parasitic infection, adhesion, or hepatic cirrhosis; a pseudochylous condition may result from the presence of leukocytes or tumor cells. Differential diagnosis of true chylous ascites depends on the presence of elevated triglyceride levels ($\geqslant$400 mg/dl) and microscopic fat globules. Cloudy or turbid fluid may indicate peritonitis due to primary bacterial infection, ruptured bowel (after trauma), pancreatitis, strangulated or infarcted intestine, or appendicitis. Bloody fluid may result from a benign or malignant tumor, hemorrhagic pancreatitis, or a traumatic tap; however, if the fluid fails to clear on continued aspiration, traumatic tap isn't the cause. Bile-stained green fluid may indicate a ruptured gallbladder, acute pancreatitis, or perforated intestine or duodenal ulcer.

An RBC count over 100/µl indicates neoplasm or tuberculosis; a count over 100,000/µl indicates intra-abdominal trauma. A WBC count over 300/µl, with more than 25% neutrophils, occurs in 90% of patients with spontaneous bacterial peritonitis and in 50% of those with cirrhosis. A high percentage of lymphocytes suggests tuberculous peritonitis or chylous ascites. Numerous mesothelial cells indicate tuberculous peritonitis.

Protein levels rise above 3 g/dl in malignancy and above 4 g/dl in tuberculosis. Peritoneal fluid glucose levels fall below 60 mg/dl in 30% to 50% of patients with tuberculous peritonitis and

peritoneal carcinomatosis. Amylase levels rise in about 90% of patients with pancreatic trauma, pancreatic pseudocyst, or acute pancreatitis, and may also rise in intestinal necrosis or strangulation. Peritoneal alkaline phosphatase levels rise to more than twice the normal serum levels in about 90% of patients with ruptured or strangulated small intestine. Peritoneal ammonia levels also exceed twice the normal serum levels in ruptured or strangulated large and small intestines, and in ruptured ulcer or appendix.

A protein ascitic fluid/serum ratio of 0.5 or greater, an LDH ascitic fluid/serum ratio over 0.6, and an ascitic fluid LDH level over 400 µ/ml suggest malignant, tuberculous, or pancreatic ascites. Any two of these findings indicates a non-hepatic cause; absence of all three usually suggests uncomplicated hepatic disease. An albumin gradient between ascitic fluid and serum over 1 g/dl indicates chronic hepatic disease; a lesser value suggests malignancy.

Cytologic examination of peritoneal fluid accurately detects malignant cells. Microbiologic examination can reveal coliforms, anaerobes, and enterococci, which can enter the peritoneum from a ruptured organ, or from infections accompanying appendicitis, pancreatitis, tuberculosis, or ovarian disease. Gram-positive cocci often indicate primary peritonitis; gram-negative organisms, secondary peritonitis. The presence of fungi may indicate histoplasmosis, candidiasis, or coccidioidomycosis.

Post-test care
□ Apply a gauze dressing to the puncture site. Make sure it's thick enough to absorb all drainage. Check the dressing frequently, whenever you check vital signs; reinforce or apply a pressure dressing, if needed.
□ Monitor vital signs until stable. If the patient's recovery is poor, check vital signs every 15 minutes, as ordered. Weigh the patient and measure abdominal girth; compare these with baseline measurements.

☐ Allow the patient to rest, and if possible, withhold treatment or procedures that may cause undue stress.

☐ Monitor urinary output for at least 24 hours, and watch for hematuria, which may indicate bladder trauma.

☐ If a large amount of fluid was aspirated, watch for signs of vascular collapse (color change, elevated pulse rate and respirations, decreased blood pressure and central venous pressure, mental changes, and dizziness). Administer fluids orally if the patient is alert and can accept them.

 ☐ Watch for signs of hemorrhage and shock, or for increasing pain and abdominal tenderness. These may indicate a perforated intestine or, depending on the site of the tap, puncture of the inferior epigastric artery, hematoma of the anterior cecal wall, or rupture of the iliac vein or bladder.

 ☐ Observe the patient with severe hepatic disease for signs of hepatic coma, which may result from loss of sodium and potassium accompanying hypovolemia. Watch for mental changes, drowsiness, and stupor. Such a patient is also prone to uremia, infection, hemorrhage, and protein depletion.

☐ Administer I.V. infusions and albumin as ordered. Check the laboratory report for electrolytes (especially sodium) and serum protein levels.

Interfering factors

☐ Failure to send the sample to the laboratory immediately or unsterile collection technique interferes with accurate testing.

☐ Injury to underlying structures during paracentesis may contaminate the sample with bile, blood, urine, or feces.

MARY C. SMOLENSKI, RN, MSN

FECAL CONTENTS

Fecal Occult Blood Test

Fecal occult blood, invisible because of its minute quantity, can be detected by microscopic analysis or by chemical tests for hemoglobin, such as the guaiac or orthotolidin test. Because small amounts of blood (2 to 2.5 ml/day) normally appear in the feces, tests for occult blood are designed to detect quantities larger than this. These tests are indicated in patients whose clinical symptoms and preliminary blood studies suggest GI bleeding. However, further tests are required to pinpoint the origin of the bleeding. Stool color correlates roughly with the site of bleeding, for example, melena usually results from hemorrhage in the esophagus or stomach. Gastric juices act to digest this blood, blackening it. Melena may also result from hemorrhage in the jejunum or ileum, provided its passage through the intestine is slow. Dark maroon stools result from hemorrhage beyond the ligament of Treitz.

Purpose

☐ To detect GI bleeding

☐ To aid early diagnosis of colorectal cancer.

Patient preparation

Explain to the patient that this test helps detect abnormal GI bleeding. Instruct him to maintain a high-fiber diet and to refrain from eating red meats, poultry, fish, turnips, and horseradish for 48 to 72 hours before the test, as well as throughout the collection period. Tell him the test requires collection of three stool specimens. (Occasionally, only a random specimen is collected.)

As ordered, withhold iron preparations, bromides, iodides, rauwolfia derivatives, indomethacin, colchicine, salicylates, phenylbutazone, steroids, and

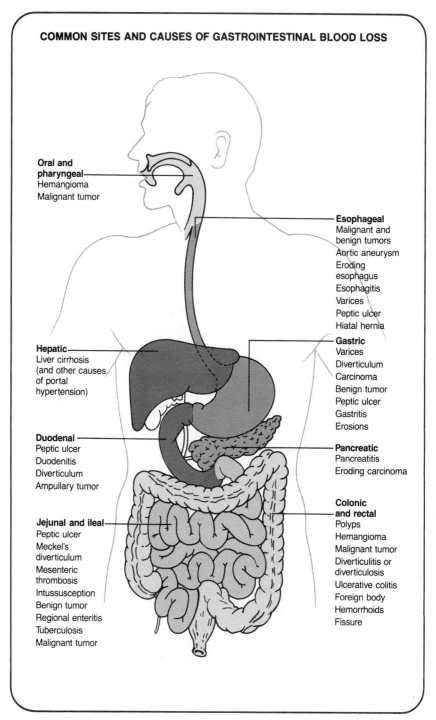

COMMON SITES AND CAUSES OF GASTROINTESTINAL BLOOD LOSS

Oral and pharyngeal
Hemangioma
Malignant tumor

Esophageal
Malignant and benign tumors
Aortic aneurysm
Eroding esophagus
Esophagitis
Varices
Peptic ulcer
Hiatal hernia

Hepatic
Liver cirrhosis (and other causes of portal hypertension)

Gastric
Varices
Diverticulum
Carcinoma
Benign tumor
Peptic ulcer
Gastritis
Erosions

Duodenal
Peptic ulcer
Duodenitis
Diverticulum
Ampullary tumor

Pancreatic
Pancreatitis
Eroding carcinoma

Jejunal and ileal
Peptic ulcer
Meckel's diverticulum
Mesenteric thrombosis
Intussusception
Benign tumor
Regional enteritis
Tuberculosis
Malignant tumor

Colonic and rectal
Polyps
Hemangioma
Malignant tumor
Diverticulitis or diverticulosis
Ulcerative colitis
Foreign body
Hemorrhoids
Fissure

TESTING FOR OCCULT BLOOD

Of the commercial screening tests for occult blood, Hematest and Hemoccult are the two most commonly used. Hematest uses orthotolidin to detect hemoglobin; Hemoccult uses guaiac. Although both tests can differentiate between normal and abnormal amounts of fecal blood, Hematest is slightly more sensitive; Hemoccult is generally more accurate and reliable. However, positive results with either test aren't conclusive.

---

ascorbic acid for 48 hours before the test and also during it. If these medications must be continued, note this on the laboratory slip.

Procedure
Collect three stool specimens or a random specimen, as ordered. Testing can take place in the laboratory or in a utility room on the nursing unit, depending on hospital policy.

First, place a small amount of stool on a piece of filter paper. Then, add two drops each of tap water, glacial acetic acid, 1:60 solution of gum guaiac in 95% ethyl alcohol, and 3% hydrogen peroxide, *or* two drops each of 0.2% orthotolidin and 0.3% hydrogen peroxide. Mix thoroughly with a tongue blade. Note the color immediately, and check it again after 5 minutes.

Be sure to obtain specimens from two different areas of each stool, to allow for variance in distribution of blood.

Precautions
□ Instruct the patient to avoid contaminating the stool specimen with toilet tissue or urine.
□ Send the specimen to the laboratory or perform the test immediately.

Findings
Normally, less than 2.5 ml of blood is present, resulting in a green reaction.

Implications of results
A dark blue reaction that appears within 5 minutes indicates that the test is positive for occult blood; a strongly positive reaction within 3 to 4 minutes is always abnormal. A faint blue reaction is weakly positive and isn't necessarily abnormal. A positive test indicates GI bleeding, which may result from many disorders, such as varices, peptic ulcer, carcinoma, ulcerative colitis, dysentery, or hemorrhagic disease. This test is particularly important for early diagnosis of colorectal cancer, since 80% of persons with this type of cancer demonstrate positive results. Further tests, such as barium swallow, analyses of gastric contents, and endoscopic procedures, are necessary to define the site and extent of bleeding.

Post-test care
As ordered, the patient may resume his usual diet and medications.

Interfering factors
□ Failure to adhere to dietary restrictions, to test the specimen immediately, or to send it to the laboratory immediately may affect test results.
□ Bleeding may result from use of iron preparations, bromides, rauwolfia derivatives, indomethacin, colchicine, phenylbutazone, or steroids.
□ Ascorbic acid (vitamin C) can interfere with accurate testing by producing normal test results even in the presence of significant bleeding.
□ Ingestion of 2 to 5 ml of blood, such as from bleeding gums, can cause abnormal results.

LOLITA M. ADRIEN, RN, BA, BSN
CLAIRE B. MAILHOT, RN, MS

Fecal Lipids

Lipids excreted in feces include mono-glycerides, diglycerides, triglycerides, phospholipids, glycolipids, soaps (fatty acids and fatty acid salts), sterols, and cholesterol esters. These lipids are derived from sloughed intestinal bacterial cells and epithelial cells, unabsorbed dietary lipids, and gastrointestinal secretions. Normally, dietary lipids emulsified by bile are almost completely absorbed in the small intestine, provided biliary and pancreatic secretions are adequate. However, excessive excretion of fecal lipids—steatorrhea—occurs in various malabsorption syndromes. Both qualitative and quantitative tests can detect excessive excretion of lipids in patients with signs of malabsorption: weight loss, abdominal distention, and scaly skin. In the qualitative test, a specimen from a random stool is stained with Sudan III dye and examined microscopically for evidence of malabsorption—undigested muscle fibers and various fats. In the quantitative test, the entire 72-hour specimen is dried and weighed; the lipids therein are extracted with a solvent, evaporated, and weighed. Only the quantitative test can confirm steatorrhea.

Purpose
□ To confirm steatorrhea.

Patient preparation
Explain to the patient that this test evaluates digestion of fats. Instruct him to abstain from alcohol and to maintain a high-fat diet (100 g/day) for 3 days before the test and during the collection period. Tell him the test requires a 72-hour stool collection.

Withhold drugs that may affect test results, as ordered. If these medications must be continued, note this on the laboratory slip.

Teach the patient how to collect a timed stool specimen, and provide him with the necessary equipment. Inform him that the laboratory requires 1 or 2 days to complete the analysis.

Procedure
Collect a 72-hour stool specimen.

Precautions
□ Don't use a waxed collection container, because the wax may become incorporated in the stool and interfere with accurate testing.
□ Tell the patient to avoid contaminating the stool specimen with toilet tissue or urine.
□ Refrigerate the collection container between defecations, and keep it tightly covered.

Values
Fecal lipids normally comprise less than 20% of excreted solids, with excretion of less than 7 g/24 hours.

Implications of results
Both digestive and absorptive disorders cause steatorrhea. Digestive disorders may affect the production and release of pancreatic lipase or bile; absorptive disorders may affect the integrity of the intestine. In pancreatic insufficiency, impaired lipid digestion may result from insufficient production of lipase. Pancreatic resection, cystic fibrosis, chronic pancreatitis, or ductal obstruction by stone or tumor may prevent the normal release or action of lipase. In impaired hepatic function, faulty lipid digestion may result from inadequate production of bile salts. Biliary obstruction, which may accompany gallbladder disease, may prevent the normal release of bile salts into the duodenum. Extensive small bowel resection or bypass may also interrupt normal enterohepatic circulation of bile salts.

Diseases of the intestinal mucosa affect normal absorption of lipids; regional ileitis and atrophy due to malnutrition cause gross structural changes in the intestinal wall, while celiac disease and tropical sprue produce mucosal abnormalities. Scleroderma, radiation enteritis, fistulas, intestinal tuberculosis, small intestine diverticula, and altered intestinal flora may also cause steatorrhea. Whipple's disease and lymphomas cause lymphatic obstruction that may inhibit fat absorption.

Post-test care
As ordered, the patient may resume his usual diet and medications withheld before the test.

Interfering factors
□ The following substances may produce inaccurate test results by inhibiting absorption or affecting chemical digestion: azathioprine, bisacodyl, cholestyramine, kanamycin, neomycin, colchicine, aluminum hydroxide, calcium carbonate, alcohol, potassium chloride, and mineral oil.

□ Failure to observe pretest instructions pertaining to diet and ingestion of alcohol, use of a waxed collection container, contamination of the sample, and incomplete stool specimen collection (total weight less than 300 g) interfere with accurate testing.

LOLITA M. ADRIEN, RN, BA, BSN
CLAIRE B. MAILHOT, RN, MS

Fecal Urobilinogen

Urobilinogen, the end product of bilirubin metabolism, is a brown pigment formed by bacterial enzymes in the small intestine. It's excreted in feces or reabsorbed into portal blood, where it is returned to the liver and reexcreted in bile; a small amount of urobilinogen is also excreted in urine. Because bilirubin metabolism depends on a properly functioning hepatobiliary system and a normal erythrocyte life span, measurement of fecal urobilinogen is a useful indicator of hepatobiliary and hemolytic disorders. However, this test is rarely performed, since serum bilirubin and urine urobilinogen can be measured more easily.

Purpose
□ To aid diagnosis of hepatobiliary and hemolytic disorders.

Patient preparation
Explain to the patient that this test evaluates function of the liver and bile ducts or detects RBC disorders. Inform him that he needn't restrict food or fluids before the test. Tell him the test requires collection of a random stool specimen.

Withhold broad-spectrum antibiotics, sulfonamides, and salicylates for 2 weeks before the test, as ordered. If these medications must be continued, note this on the laboratory slip.

Procedure
Collect a random stool specimen.

Precautions
□ Tell the patient not to contaminate the stool specimen with toilet tissue or urine.
□ Use a light-resistant collection container, since urobilinogen breaks down to urobilin on exposure to light.
□ Send the specimen to the laboratory immediately. If transport or testing is delayed more than 30 minutes, refrigerate the specimen; if testing is being performed by an outside laboratory, freeze the specimen.

Values
Normally, fecal urobilinogen values range from 50 to 300 mg/24 hours.

Implications of results
Low levels or absence of urobilinogen in the feces indicates obstructed bile flow—the result of intrahepatic disorders—such as hepatocellular jaundice due to cirrhosis or hepatitis—extrahepatic disorders—such as tumor of the head of the pancreas, the ampulla of Vater, or the bile duct—and choledocholithiasis. Low fecal urobilinogen levels are also characteristic of depressed erythropoiesis, as in aplastic anemia.

Elevated fecal urobilinogen levels are typical in hemolytic jaundice, thalassemia, and hemolytic, sickle cell, and pernicious anemias.

Post-test care
Resume administration of medications withheld before the test, as ordered.

Interfering factors
□ Broad-spectrum antibiotics can depress fecal urobilinogen levels by inhibiting bacterial growth in the colon. Sulfonamides, which react with the reagent

used by the laboratory in this test, and large doses of salicylates can raise fecal urobilinogen levels.

☐ Failure to use a light-resistant collec-

tion container or contamination of the specimen prevents accurate testing.

LOLITA M. ADRIEN, RN, BA, BSN
CLAIRE B. MAILHOT, RN, MS

ENDOSCOPY

Esophagogastroduodenoscopy

Esophagogastroduodenoscopy is the visual examination of the lining of the esophagus, the stomach, and the upper duodenum using a flexible fiberoptic endoscope. It's indicated in patients with hematemesis, melena, or substernal or epigastric pain, and in postoperative patients with recurrent or new symptoms. This procedure is generally safe, but can cause perforation of the esophagus, stomach, or duodenum, especially if the patient is restless or uncooperative.

Esophagogastroduodenoscopy eliminates the need for extensive exploratory surgery and can detect small or surface lesions missed by radiography. It also permits laboratory evaluation of abnormalities first detected by radiography, since the scope provides a channel for biopsy forceps or a cytology brush. Similarly, it allows removal of foreign bodies by suction (for small, soft objects) or by electrocautery snare or forceps (for large, hard objects).

Purpose
☐ To diagnose inflammatory disease, malignant and benign tumors, ulcers, Mallory-Weiss syndrome, and structural abnormalities
☐ To evaluate the stomach and duodenum postoperatively
☐ To obtain emergency diagnosis of duodenal ulcer or esophageal injury, such as that caused by ingestion of chemicals.

Patient preparation
Explain to the patient that this procedure

permits visual examination of the lining of the esophagus, the stomach, and the upper duodenum. Instruct him to fast for 6 to 12 hours before the test. Tell him that the test requires that a flexible instrument be passed through his mouth, who will perform this procedure and where, and that it takes about 30 minutes. (If an emergency esophagogastroduodenoscopy is to be performed, tell the patient that stomach contents are aspirated through a nasogastric tube.) Also, inform him that a blood sample may be drawn before the procedure.

Inform the patient that a bittertasting local anesthetic will be sprayed into his mouth and throat to calm the gag reflex, and that his tongue and throat may feel swollen, making swallowing seem difficult. Advise him to let the saliva drain from the side of his mouth; a suction machine may be used to remove saliva, if necessary. If the patient has teeth, tell him a mouth guard will be inserted to protect his teeth and the endoscope; assure him that the mouth guard won't obstruct his breathing. Inform him that he'll receive a sedative before the endoscope is inserted to help him relax, but that he'll remain conscious. If the procedure is being done on an outpatient, advise the patient to arrange for transportation home, since he may feel drowsy from the sedative.

Tell the patient he may experience pressure in the stomach as the endoscope is moved about, and a feeling of fullness when air or carbon dioxide is insufflated (insufflation distends and flattens the stomach walls to aid their visualization). If the patient is apprehensive, administer meperidine or another analgesic I.M. about 30 minutes before the test, as ordered; also, as ordered, administer atropine sulfate subcutaneously at this time, to decrease gastrointestinal secretions, which would interfere with test results.

Make sure the patient or responsible member of the family has signed a consent form. Check the patient's history for hypersensitivity to the medications and anesthetic ordered for the test.

Just before the procedure, instruct the patient to remove dentures, eyeglasses, necklaces, hairpins, combs, and constricting undergarments.

Procedure

Obtain baseline vital signs, and leave the blood pressure cuff in place for monitoring throughout the procedure. Then, ask the patient to hold his breath while his mouth and throat are sprayed with a local anesthetic. The patient is given an emesis basin to spit out saliva and is provided with tissues to wipe excess saliva from his mouth. Since the anesthetic spray causes the patient to lose some control of his secretions and increases the risk of aspiration, encourage him to let saliva drain from the side of his mouth.

After the patient is placed in a left lateral position, his head is bent forward and he is asked to open his mouth. The examiner inserts his finger into the mouth and guides the tip of the endoscope alongside his finger, to the back of the throat. The rubber tip is deflected downward with the left index finger, and the endoscope is advanced. As the endoscope passes through the posterior pharynx and the cricopharyngeal sphincter, the patient's head is slowly extended to aid advancement of the scope. The patient's chin must be kept at midline. The endoscope is then passed along the esophagus under direct vision. When the endoscope is well into the esophagus (about 12″ [30 cm]), the patient's head is positioned with his chin toward the table, so saliva can drain out of his mouth.

When examination of the esophagus and the cardiac sphincter is completed, the endoscope is rotated clockwise with the tip angled upward, and is advanced into the stomach. After the lining of the stomach is examined completely, including the gastric side of the cardiac and pyloric sphincters, the endoscope is advanced into the duodenum. Following this examination, the endoscope is slowly withdrawn, and suspicious areas of the gastric and esophageal lining are reexamined.

During the examination, air may be instilled into the gastrointestinal tract to open the bowel lumen and flatten tissue folds, water instilled to rinse material or fluid from the lens, and suction applied to remove unnecessary insufflated air or secretions. A camera may be attached to the endoscope to photograph areas for later study, or a measuring tube passed through the endoscope to determine the size of a lesion. Biopsy forceps to obtain a tissue specimen, or a cytology brush to obtain cells may also be passed through the scope. Tissue specimens are immediately placed in a specimen bottle containing 10% formaldehyde solution; cell specimens are smeared on glass slides and placed in a Coplin jar containing 95% ethyl alcohol.

Precautions

□ Esophagogastroduodenoscopy is usually contraindicated in patients with Zenker's diverticulum, large aortic aneurysm, or recent ulcer perforation.

□ Esophagogastroduodenoscopy should not be performed within 2 days after an upper gastrointestinal series, because barium retention hinders visual examination.

□ Observe closely for medication side effects: respiratory depression, apnea, hypotension, excessive diaphoresis, bradycardia, and laryngospasm. Have available emergency resuscitation equipment and a narcotic antagonist, such as naloxone or levallorphan tartrate. Be prepared to intervene, as necessary.

□ If tissue or cell specimens are obtained during the procedure, label and send them to the appropriate laboratory immediately.

Findings

The smooth mucosa of the esophagus is

normally yellow-pink and is marked by a fine vascular network. A pulsation on the anterior wall of the esophagus between 8″ and 10″ (20 and 25 cm) from the incisor teeth represents the aortic arch. The orange-red mucosa of the stomach begins at the "Z" line, an irregular transition line slightly above the esophagogastric junction. Unlike the esophagus, the stomach has rugal folds, and its blood vessels aren't visible beneath the gastric mucosa. The reddish mucosa of the duodenal bulb is marked by a few shallow longitudinal folds. However, the mucosa of the distal duodenum has prominent circular folds, is lined with villi, and appears velvety.

Implications of results

Esophagogastroduodenoscopy, with the results of histologic and cytologic tests, may indicate acute or chronic ulcers, benign or malignant tumors, and inflammatory disease, including esophagitis, gastritis, and duodenitis. This test may demonstrate diverticula, varices, Mallory-Weiss syndrome, esophageal rings, esophageal and pyloric stenoses, and esophageal hiatal hernia. Although esophagogastroduodenoscopy can evaluate gross abnormalities of esophageal motility, such as occurs in achalasia, manometric studies are more accurate.

Post-test care

□ Observe the patient for possible perforation. Perforation in the cervical area of the esophagus produces pain on swallowing and with neck movement; thoracic perforation causes substernal or epigastric pain that increases with breathing or with movement of the trunk; diaphragmatic perforation produces shoulder pain and dyspnea; gastric perforation causes abdominal or back pain, cyanosis, fever, or pleural effusion.

□ Check vital signs every 15 minutes for 4 hours, every hour for 4 hours, then every 4 hours.

□ Withhold food and fluids until the gag reflex returns. Test the gag reflex by touching the back of the throat with a tongue blade. When the gag reflex returns—usually in 1 hour—allow fluids and a light meal, as ordered.

□ Tell the patient he may burp some insufflated air and may have a sore throat

ESOPHAGEAL TOPOGRAPHY

Incisor teeth

23 centimeters

Aortic arch

Z line

This diagram of the esophagus and part of the stomach shows the approximate location of the aortic arch and the Z line, an irregular boundary where the smooth esophageal mucosa changes abruptly to the furrowed lining of the stomach.

for 3 or 4 days. Provide throat lozenges and warm saline gargles to ease his discomfort.

□ If the patient experiences soreness at the I.V. site, apply warm soaks.

□ Be sure the outpatient has transportation home, since he shouldn't drive for 12 hours due to drowsiness from sedation. Instruct him to watch for persistent difficulty in swallowing, and for pain, fever, black stools, or vomiting blood. Tell him to notify the doctor immediately if any of these complications develop.

Interfering factors

Failure to adhere to dietary restrictions or to send specimens to the laboratory immediately may interfere with accurate determination of test results.

MAE E. PAULFREY, RN, MN

Colonoscopy

Colonoscopy is the visual examination of the lining of the large intestine with a flexible fiberoptic endoscope. This test is indicated for patients with histories of constipation and diarrhea, persistent rectal bleeding, or lower abdominal pain when results of proctosigmoidoscopy and the barium enema test prove negative or inconclusive. The colonoscope is available in 42" to 72" (105 to 180 cm) lengths and contains a bundle of glass fibers that transmit light. It is inserted anally and is advanced through the large intestine under direct vision, using the scope's optical system. Fluoroscopy and abdominal palpation may facilitate passage of the endoscope through the bends in the large intestine. Colonoscopy is usually a safe procedure but can cause perforation of the large intestine, excessive bleeding, and retroperitoneal emphysema.

Purpose

□ To detect or evaluate inflammatory and ulcerative bowel disease

□ To locate the origin of lower gastrointestinal bleeding

□ To aid diagnosis of colonic strictures and benign or malignant lesions

□ To evaluate the colon postoperatively for recurrence of polyps or malignant lesions.

Patient preparation

Explain to the patient that this test permits examination of the lining of the large intestine. Instruct him to maintain a clear liquid diet for 48 hours before the test. Tell him the test requires that a flexible instrument be passed through his anus, who will perform the test and where, and that the procedure generally takes 30 to 60 minutes.

Tell the patient that the large intestine must be thoroughly cleansed to be clearly visible. Give him a laxative, such as 10 oz (300 ml) of magnesium citrate or 3 tbsp (45 ml) of castor oil, in the evening, and a warm tap-water or sodium biphosphate enema 3 to 4 hours before the test, as ordered, until the return is clear. Don't administer a soapsuds enema, since this irritates the mucosa and stimulates mucous secretions that may hinder the examination.

Inform the patient that he may receive a sedative I.M. or I.V. to help him relax. Assure him that the colonoscope is well lubricated to ease its insertion, that it initially feels cool, and that he may feel an urge to defecate when it's inserted and advanced. Instruct him to breathe deeply and slowly through his mouth to relax the abdominal muscles.

Explain to the patient that air may be introduced into the large intestine through the colonoscope to distend the intestinal wall and provide a better view of the lining and to facilitate the instrument's advance. Tell him that flatus normally escapes around the instrument due to air insufflation, and that he shouldn't attempt to control it. Tell him that a suction machine may remove any blood or liquid feces that obscure vision, but that this won't cause any discomfort.

Make sure the patient or responsible member of the family has signed a con-

PERFORMING FIBEROPTIC COLONOSCOPY

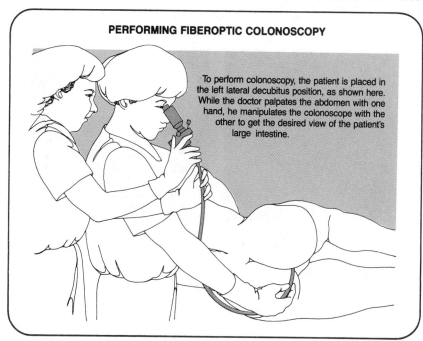

To perform colonoscopy, the patient is placed in the left lateral decubitus position, as shown here. While the doctor palpates the abdomen with one hand, he manipulates the colonoscope with the other to get the desired view of the patient's large intestine.

sent form. Check the patient's vital signs 30 minutes before the test; if they're stable, administer the sedative, as ordered.

Procedure

Place the patient on his left side, with his knees flexed, and drape him. Instruct him to breathe deeply and slowly through his mouth as the doctor inserts his gloved, lubricated index finger into the anus and rectum, and palpates the mucosa. After a water-soluble lubricant has been applied to the patient's anus and to the tip of the colonoscope, tell the patient the colonoscope is about to be inserted.

Following insertion of the colonoscope through the patient's anus, a small amount of air is insufflated to locate the bowel lumen. The scope is advanced through the rectum into the sigmoid colon under direct vision. When the instrument reaches the descending sigmoid junction, assist the patient to a supine position to aid the scope's advance, if necessary; this position may also be assumed to negotiate the splenic flexure. After the scope has passed the splenic flexure, it is advanced through the transverse colon, through the hepatic flexure, and passed into the ascending colon and cecum. Abdominal palpation or fluoroscopy may guide the colonoscope through the large intestine. (If the tip of the scope becomes lodged in the colon, fluoroscopy is especially helpful for locating the tip and adjusting the angle of entry.) During the examination, suction may be used to remove blood or excessive secretions that obscure vision.

Biopsy forceps or a cytology brush may be passed through a channel in the colonoscope to obtain specimens for histologic and cytologic examinations, respectively; an electrocautery snare may be used to remove polyps. If the examiner removes a tissue specimen, immediately place it in a specimen bottle containing 10% formalin; immediately place cytology smears in a Coplin jar containing 95% ethyl alcohol.

Precautions

☐ Colonoscopy is contraindicated in patients who have ischemic bowel disease,

NORMAL AND ABNORMAL COLONOSCOPY VIEWS

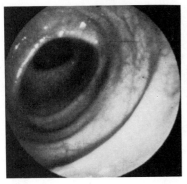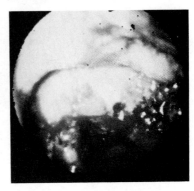

These two views, taken with a fiberoptic colonoscope, show a normal descending colon (left) and a colon with cancer (right).

acute diverticulitis, peritonitis, fulminant granulomatous colitis, or fulminant ulcerative colitis.

 □ Watch closely for side effects of the sedative, such as respiratory depression, hypotension, excessive diaphoresis, bradycardia, and confusion. Have available emergency resuscitation equipment and a narcotic antagonist, such as naloxone, for intravenous use, if necessary.

□ If the doctor has obtained a tissue or cell specimen, send it to the appropriate laboratory immediately.

□ If a polyp is removed but not retrieved during the examination, give enemas and strain stools, as ordered, to retrieve it.

Findings

Normally, the mucosa of the large intestine beyond the sigmoid colon appears light pink-orange and is marked by semilunar folds and deep tubular pits. Blood vessels are visible beneath the intestinal mucosa, which glistens from mucous secretions.

Implications of results

Visual examination of the large intestine, coupled with histologic and cytologic tests results, may indicate proctitis, granulomatous and ulcerative colitis, Crohn's disease, and malignant or benign lesions. Such examination alone can detect diverticular disease or the site of lower gastrointestinal bleeding.

Post-test care

 □ Observe patient closely for signs of bowel perforation: malaise, rectal bleeding, abdominal pain and distention, fever, and mucopurulent drainage. Notify the doctor immediately if such signs develop.

□ Check vital signs until stable.

□ After the patient has recovered from sedation, he may resume his usual diet.

□ Tell the patient he may pass large amounts of flatus, resulting from the air insufflated to distend the colon. Provide privacy in order to minimize embarrassment.

□ If a polyp has been removed, inform the patient that there may be some blood in his stool.

Interfering factors

□ Barium retained in the intestine from previous diagnostic studies makes accurate visual examination impossible.

□ Blood from acute colonic hemorrhage

interferes with the examination.

□ Fixation of the sigmoid colon from inflammatory bowel disease, surgery, or irradiation may inhibit passage of the colonoscope.

□ Failure to place histologic or cytologic specimens in the appropriate preservative or to send the specimens to the laboratory immediately may interfere with test results.

MAE E. PAULFREY, RN, MN

Proctosigmoidoscopy

Proctosigmoidoscopy is the endoscopic examination of the lining of the distal sigmoid colon, the rectum, and the anal canal, using two different instruments: a proctoscope and a sigmoidoscope. It's indicated in patients with recent changes in bowel habits, lower abdominal and perineal pain, prolapse on defecation, pruritus, or passage of mucus, blood, or pus in the stool.

This procedure involves three separate steps: a digital examination, sigmoidoscopy, and proctoscopy. During digital examination, the anal sphincters are dilated to detect obstruction that might hinder the passage of the endoscope. During sigmoidoscopy, a 10" to 12" (25 to 30 cm) rigid sigmoidoscope is inserted into the anus, to allow visualization of the distal sigmoid colon and rectum. (Use of a flexible sigmoidoscope also permits visualization of the descending colon.) During proctoscopy, a 2¾" (7 cm) rigid proctoscope is inserted into the anus to aid examination of the lower rectum and anal canal. At any step in this procedure, specimens may be obtained from suspicious areas of the mucosa by biopsy, lavage or cytology brush, or culture swab. Possible complications of this procedure include rectal bleeding and, rarely, bowel perforation.

Purpose

□ To aid diagnosis of inflammatory, in-

fectious, and ulcerative bowel disease

□ To diagnose malignant and benign neoplasms

□ To detect hemorrhoids, hypertrophic anal papilla, polyps, fissures, fistulas, and abscesses within the rectum and anal canal.

Patient preparation

Explain to the patient that this procedure allows visual examination of the lining of the distal sigmoid colon, the rectum, and the anal canal. Tell him the test requires passage of two special instruments through the anus, who will perform this procedure and where, and that it takes 15 to 30 minutes.

Since dietary and bowel preparation for this procedure varies considerably, follow the doctor's orders carefully. As ordered, instruct the patient to maintain a clear liquid diet for 48 hours before the test, to avoid eating fruits and vegetables before the procedure, and to fast the morning of the procedure. If special bowel preparation is ordered, explain to the patient that this clears the intestine to ensure a better view. As ordered, administer a warm tap-water or sodium biphosphate enema 3 to 4 hours before the procedure. (The procedure may be started without bowel preparation since enemas can alter intestinal markings and traumatize mucous membranes. For this reason, irritating soapsuds enemas are inappropriate before this test. If the examination is then hindered by excessive fecal matter, an enema may be ordered before the examination proceeds.)

Describe to the patient the position he'll be asked to assume—knee-chest or left lateral—and assure him that he'll be adequately draped to minimize embarrassment. Tell him he may be placed on a tilting table that rotates into horizontal and vertical positions, but that he'll be adequately secured to the table.

Tell the patient the doctor's finger and the instrument are well lubricated to ease insertion, that the instrument initially feels cool, and that he may experience the urge to defecate when it's inserted and advanced. Inform him that

COLON ABNORMALITIES

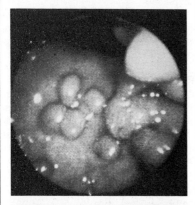

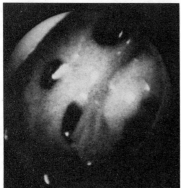

These abnormal views of the colon were taken with a proctosigmoidoscope. The top view demonstrates familial polyposis—multiple adenomatous growths with high malignancy potential. The bottom view shows diverticular orifices of the colon associated with muscle hypertrophy, which almost obscures the slit-like lumen (at right).

the instrument may stretch the intestinal wall and cause transient muscle spasms or a colicky lower abdominal pain. Instruct the patient to breathe deeply and slowly through his mouth to relax the abdominal muscles; this calms the urge to defecate and eases discomfort.

Explain to the patient that air may be introduced through the endoscope into the intestine to distend its walls. Tell him this causes flatus to escape around the endoscope and he shouldn't attempt to control it. Inform him that a suction machine may remove blood, mucus, or liquid feces that obscure vision, but it will cause no discomfort.

Make sure the patient or responsible member of the family has signed a consent form. Check the patient's history for barium tests within the past week, since the presence of barium in the colon makes accurate examination impossible. If the patient has rectal inflammation, about 15 to 20 minutes before the procedure, provide a local anesthetic, if ordered, to minimize discomfort.

Procedure

Place the patient in a knee-chest or left lateral position, with knees flexed, and drape him. If a left lateral position is used, a sandbag may be placed under the patient's left hip, so the buttocks project over the edge of the table. The right buttock is gently raised, and the anus and perianal region are examined under good lighting. Instruct the patient to breathe deeply and slowly through his mouth, as the doctor inserts a well-lubricated, gloved index finger into the anus and carefully palpates the anal canal for induration and tenderness. The doctor advances his finger into the rectum and palpates the rectal mucosa; the finger is withdrawn and checked for the presence of blood, mucus, or fecal matter. The sigmoidoscope is lubricated and the patient is told that the instrument is about to be inserted. The right buttock is raised, and the sigmoidoscope is inserted into the anus. As the scope is passed with steady pressure through the anal sphincters, instruct the patient to bear down as though defecating, to aid its passage. The sigmoidoscope is advanced through the anal canal into the rectum. At the rectosigmoid junction, a small amount of air may be insufflated to open the bowel lumen. The scope is then gently manipulated backward and forward to negotiate this flexure, and is advanced to its full length into the distal sigmoid colon.

As the sigmoidoscope is slowly withdrawn, air is carefully insufflated, and the intestinal mucosa is thoroughly examined. If fecal matter obscures vision, the eyepiece on the scope is removed, a cotton swab is inserted through the scope, and the bowel lumen is swabbed. (A suction machine may remove blood, excessive secretions, or liquid feces.) To obtain specimens from suspicious areas of the intestinal mucosa, the magnifying lens of the eyepiece is removed, and a biopsy forceps, a cytology brush, or a culture swab is passed through the sigmoidoscope. Polyps may also be removed for histologic examination by insertion of an electrocautery snare through the sigmoidoscope. After the specimen is obtained, it is immediately placed in a specimen bottle containing 10% formalin; cytology slides are placed in a Coplin jar containing 95% ethyl alcohol; and the culture swab is placed in a culture tube.

After the sigmoidoscope is withdrawn, the proctoscope is lubricated, and the patient is told that the proctoscope is about to be inserted. Assure him that he will experience less discomfort during passage of the proctoscope. The right buttock is raised, and the proctoscope inserted through the anus and gently advanced to its full length. The obturator is removed, and the light source is inserted through the handle of the proctoscope. As the instrument is slowly withdrawn, the rectal and anal mucosa are carefully examined. To obtain specimens from suspicious areas of the intestinal mucosa, the same steps are followed as during sigmoidoscopy. However, if a biopsy of the anal canal is required, a local anesthetic may first be administered, since this area is pain sensitive. After the examination is completed, the proctoscope is withdrawn.

If the patient has been examined in a knee-chest position, instruct him to rest in a supine position for several minutes before standing, to prevent postural hypotension.

Precautions

If a tissue specimen or culture swab has been obtained, label it and send it to the appropriate laboratory immediately.

Findings

The mucosa of the sigmoid colon appears light pink-orange and is marked by semilunar folds and deep tubular pits. The rectal mucosa appears redder due to its rich vascular network, deepens to a purple hue at the pectinate line (the anatomic division between the rectum and anus), and has three distinct valves. The lower two thirds of the anus (anoderm) is lined with smooth gray-tan skin and joins with the hair-fringed perianal skin.

Implications of results

Visual examination and palpation demonstrate abnormalities of the anal canal and rectum, including internal and external hemorrhoids, hypertrophic anal papilla, anal fissures, anal fistulas, and anorectal abscesses. However, biopsy, culture, and other laboratory tests are often necessary to detect various disorders. For example, biopsy can distinguish benign from malignant tumors and can aid diagnosis of ulcerative and ischemic colitis. X-ray films after barium enema or colonoscopy can confirm Crohn's disease and polyposis. Stool culture and serum agglutination tests demonstrate bacterial infection; culture and serologic tests, such as the VDRL (Venereal Disease Research Laboratory) test, detect syphilis.

Post-test care

□ Observe the patient closely for signs of bowel perforation—malaise, rectal bleeding, abdominal distention and pain, mucopurulent drainage, and fever) and for vasovagal attack due to emotional stress (depressed blood pressure, pallor, diaphoresis, and bradycardia). Notify the doctor immediately if such signs develop.

□ If air was introduced into the intestine, tell the patient that he may pass large amounts of flatus. Provide privacy while he rests after the test.

□ If a biopsy or polypectomy was performed, inform the patient that blood may appear in his stool.

Interfering factors
□ Barium retained in the intestine from previous diagnostic studies makes accurate visual examination impossible.
□ Large amounts of stool in the intestine hinders visual examination and the advancement of the endoscope.
□ Failure to place histologic or cytologic specimens in the appropriate preservative or to send the specimens to the laboratory immediately may interfere with accurate determination of test results.

MAE E. PAULFREY, RN, MN

CONTRAST RADIOGRAPHY

Barium Swallow
[Esophagography]

Barium swallow is the cineradiographic examination of the pharynx and the fluoroscopic examination of the esophagus after ingestion of thick and thin mixtures of barium sulfate. This test, most commonly performed as part of the upper gastrointestinal series, is indicated in patients with histories of dysphagia and regurgitation. Further testing is usually required for definitive diagnosis. However, cholangiography and the barium enema test, if ordered, should precede the barium swallow, since ingested barium may obscure anatomic detail on the radiographs.

Purpose
□ To diagnose hiatus hernia, diverticula, and varices
□ To detect strictures, ulcers, tumors, polyps, and motility disorders.

Patient preparation
Explain to the patient that this test evaluates the function of the pharynx and esophagus. Instruct him to fast after midnight before the test. If the patient's an infant, delay feeding to ensure complete digestion of barium. Tell him who will perform the test and where, and that the procedure takes approximately 30 minutes.

Describe to the patient the milkshake consistency and chalky taste of the bar-ium preparation he is required to ingest. Although it's flavored, he may find it unpleasant to swallow. Tell him he will first receive a thick mixture, then a thin one, and that he must drink 12 to 14 oz (350 to 425 ml) during the examination. Inform him that he will be placed in various positions on a tilting X-ray table, and that X-ray films will be taken. Assure him that he will be adequately secured to the table, and will be helped to supine and prone positions.

Withhold antacids, as ordered, if gastric reflux is suspected. Just before the procedure, instruct the patient to put on a hospital gown without snap closures and to remove jewelry, dentures, hairclips, or other radiopaque objects from the X-ray field.

Procedure
The patient is placed in an upright position behind the fluoroscopic screen, and his heart, lungs, and abdomen are examined. He is then instructed to take one swallow of the thick barium mixture, and the pharyngeal action is recorded, using cineradiography. (This action occurs too rapidly for adequate fluoroscopic evaluation.) The patient is then told to take several swallows of the thin barium mixture. The passage of the barium is examined fluoroscopically, and spot films of the esophageal region are taken from lateral angles and from right and left posteroanterior angles. Esophageal strictures and obstruction of the esophageal lumen by the lower esophageal ring are best detected when the patient is upright. To accentuate

small strictures or demonstrate dysphagia, the patient may be requested to swallow a special "barium marshmallow" (soft white bread that has been soaked in barium).

The patient is then secured to the radiographic table and is rotated to the Trendelenburg position, to evaluate esophageal peristalsis or demonstrate hiatus hernia and gastric reflux. Again he is instructed to take several swallows of barium, while the esophagus is examined fluoroscopically, and spot films of significant findings are taken when indicated. After the table is rotated to a horizontal position, the patient is told to take several swallows of barium so that the esophagogastric junction and peristalsis may be evaluated. The passage of the barium is then fluoroscopically observed, and spot films of significant findings are taken with the patient in supine and prone positions.

During fluoroscopic examination of the esophagus, the cardia and fundus of the patient's stomach are also carefully studied, because neoplasms in these areas may invade the esophagus and cause obstruction.

Precautions

Barium swallow is usually contraindicated in a patient with intestinal obstruction.

Findings

After the barium sulfate is swallowed, the bolus pours over the base of the tongue into the pharynx. A peristaltic wave propels the bolus through the entire length of the esophagus in about 2 seconds. When the peristaltic wave reaches the base of the esophagus, the cardiac sphincter opens, allowing the bolus to enter the stomach. After passage of the bolus, the cardiac sphincter closes. Normally, the bolus evenly fills and distends the lumen of the pharynx and esophagus, and the mucosa appears smooth and regular.

GASTROESOPHAGEAL REFLUX SCANNING

When results of a barium swallow are inconclusive, gastroesophageal reflux scanning may be done to evaluate esophageal function and detect reflux. This test delivers less radiation than a conventional barium swallow and is a much more sensitive indicator of reflux. It also allows reflux to be measured without insertion of an esophageal tube—an important consideration in testing infants, small children, and other patients for whom intubation is contraindicated.

The patient is instructed to fast after midnight before the test, to clear stomach contents that impede passage of the imaging agent. As the test begins, the patient is placed in a supine or upright position and is asked to swallow a solution containing a radiopharmaceutical, such as technetium-99m sulfur colloid (^{99m}Tc). A gamma counter placed over the patient's chest records passage of the ^{99m}Tc through the esophagus into the stomach, to determine transit time and to evaluate esophageal function. If gastroesophageal reflux is suspected, the patient is repositioned as his stomach distends, and continuous recordings visualize reflux and estimate its quantity. (Depending on hospital policy, manual pressure may be applied to the patient's upper abdomen, and recordings may be taken at specific intervals.)

Normally, ^{99m}Tc descends through the esophagus in about 6 seconds; radioactivity is then detected only in the stomach and small bowel. However, diffuse spasm of the esophagus, achalasia, or other esophageal motility disorders may prolong transit time; in gastroesophageal reflux, radioactivity may be detected in the esophagus.

Like other radionuclide studies, this scan is usually contraindicated during pregnancy and lactation. It can be modified for use in infants and children.

FRANCES W. QUINLESS, RN, PhD

Implications of results

Barium swallow may reveal hiatus hernia, diverticula, and varices. Although strictures, tumors, polyps, ulcers, and motility disorders (pharyngeal muscular disorders, esophageal spasms, and achalasia) may be detected, definitive diagnosis commonly necessitates endoscopic biopsy or, for motility disorders, manometric studies.

Post-test care

□ Check that additional spot films and repeat fluoroscopic evaluation haven't been ordered before allowing the patient to resume his usual diet.

□ Administer a cathartic, if ordered.

□ Inform the patient that stools will be chalky and light colored for 24 to 72 hours. Record description of all stools passed by the patient in the hospital. Barium retained in the intestine may harden, causing obstruction or fecal impaction. Notify the doctor if the patient hasn't expelled the barium in 2 or 3 days.

Interfering factors

None.

MAE E. PAULFREY, RN, MN

Upper Gastrointestinal and Small Bowel Series

The upper gastrointestinal (GI) and small bowel series is the fluoroscopic examination of the esophagus, stomach, and small intestine after the patient ingests barium sulfate, a contrast agent. As the barium passes through the digestive tract, fluoroscopy outlines peristalsis and the mucosal contours of the respective organs, and spot films record significant findings. This test is indicated in patients with upper GI symptoms (difficulty in swallowing, regurgitation, burning or gnawing epigastric pain), signs of small bowel disease (diarrhea, weight loss), and signs of GI bleeding (hematemesis, melena). Although this test can detect various mucosal abnormalities, subsequent biopsy is often necessary to rule out malignancy or distinguish specific inflammatory diseases. Oral cholecystography, barium enema, and routine radiography should always precede this test, since retained barium clouds anatomic detail on X-ray films.

Purpose

□ To detect hiatal hernia, diverticula, and varices

□ To aid diagnosis of strictures, ulcers, tumors, regional enteritis, and malabsorption syndrome

□ To help detect motility disorders.

Patient preparation

Explain to the patient that this procedure examines the esophagus, stomach, and small intestine through X-ray films taken after the ingestion of barium. Instruct him to maintain a low-residue diet for 2 or 3 days before the test, then to fast and avoid smoking after midnight before the test as well as during it. Tell him who will perform the procedure and where. Because the procedure takes up to 6 hours to complete, encourage the patient to bring reading material to the X-ray department.

Inform the patient that he'll be placed on an X-ray table that rotates into vertical, semivertical, and horizontal positions. Assure him that he'll be adequately secured to the table and will be assisted to supine, prone, and sidelying positions. Describe the milkshake consistency and chalky taste of the barium mixture. Although it's flavored, he may find its taste unpleasant, but tell him he must drink 16 to 20 oz (480 to 600 ml) for a complete examination. Inform him that his abdomen may be compressed to ensure proper coating of the stomach or intestinal walls with barium, or to separate overlapping bowel loops.

As ordered, withhold most oral medications after midnight, and anticholinergics and narcotics for 24 hours, since these drugs affect small intestinal motility. Antacids are also sometimes withheld for several hours if gastric reflux is suspected. Administer a cathartic and a saline or warm tap-water enema the evening before the test, as ordered.

Just before the procedure, instruct the patient to put on a hospital gown without snap closures and to remove jewelry, dentures, hairclips, or other objects that might obscure anatomic detail on the X-ray films.

Procedure

After the patient is secured in a supine position on the radiographic table, the table is tilted until the patient is erect, and the heart, lungs, and abdomen are examined fluoroscopically. The patient is then instructed to take several swallows of the barium suspension, and its passage through the esophagus is observed. (Occasionally, the patient is given a thick barium suspension, especially when esophageal pathology is strongly suspected.) During fluoroscopic examination, spot films of the esophagus are taken from lateral angles and from right and left posteroanterior angles.

When barium enters the stomach, the patient's abdomen is palpated or compressed to ensure adequate coating of the gastric mucosa with barium. To perform a double contrast examination, the patient is instructed to sip the barium through a perforated straw. As he does so, a small amount of air is also introduced into the stomach; this permits detailed examination of the gastric rugae, and spot films of significant findings are taken. The patient is then instructed to ingest the remaining barium suspension, and the filling of the stomach and emptying into the duodenum are observed fluoroscopically. Two series of spot films of the stomach and duodenum are taken from posteroanterior, anteroposterior, oblique, and lateral angles, with the patient erect and then supine.

The passage of barium into the remainder of the small intestine is then observed fluoroscopically, and spot films are taken at 30- to 60-minute intervals

> ### GASTROINTESTINAL MOTILITY STUDY
>
> When intestinal disease is strongly suspected, the gastrointestinal (GI) motility study may follow the upper GI and small bowel series. This study, which evaluates intestinal motility and the integrity of the mucosal lining, records the passage of barium through the lower digestive tract, using spot films taken at specified intervals.
>
> About 6 hours after barium ingestion, the head of the barium column is usually in the hepatic flexure; the tail, in the terminal ileum. The barium completely opacifies the large intestine 24 hours after ingestion. Since the amount of barium passing through the large intestine isn't sufficient to fully extend the lumen, spot films taken 24, 48, or 72 hours after barium ingestion prove inferior to the barium enema. However, when spot films suggest intestinal abnormalities, the barium enema and colonoscopy can provide more specific, confirming diagnostic information.

until the barium reaches the ileocecal valve and the region around it. If abnormalities in the small intestine are detected, the area is palpated and compressed to help clarify the defect, and a spot film is taken. When the barium enters the cecum, the examination is ended.

Precautions

The upper GI and small bowel series is contraindicated in patients with obstruction or perforation of the digestive tract. In such patients, barium may intensify the obstruction or seep into the abdominal cavity.

Findings

After the barium suspension is swallowed, it pours over the base of the tongue into the pharynx, and is propelled by a peristaltic wave through the entire length of the esophagus in about 2 seconds. The bolus evenly fills and distends the lumen of the pharynx and esophagus, and the mucosa appears smooth and regular. When the peristaltic wave reaches the base of the esophagus, the cardiac sphincter opens, allowing the bolus to enter the stomach. After passage of the bolus, the cardiac sphincter closes.

As barium enters the stomach, it outlines the characteristic longitudinal folds called rugae, which are best observed using the double-contrast technique. When the stomach is completely filled with barium, its outer contour appears smooth and regular without evidence of flattened, rigid areas suggestive of intrinsic or extrinsic lesions.

After barium enters the stomach, it quickly empties into the duodenal bulb through relaxation of the pyloric sphincter. Although the mucosa of the duodenal bulb is relatively smooth, circular folds become apparent as barium enters the duodenal loop. These folds deepen and become more numerous in the jejunum. Barium temporarily lodges between these folds, producing a speckled pattern on the X-ray film. As barium enters the ileum, the circular folds become less prominent and, except for their broadness, resemble those in the duodenum. The film also shows that the diameter of the small intestine tapers gradually from the duodenum to the ileum.

Implications of results

X-ray studies of the esophagus may reveal strictures, tumors, hiatal hernia, diverticula, varices, and ulcers (particularly in the distal esophagus). Benign strictures usually dilate the esophagus, whereas malignant ones cause erosive changes in the mucosa. Tumors produce filling defects in the column of barium, but only malignant ones change the mucosal contour. Nevertheless, biopsy is necessary for definitive diagnosis of both esophageal strictures and tumors.

Motility disorders, such as esophageal spasm, are usually difficult to detect, since spasms are erratic and transient; manometry, which measures the length and pressure of peristaltic contractions and evaluates the function of the cardiac sphincter, is generally performed to detect such disorders. However, achalasia (cardiospasm) is strongly suggested when the distal esophagus has a beaking appearance. Gastric reflux appears as a backflow of barium from the stomach into the esophagus.

X-ray studies of the stomach may reveal tumors and ulcers. Malignant tumors, usually adenocarcinomas, appear as filling defects on the X-ray film and usually disrupt peristalsis. Benign tumors, such as adenomatous polyps and leiomyomas, appear as outpouchings of the gastric mucosa and generally don't affect peristalsis. Ulcers occur most commonly in the stomach and duodenum (particularly in the duodenal bulb), and these two areas are thus examined together. Benign ulcers usually demonstrate evidence of partial or complete healing, and are characterized by radiating folds extending to the edge of the ulcer crater. Malignant ulcers, usually associated with a suspicious mass, generally have radiating folds that extend beyond the ulcer crater to the edge of the mass. However, biopsy is necessary for definitive diagnosis of both tumors and ulcers.

Occasionally, this test detects signs that suggest pancreatitis or pancreatic carcinoma. Such signs include edematous changes in the mucosa of the antrum or duodenal loop, or dilation of the duodenal loop. These findings mandate further studies for pancreatic disease, such as endoscopic retrograde cholangiopancreatography, abdominal ultrasonography, or computerized tomography.

X-ray studies of the small intestine may reveal regional enteritis, malabsorption syndrome, and tumors. Although regional enteritis may not be detected in its early stages, small ulcerations and edematous changes develop in the mucosa as the disease progresses. Edematous changes, segmentation of the barium column, and flocculation characterize malabsorption syndrome. Filling defects occur with Hodgkin's disease and lymphosarcoma.

Post-test care

□ Be sure additional radiographs haven't been ordered before allowing the patient food, fluids, and oral medications (if applicable).

□ Administer a cathartic or enema to the patient, as ordered. Tell him his stool will be lightly colored for 24 to 72 hours. Record and describe any stool passed by the patient in the hospital. Since retention of barium in the intestine may cause obstruction or fecal impaction, notify the doctor if the patient doesn't pass barium within 2 or 3 days.

☐ Encourage bed rest, since this test exhausts most patients.

Interfering factors
☐ Failure to observe restriction of diet, smoking, and medications may interfere with accurate determination of the test results.
☐ Failure to remove radiopaque objects in X-ray field and excess air within the small bowel can obscure details on the X-ray films.

MAE E. PAULFREY, RN, MN

Barium Enema
[Lower gastrointestinal examination]

Barium enema is the radiographic examination of the large intestine after rectal instillation of barium sulfate (single-contrast technique) or barium sulfate and air (double-contrast technique). It's indicated in patients with histories of altered bowel habits, lower abdominal pain, or the passage of blood, mucus, or pus in the stool. It may also be indicated after colostomy or ileostomy; in such patients, barium (or barium and air) is instilled through the stoma. Complications include perforation of the colon, water intoxication, barium granulomas, and rarely, intra- and extraperitoneal extravasation of barium and barium embolism.

The single-contrast technique provides a profile view of the large intestine; the double-contrast technique provides profile and frontal views. The latter technique best detects small intraluminal tumors (especially polyps), the early

mucosal changes of inflammatory disease, and the subtle intestinal bleeding caused by ulcerated polyps or shallow ulcerations of inflammatory disease.

Although barium enema clearly outlines most of the large intestine, proctosigmoidoscopy provides the best view of the rectosigmoid region. Barium enema should precede the barium swallow and upper gastrointestinal and small bowel series, since barium ingested in the latter procedure may take several days to pass through the gastrointestinal tract and thus may interfere with subsequent X-ray studies.

Purpose
☐ To aid diagnosis of colorectal cancer and inflammatory disease
☐ To detect polyps, diverticula, and structural changes in the large intestine.

Patient preparation
Explain to the patient that this test examines the large intestine through X-ray films taken after a barium enema. Tell him who will perform the test and where, and that the test takes 30 to 45 minutes.

 Since residual fecal material in the colon obscures normal anatomy on radiographs, carefully follow the prescribed bowel preparation. Although various diets, laxatives, and cleansing enemas may be used, remember that certain conditions, such as ulcerative colitis and active gastrointestinal bleeding, may prohibit the use of laxatives and enemas. Stress to the patient that accurate test results depend on his cooperation in the prescribed dietary restrictions and bowel preparation.

In a commonly used bowel preparation technique, instruct the patient to maintain a low-residue diet for 1 to 3 days before the test; occasionally, intake is further restricted to clear liquids the day before the test or for the evening meal. Encourage the patient to drink water or clear liquids for 12 to 24 hours before the test to ensure adequate hydration. Administer 1½ to 2 oz (45 to 60 ml) of castor oil the afternoon before the test, as ordered, then a cleansing enema (warm tap water) in the evening or early morning of the test. Repeat enemas until the solution returns clear, but give no more than three enemas. About 1 hour before the test, give the patient a light breakfast of toast and black coffee or clear tea.

Tell the patient that he'll be adequately draped during the test, and will be placed on a tilting X-ray table. Assure him that he'll be secured to the table, and will be assisted to various positions.

Inform the patient that he may experience cramping pains or the urge to defecate as the barium or air is introduced into the intestine. Instruct him to breathe deeply and slowly through his mouth to ease this discomfort. Tell him to keep his anal sphincter tightly contracted against the rectal tube; this holds the tube in position and helps prevent leakage of barium. Stress the importance of retaining the barium enema; if the intestinal walls aren't adequately coated with barium, test results may be inaccurate. Assure the patient that the barium enema is fairly easy to retain because of its cool temperature.

Approximately 15 to 20 minutes before the test, give the patient with anal inflammation a local anesthetic salve to apply, as ordered.

Procedure

After the patient is in a supine position on a tilting radiographic table, scout films of the abdomen are taken. The patient is then assisted to Sims' position, and a well-lubricated rectal tube is inserted through the anus. If the patient has anal sphincter atony or severe mental or physical debilitation, a rectal tube with a retaining balloon may be inserted. The barium is then administered slowly, and the filling process is monitored fluoroscopically. To aid filling, the table may be tilted or the patient assisted to supine, prone, and lateral decubitus positions. As the flow of barium is observed, spot films are taken of significant findings. When the intestine is filled with barium, overhead films of the abdomen

are taken. The rectal tube is withdrawn, and the patient is escorted to the toilet or provided with a bedpan and is instructed to expel as much barium as possible. After evacuation, an additional overhead film is taken to record the mucosal pattern of the intestine and to evaluate the efficiency of colonic emptying.

A double-contrast barium enema may directly follow this examination or may be performed separately. If it's performed immediately, a thin film of barium remains in the patient's intestine, coating the mucosa, and air is carefully injected to distend the bowel lumen. When the double-contrast technique is performed separately, a colloidal barium suspension is instilled, filling the patient's intestine to either the splenic flexure or the middle of the transverse colon. The suspension is then aspirated, and air is forcefully injected into the intestine. The intestine may also be filled to the lower descending colon and then air forcefully injected, without prior aspiration of the suspension.

The patient is then assisted to erect, prone, supine, and lateral decubitus positions in sequence. Barium filling is monitored fluoroscopically, and spot films are taken of significant findings. After the required films are taken, the patient is escorted to the toilet or provided with a bedpan.

Precautions

Barium enema is contraindicated in patients with tachycardia, fulminant ulcerative colitis associated with systemic toxicity and megacolon, toxic megacolon, or suspected perforation. It should be performed cautiously in patients with obstruction, acute inflammatory conditions (such as ulcerative colitis, diverticulitis), acute vascular insufficiency of the bowel, acute fulminant bloody diarrhea, and suspected pneumatosis cystoides intestinalis.

Findings

In the single-contrast enema, the intestine is uniformly filled with barium, and colonic haustral markings are clearly apparent. The intestinal walls collapse as the barium is expelled, and the mucosa has a regular, feathery appearance on the postevacuation film. In the double-contrast enema, the intestine is uniformly distended with air, with a thin layer of barium providing excellent detail of the mucosal pattern. As the patient is assisted to various positions, the barium collects on the dependent walls of the intestine by the force of gravity.

Implications of results

Although most colonic cancers occur in the rectosigmoid region and are best detected by proctosigmoidoscopy, X-ray films may reveal adenocarcinoma and, rarely, sarcomas occurring higher in the intestine. Carcinoma usually appears as a localized filling defect, with a sharp transition between the normal and the necrotic mucosa. These characteristics help distinguish carcinoma from the more diffuse lesions of inflammatory disease, but endoscopic biopsy may be necessary to confirm diagnosis.

These X-ray studies demonstrate and define the extent of inflammatory disease, such as diverticulitis, ulcerative colitis, and granulomatous colitis. Ulcerative colitis usually originates in the anal region and ascends through the intestine; granulomatous colitis usually originates in the cecum and terminal ileum, then descends through the intestine. However, biopsy may be necessary to confirm diagnosis. Barium X-ray films may also reveal saccular adenomatous polyps, broad-based villous polyps, structural changes in the intestine (such as intussusception, telescoping of the bowel, sigmoid volvulus [360° turn or greater], and sigmoid torsion [up to 180° turn]), gastroenteritis, irritable colon, vascular injury due to arterial occlusion, and selected cases of acute appendicitis.

Post-test care

☐ Be sure further X-ray studies haven't been ordered before allowing the patient food and fluids. Encourage extra intake of fluids, as ordered, since bowel preparation and the test itself can cause dehydration.

☐ Encourage rest, since this test and the bowel preparation that precedes it exhausts most patients.

☐ Since retention of barium after this test can cause intestinal obstruction or fecal impaction, administer a mild cathartic or a cleansing enema, as ordered. Tell the patient his stool will be lightly colored for 24 to 72 hours. Record and describe any stool passed by the patient in the hospital.

Interfering factors

☐ Inadequate bowel preparation impairs quality of the X-ray films.

☐ Barium swallow performed within several days before barium enema impairs quality of subsequent X-ray films.

☐ The patient's inability to retain the barium enema causes an incomplete test.

MAE E. PAULFREY, RN, MN

Hypotonic Duodenography

Hypotonic duodenography is the fluoroscopic examination of the duodenum after instillation of barium sulfate and air through an intestinal catheter. This test is indicated in patients with symptoms of duodenal or pancreatic pathology, such as persistent upper abdominal pain.

After the catheter is passed through the patient's nose into the duodenum, I.V. infusion of glucagon or I.M. injection of propantheline bromide (or other anticholinergic) induces duodenal atony. Instillation of barium and air distends the relaxed duodenum, flattening its deep circular folds; spot films then record the precise delineation of the duodenal anatomy. Although these films readily demonstrate small duodenal lesions and tumors of the head of the pancreas that impinge on the duodenal wall, differential diagnosis requires further studies.

Purpose
□ To detect small postbulbar duodenal lesions, tumors of the head of the pancreas, and tumors of the ampulla of Vater
□ To aid diagnosis of chronic pancreatitis.

Patient preparation
Explain to the patient that this test examines the duodenum and pancreas after the instillation of barium and air. Instruct him to fast from midnight before the test. Tell him who will perform the test and where, and that the procedure takes approximately 30 minutes.

Inform the patient that a tube will be passed through his nose into the duodenum to serve as a channel for the barium and air. Tell him he may experience a cramping pain as air is introduced into the duodenum. Instruct him to breathe deeply and slowly through his mouth if he experiences this pain, to help relax the abdominal muscles. If glucagon or an anticholinergic is to be administered during the procedure, describe the possible side effects of glucagon—nausea, vomiting, hives, and flushing—or of anticholinergics—dry mouth, thirst, tachycardia, urinary retention (especially in patients with prostatic hypertrophy), and blurred vision. If an anticholinergic is being administered to an outpatient, advise him to have someone accompany him home.

Just before the test, tell the patient to remove dentures, glasses, necklaces, hairpins, combs, and constricting undergarments. Then, instruct him to void.

Procedure
While the patient is in a sitting position, a catheter is passed through his nose into the stomach. Then he is placed in a supine position on the radiographic table, and the catheter is advanced into the duodenum, under fluoroscopic guidance. Glucagon I.V. is administered to the patient, which quickly induces duodenal atony for approximately 20 minutes, or an anticholinergic is injected I.M. Throughout the procedure, the patient is observed for side effects.

Barium is then instilled through the catheter, and spot films are taken of the duodenum. Some of the barium is then withdrawn and air is instilled; then additional spot films are taken. When the required films have been obtained, the catheter is removed.

Precautions
Anticholinergics are contraindicated in patients with severe cardiac disorders or glaucoma.

Findings
When barium and air distend the atonic duodenum, the mucosa normally appears smooth and even. The regular contour of the head of the pancreas also appears on the duodenal wall.

Implications of results
Irregular nodules or masses on the duodenal wall may indicate duodenal lesions, tumors of the ampulla of Vater, tumors of the head of the pancreas, or chronic pancreatitis. Differential diagnosis requires further tests, such as serum and urine amylase determinations, endoscopic retrograde cholangiopancreatography, pancreas ultrasonography, and pancreatic computerized tomography.

Post-test care
□ Watch for possible side effects after administration of glucagon or an anticholinergic. If an anticholinergic was given, be sure the patient voids within a few hours after the test. Advise the outpatient to rest in a waiting area until his vision clears (about 2 hours), unless someone can accompany him home.
□ Administer a cathartic, as ordered.
□ Tell the patient he may burp instilled air or pass flatus, and that the barium colors the stool chalky white for 24 to 72 hours. Record description of any stool passed by the patient in the hospital, and notify the doctor if the patient hasn't expelled the barium after 2 or 3 days.

Interfering factors
None.

MAE E. PAULFREY, RN, MN

Oral Cholecystography

Oral cholecystography is the radiographic examination of the gallbladder after administration of a contrast medium. It's indicated in patients with symptoms of biliary tract disease, such as upper right quadrant epigastric pain, fat intolerance, and jaundice, and is most commonly performed to confirm gallbladder disease.

After the contrast medium is ingested, it is absorbed by the small intestine, filtered by the liver, excreted in the bile, and then concentrated and stored in the gallbladder. Full gallbladder opacification usually occurs 12 to 14 hours after ingestion, and a series of X-ray films then records gallbladder appearance. Additional information is obtained by giving the patient a fat stimulus, causing the gallbladder to contract and empty the contrast-laden bile into the common bile duct and small intestine. Films are then taken to record this emptying and to evaluate patency of the common bile duct.

Oral cholecystography should precede barium studies, since retained barium may cloud subsequent X-ray films.

Purpose
☐ To detect gallstones
☐ To aid diagnosis of inflammatory disease and tumors of the gallbladder.

Patient preparation
Explain to the patient that this procedure examines the gallbladder through X-ray films taken after ingestion of a contrast medium. If ordered, instruct him to eat a meal containing fat at noon the day before the test, and a fat-free meal in the evening. The former stimulates release of bile from the gallbladder, preparing it to receive the contrast-laden bile; the latter inhibits gallbladder contraction, promoting accumulation of bile. After the evening meal, instruct the patient to restrict food and fluids, except water.

Give the patient six tablets (3 g) of iopanoic acid 2 or 3 hours after the evening meal, as ordered. Other commercial contrast agents are available (such as sodium ipodate), but iopanoic acid is most commonly used. Have the patient swallow the tablets one at a time, at 5-minute intervals, with one or two mouthfuls of water, for a total of 8 oz (240 ml) of water. Thereafter, withhold water. Tell him who will perform this procedure and where, and that it usually takes 30 to 45 minutes (possibly longer if a fat stimulus is to be given, followed by another series of films).

Tell the patient he'll be placed on an X-ray table, and that films will be taken of his gallbladder.

Check the patient's history for hypersensitivity to iodine, seafood, or contrast media used for other diagnostic tests. Inform him that the possible side effects of dye ingestion include diarrhea (common) and, rarely, nausea, vomiting, abdominal cramps, and dysuria. Tell him to report such symptoms immediately if they develop.

 Examine any emesis or diarrhea for undigested tablets. If any tablets were expelled, notify the doctor and the X-ray department.

Administer a cleansing enema the morning of the test, if ordered. This clears the gastrointestinal tract of interfering shadows that may obscure the gallbladder.

Procedure
After the patient is in a prone position on the radiographic table, the abdomen is examined fluoroscopically to evaluate gallbladder opacification, and films are taken of significant findings. The patient is then examined while in left lateral decubitus and erect positions, to detect possible layering or mobility of any filling defects, and additional films are taken.

The patient may then be given a fat stimulus, such as a high-fat meal or a synthetic fat-containing agent (for example, Bilevac). Fluoroscopy is used to observe the emptying of the gallbladder in response to the fat stimulus, and spot films are taken at 15 and 30 minutes to visualize the common bile duct. If the gallbladder empties slowly or not at all, these films are also taken at 60 minutes.

Precautions
Oral cholecystography is contraindicated in patients with severe renal or hepatic damage, or with hypersensitivity to iodine, seafood, or contrast media used for other diagnostic tests.

Findings
The gallbladder is normally opacified, and appears pear-shaped, with smooth, thin walls. Although its size is variable, its basic structure—neck, infundibulum, body, and fundus—is clearly outlined on film.

Implications of results
When the gallbladder is opacified, filling defects (typically appearing within the lumen as negative shadows that show mobility) indicate the presence of gallstones. Fixed defects, on the other hand, may indicate the presence of cholesterol polyps or a benign tumor, such as an adenomyoma.

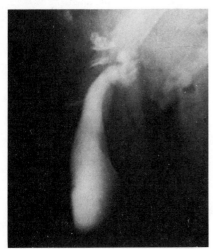

This decubitus view of a normal oral cholecysto-gram shows characteristic opacification of the pear-shaped gallbladder.

When the gallbladder fails to opacify or when only faint opacification occurs, inflammatory disease, such as cholecystitis—with or without gallstone formation—may be present. Gallstones may obstruct the cystic duct and prevent the contrast medium from entering the gallbladder; inflammation may impair the concentrating ability of the gallbladder mucosa and prevent or diminish opacification.

When the gallbladder fails to contract following stimulation by a fatty meal, cholecystitis or common bile duct obstruction may be present. If the X-ray films are inconclusive, oral cholecystography will have to be repeated the following day.

Post-test care
☐ If the test results are normal, the patient may resume his usual diet withheld before the test.
☐ Nonopacification and repeat cholecystography require continuation of a low-fat diet until definitive diagnosis can be made.
☐ If gallstones are discovered during opacification, the doctor will order an appropriate diet—usually one that restricts fat intake, to help prevent acute attacks.

Interfering factors
☐ Failure to adhere to dietary preparation and restrictions before contrast study can interfere with accurate determination of results.
☐ Failure to ingest the full dosage of contrast medium, partial loss of the contrast medium through emesis or diarrhea, inadequate absorption of the contrast medium in the small intestine, and barium retained from previous studies of the biliary tract can interfere with accurate determination of test results.
☐ Impaired hepatic function and moderate jaundice (serum bilirubin levels greater than 3 mg/dl) cause diminished excretion of the contrast medium into the bile, thereby inhibiting adequate visualization of the biliary tract.

MAE E. PAULFREY, RN, MN

Percutaneous Transhepatic Cholangiography

Percutaneous transhepatic cholangiography is the fluoroscopic examination of the biliary ducts after injection of an iodinated contrast medium directly into a biliary radicle. This test opacifies the biliary ducts without depending on the gallbladder's concentrating ability. It's therefore especially useful for evaluating patients with persistent upper abdominal pain after cholecystectomy, and for evaluating patients with severe jaundice, since impaired hepatic function often prevents uptake and excretion of the contrast medium during oral cholecystography or intravenous cholangiography.

Although computed tomography scan or ultrasonography is usually performed first when obstructive jaundice is suspected, percutaneous transhepatic cholangiography may provide the most detailed view of the obstruction; however, this invasive procedure carries a potential risk of complications that include bleeding, septicemia, bile peritonitis, extravasation of the contrast medium into the peritoneal cavity, and subcapsular injection.

In percutaneous transhepatic cholangiography, the patient's liver is punctured with a thin, flexible needle (Chiba needle) under fluoroscopic guidance, and the contrast medium is injected as the needle is slowly withdrawn. When the contrast medium enters a biliary radicle, it begins to outline the biliary tree. As it flows through the biliary ducts, the filling process is visualized by fluoroscopy. Spot films are then taken of any significant findings.

Purpose
□ To determine the cause of upper abdominal pain following cholecystectomy

□ To distinguish between obstructive and nonobstructive jaundice

□ To determine the location, the extent, and often the cause of mechanical obstruction.

Patient preparation
Explain to the patient that this procedure allows examination of the biliary ducts through X-ray films taken after injection of a contrast medium into the liver. Instruct him to fast for 8 hours before the test. Tell him who will perform the test and where, and that the procedure takes about 30 minutes.

Inform the patient that he'll be placed on a tilting X-ray table that rotates into vertical and horizontal positions during the procedure. Assure him that he will be adequately secured to the table, and assisted to supine and side-lying positions throughout the procedure.

Warn him that injection of the local anesthetic may sting the skin and produce transient pain when it punctures the liver capsule. Also, advise him that injection of the contrast medium may produce a sensation of pressure and epigastric fullness, and may cause transient upper back pain on his right side. If appropriate, advise him that a sedative will be administered just before the procedure begins, and tell him that he must rest for at least 6 hours after the procedure is completed.

Make sure the patient or responsible member of the family has signed a consent form. Check the patient's history for hypersensitivity to iodine, seafood, contrast media used in other diagnostic tests, and the local anesthetic. Although hypersensitivity reactions to the contrast medium are more acute and common with I.V. injection, describe the possible side effects of contrast administration, such as nausea, vomiting, excessive salivation, flushing, urticaria, sweating, and rarely, anaphylaxis; tachycardia and fever may also accompany intraductal injection. Also, check the patient's history for normal bleeding, clotting, and prothrombin times, and a normal platelet count. If ordered, administer 1 g of ampicillin I.V. every 4 to 6 hours for 24 hours before the procedure.

Just before the procedure, administer a sedative, if ordered.

Procedure

After the patient is placed in a supine position on the radiographic table and is adequately secured, the upper right quadrant of the abdomen is cleansed and draped, and the skin, subcutaneous tissue, and liver capsule are infiltrated with a local anesthetic. While the patient holds his breath at the end of expiration, the flexible needle is inserted under fluoroscopic guidance, through the eighth or ninth intercostal space in the midaxillary line, into the liver. The needle is passed deeply into the liver substance, then slowly withdrawn, injecting the contrast medium to locate a biliary radicle. When fluoroscopy reveals placement in a radicle, the needle is held in position and the remaining contrast is injected. Using a fluoroscope and television monitor, the opacification of the

biliary ducts is observed, and spot films of significant findings are taken with the patient in supine and lateral recumbent positions. When the required films have been taken, the needle is removed, and a sterile dressing is applied to the puncture site.

Precautions

Percutaneous transhepatic cholangiography is contraindicated in patients with cholangitis, massive ascites, uncorrectable coagulopathy, or hypersensitivity to iodine.

Findings

The biliary ducts are of normal diameter and appear as regular channels homogeneously filled with contrast medium.

Implications of results

Distinguishing between obstructive and nonobstructive jaundice hinges on whether biliary ducts are dilated or of normal size. Obstructive jaundice is associated with dilated ducts; nonobstruc-

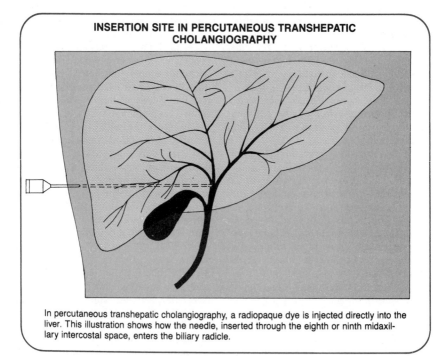

INSERTION SITE IN PERCUTANEOUS TRANSHEPATIC CHOLANGIOGRAPHY

In percutaneous transhepatic cholangiography, a radiopaque dye is injected directly into the liver. This illustration shows how the needle, inserted through the eighth or ninth midaxillary intercostal space, enters the biliary radicle.

ABNORMAL PERCUTANEOUS CHOLANGIOGRAM

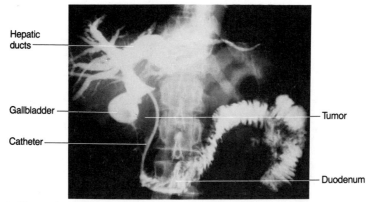

Hepatic ducts

Gallbladder

Catheter

Tumor

Duodenum

In this percutaneous cholangiogram, the dilated hepatic ducts indicate obstruction of the common bile duct by a tumor. The catheter tip has been passed through the tumor into the duodenum.

tive jaundice, with normal-sized ducts. When ducts are dilated, the obstruction site may be defined. Obstruction may result from cholelithiasis, biliary tract carcinoma, or carcinoma of the pancreas or papilla of Vater that impinges on the common bile duct, causing deviation or stricture. When ducts are of normal size and intrahepatic cholestasis is indicated, liver biopsy may be performed to distinguish among hepatitis, cirrhosis, and granulomatous disease.

Post-test care

□ Check the patient's vital signs until they're stable.

□ Enforce bed rest for at least 6 hours after the test, preferably with the patient lying on his right side, to help prevent hemorrhage.

 □ Check the injection site for bleeding, swelling, and tenderness. Watch for signs of peritonitis: chills, temperature of 102° to 103° F. (38.9° to 39.4° C.), and abdominal pain, tenderness, and distention. Notify the doctor immediately if such complications develop.

□ Tell the patient he may resume his usual diet withheld before the test.

Interfering factors

Marked obesity or gas overlying the biliary ducts may interfere with clarity of X-ray films.

MAE E. PAULFREY, RN, MN

Postoperative Cholangiography
[T-tube cholangiography]

Often immediately after cholecystectomy or common bile duct exploration, a T-shaped rubber tube is inserted into the common bile duct to facilitate drainage. Post-operative cholangiography, performed 7 to 10 days after this surgery, is the radiographic and fluoroscopic examination of the biliary ducts after the injection of contrast medium through the T-tube. The contrast flows through the biliary ducts and outlines the size and patency of the ducts, revealing any obstruction overlooked during surgery.

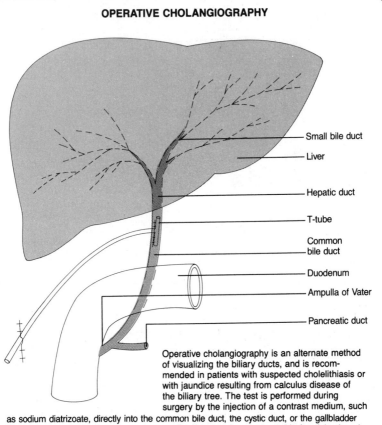

OPERATIVE CHOLANGIOGRAPHY

Small bile duct

Liver

Hepatic duct

T-tube

Common bile duct

Duodenum

Ampulla of Vater

Pancreatic duct

Operative cholangiography is an alternate method of visualizing the biliary ducts, and is recommended in patients with suspected cholelithiasis or with jaundice resulting from calculus disease of the biliary tree. The test is performed during surgery by the injection of a contrast medium, such as sodium diatrizoate, directly into the common bile duct, the cystic duct, or the gallbladder through a thin needle or catheter. If the gallbladder has been removed before injection, the contrast medium may be administered through a T-tube (shown above) inserted after cholecystectomy (operative T-tube cholangiography).

As the contrast flows through the biliary ducts, it reveals calculi and small intraluminal neoplasms, permitting the surgeon to remove them before closing the incision. Operative cholangiography can therefore eliminate the need for two surgical procedures, since gallbladder disease requiring cholecystectomy is often associated with biliary tract disease. However, this advantage must be weighed against the risks associated with contrast administration during a simple cholecystectomy.

Purpose
□ To detect calculi, strictures, neoplasms, and fistulae in the biliary ducts.

Patient preparation
Explain to the patient that this procedure permits examination of the biliary ducts through X-ray films taken after the injection of a contrast medium through the T-tube. Tell him who will perform the test and where, and that the procedure

takes approximately 15 minutes.

Although this procedure isn't painful, warn the patient he may experience a sensation of bloating in the upper right quadrant as the contrast medium is injected.

Clamp the T-tube the day before the procedure, if ordered. Since bile fills the tube after clamping, this helps prevent air bubbles from entering the ducts. Withhold the meal just before the test, and administer a cleansing enema about 1 hour before the procedure, if ordered.

Make sure the patient or responsible member of the family has signed a consent form. Check the patient's history for hypersensitivity to iodine, seafood, or contrast media used in other diagnostic tests. Sensitivity reactions to the contrast medium are more acute and more common after intravenous injection. Nevertheless, tell the patient the side effects of intraductal administration may include nausea, vomiting, excessive salivation, flushing, urticaria, sweating, and rarely, anaphylaxis.

Procedure

After the patient is in supine position on the radiographic table, the injection area of the T-tube is cleansed with sponges soaked with 70% alcohol. The T-tube is held in a vertical position, which allows trapped air to surface, and a needle attached to a long transparent catheter is carefully inserted into the end of the T-tube. Care must be taken to avoid injecting air into the biliary tree, since air bubbles may affect the clarity of the X-ray films. Approximately 5 ml of contrast medium (usually sodium diatrizoate) is injected under fluoroscopic guidance, and a spot film is taken in the anteroposterior projection. Additional injections are then administered, totaling 20 to 25 ml, and spot films and plain films are taken with the patient in supine and right lateral decubitus positions. The T-tube is then clamped, and the patient is assisted to an erect position for additional films; in this position, air bubbles may be distinguished from calculi or other pathology. A final film is taken 15 minutes after contrast injection to record the emptying of contrast-laden bile into the duodenum. If emptying is delayed, additional films may be taken at 15- or 30- minute intervals until this action is demonstrated.

Precautions

Postoperative cholangiography is contraindicated in patients who are hypersensitive to iodine.

Findings

Biliary ducts demonstrate homogeneous filling with contrast medium and are normal in diameter. When the sphincter

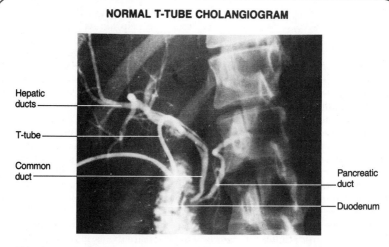

NORMAL T-TUBE CHOLANGIOGRAM

Hepatic ducts

T-tube

Common duct

Pancreatic duct

Duodenum

This photograph of a T-tube cholangiogram shows homogeneous filling of biliary ducts. These ducts are of normal diameter, and the presence of contrast medium in the duodenum shows that the ducts are also patent.

of Oddi is functioning properly and the ducts are patent, the contrast flows unimpeded into the duodenum.

Implications of results

Negative shadows or filling defects within the biliary ducts associated with dilatation may indicate calculi or neoplasms overlooked during surgery. Abnormal channels of contrast medium departing from the biliary ducts indicate fistulae.

Post-test care

□ If a sterile dressing is applied after removal of the T-tube, observe and record any drainage. Change the dressing, as necessary.

□ If the T-tube is left in place, attach it to the drainage system, as ordered.

Interfering factors

Marked obesity or gas overlying the biliary ducts may invalidate X-ray films.

MAE E. PAULFREY, RN, MN

Endoscopic Retrograde Cholangiopancreatography

Endoscopic retrograde cholangiopancreatography (ERCP) is the radiographic examination of the pancreatic ducts and hepatobiliary tree after injection of a contrast medium into the duodenal papilla. It's indicated in patients with confirmed or suspected pancreatic disease, or obstructive jaundice of unknown etiology. With the development of smaller, side-viewing endoscopes, ERCP is now being performed more frequently, especially when abdominal ultrasonography, computerized tomography, liver scanning, hypotonic duodenography, and biliary tract X-ray studies (including percutaneous transhepatic cholangiography) prove diagnostically inadequate. Complications may include cholangitis and pancreatitis.

Purpose

□ To evaluate obstructive jaundice

□ To diagnose cancer of the duodenal papilla, the pancreas, and the biliary ducts

□ To locate calculi and stenosis in the pancreatic ducts and hepatobiliary tree.

Patient preparation

Explain to the patient that this procedure permits examination of the liver, the gallbladder, and the pancreas through X-ray films taken after injection of a contrast medium. Instruct him to fast after midnight before the test. Tell him who will perform the procedure and where, and that it takes 30 to 60 minutes.

Inform the patient that a local anesthetic will be sprayed into his mouth to calm the gag reflex. Warn him that the spray has an unpleasant taste and makes the tongue and throat feel swollen, causing difficulty in swallowing. Instruct him to let saliva drain from the side of his mouth, and tell him that suction may be used to remove saliva. If the patient has teeth, tell him a mouthguard will be inserted to protect them and the endoscope; assure him that it won't obstruct his breathing.

Assure the patient that he'll receive a sedative before insertion of the endoscope, to help him relax, but that he'll remain conscious. Tell him that he'll also receive an anticholinergic or glucagon I.V. after insertion of the scope. Describe the possible side effects of anticholinergics (dry mouth, thirst, tachycardia, urinary retention, and blurred vision) or of glucagon (nausea, vomiting, hives, and flushing). Warn him that he may experience transient flushing on injection of the contrast medium. Advise him that he may have a sore throat for 3 or 4 days after the examination.

Make sure the patient or responsible member of the family has signed a consent form. Check the patient's history for hypersensitivity to iodine, seafood, or contrast media used for other diagnostic procedures.

Just before the procedure, obtain baseline vital signs. Instruct the patient to remove all metal or other radiopaque objects, and constricting undergarments. Then, tell him to void, to minimize the discomfort of urinary retention that may follow the procedure.

Procedure

An I.V. is started with 150 ml of normal saline solution. First, the local anesthetic is administered, as ordered; this usually takes effect in about 10 minutes. If a spray is used, ask the patient to hold his breath while his mouth and throat are sprayed. Then place him in a left lateral position, and give him an emesis basin; provide tissues. Since the anesthetic causes the patient to lose some control of his secretions and thus increases the risk of aspiration, encourage him to allow saliva to drain from the side of his mouth. Then, the mouthguard is inserted.

While the patient remains in the left lateral position, 5 to 20 mg of diazepam is administered I.V. When ptosis or dysarthria develops, the patient's head is bent forward, and he is asked to open his mouth. The examiner inserts his left index finger in the patient's mouth, and guides the tip of the endoscope along his finger, to the back of the patient's throat. The scope is then deflected downward with the left index finger and advanced. As the endoscope passes through the posterior pharynx and cricopharyngeal sphincter, the patient's head is slowly extended to assist the advance of the endoscope. The patient's chin must be kept midline. When the endoscope has passed the cricopharyngeal sphincter, the scope is advanced under direct vision. When it's well into the esophagus (about 12″ [30 cm]), the patient's chin is moved toward the table, so saliva can drain from the mouth. The endoscope is advanced through the remainder of the esophagus and into the stomach under direct vision. When the pylorus is located, a small amount of air is insufflated, and the tip of the endoscope is angled upward and passed into the duodenal bulb.

After the endoscope is rotated clockwise to enter the descending duodenum, the patient is assisted to prone position.

An anticholinérgic or glucagon I.V. is then administered to induce duodenal atony and to relax the ampullary sphincter. A small amount of air is insufflated, and the endoscope is manipulated until the optic lies opposite the duodenal papilla. Then, the cannula filled with contrast medium is passed through the biopsy channel of the endoscope, the duodenal papilla, and into the ampulla of Vater. The pancreas is visualized first, under fluoroscopic guidance, by injection of 2 to 5 ml of contrast medium.

The cannula is repositioned at a more cephalad angle, and the hepatobiliary tree is visualized by injection of 10 to 15 ml of contrast medium. After each injection, rapid-sequence X-ray films are taken.

The patient is instructed to remain prone while the films are developed and reviewed. If necessary, additional films may be taken. When the required radiographs have been obtained, the cannula is removed. Before the endoscope is withdrawn, a tissue specimen may be obtained or fluid aspirated for histologic and cytologic examination, respectively.

Precautions

□ ERCP is contraindicated in patients with infectious disease, pancreatic pseudocysts, stricture or obstruction of the esophagus or duodenum, and acute pancreatitis, cholangitis, or cardiorespiratory disease.

□ Vital signs are monitored, and the airway is kept patent throughout the procedure. If you assist with this procedure, watch for signs of respiratory depression, apnea, hypotension, excessive diaphoresis, bradycardia, and laryngospasm. Be sure to have available emergency resuscitation equipment and a narcotic antagonist, such as naloxone. A second nurse also assists with the procedure, as ordered.

Findings

The duodenal papilla appears as a small, red or sometimes pale erosion protruding into the lumen. Its orifice is com-

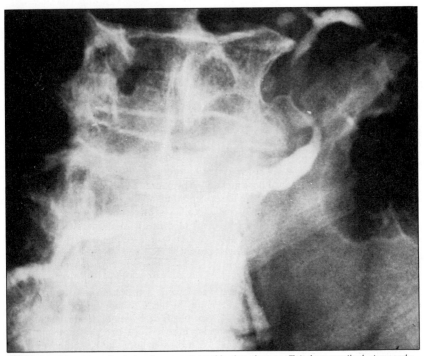

This endoscopic retrograde cholangiopancreatographic view shows a dilated pancreatic duct secondary to stenosis. Stenosis was caused by carcinoma at the head of the pancreas.

monly bordered by a fringe of white mucosa, and a longitudinal fold running perpendicular to the deep circular folds of the duodenum helps mark its location. Although the pancreatic and the hepatobiliary ducts usually unite in the ampulla of Vater and empty through the duodenal papilla, separate orifices are sometimes present.

The contrast medium uniformly fills the pancreatic duct, the hepatobiliary tree, and the gallbladder.

Implications of results

Obstructive jaundice may result from various abnormalities of the hepatobiliary tree and pancreatic duct. Examination of the hepatobiliary tree may reveal stones, strictures, or irregular deviations that suggest biliary cirrhosis, primary sclerosing cholangitis, or carcinoma of the bile ducts. Examination of the pancreatic ducts may also show stones, strictures, and irregular devia-

tions that may indicate pancreatic cysts and pseudocysts, pancreatic tumor, carcinoma of the head of the pancreas, chronic pancreatitis, pancreatic fibrosis, carcinoma of the duodenal papilla, and papillary stenosis.

Depending on test findings, definitive diagnosis may require further studies.

Post-test care

□ Observe closely for signs of cholangitis and pancreatitis. Hyperbilirubinemia, fever, and chills are the immediate signs of cholangitis; hypotension associated with gram-negative septicemia may develop later. Upper left quadrant pain and tenderness, elevated serum amylase levels, and transient hyperbilirubinemia are the usual signs of pancreatitis. Draw blood samples for amylase and bilirubin determinations, if ordered, but remember that these levels usually rise after ERCP.

□ Continue to watch for signs of respiratory depression, apnea, hypotension, excessive diaphoresis, bradycardia, and laryngospasm. Check vital signs every 15 minutes for 4 hours, every hour for 4 hours, then every 4 hours for 48 hours.

□ Withhold food and fluids until the gag reflex returns. Test the gag reflex by touching the back of the throat with a tongue blade. When the gag reflex returns, allow fluids and a light meal.

□ Discontinue or maintain I.V., as ordered.

□ Check for signs of urinary retention. Notify the doctor if the patient hasn't voided within 8 hours.

□ If the patient has a sore throat, provide soothing lozenges and warm saline gargles to ease discomfort.

Interfering factors
None.

MAE E. PAULFREY, RN, MN

Splenoportography
[Transsplenic portography]

Splenoportography is the cineradiographic examination of the splenic veins and portal system after injection of a contrast medium into the splenic pulp. It's indicated in patients with confirmed or suspected portal hypertension, and in those with cirrhosis, to stage the disease. Splenoportography generally provides clearer definition of the venous system than superior mesenteric arteriography; however, it fails to outline the portal vein and, often, the splenic vein in portal hypertension associated with reversed venous blood flow. Superior mesenteric arteriography offers the advantage of outlining the portal and splenic veins even during reversed blood flow, and causes fewer complications.

In splenoportography, splenic pulp pressure is first measured by attaching a spinal manometer filled with normal saline solution to a sheath inserted into the spleen. The contrast medium is then injected through the sheath, and cineradiography is used to record the subsequent filling of the splenic tributary veins, the splenic and portal veins, and the intrahepatic portal radicles. This test may cause excessive bleeding that requires transfusion or, occasionally, splenectomy.

Purpose
□ To diagnose or assess portal hypertension

□ To stage cirrhosis.

Patient preparation
Explain to the patient that this procedure permits examination of the veins supplying the spleen and liver through films taken after injection of a contrast medium. Instruct him to fast after the evening meal the day before the procedure. Tell him who will perform this procedure and where, and that it takes 30 to 45 minutes.

Inform the patient that he may experience a brief stinging sensation on injection of the local anesthetic and a transient flushed feeling on injection of the contrast medium. Instruct him to report upper left quadrant pain (which indicates subcapsular injection) immediately.

Make sure the patient or responsible member of the family has signed a consent form. Check the patient's history for hypersensitivity to iodine, seafood, or contrast media used in other diagnostic tests. Describe the possible side effects of contrast administration, such as nausea, vomiting, excessive salivation, flushing, urticaria, sweating, and rarely, anaphylaxis. Since these reactions usually occur 5 to 10 minutes after injection of the contrast medium, tell the patient to report such signs if they develop. Make sure platelet count and bleeding, clotting, and prothrombin times are normal.

About 30 minutes before the procedure, obtain baseline vital signs, and administer a mild sedative and an analgesic, as ordered.

Procedure

The patient is placed in a supine position on the radiographic table, with his left hand under his head. The left side of his thorax and abdomen is cleansed with antiseptics. Using fluoroscopy, the spleen is located and palpated, and a scout film is taken. After a skin wheal is made with the local anesthetic, to mark the puncture site—usually the intersection of the ninth or tenth intercostal space and the mid- or posterior axillary line—the skin

CAUSES OF PORTAL HYPERTENSION

CAUSE	COMPLICATIONS	APPEARANCE
Suprahepatic • Tricuspid valve incompetence • Hepatic vein thrombosis • Constrictive pericarditis	• Enlarged liver • Moderately enlarged spleen • Few esophageal varices	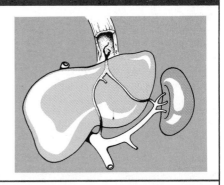
Intrahepatic • Liver cirrhosis	• Esophageal varices • Markedly enlarged spleen	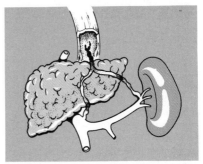
Infrahepatic • Portal vein thrombosis	• Esophageal varices • Decidedly enlarged spleen	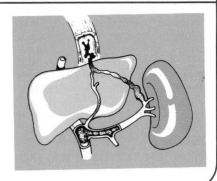

ABNORMAL SPLENOPORTOGRAM

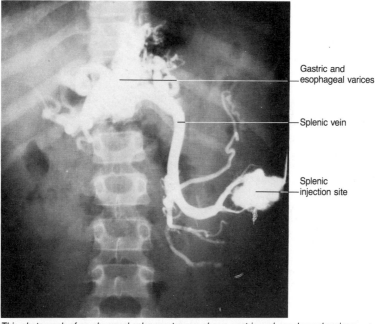

Gastric and esophageal varices

Splenic vein

Splenic injection site

This photograph of an abnormal splenoportogram shows gastric and esophageal varices associated with portal hypertension.

and subcutaneous tissue are infiltrated to the peritoneum. As the patient holds his breath midrespiration, the sheathed needle is rapidly inserted into the spleen, and the inner needle withdrawn; blood wells up slowly through the remaining sheath, if it's positioned in the spleen. The patient is then instructed to maintain shallow respirations with the sheath in place. With flexible plastic tubing, a spinal manometer filled with normal saline solution is connected to the sheath, and the splenic pulp pressure is measured. The manometer is then replaced with a syringe containing 50 ml of sodium diatrizoate, warmed to body temperature, and the sheath is taped in place. Sheath placement is checked fluoroscopically by injection of a few milliliters of contrast medium; the contrast should spread through the splenic parenchyma and into the splenic vein,

without leakage into the abdomen or subcapsular space. If the sheath is properly positioned, the patient is moved over the angiographic changer, the remaining contrast (about 40 ml) is injected, and films are ordered. When the required films have been obtained, the sheath is withdrawn, and pressure and a sterile dressing are applied to the puncture site.

Precautions

Splenoportography is contraindicated in patients with ascites, uncorrectable coagulopathy, splenomegaly due to infection, markedly impaired liver or kidney function, and hypersensitivity to iodine.

Findings

Splenic pulp pressure is normally 50 to 180 mmH$_2$O (3.5 to 13.5 mmHg). After the contrast medium is injected into the splenic pulp, it outlines splenic tributary veins (splenography), then drains into the splenic and portal veins; venous flow is normally contained within these two vessels, without diversion into collateral veins. The contrast outlines the intrahepatic portal radicles (hepatography), with the radicles branching in an acute and homogeneous fashion throughout the liver. When the radicles empty, a dense hepatogram results.

Implications of results

In portal hypertension, splenic pulp pressure ranges from 200 to 450 mmH$_2$O (15 to 34 mmHg). The presence of collateral veins, often associated with esophageal varices, splenomegaly, and in some cases, hepatomegaly—can also indicate portal hypertension resulting from intra- or extrahepatic obstruction to portal venous flow. Results may also show thrombosis or occlusion in the splenic and portal veins, provided venous flow isn't reversed.

In early-stage cirrhosis, a normal splenogram is characteristic, but emptying of the intrahepatic radicles is delayed. As cirrhosis progresses, collateral veins develop, the intrahepatic radicles become angular and shortened, and emptying is again delayed. In advanced cirrhosis, venous blood flow reverses, preventing visualization of the portal and, usually, the splenic veins. Numerous collateral veins in the hilum of the spleen and the immediate retroperitoneum are also characteristic. Actually, the presence of such collateral veins on a film that fails to show the portal vein generally indicates portal hypertension. However, superior mesenteric arteriography is then appropriate to confirm portal vein occlusion or thrombosis.

Post-test care

☐ Check vital signs every 15 minutes for 1 hour, every 30 minutes for 2 hours, then every hour for 4 hours until stable. Observe for bleeding, swelling, and tenderness at the puncture site, and notify the doctor if such signs develop.

☐ Instruct the patient to lie on his left side for 24 hours to minimize the risk of bleeding. Advise an additional 24 hours of bed rest.

☐ As ordered, the patient may resume his usual diet withheld before the test. Encourage fluids to promote excretion of the contrast medium.

☐ Draw a blood sample for hematocrit determination every 8 to 12 hours until hematocrit levels stabilize.

Interfering factors

None.

MAE E. PAULFREY, RN, MN

Celiac and Mesenteric Arteriography

Celiac and mesenteric arteriography is the radiographic examination of the abdominal vasculature after intraarterial injection of contrast medium through a catheter. Most commonly, the catheter is passed through the femoral artery into the aorta, then, using fluoroscopy, is positioned in the celiac, superior mesenteric, or inferior mesenteric artery. Injection of contrast medium into one or more of these arteries provides a map of abdominal vasculature; injection into specific arterial branches, called superselective angiography, permits detailed visualization of a particular area. As the contrast medium flows through the abdominal vasculature, serial radiographs outline abdominal vessels in the arterial, capillary, and venous phases of perfusion. Complications associated with this test include hemorrhage, venous and intracardiac thrombosis, cardiac arrhythmia, and emboli caused by dislodging atherosclerotic plaques.

Celiac and mesenteric arteriography is indicated when endoscopy is unable to locate the source of gastrointestinal bleeding, or when barium studies, ultrasonography, and nuclear medicine or computerized tomography scanning prove inconclusive in evaluating neoplasms.

It's also used to evaluate cirrhosis and portal hypertension (especially when a portacaval shunt is being considered); to evaluate vascular damage, particularly in the spleen and liver, after abdominal trauma; and to detect vascular abnormalities. Since arteriography can demonstrate the portal vein even when portal venous flow is reversed, it is used more often than splenoportography.

Purpose
□ To locate the source of gastrointestinal bleeding
□ To help distinguish between benign and malignant neoplasms
□ To evaluate cirrhosis and portal hypertension
□ To evaluate vascular damage after abdominal trauma
□ To detect vascular abnormalities.

Patient preparation
Explain to the patient that this test examines the abdominal blood vessels after injection of a contrast medium. Instruct him to fast for 8 hours before the test.

Inform the patient that he will receive a local anesthetic and that he may feel a brief, stinging sensation as it is injected. He may also feel pressure when the femoral artery is palpated, but the local anesthetic will minimize the pain when the needle is introduced into the artery. Tell him he may feel a transient burning as the contrast medium is injected, and that he may experience a transient headache, a salty taste, and nausea and vomiting.

Tell the patient that the X-ray equipment makes a loud, clacking sound as the films are taken. Instruct him to lie still during the test, to avoid blurring the films, and inform him that restraints may be used to help him maintain this position. Warn him that he may feel some temporary stiffness after the test from lying still on the hard, flat X-ray table. Tell him who will perform the test and where, and that it takes 30 minutes to 3 hours, depending on the number of vessels studied.

Administer a cathartic the day before

ANGIOGRAPHY FOR CONTROLLING GI BLEEDING

When conservative measures, such as blood transfusion, fail to control GI bleeding, angiography can provide a safe, effective alternative. Once the site of bleeding is identified, vasopressin infusion or arterial embolization can usually control bleeding.

In vasopressin infusion, the angiographic catheter is positioned in the appropriate artery, and vasopressin is infused slowly. After 20 minutes, a radiograph shows the effectiveness of vasopressin, and the rate of infusion may then be changed, as appropriate, to curtail bleeding. Selective vasopressin infusion is generally effective in controlling hemorrhagic gastritis, most intestinal bleeding, and bleeding from Mallory-Weiss lacerations and stress ulcers. It is less consistently effective in controlling bleeding from gastric ulcers, and rarely effective in controlling bleeding from duodenal ulcers. This technique should be used cautiously in patients with coronary artery disease, since its side effects include arrhythmias and fluid retention.

If vasopressin infusion fails to control GI bleeding, or if bleeding results from gastric or duodenal ulcers, arterial embolization may prove effective. In this technique, the angiographic catheter is positioned in the appropriate artery and embolic material, such as an epsilon-aminocaproic acid (Amicar) clot or absorbable gelatin sponge (Gelfoam) is injected through the catheter. X-ray films are taken to assess the placement of embolization. Additional material may be injected, if necessary. This technique shouldn't be used after gastric or intestinal surgery, since it exaggerates the risk of infarction.

---

the test, as ordered, and make sure the patient or responsible member of the family has signed a consent form. Check the patient's history for hypersensitivity to iodine, shellfish, or the contrast medium. Make sure blood studies (hemoglobin, hematocrit, clotting time, prothrombin time, activated partial thromboplastin time, and platelet count) have been completed. Just before the procedure, instruct the patient to put on a hospital gown and to remove jewelry and other objects that might obscure anatomic detail on X-ray films. Tell the patient to void, then record baseline vital signs. Administer a sedative, if ordered.

Procedure

After placing the patient in supine position on the radiographic table, an I.V. infusion of 5% dextrose in water is started to maintain hydration and to permit emergency administration of medication. Scout films of the patient's abdomen are taken, and the peripheral pulses are palpated and marked. The puncture site is cleansed with an antiseptic and the skin wiped with alcohol, and the local anesthetic is injected. Then, the femoral artery is located by palpation, and the needle is gently inserted until a pulsing blood flow is obtained. A guide wire is passed through the needle into the aorta,

then the needle is removed, leaving the guide wire in place. After the angiographic catheter is inserted over the guide wire, catheter placement is checked fluoroscopically or radiographically, and the guide wire is withdrawn. Then the catheter is advanced into one of the major arteries—celiac, superior mesenteric, or inferior mesenteric—under fluoroscopic guidance. After correct placement of the catheter is verified, an automatic injector is attached to the catheter. As the contrast medium is injected, a series of films are taken in rapid sequence.

After injecting one or more major ar-

TYPES OF ARTERIAL ENCASEMENT

When a tumor invades or encases nearby arteries, it distorts their regular, channel-like appearance into serrated, serpiginous, or smooth forms.

In *serrated encasement,* the arterial walls become jagged and irregular. This condition only occurs with cancer and is not present in other diseases.

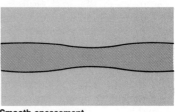

Serrated encasement

In *serpiginous encasement,* the arterial channel itself becomes irregular. This condition usually indicates cancer but may also result from severe fibrosis.

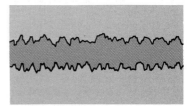

Serpiginous encasement

In *smooth encasement,* the arterial channel narrows. This condition may or may not indicate cancer.

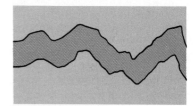

Smooth encasement

teries, superselective catheterization may be performed. Using fluoroscopy, the catheter is repositioned in a specific branch of a major artery, contrast medium is injected, and rapid-sequence films are ordered. If necessary, several specific branches may be catheterized.

After filming, the catheter is withdrawn, and firm pressure is applied to the puncture site for about 15 minutes. The site is observed for hematoma formation, a pressure dressing is applied, and peripheral pulses are checked.

Precautions

 ☐ Celiac and mesenteric arteriography should be performed cautiously in patients with coagulopathy.

 ☐ Most reactions to the contrast medium occur within a half-hour. Watch carefully for cardiovascular shock or arrest, hives, flushing, laryngeal stridor, or urticaria.

Findings

X-ray films show the three phases of perfusion—arterial, capillary, and venous. The arteries normally taper regularly, becoming gradually smaller with subsequent divisions. The contrast medium then spreads evenly within the sinusoids. The portal vein appears 10 to 20 seconds after the injection, as the contrast medium empties from the spleen into the splenic vein or from the intestine into the superior mesenteric vein, and further into the portal vein.

Implications of results

Gastrointestinal (GI) hemorrhage appears on the angiogram as the extravasation of contrast medium from the damaged vessels. Upper GI hemorrhage can result from conditions such as Mallory-Weiss syndrome, gastric or peptic ulcer, hemorrhagic gastritis, and eroded hiatal hernia. Esophageal hemorrhage rarely appears on the angiogram, since the contrast medium usually fails to fill the esophageal vein. Lower GI hemorrhage can result from condi-

ARTIFICIAL ARTERIAL EMBOLIZATION

The two most commonly used artificial clotting agents for arterial embolization are epsilon-aminocaproic acid (Amicar) and absorbable gelatin sponge (Gelfoam). To use Amicar, the doctor first draws 9 ml of blood from an aortic catheter into a syringe containing 1 ml of Amicar. In the syringe, the Amicar acts on the blood, and a clot forms in about 30 minutes. At this time a 0.5 ml aliquot is removed from the clot, placed in a tuberculin syringe containing 0.5 ml of unheparinized saline solution, and is injected into the catheter that has been placed in the artery requiring embolization. On injection, the clot fragments and occludes the artery and several branches. Amicar clots dissolve within 24 hours in the branches but last longer in the damaged vessel.

Gelfoam comes from the manufacturer in squares that can be cut into 4-mm cubes. The cubes are placed in normal saline solution to make them pliable. Then, they are injected in a manner similar to the Amicar clot. Gelfoam remains intact for longer than 24 hours, resulting in the development of collateral circulation within the area ordinarily supplied by the occluded artery.

tions such as bleeding diverticula and angiodysplasia.

Abdominal neoplasms—carcinoid tumors, adenomas, leiomyomas, angiomas, and adenocarcinomas—can disrupt the normal vasculature in several ways. Neoplasms can invade or encase nearby arteries and veins, distorting their regular channel-like appearance and, in late stages, displacing them. Vessels within the neoplasm, known as neovasculature, appear as abnormal vascular areas. Areas of necrosis appear as puddles of contrast medium. Contrast medium may also remain in the neoplasm longer during capillary perfusion, producing a tumor blush or stain on the angiogram. Arteriovenous shunting may also be present, depending on the size and location of the tumor. Since these characteristics aren't uniformly present in all neoplasms, combinations of these characteristics can often distinguish between benign and malignant neoplasms.

In early or mild cirrhosis, portal venous flow to the liver remains relatively unaffected, and the hepatic artery and its branches appear normal. As this disease progresses, portal venous flow diminishes, the hepatic artery and its branches become dilated and tortuous, and collateral veins develop. In advanced cirrhosis, portal venous flow reverses. However, the portal vein still appears on the X-ray film, which may also show thrombi.

Abdominal trauma often causes splenic and, less often, hepatic injury. Splenic rupture often displaces intrasplenic arterial branches, and contrast medium leaks from splenic arteries into the splenic pulp. When rupture occurs without subcapsular hematoma, the spleen usually maintains its normal size. However, in subcapsular hematoma, the spleen enlarges to displace the splenic artery and vein; the subcapsular hematoma itself appears as a large, avascular mass that stretches intrasplenic arteries and compresses the splenic pulp away from the capsule.

Hepatic injury causes similar vascular distortion, such as displacement of the common hepatic artery and extrahepatic branches. Intrahepatic and subcapsular hematomas displace and stretch intrahepatic arteries. As the hepatic vascular supply is disrupted, arteriovenous fistula may develop between the hepatic artery and the portal vein.

Various abnormalities affecting the diameter and course of an artery may appear on the angiogram. Atherosclerotic plaques or atheromas—lipid deposits on the intima—narrow the arterial lumen and may even occlude it, with formation of collaterals. Other identifiable vascular abnormalities include aneurysm, thrombus, and embolus.

Post-test care

□ Instruct the patient to lie flat, and enforce bed rest for at least 12 hours after the test.

□ Monitor vital signs, as ordered, until stable, and check peripheral pulses. Note the color and temperature of the leg that was used for the test.

□ Check the puncture site for bleeding and hematoma. (A sandbag may be placed over the site for the first 2 to 4 hours to prevent bleeding.) If bleeding develops, apply pressure to the site; if bleeding continues or is excessive, notify the doctor. If a hematoma develops, apply warm soaks.

□ Ask the doctor if the patient can resume his usual diet. If the patient isn't receiving I.V. infusions, encourage intake of fluids, to speed excretion of the contrast medium.

Interfering factors

None.

MAE E. PAULFREY, RN, MN

NUCLEAR MEDICINE

Liver-spleen Scanning

In this test, a rectilinear scanner or gamma camera records the distribution of radioactivity within the liver and spleen after I.V. injection of a radioactive colloid. The colloid most commonly used, technetium sulfide-99m (^{99m}Tc), concentrates in the reticuloendothelial cells through phagocytosis. About 80% to 90% of the injected colloid is taken up by Kupffer's cells in the liver, 5% to 10% by the spleen, and 3% to 5% by bone marrow. A rectilinear scanner records this distribution by scanning back and forth over the liver and spleen; the gamma camera images either organ instantaneously without scanning.

Liver-spleen scanning is indicated in patients with palpable abdominal masses to demonstrate hepatomegaly or splenomegaly, and in those with suspected hematoma after abdominal trauma. It's generally the most reliable screening test *for detecting hepatocellular disease, hepatic metastases, and focal disease, such as tumors, cysts, and abscesses. However, such scanning demonstrates focal disease nonspecifically as a cold spot (a defect that fails to take up the colloid) and may fail to detect focal lesions smaller than ¾" (2 cm) in diameter. Although clinical signs and symptoms may aid diagnosis, liver-spleen scanning frequently requires confirmation by ultrasonography, computerized tomography, gallium scanning, or biopsy.*

Purpose

□ To screen for hepatic metastases and hepatocellular disease, such as cirrhosis and hepatitis

□ To detect focal disease, such as tumors, cysts, and abscesses in the liver and spleen

□ To demonstrate hepatomegaly, splenomegaly, and splenic infarcts

□ To assess the condition of the liver and spleen after abdominal trauma.

Patient preparation

Explain to the patient that this procedure permits examination of the liver and spleen through scintigraphs or scans taken after I.V. injection of a radioactive substance. Inform him that he needn't restrict food or fluids before the test. Tell him who will perform the test and where, that he may experience transient discomfort from the needle puncture, and that the test takes about 1 hour.

Be sure the patient isn't scheduled for more than one radionuclide scan on the same day. Assure him that the injection isn't dangerous, since the test substance contains only trace amounts of radioactivity, and that allergic reactions to it are rare. Tell him the uptake probe and detector head of the gamma camera may touch his abdomen (if appropriate), but that this isn't dangerous; or inform him that the rectilinear scanner will make a soft, irregular clicking noise as it moves across his abdomen. Advise the patient that he'll be asked to lie still and to breathe quietly

during the procedure, to ensure images of good quality; he may also be asked to hold his breath briefly. This technique helps to evaluate liver mobility and pliability.

Procedure

The ⁹⁹ᵐTc is injected I.V., and after 10 to 15 minutes, the patient's abdomen is scanned with the patient placed in supine, left and right lateral, left and right anterior oblique, and prone positions, to ensure optimal visualization of the liver and spleen. The left anterior oblique position provides the best view of the spleen separate from the left lobe of the liver. With the patient supine, liver mobility and pliability may be evaluated by marking the costal margin and scanning as the patient breathes deeply. Since the liver normally moves and changes shape with deep breathing, fixation suggests pathology.

After the required scintigraphs have been taken, they are reviewed for clarity before the patient is allowed to leave. If necessary, additional views are obtained.

Precautions

Liver-spleen scanning is usually contraindicated in children, and during pregnancy and lactation.

Findings

Since the liver and spleen contain equal numbers of reticuloendothelial cells, both organs normally appear equally bright on the image. However, distribution of radioactive colloid is generally more uniform and homogeneous in the spleen than in the liver. The liver has various normal indentations and impressions, such as the gallbladder fossa and falciform ligament, that may mimic focal disease.

Implications of results

Although liver-spleen scanning may fail to detect early hepatocellular disease, it shows characteristic, distinct patterns as such disease progresses. The most prominent sign of hepatocellular disease is a shift of the radioactive colloid, caused by reduced hepatic blood flow and impaired function of Kupffer's cells. This inhibits distribution of the colloid in the liver, causing it to appear uniformly decreased or patchy. The spleen and bone marrow then take up the abnormally large amounts of the colloid unabsorbed

IDENTIFYING LIVER INDENTATIONS IN NUCLEAR IMAGING

In nuclear imaging, normal indentations and impressions may be mistaken for focal lesions. These drawings of the liver—anterior view and posterior view—identify the contours and impressions that may be misread.

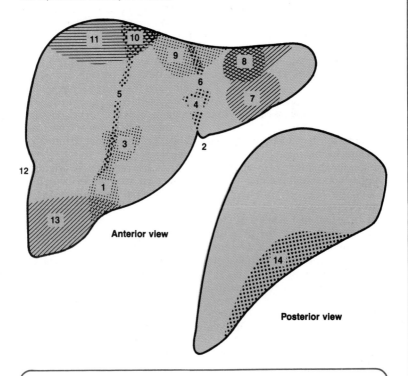

Anterior view

Posterior view

Key:

1 - gallbadder fossa
2 - ligamentum teres and falciform ligament
3 - hilum, main branching of the portal vein
4 - pars umbilicus portion, left portal vein
5 - variable stripe of lobar fissure between right and left lobes
6 - variable stripe of segmental fissure, left lobe

7 - thinning of left lobe
8 - impression of pectus excavatum
9 - cardiac impression
10 - hepatic veins and inferior vena cava
11 - shielding from right female breast
12 - Harrison's groove or costal impression
13 - impression of hepatic flexure of colon
14 - right renal impression

Adapted with permission from Alexander R. Margulis and Joachim H. Burhenne, *Alimentary Tract Radiology: Abdominal Imaging*, Vol. III (St. Louis: C.V. Mosby Co., 1979).

by the liver, thus concentrating more radioactivity than the liver, and appear brighter on the scan. This same distribution pattern (colloid shift) also accompanies portal hypertension due to extrahepatic causes.

Hepatitis and cirrhosis are both associated with hepatomegaly and a colloid shift, but certain characteristics help distinguish them. In hepatitis, distribution of the colloid is usually uniformly decreased; in cirrhosis, it's patchy. Splenomegaly is typical in cirrhosis but not in hepatitis.

Metastasis to the liver or spleen may appear on the scan as a focal defect and requires biopsy to confirm diagnosis. Liver metastasis usually originates in the gastrointestinal or genitourinary tract, the breasts, or the lungs, and is more common than metastasis to the spleen. After metastasis is confirmed, serial liver-spleen studies are useful to evaluate effectiveness of therapy.

Because cysts, abscesses, and tumors fail to take up the radioactive colloid, they appear on the scan as solitary or multiple focal defects. Hepatic cysts may appear as solitary defects; polycystic hepatic disease, as multiple defects. Splenic cysts are rarer than hepatic cysts and may have a parasitic or nonparasitic origin. Ultrasonography can confirm hepatic or splenic cysts.

Intrahepatic abscesses are usually pyogenic or amebic. Subphrenic abscesses, located beneath the diaphragm, may distort the dome of the right lobe. Splenic abscesses are characteristic in bacterial endocarditis. All abscesses require gallium scanning or ultrasonography to confirm diagnosis.

Benign hepatic tumors—such as hemangiomas, adenomas, and hamartomas—require confirming biopsy or flow studies. Primary malignant tumors, such as hepatomas, also require biopsy. Benign splenic tumors are rare and include hemangiomas, fibromas, myomas, and hamartomas. Primary malignant splenic tumors are also rare, except in lymphoreticular malignancies such as Hodgkin's disease. Splenic tumors also

---

FLOW STUDIES

In contrast to liver-spleen scanning, which provides static nuclear images, flow studies (dynamic scintigraphy) record in rapid sequence the stages of perfusion after I.V. injection of a radionuclide, such as technetium sulfide-99m. Since flow studies demonstrate the vascularity of a nonspecific focal defect, they sometimes help distinguish among metastases, tumors, cysts, and abscesses.

In flow studies, a hot defect demonstrates early, increased uptake of the radionuclide when compared to the surrounding parenchyma, and then appears as a filling defect, or cold spot, on later routine images. Cysts and abscesses, which are avascular, fail to take up the radionuclide; hemangiomas appear characteristically hot, due to their enlarged vessels. Tumors and metastases are generally more difficult to evaluate, since their vascularity is more variable. Although vascular metastases may appear hot, most metastases demonstrate poor uptake of the radionuclide. Hepatomas can also appear hot or can show perfusion similar to normal parenchyma.

---

require biopsy to confirm diagnosis. Although focal disease usually inhibits uptake of radioactive colloid, both obstruction of the superior vena cava and Budd-Chiari syndrome cause markedly increased uptake.

Liver-spleen scanning can verify palpable abdominal masses and differentiates between splenomegaly and hepatomegaly. An upper left quadrant mass may result from splenomegaly, or from hepatomegaly if the liver is grossly extended across the abdomen. An upper right quadrant mass may result from hepatomegaly; a lower right quadrant mass may be a Riedel's lobe or a large dependent gallbladder. Splenic infarcts, often associated with bacterial endocarditis and massive splenomegaly, appear as peripheral defects, with decreased and irregular colloid distribution. Scanning can assess hepatic or splenic injury after abdominal trauma. Intrahepatic hematoma appears as a focal defect; subcapsular hematoma, as a lentiform defect on the periphery of the liver; hepatic laceration, as a linear defect. Splenic hematoma appears as a focal defect; sub-capsular hematoma, as a lentiform defect on the periphery; hepatic laceration as a linear defect. Splenic hematoma appears as a focal defect in or next to the spleen and may transect it.

Post-test care
Watch for anaphylactoid or pyrogenic re-actions that may result from a stabilizer, such as dextran or gelatin, added to ^{99m}Tc.

Interfering factors
Radionuclides administered in other studies on the same day can interfere with liver-spleen imaging.
MAE E. PAULFREY, RN, MN

COMPUTED TOMOGRAPHY

Computed Tomography of the Biliary Tract and Liver

In computed tomography (CT) of the biliary tract and liver, multiple X-rays pass through the upper abdomen and are measured while detectors record differences in tissue attenuation. A computer reconstructs this data as a three-dimensional image on a television screen. Since soft tissue appearance varies with tissue attenuation, CT accurately distinguishes the biliary tract and the liver if the ducts are large. Use of I.V. contrast media during CT can accentuate different densities.

CT images can specify focal defects detected by liver-spleen scanning as solid, cystic, inflammatory, and vascular lesions; however, biopsy may be necessary to rule out malignancy or to distinguish between metastatic and primary tumors. CT can also detect suspected hematoma after abdominal trauma, and can determine the type of jaundice.

Although CT and ultrasonography both detect biliary tract and liver disease equally well, the latter technique is performed more often. CT is more expensive than ultrasonography and involves patient exposure to moderate amounts of radiation. However, it's the test of choice in patients who are obese and in those
with livers positioned high under the rib cage, since bone and excessive fat hinder ultrasound transmission.

Barium studies should precede this test by at least 4 days, since barium may hinder visualization.

Purpose
□ To detect intrahepatic tumors and abscesses, subphrenic and subhepatic abscesses, cysts, and hematomas
□ To distinguish between obstructive and nonobstructive jaundice.

Patient preparation
Explain to the patient that this test helps detect biliary tract and liver disease. Instruct him to fast after midnight before the test. Tell him who will perform the test and where, and that it takes approximately 1½ hours.

Inform the patient that he'll be placed on an adjustable table, which is positioned inside a scanning gantry. Assure him that the test will be painless. Tell him he'll be asked to remain still during the test and to hold his breath when instructed. Stress the importance of remaining still during the test, because movement can cause artifacts, thereby prolonging the test and limiting its accuracy. If I.V. contrast medium is being used, inform the patient that he may experience transient discomfort from the needle puncture and a localized feeling of warmth on injection. Tell the patient to report immediately nausea, vomiting, dizziness, headache, and urticaria.

Make sure the patient or responsible

member of the family has signed a consent form. Check the patient's history for hypersensitivity to iodine, seafood, or the contrast media used in other diagnostic tests. If ordered, give him 300 to 400 ml of gastrografin about 10 minutes before the test.

Procedure
The patient is placed in supine position on a radiographic table, and the table is positioned within the opening in the scanning gantry. A series of transverse X-ray films are taken and recorded on magnetic tape. This information is reconstructed by a computer and appears as images on a television screen. These images are studied, and selected ones are photographed. When the first series of films is completed, the images are reviewed. Then, contrast enhancement may be ordered. After the contrast medium is injected, a second series of films is taken, and the patient is carefully observed for allergic reaction.

Precautions
CT of the biliary tract and liver is usually contraindicated during pregnancy and, if I.V. contrast medium is used, in patients with hypersensitivity to iodine or with severe renal or hepatic disease.

Findings
Normally, the liver has a uniform density that's slightly greater than that of the pancreas, kidneys, and spleen. Linear and circular areas of slightly lower density, representing hepatic vascular structures, may interrupt this uniform appearance. The portal vein is usually visible; the hepatic artery usually isn't. I.V. contrast medium enhances both vascular structures and the liver parenchyma, and they become isodense.

Intrahepatic biliary radicles are normally not visible, but the common hepatic and bile ducts are occasionally visible as low-density structures. Since bile has the same density as water, use of I.V. contrast aids visualization of the biliary tract by enhancing surrounding parenchyma and vascular structures.

Like the biliary ducts, the gallbladder is visible as a round or elliptic low-density structure. A contracted gallbladder may be impossible to visualize.

Implications of results
Most focal hepatic defects appear less dense than the normal parenchyma, and CT can detect small lesions. Use of rapid-sequence scanning with I.V. contrast medium helps distinguish between the two, since the normal parenchyma shows greater enhancement than focal defects. Primary and metastatic neoplasms may appear as well-circumscribed or poorly defined areas of slightly lower density than the normal parenchyma. However, some lesions have the same density as the liver parenchyma and may thus prove undetectable. Neoplasms that are especially large may distort the liver's contour. Hepatic abscesses appear as relatively low-density, homogeneous areas, usually with well-defined borders. Hepatic cysts appear as sharply defined round or oval structures, and have a density lower than abscesses and neoplasms.

The density of a hepatic hematoma varies with its age. A fresh clot is as dense as or slightly denser than the normal parenchyma; a resolving clot is of slightly lower density than the normal parenchyma. Intrahepatic hematomas vary in shape; subcapsular hematomas are usually crescent-shaped and compress the liver away from the capsule.

In distinguishing between obstructive and nonobstructive jaundice, dilatation of the biliary ducts indicates the former; absence of dilatation, the latter. Dilated intrahepatic bile ducts appear as low-density linear and circular branching structures. Dilatation of the common hepatic duct, common bile duct, and gallbladder may also be apparent, depending on the site and severity of obstruction. Use of an I.V. contrast medium helps detect biliary dilatation, especially when the ducts are only slightly dilated.

CT can usually identify the cause of obstruction, such as calculi or pancreatic carcinoma. However, when the site of obstruction must be located before surgery, percutaneous transhepatic cholangiography or, less commonly, endoscopic retrograde cholangiopancreatography may also be performed.

Post-test care

The patient may resume his usual diet.

Interfering factors

☐ Use of P.O. or I.V. contrast media that are excreted in the bile in previous diagnostic studies can interfere with detection of biliary dilatation, since they may cause the biliary tract to appear as dense as the surrounding parenchyma.

☐ Barium studies performed within 4 days before CT may obscure the test results.

FRANCES W. QUINLESS, RN, PhD

Computed Tomography of the Pancreas

In computed tomography (CT) of the pancreas, multiple X-rays penetrate the upper abdomen and are measured, while a detector records the differences in tissue attenuation. A computer then reconstructs this data as a three-dimensional image on a television screen. Since attenuation varies with tissue density, CT accurately distinguishes the pancreas, and surrounding organs and vessels if enough fat is present between the structures. Use of an I.V. or P.O. contrast medium can accentuate differences in tissue density.

CT of the pancreas is indicated in patients with signs and symptoms of pancreatic carcinoma (weight loss, jaundice, gnawing epigastric pain radiating to the back); in patients with pancreatitis, to detect and evaluate its complications; or in patients wtih suspected pancreatitis, when radiologic and biochemical tests prove inconclusive. CT can't detect tumors too small to alter pancreatic size and

shape, and may fail to distinguish between carcinoma and pancreatitis.

Purpose

☐ To detect pancreatic carcinoma or pseudocysts

☐ To detect or evaluate pancreatitis

☐ To distinguish between pancreatic disorders and disorders of the retroperitoneum.

Patient preparation

Explain to the patient that this test helps detect disorders of the pancreas. Instruct him to fast after midnight before the test. Tell him who will perform the test and where, and that it takes about 1½ hours.

Inform the patient that he'll be placed on an adjustable table that is positioned inside a scanning gantry. Assure him that, although the test equipment looks formidable, the procedure is painless. Tell him he'll be asked to remain still during the test and to hold his breath at certain times. Inform him that he may be given a contrast medium I.V. or P.O. or both to aid visualization of the pancreas. Describe the possible side effects of the contrast—nausea, flushing, dizziness, and sweating—and tell the patient to report them if they develop.

Make sure the patient or responsible member of the family has signed a consent form. Check the patient's history for recent barium studies and for hypersensitivity to iodine, seafood, or the contrast media used in other diagnostic tests. Give calcium phosphate or gastrografin, as ordered, to clearly define and demarcate the stomach and intestines.

Procedure

The patient is placed in supine position on a radiographic table, and the table is positioned within the opening in the scanning gantry. A series of transverse X-rays is taken and recorded on magnetic tape. The varying tissue absorption is calculated by a computer, and the information is reconstructed as images on a television screen. These images are studied, and selected ones are photographed. After the first series of films is

NORMAL CT SCAN OF THE PANCREAS

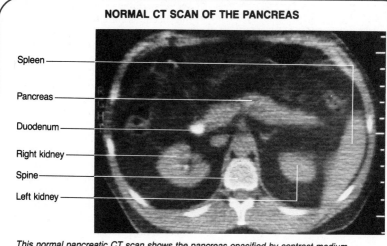

Spleen

Pancreas

Duodenum

Right kidney

Spine

Left kidney

This normal pancreatic CT scan shows the pancreas opacified by contrast medium.

completed, the images are reviewed. Then contrast enhancement may be ordered. After the contrast medium is administered, another series of films is taken, and the patient is observed for an allergic reaction—itching, hypotension, hypertension, diaphoresis, or dyspnea.

Precautions
CT of the pancreas is contraindicated during pregnancy and, if a contrast medium is used, in patients with hypersensitivity to iodine or with severe renal or hepatic disease.

Findings
The pancreas generally lies obliquely across the upper abdomen, and its parenchyma demonstrates a uniform density (particularly if an I.V. contrast medium is used). The gland normally thickens from tail to head and generally has a smooth surface. Contrast administered P.O. opacifies the adjacent stomach and duodenum, and helps outline the pancreas, particularly in persons with little peripancreatic fat, such as children and very thin adults.

Implications of results
Since the tissue density of pancreatic car-cinoma resembles that of the normal parenchyma, changes in pancreatic size and shape help demonstrate carcinoma and pseudocysts. Usually, carcinoma first appears as a localized swelling of the head, body, or tail of the pancreas, and may spread to obliterate the fat plane, dilate the main pancreatic duct and common bile duct by obstructing them, and produce low-density focal lesions in the liver, from metastasis. Use of an I.V. contrast medium helps detect metastases by opacifying the pancreatic and hepatic parenchyma.

Adenocarcinoma and islet cell tumor are the most common carcinomas of the pancreas. Cystadenomas and cystadenocarcinomas, usually multilocular, occur most frequently in the body and tail of the pancreas, and appear as low-density focal lesions marked by internal septa. P.O. contrast medium helps distinguish between bowel loops and tumors in the tail of the pancreas.

Acute pancreatitis, either edematous (interstitial) or necrotizing (hemorrhagic), produces diffuse enlargement of the pancreas. In acute edematous pancreatitis, the density of the parenchyma is uniformly decreased. In acute necrotizing pancreatitis, the density is non-

PANCREATIC COMPUTED TOMOGRAPHY

Computed tomography (CT) is replacing ultrasonography as the test of choice for pancreatic examination. Ultrasonography costs less and involves less risk for the patient, but it is also somewhat less accurate.

In retroperitoneal disorders—and specifically when pancreatitis is suspected—CT scanning goes beyond ultrasonography by showing the general swelling that accompanies acute inflammation of the gland. In chronic cases, CT scanning easily detects calcium deposits often missed by simple radiography, particularly in patients who are obese.

Besides detecting tumors, cysts, and abscesses, CT can also distinguish between benign and malignant tumors, because of its unique sensitivity to variations in tissue density. Although less reliable in the early detection of pancreatic carcinomas, CT scanning can spot presymptomatic warning signs, such as localized swelling in the head, body, or tail of the gland.

uniform due to the presence of both necrosis and hemorrhage. The areas of tissue necrosis have diminished density. In acute pancreatitis, inflammation often spreads into the peripancreatic fat and blurs the margin of the gland. Ab-

scesses, phlegmons, and pseudocysts may occur as complications of acute pancreatitis. Abscesses, either within or outside the pancreas, appear as low-density areas and are most readily detected when they contain gas. Pseudocysts, which may be unilocular or multilocular, appear as sharply circumscribed, low-density areas that may contain debris. Ascites and pleural effusion may also be apparent in acute pancreatitis.

In chronic pancreatitis, the pancreas may appear normal, enlarged (localized or generalized), or atrophic, depending on the severity of the disease. Calcification of the ducts and dilatation of the main pancreatic duct are characteristic. Pseudocysts, obliteration of the fat plane, and secondary complications (such as biliary obstruction) may occur.

Post-test care
The patient may resume his usual diet.

Interfering factors
☐ Barium retained in the gastrointestinal tract may obscure visualization.
☐ Excessive movement by the patient during scanning may produce artifacts.
☐ Excessive peristaltic movement during scanning may produce artifacts.
FRANCES W. QUINLESS, RN, PhD

ULTRASONOGRAPHY

Ultrasonography of the Gallbladder and the Biliary System

In ultrasonography of the gallbladder and the biliary system, a focused beam of high-frequency sound waves passes into the upper right quadrant of the abdomen, creating echoes that vary with changes in tissue density. When these echoes are converted to electrical energy and amplified by a transducer, they appear on an oscilloscope screen as a pattern of spikes or dots. This pattern reveals the size, shape, and position of the gallbladder and may outline a portion of the biliary system. Ultrasonography can also evaluate the gallbladder after injection of sincalide, a hormonal analogue that causes the organ to contract and expel bile. Although oral cholecystography is frequently performed first in diagnosing cholelithiasis or cholecystitis, ultrasonography is used if cholecystography is inconclusive or doesn't adequately visualize the gallbladder. Since the accuracy of ultrasonography doesn't depend on hepatic and gallbladder function, it's especially use-

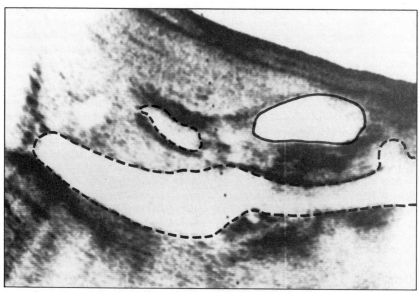

This ultrasonogram is a longitudinal view of a normal gallbladder (solid color line) and the extrahepatic bile duct (dotted color line). Also shown is the inferior vena cava (dotted black line).

ful for evaluating patients with elevated serum bilirubin levels when contrast radiography may prove ineffective. It's the procedure of choice for evaluating jaundice (since it readily distinguishes between obstructive and nonobstructive types) and for emergency diagnosis of patients with signs of acute cholecystitis, such as upper right quadrant pain, with or without local tenderness.

Purpose
☐ To confirm diagnosis of cholelithiasis
☐ To diagnose acute cholecystitis
☐ To distinguish between obstructive and nonobstructive jaundice.

Patient preparation
Explain to the patient that this procedure allows examination of the gallbladder and the biliary system. Instruct him to eat a fat-free meal in the evening and then to fast for 8 to 12 hours before the procedure, if possible; this promotes accumulation of bile in the gallbladder and enhances ultrasonic visualization. Tell him who will perform the procedure and where, that the room may be darkened slightly to aid visualization on the os-

cilloscope screen, and that the test takes 15 to 30 minutes.

Tell the patient a transducer will pass smoothly over the upper right quadrant, in direct contact with his skin, but assure him he'll feel only mild pressure. If sincalide will be injected to stimulate gallbladder contraction, tell the patient he may experience abdominal cramping, tenesmus, nausea, dizziness, sweating, and flushing. Instruct him to remain as still as possible during the procedure, and to hold his breath when requested; this ensures that the gallbladder is in the same position for each scan.

Just before the procedure, instruct the patient to put on a hospital gown.

Procedure
The patient is placed in supine position. A water-soluble lubricant is applied to the face of the transducer, and transverse scans of the gallbladder are taken at ⅜″ (1-cm) intervals, starting at the level of the xiphoid and moving laterally to the right subcostal area. Concurrently, the organ's medial and lateral borders are mapped on the patient's skin with a marking pen; these borders are used as

guidelines for further scanning. Longitudinal oblique scans are taken at 5-mm intervals parallel to the long axis of the gallbladder marked on the patient's skin, beginning medial to the gallbladder and continuing through to its lateral border. During each scan, the patient is asked to exhale deeply and hold his breath. If the gallbladder is positioned deeply under the right costal margin, a scan may be taken through the intercostal spaces, while the patient inhales deeply and holds his breath.

The patient is then placed in a left lateral decubitus position and is scanned beneath the right costal margin. This position and scanning angle are particularly useful for displacing stones lodged in the cystic duct region, which may escape detection when the patient is supine. Scanning with the patient erect helps demonstrate mobility or fixation of suspicious echogenic areas.

Gallbladder contractibility may then be evaluated by giving the patient a fatty meal or an I.V. injection of sincalide. Administration of sincalide is usually preferred, because the patient may swallow air while eating, hindering ultrasound transmission. Within 5 to 30 minutes after injection, the gallbladder normally contracts, and the scans are repeated. When good oscilloscopic views are obtained, they are photographed for later study.

Precautions

Sincalide should not be administered to children, females who are pregnant, or patients who are hypersensitive to this medication.

Findings

The normal gallbladder is sonolucent; it appears circular on transverse scans and pear-shaped on longitudinal scans. Although the size of the gallbladder is variable, its outer walls normally appear sharp and smooth. Intrahepatic radicles seldom appear, because the flow of sonolucent bile is very fine. The cystic duct may also be indistinct—the result of folds known as Heister's valves that line

the cystic duct lumen. When visualized, the cystic duct has a serpentine appearance. The common bile duct, in contrast, has a linear appearance but is sometimes obscured by overlying bowel gas.

Implications of results

Gallstones within the gallbladder lumen or the biliary system typically appear as mobile, echogenic areas, usually associated with an acoustic shadow. The size of gallstones generally parallels the size of their shadows; gallstones 5 mm or larger usually produce shadows. However, if the gallbladder is distended with bile, gallstones as small as 1 mm can be detected. Sonolucent bile provides the ideal background for demonstrating stones, since the acoustic contrast between fluid bile and solid gallstones is great; this explains why it's sometimes difficult to detect stones in the biliary ducts, which contain much less bile. When the gallbladder is shrunken or fully impacted with gallstones, inadequate bile may again make gallstone detection difficult, and the gallbladder itself may fail to be visualized. In this case, the presence of an acoustic shadow in the gallbladder fossa indicates cholelithiasis, even though gallstones can't be seen; the presence of such a shadow in the cystic and common bile ducts can also indicate cholelithiasis.

Polyps and carcinoma within the gallbladder lumen are distinguished from gallstones by their fixity. Polyps usually appear as sharply defined, echogenic areas; carcinoma appears as a poorly defined mass, often associated with a thickened gallbladder wall.

Biliary sludge within the gallbladder lumen appears as a fine layer of echoes that slowly gravitates to the dependent portion of the gallbladder as the patient changes position. Although biliary sludge may arise without accompanying pathology, it may also result from obstruction and can predispose to gallstone formation.

Acute cholecystitis is indicated by an enlarged gallbladder with thickened, double-rimmed walls, usually accompanied by gallstones within the lumen. Similarly, in chronic cholecystitis, the walls of the gallbladder appear thickened. The organ itself, however, is generally contracted. In obstructive jaundice, ultrasonography readily demonstrates a dilated biliary system and, usually, a dilated gallbladder. Dilated intrahepatic radicles appear tortuous and irregular; a dilated gallbladder usually loses its characteristic pear shape, becoming spherical, and fails to contract after injection of sincalide.

Biliary obstruction may result from intrinsic factors, such as a gallstone or small carcinoma within the biliary system. (Ultrasonography can't distinguish between these two echogenic masses.) Or, it may result from extrinsic factors, such as a mass in the hepatic portal that compresses the cystic duct and interferes with bile drainage from the intrahepatic radicles, or from pathology in the head of the pancreas that obstructs the common bile duct; such pathology includes carcinoma and pancreatitis, although ultrasonography can't distinguish between the two. When ultrasonography fails to clearly define the site of biliary obstruction, percutaneous transhepatic cholangiography or endoscopic retrograde cholangiopancreatography should be performed.

Post-test care
□ Be sure the lubricating jelly is removed from the patient's skin.
□ As ordered, the patient may resume his usual diet.

Interfering factors
□ Patient's failure to observe pretest dietary restrictions interferes with accurate testing.
□ Overlying bowel gas or retention of barium from a preceding test hinders ultrasound transmission.
□ In a patient who is dehydrated, ultrasonography can fail to demonstrate the boundaries between organs and tissue structures, due to deficiency of body fluids.

MAE E. PAULFREY, RN, MN

Ultrasonography of the Liver

This ultrasonographic examination produces cross-sectional images of the liver by channeling high-frequency sound waves into the upper right quadrant of the abdomen. The resultant echoes are converted to electrical energy that appears as a pattern of spikes or dots on an oscilloscope screen. Since this pattern varies with tissue density, it can depict intrahepatic structures, as well as organ size, shape, and position. Liver ultrasonography is indicated in patients with jaundice of unknown etiology, with unexplained hepatomegaly and abnormal biochemical test results, with suspected metastatic tumors and elevated serum alkaline phosphatase levels, and with recent abdominal trauma. When used to complement liver-spleen scanning, ultrasonography can define cold spots—focal defects that fail to pick up the radionuclide—as tumors, abscesses, or cysts; it also provides better views of the periportal and perihepatic spaces than liver-spleen scanning. If ultrasonography fails to provide definitive diagnosis, computerized tomography, gallium scanning, or liver biopsy may provide more specific information.

Purpose
□ To distinguish between obstructive and nonobstructive jaundice
□ To screen for hepatocellular disease
□ To detect hepatic metastases and hematoma
□ To define cold spots as tumors, abscesses, or cysts.

Patient preparation
Explain to the patient that this procedure allows examination of the liver. Instruct him to fast for 8 to 12 hours before the test; this reduces bowel gas, which hinders transmission of ultrasound. Tell him

who will perform the test and where, that the room is darkened slightly to aid visualization on the oscilloscope screen, and that the test takes 15 to 30 minutes.

Tell the patient a transducer will pass smoothly over the upper right quadrant, channeling sound waves into the liver. Assure him this test isn't harmful or painful, although he may feel some mild pressure as the transducer presses against his skin. Instruct him to remain as still as possible during the procedure, and to hold his breath when requested; this technique aids visualization by displacing the liver caudally from the costal margin and the ribs.

Just before the procedure, instruct the patient to put on a hospital gown.

Procedure

The patient is placed in supine position. A water-soluble lubricant is applied to the face of the transducer, and transverse scans are taken at ⅜″ (1-cm) intervals, using a single-sweep technique between the costal margins. Although this technique easily demonstrates the left lobe of the liver and part of the right lobe,

sector scans are taken through the intercostal spaces to view the remainder of the right lobe.

Scans are taken longitudinally—from the right border of the liver to the left. For better demonstration of the right lateral dome, oblique cephalad-angled scans may be taken beneath the right costal margin. Scans are then taken parallel to the hepatic portal, at a 45° angle toward the superior right lateral dome, to examine the peripheral anatomy, portal venous system, common bile duct, and biliary tree.

During each scan, the patient is asked to hold his breath briefly in deep inspiration. When good oscilloscopic views are obtained, they are photographed for later study.

Precautions

None.

Findings

The liver normally demonstrates a homogeneous, low-level echo pattern, interrupted only by the different echo patterns of its vascular channels. Al-

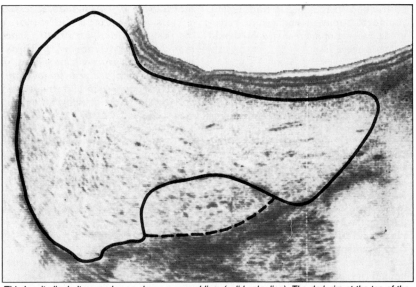

This longitudinal ultrasound scan shows a normal liver (solid color line). The dark rim at the top of the scan is the anterior abdominal wall. The structure tucked below the liver (dotted color line) is the right kidney.

though intrahepatic biliary radicles and hepatic arteries aren't apparent, portal and hepatic veins, the aorta, and the inferior vena cava do appear. Hepatic veins appear completely sonolucent, whereas portal veins have margins that are highly echogenic.

Implications of results

In obstructive jaundice, ultrasonography shows dilated intrahepatic biliary radicles and extrahepatic ducts. Conversely, in nonobstructive jaundice, ultrasonography shows a biliary tree of normal diameter.

Ultrasonographic characteristics of hepatocellular disease are generally nonspecific, and budding disorders can escape detection; liver-spleen scanning, which assesses hepatic function by evaluating the uptake of a radionuclide, is a more sensitive diagnostic tool. In cirrhosis, ultrasonography may demonstrate variable liver size; dilated, tortuous portal branches associated with portal hypertension; and an irregular echo pattern with increased echo amplitude, causing overall increased attenuation. Demonstration of splenomegaly—also associated with portal hypertension—by spleen ultrasonography or liver-spleen scanning aids diagnosis. In fatty infiltration of the liver, ultrasonography may show hepatomegaly and a regular echo pattern that, although greater in echo amplitude than that of normal parenchyma, doesn't alter attenuation.

Ultrasonographic characteristics of metastases in the liver, the most common intrahepatic neoplasm—are extremely variable; metastases may appear either hypoechoic or echogenic, poorly defined or well defined. For example, metastatic lymphomas and sarcomas are generally hypoechoic, while mucin-secreting adenocarcinoma of the colon is highly echogenic. Liver biopsy is necessary to confirm tumor type, but after the tumor is identified and treatment begun, serial ultrasonography can be used to monitor the effectiveness of therapy.

Primary hepatic tumors also present a varied appearance and may mimic metastases, requiring angiography and liver biopsy for definitive diagnosis. Hepatomas are the most common malignant tumors in adults; hepatoblastomas are most common in children. Benign tumors are far less common than malignant ones.

Abscesses usually appear as sonolucent masses with ill-defined, slightly thickened borders, and accentuated posterior wall transmission; scattered internal echoes, caused by necrotic debris, may also be present. Intrahepatic abscesses are occasionally mistaken for hematomas, necrotic metastases, or hemorrhagic cysts, since they produce similar echo patterns. Gas-containing intrahepatic abscesses, which may be echogenic, are sometimes confused with solid intrahepatic lesions. Subphrenic abscesses occur between the diaphragm and the liver, whereas subhepatic abscesses appear inferior to the liver and anterior to the upper pole of the right kidney. The presence of ascitic fluid may simulate a subhepatic abscess, but such fluid lacks internal echoes and has a more regular border.

Cysts usually appear as spherical, sonolucent areas with well-defined borders and accentuated posterior wall transmission. When a cyst can't be distinguished from an abscess or necrotic metastases, gallium scanning, computerized tomography, and angiography should be performed.

Hematomas—either intrahepatic or subcapsular—usually result from trauma. Intrahepatic hematomas appear as poorly defined, relatively sonolucent masses, and may have scattered internal echoes due to clotting; serial ultrasonography can differentiate between a hematoma and a cyst or tumor as the hematoma becomes smaller. Subcapsular hematoma may appear as a focal, sonolucent mass on the periphery of the liver or as a diffuse, sonolucent area surrounding part of the liver.

Post-test care

☐ Be sure the lubricating jelly is removed from the patient's skin.

□ The patient may resume his usual diet.

Interfering factors
□ Overlying ribs, and gas or residual barium in the stomach or colon hinder transmission of ultrasound.

□ In a patient who is dehydrated, ultrasonography may fail to demonstrate the boundaries between organs and tissue structures, due to a lack of body fluids.

MAE E. PAULFREY, RN, MN

Ultrasonography of the Spleen

In ultrasonography of the spleen, a focused beam of high-frequency sound waves passes into the upper left quadrant of the abdomen, creating echoes that vary with changes in tissue density. These echoes, when converted to electrical energy and amplified by a transducer, appear on an oscilloscope screen as a pattern of spikes or dots. This pattern represents the size, shape, and position of the spleen and surrounding viscera.

Ultrasonography is indicated in patients with an upper left quadrant mass of unknown origin; with known splenomegaly, to evaluate changes in splenic size; with upper left quadrant pain and local tenderness; and with recent abdominal trauma. Although ultrasonography can show splenomegaly, it usually doesn't identify the cause; computerized tomography (CT) can provide more specific information. However, as a supplementary diagnostic procedure after liver-spleen scanning, ultrasonography can clarify the nature of cold spots or detect focal defects not infiltrated by tracer radioisotopes.

Purpose
□ To demonstrate splenomegaly
□ To monitor progression of primary and secondary splenic disease, and to evaluate effectiveness of therapy
□ To evaluate the spleen after abdominal trauma
□ To help detect splenic cysts and subphrenic abscess.

Patient preparation
Explain to the patient that this procedure allows examination of the spleen. Instruct him to fast for 8 to 12 hours before the procedure, if possible; this reduces the amount of gas in the bowel, which if present hinders transmission of ultrasound. Tell him who will perform this test and where, that the room may be darkened slightly to aid visualization on the oscilloscope screen, and that this test takes 15 to 30 minutes.

Tell the patient a transducer will pass smoothly over the upper left quadrant, in direct contact with his skin, but assure him he will feel only mild pressure. Instruct him to remain as still as possible during the procedure, and to hold his breath when requested; this technique displaces the spleen inferiorly and thus aids visualization.

Just before the procedure, instruct the patient to put on a hospital gown.

Procedure
Since the procedure for ultrasonography varies, depending on the size of the spleen or the patient's physique, the patient is usually repositioned several times; the transducer scanning angle or path is also changed. Generally, the patient is first placed in supine position, with his chest uncovered. A water-soluble lubricant is applied to the face of the transducer, and transverse scans of the spleen are taken at ⅜″ to ¾″ (1- to 2-cm) intervals, beginning at the level of the diaphragm and moving posteriorly while the transducer is angled anteromedially. After the patient is placed in right lateral decubitus position, additional transverse scans are taken through the intercostal spaces, using a sectoring motion. A pillow may be placed under the patient's right side to help separate the intercostal spaces, making it easier to position the transducer face between

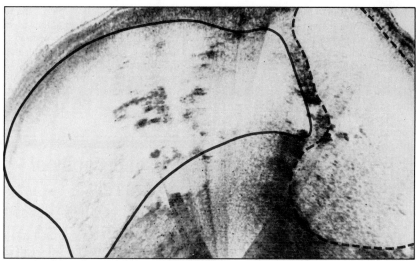

This transverse ultrasound view of the upper abdomen shows a normal liver (solid color line) and an enlarged spleen (dotted color line).

them. For longitudinal scans, the patient remains in the right lateral decubitus position, and scans are taken from the axilla toward the iliac crest. To prevent rib artifacts, oblique scans are taken by passing the transducer face along the intercostal spaces; this scan provides the best view of the splenic parenchyma. During each scan, the patient may be asked to hold his breath briefly at varying stages of inspiration. When good oscilloscopic views are obtained, they are photographed for later study.

Precautions
None.

Findings
The splenic parenchyma normally demonstrates a homogeneous, low-level echo pattern; its individual vascular channels aren't usually apparent. The superior and lateral splenic borders are clearly defined, each having a convex margin. The undersurface and medial borders, in contrast, show indentations from surrounding organs (stomach, left kidney, and pancreas). The hilar region, where the vascular pedicle enters the spleen, commonly produces an area of highly reflective echoes. The medial surface is

generally concave, a characteristic particularly useful when differentiating between upper left quadrant masses and an enlarged spleen. Even when splenomegaly is present, the spleen generally remains concave medially, unless a space-occupying lesion distorts this contour.

Implications of results
Splenomegaly is generally characterized by increased echogenicity. Enlarged vascular channels are commonly visible, especially in the hilar region. If space-occupying lesions distort the splenic contour, liver-spleen scanning should be performed, to confirm splenomegaly. However, CT can demonstrate the extent of enlargement most accurately.

Abdominal trauma may result in splenic rupture or subcapsular hematoma. In splenic rupture, ultrasonography demonstrates splenomegaly and an irregular, sonolucent area (the presence of free intraperitoneal fluid); however, these findings must be confirmed by arteriography. In subcapsular hematoma, ultrasonography shows splenomegaly, as well as the presence of a double contour, altered splenic position, and a relatively sonolucent area on the periphery of the spleen. The double contour results from blood accumulation between the splenic parenchyma and the intact splenic capsule. As the spleen enlarges, a transverse section shows its anterior margin extending more anteriorly than the aorta. Ultrasonography may prove difficult and painful after abdominal trauma, since the transducer may have to pass across fractured ribs and contusions. If so, CT should be used instead. CT offers the advantage of differentiating between blood and fluid in the peritoneal space.

In subphrenic abscess, ultrasonography shows a sonolucent area beneath the diaphragm, and the patient's clinical symptoms help differentiate between abscess and blood or fluid accumulation.

As a complementary procedure to liver-spleen scanning, ultrasonography differentiates cold spots as cystic or solid lesions. It shows cysts as spherical, sonolucent areas with well-defined, regular margins, with acoustic enhancement behind them. When ultrasonography fails to identify a cyst as splenic or extrasplenic—especially if the cyst is located in the upper pole of the left kidney and the adrenal gland, or in the tail of the pancreas—CT and arteriography are then appropriate. Ultrasonography can readily clarify cystic cold spots, but using CT with a contrast medium is superior for evaluating primary and metastatic tumors. Ultrasonography usually fails to identify tumors associated with lymphoma and chronic leukemias, since these resemble tumors of the splenic parenchyma.

Post-test care
□ Be sure the lubricating jelly is removed from the patient's skin.
□ The patient may resume his usual diet.

Interfering factors
□ Overlying ribs, an aerated left lung, or gas or residual barium in the colon or stomach may prevent visualization of the spleen.
□ In a patient who is dehydrated, ultrasonography may fail to demonstrate the boundaries between organs and tissue structures, due to a lack of body fluids.

□ Body physique affecting splenic shape, or adjacent masses displacing the spleen may be confused with splenomegaly.
□ The patient with splenic trauma may be unable to tolerate the procedure due to pain caused by the transducer moving across his abdomen.

MAE E. PAULFREY, RN, MN

Ultrasonography of the Pancreas

In this noninvasive test, cross-sectional images of the pancreas are produced by channeling high-frequency sound waves into the epigastric region, converting the resultant echoes to electrical impulses, and then displaying these impulses as a pattern of spikes or dots on an oscilloscope screen. The pattern varies with tissue density and so represents the size, shape, and position of the pancreas and surrounding viscera. Although ultrasonography cannot provide a sensitive measure of pancreatic function, it can help detect anatomic abnormalities, such as pancreatic carcinoma and pseudocysts, and can guide the insertion of biopsy needles. Since ultrasonography doesn't expose the patient to radiation, it has largely replaced hypotonic duodenography, endoscopic retrograde cholangiopancreatography, radioisotope studies, and arteriography.

Purpose
□ To aid diagnosis of pancreatitis, pseudocysts, and pancreatic carcinoma.

Patient preparation
Explain to the patient that this procedure permits examination of the pancreas. Instruct him to fast for 8 to 12 hours before the procedure; this reduces bowel gas, which hinders transmission of ultrasound. Tell him who will perform the procedure and where, that the room is darkened slightly to aid visualization on

PANCREATIC ULTRASONOGRAPHY

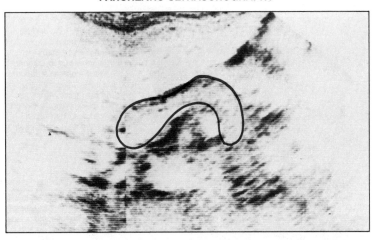

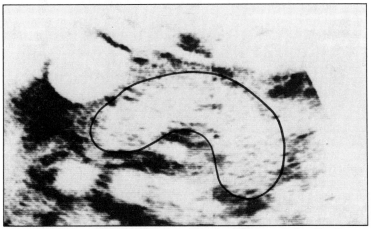

The ultrasound view on the top shows a normal pancreas. The pancreas is outlined in color. The ultrasound view on the bottom shows a diffusely enlarged pancreas due to pancreatitis. The color outline of the pancreas indicates the extent of enlargement.

the oscilloscope screen, and that this test takes 30 to 40 minutes. If the patient is a smoker, ask him to abstain before the test; this eliminates the risk of swallowing air while inhaling, which interferes with test results.

Tell the patient a transducer will pass smoothly over his epigastric region, channeling sound waves into the pancreas. Assure him this isn't harmful or painful, although he may experience mild pressure. Tell him he'll be asked to inhale deeply during scanning, and instruct him to remain as still as possible during the procedure.

Just before the procedure, instruct the patient to put on a hospital gown.

Procedure

The patient is placed in supine position. A water-soluble lubricant or mineral oil is applied to the abdomen, and with the

POSITIONING THE PATIENT FOR ULTRASONOGRAPHY OF THE PANCREAS

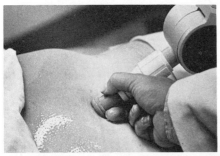

For ultrasonography of the pancreas, the patient is placed in supine position (photograph at left). A water-soluble lubricant is applied to the patient's abdomen, and the transducer is passed over the epigastric region near the xiphoid. To visualize the pancreas at other angles, the patient may need to change his position (bottom photograph).

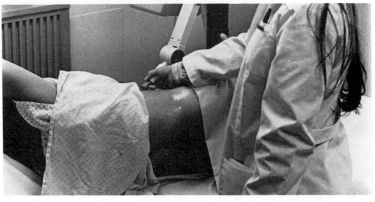

patient at full inspiration, transverse scans are taken at 1-cm intervals, starting from the xiphoid and moving caudally. Other scanning techniques include the longitudinal scan to view the head, body, and tail of the pancreas in sequence; the right anterior oblique view for the head and body of the pancreas; the oblique sagittal view for the portal vein; and the sagittal view for the vena cava. When good oscilloscopic views are obtained, they're photographed for later study.

Precautions
None.

Findings
The pancreas normally demonstrates a coarse, uniform echo pattern (reflecting tissue density) and usually appears more echogenic than the adjacent liver.

Implications of results
Ultrasonography can detect alterations in the size, contour, and parenchymal texture of the pancreas—changes that characterize pancreatic disease. An enlarged pancreas with decreased echogenicity and distinct borders suggests pancreatitis; a well-defined mass with an essentially echo-free interior indicates pseudocyst; an ill-defined mass with scattered internal echoes, or a mass in the head of the pancreas (obstructing the common bile duct) and a large non-contracting gallbladder suggest pancreatic carcinoma.

Subsequent computed tomography and biopsy of the pancreas may be necessary to confirm diagnosis suggested by ultrasonography.

Post-test care

□ Be sure the lubricating jelly is removed from the patient's skin.
□ The patient may resume his usual diet.

Interfering factors

□ Gas or residual barium in the stomach and intestine hinders ultrasound transmission.

□ In a patient who is dehydrated, ultrasonography may fail to demonstrate the boundaries between organs and tissue structures, due to a lack of body fluids.
□ Obesity interferes with ultrasound transmission, and fatty infiltration of the gland makes it difficult to delineate the pancreas from surrounding tissue.

MAE E. PAULFREY, RN, MN

Selected References

Arnell, Iris, and Nassberg, Barbara R. "A Clean, Quick Way to Administer a Barium Enema Through a Colostomy," *Nursing81* 11:81-83, February 1981.

Beck, Marjorie L. "Guiding Your Patient...a Step at a Time...Through a Colonoscopy," *Nursing81* 11:28-31, June 1981.

Brunner, Lillian S., and Suddarth, Doris S. *Textbook of Medical-Surgical Nursing,* 5th ed. Philadelphia: J.B. Lippincott Co., 1984.

Byrne, C. Judith, et al. *Laboratory Tests: Implications for Nurses and Allied Health Professionals.* Reading, Mass.: Addison-Wesley Publishing Co., 1981.

Fischbach, Frances. *A Manual of Laboratory Diagnostic Tests,* 2nd ed. Philadelphia: J.B. Lippincott Co., 1984.

Gastrointestinal Disorders. Nurse's Clinical Library. Springhouse, Pa.: Springhouse Corp., 1985.

Given, Barbara A., and Simmons, Sandra J. *Gastroenterology in Clinical Nursing,* 4th ed. St. Louis: C.V. Mosby Co., 1983.

Grossman, Zachary D., et al. *The Clinician's Guide to Diagnostic Imaging.* New York: Raven Press Pubs., 1983.

Guyton, Arthur C. *Textbook of Medical Physiology,* 6th ed. Philadelphia: W.B. Saunders Co., 1981.

Harvey, A. McGehee, ed. *The Principles and Practice of Medicine,* 21st ed. East Norwalk, Conn.: Appleton-Century-Crofts, 1984.

Henry, John Bernard, ed. *Todd-Sanford-Davidsohn Clinical Diagnosis and Management by Laboratory Methods,* vol. 1, 17th ed. Philadelphia: W.B. Saunders Co., 1984.

Lamb, Jane O. *Laboratory Tests in Clinical Nursing.* Bowie, Md.: Robert J. Brady Co., 1984.

Luckmann, Joan, and Sorensen, Karen C. *Medical-Surgical Nursing: A Psychophysiologic Approach,* 2nd ed. Philadelphia: W.B. Saunders Co., 1980.

Nursing85 Drug Handbook. Springhouse, Pa.: Springhouse Corp., 1985.

Performing GI Procedures. Nursing Photobook series. Springhouse, Pa.: Springhouse Corp., 1984.

Petersdorf, Robert G., and Adams, Raymond D., eds. *Harrison's Principles of Internal Medicine,* 10th ed. New York: McGraw-Hill Book Co., 1983.

Peterson, Walter L., et al. "Routine Early Endoscopy in Upper-Gastrointestinal-Tract Bleeding," *New England Journal of Medicine* 304(16):925-29, April 16, 1981.

Price, Sylvia, and Wilson, Lorraine. *Pathophysiology: Clinical Concepts of Disease Processes,* 2nd ed. New York: McGraw-Hill Book Co., 1982.

Ravel, Richard. *Clinical Laboratory Medicine,* 4th ed. Chicago: Year Book Medical Pubs., 1984.

Spiro, Howard M. *Clinical Gastroenterology,* 3rd ed. New York: Macmillan Publishing Co., 1983.

Tilkian, Sarko M., et al. *Clinical Implications of Laboratory Tests,* 3rd ed. St. Louis: C.V. Mosby Co., 1983.

Widmann, Frances K. *Clinical Interpretation of Laboratory Tests,* 9th ed. Philadelphia: F.A. Davis Co., 1983.

Wyngaarden, James, and Smith, Lloyd. *Cecil Textbook of Medicine,* 16th ed. Philadelphia: W.B. Saunders Co., 1982.

28 Cardiovascular System

LEARNING OBJECTIVES

After completing this chapter, the reader will be able to:

- explain the anatomy and physiology of the cardiovascular system.
- understand the action of sodium and potassium ions in cardiac electrical activity.
- state the six major test groups that identify cardiovascular dysfunction.
- discuss the importance of the cardiac series.
- identify EKG tracings of three pathologic changes occurring during myocardial infarction.
- compare the treadmill and bicycle ergometer tests.
- describe electrode placement for exercise electrocardiography.
- state the purpose of each test discussed in the chapter.
- prepare the patient physically and psychologically for each test.
- describe the procedure for performing each test.
- specify appropriate precautions for safe administration of each test.
- recognize signs of adverse reaction, and respond appropriately.
- implement appropriate post-test care.
- identify the normal findings of each test.
- discuss the implications of abnormal test results.
- list factors that may interfere with accurate test results.

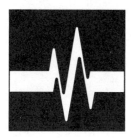

Cardiovascular System

Introduction

According to the American Heart Association, disorders of the cardiovascular system afflict nearly 30 million Americans. Since a wide range of diagnostic tests can detect many such disorders, it's important to understand the indications for each test and its clinical implications in order to prepare the patient physically and psychologically before the test, assist the doctor effectively during the test, and implement proper care after the test.

The tests for cardiovascular dysfunction fall into six major groups: cardiac enzyme analysis, radiography, graphic recording, ultrasonography, nuclear medicine, and catheterization. Cardiac enzyme analysis (covered in Chapter 4, ENZYMES) proves most useful in detecting acute myocardial infarction (MI). Radiography, including X-ray films of the heart, is one of the first diagnostic tests used to assess myocardial or vascular dysfunction. Graphic recording, such as electrocardiography, apexcardiography, or phonocardiography, is a noninvasive technique for evaluating cardiac electrical, mechanical, or acoustic activity; specially trained nurses may occasionally perform these procedures. Ultrasonography, another noninvasive technique, now holds an important place in cardiovascular testing; for example, echocardiography has superseded cardiac series fluoroscopy for most diagnostic

applications. Nuclear medicine is one of the most rapidly changing areas of diagnostic testing, partly because of the development of new radiopharmaceuticals. Catheterization is an effective invasive method for evaluating cardiac and vascular dysfunction.

Choice of a specific diagnostic test depends on the doctor's clinical suspicions, the kind of information needed, and the risk to the patient. As a rule, noninvasive tests precede invasive ones, since the invasive tests are generally more hazardous and more costly. However, invasive tests are often necessary to obtain the most diagnostic information.

The pump

The heart is the mechanism and the arteries, veins, and capillaries are the pathway by which blood circulates throughout the body. Together they act to deliver oxygen and vital nutrients to the body cells and to remove carbon dioxide and other waste products.

The heart is a hollow, muscular organ located in the mediastinum between the lungs. It is enclosed by a membranous sac called the pericardium, which consists of two layers, one inside the other: an external fibrous (parietal) layer attached to the great vessels leaving the heart, and an internal serous (visceral) sac that envelops the heart and lines the

THE HEART'S BLOOD SUPPLY

ANTERIOR

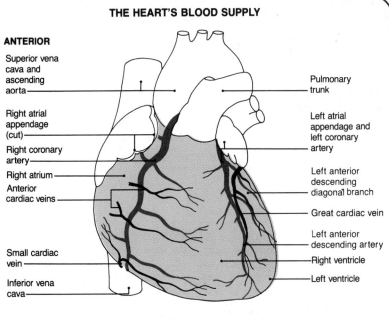

Superior vena cava and ascending aorta

Right atrial appendage (cut)

Right coronary artery

Right atrium

Anterior cardiac veins

Small cardiac vein

Inferior vena cava

Pulmonary trunk

Left atrial appendage and left coronary artery

Left anterior descending diagonal branch

Great cardiac vein

Left anterior descending artery

Right ventricle

Left ventricle

POSTERIOR

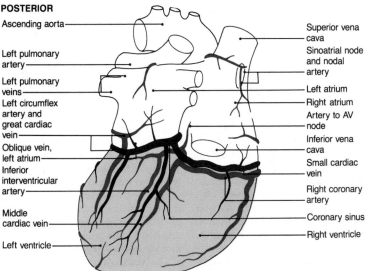

Ascending aorta

Left pulmonary artery

Left pulmonary veins

Left circumflex artery and great cardiac vein

Oblique vein, left atrium

Inferior interventricular artery

Middle cardiac vein

Left ventricle

Superior vena cava

Sinoatrial node and nodal artery

Left atrium

Right atrium

Artery to AV node

Inferior vena cava

Small cardiac vein

Right coronary artery

Coronary sinus

Right ventricle

The heart's blood supply system is shown in these schematic anterior and posterior views. Coronary angiography—a cardiac catheterization procedure—evaluates coronary artery function. Coronary artery disease results mainly from atherosclerosis, which impedes blood flow and thus interferes with the supply of oxygen and nutrients to the myocardium.

Adapted with permission from J.T. Shephard and P.M. VanHoutte, *The Human Cardiovascular System* (New York: Raven Press, Pubs., 1979).

fibrous portion. Space between these layers is filled with 10 to 50 ml of pericardial fluid, which lubricates the layers as they glide over each other during heart movement.

The heart pump is comprised of four chambers. The atria—the two smaller upper chambers—receive blood from the systemic and the pulmonary circulation. The two larger, thicker lower chambers —the ventricles—receive blood from the atria. The interventricular septum divides the heart into right and left halves. Two valves separate the atria from the ventricles: the tricuspid valve in the right side and the mitral valve in the left side of the heart. The mitral valve has two movable leaflets; the tricuspid valve has three. Two semilunar valves, each with three fibrous cusps, guard the entrances to the aortic and pulmonary arteries.

The vascular system

The vascular system comprises the arteries, arterioles, capillaries, venules, and veins. Both arteries and veins have three layers: a tunica intima (inner coat) of endothelial, connective, and elastic tissues; a tunica media (middle coat) of smooth muscle fibers, and elastic and collagenous tissue; and a tunica adventitia (external coat) of connective, smooth muscle, and elastic tissue. Capillaries consist of endothelial tissues one cell thick, while venules and arterioles have a variable composition depending on their size.

Arteries, which contain 15% of circulating blood volume, carry blood away from the heart. Normally, the aorta (the largest artery) and its branches can withstand large changes in cardiac pressure that distend them during ventricular contraction; these pressure changes are detectable as a palpable wave (pulse) in certain arteries near the skin. The aorta and other large arteries add little to total peripheral vascular resistance since they do not ordinarily impede blood flow. The arterioles largely control the degree of total peripheral resistance and, consequently, the amount of blood flow

ACTIVATING THE HEART PUMP: THE CONDUCTION SYSTEM

The heart's conduction system contains specialized muscle fibers that generate and conduct their own electrical impulses. The sinoatrial (SA) node—located in the right atrium, beneath the orifice of the superior vena cava—normally controls heart rate and is called the "pacemaker." It sends an impulse through the internodal pathways and atrial muscle to the atrioventricular (AV) node, in the lower posterior part of the right atrium, near the lumen of the coronary sinus. As an impulse passes through the atrial muscles, the atria contract. After a short delay in the AV node, the impulse continues down the His bundle—which divides into right and left bundle branches—and finally, into the subendothelial Purkinje fibers, which transmit the impulse into the ventricular myocardium, causing it to contract.

After this contraction, the myocardium repolarizes, while the ventricles relax and begin to fill with blood, in preparation for the next impulse from the SA node. Evidence of this conduction of electric currents through the heart may be picked up on the skin surface and graphically recorded by the electrocardiogram (EKG).

The SA node discharges 60 to 100 impulses/minute. If it fails to generate the expected impulses, the AV node can also discharge, but at a slower rate of 40 to 60 impulses/minute. If both nodes fail to discharge, the Purkinje fibers can discharge at a rate of 15 to 40 impulses/minute. The ability of the heart to spontaneously generate and maintain its own impulse rate is known as *automaticity.* When any part of the heart other than the SA node takes over to pace the heart, this part is known as an ectopic pacemaker. If the electrical impulse is too weak, it won't excite the muscle fiber at all; if it's strong enough to cause the fiber to reach its electrical threshold potential, excitation occurs. The current then spreads to neighboring fibers by virtue of the low resistance of their cell walls, and the entire muscle mass reacts as a unit. This response is called the "all-or-nothing" principle.

to and in the tissues by their ability to dilate and contract.

The veins carry blood toward the heart and contain 50% of total circulating blood volume. The superior and inferior venae cavae, which empty into the right atrium, are the body's largest veins. In the venous system, pressure changes only slightly with vessel dilatation or constriction. However, total circulating blood volume, heart and lung function, venomotor tone, and the condition of the one-way venous valves in the limbs may affect the capacitance and the pressure of the venous system.

In the coronary circulation, blood flow occurs mainly during diastole, and depends directly on the perfusion pressure (the pressure gradient between the coronary arteries and the right atrium). Coronary blood flow may diminish if aortic pressure decreases or right heart pressure increases. It may also be influenced by tachycardias, which reduce diastolic flow time, and by conditions that reduce diastolic perfusion pressure, such as hypotension.

Coronary circulation constitutes 5% of total cardiac output in the resting heart. It uses 70% of the arterial oxygen. Increased oxygen demand requires increased coronary blood flow, since the heart extracts virtually all oxygen from the blood, even at rest.

Radiographic tests

Cardiac radiography permits visualization of the position, size, and contour of the heart and great vessels of the circulatory system. Chest X-ray films can show enlargement of the heart, interstitial and alveolar edema, aortic dilatation, left heart failure, and intracardiac calcifications.

Cardiac series (chest fluoroscopy) allows visualization of the heart's motion and the pulsations of the heart and great vessels during systole and diastole, and helps detect and confirm malfunctions of prosthetic heart valves. Although used extensively in the past, the cardiac series has been largely replaced by echocardiography.

Lower limb venography, the injection of a contrast medium into the veins to permit their visualization on film, may confirm deep vein thrombosis (DVT), identify the causes of leg edema, and assess vascular status before surgery. However, this test's usefulness must be weighed against the potential risks of radiation exposure. For example, for a patient with suspected DVT, the test's benefits outweigh the risks.

Graphic recording

Electrocardiography—the most frequently performed graphic recording

---

THE CARDIAC CYCLE

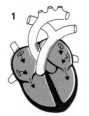 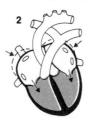 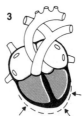 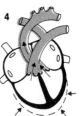

These schematic drawings show events during a single cardiac cycle.

Period of rapid ventricular filling (1): Unoxygenated blood returning from the tissues enters the right atrium at the same time that oxygenated blood from the lungs enters the left atrium. The atria and ventricles are passively filled.

Atrial kick (2): About 70% of incoming blood flows through the atria directly into the ventricles before the atria contract; when they do, they force an additional 30% of blood into the ventricles—the atrial kick.

Period of isovolumic contraction (3): The ventricles begin contracting before emptying.

Period of ejection (4): The ventricles contract, pushing the unoxygenated blood into pulmonary arteries and the oxygenated blood into the aorta.

Adapted with permission from M. Jackle and M. Halligan, *Cardiovascular Problems: A Critical Care Nursing Focus* (Bowie, Md.: Robert J. Brady Co.), 1980.

COMMON INDICATIONS FOR ARTERIOGRAPHY

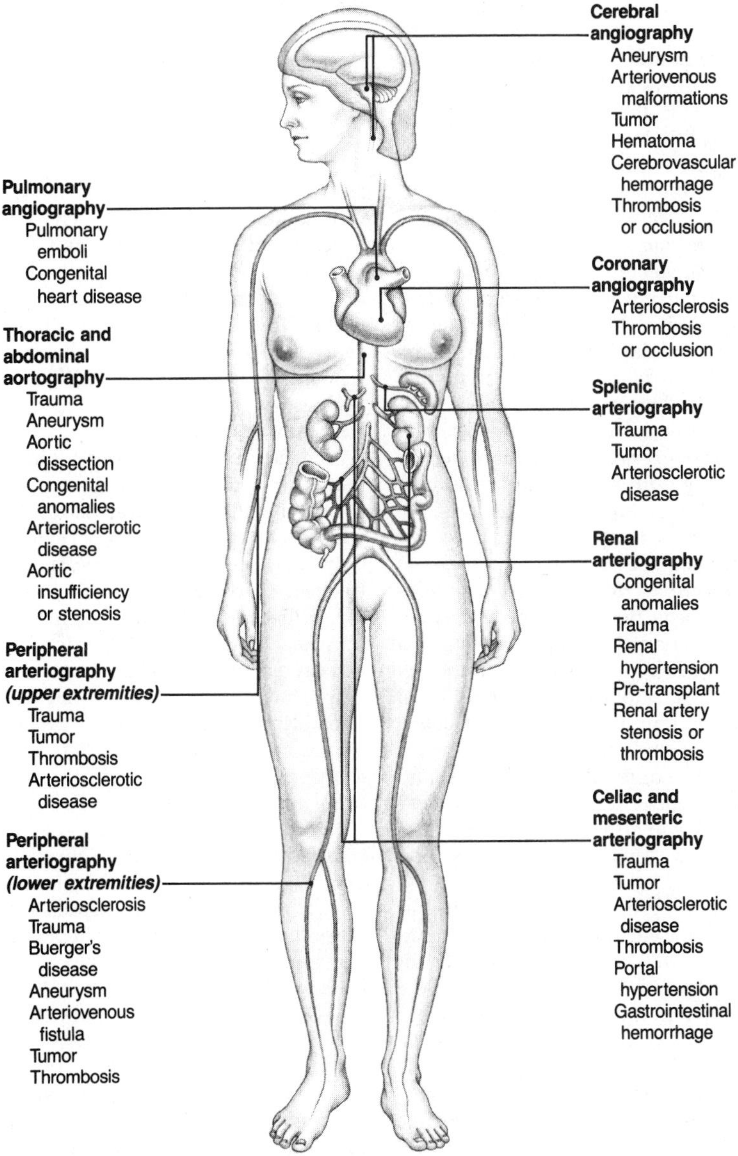

Cerebral angiography
Aneurysm
Arteriovenous malformations
Tumor
Hematoma
Cerebrovascular hemorrhage
Thrombosis or occlusion

Coronary angiography
Arteriosclerosis
Thrombosis or occlusion

Splenic arteriography
Trauma
Tumor
Arteriosclerotic disease

Renal arteriography
Congenital anomalies
Trauma
Renal hypertension
Pre-transplant
Renal artery stenosis or thrombosis

Celiac and mesenteric arteriography
Trauma
Tumor
Arteriosclerotic disease
Thrombosis
Portal hypertension
Gastrointestinal hemorrhage

Pulmonary angiography
Pulmonary emboli
Congenital heart disease

Thoracic and abdominal aortography
Trauma
Aneurysm
Aortic dissection
Congenital anomalies
Arteriosclerotic disease
Aortic insufficiency or stenosis

Peripheral arteriography (upper extremities)
Trauma
Tumor
Thrombosis
Arteriosclerotic disease

Peripheral arteriography (lower extremities)
Arteriosclerosis
Trauma
Buerger's disease
Aneurysm
Arteriovenous fistula
Tumor
Thrombosis

Arteriography (often called angiography) is the radiographic examination of one or more arteries after injection of a contrast medium into the femoral artery or, less frequently, into the brachial or carotid artery. Although indications for this test vary, depending on the artery being studied, arteriography can demonstrate blood flow status, aneurysm formation, collateral circulation, vascular anomaly, tumor, or hemorrhage.

test—records the conduction, magnitude, and duration of the electrical activity of the heart. It identifies rhythm disturbances, conduction abnormalities and electrolyte imbalances, and contributes information about the size of the heart chambers and the relative position of the heart in the chest. The electrocardiogram (EKG) is useful in documenting the diagnosis and progression of MI, ischemia, and pericarditis, and in evaluating the effectiveness of artificial pacemakers and cardiotonic drugs.

Exercise electrocardiography measures the cardiovascular effects of controlled physical stress (bike riding or treadmill walking). During this test, the EKG is checked for evidence of ischemia, arrhythmias, or conduction abnormalities. The exercise EKG can help identify the cause of chest pain and plan therapy for patients with known cardiovascular disease. Both ambulatory and exercise electrocardiography must be preceded by a thorough clinical workup.

Ambulatory (Holter) electrocardiography records the heart's electrical activity for 24 hours or longer as the patient performs his usual activities and experiences normal physical and emotional stress. The ambulatory EKG can detect intermittent arrhythmias, gauge the effectiveness of antiarrhythmic drugs, and assess patient progress during recovery from MI. It can also help detect the cause of dizziness, vertigo, palpitations, and chest pain.

Apexcardiography records the pulsations over the cardiac point of maximum impulse (PMI), which is generally located in the fifth intercostal space in the midclavicular line. It's useful for identifying heart sounds and for evaluating left ventricular dysfunction, such as MI.

Phonocardiography records the normal and abnormal sounds of the cardiac cycle—including gallops, murmurs, and other heart sounds—and the vibrations of the great vessels. It aids in timing the cardiac cycle and measuring ventricular function by demonstrating systolic time intervals, and in identifying structural defects of the valves, such as mitral stenosis and regurgitation. Phonocardiography is often performed simultaneously with electrocardiography, apexcardiography, and a carotid pulse tracing.

Vectorcardiography, another noninvasive graphic recording, detects cardiac impulses through electrodes that are placed on the skin, and records a three-dimensional view of the heart showing the magnitude and direction of electrical activity. Vectorcardiography can detect conduction abnormalities, such as right or left bundle branch block and MI.

Impedance plethysmography evaluates changes in blood volume in the limbs. This procedure can confirm diagnosis of DVT, but is less reliable than venography in detecting small thrombi.

Ultrasonography

Echocardiography, a painless noninvasive test, directs ultra–high-frequency sound waves through the chest wall into the heart, which then reflects these waves to a transducer and a recording device at various frequencies, depending on the density of the cardiac tissue. It shows the movement of cardiac structures and the dimensions of heart chambers. This test evaluates cardiac structure and function, and can reveal valve deformities (mitral prolapse), tumors (left atrial myxoma), septal defects, pericardial effusion, and idiopathic hypertrophic subaortic stenosis.

Doppler ultrasonography—in which sound waves are transmitted through the skin and reflected from moving blood cells in underlying blood vessels—evaluates the major vascular network of the arms and legs and the extracranial cerebrovascular system. It helps detect DVT, peripheral arterial aneurysms, and carotid arterial occlusive disease.

Ultrasonography of the abdominal aorta is used to detect and monitor the progression of abdominal aortic aneurysms, evaluate the inferior vena cava, and locate visceral arteries.

Nuclear medicine

Thallium imaging evaluates myocardial blood flow and the status of myocardial cells after the I.V. injection of the ra-

STROKE VOLUME AND STARLING'S LAW

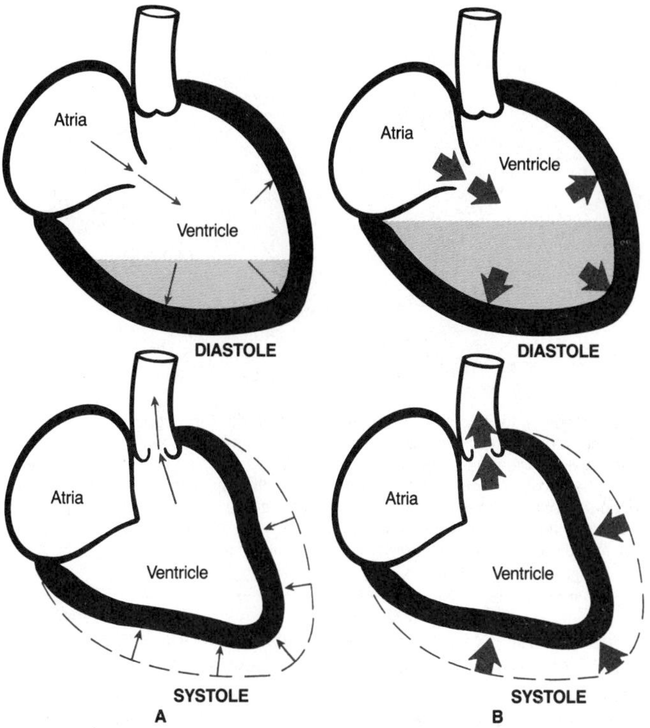

Total ventricular volume in each cardiac cycle reaches 120 to 130 ml during diastolic filling (end-diastolic volume), and falls to 50 to 60 ml as the ventricles empty during contraction; this 70-ml difference represents the *stroke volume.* The stroke volume multiplied by heart rate/minute equals cardiac output, or the volume of blood pumped in 1 minute. Normally, the cardiac output for a resting person is about 5 liters, but this amount varies with body size, heart rate, and stroke volume.

The heart's remarkable ability to deliver equal volumes of blood each minute, even when the right and left ventricles deliver very different volumes of blood per stroke, is explained by *Starling's law:* the force of contraction of each heartbeat depends on the length of the muscle fibers of the walls of the heart. Thus, if right ventricular output exceeds left ventricular output, the fibers of the left ventricle lengthen at end-diastole to increase the force of contraction. In the diagram, at (A), normal diastolic filling during diastole causes normal fiber stretch, normal contractile force, and normal stroke volume. At (B), increased filling during diastole increases fiber stretch, force of contraction, and stroke volume.

Adapted with permission from S.A. Price and L.M. Wilson, *Pathophysiology: Clinical Concepts of Disease Processes* (New York: McGraw-Hill Book Co., 1978).

dioisotope thallium-201; healthy myocardial tissue absorbs the radioisotope but ischemic or necrotic tissue does not (thus, the name cold spot scanning). This test can detect abnormalities associated with perfusion defects in the coronary arteries and myocardium. *Stress testing* after thallium injection can reveal areas of ischemia resulting from exercise.

Unlike thallium imaging, *technetium pyrophosphate scanning* reveals dam-

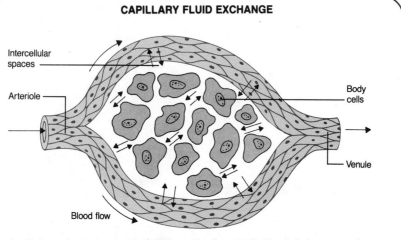

CAPILLARY FLUID EXCHANGE

Intercellular spaces

Arteriole

Body cells

Venule

Blood flow

Capillaries exchange water and metabolites with adjacent cells through their porous walls (arrows). Normally, hydrostatic pressure—produced by the pumping action of the heart—is higher in the capillary than the surrounding intercellular fluid, which encourages the outflow of water from the capillary. The outflow of water is opposed by colloid osmotic pressure—relative concentrations of proteins inside and outside the capillary membrane—which normally encourages the inflow of water. The balance between these two pressures regulates the quantity and direction of water flow across the capillary membrane.

aged myocardial tissue as hot spots—areas where the radioisotope technetium pyrophosphate accumulates. The test helps to detect acute MI and define its location and size.

Blood pool imaging, in which a radioisotope is tagged to RBCs or albumin and injected I.V., outlines the heart cavities to detect left ventricular regional wall motion abnormalities (commonly seen after MI). In this test, a scintillation camera records the first pass of the radioisotope through the heart; then, in subsequent gated or timed imaging, the camera records two or more points in the cardiac cycle, allowing study of left ventricular function. Blood pool imaging also aids diagnosis of left ventricular aneurysm, cardiomyopathies, and intracardiac shunts.

Catheterization

Cardiac catheterization is the insertion of a catheter into the right or left side of the heart and the injection of contrast medium to permit visualization of car-

diac contraction and cardiac structures. Left heart catheterization helps evaluate aortic and mitral valve function, measurement of cardiac output, and coronary artery patency; right heart catheterization permits evaluation of pulmonary and tricuspid valve function, and measurement of cardiac output, right heart pressures, and pulmonary capillary wedge pressure (PCWP). The test can demonstrate valvular efficiency or defects, assess the causes of chest pain, detect congenital heart defects, and help evaluate candidates for coronary artery surgery. It's usually contraindicated in patients with acute MI, and acute debilitating conditions.

In *His bundle electrography,* an electrode-tipped catheter is passed into the right atrium and ventricle to record and study the activity of the heart's conduction system. This test allows precise location of bundle branch blocks, detection of arrhythmias, and evaluation of the effects of antiarrhythmic drugs. This test is contraindicated in patients with severe coagulopathy and acute pulmonary embolism.

Pulmonary artery catheterization permits measurement of PCWP after passage of a balloon-tipped, flow-directed catheter into a small branch of the pulmonary artery; the PCWP reflects both left atrial and left ventricular end-diastolic pressure. This test, performed primarily on patients who have suffered an acute myocardial infarction, helps assess left ventricular failure and monitors the effects of therapy after complications develop. This test should be performed cautiously in patients with left bundle branch block.

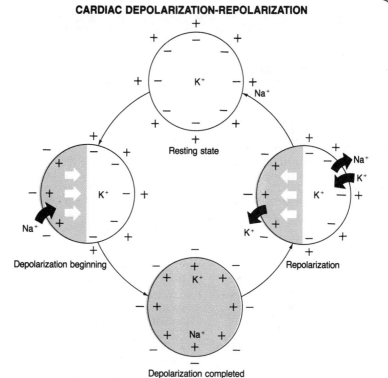

CARDIAC DEPOLARIZATION-REPOLARIZATION

Resting state

Depolarization beginning

Repolarization

Depolarization completed

Heart muscle cells are arranged so that they act together as a single network. Alternating waves of electrical activity—depolarization and repolarization involving exchange of sodium (Na$^+$) and potassium (K$^+$) ions across the cell membrane—flow through this network. During depolarization, the cells are stimulated and the muscle contracts; during repolarization, the muscle relaxes. The diagram above shows what goes on at the cellular level.

During the resting (polarized) state, the number of positive charges outside the cell membrane equals the number of negative ones inside it. The concentration of sodium ions is greater outside the cell than inside it, while potassium concentration is greater inside than outside. A stimulus from the sinoatrial node briefly reverses this ionic status and causes depolarization. Sodium ions move from outside to inside the cell until the charges on the inner and outer surfaces are reversed and the membrane is fully depolarized. Immediately after the cell is fully depolarized, potassium ions begin to flow from inside to outside the cell, and the cell repolarizes. It returns to its resting state through the action of an ion-transport mechanism called the sodium-potassium pump, which is fueled by energy from adenosine triphosphate as it's changed to adenosine diphosphate by the enzyme adenosinetriphosphatase.

Miscellaneous tests

The *cold stimulation test for Raynaud's syndrome,* performed by immersing a patient's hand in ice water and checking digital temperatures after removing the hand from the water, can verify Raynaud's syndrome in patients in whom arterial-tree occlusion is absent.

Pericardial fluid analysis, performed after needle aspiration of fluid from the pericardial sac, helps detect the cause of pericardial effusion. After aspiration, the fluid specimen is sent to the laboratory for biochemical analysis and bacterial culture.

REGINA DALEY FORD, RN, BSN, MA

RADIOGRAPHY

Cardiac Radiography

Among the most frequently used tests for evaluating cardiac disease and its effects on the pulmonary vasculature, cardiac radiography provides images of the thorax, mediastinum, heart, and lungs. In a routine evaluation, posteroanterior and left lateral views are taken. The posteroanterior view is preferable to the anteroposterior view because it places the heart slightly closer to the plane of the film, giving a sharper, less-distorted image. Using portable equipment, cardiac radiographs may be taken of patients who are bedridden, but such equipment can provide only anteroposterior views.

Purpose

☐ To help detect cardiac disease and abnormalities that change the size, shape, or appearance of the heart and lungs
☐ To ensure correct positioning of pulmonary artery and cardiac catheters, and of pacemaker wires.

Patient preparation

Explain to the patient that this test reveals the size and shape of the heart. Tell him who performs the test and where. Reassure him that the test employs little radiation and is harmless.

Instruct the patient to remove jewelry and other metal objects, and clothing above his waist, and to put on a hospital gown with ties instead of metal snaps.

Procedure

Posteroanterior view: The patient stands erect about 6' (1.82 m) from the X-ray machine, with his back to the machine and his chin resting on top of the film cassette holder. The holder is adjusted to slightly hyperextend the patient's neck. The patient places his hands on his hips, with his shoulders touching the holder, and centers his chest against it. Then he is asked to take a deep breath and hold it during the X-ray film exposure.

Left lateral view: The patient is positioned with his arms extended over his

---

THE CARDIAC SERIES

Now superseded by echocardiography for most diagnostic purposes, the cardiac series remains useful for comprehensive examination of heart action. Using X-rays, it provides a constant image of the heart in motion on a fluoroscope. By examining the beating heart from four directions, the test permits observation of cardiac pulsations, assessment of heart chamber structural abnormalities (such as aneurysm and congenital heart disease), detection of aortic and mitral valve calcification, and evaluation of prosthetic valve function. When performed with a barium swallow, the cardiac series highlights abnormal deviation of esophageal contours (possibly caused by left atrial enlargement) or makes abnormalities of the aortic arch more visible. Views may be preserved for later study on spot films or motion pictures.

Since the cardiac series entails exposure to 15 to 20 times more radiation than the cardiac X-ray films, it may be contraindicated in some patients, especially pregnant women. If this test is necessary during pregnancy, the patient's pelvic and abdominal areas must be adequately shielded during the test.

head and his left torso flush against the cassette and centered. Then he is asked to take a deep breath and hold it during the X-ray film exposure.

Anteroposterior view of a bedridden patient: The head of the bed is elevated as much as possible, and the patient is assisted to upright position, to reduce visceral pressure on the diaphragm and other thoracic structures. The film cassette is centered under the patient's back. Although the distance between the patient and the X-ray machine may vary, the path between the two should be clear. The patient is instructed to take a deep breath and hold it during the X-ray film exposure.

Precautions
□ Cardiac radiography is usually contraindicated during the first trimester of pregnancy. If it is performed during pregnancy, a lead shield or apron should cover the abdomen and pelvic area during the X-ray exposure.
□ When testing an ambulatory patient, make sure the radiographic order stipulates a posteroanterior view and not an anteroposterior view. Include on the order any pertinent findings from previous cardiac radiographs, as well as the indication for this test.
□ When testing a bedridden patient, be sure anyone else in the room is protected from X-rays by a lead shield, a room divider, or sufficient distance.

Findings
Normally, in the posteroanterior view, the thoracic cage appears at least twice as wide as the heart. However, in the anteroposterior view, relative heart size and position may look different, and the cardiac silhouette and vascular markings may increase.

If cardiac radiography is performed to evaluate the position of cardiac catheters and pacemakers, the films should confirm accurate placement.

Implications of results
Cardiac X-ray films must be evaluated in light of the patient's history, physical ex-

FORCED INSPIRATION GIVES ACCURATE RESULTS

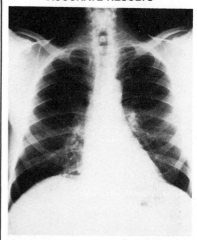

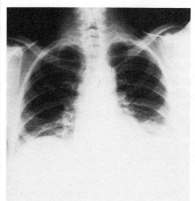

Both photographs show cardiac radiographs of healthy persons. In the X-ray film at top, the person breathed deeply and held it during radiography; in the film at bottom, the person failed to hold his breath, causing the film to show what looks like an enlarged heart.

amination, electrocardiography results, and results of previous radiographic tests for cardiac abnormalities.

An abnormal cardiac silhouette usually reflects left or right ventricular or left atrial enlargement. In left ventricular enlargement, the posteroanterior view shows a rounded, convex left heart border, with lateral extension of the lower

CARDIAC ABNORMALITIES REVEALED BY CHEST RADIOGRAPHY

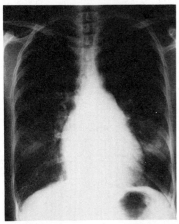

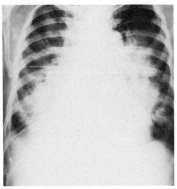

The X-ray film at top—a posteroanterior view—shows double density behind the right heart, indicating left atrial enlargement. Sometimes this enlargement may also raise the left main stem bronchus. The X-ray film at bottom shows congestive heart failure, with pulmonary edema and right pleural effusion.

atrium, straightening of left heart border, elevation of left main bronchus, and rarely, lateral extension of the right heart border superior to the right ventricle; the lateral view shows a posterior bulge at the level of the left atrium.

In the posteroanterior view, dilatation of pulmonary venous shadows in the superior lateral aspect of the hilus, and vascular shadows horizontally and inferiorly along the margin of the right heart may be the first signs of pulmonary vascular congestion. Chronic pulmonary venous hypertension produces an antler pattern, caused by dilated superior pulmonary veins and normal or constricted inferior pulmonary veins. Acute alveolar edema may produce a butterfly appearance, with increased densities in central lung fields; interstitial pulmonary edema, a cloudy or cotton-puff appearance.

Post-test care
None.

Interfering factors
☐ Patient failure to maintain inspiration or to remain motionless during the test interferes with clarity of the image.
☐ If the patient's chest isn't centered on the film cassette, the costophrenic angle may not be visible on the X-ray film.
☐ Thoracic deformity, such as scoliosis, affects radiographic interpretation.
☐ Over- or underexposed X-ray films can invalidate the test.

ARLENE STRONG, RN, MN

Lower Limb Venography
[Ascending contrast phlebography]

Venography is the radiographic examination of a vein and is often used to assess the condition of the deep leg veins after injection of a contrast medium. It's

left border; the lateral view shows posterior bulging of the left ventricle. In right ventricular enlargement, the view shows secondary prominence of the pulmonary artery segment at the left heart border; the lateral view shows anterior bulging in the region of the right ventricular outflow tract.

In left atrial enlargement, the view shows double density of enlarged left

the definitive test for deep vein thrombosis (DVT), an acute condition marked by inflammation and thrombus formation in the deep veins of the legs. Such thrombi usually develop in valve pockets—venous junctions or sinuses of the calf muscle—travel to the deep calf veins and, if untreated, may occlude the popliteal, femoral, and iliac vein systems. This condition may lead to pulmonary embolism, a potentially lethal complication. Predisposing factors to DVT include vein wall injury, prolonged bed rest, coagulation abnormalities, surgery, childbirth, and use of oral contraceptives, such as estrogen.

Venography shouldn't be used for routine screening since it exposes the patient to relatively high doses of radiation and can cause complications, such as phlebitis, local tissue damage, and occa-sionally, DVT itself. It's also expensive and isn't easily repeated. A combination of three noninvasive tests—Doppler ultrasonography, impedance plethysmography, and ^{125}I fibrinogen scan—provides an acceptable though less accurate alternative to venography.

Purpose

□ To confirm diagnosis of DVT
□ To distinguish clot formation from venous obstruction (a large tumor of the pelvis impinging on the venous system, for example)
□ To evaluate congenital venous abnormalities
□ To assess deep vein valvular competence (especially helpful in identifying underlying causes of leg edema)
□ To locate a suitable vein for arterial bypass grafting.

ABNORMAL VENOGRAMS

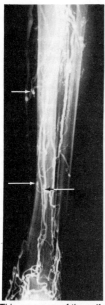 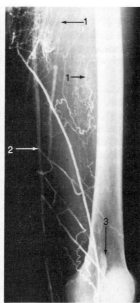 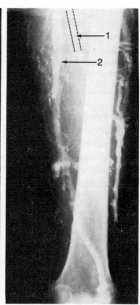

This venogram of the calf shows incompetent veins (arrows).

This venogram of the thigh shows development of collateral veins (1), filling of some superficial veins (2), and obstruction of the popliteal vein (3).

This venogram of the thigh shows a filling defect due to a thrombus (1) and backflow from a blockage of the iliac veins (2).

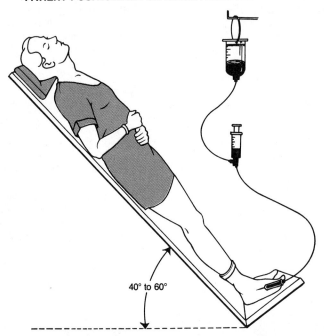

PATIENT POSITIONING FOR LOWER LIMB VENOGRAPHY

40° to 60°

In lower limb venography, the patient lies on an X-ray table inclined 40 ° to 60 °, while keeping his weight off the leg being tested. Fluoroscopy monitors the progress of the contrast medium, and spot films are taken as the contrast circulates through the venous system of the leg.

Patient preparation

Explain to the patient that this test helps detect abnormal conditions in the veins of the legs. Instruct him to restrict food and to drink only clear liquids for 4 hours before the test. Tell him who will perform the test and where, and that it takes 30 to 45 minutes. Warn him that he may feel a transient burning sensation in his leg on injection of the contrast medium, and some discomfort during the procedure.

Make sure the patient or responsible family member has signed a consent form. Check the patient's history for hypersensitivity to iodine or iodine-containing foods, or to contrast media used in previous diagnostic tests. Reassure the patient that complications from the contrast medium are rare, but tell him to report nausea, severe burning or itching, constriction in the throat or chest, or dyspnea immediately. If ordered, restrict anticoagulant therapy.

Just before the test, instruct the patient to void, to remove all clothing below the waist, and to put on a hospital gown. If ordered, give the patient who is anxious or uncooperative a mild sedative.

Procedure

The patient is positioned on a tilting radiographic table so that the leg being tested doesn't bear any weight. The patient is instructed to relax this leg and keep it still; a tourniquet may be tied around the ankle to expedite venous filling. Then, normal saline solution is injected into a superficial vein in the dorsum of the patient's foot. Once correct needle placement is achieved, 100 to 150 ml of contrast medium is slowly injected (90 seconds to 3 minutes) and the presence of extravasation is checked. (If a suitable superficial vein can't be found, due to edema, a surgical cutdown of the vein may be performed.) Using a fluoroscope, the distribution of the contrast medium is monitored, and spot films are taken from the anteroposterior and oblique projections, and over the thigh and femoroiliac regions. Then, overhead films are taken of the calf, knee, thigh, and femoral area.

After filming, the patient is repositioned horizontally, the leg being tested is quickly elevated, and normal saline solution infused to flush the contrast medium from the veins. The fluoroscope is checked to confirm complete emptying. Then the needle is removed, and an adhesive bandage is applied to the injection site.

Precautions

Since most allergic reactions to the contrast medium occur within 30 minutes of injection, carefully observe for signs of anaphylaxis: flushing, hives, urticaria, laryngeal stridor.

Findings

A normal venogram shows steady opacification of the superficial and deep vasculature with no filling defects.

Implications of results

A venogram that shows consistent filling defects on repeat views, abrupt termination of a column of contrast material, unfilled major deep veins, or diversion of flow (through collaterals, for example) is diagnostic of DVT.

Post-test care

☐ Monitor vital signs until stable; check the pulse rate on the dorsalis pedis, popliteal, and femoral arteries.

☐ Administer analgesics, as ordered, to counteract the irritating effects of the contrast medium.

☐ Watch for hematoma, redness, bleeding, or infection (especially if a cutdown

of the vein was performed) at the puncture site, and replace the dressing when necessary. Notify the doctor if complications develop.

☐ If the venogram indicates DVT, initiate therapy (heparin infusion, bed rest, leg elevation or support, blood chemistry tests), as ordered.

☐ As ordered, the patient may resume

RADIONUCLIDE VENOGRAPHY

Although venography accurately detects deep vein thrombosis (DVT), it's an expensive and sometimes hazardous invasive test, since the injection can cause localized clots. Currently, radionuclide tests, such as the ^{125}I fibrinogen scan, screen for DVT or attempt to detect the disorder in a patient who is too ill for venography or is hypersensitive to the contrast medium. In the ^{125}I fibrinogen scan, labeled fibrinogen injected I.V. collects at sites of active thrombus formation. A scintillation counter records radioactivity at several sites on the calf and thigh after 6, 24, 48, and 72 hours (the time required for the isotope to concentrate in possible thrombi).

An increase of more than 20% in radioactivity between any adjacent sites on the same leg, from results of previous scans or from a corresponding scan on the opposite leg, suggests DVT; an abnormality that persists for more than 24 hours confirms DVT.

The ^{125}I fibrinogen scan is highly sensitive to calf vein thrombi in a patient at high risk, but proves insensitive to groin and pelvic thrombi because of high background radiation from large veins and arteries, and unfavorable anatomic relationships; this is a major limitation since large thrombi can originate in the groin and pelvis, especially after local trauma, such as hip surgery.

Lugol's solution is administered for a week before and a week after this test, to keep the radioactive iodine out of the thyroid gland. The sodium pertechnetate ^{99m}Tc scan, another radionuclide test, can detect peripheral vascular disease—usually in the veins, less often in the arteries. When tagged to albumin, the isotope can image both the lower leg and pulmonary veins. Xenon-133 (^{133}Xe) washout and radioactive centrosome tests, used in research, evaluate peripheral arterial blood flow in the lower legs.

usual diet and medications.

Interfering factors
□ If the patient places weight on the leg being tested, the contrast medium may fail to fill the leg veins.

□ Movement of the leg being tested, excessive tourniquet constriction, insufficient injection of contrast medium, or delay between injection and radiography interfere with accurate testing.

BARBARA MADIGAN, RN, MSN

GRAPHIC RECORDING

Electrocardiography

Electrocardiography, the most frequently used test for evaluating cardiac status, graphically records the electrical current (electrical potential) generated by the heart. This current radiates from the heart in all directions and, on reaching the skin, is measured by electrodes connected to an amplifier and strip chart recorder. The standard resting (scalar) electrocardiogram (EKG) uses 5 electrodes to measure the electrical potential from 12 different leads: the standard limb leads (I, II, III), the augmented limb leads (AVR, AVL, and AVF), and the precordial, or chest, leads (V₁ through V₆).

EKG tracings normally consist of three identifiable waveforms: the P wave, the QRS complex, and the T wave. The P wave depicts atrial depolarization; the QRS complex, ventricular depolarization; and the T wave, ventricular repolarization. Although the EKG records only about 50 to 100 of the more than 100,000 cardiac cycles that occur in 24 hours, it's extremely useful for detecting the presence and location of myocardial infarction (MI), ischemia, conduction delay, chamber enlargement, or arrhythmias.

Purpose
□ To help identify primary conduction abnormalities, cardiac arrhythmias, cardiac hypertrophy, pericarditis, electrolyte imbalance, myocardial ischemia, and the site and extent of MI
□ To monitor recovery from MI
□ To evaluate the effectiveness of cardiac medication (cardiac glycosides, antiar-

rhythmics, antihypertensives, and vasodilators)
□ To observe pacemaker performance.

Patient preparation
Explain to the patient that this test evaluates the heart's function by recording its electrical activity. Inform him that he needn't restrict food or fluids before the test. Tell him who will perform the test and where, and that the procedure takes about 15 minutes.

Inform the patient that electrodes will be attached to his arms, legs, and chest, and that he may experience mild discomfort during the preparation of these sites. Tell him he'll be asked to lie still, to relax, and to breathe normally during the procedure. Advise him not to talk during the test, since the sound of his voice may distort the EKG tracing.

Check the patient's history for cardiac medication, and note any current therapy on the test request form.

Equipment
EKG machine with amplifier and strip chart recorder/five lead wires/four limb lead electrodes, with rubber straps/one suction cup chest electrode/conductive jelly (a pad soaked in alcohol or normal saline solution may be used in place of conductive jelly for the limb leads)/4″ x 4″ gauze pads/towel.

Procedure
The patient is instructed to remove all clothing to the waist and to expose both legs for electrode placement; the female patient's chest is draped until precordial leads are applied. Electrode sites are cleansed with alcohol and wiped dry. If

THE STANDARD 12-LEAD ELECTROCARDIOGRAM

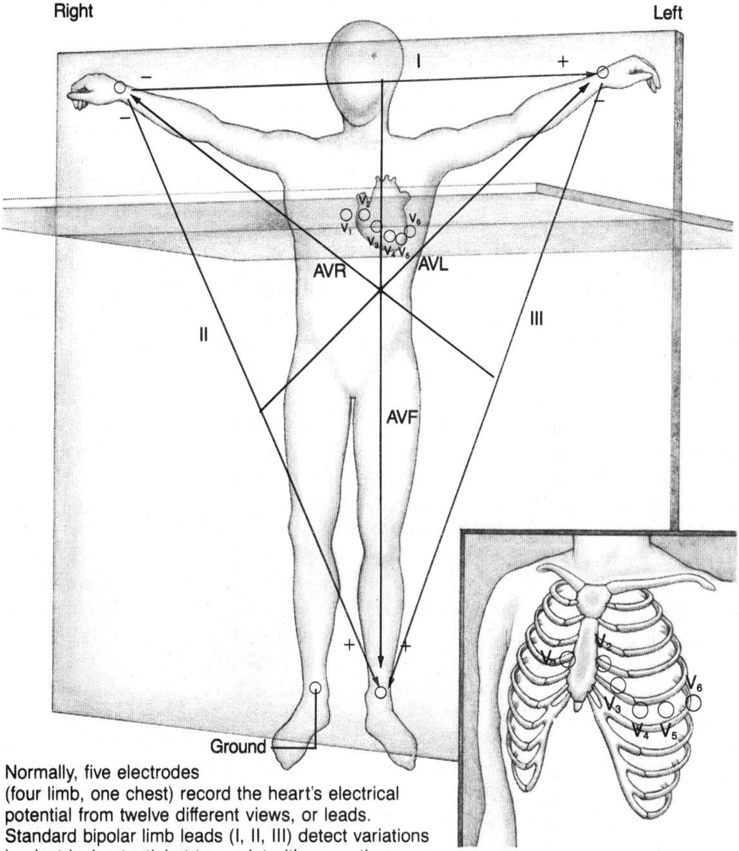

Right

Left

I

AVR   AVL

II   III

AVF

Ground

Normally, five electrodes (four limb, one chest) record the heart's electrical potential from twelve different views, or leads. Standard bipolar limb leads (I, II, III) detect variations in electrical potential at two points (the negative pole and the positive pole) and record the difference. When current flows toward the positive pole, the EKG wave deflects upward; when it flows toward the negative pole, the wave inverts. (The arrows, called Einthoven's reference lines, form a triangle indicating the direction electrical current moves to produce a positive [upward] deflection.)

Lead I connects the left and the right arms, and the EKG tracing shows an upward deflection since the left arm is positive and the right arm negative. Lead II connects the left leg and right arm, and the tracing deflects upward since the left leg is positive and the right arm negative. Lead III connects the left leg and left arm, and the tracing deflects upward since the left leg is positive and the left arm negative.

The unipolar augmented limb leads (AVR, AVL, and AVF), which use the same electrode placement as standard limb leads, measure electrical potential between one augmented limb lead and the electrical midpoint of the remaining two leads (determined electronically by the EKG machine). Both standard and augmented leads measure electrical potential while viewing the heart from the front, in a vertical plane.

The six unipolar chest leads (V_1 through V_6) view the electrical potential from a horizontal plane that helps locate pathology in the lateral, anterior, and posterior walls of the heart. The EKG machine averages the electrical potentials of all three limb lead electrodes (I, II, III) and compares this average with the electrical potential of the chest electrode. Recordings made with the V connection show electrical potential variations that occur under the chest electrode as its position is changed.

necessary, precordial areas are shaved.

The patient is placed in supine position. Care should be taken that his feet don't touch the bed's footboard, to prevent leakage that distorts the EKG tracing. Flat, fleshy, hairless sites on the arms and legs—usually the inner forearm and the inner calf just above the ankle—are selected for electrode placements. After each electrode site is cleaned and shaved (if necessary), conductive jelly is applied. Limb electrodes are secured with a rubber strap; the strap should not be tightened excessively, since muscle spasms may distort the recording. Leg electrodes are positioned so their connector ends point upward, to minimize bending or straining the wires.

Each electrode is color-coded and is matched to a corresponding lead wire: white (right arm), black (left arm), green (right leg), red (left leg), and brown (chest). Generally, lead wires are also coded with initials. The wire and electrode are connected by inserting the lead wire prong into the terminal post and tightening the screw.

After the paper supply in the EKG machine is checked, the power switch is turned on, and the stylus is centered on the paper. The machine is set to record; the stylus will draw a straight baseline. Paper speed is adjusted to 25 mm/second, and the machine is calibrated. To provide a consistent frame of reference throughout the procedure, the machine should be calibrated after running each lead.

The lead selector is turned to lead I, and the EKG sequence begins to record. The machine is run for about 6 seconds for each lead from I through AVF. Before each lead run, the lead name is written on the paper, or the marking button is pushed on the machine, using a series of dots and dashes to mark the leads.

After completing the AVF run, the lead selector is turned to a neutral position before running precordial leads V_1 to V_6. This keeps the stylus from swinging wildly and possibly damaging the paper. To determine the proper placement for leads V_1 to V_6, it is first necessary to locate the second intercostal space directly to the right of Louis' angle—the articulation between the manubrium and the body of the sternum, usually felt as a notch. Then two or more intercostal spaces are counted down: the V_1 position is at the fourth intercostal space to the right of the sternum; V_2 is at the fourth intercostal space to the left of the sternum; V_4 is at the left midclavicular line in the fifth intercostal space; V_3 is midway between V_2 and V_4; V_5 follows V_4 in a straight line to the anterior axillary line; and V_6 follows V_4 in a straight line to the left midaxillary line. Mark these positions on the patient with a marking pen to ensure that future EKGs can be taken from the same positions.

The chest lead wire is connected to the suction cup of the electrode, and the cup is pressed to the V_1 chest position. To minimize artifacts, enough conductive jelly is applied to produce efficient suction and low skin resistance. The patient is asked to breathe normally; if respiration distorts the recording, he is instructed to hold his breath briefly. The lead selector is turned to V, the stylus is centered, and a V_1 strip is recorded for 6 seconds. The lead is identified by writing on the paper or using a marking code. The lead selector is returned to a neutral position, and the suction cup is moved from the V_1 to the V_2 chest position. Then, the selector is turned to V again, the stylus centered, the paper marked, and the V_2 strip recorded for 6 seconds. This procedure is repeated through V_6, always turning the lead selector to neutral before moving the suction cup.

After completing V_6, a rhythm strip may be run on lead II for at least 6 seconds. To end the recording, the lead selector is again standardized.

With some EKG machines, such as the three-channel types that record from three leads at once, the procedure is slightly different. After the six chest electrodes and standard limb leads are positioned, the machine automatically records and marks the 12 lead strips in correct sequence.

Each EKG strip should be labeled with

NORMAL EKG WAVEFORMS

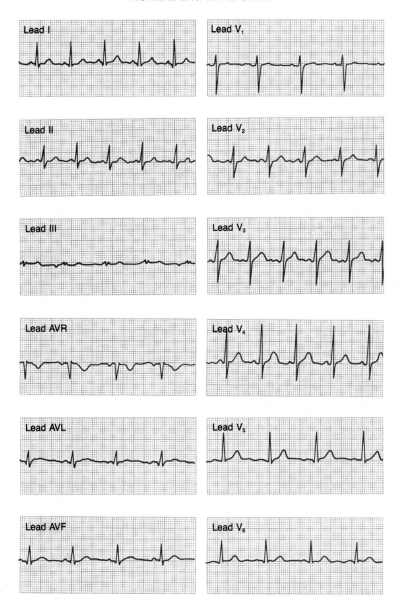

Lead I

Lead II

Lead III

Lead AVR

Lead AVL

Lead AVF

Lead V₁

Lead V₂

Lead V₃

Lead V₄

Lead V₅

Lead V₆

Since each lead takes a different view of heart activity, it generates its own characteristic tracing. The traces shown here are representative of each of the 12 leads. Leads AVR, V_1, V_2, and V_3 normally show strong negative deflections below the baseline. Negative deflections indicate current is flowing away from the positive electrode; positive deflections, that the current's flowing toward the positive electrode.

SOME ABNORMAL EKG WAVEFORMS

PREMATURE VENTRICULAR CONTRACTION—LEAD V₁

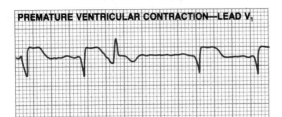

Premature ventricular contractions (PVCs) originate in an ectopic focus of the ventricular wall. They can be unifocal (having the same single focus), as shown in this tracing from lead V_1, or they can be multifocal, arising from more than one ectopic focus. In PVCs, the P wave is lacking, and the QRS complex shows considerable distortion, usually deflecting in the opposite direction from the patient's normal QRS. The T wave also deflects in the opposite direction from the QRS complex, and the PVC usually precedes a compensatory pause. Some examples of abnormalities causing PVCs include electrolyte imbalance (especially hypokalemia), old myocardial infarction, hypoxia, and drug toxicity (digitalis, beta-adrenergics).

FIRST-DEGREE HEART BLOCK—LEAD V₁

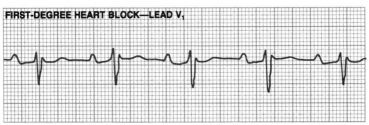

First-degree heart block—the most common conduction disturbance—occurs in healthy hearts as well as in diseased hearts and usually is clinically insignificant. It's often characteristic in elderly patients with chronic degeneration of the cardiac conduction system, and occasionally occurs in patients receiving digitalis and antiarrhythmic drugs, such as procainamide or quinidine. In children, first-degree heart block may be the earliest sign of acute rheumatic fever. In this lead V_1 tracing, the interval between the P wave and QRS complex (the P-R interval) exceeds 0.20 seconds.

HYPOKALEMIA—LEAD V₁

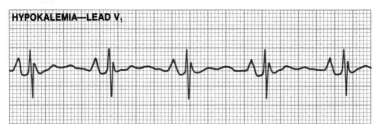

Hypokalemia is a common type of electrolyte imbalance, resulting from low blood potassium levels, that affects the electrical activity of the myocardium. Mild hypokalemia may cause only muscle weakness and fatigue, and possibly atrial or ventricular irritability; a severe condition causes pronounced muscle weakness, paralysis, atrial tachycardia with varying degress of block, and PVCs that may progress to ventricular tachycardia and fibrillation.

Early signs of hypokalemia, as shown on this V_1 tracing, include prominent U waves, a prolonged Q-U interval, and flat or inverted T waves. Usually T waves do not flatten or invert until potassium depletion becomes severe.

STAGES OF MYOCARDIAL INFARCTION

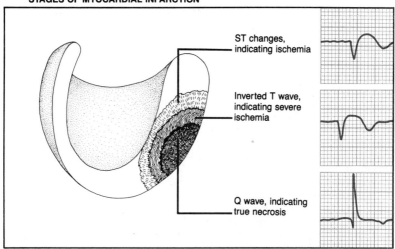

Myocardial infarction produces typical EKG changes in several leads at once, enabling the doctor to determine accurately the location and extent of tissue damage. Myocardial infarction causes three changes: an inner zone of tissue necrosis, a surrounding zone of inflamed tissue, and an outer zone of ischemia (see diagram). As the infarction progresses, the first EKG change is an elevated ST segment, which indicates formation of an ischemic zone. Then the T wave begins to flatten and finally inverts, and enlarged Q waves appear, indicating developing necrosis— a true infarction. (Abnormal Q waves should be larger than one small square on the chart— 0.04 second by 0.1 millivolt.) The T wave may stay inverted for the rest of the patient's life, or it can revert to normal, while the deep Q wave remains as a permanent indicator of necrosis. The infarction can be located by studying the characteristic ST, T, and Q wave changes in various lead combinations. In the three tracings shown below, the ST segments elevated in leads I, II, and AVF indicate an infarction in the inferior (diaphragmatic) area of the heart.

EKG CHANGES WITH AN INFERIOR INFARCTION

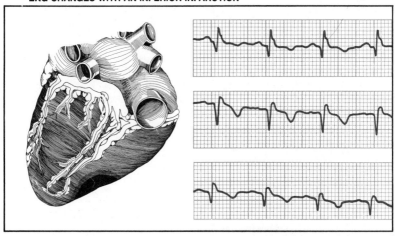

the patient's name and room number (if applicable), the date and time of the procedure, and the doctor's name.

Precautions

☐ The recording equipment and other nearby electrical equipment should be properly grounded to prevent electrical interference that distorts EKG recording.

☐ Double-check color codes and lead markings to be sure connectors match.

☐ Check to be sure suction cups are firmly attached, and reattach electrodes if loose skin contact is suspected.

☐ Be sure the patient is quiet and motionless during the test, since talking or limb movement distorts the recordings.

☐ If a patient experiences chest pains during a lead run, note it on the EKG strip involved. If he has a pacemaker in place, electrocardiography may be performed with or without a magnet. Indicate the presence of a pacemaker and whether or not a magnet is used. (Many pacemakers function only when the heartbeat falls below a preset rate; a magnet makes the pacemaker fire regularly, which permits evaluation of pacemaker performance.)

Findings

The lead II waveform, known as the rhythm strip, depicts the heart's rhythm more clearly than any other waveform. In lead II, the normal P wave does not exceed 2.5 mm (0.25 millivolt) in height or last longer than 0.11 second. The P-R interval, which includes the P wave plus the PR segment, persists for 0.12 to 0.2 second for cardiac rates over 60 beats/minute. The Q-T interval varies with the cardiac rate and lasts 0.52 to 0.4 second for rates above 60; the voltage of the R wave in the V_1 through V_6 leads doesn't exceed 27 mm. The total QRS interval lasts 0.06 to 0.1 second.

The chart on page 883 shows normal waveforms for all 12 EKG leads.

Implications of results

An abnormal EKG may show MI, right or left ventricular hypertrophy, arrhythmias, right or left bundle branch block, ischemia, conduction defects or pericarditis, electrolyte abnormalities (such as hypokalemia), or the effects of cardioactive drugs. Sometimes an EKG may reveal abnormal waveforms only during episodes of symptoms such as angina or during exercise (see EXERCISE ELECTROCARDIOGRAPHY and AMBULATORY ELECTROCARDIOGRAPHY). Some common abnormal EKG patterns appear in the tracings on pages 884 and 885.

Post-test care

Disconnect the equipment, and wash the conductive jelly from the patient's skin with a damp cloth.

Interfering factors

☐ Mechanical difficulties, such as EKG machine malfunction, inadequate or ineffective conductive jelly, or electromag-

---

TESTING PACEMAKER FUNCTION

Using the EKG machine and a magnet, you can easily test your patient's pacemaker. Set up a 12-lead EKG, and run and mark strips for leads I and II. Then, set the selector to lead II, and hold the magnet about 1″ (2.5 cm) above the pacemaker site (some magnets may be placed on the skin). If the pacemaker is functioning properly, the magnet causes it to fire regularly. In some pacemakers, the magnet rate is normally faster than the set rate. Check the patient's pacemaker ID card to identify the normal rate.

Run a strip for about 1 minute indicating that a magnet was used. Then, set aside the magnet, and run the other 10 leads. Determine the pacemaker rate by calculating the distance between each spike instead of between each QRS complex. If the pacemaker doesn't maintain a regular rate, notify the doctor.

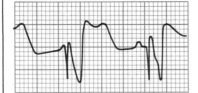

The lead II waveform illustrated above shows a regular 75 beat/minute rate. Notice the spike preceding the QRS complex; this indicates that the pacemaker has fired.

netic interference, can produce artifacts.
□ Improper placement of electrodes, patient movement or muscle tremor, strenuous exercise before the test, or medication reactions can produce inaccurate test results.

ARLENE STRONG, RN, MN

Exercise Electrocardiography
[Stress test]

Exercise electrocardiography evaluates heart action during physical stress—to test cardiac reaction to increased demand for oxygen—and so provides important diagnostic information that can't be obtained from resting electrocardiography alone. An electrocardiogram (EKG) and blood pressure readings are taken while the patient walks on a treadmill or pedals a stationary bicycle, and his response to a constant or an increasing workload is observed. Unless complications develop, the test continues until the patient reaches the target heart rate (determined by an established protocol) or experiences chest pain or fatigue. The patient with recent myocardial infarction (MI) or coronary artery surgery may walk the treadmill at a slow pace to determine his activity tolerance before discharge from the hospital.

The risk of MI during exercise electrocardiography is less than 1 in 500; the risk of death, less than 1 in 10,000.

Purpose
□ To help diagnose the cause of chest pain or other possible cardiac pain
□ To determine the functional capacity of the heart after surgery or MI
□ To screen for asymptomatic coronary artery disease (particularly in men over age 35)
□ To help set limitations for an exercise program
□ To identify cardiac arrhythmias that develop during physical exercise
□ To evaluate the effectiveness of antiarrhythmic or antianginal therapy.

Patient preparation
Explain to the patient that this test records the heart's electrical activity and performance under stress. Instruct him not to eat, smoke, or drink alcoholic or caffeinic beverages for 3 hours before the test, but to continue any drug regimen unless the doctor directs otherwise. Tell him who will perform the test and where, and that a doctor will be available in the testing area at all times.

Inform the patient that the test will cause him to feel fatigued, slightly breathless, and sweaty, but assure him that it has few risks; he may, in fact, stop the test if he experiences extreme fatigue or chest pain.

Advise the patient to wear comfortable socks and shoes, and loose, lightweight shorts or slacks during the procedure; men usually don't wear a shirt during the test, and women generally wear a bra and a lightweight short-sleeved blouse or a patient gown with a front closure. Inform the patient that several areas on his chest and, possibly, on his back will be cleansed, shaved (if necessary), and abraded to prepare the skin for the electrodes. Reassure him he won't feel any current from the electrodes, but the electrode sites may itch slightly. Mention that his blood pressure and heart rate will be checked periodically throughout the procedure.

If the patient is scheduled for a multistage *treadmill test,* explain that the speed and incline of the treadmill increase at predetermined intervals, and tell him he'll be informed of each adjustment. If he's scheduled for a *bicycle ergometer test,* explain that the resistance he experiences in pedaling increases gradually as he tries to maintain a specific speed. Encourage him to report his feelings during the test. Tell him his blood pressure and EKG will be monitored for 10 to 15 minutes after the test.

Check the patient's history for a recent physical examination (within 1 week)

COMPARING TWO EXERCISE TESTS: THE TREADMILL AND BICYCLE ERGOMETER

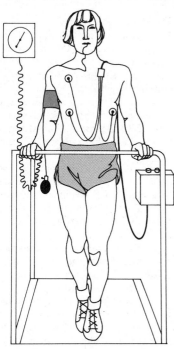

ADVANTAGES
- standardized and most reproducible
- walking is a familiar activity
- constant work rate
- attains highest maximum oxygen uptake
- involves muscles commonly used; less chance of fatigue

DISADVANTAGES
- possibility of patient losing balance and falling off
- workload depends on weight; as weight increases, work load increases
- less easy to obtain blood pressure readings and EKG recordings since upper body's in motion
- expensive
- noisy, making communication with patient more difficult

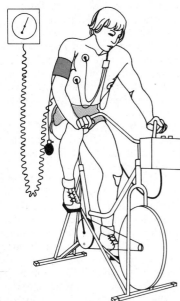

ADVANTAGES
- workload doesn't depend on weight
- easy to obtain blood pressure readings and EKG recordings since upper body remains relatively still
- less expensive

DISADVANTAGES
- constant rate of pedaling required to maintain power
- frequent calibration necessary
- bicycle exercise induces greater stress
- attains lower maximum oxygen uptake
- involves muscles less commonly used; greater chance of fatigue

and for baseline 12-lead EKG results. Make sure the patient or a responsible family member has signed a consent form.

Procedure
The electrode sites are shaved, if necessary, and the skin is thoroughly cleansed with an alcohol swab. The superficial epidermal cell layer and excess skin oils are removed with a gauze pad, fine sandpaper, or dental burr; adequately prepared sites appear slightly red.

Chest electrodes are placed according to the lead system selected and are secured with adhesive tape or a rubber belt. The lead wire cable is placed over the patient's shoulder and the lead wire box is placed on his chest. The cable is secured by pinning it to the patient's clothing or taping it to his shoulder or back. Then, the lead wires are connected to the chest electrodes.

The monitor is started, and a stable baseline tracing is obtained. A baseline rhythm strip is checked for arrhythmias. A blood pressure reading is taken, and the patient is auscultated for presence of S_3 or S_4 gallops, or rales.

Treadmill test: The treadmill is turned on to a slow speed, and the patient is shown how to step onto it and how to use the support railings to maintain balance, but not to support weight. Then, the treadmill is turned off. The patient is instructed to step onto the treadmill, and it is turned on to slow speed until the patient gets used to walking on it.

Bicycle ergometer test: The patient is instructed to sit on the bicycle. The seat and handlebars are adjusted, if necessary, so that he can pedal the bike comfortably. The patient is instructed not to grip the handlebars tightly, but to use them only for maintaining balance, and to pedal until he reaches the desired speed, as shown on the speedometer.

In both tests, a monitor is observed continuously for changes in the heart's electrical activity. The rhythm strip is checked at preset intervals for arrhythmias, premature ventricular contrac-

tions (PVCs), or ST segment changes. The test level and the elapsed time into the test level are marked on each strip. Blood pressure is monitored at predetermined intervals—usually at the end of each test level—and changes in systolic readings are noted. Some common responses to maximal exercise are dizziness, lightheadedness, leg fatigue, dyspnea, diaphoresis, and a slightly ataxic gait. If symptoms become severe, the test is stopped. Usually, testing stops when the patient reaches the target heart rate. As the treadmill speed slows, he may be instructed to continue walking for several minutes to prevent nausea or dizziness. Then, the treadmill is turned off, the patient is helped to a chair, and his blood pressure and EKG are monitored for 10 to 15 minutes.

Precautions
□ Since exercise electrocardiography places considerable stress on the heart, it may be contraindicated in patients with ventricular or dissecting aortic aneurysm, uncontrolled arrhythmias, pericarditis, myocarditis, severe anemia, uncontrolled hypertension, unstable angina, and congestive heart failure.
□ Stop the test immediately if the EKG shows three consecutive PVCs, if systolic blood pressure falls below resting level, if heart rate falls to 10 beats/minute below resting level, or if the patient becomes exhausted. Depending on the patient's condition, the test may be stopped if the EKG shows bundle branch block, ST segment depression that exceeds 3 mm, or frequent or complicated PVCs; if blood pressure fails to rise above resting level; if systolic pressure exceeds 220 mmHg; or if the patient experiences angina. Rarely, persistent ST segment elevation may indicate transmural myocardial ischemia and should end the test.

Findings
In a normal exercise EKG, the P, QRS, and T waves and the ST segment change slightly; slight ST segment depression occurs in some patients, especially women. Heart rate rises in direct pro-

ELECTRODE PLACEMENT FOR EXERCISE ELECTROCARDIOGRAPHY

TYPE	LEAD	ELECTRODE PLACEMENT	
Three-electrode monitor	Lead II	Positive (+): left side of chest, lowest palpable rib, midclavicular Negative (−): right shoulder, below clavicular hollow Ground (G): left shoulder, below clavicular hollow	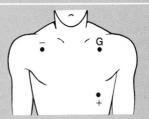
	MCL₁	Positive (+): right sternal border, lowest palpable rib Negative (−): left shoulder, below clavicular hollow Ground (G): right shoulder, below clavicular hollow	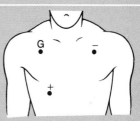
	MCL₆	Positive (+): left side of chest, lowest palpable rib, midclavicular Negative (−): left shoulder, below clavicular hollow Ground (G): right shoulder, below clavicular hollow	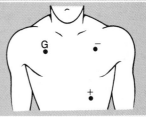
Five-electrode monitor	V₁ through V₆	Positive (+): left side of chest, just below lowest palpable rib Negative (−): right shoulder, midclavicular Ground (G): right side of chest, just below lowest palpable rib Inactive (I): left shoulder, midclavicular Chest V₁: fourth intercostal space to right of sternum Chest V₂: fourth intercostal space to left of sternum Chest V₃: halfway between V₂ and V₄ Chest V₄: fifth intercostal space, midclavicular, left side Chest V₅: halfway between V₄ and V₆ Chest V₆: same line as V₅ at midaxillary line	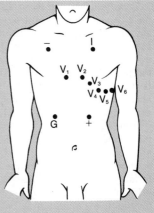

If you're working with a three-electrode monitor, you can establish the three standard leads (I, II, III) and the three augmented limb leads (AVR, AVL, AVF). However, if you want to obtain readings similar to the V₁ and V₆ chest leads, you can use modified chest leads (MCL₁, MCL₆). If you're using a five-electrode monitor, the most sensitive of these recording devices, you can record standard and augmented leads as well as six chest leads.

portion to the workload and metabolic oxygen demand; systolic blood pressure also rises as workload increases. The normal patient attains the endurance levels predicted by his age and the appropriate exercise protocol.

Implications of results

Although criteria for judging test results vary, two findings strongly suggest an abnormality: a flat or downsloping ST segment depression of 1 mm or more for at least 0.08 second after the junction of the QRS and ST segments (J point); and a markedly depressed J point, with an upsloping but depressed ST segment of 1.5 mm below the baseline 0.08 second after the J point. Initial ST segment depression on the resting EKG must be further depressed by 1 mm during ex-

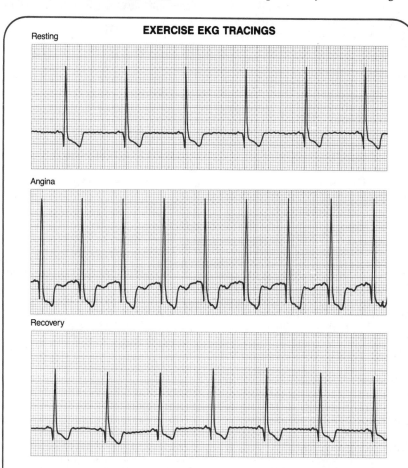

EXERCISE EKG TRACINGS

Resting

Angina

Recovery

These tracings are from an abnormal exercise EKG obtained during a treadmill test performed on a patient who had just undergone a triple coronary artery bypass graft. The first tracing shows the heart at rest, blood pressure 124 over 80. In the second tracing, the patient worked up to a 10% grade at 1.7 mph before experiencing angina at 2 minutes 25 seconds. The tracing shows a depressed ST segment; heart rate was 85, blood pressure 140 over 70. The third tracing shows the heart at rest 6 minutes after the test; blood pressure was 140 over 90.

(Tracings courtesy of Arlene Strong, RN, MN)

ercise to be considered abnormal.

Hypotension resulting from exercise, ST depression of 3 mm or more, down-sloping ST segments, and ischemic ST segments appearing within the first 3 minutes of exercise and lasting 8 minutes into the post-test recovery period may indicate multivessel or left coronary artery disease. ST segment elevation may indicate dyskinetic left ventricular wall motion or severe transmural ischemia.

The predictive value of this test for coronary artery disease varies with the patient's history and sex; however, false-negative and false-positive test results are common. To detect coronary artery disease accurately, thallium imaging and stress testing, exercise multiple-gated acquisition scanning (see CARDIAC BLOOD POOL IMAGING), or coronary angiography (see CARDIAC CATHETERIZATION) may be necessary.

Post-test care

□ Assist the patient to a chair, and continue monitoring heart rate and blood pressure for 10 to 15 minutes or until the EKG returns to baseline.

□ Auscultate for the presence of S_3 or S_4 gallops. Frequently, an S_4 gallop develops after exercise, due to increased blood flow volume and turbulence. However, an S_3 gallop is more significant than an S_4 gallop, indicating transient left ventricular dysfunction.

□ Remove all chest electrodes, and clean the electrode sites. Tell the patient to wait at least 1 hour before showering. Caution him to use warm water; hot water may cause him to faint or feel dizzy.

□ Instruct the patient to resume usual diet discontinued before the test.

Interfering factors

□ Patient failure to observe pretest restrictions hinders the heart's ability to respond to stress.

□ Use of beta-blockers may make test results difficult to interpret.

□ Inability to exercise to the target heart rate because of fatigue or uncooperativeness interferes with accurate testing.

□ Wolff-Parkinson-White syndrome

(anomalous atrioventricular excitation), electrolyte imbalance, and digitalis may cause false-positive results.

□ Conditions that cause left ventricular hypertrophy (congenital abnormalities, hypertension) may interfere with testing for ischemia.

ARLENE STRONG, RN, MN

Ambulatory Electrocardiography
[Holter monitoring, ambulatory monitoring]

Ambulatory electrocardiography, commonly called Holter monitoring after the scientist who developed the technique, is the continuous recording of heart activity as the patient follows his normal routine. In this test, which is usually performed for 24 hours or about 100,000 cardiac cycles, the patient wears a small reel-to-reel or cassette tape recorder connected to electrodes placed on his chest, and keeps a diary of his activities and any associated symptoms. At the end of the recording period, the tape is analyzed by a microcomputer and a report is printed, permitting correlation of cardiac irregularities, such as arrhythmias and ST segment changes, with the activities in the patient's diary.

Although ambulatory electrocardiography isn't a substitute for coronary care unit surveillance, it can detect sporadic arrhythmias missed by an exercise or resting electrocardiogram (EKG). It can also evaluate the status of a patient recuperating from an acute myocardial infarction (MI); in such a patient, monitoring may uncover electrical instability or ischemia that delays hospital discharge, or requires a change in therapy, additional therapy, or a revised rehabilitation plan.

Patient-activated monitors can be worn for 5 to 7 days. With these devices, the

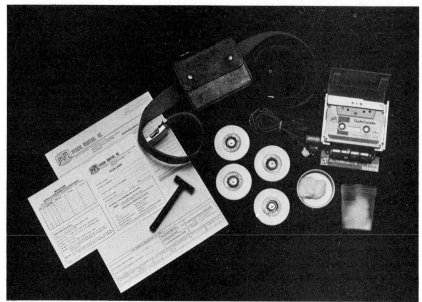

A portable cassette recorder, carried by a patient as he goes through his daily routine, monitors as many as 100,000 cardiac cycles over a 24-hour period. Basic equipment includes a set of electrodes, the monitor and belt, and a patient diary in which all activities are recorded, especially those that bring on arrhythmias.

patient manually initiates recording of heart activity only when he experiences symptoms. Intermittent monitoring, triggered only by an unusual heart rhythm, is used in cardiac research.

Purpose
□ To detect cardiac arrhythmias
□ To evaluate chest pain
□ To evaluate cardiac status after acute MI or pacemaker implantation
□ To evaluate effectiveness of antiarrhythmic drug therapy
□ To assess and correlate dyspnea, CNS symptoms—such as syncope and lightheadedness—and palpitations with actual cardiac events and the patient's activities.

Patient preparation
Explain to the patient that this test helps determine how the heart responds to normal activity or, if appropriate, to cardioactive medication. Inform him that monitoring requires attachment of electrodes to his chest, that his chest may be

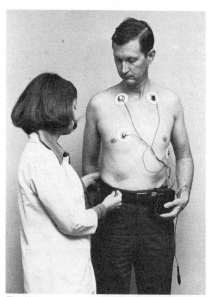

The Holter monitor is worn on a belt at the waist, as shown above. The belt should be adjusted so it fits comfortably, but not so loose that the monitor's weight pulls on the electrodes secured to the patient's chest.

shaved, and that he may experience some discomfort during preparation of the electrode sites. Tell him that it also requires him to wear a small tape recorder for 24 hours (for 5 to 7 days if a patient-activated monitor is being used). Mention that a shoulder strap or a special belt will be provided to carry the recorder, which weighs about 2 lb (0.9 kg). Show him how to position the recorder when he lies down.

Encourage the patient to continue his routine activities during the monitoring period. Stress the importance of logging his usual activities (walking, stair-climbing, urinating, sleeping, sexual activity, for example), emotional upsets, physical symptoms (dizziness, palpitations, fatigue, chest pain, and syncope), and ingestion of medication; show the patient a sample diary. If applicable to the monitor, demonstrate how to mark the tape at onset of symptoms. (If a patient-activated monitor is being used, show the patient how to press the event button to activate the monitor if he experiences any unusual sensations.)

Advise the patient to wear loose-fitting clothing with front-buttoning tops during monitoring. Instruct him not to tamper with the monitor or to disconnect the lead wires or electrodes. If he must bathe, advise a sponge bath, since equipment mustn't get wet. Tell him to avoid magnets, metal detectors, high-voltage areas, and electric blankets. Show him how to check the recorder to make sure it's working properly. Explain that, if the monitor light flashes, one of the electrodes may be loose and that he should depress the center of each one. Tell him to notify you if one comes off.

If the patient won't be returning to the office or hospital immediately after the monitoring period, show him how to remove and store the equipment. Remind him to bring the diary when he returns.

Procedure

The electrode sites are shaved, if necessary, cleansed with an alcohol swab, and gently abraded until they redden. After the backings are peeled off, the electrodes are applied to the correct sites; the sides and bottom of each electrode are pressed firmly to ensure that the adhesive portion of the electrode is securely fastened to the skin. Then, the center of the electrode is pressed lightly to make good contact between the jelly and the patient's skin. The electrode cable should be securely attached to the monitor. The monitor and case is positioned as the patient will wear it, then the lead wires are attached to the electrodes. Care should be taken that there isn't too much slack or pull on the wires. After a new or fully charged battery is installed into the recorder, the tape is inserted and the recorder is turned on. The electrode attachment circuit is tested by connecting the recorder to a standard EKG machine. Watch for artifacts while the patient moves normally (stands, sits).

Precautions

To eliminate muscle artifact, make sure the lead cable is firmly plugged in. Check that electrodes aren't placed over large muscle masses, such as the pectorals.

Findings

When compared with the patient's diary, the normal EKG pattern shows no significant arrhythmias or ST segment changes. Changes in heart rate normally occur during various activities.

Implications of results

Abnormalities of the heart detected by ambulatory electrocardiography include premature ventricular contractions (PVCs), conduction defects, tachyarrhythmias, bradyarrhythmias, and brady-tachyarrhythmia syndrome. Arrhythmias may be associated with dyspnea and CNS symptoms, such as dizziness and syncope.

During recovery from an MI, this test can monitor for PVCs to help determine the prognosis and the effectiveness of drug therapy.

ST-T wave changes associated with ischemia may coincide with chest pain or increased patient activity. ST segment changes associated with an acute MI require careful study, since smoking, eating, postural changes, certain drugs, Wolff-Parkinson-White syndrome, bundle branch block, myocarditis, myocardial hypertrophy, anemia, hypoxemia, and abnormal hemoglobin binding can produce a similar tracing on the EKG. Monitoring the MI patient 1 to 3 days before discharge and again 4 to 6 weeks after discharge, may detect ST-T wave changes associated with ischemia or arrhythmias; such information aids patient therapy and rehabilitation, and refines prognosis. Monitoring a patient with an artificial pacemaker may detect an arrhythmia, such as bradycardia, that the pacemaker fails to override.

Although ambulatory electrocardiography correlates patient symptoms and EKG changes, it doesn't always identify their causes. If initial monitoring proves inconclusive, the test may be repeated.

Post-test care
Remove all chest electrodes, and clean the electrode sites.

Interfering factors
□ Failure to apply the electrodes correctly can cause muscle or movement artifact.

□ Patient failure to carefully record daily activities and symptoms, or to maintain normal routine, interferes with accurate testing.

□ If a patient-activated monitor is used, patient failure to turn on the monitor during symptoms interferes with accurate testing.

□ Physiologic variation in frequency and severity of arrhythmias may cause an arrhythmia to be missed on the 24-hour ambulatory EKG.

ARLENE STRONG, RN, MN

Apexcardiography

Apexcardiography is the graphic recording of chest movement caused by low-frequency precordial cardiac pulsations. A transducer placed on the patient's chest at the cardiac apex picks up these pulsations and converts them from kinetic to electrical energy. A recorder then converts this electrical energy into waveforms, or apexcardiograms (ACGs), that depict cardiac events during systole and diastole.

Apexcardiography alone usually doesn't provide sufficient information to make an accurate diagnosis; however, when it's performed simultaneously with electrocardiography, phonocardiography, or carotid and/or jugular pulse tracings, it aids diagnosis of cardiac abnormalities, especially left ventricular dysfunction, and helps identify heart sounds.

Purpose
□ To aid evaluation of left ventricular function

□ To help identify effects of ventricular enlargement, infarction, and/or ischemia; ventricular aneurysm; and pericarditis

□ To aid identification of heart sounds.

Patient preparation
Explain to the patient that this test records movements of the chest wall caused by the heart's pumping action. Advise him that he needn't restrict food or fluids. Tell him who will perform the test and where, and that it takes approximately 15 minutes. Reassure him that the test, performed simultaneously with electrocardiography, is safe and painless. When appropriate, tell him that phonocardiography and pulse wave tracings will also be performed.

Inform the patient that he'll lie on his left side during the procedure, and that electrodes will be attached to his arms and legs for electrocardiography. Tell him that the transducer will then be positioned over the heart, and held in place by an elastic strap or stand. Inform him that he'll be instructed to breathe slowly or to hold his breath so that respiratory variations don't distort test results, and that he may be asked to do isometric

READING AN APEXCARDIOGRAM

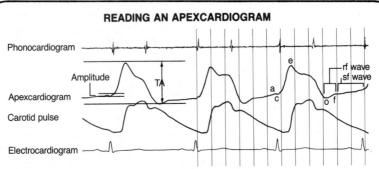

Phonocardiogram

Amplitude   TA

Apexcardiogram

Carotid pulse

Electrocardiogram

e

a
c

rf wave
sf wave

o f

This illustration shows a normal apexcardiogram (ACG), accompanied by a simultaneous phonocardiogram, carotid pulse wave tracing, and electrocardiogram. The ACG waveform provides the following information about the cardiac cycle:
a wave: atrial systole (normally less than 15% of total apical amplitude [TA]); ventricular filling
c point: isovolumetric ventricular systole
e point: ventricular systole; aortic valve opens
o point: mitral valve opens (approximate time)
rf wave: rapid ventricular filling
f point: marks change from rapid to slow ventricular filling
sf wave: slow, passive ventricular filling.

(muscle-clenching) hand-grip exercises. Advise the patient not to talk or move during the procedure, unless asked to do so; this helps ensure a clear recording.

Just before the procedure, instruct the patient to remove any metallic objects above the sites where the electrodes are to be placed.

Procedure

After the patient is placed in left oblique position, electrocardiography electrodes are attached to the arms and legs for continuous recording throughout the procedure. The patient's chest wall is palpated to locate the point of maximum impulse (PMI), and the transducer to which conductive jelly has been applied is placed on the PMI, making sure it doesn't interfere with chest wall motion. During the recordings, the patient is asked to breathe in and out slowly, to hold his breath, and to do isometric hand-grip exercises; these exercises increase systemic resistance, and the resultant recordings demonstrate their effect on ventricular function. When the recordings are completed, the transducer and electrodes are removed.

Precautions

None.

Findings

The components of the ACG waveform include the a wave, c point, e point, o point, rf wave, f point, sf wave, and stasis. The illustration on this page shows a normal ACG waveform and describes what each component represents in the cardiac cycle.

Implications of results

Absence of the a wave characterizes atrial fibrillation and mitral stenosis; a series of small a waves characterizes atrial flutter. Abnormally large a waves may occur in systemic hypertension, aortic valve stenosis, and idiopathic hypertrophic subaortic stenosis. Abnormal a wave configuration during isometric exercises may indicate a latent left ventricular abnormality.

A late systolic apical impulse, or systolic bulge, is characteristic in left ventricular aneurysm, ischemia, or infarction, and may occur in systemic hypertension, aortic stenosis, primary myocardial disease, and coronary artery disease. The slope of the rf wave, which is normally steep due to rapid ventricular filling, decreases in mitral stenosis but may increase in myocardial failure, mitral regurgitation, and constrictive pericarditis. Abnormal ACG results should be correlated with results from phonocardiography, electrocardiography, and carotid and/or jugular pulse tracings. Additional tests, such as echocardiography and cardiac catheterization, may be needed to clarify or confirm results.

Post-test care
Be sure the conductive jelly is removed from the patient's skin.

Interfering factors
□ Respiratory excursions can distort recordings.
□ Incorrect patient positioning, transducer placement, or transducer tension can distort recordings.
ARLENE STRONG, RN, MN

Phonocardiography

Phonocardiography graphically records heart sounds—audible vibrations produced as blood courses through the heart and great vessels. This test is valuable for locating and timing abnormal heart sounds detected on auscultation and diagnosing valvular abnormalities. During phonocardiography, microphones are placed on the patient's chest, usually at the apex and the base of the heart. A transducer in each microphone picks up heart sounds, amplifies them, converts them to electrical impulses, and relays these impulses to a recorder, which produces a graph of heart sounds in waveform—a phonocardiogram (PCG).

Phonocardiography is usually performed simultaneously with electrocardiography, carotid and/or jugular pulse wave tracings, and apexcardiography. Together these tests permit precise timing of heart sounds and cardiac events.

Purpose
□ To aid the precise timing of cardiac events
□ To aid calculation of systolic time intervals
□ To help diagnose valvular abnormalities and other cardiac disorders.

Patient preparation
Explain to the patient that this test times heart sounds and helps diagnose cardiac abnormalities. Advise him that he needn't restrict food or fluids. Tell him who will perform the test and where and that it takes about 15 to 30 minutes. Reassure

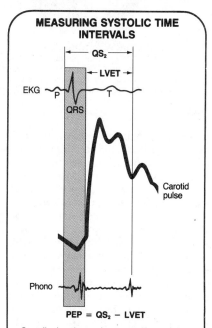

MEASURING SYSTOLIC TIME INTERVALS

$$PEP = QS_2 - LVET$$

Systolic time intervals are made up of the pre-ejection period (PEP), left ventricular ejection time (LVET), and total electromechanical systole (QS_2). As shown above, they can be measured by correlating the results from three simultaneously performed tests: phonocardiography, electrocardiography, and carotid pulse wave tracing. The PEP:LVET ratio reflects the efficiency of left ventricular contraction, and thus helps identify cardiac abnormalities. For example, in left ventricular dysfunction, PEP increases and LVET decreases; conversely, in hypertension, PEP decreases and LVET increases.

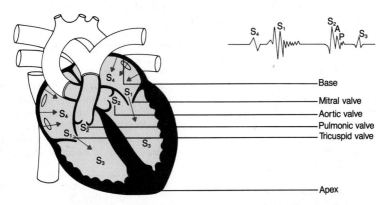

UNDERSTANDING HEART SOUNDS

S_4 S_1 S_2 S_3
A
P

Base
Mitral valve
Aortic valve
Pulmonic valve
Tricuspid valve

Apex

Although the physiologic cause of heart sounds hasn't been clearly defined, S_1 probably results from closure of the mitral and tricuspid valves; S_2, closure of the aortic and pulmonic valves; S_3, early rapid filling of the ventricles with limited distensibility; and S_4, atrial contraction against increasing ventricular resistance, as shown above. The accompanying phonocardiogram shows the S_3 and S_4 sounds in relation to the S_1 and S_2 sounds.

the patient that the procedure is safe and painless. Mention that additional tests (electrocardiography, carotid and/or jugular pulse wave tracings, and apexcardiography) are usually performed simultaneously with phonocardiography.

Inform the patient that small microphones will be placed on his chest and secured with straps. If the patient's chest is hairy, mention that it may be shaved before the microphones are applied, to ensure a clear recording. Instruct the patient to remain still and quiet during the test, except when asked to change position, perform isometric exercises (hand grip) and Valsalva's maneuver, or slowly breathe in and out or hold his breath. Tell him he may be asked to inhale a drug with a slightly sweet odor (amyl nitrite). Although this drug may increase heart rate and produce flushing, dizziness and palpitations, assure the patient that these effects soon subside. Instruct him to report any chest discomfort immediately.

Procedure

The patient is placed in supine position and is prepared for electrocardiography, apexcardiography, and carotid and/or jugular pulse wave tracing. Then the apex and base of the heart are located with a stethoscope, and microphones are strapped to the patient's chest. Both sites may be recorded simultaneously, or the base site may be recorded first; 4 complete cardiac cycles are recorded in patients with sinus rhythm, 7 to 10 cycles in those with cardiac arrhythmias.

To record changes in heart sounds under different conditions, the patient may be asked to assume various positions (supine, upright, and left lateral oblique), to breath in and out slowly or to hold his breath, to perform isometric exercises, or to inhale amyl nitrite.

Precautions

None.

Findings

A normal PCG has a smooth baseline interrupted by vibrations from the major heart sounds. The first and second heart sounds, S_1 and S_2, generate the strongest vibrations, which appear as spikes above and below the baseline. S_1 splitting normally results from the sequential closing of the mitral and tricuspid valves. S_2 splitting into aortic and pulmonic components is best heard during inspiration.

The third and fourth heart sounds, S_3 and S_4, generate weaker vibrations than the S_1 and S_2. S_3, or ventricular gallop, occurs after the aortic valve closes, and may be normal in children and in adults with high cardiac output; it results from unusually rapid or large-volume early diastolic ventricular filling. S_4, or atrial gallop, occurs after the onset of the P wave and may sometimes occur under normal conditions.

JUGULAR AND CAROTID PULSE WAVE TRACINGS

Jugular and carotid pulse wave tracings graphically record low-frequency vibrations from the jugular vein and carotid artery, which reflect the heart's pulsations during diastole and systole. A transducer placed over either the jugular vein or carotid artery, 1 to 2 cm below the jaw, picks up these vibrations and converts them from kinetic to electrical energy. A recorder then shapes this electrical energy into pulse wave tracings.

The superior vena cava connects the jugular vein and the right atrium. Since no valves interrupt this pathway, pressure changes in the right atrium caused by diastole and systole are reflected in the jugular vein. Jugular pulse wave tracings can thus help identify right-sided heart failure, causing increased right atrial pressure, and tricuspid valve disorders. In contrast, carotid pulse wave tracings primarily reflect events on the left side of the heart, especially changes in the aortic pulse. When blood's ejected from the left ventricle, aortic pressure rises; this pressure change is immediately reflected in the carotid artery. Carotid pulse wave tracings can thus help identify aortic valve disease, idiopathic hypertrophic subaortic stenosis, left ventricular failure, and hypertension.

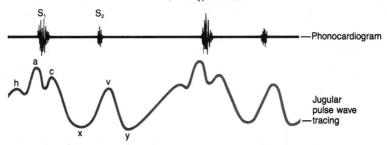

The jugular pulse wave tracing normally has three positive waves (a, c, and v) and two negative waves (x and y). The a wave shows right atrial contraction, usually as a dominant positive wave; the c wave, right ventricular contraction causing bulging of the tricuspid valve into the atrium; the x wave, right atrial relaxation; the v wave, passive filling of the right atrium; the y wave, opening of the tricuspid valve and emptying of the right atrium; and the h wave, conclusion of right ventricular filling.

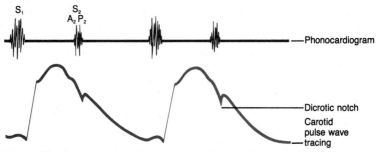

The carotid pulse wave tracing normally has a prominent positive wave coinciding with systole, and a smaller positive wave coinciding with diastole. The characteristic dicrotic notch marks the closure of the aortic (A_2) and pulmonic valves (P_2).

Implications of results

Phonocardiography performed simultaneously with electrocardiography, pulse wave tracings (carotid and jugular pulses), and apexcardiography can reveal valvular disorders, hypertrophic cardiomyopathies, and left ventricular failure. Together these recordings permit measurement of systolic time intervals, which may also help evaluate left ventricular function.

Increased S_1 intensity may indicate tricuspid or mitral stenosis, or tachycardia associated with heightened ventricular contractility. Conversely, decreased S_1 intensity may indicate pericardial effusion, impaired left ventricular function in association with myocarditis, or first-degree atrioventricular block. Widened S_1 splitting usually indicates right bundle branch block. During inspiration, widened S_2 splitting results from conditions associated with right ventricular overload and decreased pulmonary vascular resistance; during expiration, this splitting may indicate such conditions as right bundle branch block and pulmonary embolism. Narrowed S_2 splitting during inspiration accompanies increased pulmonary vascular resistance.

Although both S_3 and S_4 can occur in healthy persons, their presence often signifies cardiac abnormality. The presence of S_3 in persons over age 40 may indicate ventricular decompensation due to atrioventricular valve regurgitation, or other causes of increased ventricular filling. The presence of S_4 may result from systemic or pulmonary hypertension, aortic stenosis, hypertrophic cardiomyopathies, or coronary artery disease.

Isometric exercises can accentuate murmurs and make S_3 and S_4 easier to identify. Hand-grip exercises accentuate murmurs associated with aortic and mitral valve regurgitation. Valsalva's maneuver accentuates systolic murmurs associated with hypertrophic cardiomyopathy or mitral valve prolapse.

Post-test care

None.

Interfering factors

□ Incorrect placement of or pressure on the microphone, background noise, or patient movement (muscle tremors, shivering) interfere with accurate determination of test results.
□ Obesity makes heart sounds difficult to detect.

ARLENE STRONG, RN, MN

Vectorcardiography

Similar to electrocardiography, vectorcardiography records variations in electrical potential during the cardiac cycle. However, vectorcardiography—unlike electrocardiography—uses two simultaneously recorded lead axes to construct a three-dimensional view of the heart. Vectors, which are composites of electrical potential, possess direction, magnitude, and polarity and are measured along three axes: the X, or horizontal, axis; the Y, or vertical, axis; and the Z, or sagittal, axis. Simultaneous recording of X and Y axes produces the frontal plane; of X and Z axes, the horizontal plane; and of Z and Y axes, the sagittal plane.

In vectorcardiography, electrodes applied to the patient's skin transmit the heart's electrical impulses to a vectorcardiograph. This instrument displays the three vector loops—P, QRS, and T— on its oscilloscope screen, permitting photographic or direct graphic recording of results. These loops represent one complete cardiac cycle, and correspond to the P wave, QRS complex, and T wave of the electrocardiogram (EKG).

Although vectorcardiography is more commonly used in research and teaching than in a clinical setting, it does prove useful in clarifying questionable EKG results, especially in patients with hypertrophy, bundle branch block, myocardial infarction (MI), or combinations of these disorders. However, its clinical application is limited because of its high

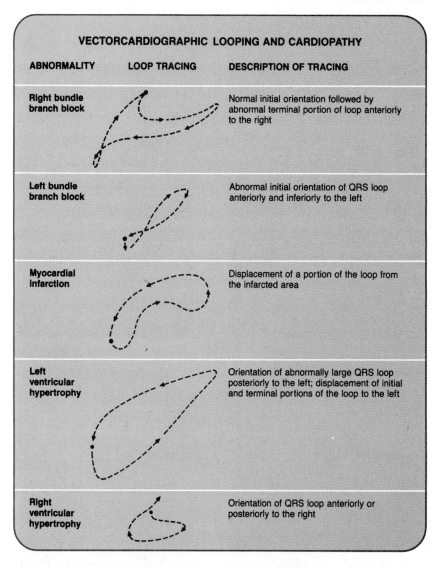

VECTORCARDIOGRAPHIC LOOPING AND CARDIOPATHY

ABNORMALITY	LOOP TRACING	DESCRIPTION OF TRACING
Right bundle branch block		Normal initial orientation followed by abnormal terminal portion of loop anteriorly to the right
Left bundle branch block		Abnormal initial orientation of QRS loop anteriorly and inferiorly to the left
Myocardial infarction		Displacement of a portion of the loop from the infarcted area
Left ventricular hypertrophy		Orientation of abnormally large QRS loop posteriorly to the left; displacement of initial and terminal portions of the loop to the left
Right ventricular hypertrophy		Orientation of QRS loop anteriorly or posteriorly to the right

cost. Interpretation of the vectorcardiogram (VCG) requires great skill, and definitive standards for normal and abnormal vectors and for lead placement do not exist.

Purpose
☐ To detect ventricular hypertrophy, interventricular conduction disturbances, and MI
☐ To clarify doubtful EKG results.

Patient preparation
Explain to the patient that this test records and evaluates the heart's electrical activity. Inform him that he needn't restrict food or fluids. Tell him who will perform the test and where, that it takes about 15 minutes, and that results are usually available in 1 or 2 days. Reassure the patient that the test, which is similar to electrocardiography, is safe and painless.

HOW VECTORCARDIOGRAMS CORRESPOND TO EKGs

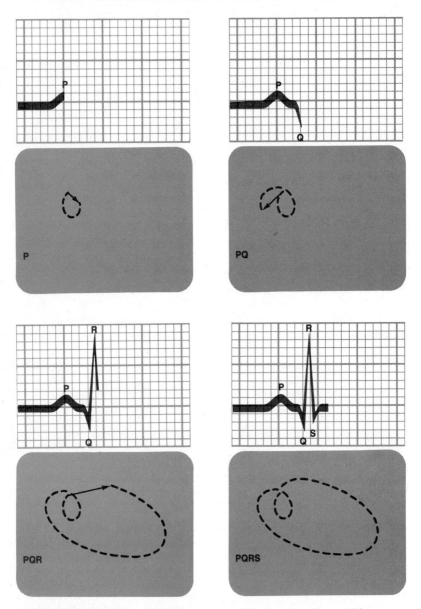

P, QRS, and T loops together represent the electrical activity of each heartbeat—atrial depolarization, ventricular depolarization, and ventricular repolarization. These VCG loops correspond to each segment of an EKG waveform, shown directly above.

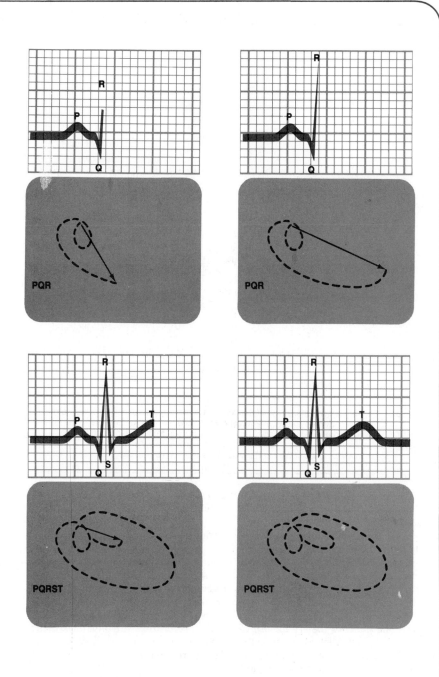

CARDIAC CONDUCTION: A THREE-DIMENSIONAL VIEW

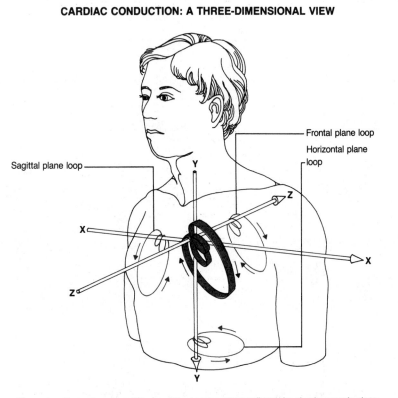

To create a three-dimensional image of the heart, vectorcardiography simultaneously views the heart from two of three planes: the frontal plane (produced from X and Y axes), the horizontal plane (produced from X and Z axes), and the sagittal plane (produced from Z and Y axes). By viewing the heart from two of these planes simultaneously, the VCG machine displays vector loops of the heart's electrical activity on its oscilloscope screen.

Tell the patient that electrodes to which conductive jelly has been applied will be secured to his chest, left leg, back, and nape of the neck or forehead (Frank system). The number and placement of electrodes varies depending on the system selected to be used. Encourage the patient to relax, and instruct him to breathe quietly, avoid talking, and remain still during the test.

Check the patient's history for use of cardioactive drugs, such as antiarrhythmics. If such medications are being administered, note this on the test request form. Just before the test, instruct the patient to put on a hospital gown and to remove any metallic objects above the waist.

Procedure

The patient is placed in supine or sitting position, and the electrodes are secured at the appropriate sites. (Care should be taken not to wrinkle the skin or squeeze the underlying muscles.) The VCG machine is turned on, and the desired number of recordings are obtained. After completing the recordings, the electrodes are removed.

Precautions

None.

Findings

Since the left atrium and left ventricle dominate the electrical field, most vectors represent forces on the left side of the heart. The appearance of the VCG itself may vary with age and sex; the shape of the loops, the spacing of the dashes, and the direction of the arrows have significance in evaluating the heart's electrical activity. Normally, three distinct loops (P, QRS, and T) are present, each representing an event in the cardiac cycle. The chart on pages 902 and 903 depicts the relationship of the VCG to the EKG and the chart on page 901 shows abnormal VCG loops.

Implications of results

Although vectorcardiography requires correlation with patient history, physical examination, and other diagnostic tests, it proves most valuable in evaluating ventricular abnormalities, which are best represented by changes in the prominent QRS loop; this loop can be considered a composite of three or four vectors—each vector signifying an abrupt change in direction. Changes in the direction of each or all vectors help identify ventricular hypertrophy, bundle branch blocks, and MI; however, demonstration of direction changes in the frontal and sagittal planes may be necessary to detect hemiblocks and inferior infarction. In addition, measurement of the angle formed by the T and QRS loops aids diagnosis of myocardial ischemia, ventricular hypertrophy and strain, and metabolic disturbances.

The chart on page 901 shows loop configurations in the horizontal plane, representing common cardiac abnormalities.

Post-test care

Be sure the conductive jelly is removed from the patient's skin.

Interfering factors

□ Cardioactive drugs, such as antiarrhythmics or digitalis glycosides, can alter test results.
□ Incorrect placement of electrodes or excessive patient movement during the test can produce inaccurate results.
□ In patients with a heavy body build, the QRS loop may simulate right ventricular hypertrophy.

ARLENE STRONG, RN, MN

Impedance Plethysmography
[Occlusive impedance phlebography]

Impedance plethysmography—a reliable, widely used, noninvasive test for measuring venous flow in the limbs— aims principally to detect deep vein thrombosis (DVT) in the leg. Electrodes from a plethysmograph are applied to the patient's leg to record changes in electrical resistance (impedance) caused by blood volume variations—the result of respiration or venous occlusion. If a pressure cuff applied to the thigh is inflated to temporarily occlude venous return without interfering with arterial blood flow, blood volume in the calf distal to the cuff normally increases. However, in DVT, blood volume increases less than expected, because the veins are already at capacity and cuff release causes an abnormally slow return of blood volume to physiologic levels.

This test is especially sensitive for DVT in the popliteal and iliofemoral venous systems. It's less sensitive for calf vein clots or partially occlusive thrombi, since these are less likely to cause detectable obstruction in veins below the knee.

Purpose

□ To detect DVT in the proximal deep veins of the leg
□ To screen patients at high risk for thrombophlebitis
□ To evaluate patients with suspected pulmonary embolism (since most pulmonary emboli are complications of DVT in the leg).

Patient preparation

Explain to the patient that this test helps detect DVT. Inform him that he needn't restrict food, fluids, or medications. Tell him the test requires that both legs be tested and that three to five tracings may be made for each leg; who will perform the test and where; and that it takes 30 to 45 minutes. Assure him that the test is painless and safe.

Emphasize that accurate testing requires that leg muscles be relaxed and breathing be normal. Reassure him that if he experiences pain that may interfere with leg relaxation, a mild analgesic will be administered, as ordered.

Just before the test, instruct the patient to void and to put on a hospital gown.

Procedure

The patient is placed in supine position with the leg being tested elevated 30° to 35°, to promote venous drainage (the calf should be above heart level). He is asked to flex his knee slightly and to rotate his hips by shifting weight to the same side as the leg being tested.

After the electrodes (connected to the plethymosgraph) have been loosely attached to the calf, about 3″ to 4″ (7.5 to 10 cm) apart, the pressure cuff (connected to an air pressure system) is wrapped snugly around the thigh—about 2″ (5 cm) above the knee. Then the pressure cuff is inflated with 45 to 60 cm of water, allowing full venous distention without interfering with arterial blood flow. Pressure is maintained for 45 seconds or until the tracing stabilizes. (In a patient with reduced arterial blood flow, pressure is maintained for 2 minutes or longer to permit complete venous filling, then the cuff pressure is rapidly deflated.)

The strip chart tracing, which records the increase in the venous volume following cuff inflation and the decrease in venous volume 3 seconds after deflation, is checked. The test is repeated for the other leg. If necessary, three to five tracings for each leg are obtained to confirm full venous filling and outflow; the tracing showing the greatest rise and fall

in venous volume is used as the test result. If the result is ambiguous, the position of the patient's leg, and cuff and electrode placement are checked.

Precautions

None.

Findings

Temporary venous occlusion normally produces a sharp rise in venous volume; release of the occlusion produces rapid venous outflow. The chart in the color section in this chapter shows a typical normal tracing.

Implications of results

When clots in a major deep vein obstruct venous outflow, the pressure in the distal leg (calf) veins rises, and these veins become distended. Such veins are unable to expand further when additional pressure is applied with an occlusive thigh cuff. Blockage of major deep veins also decreases the rate at which blood flows from the leg. Therefore, if significant thrombi are present in a major deep vein of the lower leg (popliteal, femoral, or iliac), both calf vein filling and venous outflow rate are reduced.

Post-test care

Be sure the conductive jelly is removed from the patient's skin.

Interfering factors

☐ Decreased peripheral arterial blood flow resulting from shock, increased vasoconstriction, low cardiac output, or arterial-tree occlusive disease may interfere with test results.

☐ Extrinsic venous compression, such as from pelvic tumors, large hematomas, or constricting clothing or bandages, may alter test results.

☐ Patient failure to relax leg muscles completely or to breathe normally may interfere with accurate determination of test results.

☐ Coldness of extremities due to environmental factors can interfere with accurate readings.

BARBARA MADIGAN, RN, MSN

ULTRASONOGRAPHY

Echocardiography

This widely used, noninvasive test examines the size, shape, and motion of cardiac structures and is useful for evaluating patients with chest pain, enlarged cardiac silhouettes on X-ray films, electrocardiographic changes unrelated to coronary artery disease, and abnormal heart sounds on auscultation. In echocardiography, a special transducer placed at an acoustic window (an area where bone and lung tissue are absent) on the patient's chest directs ultra–high-frequency sound waves toward cardiac structures, which reflect these waves. The transducer picks up the echoes, converts them to electrical impulses, and relays them to an echocardiography machine for display on an oscilloscope screen and for recording on a strip chart or videotape. Electrocardiography and phonocardiography may be performed simultaneously to time events in the cardiac cycle.

The techniques most commonly used in echocardiography are M-mode (motion-mode) and two-dimensional (cross-sectional). In M-mode echocardiography, a single pencil-like ultrasound beam strikes the heart, producing an ice pick or vertical view of cardiac structures; this method is especially useful for precisely recording the motion and dimensions of intracardiac structures. In two-dimensional echocardiography, the ultrasound beam rapidly sweeps through an arc, producing a cross-sectional or fan-shaped view of cardiac structures; this technique is useful for recording lateral motion and providing the correct spatial relationship between cardiac structures. Often, these techniques complement each other.

Unlike highly standardized tests, such as electrocardiography and cardiac radiography, special skill is needed to per-

form the test and to interpret the results.

Purpose

☐ To diagnose and evaluate valvular abnormalities
☐ To measure the size of the heart's chambers
☐ To evaluate chambers and valves in congenital heart disorders
☐ To aid diagnosis of hypertrophic and related cardiomyopathies
☐ To detect atrial tumors
☐ To evaluate cardiac function or wall motion after myocardial infarction
☐ To detect pericardial effusion.

Patient preparation

Explain to the patient that this test evaluates the size, shape, and motion of various cardiac structures. Inform him that he needn't restrict food or fluids before the test. Tell him who will perform the test and where, and that it usually takes 15 to 30 minutes. Reassure him that the test is safe and painless. Explain that the room may be darkened slightly to aid visualization on the oscilloscope screen, and that other procedures (electrocardiography and phonocardiography) may be performed simultaneously.

Tell the patient that conductive jelly will be applied to his chest and a dime-sized transducer placed directly over it. Since pressure is exerted to keep the transducer in contact with the skin, warn the patient that he may feel a slight discomfort. Explain that the transducer is angled to observe different parts of the heart, and that he may be repositioned on his left side during the procedure.

Inform the patient that he may be asked to breathe in and out slowly, to hold his breath, or to inhale a gas with a slightly sweet odor (amyl nitrite), while changes in heart function are recorded. Describe the possible side effects of amyl nitrite (dizziness, flushing, and tachycardia), but assure the patient that such symptoms quickly subside. Instruct the

REAL-TIME ECHOCARDIOGRAMS

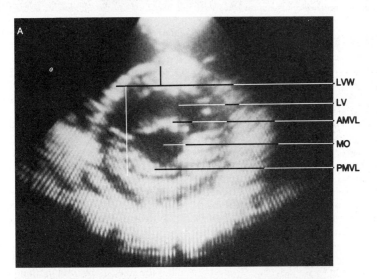

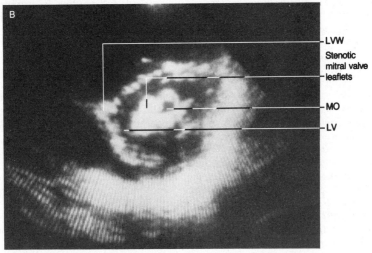

Short-axis cross-sectional mitral valve echocardiograms from a normal patient (A) and a patient with mitral stenosis (B). In the latter, note the greatly reduced mitral valve orifice due to stenotic, calcified valve leaflets.

KEY

LVW	=	Left wall
LV	=	Left ventricle
AMVL	=	Anterior mitral valve leaflet
PMVL	=	Posterior mitral valve leaflet
MO	=	Mitral orifice

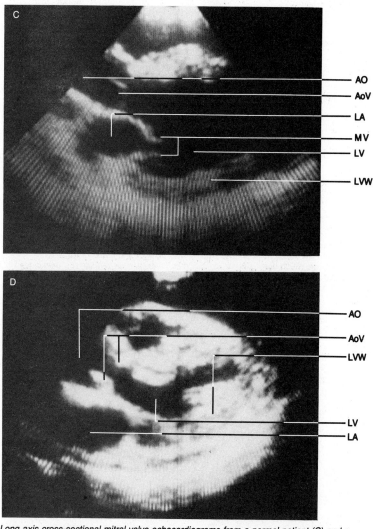

Long axis cross-sectional mitral valve echocardiograms from a normal patient (C) and a patient with idiopathic hypertrophic subaortic stenosis (D). Note the markedly thickened left ventricular wall in the latter.

KEY
    Ao = Aorta
   AoV = Aortic valve
  LVW = Left ventricular wall
    LV = Left ventricle
    LA = Left atrium

M-MODE ECHOCARDIOGRAMS

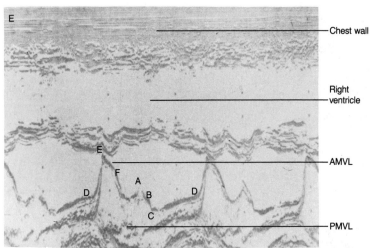

In this normal motion-mode echocardiogram of the mitral valve, valve movement appears as a characteristic lopsided M-shaped tracing. The anterior and posterior mitral valve leaflets separate (D) in early diastole, quickly reach maximum separation (E), then close during rapid ventricular filling (E-F). Leaflet separation varies during mid-diastole, and the valve opens widely again (A) following atrial contraction. The valve starts to close with atrial relaxation (A-B) and is completely closed during the start of ventricular systole (C). The steepness of the slope E-F indirectly shows the speed of ventricular filling, which is normally rapid.

KEY
AMVL = Anterior mitral valve leaflet   **PMVL** = Posterior mitral valve leaflet

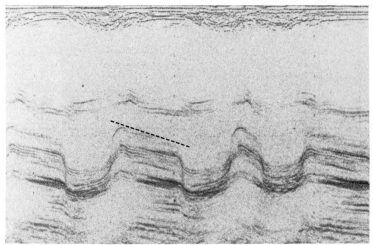

Mitral stenosis is evident in this abnormal echocardiogram. The E-F slope (dashed line) is very shallow, indicating slowed left ventricular filling.

patient to remain still during the test, since movement may distort results.

Procedure

The patient is placed in supine position. Conductive jelly is applied to the third or fourth intercostal space to the left of the sternum, and the transducer is placed directly over it. The transducer is systematically angled to direct ultrasonic waves at specific parts of the patient's heart. During the test, the oscilloscope screen, which displays the returning echoes, is observed; significant oscilloscopic findings are recorded on a strip chart recorder (M-mode echocardiography) or on a videotape recorder (two-dimensional echocardiography).

For a different view of the heart, the transducer is placed beneath the xiphoid process or directly above the sternum. Or for a left lateral view, the patient may be positioned on his left side. To record heart function under various conditions, the patient is asked to inhale and exhale slowly, to hold his breath, or to inhale amyl nitrite.

Precautions

None.

Findings

An echocardiogram can reveal both the motion pattern and structure of the four cardiac valves. Anterior and posterior mitral valve leaflets normally separate in early diastole, with the anterior leaflet moving toward the chest wall and the posterior leaflet moving away from it. The leaflets attain maximum excursion rapidly, then move toward each other during ventricular diastole; after atrial contraction, they come together and remain so during ventricular systole. On an M-mode echocardiogram, the leaflets appear as two fine lines within the echo-free, blood-filled left ventricular cavity.

The aortic valve cusps lie between the parallel walls of the aortic root, which move anteriorly during systole and posteriorly during diastole. During ventricular systole, these cusps separate and appear as a boxlike configuration on an M-mode echocardiogram. They remain open throughout systole and normally demonstrate a characteristic fine fluttering motion. During diastole, the cusps come together and appear as a single or double line within the aortic root on an M-mode echocardiogram.

An echocardiogram can also show the tricuspid and pulmonary valves. The motion of the tricuspid valve resembles that of the mitral valve; the motion of the pulmonary valve—particularly the posterior cusp—is quite different. During diastole, this cusp gradually moves posteriorly; during atrial systole, it's displaced posteriorly; and during ventricular systole, it quickly moves posteriorly. During right ventricular ejection, the cusp moves anteriorly, attaining its most anterior position during diastole.

An echocardiogram can also help evaluate both the left and the right ventricles. The left ventricular cavity normally appears as an echo-free space between the interventricular septum and the posterior left ventricular wall. Echoes produced by the chordae tendineae and the mitral leaflet appear within this cavity. The right ventricular cavity normally appears as an echo-free space between the anterior chest wall and the interventricular septum.

Implications of results

Valvular abnormalities readily appear on the echocardiogram. In mitral stenosis, the valve narrows abnormally due to the leaflets' thickening and disordered motion. Instead of moving in opposite directions during diastole, both mitral valve leaflets move anteriorly. In mitral valve prolapse, one or both leaflets balloon into the left atrium during systole.

Aortic valve abnormalities—especially aortic insufficiency—can also affect the mitral valve, since the anterior mitral leaflet is just below the aortic cusps. When blood regurgitates through the aortic valve during diastole, it strikes this leaflet, causing the flutter seen in M-mode. Although the aortic valve may appear normal, this characteristic flutter-

COMPARING M-MODE AND TWO-DIMENSIONAL ECHOCARDIOGRAPHY

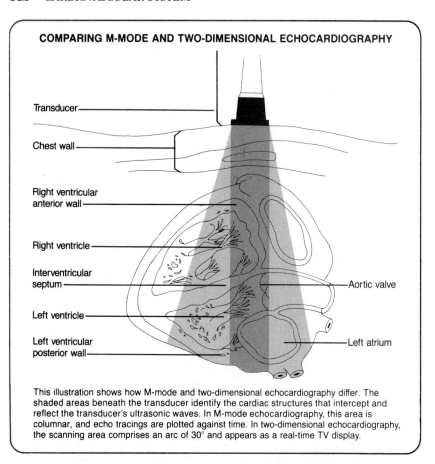

Transducer

Chest wall

Right ventricular anterior wall

Right ventricle

Interventricular septum

Left ventricle

Left ventricular posterior wall

Aortic valve

Left atrium

This illustration shows how M-mode and two-dimensional echocardiography differ. The shaded areas beneath the transducer identify the cardiac structures that intercept and reflect the transducer's ultrasonic waves. In M-mode echocardiography, this area is columnar, and echo tracings are plotted against time. In two-dimensional echocardiography, the scanning area comprises an arc of 30° and appears as a real-time TV display.

ing confirms aortic insufficiency. In stenosis due to conditions such as rheumatic fever or bacterial endocarditis, the aortic valve thickens and thus generates more echoes. However, in rheumatic fever, the valve may thicken slightly and allow normal motion during systole, or it may thicken severely and curtail motion. In bacterial endocarditis, valve motion is disrupted, and shaggy or fuzzy echoes usually appear on or near the valve.

Other chamber or valve abnormalities may indicate a congenital heart disorder, such as aortic stenosis, which may require further tests. A large chamber size may indicate cardiomyopathy, valvular disorders, or congestive heart failure; a small chamber, restrictive pericarditis.

Idiopathic hypertrophic subaortic stenosis can also be identified by the echocardiogram, with systolic anterior motion of the mitral valve and asymmetric septal hypertrophy.

Left atrial tumor is usually on a pedicle, and can thus shift in and out of the mitral opening. During diastole, the tumor appears as a mass of echoes against the anterior mitral valve leaflet; during ventricular systole, these echoes shift back into the body of the atrium.

In coronary artery disease, ischemia or infarction may cause absent or paradoxical motion in ventricular walls that normally move together and thicken during systole. These affected areas may also fail to thicken or may become thinner, particularly if scar tissue is present.

The echocardiogram is especially sensitive in detecting pericardial effusion. Normally, the epicardium and pericardium are continuous membranes, and thus produce a single or near-single echo. When fluid accumulates between these membranes, it causes an abnormal echo-free space to appear. In large effusions, pressure exerted by excess fluid can restrict pericardial motion. An echocardiogram should be correlated with clinical history, physical examination, and results of additional tests.

Post-test care
Remove conductive jelly from the skin.

Interfering factors
☐ Incorrect transducer placement and excess movement interfere with results.
☐ Patients with thick chests, chronic obstructive lung disease, or chest wall abnormalities may be difficult to test.

ARLENE STRONG, RN, MN

Doppler Ultrasonography

This noninvasive test evaluates blood flow in the major veins and arteries of the arms and legs and in the extracranial cerebrovascular system. Developed as an alternative to arteriography and venography, Doppler ultrasonography is safer, less costly, and requires a shorter test period than invasive tests. Although this test has a 95% accuracy rate in detecting arteriovenous disease that significantly impairs blood flow (at least 50%), it may fail to detect mild arteriosclerotic plaques and smaller thrombi, and generally fails to detect major calf vein thrombosis.

In Doppler ultrasonography, a hand-held transducer directs high-frequency sound waves to the artery or vein being tested. The sound waves strike moving RBCs and are reflected back to the transducer at frequencies that correspond to the velocity of blood flow through the vessel. The transducer then amplifies the sound waves to permit direct listening and graphic recording of blood flow.

Measurement of systolic pressure during this test helps detect the presence, location, and extent of peripheral arterial occlusive disease. Observation of changes in sound wave frequency during respiration helps detect venous occlusive disease, since venous blood flow normally fluctuates with respiration. Use of compression maneuvers also helps detect occlusion of the veins as well as occlusion or stenosis of carotid arteries.

Pulse volume recorder (PVR) testing may be performed along with Doppler ultrasonography to yield a quantitative recording of changes in blood volume or flow in an extremity or organ.

Purpose
☐ To aid diagnosis of chronic venous insufficiency, and superficial and deep vein thromboses (popliteal, femoral, iliac)
☐ To aid diagnosis of peripheral artery disease and arterial occlusion
☐ To monitor patients who have had arterial reconstruction and bypass grafts
☐ To detect abnormalities of carotid artery blood flow associated with such conditions as aortic stenosis
☐ To evaluate possible arterial trauma.

Patient preparation
Explain that this test helps evaluate blood flow in the arms and legs or neck. Tell the patient who will perform the test and that it takes about 20 minutes.

Reassure the patient that the test doesn't involve risk or discomfort. Tell him he'll be asked to move his arms to different positions and to perform breathing exercises as measurements are taken, to vary blood flow during the exam. Check with the vascular laboratory to determine if special equipment will be used and if special instructions are necessary. Explain that a small ultrasonic probe resembling a microphone is placed at various sites along specific veins and/or arteries, and that blood pressure is checked at several sites.

Procedure

Water-soluble conductive jelly is applied to the tip of the transducer to provide coupling between the skin and the transducer.

For *peripheral arterial evaluation,* always performed bilaterally, the usual test sites in the leg include the common femoral, superficial femoral, popliteal, posterior tibial, and dorsalis pedis arteries; in the arm, the subclavian, brachial, radial, ulnar, and occasionally, the palmar arch and digital arteries.

The patient is instructed to remove all clothing above or below the waist, de-

pending on the test site. After he is placed in supine position on the examining table or bed, with his arms at his sides, brachial blood pressure is measured, and the transducer is placed at various points along the test arteries. The signals are monitored and the waveforms recorded for later analysis.

Segmental limb blood pressure is obtained to localize arterial occlusive disease. For lower extremity tests, a blood pressure cuff is wrapped around the calf, pressure readings are obtained, and waveforms recorded from the dorsalis pedis and posterior tibial arteries. Then, the cuff is wrapped around the thigh, and waveforms are recorded at the popliteal artery. For upper extremity tests,

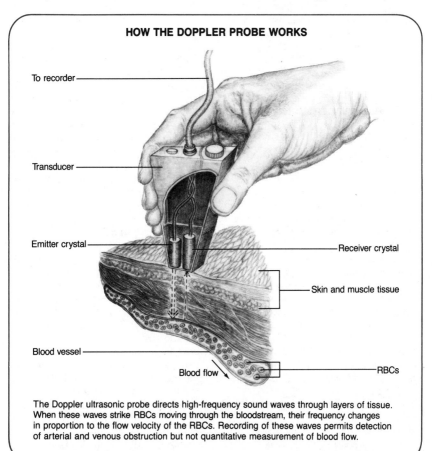

HOW THE DOPPLER PROBE WORKS

To recorder

Transducer

Emitter crystal — Receiver crystal

— Skin and muscle tissue

Blood vessel

Blood flow — RBCs

The Doppler ultrasonic probe directs high-frequency sound waves through layers of tissue. When these waves strike RBCs moving through the bloodstream, their frequency changes in proportion to the flow velocity of the RBCs. Recording of these waves permits detection of arterial and venous obstruction but not quantitative measurement of blood flow.

a blood pressure cuff is wrapped around the forearm, and pressure readings are taken, and waveforms recorded over both the radial and the ulnar arteries. Then, the cuff is wrapped around the upper arm, pressure readings are taken, and waveforms are recorded with the transducer over the brachial artery.

Blood pressure readings and waveform recordings are repeated with the arm in extreme hyperextension and hyperabduction to check for possible compression factors that may interfere with arterial blood flow. The upper extremity examination is performed on one arm, with the patient first supine, then sitting; it's then repeated on the other arm.

For *peripheral venous evaluation,* usual test sites in the leg include the popliteal, superficial femoral, and common femoral veins, and the posterior tibial vein at the ankle; in the arm, the brachial, axillary, subclavian, and jugular veins, and occasionally, the inferior and superior vena cava.

The patient is instructed to remove all clothing above or below the waist, depending on the test site. He is placed in supine position and instructed to breathe normally. The transducer is placed over the appropriate vein, waveforms are recorded, and respiratory modulations noted.

Proximal limb compression maneuvers are performed and augmentation noted after release of compression, to evaluate venous valve competency. Changes in respiration are monitored. For lower extremity tests, the patient is asked to perform a Valsalva's maneuver, and venous blood flow is recorded. The procedure is repeated for the other arm or leg.

For *extracranial cerebrovascular evaluation,* usual test sites include the supraorbital, common carotid, external carotid, internal carotid, and vertebral arteries.

The patient is placed in supine position on the examining table or bed, with a pillow beneath his head for support. Brachial blood pressure is then recorded, using the Doppler probe. Next,

the transducer is positioned over the test artery, and blood flow velocity is monitored and recorded. The influence of compression maneuvers on blood flow velocity is measured, and the procedure is repeated on the opposite side.

Precautions
Don't place the Doppler probe over an open or draining lesion.

Findings
Arterial waveforms of the arms and legs are multiphasic, with a prominent systolic component and one or more diastolic sounds. The ankle-arm pressure index (API)—the ratio between ankle systolic pressure and brachial systolic pressure—is normally equal to or greater than 1. (The API is also known as arterial ischemia index, the ankle/brachial index, or the pedal/brachial index.) Proximal thigh pressure is normally 20 to 30 mmHg higher than arm pressure, but pressure measurements at adjacent sites are similar. In the arms, pressure readings should remain unchanged despite postural changes.

Venous blood flow velocity is normally phasic with respiration, and is of a lower pitch than arterial flow. Distal compression or release of proximal limb compression increases blood flow velocity. In the legs, abdominal compression eliminates respiratory variations, but release increases blood flow; a Valsalva's maneuver also interrupts venous flow velocity.

In cerebrovascular testing, a strong velocity signal is present. In the common carotid artery, blood flow velocity increases during diastole, due to low peripheral vascular resistance of the brain. The direction of periorbital arterial flow is normally anterograde out of the orbit.

Implications of results
Arterial stenosis or occlusion diminishes the blood flow velocity signal, with no diastolic sound and a less prominent systolic component distal to the lesion. At the lesion, the signal is high-pitched and, occasionally, turbulent. If complete oc-

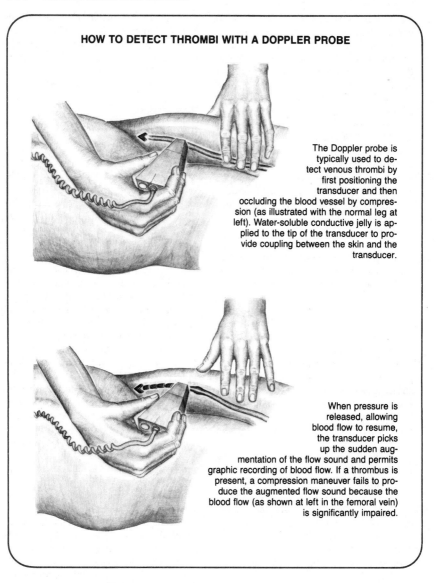

HOW TO DETECT THROMBI WITH A DOPPLER PROBE

The Doppler probe is typically used to detect venous thrombi by first positioning the transducer and then occluding the blood vessel by compression (as illustrated with the normal leg at left). Water-soluble conductive jelly is applied to the tip of the transducer to provide coupling between the skin and the transducer.

When pressure is released, allowing blood flow to resume, the transducer picks up the sudden augmentation of the flow sound and permits graphic recording of blood flow. If a thrombus is present, a compression maneuver fails to produce the augmented flow sound because the blood flow (as shown at left in the femoral vein) is significantly impaired.

clusion is present and collateral circulation has not taken over, the velocity signal may be absent.

A pressure gradient exceeding 20 to 30 mmHg at adjacent sites of measurement in the leg may indicate occlusive disease. Specifically, low proximal thigh pressure signifies common femoral or aorto-iliac occlusive disease. An abnormal gradient between the proximal thigh and the above- or below-knee cuffs indicates superficial femoral or popliteal artery occlusive disease; an abnormal gradient between the below-knee and ankle cuffs, tibiofibular disease. Abnormal gradients of arm and forearm pressure readings may indicate brachial artery occlusion.

An abnormal API is directly proportional to the degree of circulatory impairment: mild ischemia, 1 to 0.75; claudication, 0.75 to 0.50; pain at rest, 0.50 to 0.25; and pregangrene, 0.25 to 0.

If venous blood flow velocity is unchanged by respirations, doesn't increase in response to compression or Valsalva's maneuvers, or is absent, venous thrombosis is indicated. In chronic venous insufficiency and varicose veins, the flow velocity signal may be reversed. Confirmation of results may require venography.

Inability to identify Doppler signals during cerebrovascular examination implies total arterial occlusion. Reversed periorbital arterial flow indicates significant arterial occlusive disease of the extracranial internal carotid artery; in addition, the audible signal may take on the acoustic characteristics of a normal peripheral artery. Stenosis of the internal carotid artery causes turbulent signals. Collateral circulation can be assessed by compression maneuvers.

Oculoplethysmography, carotid phonoangiography, or carotid imaging can further evaluate cerebrovascular disease. Retrograde blood velocity in the vertebral artery can indicate subclavian steal syndrome. Weak velocity signal on comparison of contralateral vertebral arteries can indicate diffuse vertebral artery disease.

Post-test care
Be sure the conductive jelly is removed from the patient's skin.

Interfering factors
If the patient is uncooperative, test results may be invalid.

NANCY L. MAULDIN, RN

Ultrasonography of the Abdominal Aorta

In this safe, noninvasive test, a transducer directs high-frequency sound waves into the abdomen over a wide area from the xiphoid process to the umbilical region. The sound waves, echoing to the transducer from interfaces between tissue of different densities (acoustic interfaces), are transmitted as electrical impulses and displayed on an oscilloscope or television screen, to reveal internal organs, the vertebral column, and, most importantly, the size and course of the abdominal aorta and other major vessels.

Ultrasonography helps confirm a suspected aortic aneurysm and is the method of choice for determining its diameter. Several scans may be performed to detect expansion of a known aneurysm, because the risk of rupture is highest when aneurysmal diameter is 7 cm or greater. However, angiography is indicated preoperatively to visualize the extent of atherosclerotic changes and to discover anatomic anomalies, such as three renal arteries. It's also indicated when diagnosis is unclear. Once an aneurysm is detected, ultrasonography is used every six months to monitor changes in patient status.

Purpose
□ To detect and measure suspected abdominal aortic aneurysm
□ To measure and detect expansion of known abdominal aortic aneurysm.

Patient preparation
Explain to the patient that this test allows examination of the abdominal aorta. Instruct him to fast for 12 hours before the test, to minimize bowel gas and motility. Tell him who will perform the test and where, that the room light may be reduced to improve visualization, and that the test takes 30 to 45 minutes.

Tell the patient that mineral oil or a gel will be applied to his abdomen and will feel cool. Explain that a transducer will pass over his skin, from the costal margins to the umbilicus or slightly below, directing inaudible sound waves into the abdominal vessels and organs. Assure him that this is safe and painless but that he will feel slight pressure. If he

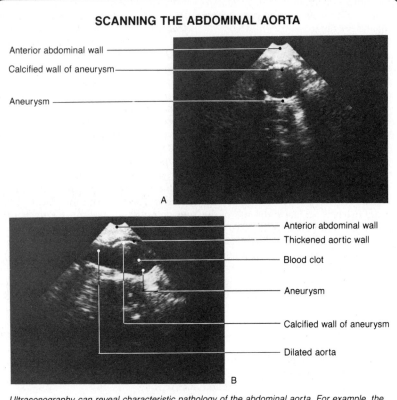

SCANNING THE ABDOMINAL AORTA

Anterior abdominal wall

Calcified wall of aneurysm

Aneurysm

A

Anterior abdominal wall

Thickened aortic wall

Blood clot

Aneurysm

Calcified wall of aneurysm

Dilated aorta

B

Ultrasonography can reveal characteristic pathology of the abdominal aorta. For example, the cross-sectional view of one patient (A) reveals calcification at the aneurysm site. The longitudinal view of another patient (B) reveals a thickened aortic wall as well as calcification. A blood clot appears in the aneurysm, and the aorta is slightly dilated.

has a known aneurysm, reassure him that the sound waves will not cause it to rupture. Instruct him to remain still during scanning and to hold his breath when requested.

If ordered, give simethicone to reduce bowel gas. Just before the test, instruct the patient to put on a hospital gown.

Procedure
The patient is placed in a supine position, and acoustic coupling gel or mineral oil is applied to his abdomen. Longitudinal scans are made at 0.5- to 1-cm intervals left and right of the midline until the entire abdominal aorta is outlined. Transverse scans are made at 1- to 2-cm intervals from the xiphoid to the bifurcation at the common iliac arteries. The patient may be placed in right and left lateral positions. Appropriate views are photographed or videotaped.

Precautions
None.

Findings
In adults, the normal abdominal aorta tapers from about 2.5 to 1.5 cm in diameter along its length from the diaphragm to the bifurcation. It descends through the retroperitoneal space, anterior to the vertebral column and slightly left of the midline. Four of its major branches are usually well visualized: the celiac trunk, the renal arteries, the su-

perior mesenteric artery, and the common iliac arteries.

Implications of results
Luminal diameter of the abdominal aorta greater than 4 cm is aneurysmal; over 7 cm, aneurysmal with high risk of rupture.

Post-test care
☐ Remove the acoustic coupling gel from the patient's skin.
☐ Instruct the patient to resume his usual diet and medications.

☐ Aneurysms may expand and dissect rapidly, so check the patient's vital signs frequently. Remember that sudden onset of constant ab-

dominal or back pain accompanies rapid expansion of the aneurysm; sudden, excrutiating pain with weakness, sweating, tachycardia, and hypotension signals rupture.

Interfering factors
☐ Bowel gas and motility, excessive body movement, surgical wounds, and severe dyspnea may prevent adequate imaging.
☐ Residual barium from gastrointestinal contrast studies within the past 24 hours and air introduced during endoscopy within the past 12 to 24 hours hinder ultrasound transmission.
☐ In obese patients, mesenteric fat may impair transmission of ultrasound waves during testing.

PATRICIA L. BAUM, RN, BSN

NUCLEAR MEDICINE

Technetium Pyrophosphate Scanning

[Hot spot myocardial imaging, infarct avid imaging]

Technetium pyrophosphate scanning is used to detect recent myocardial infarction (MI) and to determine its extent. In this test, an I.V. tracer isotope (technetium-99m pyrophosphate) accumulates in damaged myocardial tissue (possibly by combining with calcium in the damaged myocardial cells), where it forms a hot spot on a scan made with a scintillation camera. Such hot spots first appear within 12 hours of infarction, are most apparent after 48 to 72 hours, and usually disappear after 1 week. Hot spots that persist longer than 1 week usually suggest ongoing myocardial damage.

This test is most useful for confirming recent MI in patients suffering from obscure cardiac pain (postoperative car-

diac patients), when electrocardiograms (EKGs) are equivocal (as with left bundle-branch block or old myocardial scars, for example) or when serum enzyme tests are unreliable.

Purpose
☐ To confirm recent MI
☐ To define the size and location of a recent MI
☐ To assess prognosis after acute MI.

Patient preparation
Explain to the patient that this test helps determine if any areas of the heart muscle are injured. Inform him that he needn't restrict food or fluids. Tell him who will perform the test and where, and that it takes 30 to 60 minutes.

Inform the patient that he'll receive a tracer isotope I.V. 2 or 3 hours before the procedure, and that multiple images of his heart will be made. Reassure him that the injection causes only transient discomfort, that the scan itself is painless, and that the test involves less exposure to radiation than chest radiography. Instruct him to remain quiet and motionless while he's being scanned,

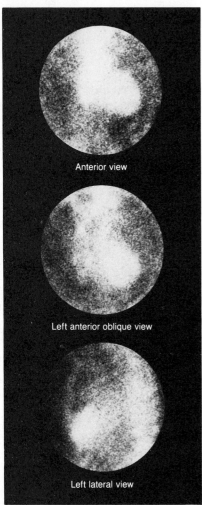

Anterior view

Left anterior oblique view

Left lateral view

In this case of acute anterior myocardial infarction, newly damaged heart tissue collects technetium pyrophosphate and thus appears bright, or "hot," on the scan.

but assure him that he can talk and move about between views.

Make sure the patient or responsible member of the family has signed a consent form.

Procedure
Usually, 20 mCi of technetium-99m pyrophosphate are injected into the antecubital vein. After 2 or 3 hours, the patient is placed in supine position, and electrocardiography electrodes are attached for continuous monitoring during the test. Generally, scans are taken with the patient in several positions, including anterior, left anterior oblique, right anterior oblique and left lateral. Each scan takes 10 minutes.

Precautions
None.

Findings
A normal technetium scan shows no accumulation of the isotope in the myocardium.

Implications of results
The isotope is taken up by the sternum and ribs, and the activity of these is compared with that in the heart; 2^+, 3^+, and 4^+ activity (equal to or greater than bone) indicate a positive myocardial scan. The technetium scan can reveal areas of isotope accumulation, or hot spots, in damaged myocardium, particularly 48 to 72 hours after onset of acute MI; however, hot spots are apparent as early as 12 hours after acute MI. In most patients with MI, hot spots disappear after 1 week; in some, they persist for several months if necrosis continues in the area of infarction. Knowing where the infarct is located makes it possible to anticipate complications and to plan patient care. About one fourth of patients with unstable angina pectoris show hot spots due to subclinical myocardial necrosis, and may require coronary arteriography and bypass grafting.

Post-test care
None.

Interfering factors
In about 10% of patients studied with technetium pyrophosphate scanning, isotope accumulations may result from ventricular aneurysm associated with dystrophic calcification, pulmonary neoplasm, recent cardioversion, and from valvular heart disease associated with severe calcification.

BARBARA BOYD EGOVILLE, RN, MSN

Thallium Imaging

[Cold spot myocardial imaging, thallium scintigraphy]

This test evaluates myocardial blood flow after I.V. injection of the radioisotope thallium-201 (thallous chloride Tl 201, or $^{201}TlCl$). Thallium, the physiologic analogue of potassium, concentrates in healthy myocardial tissue but not in necrotic or ischemic tissue. Hence, areas of the heart with normal blood supply and intact cells rapidly take up the isotope; areas with poor blood flow and ischemic cells fail to take up the isotope and appear as cold spots on a scan.

This test is performed in a resting state or after stress (treadmill exercise). Resting imaging can detect acute myocardial infarction (MI) within the first few hours of symptoms but does not distinguish an old from a new infarct. Stress imaging, performed after the patient exercises on a treadmill until he experiences angina or rate-limiting fatigue, can assess known or suspected coronary artery disease and can evaluate the effectiveness of antianginal therapy or balloon angioplasty and the patency of grafts after coronary artery bypass surgery. Complications of stress testing include arrhythmias, angina pectoris, and MI.

Purpose
☐ To assess myocardial scarring and perfusion
☐ To demonstrate the location and extent of acute or chronic MI, including transmural and postoperative infarction (resting imaging)
☐ To diagnose coronary artery disease (stress imaging)
☐ To evaluate the patency of grafts after coronary artery bypass surgery
☐ To evaluate the effectiveness of antianginal therapy or balloon angioplasty (stress imaging).

Patient preparation
Explain to the patient that these tests help determine if any areas of the heart muscle aren't receiving an adequate supply of blood. For stress imaging, instruct him to restrict alcohol, tobacco, and unprescribed medications for 24 hours before the test, and to have nothing by mouth for 3 hours before the test (he may eat a light meal earlier). Tell him who will perform the test and where; that initial testing takes 45 to 90 minutes; and that additional scans may be required.

Tell the patient he will receive a radioactive tracer I.V., and that multiple images of his heart will be scanned. Warn him that he may experience discomfort from skin abrasion during preparation for electrode placement. Reassure him that there is no known radiation danger from the isotope.

Make sure the patient or responsible member of the family has signed a consent form. For stress imaging, instruct the patient to wear walking shoes during the treadmill exercise and to report fatigue, pain, or shortness of breath immediately.

Procedure
Stress imaging: The patient, wired with electrodes, walks on a treadmill at a regulated pace that's gradually increased, while the electrocardiogram (EKG), blood pressure, and heart rate are monitored. When the patient reaches peak stress, the examiner injects 1.5 to 3 mCi of thallium into the antecubital vein and flushes it with 10 to 15 ml of normal saline solution. The patient exercises an additional 45 to 60 seconds to permit circulation and uptake of the isotope, then lies on his back under the scintillation camera. If the patient is asymptomatic, the precordial leads are removed. Scanning begins after 3 to 5 minutes with the patient in anterior, 45° and 60° left anterior oblique, and left lateral positions. Additional scans may be taken after the patient rests 3 to 6 hours.

Resting imaging: Within the first few hours of symptoms of MI, the patient receives an injection of thallium I.V. Scan-

THALLIUM SCANS OF THE HEART

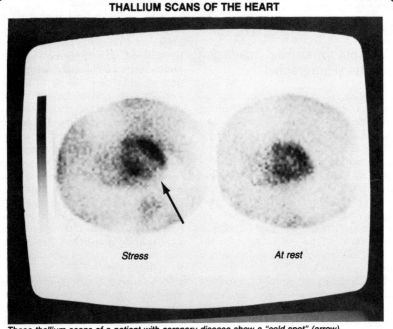

Stress   At rest

These thallium scans of a patient with coronary disease show a "cold spot" (arrow), indicating stress-induced ischemia after treadmill exercise. The scan at right shows the same heart at rest after the test; the spot has disappeared.

ning begins after 3 to 5 minutes, with the patient positioned as above.

Precautions
□ Contraindications to stress imaging include impaired neuromuscular function, pregnancy, locomotor disturbances, acute MI and myocarditis, aortic stenosis, acute infection, unstable metabolic conditions (such as diabetes), digitalis toxicity, and recent pulmonary infarction.

 □ Stress imaging is stopped at once if the patient develops chest pain, dyspnea, fatigue, syncope, hypotension, ischemic EKG changes, significant arrhythmias, or critical signs (pallor, clammy skin, confusion, or staggering gait).

Findings
Imaging should reveal characteristic

distribution of the isotope throughout the left ventricle and no visible defects (cold spots).

Implications of results
Persistent defects generally indicate MI; transient defects (present during peak exercise but not after 3- to 6-hour rest) usually indicate ischemia from coronary artery disease. After coronary artery bypass surgery, improved regional perfusion suggests patency of the graft. Increased perfusion after ingestion of antianginal drugs can demonstrate their effectiveness in relieving ischemia. Improved perfusion after balloon angioplasty suggests increased coronary flow.

Post-test care
If the patient must return for further scanning, tell him to rest in the interim. Restrict his diet to clear liquids before redistribution studies.

Interfering factors

□ Cold spots—although usually due to coronary artery disease—may result from sarcoidosis, myocardial fibrosis, cardiac contusion, attenuation due to soft tissue and artifacts (for example, diaphragm, breast, implants, electrodes), apical cleft, and coronary spasm.

□ Absence of cold spots in the presence of coronary artery disease may result from insignificant obstruction, inadequate stress, delayed imaging, single-vessel disease (particularly the right or left circumflex coronary arteries), and collateral circulation.

PAULA BRAMMER VETTER, RN, BSN, CCRN

Cardiac Blood Pool Imaging

Cardiac blood pool imaging evaluates regional and global ventricular performance after I.V. injection of human serum albumin or RBCs tagged with the isotope technetium-99m (^{99m}Tc) pertechnetate. In first-pass imaging, a scintillation camera records the radioactivity emitted by the isotope in its initial pass through the left ventricle. Higher counts of radioactivity occur during diastole because there is more blood in the ventricle; lower counts occur during systole as the blood is ejected. The portion of isotope ejected during each heartbeat can then be calculated to determine the ejection fraction; the presence and size of intracardiac shunts can also be determined.

Gated cardiac blood pool imaging, performed after first-pass imaging or as a separate test, has several forms; however, most use signals from an electrocardiogram (EKG) to trigger the scintillation camera. In two-frame gated imaging, the camera records left ventricular end-systole and end-diastole for 500 to 1,000 cardiac cycles; superimposition of these gated images allows assessment of left ventricular contraction

to find areas of dyskinesia or akinesia. In multiple-gated acquisition (MUGA) scanning, the camera records 14 to 64 points of a single cardiac cycle, yielding sequential images that can be studied like motion picture films to evaluate regional wall motion and determine the ejection fraction and other indices of cardiac function. In the stress MUGA test, the same test is performed at rest and after exercise to detect changes in ejection fraction and cardiac output. In the nitro MUGA test, the scintillation camera records points in the cardiac cycle after the sublingual administration of nitroglycerin, to assess its effect on ventricular function.

Blood pool imaging is more accurate and involves less risk to the patient than left ventriculography in assessing cardiac function.

Purpose

□ To evaluate left ventricular function

□ To detect aneurysms of the left ventricle and other myocardial wall-motion abnormalities (areas of akinesia or dyskinesia)

□ To detect intracardiac shunting.

Patient preparation

Explain to the patient that this test permits assessment of the heart's left ventricle. Advise him he needn't restrict food or fluids. Tell him who will perform the test and where; that he will receive an I.V. injection of a radioactive tracer; and that a detector positioned above his chest will record the circulation of this tracer through the heart. Reassure him that the tracer poses no radiation hazard and rarely produces side effects. Inform him that he may experience transient discomfort from the needle puncture, but that the imaging itself is painless. Instruct him to remain silent and motionless during imaging, unless otherwise instructed. Make sure the patient or responsible family member has signed a consent form.

Procedure

The patient is placed in supine position

beneath the detector of a scintillation camera, and 15 to 20 mCi of albumin or RBCs tagged with technetium-99m pertechnetate are injected. For the next minute, the scintillation camera records the first pass of the isotope through the heart, for subsequent localization of the aortic and mitral valves. Then, using an EKG, the camera is gated for selected 60-millisecond intervals, representing end-systole and end-diastole, and 500 to 1,000 cardiac cycles are recorded on X-ray or Polaroid film. To observe septal and posterior wall motion, the patient may be assisted to modified left anterior oblique position; or he may be assisted to right anterior oblique position and given 0.4 mg of nitroglycerin sublingually. The scintillation camera then records additional gated images to evaluate abnormal contraction in the left ventricle.

The patient may be asked to exercise as the scintillation camera records gated images.

Precautions
Cardiac blood pool imaging is contraindicated during pregnancy.

Findings
Normally, the left ventricle contracts symmetrically, and the isotope appears evenly distributed in the scans. The normal ejection fraction is 55% to 65%.

Implications of results
Patients with coronary artery disease usually have asymmetric blood distribution to the myocardium, which produces segmental abnormalities of ventricular wall motion; such abnormalities may also result from preexisting conditions, such as myocarditis. In contrast, patients with cardiomyopathies show globally reduced ejection fractions. In patients with left-to-right shunts, the recirculating radioisotope prolongs the downslope of the curve of scintigraphic data; early arrival of activity in the left ventricle or aorta signifies a right-to-left shunt.

Post-test care
None.

Interfering factors
None.

BARBARA BOYD EGOVILLE, RN, MSN

CATHETERIZATION

Cardiac Catheterization

Simply stated, cardiac catheterization is the passing of a catheter into the right or the left side of the heart. Catheterization can determine blood pressure and blood flow in the chambers of the heart, permit collection of blood samples, or record films of the heart's ventricles (contrast ventriculography) or arteries (coronary arteriography or angiography).

In left heart catheterization, a catheter is inserted into an artery in the antecubital fossa or into the femoral artery through a puncture or cutdown procedure and, guided by fluoroscopy, the catheter is advanced retrograde through the aorta into the coronary artery orifices and/or left ventricle. Then, injection of a contrast medium into the ventricle permits radiographic visualization of the ventricle and the coronary arteries, and filming (cineangiography) of heart activity. Left heart catheterization assesses the patency of the coronary arteries, mitral and aortic valve function, and left ventricular function; it aids diagnosis of left ventricular enlargement, aortic stenosis and regurgitation, aortic root enlargement, mitral regurgitation, aneurysm and intracardiac shunt.

In right heart catheterization, the

RIGHT AND LEFT HEART CATHETERIZATION

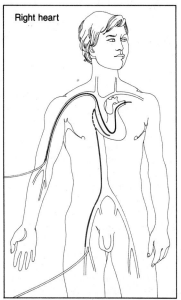

Right heart

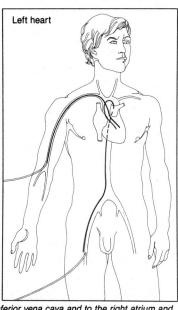

Left heart

The catheter is inserted through veins to the inferior vena cava and to the right atrium and ventricle for right-side catheterization, and through arteries to the aorta and into the coronary artery orifices and/or left ventricle for left-side catheterization. Note that both approaches use the antecubital and femoral vessels.

catheter is inserted into an antecubital vein or into the femoral vein and advanced through the inferior vena cava or right atrium into the right side of the heart, and into the pulmonary artery. Right heart catheterization assesses tricuspid and pulmonary valve function and pulmonary artery pressures.

Catheterization permits blood pressure measurement in the heart chambers to determine valve competency and cardiac wall contractility, and to detect intracardiac shunts. If thermodilution catheters are used, it allows calculation of cardiac output.

Purpose

☐ To evaluate valvular insufficiency or stenosis, septal defects, congenital anomalies, myocardial function and blood supply—and cardiac wall motion.

Patient preparation

Explain to the patient that this test evaluates the function of the heart and its vessels. Instruct him to restrict food and fluids for at least 6 hours before the test. Tell him who will perform the test and where, and that it takes 2 to 3 hours. Inform him that he may receive a mild sedative, but will remain conscious during the procedure.

Inform the patient he'll be strapped to a padded table, and the table may be tilted so his heart can be examined from different angles. Warn the patient that the catheterization team wears gloves, masks, and gowns to protect him from infection, and that the changing X-ray plates and advancing film make a clacking noise. Inform him that he will have an I.V. needle inserted in his arm to allow administration of medication. As-

NORMAL PRESSURE CURVES

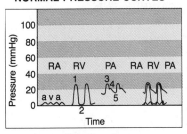

RIGHT HEART CHAMBERS
Two pressure complexes are represented for each chamber. Complexes at far right in this diagram represent simultaneous recordings of pressures from the right atrium, right ventricle, and pulmonary artery. The numbered tracings are: 1, RV peak systolic pressure; 2, RV end-diastolic pressure; 3, PA peak systolic pressure; 4, PA dicrotic notch; 5, PA diastolic pressure.

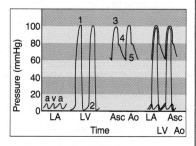

LEFT HEART CHAMBERS
Overall pressure configurations are similar to those of the right heart, but left heart pressures are significantly higher, because systemic flow resistance is much greater than pulmonary resistance.

KEY

PA	= Pulmonary artery
RV	= Right ventricle
RA	= Right atrium
a wave	= Contraction
v wave	= Passive filling
LV	= Left ventricle
LA	= Left atrium
Asc Ao	= Ascending aorta

From H. Kasparian et al., "Interpreting Cardiac Catheterization Data," *Postgraduate Medicine,* 57:4:66 (April 1975).

sure him the electrocardiography electrodes attached to his chest during the procedure cause no discomfort.

Tell the patient that the catheter is inserted into an artery or vein in his arm or leg and if the skin above the vessel is hairy, it will be shaved and cleansed with an antiseptic. Tell him he'll experience a transient stinging sensation when a local anesthetic is injected to numb the incision site for catheter insertion, and he may feel pressure as the catheter moves along the blood vessel; assure him these sensations are normal. Inform him that injection of a contrast medium through the catheter may produce a hot, flushing sensation or nausea that quickly passes; instruct him to follow directions to cough or breathe deeply. Tell him that he'll be given medication if he experiences chest pain during the procedure and may also receive nitroglycerin periodically to dilate coronary vessels and aid visualization. Assure him complications, such as myocardial infarction (MI) or thromboemboli, are rare.

Make sure the patient or responsible member of the family has signed a consent form. Check patient hypersensitivity to shellfish, iodine, or the contrast media used in other diagnostic tests; notify the doctor if such hypersensitivities exist. If the patient's scheduled for right heart catheterization, discontinue any anticoagulant therapy, as ordered, to reduce the risk of complications from venous bleeding. If he's scheduled for left heart catheterization, begin or continue anticoagulant therapy, as ordered, to reduce the risk of arterial catheter-tip clotting. Just before the procedure, tell the patient to void and put on a hospital gown.

Procedure

The patient is placed in supine position on a tilt-top table and secured by restraints. Electrocardiogram (EKG) leads are applied for continuous monitoring and an I.V. line, if not already in place, is started, with 5% dextrose in water or normal saline solution at keep-vein-open (K.V.O.) rate. After the local anesthetic is injected at the catheterization site, a small incision or percutaneous puncture is made into the artery or vein, depending on whether left-side or right-side studies are to be performed, and the catheter is passed through the needle into the vessel; the catheter is guided to the cardiac chambers or coronary arteries using fluoroscopy. When the catheter is in place, the contrast medium is injected through it to visualize the cardiac vessels and structures.

The patient may be asked to cough or breathe deeply. Coughing helps counteract nausea or light-headedness caused by the contrast medium and can correct arrhythmias produced by its depressant effect on the myocardium; deep breathing can ease catheter placement into the pulmonary artery or the wedge position and moves the diaphragm downward, making the heart easier to visualize. During the procedure, the patient may be given nitroglycerin to eliminate catheter-induced spasm or measure its effect on the coronary arteries. Ergonovine maleate, a vasoconstrictor, may be administered to provoke coronary artery spasm (a risky but valuable test in Prinzmetal's angina).

The heart rate and rhythm, respiration, pulse rate, and blood pressure are monitored frequently during the procedure. After completing the procedure, the catheter is removed and a pressure dressing is applied to the incision site.

Precautions
□ Coagulopathy, poor renal function, or debilitation usually contraindicates both left and right heart catheterization. Unless a temporary pacemaker is inserted to counteract induced ventricular asystole, left bundle branch block contraindicates right heart catheterization. Acute MI once contraindicated left-heart catheterization. Now, many doctors perform catheterization and surgically bypass blocked vessels during acute ischemic episodes to prevent myocardial necrosis.
□ If the patient has valvular heart disease, prophylactic antibiotic therapy

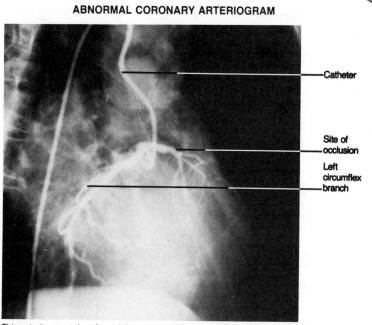

ABNORMAL CORONARY ARTERIOGRAM

Catheter

Site of occlusion

Left circumflex branch

This arteriogram taken from right anterior oblique position shows occlusion of the left anterior descending artery.

COMPLICATIONS OF CARDIAC CATHETERIZATION

Because cardiac catheterization is an invasive test usually done on high-risk patients, it imposes more patient risk than most other diagnostic tests. Although the incidence of such complications is low, they are potentially life-threatening and require careful observation during the procedure.

Keep in mind that some complications are common to *both* left-heart and right-heart catheterization; others result only from catheterization of one side. In either case, complications require that you notify the doctor and carefully document the complication and its treatment.

LEFT- OR RIGHT-SIDE CATHETERIZATION

COMPLICATION	SIGNS AND SYMPTOMS	NURSING CONSIDERATIONS
Myocardial infarction *Possible causes:* • Emotional stress induced by procedure • Blood clot dislodged by catheter tip travels to a coronary artery (left-side catheterization only) • Air embolism	• Chest pain, possibly radiating to left arm, back, and/or jaw • Cardiac arrhythmias • Diaphoresis, restlessness, and/or anxiety • Thready pulse • Fever • Peripheral cyanosis, causing cool skin	• Keep resuscitation equipment available. • Give oxygen or other drugs, as ordered. • Monitor patient continuously, as ordered.
Arrhythmias *Possible cause:* • Cardiac tissue irritated by catheter	• Irregular heartbeat • Irregular apical pulse • Palpitations	• Monitor patient continuously, as ordered. • Administer antiarrhythmic drugs, if ordered.
Cardiac tamponade *Possible cause:* • Perforation of heart wall by catheter	• Sudden shock • Arrhythmias • Increased heart rate • Decreased blood pressure • Chest pain • Diaphoresis and cyanosis • Distant heart sounds	• Give oxygen, if ordered. • Prepare patient for emergency surgery, if ordered. • Monitor patient continuously, as ordered. • Keep emergency equipment available.
Infection (systemic) *Possible causes:* • Poor aseptic technique • Catheter contaminated during manufacture, storage, or use	• Fever • Increased pulse rate • Chills and tremors • Unstable blood pressure	• Collect urine, sputum, and blood samples for culture, as ordered. • Monitor vital signs.
Hypovolemia *Possible cause:* • Diuresis from angiography contrast medium	• Increased urinary output • Hypotension	• Replace fluids by giving patient 1 or 2 glasses of water every hour, or maintain I.V. at a rate of 150 to 200 ml/hr, as ordered. • Monitor fluid intake and output closely. • Monitor vital signs.

COMPLICATIONS OF CARDIAC CATHETERIZATION (continued)

LEFT- OR RIGHT-SIDE CATHETERIZATION

COMPLICATION	SIGNS AND SYMPTOMS	NURSING CONSIDERATIONS
Pulmonary edema *Possible cause:* • Excessive fluid administration	• Early stage: tachycardia, tachypnea, dependent rales, diastolic (S_3) gallop • Acute stage: dyspnea; rapid, noisy respirations; cough with frothy, blood-tinged sputum; cyanosis with cold, clammy skin; tachycardia; hypertension	• Administer oxygen, as ordered. • Give medication (digitalis, diuretics, morphine), as ordered. • Restrict fluids and insert a Foley catheter. • Monitor the patient continuously, as ordered. • Maintain the patient's airway, and keep him in semi-Fowler's position. • Apply rotating tourniquets, as ordered. • Keep resuscitation equipment available.
Hematoma or blood loss at insertion site *Possible cause:* • Bleeding at insertion site from vein or artery damage	• Bloody dressing • Limb swelling • Decreased blood pressure • Increased heart rate	• Elevate limb, and apply direct manual pressure. • When the bleeding's stopped, apply a pressure bandage. • If bleeding continues, or if vital signs are unstable, notify doctor.
Reaction to contrast medium *Possible cause:* • Allergy to iodine	• Fever • Agitation • Hives • Itching • Decreased urinary output, indicating kidney failure	• Administer antihistamines to relieve itching, as ordered. • Administer diuretics to treat kidney failure, as ordered. • Monitor fluid intake and output closely.
Infection at insertion site *Possible cause:* • Poor aseptic technique	• Swelling, warmth, redness, and soreness at site • Purulent discharge at site	• Obtain drainage sample for culture. • Clean site, and apply antimicrobial ointment, if ordered. Cover site with sterile gauze pad. • Review and improve aseptic technique.

COMPLICATIONS OF CARDIAC CATHETERIZATION *(continued)*

LEFT-SIDE CATHETERIZATION

COMPLICATION	SIGNS AND SYMPTOMS	NURSING CONSIDERATIONS
Arterial embolus or thrombus in limb *Possible causes:* • Injury to artery during catheter insertion, causing blood clot • Plaque dislodged from artery wall by catheter	• Slow or faint pulse distal to insertion site • Loss of warmth, sensation, and color in arm or leg distal to insertion side	• Notify doctor. He may perform an arteriotomy and Fogarty catheterization to remove embolus or thrombus. • Protect affected arm or leg from pressure. Keep it at room temperature, and maintain at a level or slightly dependent position. • Administer a vasodilator, such as papaverine, to relieve painful vasospasm, if ordered.
Cerebrovascular accident (CVA) *Possible cause:* • Blood clot or plaque dislodged by catheter tip travels to brain	• Hemiplegia • Aphasia • Lethargy • Confusion, or decreased level of consciousness	• Monitor vital signs closely. • Keep suctioning equipment nearby. • Administer oxygen, as ordered.

RIGHT-SIDE CATHETERIZATION

COMPLICATION	SIGNS AND SYMPTOMS	NURSING CONSIDERATIONS
Thrombophlebitis *Possible cause:* • Vein damaged during catheter insertion	• Vein is hard, sore, cordlike, and warm. Vein may look like a red line above catheter insertion site. • Swelling at site	• Elevate arm or leg, and apply warm, wet compresses. • Administer anticoagulant or fibrinolytic drugs, if ordered.
Pulmonary embolism *Possible cause:* • Blood clot or plaque dislodged by catheter tip travels to lungs	• Shortness of breath • Tachypnea • Increased heart rate • Chest pain	• Place patient in high Fowler's position. • Administer oxygen, if ordered. • Monitor vital signs.
Vagal response *Possible causes:* • Vagus nerve endings irritated in sinoatrial node, atrial muscle tissue, or atrioventricular junction • Complete heart block	• Hypotension • Decreased heart rate • Nausea	• Monitor heart rate closely. • Administer atropine, if ordered. • Keep patient supine and quiet. • Give liquids.

may be indicated to guard against subacute bacterial endocarditis.

Findings

Cardiac catheterization should reveal no abnormalities of heart chamber size and configuration, wall motion and thickness, direction of blood flow and valve motion; the coronary arteries should have a smooth and regular outline. The graph on page 926 shows normal pressure events during a single cardiac cycle. The chart on page 932 shows upper limits of normal chamber and vessel pressures in a recumbent adult: higher pressures than these are significant; lower pressures, except in shock, usually aren't.

A normal ejection fraction (60% to 70%) is a good indicator for successful cardiac surgery.

Implications of results

Common abnormalities and defects confirmable by cardiac catheterization include coronary artery disease, myocardial incompetency, valvular heart disease, and septal defects.

In *coronary artery disease*, catheterization shows constriction of the lumen of the coronary arteries. Constriction greater than 70% is especially significant, particularly in proximal lesions. Narrowing of the left main coronary artery and occlusion or narrowing high in the left anterior descending artery is often an indication for revascularization surgery. (This lesion responds best to coronary bypass grafting.)

Impaired wall motion can indicate *myocardial incompetency* from coronary artery disease, aneurysm, cardiomyopathy, or congenital anomalies. Comparing the size of the left ventricle in systole and diastole helps assess the efficiency of cardiac muscular contraction, segmental wall motion, chamber size, and ejection fraction (comparison of the amount of blood pumped out of the left ventricle during systole with the amount of blood remaining at end diastole). An ejection fraction under 35% generally increases the risk of complications and decreases the probability of successful surgery.

Valvular heart disease is indicated by a gradient, or difference in pressures above and below a heart valve. For example, systolic pressure measurements on both sides of a stenotic aortic valve show a gradient across the valve. The higher the gradient, the greater the degree of stenosis. If left ventricular systolic pressure measures 200 mmHg and aortic systolic pressure is 120 mmHg, the gradient across the valve is 80 mmHg. Since these pressures should normally be equal during systole when the aortic valve is open, a gradient of this magnitude indicates the need for corrective surgery. Incompetent valves can be visualized in ventriculography by watching retrograde flow of the contrast medium across the valve during systole.

Septal defects (both atrial and ventricular) can be confirmed by measuring blood oxygen content in both sides of the heart. Elevated blood oxygen on the right side indicates a left-to-right atrial or ventricular shunt; decreased oxygen on the left side indicates a right-to-left shunt.

Cardiac output can be measured by analyzing blood oxygen levels in the cardiac chambers; by injecting contrast medium into the venous circulation and measuring its concentration as it moves past a thermodilution catheter; or by drawing blood from cardiac chambers.

Post-test care

□ Monitor vital signs every 15 minutes for the first hour after the procedure, then every hour until stable. If unstable, check every 5 minutes and notify the doctor.

□ Observe the insertion site for a hematoma or blood loss, and replace the pressure dressing, as needed.

□ Check the patient's color, skin temperature, and peripheral pulse below the puncture site.

□ Enforce bed rest for 8 hours. If the femoral route was used for catheter insertion, keep the patient's leg extended for 6 to 8 hours; if the antecubital fossa was used, keep the patient's arm extended for at least 3 hours.

UPPER LIMITS OF NORMAL PRESSURES IN CARDIAC CHAMBERS AND GREAT VESSELS IN RECUMBENT ADULTS

Chamber or vessel	Pressure (mmHg)
Right atrium	6 (mean)
Right ventricle	30/6*
Pulmonary artery	30/12* (mean, 18)
Left atrium	12 (mean)
Left ventricle	140/12*
Ascending aorta	140/90* (mean, 105)
Pulmonary artery wedge	Almost identical (± 1 to 2 mmHg) to left atrial mean pressure.

*Peak systolic and end-diastolic.

Adapted with permission from H. Kasparian, et al., "Interpreting Cardiac Catheterization Data," *Postgraduate Medicine*, 57:4: 67, April 1975.

☐ Review with the doctor resuming administration of medications withheld before the test. Administer analgesics, as ordered.

☐ Unless the patient is scheduled for surgery, encourage intake of fluids high in potassium, such as orange juice, to counteract the diuretic effect of the contrast medium.

☐ Make sure a post-test EKG is scheduled to check for possible myocardial damage.

Interfering factors

☐ Improperly functioning equipment or poor technique interferes with accurate testing.

☐ Patient anxiety increases the heart rate and cardiac chamber pressures.

PAULA BRAMMER VETTER, RN, BSN, CCRN

His Bundle Electrography

His bundle electrography permits measurement of discrete conduction intervals by recording electrical conduction during the slow withdrawal of a bipolar or tripolar electrode catheter from the right ventricle through the His bundle to the sinoatrial node. The catheter is introduced into the femoral vein and passed through the right atrium and across the septal leaflet of the tricuspid valve.

The His bundle electrogram can localize disturbances within the atrioventricular conduction system. When an ectopic site takes over as pacemaker of the heart, the electrogram can help pinpoint its origin. The test also aids diagnosis of syncope, evaluates a candidate for permanent artificial pacemaker implantation, and helps select or evaluate antiarrhythmic drugs.

Possible complications of His bundle electrography include arrhythmias, phlebitis, pulmonary emboli, thromboemboli, and catheter-site hemorrhage.

Purpose

☐ To diagnose arrhythmias and conduction anomalies

☐ To determine the need for implanted pacemakers and cardioactive drugs, and to evaluate their effects on the conduction system and ectopic rhythms

☐ To locate the site of a bundle branch block, especially in asymptomatic patients with conduction disturbances.

Patient preparation

Explain to the patient that this test evaluates the heart's conduction system. Instruct him to restrict food and fluids for at least 6 hours before the test. Tell him who will perform the test and where, and that it takes 1 to 3 hours.

Inform the patient that after the groin area is shaved, a catheter will be inserted into the femoral vein, and that an I.V. line may be started. Tell him that, while he'll receive a local anesthetic, he may still feel some pressure upon catheter insertion. Inform him that he'll be conscious during the test, and urge him to report any discomfort or pain.

Make sure the patient or responsible member of the family has signed a consent form. Check the patient's history, and inform the doctor of any ongoing drug therapy. Just before the test, advise the patient to void.

Procedure

The patient is placed in supine position on a special X-ray table. Limb electrodes for EKG recording during catheterization are applied, and the insertion site is shaved, scrubbed, and sterilized. The local anesthetic is injected, and a J-tip electrode is introduced I.V. into the femoral vein (occasionally, into a vein in the antecubital fossa). Guided by the fluoroscope, the catheter is advanced until it crosses the tricuspid valve and enters the right ventricle. Then, the catheter is slowly withdrawn from the tricuspid area, and recordings of conduction intervals are made from each pole of the catheter, either simultaneously or sequentially. After recordings and measurements are completed, the catheter is removed and a pressure dressing is applied to the site.

Precautions

☐ His bundle electrography is contraindicated in patients with severe coagulopathy, recent thrombophlebitis, and acute pulmonary embolism.

☐ Be sure emergency medication is available, in case the patient develops arrhythmias during the test.

Values

Normal conduction intervals in adults: H-V interval, 35 to 55 milliseconds; A-H interval, 45 to 150 milliseconds; and P-A interval, 20 to 40 milliseconds.

Implications of results

A prolonged H-V interval can result from

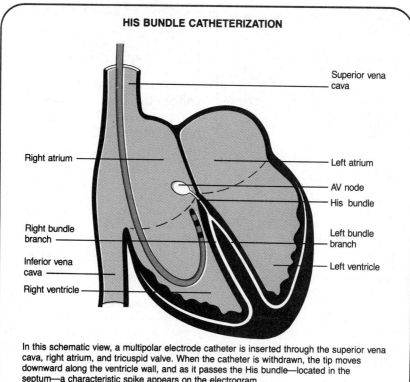

HIS BUNDLE CATHETERIZATION

Superior vena cava

Right atrium

Left atrium

AV node

His bundle

Right bundle branch

Left bundle branch

Inferior vena cava

Left ventricle

Right ventricle

In this schematic view, a multipolar electrode catheter is inserted through the superior vena cava, right atrium, and tricuspid valve. When the catheter is withdrawn, the tip moves downward along the ventricle wall, and as it passes the His bundle—located in the septum—a characteristic spike appears on the electrogram.

Adapted with permission from Mark E. Josephson and Stuart F. Seides, *Clinical Cardiac Electrophysiology: Techniques and Interpretations* (Philadelphia: Lea & Febiger, 1979).

NORMAL HIS BUNDLE ELECTROGRAM

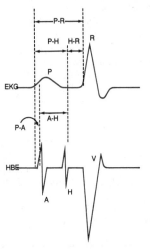

In a normal His bundle electrogram, atrial activation appears as a sharp diphasic or triphasic wave (A) during the P wave, followed by His bundle deflection (H) and ventricular activation (V). By measuring the interval between the beginning of the P wave and His bundle activation (P-H interval) or on the interval between the beginning of the atrial wave and His bundle activation (A-H interval), abnormally prolonged A-V nodal conduction can be detected.

Adapted with permission from H.H. Hecht and C.E. Kossmann, "Atrioventricular and Intraventricular Conduction," *American Journal of Cardiology*, 31:232-244.

acute or chronic disease. This interval represents the conduction time from the His bundle to the Purkinje fibers. Atrioventricular nodal (A-H interval) delays can stem from atrial pacing, chronic conduction system disease, carotid sinus pressure, recent myocardial infarction, and drugs. Intra-atrial (P-A interval) delays can result from acquired, surgically induced, or congenital atrial disease and atrial pacing.

Post-test care
☐ Monitor the patient's vital signs, as ordered—usually every 15 minutes for 1

hour, and then every hour for 4 hours. If they're unstable, check every 15 minutes, and alert the doctor. Observe for shortness of breath, chest pain, pallor, or changes in pulse rate or blood pressure. Enforce bed rest for 4 to 6 hours.

☐ Check catheter insertion site for bleeding, as ordered—usually every 30 minutes for 8 hours; apply a pressure bandage until the bleeding stops.

☐ Advise the patient he may resume his usual diet.

☐ Be sure a 12-lead resting EKG is scheduled to assess for changes.

Interfering factors
Malfunctioning recording equipment or improper catheter positioning interferes with accurate testing.

PAULA BRAMMER VETTER, RN, BSN, CCRN

Pulmonary Artery Catheterization
[Swan-Ganz catheterization, balloon flotation catheterization of the pulmonary artery, right heart catheterization]

Pulmonary artery catheterization uses a balloon-tipped, flow-directed catheter to provide intermittent occlusion of the pulmonary artery. Once the catheter is in place, this procedure permits measurement of both pulmonary artery pressure (PAP) and pulmonary artery wedge pressure (PAWP)—also known as pulmonary capillary wedge pressure. The PAWP reading accurately reflects left atrial pressure and left ventricular end-diastolic pressure, although the catheter itself never enters the left side of the heart. Such a reading is possible because the heart momentarily relaxes during diastole as it fills with blood from the pulmonary veins; at this instant, the pulmonary vasculature, left atrium, and left ventricle act as a single chamber, and all have identical pressures. Thus, changes in PAP and PAWP reflect changes in left ventricular filling pressure, permitting detection of left ventricular impairment.

In this procedure, which is usually performed at bedside in an intensive care unit, the catheter is inserted through the cephalic vein in the antecubital fossa or the subclavian (sometimes, femoral) vein. The catheter is threaded into the right atrium, the balloon is inflated, and the catheter follows the blood flow through the tricuspid valve into the right ventricle and out into the pulmonary artery.

In addition to measuring atrial and pulmonary arterial pressures, this procedure evaluates pulmonary vascular resistance and tissue oxygenation, as indicated by mixed venous oxygen content. It should be performed cautiously in patients with left bundle branch block or implanted pacemakers.

Purpose

□ To help assess right and left ventricular failure

□ To monitor therapy for complications of acute myocardial infarction, such as cardiogenic shock, pulmonary edema, fluid-related hypovolemia and hypotension, systolic murmur, unexplained sinus tachycardia, and various cardiac arrhythmias

□ To monitor fluid status in patients with serious burns, renal disease, or shock lung (noncardiogenic pulmonary edema) after open heart surgery

□ To monitor the effects of cardiovascular drugs, such as nitroglycerin and nitroprusside.

Patient preparation

Explain to the patient that this test evaluates heart function and provides information for determining appropriate therapy or for managing fluid status. Advise him that he needn't restrict food or fluids before the test. Tell him who will perform the test and where.

Inform the patient he'll be conscious during catheterization, and he may feel transient local discomfort from the administration of the local anesthetic. Tell him catheter insertion takes about 30 minutes, but the catheter will remain in place, causing little or no discomfort, for 48 to 72 hours. Instruct him to report any discomfort immediately.

Make sure the patient or responsible member of the family has signed a consent form.

Equipment

Local anesthetic (1% Xylocaine)/70% alcohol or povidone-iodine solution/antiseptic ointment/heparin/skin preparation set/sterile drape, sterile towels, and

---

MEASURING CARDIAC OUTPUT

Cardiac output—the amount of blood ejected from the right and left ventricles every 60 seconds—can be measured by a 4-lumen thermodilution catheter. One catheter lumen houses a thermistor, a pair of wires that terminate in a small bead located about 4 cm behind the catheter tip. The thermistor detects changes in blood temperature and transmits this information to a monitoring computer that calculates and displays cardiac output.

To measure cardiac output, 5 to 10 ml of cooled normal saline solution or 5% dextrose in water is injected into the proximal lumen over a period of 2 to 3 seconds. The fluid travels quickly through the right atrium and ventricle and into the pulmonary artery, where the thermistor bead records the temperature change.

Normal cardiac output is 4 to 8 liters/minute, the mean being 5 liters/minute. Cardiac output relates to body surface area, which is determined from the patient's height and weight using a nomogram. The cardiac output is divided by the figure obtained from the nomogram to get the *cardiac index*, which is a less size-dependent figure. A normal cardiac index is 2.5 to 5.0 liters/minute/m².

Decreased cardiac output and cardiac index may indicate impaired myocardial contractility due to myocardial infarction or drugs (negative inotropics, such as procainamide, quinidine, or propranolol); acidosis or hypoxia; decreased left ventricular filling pressure caused by fluid depletion; increased systemic vascular resistance from arteriosclerosis or hypertension, or valvular heart disase causing decreased blood flow from the ventricles.

Barbara Boyd Egoville, RN, MSN

tape/sterile stockinette/cutdown tray or percutaneous needle/tuberculin syringe/ 2.5-ml syringe/two-, three-, or four-lumen catheter/gloves, mask, and gown; I.V. pole; and transducer holder/strain gauge transducer with sterile dome/three 3-way stopcocks/two Sorenson Intraflo Valves/two Cobe pressure tubings/transfer pack/blood recipient set (for transfer pack), or regular I.V. tubing for pre-packaged bagged solution/pressure bag including manometer/defibrillator/emergency or code cart/4″ x 4″ gauze pads/ 500 ml normal saline solution I.V. bottle/3-0 and 4-0 silk sutures/oscilloscope/digital readout recorder.

Procedure

The flexible catheter used in this test comes in two-lumen, three-lumen, and four-lumen (thermodilution) modes and in various lengths. In the two-lumen catheter, one lumen contains the balloon, 1 mm behind the catheter tip; the other lumen, which opens at the tip, measures pressure in front of the balloon. The two-lumen catheter measures PAP and PAWP, and can be used to sample mixed venous blood and to infuse I.V. solutions. The three-lumen catheter has an additional proximal lumen that opens 30 cm behind the tip; when the tip is in the main pulmonary artery, the proximal lumen lies in the right atrium, permitting administration of fluids, or monitoring of right atrial pressure (central venous pressure). The four-lumen type includes a transistorized thermistor for monitoring blood temperature, and allows measurement of cardiac output.

Before catheterization, the equipment is set up according to the manufacturer's directions and the hospital's procedure. Then, if the insertion site is being prepared for a cutdown procedure, the patient's skin is prepared and covered with a sterile drape; or a sterile stockinette can be pulled over the arm from wrist to elbow and a hole cut in the stockinette at the insertion site.

The patient is assisted to supine position. For antecubital insertion, his arm is abducted with palm upward on an overbed table for support; for subclavian insertion, the patient is placed in supine position with his head and shoulders slightly lower than his trunk, to make the vein more accessible. If the patient can't tolerate supine position, he is assisted to semi-Fowler position. During the test, all pressures are monitored with the patient in the same position.

After the patient is positioned, the catheter balloon is checked for defects using sterile technique. Then, the catheter is introduced into the vein percutaneously or by cutdown. The catheter is directed to the right atrium, and the catheter balloon partially inflated so that venous flow carries the catheter tip through the right atrium and tricuspid valve into the right ventricle and into the pulmonary artery. While the catheter is being directed, the oscilloscope screen is observed for characteristic waveform changes, and the location of the catheter tip is found. A printout of each stage of catheter insertion is obtained for baseline information.

 As the catheter is passed into the right heart chambers, the oscilloscope screen is observed for frequent PVCs and tachycardia—the result of catheter irritation of the right ventricle. If irritation occurs, the catheter may be partially withdrawn or medication administered to suppress the arrhythmia or right bundle branch block.

To record the PAWP, the catheter balloon is carefully inflated with the specified amount of air or carbon dioxide—not fluid—using the smallest syringe possible; the catheter tip will float into the wedge position, as indicated by an altered waveform on the oscilloscope screen. If a PAWP waveform occurs with less than the recommended inflation volume, do not inflate the balloon further. After the balloon is inflated, the wedge pressure is recorded. Then, the air from the balloon is allowed to return to the syringe, which is then deflated. This allows the catheter to float back into the pulmonary artery. The oscilloscope screen is observed for a PA waveform.

FOUR-LUMEN PULMONARY ARTERY CATHETER

Thermistor hub:
Connects to the cardiac output computer to measure cardiac output.

Distal lumen hub:
Attaches to pressure line to measure pulmonary artery pressure and pulmonary artery wedge pressure. I.V. flush solution exits from the distal port.

Balloon inflation valve:
Receives the proper amount of gas (air or carbon dioxide) to inflate the balloon.

Proximal lumen hub:
Attaches to pressure line to measure right atrial central venous pressure. To measure cardiac output, disconnect from pressure line and inject solution. I.V. flush solution or injectate solution exits from proximal port.

Distal lumen port:
Rests in the pulmonary artery.

Thermistor:
Detects blood temperature changes used to measure cardiac output. Located about 1½″ (3.8 cm) from the catheter tip.

Balloon:
Expands around catheter, when inflated, without occluding distal port.

Proximal lumen port:
Rests in the right atrium.

Pulmonary artery catheters are made of pliable, radiopaque polyvinylchloride. This illustration shows a 110 cm (about 43¼ ″) catheter, marked in 10-cm increments. It has distal and proximal lumens, which are fluid-filled for pressure monitoring; a thermistor lumen, which holds the wires connecting the thermistor to the cardiac output computer; and a balloon inflation lumen with valve. As a result, this catheter can measure several pressures, as well as cardiac output.

Since catheters vary depending on their manufacturer, consult the manufacturer's manual for additional details.

The system is flushed and recalibrated.

 NURSING ALERT
The balloon catheter should not be overinflated. Overinflation could distend the pulmonary artery, causing vessel rupture. If the balloon can't be fully deflated after recording the PAWP, it shouldn't be reinflated unless the doctor is present; balloon rupture may cause a life-threatening air embolism. All connections are checked for air leaks that may have prevented balloon inflation, particularly if the patient is confused or uncooperative.

When the catheter's correct positioning and function is established, the catheter is sutured to the skin and antibiotic ointment and an airtight dressing are applied to the insertion site. A chest X-ray film is obtained, as ordered, to verify catheter placement. (The radiology department is notified before the procedure that a cath-

PULMONARY ARTERY CATHETER INSERTION

As the catheter is directed through the right heart chambers to its wedge position, it produces distinctive waveforms that are important indicators of the catheter's position in the heart on the oscilloscope screen.

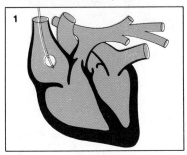

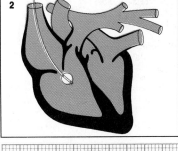

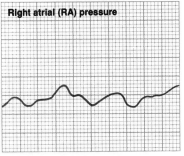

Right atrial (RA) pressure

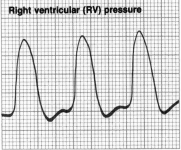

Right ventricular (RV) pressure

1. When the catheter tip reaches the right atrium from the superior vena cava, the waveform on the oscilloscope screen or readout strip looks like this. When it does, the doctor inflates the catheter's balloon, which floats the tip through the tricuspid valve into the right ventricle.

2. When the catheter tip reaches the right ventricle, the waveform looks like this.

---

eter is to be inserted.) Alarms are set on the EKG and pressure monitors. Vital signs are monitored, as ordered. PAP waveforms are documented at the beginning of each shift, and monitored frequently throughout each shift. PAWP and cardiac output are checked, as ordered (usually every 6 hours). Routine aseptic precautions are taken to prevent infection.

When the catheter is no longer needed, the patient's blood pressure and radial pulse are taken. Then, the balloon is deflated, the dressing removed, and the catheter slowly withdrawn. The EKG is monitored for arrhythmias. If any difficulty is encountered in removing the

catheter, the procedure is stopped at once and the doctor is notified immediately.

After the catheter is withdrawn, pressure, an antibiotic ointment, and a sterile dressing are applied to the insertion site. Blood pressure and radial pulse are checked.

Precautions

☐ After each PAWP reading, flush and recalibrate the monitoring system and make sure the balloon is completely deflated; if you encounter difficulty in flushing the system, notify the doctor. Maintain 300 mmHg pressure in the

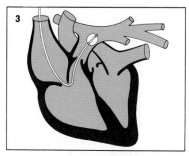

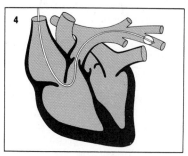

Pulmonary artery pressure (PAP)

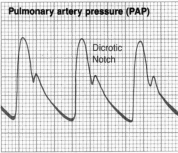

Dicrotic Notch

Pulmonary artery wedge pressure (PAWP)

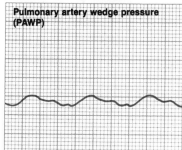

3. A waveform like this one indicates that the balloon has floated the catheter tip through the pulmonic valve into the pulmonary artery. A dicrotic notch should be visible in the waveform, indicating the closing of the pulmonic valve.

4. Blood flow in the pulmonary artery then carries the catheter balloon into one of the pulmonary artery's many smaller branches. When the vessel becomes too narrow for the balloon to pass through, the balloon wedges in the vessel, occluding it. The monitor then displays a pulmonary artery wedge pressure (PAWP) waveform like this one.

pressure bag to permit fluid flow of 3 to 6 ml/hour. Instruct the patient to extend the appropriate arm (or leg, if the catheter is inserted into femoral vein). If he develops fever while the catheter is in place, remove the catheter and send its tip to the laboratory for culture.

 □ Make sure stopcocks are properly positioned and connections are secure. Loose connections may introduce air into the system or cause blood backup, leakage of deoxygenated blood, or inaccurate pressure readings.

□ Be sure the lumen hubs are properly identified to serve the appropriate catheter ports. Don't add or remove fluids from the distal pulmonary artery port; this may cause pulmonary extravasation or damage the artery.

□ If the catheter has not been sutured to the skin, tape it securely to prevent dislodgement.

Values

Normal pressures are as follows:
Right atrial: 1 to 6 mmHg
Systolic right ventricular: 20 to 30 mmHg
End diastolic right ventricular: < 5 mmHg
Systolic PAP: 20 to 30 mmHg
Diastolic PAP: about 10 mmHg
Mean PAP: < 20 mmHg

SOLVING PROBLEMS WITH PULMONARY ARTERY LINES

PROBLEM	POSSIBLE CAUSES	SOLUTION
Dampened pressures	• Air in system	• Check Intraflow valves, stopcock, and transducer for bubbles.
	• Blood on transducer	• Flush off or change transducer.
	• Clot in system	• Aspirate blood until it thins; notify doctor.
	• Catheter kinked	• Instruct patient to cough or extend his arm to 90° angle from his body, and gently flush the catheter. If problem, obtain X-ray film.
	• Loose connection	• Check connections for security.
	• Incorrect stopcock position	• Correct stopcock position.
	• Pressure tubing too long	• Shorten distance between patient and transducer.
Transducer imbalance	• Damaged transducer	• Try another transducer.
	• Wrong amplifier	• Check transducer connection to amplifier.
	• Broken amplifier	• Change the amplifier.
	• Set at wrong level (mid-chest)	• Readjust the transducer.
Waveform drifting	• Short warm-up time	• Allow recommended time for warm-up.
	• Cable air vents kinked or coiled	• Unkink or decompress cable air vents.
False-low reading	• Dampened waveform	• See section on dampened pressures.
	• Transducer imbalance	• Place transducer at heart level.
	• Wrong calibration	• Recalibrate the monitor.
False-high reading	• Transducer imbalance	• Rebalance the transducer.
	• Flush solution administered too quickly	• Pour slow continual flush (3 to 6 ml/hour).
Configuration	• Improper catheter placement	• Try to wedge catheter. Obtain PAWP. If problem, obtain X-ray film.
	• Transducer needs to be calibrated	• Recalibrate the transducer.
	• Transducer not at RA level	• Reposition and recalibrate the transducer.
	• Transducer loosely connected to catheter	• Secure the transducer.
Drifting wedge pressure (with inflated balloon)	• Balloon overinflation	• Watch scope while inflating balloon. When waveform changes from a PA to a wedge shape, stop inflating.
	• Air in system	• Remove air from tubing and/or transducer.
PAWP pressure trace unobtainable	• Incorrect amount of balloon air	• Deflate, start again slowly. Check for air to refill syringe during balloon deflation.
	• Ruptured balloon	• With no resistance to inflation, stop inflation. Notify doctor.

PAWP: 6 to 12 mmHg
Left atrial: about 10 mmHg

Implications of results

An abnormally high right atrial pressure can indicate pulmonary disease, right heart failure, fluid overload, cardiac tamponade, tricuspid stenosis and regurgitation, or pulmonary hypertension.

Elevated right ventricular pressure can result from pulmonary hypertension, pulmonary valvular stenosis, right ventricular failure, pericardial effusion, constrictive pericarditis, chronic congestive heart failure, or ventricular septal defects.

An abnormally high PAP is characteristic in increased pulmonary blood flow, such as in a left-to-right shunt secondary to atrial or ventricular septal defect; increased pulmonary arteriolar resistance, such as in pulmonary hypertension or mitral stenosis; chronic obstructive pulmonary disease; pulmonary edema or embolus; and left ventricular failure from any cause. Pulmonary artery systolic pressure is the same as right ventricular systolic pressure. Pulmonary artery diastolic pressure is the same as left atrial pressure, except in patients with severe pulmonary disease causing pulmonary hypertension; in such patients, catheterization still provides important diagnostic information.

Elevated PAWP can result from left ventricular failure, mitral stenosis and regurgitation, cardiac tamponade, or cardiac insufficiency; depressed PAWP, from hypovolemia.

Post-test care

□ Observe the catheterization insertion site for signs of infection—redness, swelling, and discharge.

□ For 24 hours, watch for complications, such as pulmonary emboli, pulmonary artery perforation, heart murmurs, thrombi, and arrhythmias.

Interfering factors

□ Malfunctioning monitoring and recording devices, loose connections, clot formation at the catheter tip, air in the fluid column, or ruptured balloon interfere with accurate testing.

□ Incorrect catheter placement causes catheter fling—excessive catheter movement that produces a dampened pressure tracing.

□ Migration of the catheter against a vessel wall may cause constant occlusion (permanent wedging) of the pulmonary artery.

□ Mechanical ventilators with positive pressure cause increased intrathoracic pressure, which raises catheter pressure.

PAULA BRAMMER VETTER, RN, BSN, CCRN

MISCELLANEOUS TESTS

Cold Stimulation Test for Raynaud's Syndrome

The cold stimulation test demonstrates Raynaud's syndrome by recording temperature changes in the patient's fingers before and after their submersion in an ice-water bath. However, digital blood pressure recording or examination of the arteries in the arm and palmar arch

should precede this test to rule out arterial occlusive disease.

Raynaud's syndrome is an arteriospastic disorder characterized by intense episodic constriction (vasospasm) of the small cutaneous arteries and arterioles of the hands or, less often, the feet after exposure to cold or stress. In this syndrome, the skin on the fingers characteristically blanches and becomes cyanotic and hyperemic after such exposure; in some patients, color changes are variable. If the syndrome is primary, it's called Raynaud's disease; if it's sec-

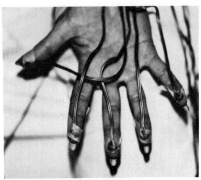

In the test for Raynaud's syndrome, thermistors taped to the fingers, as shown above, record temperature changes before and after submerging the hand in an ice-water bath.

ondary to connective tissue disorders, such as scleroderma or SLE, it's called Raynaud's phenomenon. Although the cause of Raynaud's disease is unknown, several theories attempt to explain the reduced digital blood flow: intrinsic vascular wall hypersensitivity to cold, increased vasomotor tone due to sympathetic stimulation, and antigen-antibody immune response.

Purpose
□ To detect Raynaud's syndrome.

Patient preparation
Explain to the patient that this test detects a vascular disorder. Inform him he needn't restrict food or fluids before the test. Tell him who will perform the procedure and when; that the test takes 20 to 40 minutes; and that he may experience discomfort when his hands are briefly immersed in ice water. Suggest that he remove his watch or other jewelry, and encourage him to relax.

Procedure
To minimize extraneous environmental stimuli, the test room should be neither too warm nor too cold. A thermistor is taped to each of the patient's fingers (but not so tightly as to restrict circulation), and the temperature is recorded. The patient's hands are submerged in an ice-water bath for 20 seconds. Then, he is instructed to remove his hands from the water, and the temperature of his fingers is recorded immediately and every 5 minutes thereafter until it returns to the prebath level.

Precautions
The cold stimulation test is contraindicated in patients with gangrenous fingers or open, infected wounds.

Findings
Normally, digital temperature returns to the prebath level within 15 minutes.

Implications of results
If digital temperature takes longer than 20 minutes to return to the prebath level, Raynaud's syndrome is indicated. Its benign form, Raynaud's disease, requires no specific treatment and has no serious sequelae. Its more serious form, Raynaud's phenomenon, is associated with connective tissue disorders—scleroderma, systemic lupus erythematosus, and rheumatoid arthritis—which may not be clinically apparent for several years. However, distinction between Raynaud's phenomenon and Raynaud's disease is difficult.

Post-test care
None.

Interfering factors
Excessively warm or cold test environment may cause inaccurate results.

DONNA BLACKBURN, RN
LINDA PETERSON, RN

Pericardial Fluid Analysis
[Pericardiocentesis]

Although this procedure is most useful as an emergency measure to relieve cardiac tamponade, pericardial fluid analysis provides a fluid sample to confirm diagnosis and identify the cause of pericardial effusion. However, pericardiocentesis, the needle aspiration of pericardial fluid, has both therapeutic and diagnostic purposes.

Normally, small amounts of plasma-derived fluid within the pericardium lubricate the heart, which reduces friction during expansions and contractions. Excess pericardial fluid, pericardial effusion, may accumulate after inflammation, rupture, or penetrating trauma (gunshot or stab wounds) of the pericardium. Rapidly forming effusions, such as those after penetrating trauma, may induce cardiac tamponade—a potentially lethal syndrome marked by increased intrapericardial pressure that prevents complete ventricular filling and thus reduces cardiac output. Slowly forming effusions, such as those in pericarditis, generally pose less immediate danger since they allow the pericardium more time to adapt to the accumulating fluid.

Pericardiocentesis should be performed cautiously because of the risk of potentially fatal complications, such as laceration of a coronary artery or of the myocardium; its other complications include ventricular fibrillation or vasovagal arrest, pleural infection, and accidental puncture of the lung, liver, or stomach. If possible, echocardiography should determine the effusion site before pericardiocentesis is performed, to minimize the risk of complications. Generally, surgical drainage and biopsy are safer procedures.

Purpose

☐ To assist in identifying the cause of pericardial effusion and to help determine appropriate therapy.

Patient preparation

Explain to the patient that this test detects excessive fluid around the heart, and its cause, and helps determine appropriate therapy. Inform him he needn't restrict food or fluids before the test. Tell him who will perform the test and where, and that it takes 10 to 20 minutes.

Inform the patient that a local anesthetic will be injected before the aspiration needle is inserted. Although fluid aspiration isn't painful, warn him that he may experience pressure upon insertion of the needle into the pericardial sac. Advise him that he may be asked to briefly hold his breath to aid needle insertion and placement.

Tell the patient that an I.V. line will be started at keep-vein-open (K.V.O.) rate (20 ml/hour) just before the procedure, and that premedication (such as diazepam) will be administered, as ordered. Assure him that someone will remain with him during the test, and that his pulse and blood pressure will be monitored after the procedure.

Check the patient's history for current antibiotic usage, and record such usage on the test request form. Make sure the patient or a responsible member of the family has signed a consent form. If pericardiocentesis is performed to relieve cardiac tamponade and the patient is in shock, explain the test to the family.

Equipment

Prepackaged pericardiocentesis tray, or 70% alcohol or povidone-iodine solution/ 1% procaine or 1% lidocaine for local anesthetic/sterile needles—25G for anesthetic and 14G, 16G, and 18G 4″ or 5″ cardiac needles/50-ml syringe with Luer-Lok tip/7-ml sterile test tubes—one red-top, one green-top (heparin), and one lavender-top (EDTA)/sterile specimen container for culture/vial of heparin 1:1,000/4″ x 4″ gauze pads/bandage/three-way stopcock/EKG machine or bedside monitor/Kelly clamp/alligator clips/defibrillator and emergency drugs.

Procedure

The patient is placed in supine position with the thorax elevated 60°. When he is comfortable and well-supported, he is instructed to remain still during the procedure. After the skin is prepared with alcohol or povidone-iodine solution from the left costal margin to the xiphoid process, the local anesthetic is admin-

ASPIRATING PERICARDIAL FLUID

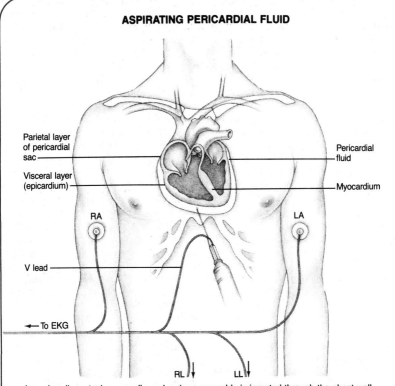

Parietal layer
of pericardial
sac

Pericardial
fluid

Visceral layer
(epicardium)

Myocardium

RA

LA

V lead

To EKG

RL

LL

In pericardiocentesis, a needle and syringe assembly is inserted through the chest wall into the pericardial sac, as illustrated above. Electrocardiographic monitoring, with a lead wire attached to the needle and electrodes placed on the limbs (right arm [RA], right leg [RL], left arm [LA], and left leg [LL]), helps ensure proper needle placement and avoids damage to the heart.

istered at the insertion site.

With the three-way stopcock open, a 50-ml syringe is aseptically attached to one end and the cardiac needle to the other end. Using an alligator clip, the EKG lead wire is attached to the hub of the needle. Then, the EKG machine is set to lead V, and turned on. (Or, the patient is connected to a bedside monitor.) The needle is inserted through the chest wall into the pericardial sac maintaining gentle aspiration until fluid appears in the syringe. The needle is angled 35° to 45° toward the tip of the right scapula between the left costal margin and the xiphoid process; this subxiphoid approach minimizes the risk of lacer-

ating the coronary vessels or the pleura. Once the needle is properly positioned, a Kelly clamp is attached to the needle at the skin surface so it won't advance further. While the fluid is being aspirated, the specimen tubes are labeled and numbered. When the needle is withdrawn, pressure is applied *immediately* to the site with sterile gauze pads for 3 to 5 minutes, then a bandage is applied.

Precautions

□ Ensure that the EKG machine is properly grounded to prevent accidental ventricular fibrillation.

□ Carefully observe the EKG

tracing during insertion of the cardiac needle; an ST segment elevation indicates that the needle has reached the epicardial surface and should be retracted slightly; an abnormally shaped QRS may indicate perforation of the myocardium. Premature ventricular contractions usually indicate that the needle has touched the ventricular wall.

☐ Watch for grossly bloody aspirate—a sign of inadvertent puncture of a cardiac chamber.

☐ Be sure to use specimen tubes with the proper additives. Although fibrin isn't a normal component of pericardial fluid, it does appear in fluid in some pericardial diseases and in carcinoma, and clotting is possible.

☐ If bacterial culture and sensitivity tests are scheduled, record any antibiotic therapy on the laboratory slip. If anaerobic organisms are suspected, consult the laboratory concerning the proper collection technique to avoid exposing the aspirate to air. The aspirate may be placed in an anaerobic collection tube or the syringe may be filled completely, displacing all air, and the collection tube capped tightly with a sterile rubber tip.

☐ Send all specimens to the laboratory immediately.

Findings

Normally, 10 to 50 ml of sterile fluid is present in the pericardium. Pericardial fluid is clear and straw-colored, without evidence of pathogens, blood, or malignant cells. It normally contains less than 1,000 WBCs/mm³. Its glucose concentration approximately equals the levels in whole blood.

Implications of results

Generally, pericardial effusions are classified as transudates or exudates. Transudates are protein-poor effusions that usually arise from mechanical factors altering fluid formation or resorption, such as increased hydrostatic pressure, decreased plasma oncotic pressure, or obstruction of the pericardial lymphatic drainage system by a tumor.

Most exudates result from inflammation and contain large amounts of protein. In these effusions, inflammation damages the capillary membrane, allowing protein molecules to leak into the pericardial fluid. Effusions can be characteristic in pericarditis, neoplasms, acute myocardial infarction, tuberculosis, rheumatoid disease, and systemic lupus erythematosus.

An elevated WBC count or neutrophil fraction may also accompany inflammatory conditions, such as bacterial pericarditis; a high lymphocyte fraction may indicate fungal or tuberculous pericarditis.

Turbid or milky effusions may result from the accumulation of lymph or pus in the pericardial sac, or from tuberculosis or rheumatoid disease.

Bloody pericardial fluid may indicate hemopericardium, hemorrhagic pericarditis, or a traumatic tap. Hemopericardium, the accumulation of blood in the pericardium, may result from myocardial rupture after infarction or aortic rupture secondary to dissecting aortic aneurysm or thoracic trauma. In hemopericardium, the fluid has a hematocrit level similar to that of whole blood; in hemorrhagic pericarditis, it has a relatively low hematocrit and doesn't clot on standing. Hemorrhagic effusions may indicate malignancies, Dressler's syndrome, closed chest trauma, or postcardiotomy syndrome. A traumatic tap is easily distinguished from hemopericardium or hemorrhagic pericarditis, since the fluid becomes progressively clearer.

Glucose concentrations below whole blood levels may reflect increased local metabolism due to malignancy, inflammation, or infection. Possible causes of bacterial pericarditis include *Staphylococcus aureus*, *Hemophilus influenzae*, and various gram-negative organisms; possible causes of granulomatous pericarditis include *Mycobacterium tuberculosis* or various fungal agents; and causes of viral pericarditis include coxsackieviruses, echoviruses, and others.

Post-test care

☐ Check blood pressure readings, pulse,

DIAGNOSING PERICARDIAL EFFUSION

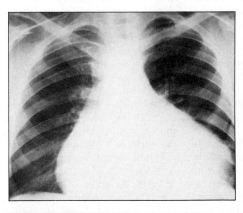

Various tests, such as chest radiography and M-mode echocardiography, aid diagnosis of pericardial effusion. In the chest X-ray film at left, the bulging white area in the center represents an enlarged pericardial sac, resulting from pericardial effusion. In the M-mode echocardiogram below, the wide light area at the bottom indicates accumulation of excess pericardial fluid. To determine the cause of such accumulation, pericardial fluid can be drawn off by pericardiocentesis to allow pericardial fluid analysis.

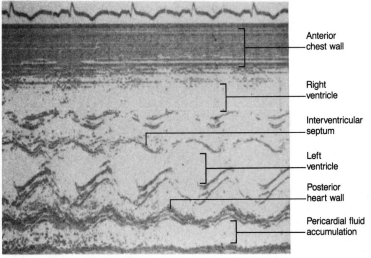

Anterior chest wall

Right ventricle

Interventricular septum

Left ventricle

Posterior heart wall

Pericardial fluid accumulation

respiration, and heart sounds every 15 minutes until stable, then every ½ hour for 2 hours, every hour for 4 hours, and every 4 hours thereafter. Reassure the patient such monitoring is routine.

□ Be alert for respiratory or cardiac distress. Watch especially for signs of cardiac tamponade: muffled and distant heart sounds, distended neck veins, paradoxical pulse, and shock. Cardiac tamponade may result from rapid reaccumulation of pericardial fluid or puncture of a coronary vessel causing bleeding into the pericardial sac.

Interfering factors

□ Failure of aseptic technique can impair microbiologic analysis of the sample, since skin contaminants may be isolated and mistaken for causative organisms. Antibiotic therapy can prevent isolation of the causative organism.
□ Failure to use the proper additives in test tubes interferes with accurate determination of test results.

SUSAN A. KAYES, SM(ASCP)
PAULA BRAMMER VETTER, RN, BSN, CCRN

Selected References

Andreoli, Kathleen G., and Fowkes, Virginia K. *Comprehensive Cardiac Care: A Text for Nurses, Physicians and Other Health Practitioners,* 5th ed. St. Louis: C.V. Mosby Co., 1983.

Babb, J.D., and Leaman, D.M. "Risk of Cardiac Catheterization Today," *Journal of Cardiovascular Medicine* 941-48, October 1980.

Benchimol, Albert O. *Non-invasive Diagnostic Techniques in Cardiology,* 2nd ed. Baltimore: Williams & Wilkins Co., 1981.

Bergan, John J., and Yao, J.S. eds. *Venous Problems.* Chicago: Year Book Medical Pubs., 1978.

Braunwald, Eugene. *Heart Disease: A Textbook of Cardiovascular Medicine.* Philadelphia: W.B. Saunders Co., 1980.

Conover, Mary H. *Understanding Electrocardiography: Physiological and Interpretive Concepts,* 3rd ed. St. Louis: C.V. Mosby Co., 1980.

Fowler, Noble O., ed. *Cardiac Diagnosis and Treatment,* 3rd ed. Philadelphia: J.B. Lippincott Co., 1980.

Ganong, William F. *Review of Medical Physiology,* 11th ed. Los Altos, Calif.: Lange Medical Publications, 1983.

Grossman, William, ed. *Cardiac Catheterization and Angiography,* 2nd ed. Philadelphia: Lea & Febiger, 1980.

Grossman, Zachary D., et al. *The Clinician's Guide to Diagnostic Imaging.* New York: Raven Press Publications, 1983.

Guyton, Arthur C. *Textbook of Medical Physiology,* 6th ed. Philadelphia: W.B. Saunders Co., 1981.

Harvey, A. McGehee, et al. *The Principles and Practice of Medicine,* 21st ed. East Norwalk, Conn.: Appleton-Century-Crofts, 1984.

Haughey, Cynthia. "Preparing Your Patient for Echocardiography," *Nursing84* 14:68-71, May 1984.

Haughey, Cynthia. "Understanding Ultrasonography," *Nursing81* 11:100-04, April 1981.

Hudson, Barbara. "Sharpen Your Assessment Skills with the Doppler Ultrasound Stethoscope," *Nursing83* 13:55-57, May 1983.

Hurst, J. Willis, et al., *The Heart,* 5th ed. New York: McGraw-Hill Book Co., 1982.

Josephson, Mark E., and Seides, Stuart F. *Clinical Cardiac Electrophysiology: Techniques and Interpretations.* Philadelphia:

Lea & Febiger, 1979.

Juergens, John L., et al. *Allen-Barker-Hines Peripheral Vascular Diseases,* 5th ed. Philadelphia: W.B. Saunders Co., 1980.

Karnes, Nancy J. "Premature Ventricular Contractions: When to Sound the Alarm," *Nursing84* 14:34-39, June 1984.

Kennedy, Harold L. *Ambulatory Electrocardiography: Including Holter Recording Technology.* Philadelphia: Lea & Febiger, 1981.

Lamb, Jane O. *Laboratory Tests in Clinical Nursing.* Bowie, Md.: Robert J. Brady Co., 1984.

Pantaleo, Nancy, et al. "Thallium Myocardial Scintigraphy and Its Use in the Assessment of Coronary Artery Disease," *Heart and Lung* 10(1):61-70, January/February 1981.

Petersdorf, Robert G., and Adams, Raymond D. eds. *Harrison's Principles of Internal Medicine,* 10th ed. New York: McGraw-Hill Book Co., 1983.

Reading EKGs Correctly, 2nd ed. New Nursing Skillbook series. Springhouse, Pa.: Springhouse Corp., 1984.

Rogers, William J. "Current Concepts in Evaluation of Coronary Artery Disease," *Hospital Medicine,* 10-21, March 1980.

Soin, Jagneet S., and Brooks, Harold L. *Nuclear Cardiology for Clinicians.* Mount Kisco, N.Y.: Futura Publishing Co., 1980.

Teasley, Deborah. "Don't Let Cardiac Catheterization Strike Fear in Your Patient's Heart," *Nursing82* 12:52-55, March 1982.

Using Monitors. Nursing Photobook series. Springhouse, Pa.: Springhouse Corp., 1981.

Vandenbelt, Ronald J., et al. *Cardiology—A Clinical Approach.* Chicago: Year Book Medical Pubs., 1979.

Visalli, Florence, and Evans, Patricia. "The Swan-Ganz Catheter: A Program for Teaching Safe, Effective Use," *Nursing81* 11(1):42-47, January 1981.

Wenger, Nanette K., et al. *Cardiology for Nurses.* New York: McGraw-Hill Book Co., 1980.

Wheeler, H. Brownwell. "A Modern Approach to Diagnosing Deep Venous Thrombosis," *Journal of Cardiovascular Medicine* 5:3, March 1980.

Zeluff, G.W., et al. "Evaluation of Coronary Arteries and Myocardium by Radionuclide Imaging," *Heart and Lung* 9(2):344-47, March/April 1980.

29 Urinary System

LEARNING OBJECTIVES

After completing this chapter, the reader will be able to:
- name two groups of diagnostic tests used to detect and evaluate urologic abnormalities.
- explain the anatomy and physiology of the urinary system.
- state the characteristics of cysts and tumors that permit differentiation by nephrotomography.
- state the purpose of each test discussed in the chapter.
- prepare the patient physically and psychologically for each test.
- describe the procedure for performing each test.
- specify appropriate precautions for safe administration of each test.
- recognize signs of adverse reaction and respond appropriately.
- implement appropriate post-test care.
- state the normal values for each test.
- discuss the implications of abnormal test results.
- list factors that may interfere with accurate test results.

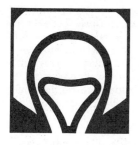

Urinary System

Introduction

Two groups of diagnostic tests exist for the detection and evaluation of urologic abnormalities in the urinary system. One group of tests analyzes the properties of urine, the end product of the urinary system; these tests, which include the invaluable routine urinalysis, are discussed in other chapters (see chapters 12 and 15). The other group of tests—which are detailed in this chapter—are used to study the structures and functions of the components of the urinary system.

Structure of the kidneys

The urinary system consists of the kidneys, ureters, bladder, and urethra. The kidneys are reddish-brown, bean-shaped organs situated in the back of the abdomen, flanking the vertebral column. Each kidney is about 4″ to 5″ (10 to 12.5 cm) long, 3″ (7.5 cm) wide, a little more than 1″ (2.5 cm) thick, and weighs 4 to 6 oz (113 to 170 g). It has an upper and a lower pole, anterior and posterior surfaces, convex lateral margins, and concave medial margins (or *hila*) that open into a fat-filled pocket called the renal sinus, through which pass the renal blood vessels, nerves, and pelvis. A fibrous capsule encloses the kidney and is continuous with internal connective tissues, which also line the sinus and calyces of the renal pelvis.

The kidneys are comprised of the *cortex* and the *medulla*. The outer cortical substance is light and granular, while the inner medullary substance is dark and striated. Both the cortex and the medulla contain uriniferous tubules—*nephrons*—and collecting tubules. Each nephron is made up of a renal corpuscle and a renal tubule. Each kidney contains about a million of these functional units.

The cortex, containing vascular glomeruli and convoluted tubules, forms a series of arches, supported on renal columns extending toward the central sinus. The arches and columns enclose the medulla, forming *renal pyramids* (8 to 12 per kidney). The bases of these pyramids project toward the cortex and their apices, ending in *papillae* toward the sinus. The minor calyces cap these papillae, collecting the urine that oozes through them. Urine drains from the minor calyces into three major calyces, which empty into the renal pelvis and from there into the ureter.

Renal blood supply

Blood flows from the aorta into the two renal arteries, each of which divides into two main branches. Just outside the sinus these main branches subdivide into more branches, to supply blood to the entire kidney. These branches are end arteries without anastomoses, so if one of them is obstructed, the result is infarction of the segment it supplies. Straight *inter-*

lobular arteries, too small to be seen with the unaided eye, supply blood to the renal columns and cortical arches. Each of these tiny arteries, in turn, supplies a group of lobules with a series of fine, twiglike *afferent arterioles.*

These minute arterioles enter the renal corpuscle, break into capillary tufts or glomeruli, and emerge as *efferent arterioles,* each of which ends in a *capillary intertubular plexus* along the convoluted tubules of its own nephron. The arterial and venous sets of capillaries are called *vasa recta* because they run parallel to the straight tubules. Venous blood from the cortex and the medulla returns to the interlobular veins and retraces the course of the arterial branches back to the sinus, ending in the renal vein.

Ureters and bladder

The ureters are narrow, muscular tubes that transport urine from the kidneys to the bladder. They are 10″ to 11″ (25 to 27.5 cm) long and nearly ¼″ (5 mm) in diameter. The renal pelvis narrows to form the top of the ureters; the tubes terminate at the posterior aspect of the bladder. The ureters enter the bladder wall obliquely, so that the ureteral openings in the bladder are normally only about 1″ (2.5 cm) apart.

An expansile, muscular sac, the bladder lies in the space between the pubic bones and the rectum, and serves as a reservoir for urine. When empty, the bladder has an apex (behind the symphysis pubis), a base, a superior aspect, and two inferolateral aspects. The base of the bladder faces downward and backward in both sexes. In males, the ampullae of the vas, the seminal vesicles, and the rectovesical fascia separate the base from the rectum. In females, the uterus and vagina intervene. Superiorly, the peritoneum loosely covers the bladder, with loops of intestine above it in males and the uterus over it in females. Inferolaterally, in both males and females, the bladder abuts the pubic bones, and the internal obturator and levator ani muscles.

The bladder comprises two basic parts: the *trigone* and the *detrusor muscle.* The trigone occupies the space between the internal urethral orifice and the two ureteral openings. The detrusor muscle—a meshwork of muscular fibers—forms most of the bladder wall, encircling the neck of the bladder and running inferiorly adjacent to the proximal urethra.

Urethra

In an adult male, the urethra is an S-shaped tube about 9″ (22.5 cm) long, extending from the internal urethral orifice through the prostate gland, the deep perineal pouch, and the corpus spongiosum of the penis. The urethra is anatomically divided into three sections: the prostatic urethra (about 2½″ [6 cm] long), the membranous urethra (about ½″ to ¾″ [1.5 to 2 cm] long), and the spongy (or cavernous) urethra (about 6″ [15 cm] long). The first two sections, which easily become infected because of their vascularity and lymph drainage, are clinically considered as one part—the *prostatic urethra.* The membranous segment—the thin-walled, least mobile part of the urethra—is susceptible to injury on catheterization or pelvic fracture. The male urethra serves as a conduit for urine and for the products of the genital system.

In an adult female, the urethra serves one function: to conduct urine out of the body. The female urethra is only 1½″ (4 cm) long and can dilate to a diameter of ¼″ (5 mm). It runs downward and forward, from the neck of the bladder to the pudendal cleft, with a slight anterior concavity behind the symphysis pubis. The lower fibers of the urethral sphincter muscle bind the urethra tightly to the anterior vaginal wall, in which it is embedded. The epithelial lining of the urethra, subject to diverse hormonal activity, undergoes postmenopausal attrition along with adjacent structures. Adventitious organisms commonly colonize the external meatus because it's so close to the vagina and the rectum, which largely accounts for the higher incidence of urinary tract infections in females.

Diagnostic applications

The diagnostic tests discussed in this chapter are recommended after a complete history and physical examination have established the presence of clinical abnormalities associated with urologic disease. For example, the patient may complain of hematuria or flank pain, and the history may reveal urgency or frequency of urination, dysuria, nocturia, enuresis, or incontinence. Physical examination may detect fever, hypertension, and weight gain related to fluid retention. Associated changes in skin color and texture may include pallor, jaundice, excoriation, infection, pitting edema, easy bruising, and urate crystals. Ocular changes may reflect hemorrhage, exudates, and papilledema. Abnormal oral findings include stomatitis and a fetid breath odor. Fluid retention may also cause edema in the eyelids, face, abdomen, arms, and legs. Palpation of the abdomen may reveal tender or enlarged kidney masses or a distended bladder. Examination of the genitalia may reveal phimosis, paraphimosis, or testicular masses; a rectal examination may reveal prostatic hypertrophy.

The tests

Diagnostic testing of a patient with urinary symptoms generally begins with *kidney-ureter-bladder* (KUB) *radiography,* which supplies information on the urinary tract, including kidney structure, size, and position.

Nephrotomography allows examination of a single slice or plane of renal tissue. Levels anterior and posterior to the selected plane are blurred, highlighting a specific area.

Renal computed tomography supplies a three-dimensional, cross-sectional view of the kidneys that has greater detail than any other urologic test.

Renal ultrasonography, often used with excretory urography, is especially helpful in differentiating between a solid tumor and a simple, fluid-filled cyst.

Lesions such as urethral strictures and calculi, as well as prostatic urethral disease and bladder disease, may be confirmed by *cystourethroscopy.* This procedure, performed under a local or general anesthetic, involves the passage of a rigid fiberoptic instrument transurethrally into the bladder to visually inspect vesicourethral structures.

In *retrograde urethrography,* a Foley catheter is inserted just far enough to permit contrast medium instillation into the urethra, to outline its structure.

In *retrograde cystography,* bladder structure is evaluated by the instillation of a contrast medium into the bladder, through a Foley catheter. Several urologic tests use contrast media to outline organ structure and help identify abnormalities such as calculi and cysts.

When disease severely affects renal function, *retrograde ureteropyelography* may be indicated for more accurate assessment. In this test, contrast medium is introduced into the renal pelvis in retrograde fashion, which allows intense opacification of the collecting system and ureters.

Antegrade pyelography examines the kidney by assessing the pressure and composition of urine drawn directly from it. Then contrast medium is injected into the kidney to detect obstructions.

Excretory urography, commonly referred to as intravenous pyelography, is the radiographic examination of the kidneys, ureters, and bladder after I.V. administration of a contrast medium. The effectiveness of this procedure depends on renal capacity to concentrate and excrete the contrast medium.

In *radionuclide renal imaging,* radionuclides administered I.V. filter through the kidneys at a specific rate and concentration, providing valuable information about the effectiveness of renal perfusion and function.

Renal angiography evaluates the efficiency of renal circulation and perfusion, and clearly outlines the renal parenchyma to help determine the cause of renovascular hypertension.

Renal venography can detect abnormalities of the renal veins and tributaries, such as thrombosis.

THE URINARY SYSTEM

THE KIDNEY: CORONAL SECTION

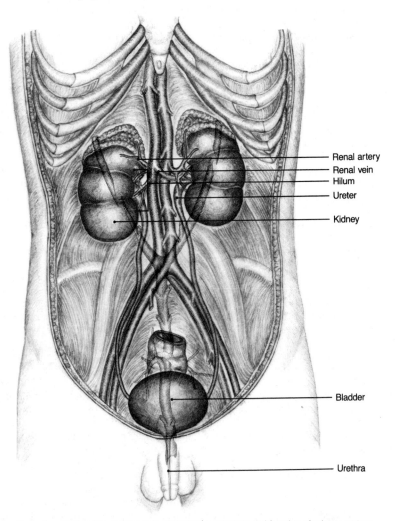

Renal artery
Renal vein
Hilum
Ureter

Kidney

Bladder

Urethra

Tests described in this chapter help evaluate the structure and function of urinary system components—kidneys, ureters, bladder, and urethra. The kidneys house over 2 million uriniferous tubules (nephrons and collecting tubules) that perform the vital renal functions: cleansing the blood of metabolic wastes and regulating the retention of substances required to preserve the body's fluid, electrolyte, and acid-base balances. The glomerulus, a tuft of capillaries within each nephron's renal corpuscle, accomplishes the actual filtration of fluids and solutes from the blood, and the renal tubule functions to reabsorb needed fluids and secrete excess electrolytes. The end product that reaches the collecting tubule is urine.

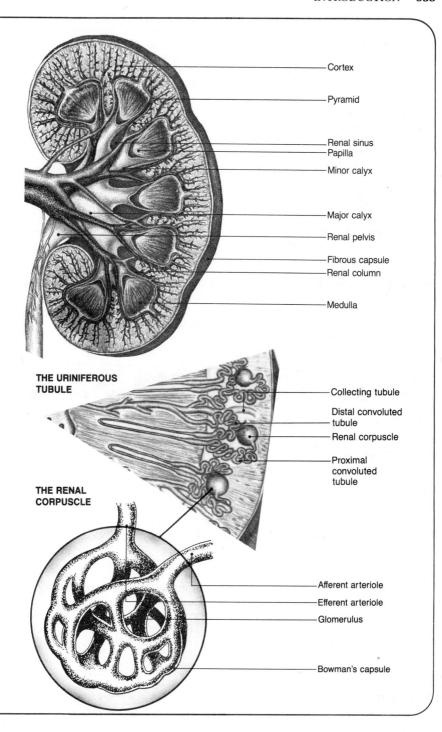

Cortex

Pyramid

Renal sinus
Papilla

Minor calyx

Major calyx

Renal pelvis

Fibrous capsule
Renal column

Medulla

THE URINIFEROUS TUBULE

Collecting tubule

Distal convoluted tubule

Renal corpuscle

Proximal convoluted tubule

THE RENAL CORPUSCLE

Afferent arteriole

Efferent arteriole

Glomerulus

Bowman's capsule

A simple noninvasive test, *uroflowmetry* evaluates urine flow to detect lower urinary tract dysfunction or obstruction.

Cystometry evaluates bladder function after instillation of normal saline solution or water, or insufflation of a gas.

To determine how well the bladder and sphincter muscle interact, *external sphincter electromyography* can measure their activity with electrodes.

Voiding cystourethrography involves injection of a contrast medium, to evaluate urethral function during voiding and to diagnose vesicoureteral reflux.

The *Whitaker test* detects obstructions and determines the need for surgery by measuring urine pressure and flow in the kidneys, ureters, and bladder.

Nursing considerations

When caring for a patient who is scheduled for or who has undergone urologic testing, remember these points:

□ Make sure the fluid intake of a patient with a suspected urinary tract lesion is adequate (except when underlying medical conditions dictate fluid restriction). Adequate hydration is also necessary to help flush out contrast medium.

□ Administer a laxative, as ordered, to a patient scheduled for radiographic tests, since overlying gas or feces in the lumen of the gastrointestinal tract may interfere with the quality of X-ray films.

□ After an invasive procedure, such as retrograde cystography, monitor fluid intake and output. Inability to void may necessitate catheterization. Notify the doctor if hematuria persists after the third voiding.

□ Watch for signs of urinary sepsis (such as fever, chills, or hypotension) after any test (such as cystourethroscopy) that involves urinary system instrumentation.

□ Because many urologic tests are embarrassing to the patient, minimize his anxiety by clearly describing the procedures he'll undergo.

PATRICE M. NASIELSKI, RN

STRUCTURAL TESTS

Kidney-Ureter-Bladder Radiography

[Scout film or flat plate of the abdomen]

Usually the first step in diagnostic testing of the urinary system, kidney-ureter-bladder (KUB) radiography surveys the abdomen to determine the position of the kidneys, ureters, and bladder, and to detect gross abnormalities. This test does not require intact renal function and may aid differential diagnosis of urologic and gastrointestinal diseases, which often produce similar signs and symptoms. However, a KUB has many limitations and nearly always must be followed by more elaborate tests, such as excretory urography or renal computed tomography. KUB should not follow recent instillation of barium, which obscures the urinary system.

Purpose

□ To evaluate the size, structure, and position of the kidneys

□ To screen for abnormalities, such as calcifications, in the region of the kidneys, ureters, and bladder.

Patient preparation

Explain to the patient that this test shows the position of the urinary system organs and helps detect abnormalities in them. Inform him that he needn't restrict food or fluids. Tell him who will perform the test and where, and that it takes only a few minutes.

Procedure

The patient is placed in supine position in correct body alignment, on a radiographic table. His arms are extended overhead, and the iliac crests are checked for symmetrical positioning. A single radiograph is taken.

Precautions

The male patient should have gonadal shielding to prevent irradiation of the testes. The female patient's ovaries can't be shielded because they're located too close to the kidneys, ureters, and bladder.

Findings

The shadows of the kidneys appear bilaterally, the right slightly lower than the left. Both kidneys should be approximately the same size, with the superior poles tilted slightly toward the vertebral column, paralleling the shadows (or stripes) produced by the psoas muscles. The ureters aren't usually visible unless an abnormality, such as calcification, is present. Visualization of the bladder depends on the density of its muscular wall and on the amount of urine in the bladder. Generally, a shadow of the bladder can be seen but not as clearly as those of the kidneys.

Implications of results

Bilateral renal enlargement may result from polycystic disease, multiple myeloma, lymphoma, amyloidosis, hydronephrosis, or compensatory hypertrophy. Tumor, cyst, or hydronephrosis may cause unilateral enlargement. Abnormally small kidneys may suggest end-stage glomerulonephritis or bilateral atrophic pyelonephritis. An apparent decrease in the size of one kidney suggests possible congenital hypoplasia, atrophic pyelonephritis, or ischemia. Renal displacement may be due to a retroperitoneal tumor, such as an adrenal tumor. Obliteration or bulging of a portion of the psoas muscle stripe may result from tumor, abscess, or hematoma.

Congenital anomalies, such as abnormal location or absence of a kidney, may be detected. Horseshoe kidney may be suggested by renal axes that parallel the vertebral column, especially if the inferior poles of the kidneys cannot be clearly distinguished. A lobulated edge or border may suggest polycystic kidney disease or patchy atrophic pyelonephritis.

Opaque bodies may reflect calculi or vascular calcification due to aneurysm or atheroma; opacification may also suggest cystic tumors, fecaliths, foreign bodies, or abnormal fluid collection. Calcifications may appear anywhere in the urinary system, but positive identi-

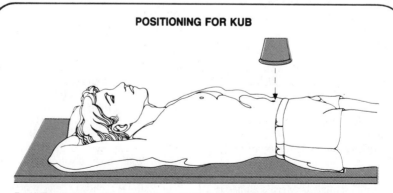

POSITIONING FOR KUB

For KUB radiography, the patient is instructed to lie in a supine position with his arms extended over his head. To prevent motion and ensure a quality image on the film, he is asked to lie very still for the few seconds it takes to make the exposure. An obese patient may be asked to exhale and then hold his breath during the brief procedure. As an added precaution, gonadal shielding should be used for the male patient.

fication requires further testing. The lone exception is staghorn calculus, which forms a perfect cast of the renal pelvis and calyces.

Post-test care
None.

Interfering factors
□ Gas, feces, contrast medium, or foreign bodies in the intestine may obscure the urinary system.

□ Calcified uterine fibromas or ovarian lesions may prevent clear visualization of the kidneys, ureters, and bladder.

□ Obesity or ascites may result in a radiograph of poor quality.

PATRICE M. NASIELSKI, RN

Nephrotomography

In nephrotomography, special films are exposed before and after opacification of the renal arterial network and parenchyma with contrast medium. The resulting tomographic slices clearly delineate various linear layers of the kidneys, while blurring structures in front of and behind these selected planes. Nephrotomography can be performed as a separate procedure or as an adjunct to excretory urography. Nephrotomography is particularly helpful in visualizing space-occupying lesions suggested by excretory urography or retrograde ureteropyelography. Additional films are exposed to define the thickness of the wall of the mass and its interior. Other tests that may resolve nephrotomographic findings include renal angiography and radionuclide renal imaging.

Purpose
□ To differentiate between a simple renal cyst and a solid neoplasm
□ To assess renal lacerations as well as post-traumatic nonperfused areas of the kidneys
□ To localize adrenal tumors when lab-

oratory tests indicate their presence.

Patient preparation
Explain to the patient that this test provides images of sections or layers of the kidney tissues and blood vessels. Instruct him to fast for 8 hours before the test. Tell him who will perform the test and where, and that the test takes less than 1 hour.

Inform the patient that he'll be positioned on an X-ray table, and that he'll hear loud, clacking sounds as the films are exposed. Tell him he may experience transient side effects from the injection of the contrast medium—usually a burning or stinging sensation at the injection site, flushing, and a metallic taste.

Make sure the patient or responsible member of the family has signed a consent form. Check the patient's history for hypersensitivity to iodine or iodine-containing foods or to contrast media used in other diagnostic tests. If the patient has a history of sensitivity, inform the doctor so he can provide anti-allergenic prophylaxis (such as diphenhydramine).

Equipment
X-ray table/X-ray and tomographic equipment/contrast medium/infusion set and equipment.

Procedure
The test may be performed using either the infusion method or the bolus method. The former is currently the method of choice, because it allows for repeating poorly defined tomograms without additional infusion of contrast. Complications resulting from either technique are minor and infrequent. Regardless of the technique used, first a plain film of the kidneys is exposed, to provide general information about position, size, and shape, and preliminary anteroposterior tomograms are made to determine tomographic levels. Posterior oblique tomograms are made to rule out the presence of radiopaque renal calculi, which would be masked by the contrast.

Infusion method: After test tomograms are reviewed, five vertical slices of renal parenchyma 1 cm apart are selected for filming. Contrast medium is then administered through the antecubital vein—the first half in 4 to 5 minutes (rapid phase) and the second half in the following 8 to 10 minutes (slow phase). Serial tomograms are made as soon as the slow phase begins.

Bolus method: After test tomograms are reviewed, circulation time from arm to tongue is determined by injecting a bolus of a bitter-tasting agent (dehydrocholic acid or sodium dehydrocholate) into the antecubital vein. Arm-to-tongue circulation time is close to arm-to-kidney circulation time (10 to 14 seconds). With the needle still in place, a loading dose of a conventional urographic contrast medium is injected, to perform excretory urography.

Five minutes after this injection, a loading dose of a contrast medium (such as Renografin-76 or Hypaque-M 75%) is quickly injected—within 2 seconds—to ensure a high concentration of the contrast in the kidneys. A multifilm tomographic cassette, exposed at the predetermined arm-to-kidney circulation time, visualizes the main renal vessels and possible vessels within tumors. A series of individual tomograms measuring 1 cm are then made in rapid succession—less than 2 minutes—through the opacified kidneys.

Although the bolus method produces exposures that are as good as, if not better than, those obtained by the infusion technique, it requires almost perfect timing. If the exposures are poor, the bolus method requires a second infusion of contrast, because the kidneys clear the contrast medium quickly.

Precautions
Although not strictly contraindicated, nephrotomography should be performed with extreme caution in patients with hypersensitivity to iodine-based compounds or in those with severe cardiovascular disease or multiple myeloma.

Findings
The size, shape, and position of the kidneys appear within normal range, with no space-occupying lesions or other abnormalities.

Implications of results
Among the abnormalities detectable through nephrotomography are simple cysts and solid tumors, renal sinus-related lesions, ectopic renal lobes, adrenal tumors, areas of nonperfusion, and renal lacerations following trauma.

Post-test care
□ If a hematoma develops at the injection

SIMPLE CYST OR SOLID TUMOR: DIFFERENTIAL DIAGNOSIS IN NEPHROTOMOGRAPHY

FEATURE	CYST	TUMOR
Consistency	Homogeneous	Irregular
Contact with healthy renal tissue	Sharply distinct	Poorly resolved
Density	Radiolucent	Variable radiolucent patches (or same as normal renal parenchyma)
Shape	Spherical	Variable
Wall of lesion	Thin and well-defined	Thick and irregular

site, apply warm soaks.

☐ Monitor vital signs and urinary output for 24 hours after the test.

☐ Observe for signs of post-test allergic reaction (flushing, nausea, urticaria, and sneezing).

Interfering factors

Pretest upper or lower gastrointestinal series, or residual barium from a recent barium enema may obscure sharp delineation of the kidneys.

FRANK LOWELL BROWN, CUT

Renal Computed Tomography

Renal computed tomography (CT) provides a useful image of the kidneys made from a series of tomograms or cross-sectional slices, which are then translated by a computer and displayed on an oscilloscope screen. The image density reflects the amount of radiation absorbed by renal tissue and permits identification of masses and other lesions. An I.V. contrast medium may be injected to accentuate the renal parenchyma's density and help differentiate renal masses. This highly accurate test is usually performed to investigate diseases found by other diagnostic procedures, such as excretory urography. It may also precede percutaneous biopsy, to guide needle placement, or may follow a kidney transplant, to determine the kidney's size and location in relation to the bladder. In addition, it can localize renal or perinephric abscesses for drainage.

Purpose

☐ To detect and evaluate renal pathology, such as tumor, obstruction, calculi, polycystic kidney disease, congenital anomalies, and abnormal fluid accumulation around the kidneys

☐ To evaluate the retroperitoneum.

Patient preparation

Explain to the patient that this test permits examination of the kidneys. If contrast enhancement is not scheduled, inform the patient that he needn't restrict food or fluids. If contrast enhancement will be performed, instruct him to fast for 4 hours before the test. Tell him who will perform the test and where, and that the procedure takes about an hour, depending on the reason for the scan and the area to be evaluated.

Inform the patient that he'll be positioned on an X-ray table, and that a scanner will take films of his kidneys. Warn him that the scanner will make loud, clacking sounds as it rotates around his body. Tell him he may experience transient side effects, such as flushing and headache, following injection of the contrast medium.

Make sure the patient or responsible member of the family has signed a consent form. Check the patient's history for hypersensitivity to shellfish, iodine, or the contrast media used in other diagnostic tests. Inform the doctor of any sensitivities.

Just before the procedure, instruct the patient to put on a hospital gown and to remove any metallic objects that could interfere with the scan. Administer a pretest sedative, as ordered.

Equipment

Total body CT scanner/contrast medium/ I.V. infusion setup/syringes and needles.

Procedure

The patient is placed in supine position on the scanning table and secured with straps. The table is moved into the scanner, and the patient is instructed to lie still. The scanner is operated from an adjacent room where the patient can be heard and observed. When the scanner is turned on, it rotates around the patient, taking multiple images at different angles within each cross-sectional slice.

When one series of tomograms is complete, contrast enhancement may be performed. An I.V. contrast medium is administered, and the patient is ob-

ABNORMAL RENAL CT SCAN

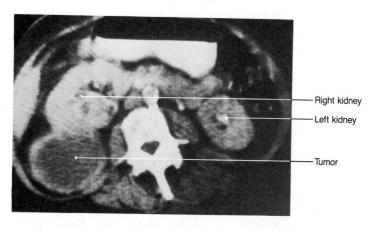

Right kidney

Left kidney

Tumor

Computerized tomography (photograph above) reveals a renal adenocarcinoma that has displaced and distorted the right kidney and exceeds it in size. The left kidney appears normal, the spine is sharp and white at the center of the photograph, and the stomach equally clear at the top. This common tumor, also called hypernephroma, accounts for 75% of renal malignancies.

served for allergic reactions, such as respiratory difficulty and urticaria or other skin eruption. Another series of tomograms is then taken. Information from the scan is stored on a disk or on magnetic tape, fed into a computer, and converted into an image for display on an oscilloscope screen. Radiographs and photographs are taken of selected views.

Precautions
Watch for signs of hypersensitivity to contrast medium if contrast enhancement is required.

Findings
Normally, the density of the renal parenchyma is slightly higher than that of the liver, but less dense than bone, which appears white on a CT scan. The density of the collecting system is generally low (black), unless contrast medium is used to enhance it to a higher (whiter) density. The position of the kidneys is evaluated according to the surrounding structures; the size and shape of the kidneys are determined by counting cuts

between the superior and inferior poles and following the contour of the renal outline.

Implications of results
Renal masses appear as areas of different density than normal parenchyma, possibly altering the kidneys' shape or projecting beyond their margins. Renal cysts, for example, appear as smooth, sharply defined masses, with thin walls and a lower density than normal parenchyma. Tumors such as renal cell carcinoma, however, are usually not as well delineated; they tend to have thick walls and nonuniform density. With contrast enhancement, solid tumors show a higher density than renal cysts but lower density than normal parenchyma. Tumors with hemorrhage, calcification, or necrosis show higher densities. Vascular tumors are more clearly defined with contrast enhancement. Adrenal tumors are confined masses, usually detached from the kidneys and from other retroperitoneal organs.

Renal CT may also identify other abnormalities, including obstructions, calculi, polycystic kidney disease, congenital anomalies, and abnormal accumulations of fluid around the kidneys, such as hematomas, lymphoceles, and abscesses. After nephrectomy, CT can detect abnormal masses, such as recurrent tumors, in a renal fossa that should be empty.

Post-test care

If the procedure was performed with contrast enhancement, observe the patient for hypersensitivity to the contrast medium, and tell him he may resume his usual diet.

Interfering factors

□ Patient failure to lie still during the scan results in blurred images.

□ Artifacts may be caused by many factors, such as recent contrast studies, foreign bodies, catheters, and surgical clips.

FRANK LOWELL BROWN, CUT

Renal Ultrasonography

In this test, high-frequency sound waves (usually 1 to 5 million cycles/second) are transmitted from a transducer through the kidneys and perirenal structures. The resulting echoes, amplified and converted into electrical impulses, are displayed on an oscilloscope screen as anatomic images. Usually performed with other urologic tests, renal ultrasonography can detect abnormalities or clarify those detected by other tests. A safe, painless procedure, it's especially valuable when excretory urography is ruled out—for example, by hypersensitivity to the contrast medium or the need for serial examinations. Unlike excretory urography, this test is not dependent on renal function and therefore can be useful in patients with renal failure. Eval-

uation of urologic disorders may also include ultrasonography of the ureter, bladder, and gonads.

Purpose

□ To determine the size, shape, and position of the kidneys, their internal structures, and perirenal tissues

□ To evaluate and localize urinary obstruction and abnormal accumulation of fluid

□ To assess and diagnose complications following kidney transplantation.

Patient preparation

Explain to the patient that this test helps detect abnormalities in the kidneys. Inform him that he needn't restrict food or fluids. Tell him who will perform the test and where, and that it takes about 30 minutes. Reassure him that the test is safe and painless; in fact, it may feel like a back rub.

Just before the procedure, instruct the patient to put on a hospital gown.

Equipment

Ultrasound transducer and jelly/cathode ray tube and amplifier/oscilloscope/Polaroid camera/dynamic or real-time imaging equipment.

Procedure

The patient is placed in prone position, and the area to be scanned is exposed. Ultrasound jelly is applied to the area before the scanning begins. First, the longitudinal axis of the kidneys is located, using measurements from excretory urography or by performing transverse scans through the upper and lower renal poles. These points are marked on the skin and connected with straight lines. Sectional images (1 to 2 cm apart) can then be obtained by moving the transducer longitudinally and transversely or at any other angle required. During the test, the patient may be asked to breathe deeply to assess the kidneys' movement during respiration.

Precautions

None.

Findings

The kidneys are located between the superior iliac crests and the diaphragm. The renal capsule should be outlined sharply; the cortex should produce more echoes than the medulla. In the center of each kidney, the renal collecting systems appear as irregular areas of higher density than surrounding tissue. The renal veins and, depending on the scanner, some internal structures can be visualized. If the bladder is also being evaluated, its size, shape, position, and urine content can be determined.

Implications of results

Cysts are usually fluid-filled, circular structures that don't reflect sound waves. Tumors produce multiple echoes and appear as irregular shapes. Abscesses found within or around the kidneys usually echo sound waves poorly; their boundaries are slightly more irregular than those of cysts. A perirenal abscess may displace the kidney anteriorly.

Generally, acute pyelonephritis and glomerulonephritis aren't detectable unless the renal parenchyma is significantly scarred and atrophied. In such patients, the renal capsule appears irregular and the kidney may appear smaller than normal; also, an increased number of echoes may arise from the parenchyma, due to fibrosis.

In patients with hydronephrosis, renal ultrasonography may show a large, echo-free, central mass that compresses the renal cortex. Calyceal echoes are usually circularly diffused and the pelvis significantly enlarged. This test can also detect congenital anomalies, such as horseshoe, ectopic, or duplicated kidneys. Ultrasonography clearly detects renal hypertrophy.

Following renal transplantation, compensatory hypertrophy of the transplanted kidney is normal but an acute increase in size indicates rejection of the transplant.

This test allows identification of abnormal accumulations of fluid within or around the kidneys that sometimes arise from an obstruction. It also allows evaluation of perirenal structures, and can identify abnormalities of the adrenal glands, such as tumors, cysts, and adrenal dysfunction. However, a normal adrenal gland is difficult to define ultrasonically because of its small size.

Renal ultrasonography can detect changes in the shape of the bladder that result from masses and can assess urine volume. Increased urine volume or residual urine postvoiding may indicate bladder dysfunction.

Post-test care

Be sure ultrasound jelly is removed from the patient's skin.

Interfering factors

None.

FRANK LOWELL BROWN, CUT

Cystourethroscopy

Cystourethroscopy, a test that combines two endoscopic techniques, allows visual examination of the bladder and the urethra. One of the instruments used in this test is the cystoscope, which has a fiberoptic light source, a magnification system, a right-angled telescopic lens, and an angled beak, for smooth passage into the bladder. The other instrument, the urethroscope or the panendoscope, is similar but has a straight-ahead lens and is used for examination of the bladder neck and the urethra. Usually a common sheath is inserted into the urethra, through which a cystoscope or urethroscope may be passed to obtain the desired view. This is less traumatic for the patient and permits a readily available channel for additional invasive procedures, such as biopsy, lesion resection, collection of calculi, or passage of a ureteral catheter to the renal pelvis, for pyelography.

Kidney-ureter-bladder radiography and excretory urography usually precede cystourethroscopy.

Purpose

To diagnose and evaluate urinary tract disorders.

Patient preparation

Explain to the patient that this test permits examination of the bladder and the urethra. Unless a general anesthetic has been ordered, inform the patient that he needn't restrict food or fluids. If a general anesthetic will be administered, instruct the patient to fast for 8 hours before the test. Tell him who will perform the test and where, and that it takes about 20 to 30 minutes. Inform him that he may experience some discomfort after the procedure, including a slight burning when he urinates.

Make sure the patient or responsible member of the family has signed a consent form. Just before the procedure, administer a sedative, as ordered, and instruct the patient to urinate.

Equipment

Cystourethroscope (components include sheath, cystoscope, and urethroscope)/light source/Bougies á boule (for urethral calibration)/sounds (for urethral dilatation)/filiforms and followers (for severe stricture)/preparatory tray/local anesthetic set/irrigating solution and administration set/sterile gloves, gown, and drape/sterile specimen containers.

Procedure

After general or regional anesthetic (as required) has been administered, the patient is placed in lithotomy position on a cystoscopic table. The genitalia are cleansed with an antiseptic solution, and the patient is draped. (Local anesthetic is instilled at this point.)

As the first step in cystourethroscopy, most urologists prefer to visually examine the urethra as they move the instrument toward the bladder. To do this,

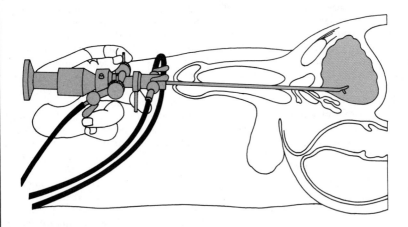

VIEWING THE URINARY SYSTEM WITH A CYSTOURETHROSCOPE

This cross-sectional illustration shows urologic examination with a cystourethroscope, a device for direct visualization of the tissues of the lower urinary tract. The sheath of the cystourethroscope permits passage of various auxiliary instruments for illuminating the urethra, bladder, and ureters. This instrument also provides a channel for minor surgical procedures, commonly including biopsies; excision of small lesions of the bladder, urethra, and prostate; removal of calculi; catheterization of the ureters, for retrograde pyelography; and dilatation of a constricted urethra. Cystourethroscopic examination and its accompanying procedures can guide therapy decisions and can sometimes eliminate the need for open surgery.

a urethroscope is inserted into the well-lubricated sheath (instead of an obturator), and both are passed gently through the urethra into the bladder. The urethroscope is then removed, and a cystoscope inserted through the sheath into the bladder. After the bladder is filled with irrigating solution, the scope is rotated to inspect the entire surface of the bladder wall and ureteral orifices with the right-angled telescopic lens. The cystoscope is then removed, the urethroscope reinserted, and both the urethroscope and the sheath are slowly withdrawn, permitting examination of the bladder neck and the various portions of the urethra, including the internal and external sphincters.

During cystourethroscopy, a urine specimen is routinely taken from the bladder for culture and sensitivity testing, and residual urine is measured. If a tumor is suspected, a urine specimen is sent to the laboratory for cytologic examination; if a tumor is found, biopsy may be performed. If a urethral stricture is present, urethral dilatation may be necessary before cystourethroscopy.

If the patient has received only a local anesthetic, he may complain of a burning sensation when the instrument is passed through the urethra. He may also feel an urgent need to urinate as the bladder is filled with irrigating solution. The patient should be reassured that these sensations are common and generally transient.

Precautions
Cystourethroscopy is contraindicated in patients with acute forms of urethritis, prostatitis, or cystitis, since instrumentation can lead to sepsis.

Findings
The urethra, bladder, and ureteral orifices appear normal in size, shape, and position. The mucosa lining the lower urinary tract should appear smooth and shiny, with no evidence of erythema, cysts, or other abnormalities. The bladder should be free of obstructions, tumors, and calculi.

Implications of results
One of the most common abnormal findings in cystourethroscopy is an enlarged prostate gland in older men. In both males and females, urethral stricture, calculi, tumors, diverticula, ulcers, and polyps are also common findings. In addition, this test may detect bladder wall trabeculation and various congenital anomalies, such as ureteroceles, duplicate ureteral orifices, or urethral valves in children.

Post-test care
☐ Monitor vital signs every 15 minutes for the first hour after the test, then every hour until they stabilize.

☐ Instruct the patient to drink fluids freely and to take the prescribed analgesic. Reassure him that burning and frequency will soon subside.

☐ Administer antibiotics, as ordered, to prevent bacterial sepsis due to urethral tissue trauma.

☐ Report flank or abdominal pain, chills, fever, or low urinary output to the doctor immediately.

☐ Record intake and output for 24 hours, and observe the patient for distention. If the patient doesn't void within 8 hours after the test, or if bright red blood continues to appear after three voidings, notify the doctor.

☐ Instruct the patient to abstain from alcohol for 48 hours.

Interfering factors
None.

FRANK LOWELL BROWN, CUT

Retrograde Urethrography

Used almost exclusively in males, this radiographic study is performed during instillation or injection of a contrast medium into the urethra, permitting visualization of its membranous, bulbar, and penile portions. *Clinical indications for retrograde urethrography include outlet obstructions, congenital anomalies, and urethral lacerations or other trauma. This test may also be performed on patients who require a follow-up examination after surgical repair of the urethra. Although visualization of the anterior portion of the urethra is excellent with this test alone, the posterior portion is more effectively outlined by retrograde urethrography in tandem with voiding cystourethrography.*

Purpose
□ To diagnose urethral strictures, lacerations, and diverticula, and congenital anomalies.

Patient preparation
Explain to the patient that this test helps diagnose urethral structural problems. Inform him that he needn't restrict food or fluids. Tell him who will perform the test and where, and that it takes about 30 minutes.

Inform the patient that he may experience some discomfort when the catheter is inserted and when the contrast medium is instilled through the catheter. Tell him he'll hear loud, clacking sounds as the X-ray films are made.

Make sure the patient or responsible member of the family has signed a consent form. Check the patient's history for hypersensitivity to iodine-based contrast media or iodine-containing foods, such as shellfish. Inform the doctor of any sensitivities.

Just before the procedure, administer a sedative, as ordered, and instruct the patient to void before leaving the unit.

Equipment
X-ray machine and table/penile clamp/ 50-ml syringe with tapered universal adapter/Foley catheter/1″ roller gauze/ contrast medium (half-strength preparation).

Procedure
The male patient is placed in a recumbent position on the examining table. Anteroposterior exposures of the bladder and urethra are made, and the resulting films studied for radiopaque densities, foreign bodies, or stones. The glans and meatus are cleansed with an antiseptic solution. The catheter is filled with the contrast medium before insertion, to eliminate air bubbles. Although no lubricant should be used, the tip of the catheter may be dipped in sterile water to facilitate insertion.

The catheter is inserted until the balloon portion is inside the meatus; the balloon is then inflated with 1 to 2 ml of water, which prevents the catheter from slipping during the procedure.

The patient then assumes the right posterior oblique position, with his right thigh drawn up to a 90° angle and the penis placed along its axis. The left thigh is extended. The contrast medium is then injected through the catheter. After three fourths of the contrast has been injected, the first X-ray film is exposed, while the rest of the contrast is injected. Left lateral oblique views may also be taken. Fluoroscopic control may be helpful, especially for evaluating urethral injury.

In females, this test may be used when urethral diverticula are suspected. A double-balloon catheter is used, which occludes the bladder neck from above and the external meatus from below. In children, the procedure is the same as for adults, except that a smaller catheter is used.

Precautions
Retrograde urethrography should be performed cautiously in the presence of urinary tract infection.

Findings
The membranous, bulbar, and penile portions of the urethra—and occasionally the prostatic portion—appear normal, in size, shape, and course.

Implications of results
Radiographs obtained during retrograde urethrography may show the following abnormalities: urethral diverticula, fistulas, strictures, false passages, calculi,

and lacerations; congenital anomalies, such as urethral valves and perineal hypospadias; and rarely, tumors (in less than 1% of patients).

Post-test care
Watch for chills and fever related to extravasation of contrast medium into the general circulation for 12 to 24 hours after retrograde urethrography. Also observe for signs of sepsis and allergic manifestations.

Interfering factors
None.

FRANK LOWELL BROWN, CUT

Retrograde Cystography

Retrograde cystography involves the instillation of contrast medium into the bladder, followed by radiographic examination. This procedure is used to diagnose bladder rupture without urethral involvement, since it can determine the location and extent of the rupture. Other indications for retrograde cystography include neurogenic bladder, recurrent urinary tract infections (especially in children), suspected vesicoureteral reflux, and vesical fistulas, diverticula, and tumors. This test is also performed when cystoscopic examination is impractical, as in male infants, or when excretory urography has not adequately visualized the bladder. Voiding cystourethrography is often performed concomitantly.

Purpose
To evaluate the structure and integrity of the bladder.

Patient preparation
Explain to the patient that the test permits radiographic examination (or X-ray films) of the bladder. Inform him that he needn't restrict food or fluids. Tell him who will perform the test and where, and that the procedure takes about 30 to 60 minutes.

Inform the patient that he may experience some discomfort when the catheter is inserted and when the contrast medium is instilled through the catheter. Tell him he'll hear loud, clacking sounds as the X-ray films are made.

Make sure the patient or responsible family member has signed a consent form. Check the patient's history for hypersensitivity to contrast media used in other diagnostic tests. Inform the doctor if such a sensitivity is present.

Equipment
X-ray equipment/drip infusion set or syringes/standard contrast medium/urethral Foley catheters.

Procedure
The patient is placed in supine position on the examining table, and a preliminary kidney-ureter-bladder radiograph is taken. This radiograph is developed immediately and scrutinized for renal shadows, calcifications, contours of the bone and psoas muscles, and gas patterns in the lumen of the gastrointestinal tract.

The bladder is then catheterized, and 200 to 300 ml of contrast medium (50 to 100 ml in an infant) is instilled, by gravity or gentle syringe injection. The catheter is then clamped.

With the patient supine, an anteroposterior film is taken. The patient is then tilted to one side, then the other, and two posterior oblique (and sometimes lateral) views are taken. If the patient's condition permits, he is placed in the jackknife position, and a posteroanterior film is taken. A space-occupying vesical lesion may require additional exposures. Rarely, to enhance visualization, 100 to 300 ml of air may be insufflated into the bladder by syringe after removal of the contrast medium (double contrast technique).

The catheter is then unclamped, the bladder fluid allowed to drain, and a

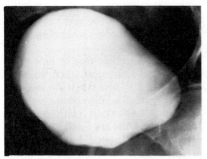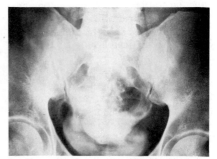

A normal retrograde cystogram (left) contrasts sharply with one showing a ruptured bladder (right). In the photograph on the right, the bladder, usually smooth and rounded when filled, has collapsed downward on itself, against the pelvic floor, and contrast material has extravasated upward into the peritoneal cavity from the tear in the bladder wall.

radiograph obtained to detect urethral diverticula, fistulous tracts into the vagina, or intra- or extraperitoneal extravasation of the contrast medium.

Precautions

□ Retrograde cystography is contraindicated during exacerbation of an acute urinary tract infection or in the presence of obstruction that prevents passage of a urinary catheter.

□ This test would not be performed in the presence of urethral evulsion or transection, unless catheter passage and flow of contrast medium were monitored fluoroscopically.

Findings

Retrograde cystography shows a bladder with normal contours, capacity, integrity, and urethrovesical angle, with no evidence of tumor, diverticula, or rupture. Vesicoureteral reflux should be absent. The bladder should not be displaced or externally compressed; the bladder wall should be smooth, not thick.

Implications of results

Retrograde cystography can identify vesical trabeculae or diverticula, space-occupying lesions (tumors), calculi or gravel, blood clots, high- or low-pressure vesicoureteral reflux, and hypo- or hypertonic bladder.

Post-test care

□ Monitor vital signs every 15 minutes for the first hour, every 30 minutes during the second hour, then every 2 hours for up to 24 hours.

□ Record the time of the patient's voidings, and the color and volume of the urine. Observe for hematuria. If it persists after the third voiding, notify the doctor.

□ Watch for signs of urinary sepsis from urinary tract infection (chills, fever, elevated pulse and respiration rates, hypotension) or similar signs related to extravasation of contrast medium into the general circulation.

Interfering factors

Residual barium from recent diagnostic tests or the presence of feces or gas in the bowel may produce cloudy images and interfere with test results.

FRANK LOWELL BROWN, CUT

Retrograde Ureteropyelography

Retrograde ureteropyelography allows radiographic examination of the renal collecting system after injection of a contrast medium through a ureteral catheter during cystoscopy. The contrast medium is usually iodine-based, and although some of it may be absorbed through the mucous membranes, this test is preferred for patients with hypersensitivity to iodine (in whom I.V. administration of an iodine-based contrast medium, as in excretory urography, is contraindicated). This test is also indicated when visualization of the renal collecting system by excretory urography is inadequate due to inferior films or marked renal insufficiency, since retrograde ureteropyelography is not influenced by impaired renal function.

Purpose

□ To assess the structure and integrity of the renal collecting system (calyces, renal pelvis, and ureter).

Patient preparation

Explain to the patient that this test permits visualization of the urinary collecting system. If a general anesthetic is ordered, instruct him to fast for 8 hours before the test. Generally, he should be well hydrated to ensure adequate urine flow. Tell him who will perform the test and where, and that it takes about 1 hour.

Inform the patient that he'll be positioned on an examining table, with his legs in stirrups, and that the position may be tiring. If he will be awake throughout the procedure, tell him he may feel pressure as the instrument is passed and a pressure sensation in the kidney area when the contrast medium is introduced. Also, he may feel an urgency to void.

Make sure the patient or responsible member of the family has signed a consent form.

Just before the procedure, administer premedication, as ordered.

Equipment

Cystoscopy setup/ureteral catheters/10-ml syringes, with ureteral adapters/X-ray equipment/contrast medium/tilt table with stirrups.

Procedure

The patient is placed in lithotomy position. Care must be taken to avoid pressure points or impairment to circulation while his legs are in the stirrups. After the patient is anesthetized, the urologist first performs a cystoscopic examination. After visual inspection of the bladder, one or both ureters are catheterized with opaque catheters, depending on the condition or abnormality suspected. Radiographic monitoring allows correct positioning of the catheter tip in the renal pelvis.

The renal pelvis is emptied by gravity drainage or aspiration. About 4 or 5 ml of contrast medium (half-strength preparation) is then injected slowly through the catheter, using the syringe fitted with a special adapter. When adequate filling and opacification have occurred, anteroposterior radiographic films are taken and immediately developed. Lateral and oblique films can be taken, as needed, after the injection of more contrast.

After the radiographs of the renal pelvis are examined, a few more milliliters of contrast medium are injected to outline the ureters, as the catheter is slowly withdrawn. Delayed films (10 to 15 minutes after complete catheter removal) are then taken to check for retention of the contrast medium, indicating urinary stasis. If ureteral obstruction is present, the ureteral catheter may be kept in place and, together with a Foley catheter, connected to a gravity drainage system until post-test urinary flow is corrected or returns to normal.

Precautions

Retrograde ureteropyelography must be done carefully in the presence of urinary stasis caused by ureteral obstruction, to prevent further injury to the ureter.

Findings

Following a normal cystoscopic examination, ureteral catheterization, and injection of contrast medium through the catheters, opacification of the renal pelves and calyces should occur immediately. Normal structures should be outlined clearly and should appear symmetrical in bilateral testing. Ureters should fill uniformly and appear normal in size and

SITES AND TYPES OF OBSTRUCTION INDICATED BY URETEROPYELOGRAPHY

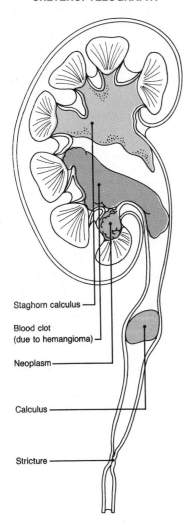

Staghorn calculus

Blood clot
(due to hemangioma)

Neoplasm

Calculus

Stricture

Ureteropyelography may detect obstruction to the flow of urine in the calices, pelvis, or ureter of the renal collecting system. Such obstruction results from stricture, neoplasm, blood clot, or calculi, as shown above. Small calculi may remain in the calices and pelvis or pass down the ureter. A staghorn calculus (a cast of the calyceal and pelvic collecting system) may form from a stone that stays in the kidney.

course. Inspiratory and expiratory exposures, when superimposed, normally create two outlines of the renal pelvis 2 cm apart.

Implications of results

Incomplete or delayed drainage reflects an obstruction, most commonly at the ureteropelvic junction. Enlargement of the components of the collecting system or delayed emptying of contrast medium may indicate obstruction due to tumor, blood clot, stricture, or calculi. Perinephric inflammation or suppuration often causes fixation of the kidney on the same side, resulting in a single sharp radiographic outline of the collecting system when inspiratory and expiratory exposures are superimposed. Upward, downward, or lateral renal displacement can result from renal abscess or tumor or from perinephric abscess. Neoplasms can cause displacement of either pole or of the entire kidney.

Post-test care

□ Check vital signs every 15 minutes for the first 4 hours, every hour for the next 4 hours, then every 4 hours for 24 hours.
□ Monitor fluid intake and urinary output for 24 hours. Observe each specimen for hematuria. Gross hematuria or hematuria after the third voiding is abnormal and should be reported. Notify the doctor if the patient doesn't void for 8 hours after the procedure, or immediately if the patient feels distress and his bladder is distended. Urethral catheterization may be necessary.
□ Be especially attentive to catheter output if ureteral catheters have been left in place, since inadequate output may reflect catheter obstruction, requiring irrigation by the doctor. Protect ureteral catheters from dislodgement.
□ Administer analgesics, as ordered, tub baths, and increased fluid intake for dysuria, which commonly occurs after retrograde ureteropyelography.
□ Watch for and report severe pain in the area of the kidneys, as well as any signs of sepsis (such as chills, fever, and hypotension).

Interfering factors

Previous contrast studies or the presence of feces or gas in the bowel impairs quality of the radiograph and hinders accurate interpretation.

FRANK LOWELL BROWN, CUT

Antegrade Pyelography

This radiographic procedure allows examination of the upper collecting system when ureteral obstruction rules out retrograde ureteropyelography or when cystoscopy is contraindicated. It depends on percutaneous needle puncture for injection of contrast medium into the renal pelvis or calyces. Antegrade pyelography also is indicated when excretory urography or renal ultrasonography demonstrates hydronephrosis and the need for therapeutic nephrostomy. After completion of radiographic studies, a nephrostomy tube can be inserted to provide temporary drainage or access for other therapeutic or diagnostic procedures.

Renal pressure can be measured during the procedure. Also, urine can be collected for cultures and cytologic studies and for evaluation of renal functional reserve before surgery.

Purpose

☐ To evaluate obstruction of the upper collecting system by stricture, stone, clot, or tumor
☐ To evaluate hydronephrosis revealed during excretory urography or ultrasonography and to enable placement of a percutaneous nephrostomy tube
☐ To evaluate the function of the upper collecting system after ureteral surgery or urinary diversion
☐ To assess renal functional reserve before surgery.

Patient preparation

Explain to the patient that this test allows radiographic examination of the kidney. Instruct him to fast, if ordered, for 4 hours before the test. However, instruct him to continue to drink fluids (antegrade pyelography is most easily performed in dilated collecting systems). Tell the patient who will perform the test and where, and that it will take approximately 1 hour.

Inform the patient that a needle will be inserted into the kidney after he is given a sedative and a local anesthetic. Explain that urine may be collected from the kidney for testing and that, if necessary, a tube will be left in the kidney for drainage. Tell him that he may feel mild discomfort during injection of the local anesthetic and contrast medium and that he may also feel transient burning and flushing from the contrast medium. Warn him that the X-ray machine makes loud clacking sounds as films are taken.

Check the patient's history for hypersensitivity reactions to contrast media. Report any such sensitivities to the doctor. Also check the history and recent coagulation studies for indications of bleeding disorders.

Make sure that the patient or a responsible family member has signed an appropriate consent form. Just before the procedure, administer a sedative, as ordered.

Equipment

X-ray equipment, including a fluoroscope and possibly ultrasound equipment/percutaneous nephrostomy tray/manometer/preparatory tray/gloves and sterile containers for specimens/syringes and needles/contrast medium/local anesthetic/emergency resuscitation equipment.

Procedure

The patient is placed prone on the X-ray table. The skin over the kidney is cleansed with antiseptic solution, and a local anesthetic is injected.

Previous urographic films or ultrasound recordings are studied for anatomic landmarks. (It's important to determine if the kidney to be studied is in normal position. If not, the angle of the needle entry must be adjusted during percutaneous puncture.) Under guidance of fluoroscopy or ultrasound, the percutaneous needle is inserted below the 12th rib at the level of the transverse process of the 2nd lumbar vertebra. Aspiration of urine confirms that the needle has reached the dilated collecting system (usually 7 to 8 cm below the skin surface in adults).

Flexible tubing is connected to the needle to prevent displacement during the procedure. If intrarenal pressure is to be measured, the manometer is connected to the tubing as soon as it's in place. Urine specimens are then taken if needed.

An amount of urine, equal to the amount of contrast medium to be injected, is withdrawn to prevent overdistention of the collecting system. The contrast medium is injected under fluoroscopic guidance. Posteroanterior, oblique, and anteroposterior radiographs are taken. Ureteral peristalsis is observed on the fluoroscope screen to evaluate obstruction. A percutaneous nephrostomy tube is inserted at this time if drainage is needed because of increased renal pressure, dilatation, or intrarenal reflux. If drainage is not needed, the catheter is withdrawn and a sterile dressing is applied.

Precautions
□ Antegrade pyelography is contraindicated in patients with bleeding disorders.
□ Watch for signs of hypersensitivity to the contrast medium.

Findings
After injection of contrast medium, the upper collecting system should fill uniformly and appear normal in size and course. Normal structures should be outlined clearly.

Implications of results
Enlargements of the upper collecting system and parts of the ureteropelvic junction indicate obstruction. Antegrade pyelography shows the degree of dilatation, clearly defines obstructions, and demonstrates intrarenal reflux. In hydronephrosis, the ureteropelvic junction shows marked distention. Results of recent surgery or urinary diversion will be obvious; for example, a ureteral stent or a dilated stenotic area will be clearly visualized.

Intrarenal pressures that exceed 20 cmH_2O indicate obstruction. Cultures or cytologic studies of urine specimens taken during antegrade pyelography can confirm antegrade pyelonephrosis or malignancy.

Post-test care
□ Check vital signs every 15 minutes for the first hour, every 30 minutes for the second hour, and every 2 hours for the next 24 hours.
□ Check dressings for bleeding, hematoma, or urine leakage at the puncture site at each check of vital signs. For bleeding, apply pressure. For a hematoma, apply warm soaks. Report urine leakage to the doctor.
□ Monitor fluid intake and urine output for 24 hours. Notify the doctor if the patient doesn't void within 8 hours. Observe each specimen for hematuria. Report hematuria if it persists after the third voiding.

□ Watch for and report signs of sepsis or extravasation of contrast medium (chills, fever, rapid pulse or respirations, hypotension).
□ Also watch for and report signs that adjacent organs have been punctured: pain in the abdomen or flank, or pneumothorax (sudden onset of pleuritic chest pain, dyspnea, tachypnea, decreased breath sounds on the affected side, tachycardia).
□ If a nephrostomy tube is inserted, check to be sure that it is patent and draining well.
□ Administer antibiotics for several days after the procedure, as ordered, to prevent infection. Administer analgesics as ordered.

Interfering factors

Recently performed barium procedures or the presence of feces or gas in the bowel can impair the visualization of the kidney, inhibiting accurate results.

ELLEN SHIPES, RN, ET, MN, MEd

STRUCTURAL & FUNCTIONAL TESTS

Excretory Urography

[Intravenous pyelography]

The cornerstone of a urologic workup, this test allows visualization of the renal parenchyma, calyces, and pelvis, as well as the ureters, bladder and, in some cases, the urethra, following I.V. administration of a contrast medium. Known traditionally as intravenous pyelography, this common and extremely useful procedure is more accurately called excretory urography, because it shows the entire urinary tract—not just the renal pelvis, as the prefix pyelo *implies. Clinical indications for this test include suspected renal or urinary tract disease, space-occupying lesions, congenital anomalies, or trauma to the urinary system.*

Purpose

□ To evaluate the structure and excretory function of the kidneys, ureters, and bladder

□ To support a differential diagnosis of renovascular hypertension.

Patient preparation

Explain to the patient that this test helps to evaluate the structure and function of the urinary tract. Be sure the patient is well hydrated, then instruct him to fast for 8 hours before the test. Tell him who will perform the test and where.

Inform the patient that he may experience a transient burning sensation and metallic taste when the contrast medium is injected. Tell him to report any other sensations he may experience. Warn him that the X-ray machine will make loud, clacking sounds during the test.

Make sure the patient or responsible member of the family has signed a consent form. Check the patient's history for hypersensitivity to iodine, iodine-containing foods, or contrast media containing iodine. If the patient has such a history, notify the doctor. Administer a laxative, as ordered, the night before the test, to minimize poor resolution of X-ray films due to feces and gas in the gastrointestinal tract.

Equipment

Contrast medium (sodium diatrizoate or iothalamate, or meglumine diatrizoate or iothalamate)/50-ml syringe (or I.V. container and tubing)/19G to 21G needle, catheter, or butterfly needle/venipuncture equipment (tourniquet, antiseptic, adhesive bandage)/X-ray table/X-ray and tomographic equipment/emergency resuscitative equipment.

Procedure

The patient is placed in supine position on the radiographic table. A kidney-ureter-bladder radiograph is exposed, developed, and studied for gross abnormalities of the urinary system. In the absence of any such abnormality, contrast medium is injected (dosage varies according to age), and the patient is observed for signs of hypersensitivity (flushing, nausea, vomiting, hives, or dyspnea). The first radiograph, visualizing the renal parenchyma, is obtained about 1 minute after the injection, possibly supplemented by tomography if small space-occupying masses like cysts or tumors are suspected. Films are then exposed at regular intervals—usually 5, 10, and 15 or 20 minutes after the injection. Ureteral compression is performed after the 5-minute film is exposed. This can be accomplished through in-

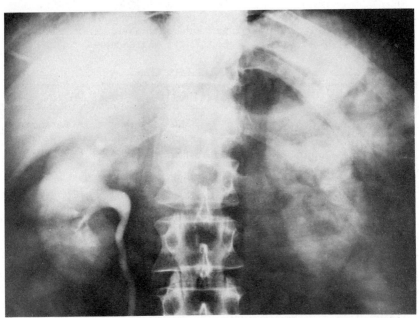

In a patient with suspected renovascular hypertension (photograph above), an excretory urogram taken 8 minutes after injection of the contrast medium shows normal filling of the right kidney but delayed opacification of left renal calices, pelvis, and ureter. This impaired excretion of the contrast material commonly results from narrowing of the renal artery feeding the subject kidney. Constriction hinders blood flow to the glomerulus, and leads to increased renal absorption of water and decreased urinary output. Demonstration of delayed caliceal opacification can differentiate between unilateral renovascular hypertension and essential hypertension.

flation of two small rubber bladders placed on the abdomen on both sides of the midline, secured by a flannel fastener wrapped around the patient's torso. The inflated bladders occlude the ureters, without causing the patient discomfort, and facilitate retention of the contrast medium by the upper urinary tract. (Ureteral compression is contraindicated by ureteral calculi, aortic aneurysm, or recent abdominal trauma or surgical procedure.) After the 10-minute film is exposed, ureteral compression is released. As the contrast flows into the lower urinary tract, another film is taken of the lower halves of both ureters and then, finally, one is taken of the bladder.

At the end of the procedure, the patient voids, and another film is made immediately to visualize residual bladder content or mucosal abnormalities of the bladder or urethra.

Precautions

Premedication with corticosteroids may be indicated for patients with severe asthma or a history of sensitivity to the contrast medium.

Findings

The kidneys, ureters, and bladder show no gross evidence of soft- or hard-tissue lesions. Prompt visualization of the contrast medium in the kidneys demonstrates bilateral renal parenchyma and pelvocalyceal systems of normal conformity. The ureters and bladder should be outlined, and the postvoiding radiograph should show no mucosal abnormalities and minimal residual urine.

Implications of results

Excretory urography can demonstrate many abnormalities of the urinary system, including renal or ureteral calculi; abnormal size, shape, or structure of kidneys, ureters, or bladder; supernumerary or absent kidney; polycystic kidney disease associated with renal hypertrophy; redundant pelvis or ureter; space-occupying lesion; pyelonephritis; renal tuberculosis; hydronephrosis; and renovascular hypertension.

Post-test care
□ If a hematoma develops at the injection site, ease the patient's discomfort by applying warm soaks.
□ Observe for delayed reactions to the contrast medium.

Interfering factors
End-stage renal disease, fecal matter or gas in the colon, insufficient injection of contrast medium, or a recent barium enema or gastrointestinal or gallbladder series may produce films of poor quality that cannot be interpreted accurately.

FRANK LOWELL BROWN, CUT

Radionuclide Renal Imaging

This test, involving I.V. injection of a radionuclide, followed by scintiphotography, can provide a wealth of information for evaluating the kidneys. Observing the uptake concentration and transit of the radionuclide during this test allows assessment of renal blood flow, nephron and collecting system function, and renal structure. Depending on the patient's clinical presentation, this procedure may include dynamic scans to assess renal perfusion and function or static scans to assess structure. The radioisotope injected depends on the specific information required and the examiner's preference. However, this procedure often includes double isotope technique to obtain a sequence of perfusion and function studies, followed by static images. This test may also be substituted for excretory urography in patients with hypersensitivity to contrast agents.

Purpose
□ To detect and assess functional and structural renal abnormalities (such as lesions), renovascular hypertension, and acute and chronic disease (such as pyelonephritis and glomerulonephritis)
□ To assess renal transplantation or renal injury due to trauma and obstruction of the urinary tract.

Patient preparation
Explain to the patient that this test permits evaluation of structure, blood flow, and function of the kidneys. Tell him who will perform the test and where, and that it takes about 1½ hours. (If static scans have been ordered, there will be a delay of several hours before the images are taken.)

Inform the patient that he'll receive an injection of a radionuclide, and that he may experience transient flushing and nausea. Emphasize that only a small amount of radionuclide is administered, and that it's usually excreted within 24 hours. Tell him several series of films will be taken of his bladder.

Make sure the patient or responsible member of the family has signed a consent form. Be sure the patient isn't scheduled for other radionuclide scans on the same day as this test. If the patient receives an antihypertensive, ask the doctor if it should be withheld before the test. Women who are pregnant and young children may receive SSKI (supersaturated solution of potassium iodide) 1 to 3 hours before the test, to block thyroid uptake of iodine.

Equipment
Computerized gamma scintillation camera/^{99m}Tc-DTPA (technetium and diethylenetriaminepentaacetic acid) for perfusion study/^{131}I-orthoiodohippurate (Hippuran) for function study/oscilloscope/magnetic tape/I.V. equipment.

Procedure
The patient is commonly placed in prone position so posterior views may be ob-

tained. If the test is being performed to evaluate transplantation, the patient is positioned supine, for anterior views. The exact position isn't critical, but the patient should be instructed not to change his position.

A perfusion study (radionuclide angiography) is performed first, to evaluate renal blood flow. ^{99m}Tc-DTPA is administered I.V., and rapid-sequence photographs (one per second) are taken for 1 minute. Next, a function study is performed to measure the transit time of the radionuclide through the kidneys' functional units. After ^{131}I-orthoiodohippurate is administered I.V., images are obtained at a rate of one per minute for 20 minutes. Alternately, this entire procedure is recorded on computer-compatible magnetic tape. Concurrently, renogram curves may be plotted. Finally, static images are obtained 4 or more hours later, after the radionuclide has drained through the pelvocaliceal system. No additional contrast is required.

Precautions
None.

Findings
Since 25% of cardiac output goes directly to the kidneys, renal perfusion should be evident immediately following uptake of the radionuclide (^{99m}Tc-DTPA) in the abdominal aorta. Within 1 to 2 minutes, a normal pattern of renal circulation should appear. The radionuclide should delineate the kidneys simultaneously, symmetrically, and with equal intensity.

^{131}I-orthoiodohippurate, administered for the function study, rapidly outlines the kidneys, which should be normal in size, shape, and position, and also defines the collecting system and bladder. Maximum counts of the radionuclide in the kidneys occur within 5 minutes after injection (and within 1 minute of each other), and should fall to approximately one third or less of the maximum counts of the same kidney within 25 minutes. Within this time, the function of both kidneys can be compared as the concentration of radionuclide shifts from the

cortex to the pelvis and, finally, to the bladder.

Renal function is best evaluated by comparing these images to the renogram curves. Total function is considered normal when the effective renal plasma flow is 420 ml/minute or greater and the percentage of the dose excreted in the urine at 30 to 35 minutes is greater than 66%.

Implications of results
Images from the perfusion study can identify impeded renal circulation, such as that arising from trauma and renal artery stenosis or renal infarction. These conditions may occur in patients with renovascular hypertension and abdominal aortic disease. Because malignant renal tumors are usually vascular, these images can help differentiate tumors from cysts. In evaluating a transplant, abnormal perfusion may indicate obstruction of the vascular grafts. The function study can detect abnormalities of the collecting system and extravasation of the urine. Markedly decreased tubular function causes reduced radionuclide activity in the collecting system; outflow obstruction causes decreased radionuclide activity in the tubules, with increased activity in the collecting system. This test can also define the level of ureteral obstruction.

Static images can demonstrate lesions, congenital abnormalities, and traumatic injury. These images also detect space-occupying lesions within or surrounding the kidney, such as tumors, infarcts, and inflammatory masses (abscesses, for example); they can also identify congenital disorders, such as horseshoe kidney and polycystic kidney disease. They can define regions of infarction, rupture, or hemorrhage after trauma.

A lower than normal total concentration of the radionuclide, as opposed to focal defects, suggests a diffuse renal disorder, such as acute tubular necrosis, severe infection, or ischemia. In a patient who has had a kidney transplant, decreased radionuclide uptake generally indicates organ rejection. Failure of visualization may indicate congenital ec-

RADIONUCLIDE RENOGRAPHY

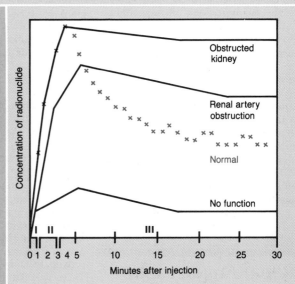

Key:
I = Vascular phase
II = Tubular phase
III = Excretory phase

ISOTOPE RENOGRAM CURVES

Commonly performed with the kidney function study following the administration of
131I-orthoiodohippurate I.V., this test provides a curve illustrating renal activity. Known as a
renogram, this curve represents uptake, transit, and excretion time of the radionuclide
by each kidney.

After the kidneys are located by a plain film of the kidney region or a kidney-ureter-
bladder radiograph, detectors placed posteriorly at each kidney record radiation counts,
which when plotted form a curve over minute integrals. The amount of radiation detected
over certain periods of time and the shape of the curve have diagnostic significance.
The illustration above, however, shows a normal absorption and excretion curve for one
normal kidney (string of red markers) compared with examples of possible curves associated
with renal pathology (solid lines). For example, an obstructed kidney absorbs but fails to
excrete the radionuclide; a kidney with a constricted renal artery takes up the radionuclide
more slowly and to a lesser degree than normal, and excretes it more slowly; a nonfunctioning kidney fails to absorb the radionuclide, so the radiation counter detects only
background radiation.

Renal uptake is represented by an initial sharp rise in the curve. Known as the vascular
phase, this filling of the renal and perirenal space usually occurs within 30 to 45 seconds
following radionuclide administration. Renal transit time, the tubular phase, occurs next and
is seen as a slower rise in the curve that lasts for 2 to 5 minutes. Finally, the excretory
phase represents drainage of the radionuclide from the kidneys.

Although certain curves are characteristic of specific disorders, the curve represents
activity of the entire kidney and doesn't distinguish between its different areas. Consequently,
renographic findings must be correlated with the patient's clinical status and results from
other urologic tests. When analyzed and correlated with images from the kidney function
study, however, the renogram can provide valuable diagnostic information. It is also invaluable
for comparing the transit time of both kidneys pre- and post-treatment.

Normal renogram supplied by Marc S. Lapayowker, M.D., Temple University, Philadelphia, Pa.; abnormal curve reprinted with
permission from J. Stewart Cameron, et al, *Nephrology for Nurses: A Modern Approach to the Kidney* (2d ed.; Garden
City, N.Y.: Medical Examination Publishing Co., 1976).

topia or aplasia.

Definitive diagnosis usually requires the combined analysis of static images, perfusion studies, and function studies.

Post-test care
Instruct the patient to flush the toilet immediately after each voiding for 24 hours, as a radiation precaution.

Interfering factors
□ In patients with hypertension, antihypertensives may interfere with test results by masking the cause of the abnormalities.

□ Scans of different organs performed on the same day may interfere with one another.

FRANK LOWELL BROWN, CUT

Renal Angiography

Renal angiography permits radiographic examination of the renal vasculature and parenchyma following arterial injection of a contrast medium. As the contrast pervades the renal vasculature, rapid-sequence radiographs show the vessels during three phases of filling: arterial, nephrographic, and venous. This procedure virtually always follows standard bolus aortography, which shows individual variations in number, size, and condition of the main renal arteries, aberrant vessels, and the relationship of the renal arteries to the aorta.

Clinical indications for renal angiography include renal masses, pseudotumors, unilateral or bilateral kidney enlargement, nonfunctioning kidneys in patients with acute renal failure, positive urograms in patients with renovascular hypertension, vascular malformations, and intrarenal calcifications of unexplained etiology.

Purpose
□ To demonstrate the configuration of

total renal vasculature before surgical procedures

□ To determine the cause of renovascular hypertension, such as from stenosis, thrombotic occlusions, emboli, and aneurysms

□ To evaluate chronic renal disease or renal failure

□ To investigate renal masses and renal trauma

□ To detect complications following renal transplantation, such as a nonfunctioning shunt or rejection of the donor organ.

Patient preparation
Explain to the patient that this test permits visualization of the kidneys, blood vessels, and functional units, and aids in diagnosing renal disease or masses. Instruct him to fast for 8 hours before the test. Tell him who will perform the test and where, and that it takes approximately 1 hour.

Describe the procedure to the patient, and inform him that he may experience transient discomfort (flushing, burning sensation, and nausea) during injection of the contrast medium.

Make sure the patient or responsible member of the family has signed a consent form. Check the patient's history for hypersensitivity to iodine-based contrast media or iodine-containing foods, such as shellfish. If the patient has a history of sensitivity, inform the doctor so he can prescribe prophylactic antiallergenics (diphenhydramine or steroids) or have them available during the procedure.

As ordered, administer medication (usually a sedative and a narcotic analgesic) before the test. Instruct the patient to put on a hospital gown and to remove all metallic objects that may interfere with test results. The patient should void before leaving the unit.

Equipment
Image-intensified fluoroscope, with television monitor/high-powered X-ray equipment/pressure-injection device/rapid cassette changer/polyethylene radiopaque vascular catheters/flexible guide wire/contrast material (such as Hy-

paque, Renografin, Conray, or Iso-paque)/preparation tray, with 70% alcohol or povidone-iodine solution/ emergency resuscitative equipment.

Procedure

The patient is placed in supine position, and a peripheral I.V. infusion is started. The skin over the arterial puncture site is cleansed with antiseptic solution, and a local anesthetic is injected. Using the Seldinger technique, the femoral artery is punctured and, under fluoroscopic visualization, cannulated. (If a femoral pulse is absent or the artery is convoluted or plaque-ridden, percutaneous transax-illary, transbrachial, or translumbar catheterization may be performed instead.) After passing the flexible guide wire through the artery, the cannula is withdrawn, leaving several inches of wire in the lumen. Next, a polyethylene catheter is passed over the wire and advanced, under fluoroscopic guidance, up the femoroiliac vessels to the aorta. At this juncture, the contrast medium is injected, and screening aortograms are taken before proceeding. On completion of the aortographic study, a renal catheter is exchanged for the former one. The guide wire is removed, and the catheter is flushed with heparinized saline solution to prevent clotting in the catheter tip.

To determine the position of the renal arteries and ensure that the tip of the catheter is in the lumen, a test bolus of contrast (about 1 ml) is injected immediately. This prevents subintimal injection or arterial spasm that may mimic a renal artery lesion. If the patient has no adverse reaction to the contrast, 20 to 25 ml of contrast is injected just below the origin of the renal arteries so it

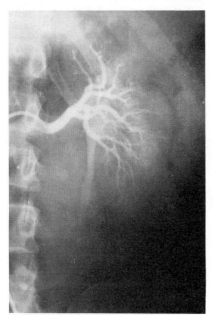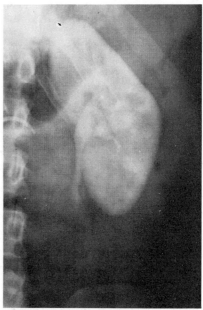

These renal angiograms show a normal kidney in arterial (left photograph) and nephrographic (right photograph) stages of filling, with the catheter visible over the spine. In the arterial phase, contrast material clearly delineates the trunk and branches of the arterial tree. The nephrographic phase demonstrates movement of the contrast from renal arteries and its diffusion throughout the renal capillary structure, with greatest concentration in the pyramids and cortex. Abnormal conditions might produce local retention of contrast matter (indicating arterial stenosis), bead-and-string filling pattern (arterial dysplasia), displacement or irregular branching of vessels, or unusual diffusion of contrast (invasion by tumor or cyst).

doesn't reach the mesenteric vessels first, obscuring the renal arteries. After this injection, a series of rapid-sequence X-ray films of the filling of the renal vascular tree is exposed.

If additional selective studies are required, the catheter remains in place while the films are examined. If the films are satisfactory, the catheter is removed, and a sterile sponge is firmly applied to the puncture site for 15 minutes. Before the patient is returned to his room, the puncture site is observed for hematoma.

Precautions
Renal angiography is contraindicated during pregnancy and in patients with bleeding tendencies, allergy to contrast media, and renal failure due to end-stage renal disease.

Findings
Renal arteriographs show normal arborization of the vascular tree and normal architecture of the renal parenchyma.

Implications of results
Renal tumors usually show hypervascularity; renal cysts typically appear as clearly delineated, radiolucent masses. Renal artery stenosis caused by arteriosclerosis produces a noticeable constriction in the blood vessels, usually within the proximal portion of its length; this is a crucial finding in confirming renovascular hypertension. Renal artery dysplasia, unlike renal artery stenosis, usually affects the middle and distal portions of the vessel. Alternating aneurysms and stenotic regions give this rare disorder a characteristic beads-on-a-string appearance.

In renal infarction, blood vessels may appear to be absent or cut off, the normal tissue replaced by scar tissue. Another typical finding is the appearance of triangular areas of infarcted tissue near the periphery of the affected kidney. The kidney itself may appear shrunken due to tissue scarring. Other disorders that may be discovered through renal angiography include renal artery aneurysms (saccular or fusiform), renal arteriovenous fistula with abnormal widening of and direct passage between the renal artery and renal vein. Destruction, distortion, and fibrosis of renal tissue with areas of reduced and tortuous vascularity may be noted in severe or chronic pyelonephritis, and an increase in capsular vessels with abnormal intrarenal circulation may indicate renal abscesses or inflammatory masses.

When angiography is used to evaluate renal trauma, it may detect intrarenal hematoma, parenchymal laceration, shattered kidney, and areas of infarction. Renal angiography may also be useful in distinguishing pseudotumors from tumors or cysts, in evaluating the volume of residual functioning renal tissue in hydronephrosis, and in evaluating donors and recipients before and after renal transplantation.

Post-test care
□ Keep the patient flat in bed for 8 to 12 hours and nonambulatory for a total of 24 hours.
□ Check vital signs every 15 minutes for 1 hour, every ½ hour for 2 hours, then every hour until they stabilize. Monitor popliteal and dorsalis pedis pulses for adequate perfusion at least every hour for 4 hours.
□ Watch for bleeding or hematomas at the injection site. Keep the pressure dressing in place, and check for bleeding every 30 minutes for 2 hours and then every hour for 4 hours. If bleeding occurs, notify the doctor, and apply direct pressure to the site.

Interfering factors
□ Recent contrast studies (such as a barium enema or an upper gastrointestinal series) may produce a cloudy radiographic image and interfere with accurate interpretation of test results.
□ Patient movement during the test may impair the quality of the radiographs.
□ The presence of feces and gas in the gastrointestinal tract may impair clarity of the radiographs and hinder accurate interpretation of results.

FRANK LOWELL BROWN, CUT

Renal Venography

This relatively simple procedure allows radiographic examination of the main renal veins and their tributaries. In this test, contrast medium is injected by percutaneous catheter passed through the femoral vein and inferior vena cava into the renal vein. Indications for renal venography include renal vein thrombosis, tumor, and venous anomalies. This test helps distinguish renal parenchymal disease and aneurysms from pressure exerted by an adjacent mass. When other diagnostic tests yield ambiguous results, renal venography can definitively differentiate renal agenesis from a small kidney.

Renal venography is also useful in assessing renovascular hypertension. Blood samples can be collected from renal veins during the procedure, and renin assays of the samples can differentiate essential renovascular hypertension from hypertension due to unilateral renal lesions.

Purpose
□ To detect renal vein thrombosis
□ To evaluate renal vein compression due to extrinsic tumors or retroperitoneal fibrosis
□ To assess renal tumors and detect invasion of the renal vein or inferior vena cava
□ To detect venous anomalies and defects
□ To differentiate renal agenesis from a small kidney
□ To collect renal venous blood samples for evaluation of renovascular hypertension.

Patient preparation
Explain to the patient that this test permits radiographic study of the renal veins. If ordered, instruct him to fast for 4 hours before the test. Tell him who will perform the test and where, and that it takes about 1 hour.

Inform the patient that a catheter will be inserted into a vein in the groin area after he is given a sedative and a local anesthetic. Tell him that he may feel mild discomfort during injection of the local anesthetic and contrast medium and that he may feel transient burning and flushing from the contrast medium. Warn him that the X-ray equipment will make loud clacking noises as the films are taken.

Check the patient's history for hypersensitivity to contrast media, iodine, or iodine-containing foods, such as shellfish. Report any sensitivities to the doctor. Check the patient's history and any coagulation studies for indications of bleeding disorders.

If renin assays will be done, check the patient's diet and medications, and consult with the doctor. As ordered, restrict the patient's salt intake and discontinue antihypertensive drugs, diuretics, estrogen, and oral contraceptives.

Make sure the patient or a responsible family member has signed a consent form. Just before the procedure, administer a sedative, as ordered.

Equipment
X-ray equipment/renal venography tray with flexible guide wires, polyethylene radiopaque vascular catheters, needle and cannula or 18G Becton Dickinson needle, three-way stopcock, and flexible tubing/preparatory tray/syringes and needles/contrast medium/local anesthetic/emergency resuscitation equipment.

Procedure
The patient is placed in a supine position on the X-ray table, with his abdomen centered over the film. The skin over the right femoral vein near the groin is cleansed with antiseptic solution and draped. A local anesthetic is injected, and the femoral vein is cannulated. Under fluoroscopic guidance, a guide wire is threaded a short distance through the cannula, which is then removed. A catheter is passed over the wire into the inferior vena cava.

When catheterization of the femoral

vein is contraindicated, the right antecubital vein is punctured, and the catheter is inserted and advanced through the right atrium of the heart into the inferior vena cava.

A test bolus of contrast medium is injected to determine that the vena cava is patent. If so, the catheter is advanced into the right renal vein and contrast medium is injected. The volume, usually 20 to 40 ml, depends on indications for the procedure. When studies of the right renal vasculature are completed, the catheter is withdrawn into the vena cava, rotated, and guided into the left renal vein.

If visualization of the renal venous tributaries is indicated, epinephrine can be injected into the ipsilateral renal artery by catheter before contrast medium is injected into the renal vein. Epinephrine temporarily blocks arterial flow and allows filling of distal intrarenal veins. Obstructing the artery briefly with a balloon catheter is an alternative method that produces the same effect.

After anteroposterior films are made, the patient is placed prone for posteroanterior films. If renin assays are indicated, blood samples are withdrawn under fluoroscopy within 15 minutes after venography is completed. The catheter is removed and a dressing applied.

Precautions

☐ Renal venography is contraindicated in severe thrombosis of the inferior vena cava.

☐ The guide wire and catheter should be advanced carefully if severe renal vein thrombosis is suspected.

☐ Watch for signs of hypersensitivity to contrast medium.

Findings

After injection of contrast medium, opacification of the renal vein and tributaries should occur immediately.

Normal renin content of venous blood in a supine adult is 1.5 to 1.6 ng/ml/hr.

Implications of results

Occlusion of the renal vein near the inferior vena cava or the kidney indicates renal vein thrombosis. If the clot is outlined by contrast medium, it may look like a filling defect. However, a clot can usually be identified because it is within the lumen and less sharply outlined than a filling defect. Collateral venous channels, which opacify with retrograde filling during contrast injection, often surround the occlusion. Complete occlusion prolongs transit of the contrast medium through the renal veins.

A filling defect of the renal vein may indicate obstruction or compression by extrinsic tumor or retroperitoneal fibrosis. A renal tumor that invades the renal vein or inferior vena cava usually produces a filling defect with a sharply defined border.

Venous anomalies are indicated by opacification of abnormally positioned or clustered vessels. Absence of a renal vein differentiates renal agenesis from a small kidney.

Elevated renin content in renal venous blood usually indicates essential renovascular hypertension when assay results correspond for both kidneys. Elevated renin levels in one kidney indicate a unilateral lesion and usually require further evaluation by arteriography.

Post-test care

☐ Check vital signs and distal pulses every 15 minutes for the first hour, every 30 minutes for the second hour, then every 2 hours for 24 hours.

☐ Check the puncture site for bleeding or hematoma; if a hematoma develops, apply warm soaks.

 ☐ Report signs of vein perforation, embolism, and extravasation of contrast medium. These include chills, fever, rapid pulse and respiration, hypotension, dyspnea, and chest, abdominal, or flank pain. Also report complaints of paresthesias or pain in catheterized limb—symptoms of nerve irritation or vascular compromise.

☐ Administer a sedative and antibiotics, as ordered.

☐ Instruct the patient to resume his usual

diet and any medications that were discontinued before the test.

Interfering factors

□ Recent contrast studies or the presence of feces or gas in the bowel impairs visualization of the renal veins.

□ Failure to restrict salt, antihypertensive drugs, diuretics, estrogen, and oral contraceptives can interfere with renin assay results.

ELLEN SHIPES, RN, ET, MN, MEd

URODYNAMIC TESTS
Uroflowmetry

This simple noninvasive test uses a uroflowmeter to detect and evaluate dysfunctional voiding patterns. The uroflowmeter, contained in a funnel into which the patient voids, measures flow rate (volume of urine voided per second), continuous flow (time of measurable flow), and intermittent flow (total voiding time, including any interruptions).

Several types of uroflowmeters are available: rotary disc, electromagnetic, spectrophotometric, and gravimetric systems. The gravimetric system, which weighs urine as it's voided and plots the weight against time, is the simplest to use and is widely available.

Purpose
□ To evaluate lower urinary tract function
□ To demonstrate bladder outlet obstruction.

Patient preparation
Explain to the patient that this test evaluates his pattern of urination. Advise him not to urinate for several hours before the test and to increase fluid intake so he'll have a full bladder and a strong urge to void. Tell him who will perform the test and where, and that it will take 10 to 15 minutes. Instruct him to remain still while voiding during the test to help ensure accurate results.

Assure the patient that he will have complete privacy during the test; many people have difficulty voiding in the presence of others. As ordered, discontinue drugs that may affect bladder and sphincter tone.

Equipment
Commode chair with funnel containing a uroflowmeter/beaker to hold urine/transducer/start and flow cables/data recording module.

Procedure
The test procedure is the same with all types of equipment. A male patient is asked to void while standing; a female patient, while sitting. The patient is asked to avoid straining to empty the bladder. Cable connections are checked, and the patient is left alone.

The patient pushes the start button on the commode chair, counts for 5 seconds (1 one-thousand, 2 one-thousand, etc.), and voids. When finished, he counts for 5 seconds and pushes the button again. The volume of urine voided is then recorded and plotted as a curve over the time of voiding. The patient's position and the route of fluid intake (oral or intravenous) are noted.

Precautions
□ The transducer must be level, and the beaker must be centered beneath the funnel.
□ The beaker must be large enough to hold all urine; overflow can invalidate results and damage the transducer.

Values
Flow rate varies according to the patient's age and sex, and the volume of urine voided. Normal values are listed below for minimum volumes needed to obtain adequate recordings.

CHARACTERISTIC UROFLOW CURVES

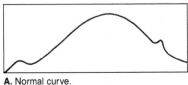

A. Normal curve.

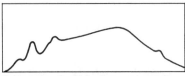

B. Normal peak with hesitancy may result from the patient's embarrassment or advanced age.

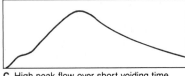

C. High peak flow over short voiding time may indicate incontinence.

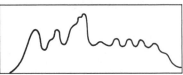

D. Many peaks over normal voiding time indicate abdominal straining and detrusor muscle weakness.

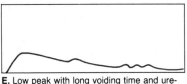

E. Low peak with long voiding time and urethral dribbling indicates obstruction.

Age	Minimum volume (ml)	Male (ml/sec)	Female (ml/sec)
4 to 7	100	10	10
8 to 13	100	12	15
14 to 45	200	21	18
46 to 65	200	12	15
66 to 80	200	9	10

Implications of results

Increased flow rate indicates reduced urethral resistance, which may be associated with external sphincter dysfunction. A high peak on the curve plotted over the voiding time indicates decreased outflow resistance, which may be due to stress incontinence. Decreased flow rate indicates outflow obstruction or hypotonia of the detrusor muscle. More than one distinct peak in a normal curve indicates abdominal straining, which may be due to pushing against an obstruction to empty the bladder. (See *Characteristic Uroflow Curves.*)

Post-test care

Instruct the patient to resume any medications that were discontinued before the test.

Interfering factors

□ Drugs that affect bladder and sphincter tone, such as urinary spasmolytics and anticholinergics, will alter test results.

□ Strong drafts can affect transducer function.

□ If the patient moves while seated on the commode chair, flow recording may be inaccurate.

□ The presence of toilet tissue in the beaker will invalidate test results.

□ If the patient strains to void, test results will be altered.

ELLEN SHIPES, RN, ET, MN, MEd

Cystometry

Cystometry assesses the bladder's neuromuscular function by measuring efficiency of the detrusor muscle reflex, intravesical pressure and capacity, and the bladder's reaction to thermal stimulation. It's especially useful for detecting the cause of involuntary bladder contractions in an unstable bladder. Cystometry alone can give ambiguous results. Consequently, cystometry results should always be supported by results of other tests of the urinary system, such as cystourethrography, excretory urography, and voiding cystourethrography.

Cystometry can be performed by the instillation of physiologic saline solution or sterile water, or by the insufflation of a gas. In either method, characteristics of the urinary stream and bladder reaction to thermal stimulation may furnish accurate pathophysiologic information.

In chronic urinary tract infections, adjustments can be made to allow accurate interpretation of results, and the procedure is less likely to cause complications.

Purpose
□ To evaluate detrusor muscle function and tonicity
□ To help determine the cause of bladder dysfunction.

Patient preparation
Explain to the patient that this test evaluates bladder function, especially detrusor muscle function relating to the development of the urgency to void and the ability to suppress voiding. Inform him that he needn't restrict food or fluids. Tell him who will perform the test and where, and that the procedure takes about 40 minutes, unless additional testing is required.

Describe the procedure to the patient. Inform him that he'll feel a strong urge to void during the test, and that the procedure may be embarrassing and uncomfortable.

Make sure the patient or responsible member of the family has signed a consent form. Also check the patient's medication history for drugs (such as antihistamines) that may affect test results. Just before the procedure, ask the patient to urinate.

Equipment
Four-channel gas cystometer/set of catheters.

Procedure
The patient is placed in the supine position on an examining table, and a catheter is then passed into the bladder to measure residual urine level. However, any difficulty with insertion of the catheter may reflect meatal or urethral obstruction.

To test the patient's response to thermal sensation, 30 ml of room temperature physiologic saline solution or sterile water is instilled into the bladder. Next, an equal volume of warm fluid (110° to 115° F.) is instilled into the patient's bladder. The patient is asked to report his sensations, such as the need to void, nausea, flushing, discomfort, and a feeling of warmth.

After the fluid is drained from the patient's bladder, the catheter is connected to the cystometer, and normal saline solution, sterile water, or gas (usually carbon dioxide) is slowly introduced into the bladder. The flow of gas is controlled automatically to the desired reading (100 ml/minute) by a four-channel cystometer. The patient is asked to indicate when he *first* feels an urge to void, then when he feels he *must* urinate. The related pressure and volume is automatically plotted on the graph. When the bladder reaches its full capacity, the patient is requested to urinate to permit the maximal intravesical voiding pressure to be recorded. The patient's bladder is then drained and, if no additional tests are required, the catheter is removed; otherwise, the catheter

CYSTOMETRY: NORMAL AND ABNORMAL FINDINGS

Since cystometry assesses micturition and vesical function, it can aid diagnosis of neurogenic bladder dysfunctions. The five main types of neurogenic bladder, as presented in the chart that begins here and continues on the following pages, result from lesions of the central or peripheral nervous systems. Uninhibited neurogenic bladder results from a lesion to the upper motor neuron and causes frequent, often uncontrollable micturition in the presence of even a small amount of urine. A complete upper motor neuron lesion characterizes reflex neurogenic bladder and causes total loss of conscious sensation and vesical control.

Normal Bladder Function

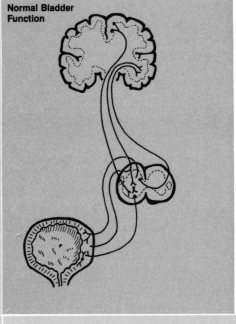

Feature or Response	
Micturition	
Start	+
Stop	+
Residual urine	0
Vesical sensation	+
First urge to void	150 to 200 ml
Bladder capacity	400 to 500 ml
Bladder contractions	0
Intravesical pressure	L
Bulbocavernosus reflex	+
Saddle sensation	+
Bethanechol test (exaggerated response)	0
Ice water test	+
Anal reflex	+
Heat sensation and pain	+

KEY: + Present/Positive   ↑ Increased   **V** Variable   **D** Delayed
        0 Absent/Negative   ↓ Decreased   **E** Early   **L** Low

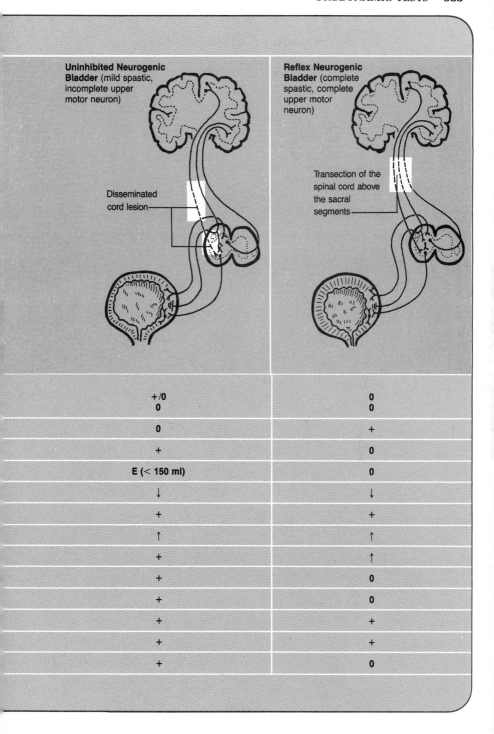

Uninhibited Neurogenic Bladder (mild spastic, incomplete upper motor neuron)

Disseminated cord lesion

Reflex Neurogenic Bladder (complete spastic, complete upper motor neuron)

Transection of the spinal cord above the sacral segments

Uninhibited Neurogenic Bladder	Reflex Neurogenic Bladder
+/0 0	0 0
0	+
+	0
E (< 150 ml)	0
↓	↓
+	+
↑	↑
+	↑
+	0
+	0
+	+
+	+
+	0

CYSTOMETRY: NORMAL AND ABNORMAL FINDINGS *(continued)*

In autonomous neurogenic bladder, a lower motor neuron lesion produces a flaccid bladder that fills without contracting. The patient can't perceive bladder fullness or initiate and maintain urination without applying external pressure. Lower motor neuron lesions can cause sensory or motor paralysis of the bladder. In sensory paralysis, the patient incurs chronic retention because he can't perceive bladder fullness. In motor paralysis, the patient has full sensation but can't initiate or control urination.

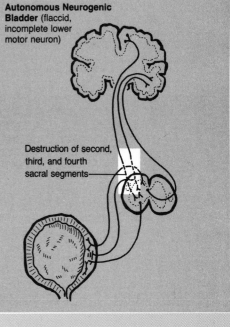

Autonomous Neurogenic Bladder (flaccid, incomplete lower motor neuron)

Destruction of second, third, and fourth sacral segments

Feature or Response

Micturition	
Start	0
Stop	0
Residual urine	+
Vesical sensation	0
First urge to void	0
Bladder capacity	↑
Bladder contractions	0
Intravesical pressure	↓
Bulbocavernosus reflex	0
Saddle sensation	0
Bethanechol test (exaggerated response)	+
Ice water test	0
Anal reflex	0
Heat sensation and pain	0

KEY: + Present/Positive   ↑ Increased   **V** Variable   **D** Delayed
        0 Absent/Negative   ↓ Decreased   **E** Early   **L** Low

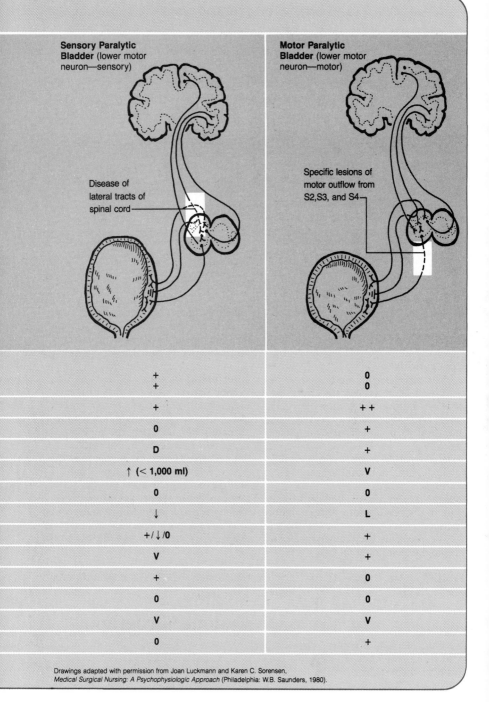

Sensory Paralytic Bladder (lower motor neuron—sensory)	Motor Paralytic Bladder (lower motor neuron—motor)
Disease of lateral tracts of spinal cord	Specific lesions of motor outflow from S2, S3, and S4
+	0
+	0
+	+ +
0	+
D	+
↑ (< 1,000 ml)	V
0	0
↓	L
+/↓/0	+
V	+
+	0
0	0
V	V
0	+

Drawings adapted with permission from Joan Luckmann and Karen C. Sorensen, *Medical Surgical Nursing: A Psychophysiologic Approach* (Philadelphia: W.B. Saunders, 1980).

SUPPLEMENTAL CYSTOMETRIC TESTS

TEST	PURPOSE	DESCRIPTION
Ice water test	Tests integrity of vesical reflex arc	After deflation of balloon catheter, 60-100 ml sterile ice water is instilled into bladder
Bulbocavernosus reflex test	Determines integrity of sacral portion of spinal cord	Insertion of gloved finger into rectum followed by squeezing of glans penis or clitoris
Saddle sensation test	Tests reflex activity of conus medullaris	Anocutaneous line of perineum is pricked or stroked with pin
Bethanechol sensitivity test	Defines patient with uninhibited and reflex type neurogenic bladders	Bethanechol chloride (2.5 mg/68 kg body weight) administered subcutaneously followed by cystometric measurement at 10, 20, and 30 minutes
Stress incontinence	Tests loss of voluntary control of vesicourethral sphincters	After filling of bladder, catheter is withdrawn and patient asked to cough, bend over, or lift heavy object

is left in place to measure urethral pressure profile or to provide supplemental findings.

Precautions
□ Cystometry is contraindicated in patients with acute urinary tract infections because uninhibited contractions may cause erroneous readings and the test may lead to pyelonephritis and septic shock.
□ Tell the patient not to strain at voiding; it can cause ambiguous cystometric readings.
□ If the patient has a spinal cord injury that has caused motor impairment, transport him on a stretcher so the test can be performed without transferring him to the examining table.

Findings and implications
The chart on pages 984 to 987 summarizes findings of cystometric testing.

Post-test care
□ Administer a sitz bath or warm tub bath if the patient experiences discomfort after the test.
□ Measure fluid intake and urinary output for 24 hours. Notify the doctor if hematuria persists after the third voiding or if the patient develops signs of sepsis (such as fever or chills).

Interfering factors
□ Poor patient response due to a misunderstanding of instructions or embarrassment may interfere with test results.
□ Inability to urinate in the supine position will interfere with test results.
□ Concurrent use of drugs that may interfere with bladder function (such as antihistamines) affect test results.
□ Inconclusive results are likely if cystometry is performed within 6 to 8 weeks after surgery for spinal cord injury.

FRANK LOWELL BROWN, CUT

Voiding Cystourethrography

In voiding cystourethrography, a contrast medium is instilled by gentle sy-

NORMAL RESPONSE
Rapid expulsion of catheter and water through urethra
Constriction of anal sphincter
Visible constriction of anal sphincter
Manometric pressure > 15 cm H_2O
No dribbling of urine from urethra (dribbling indicates stress incontinence)

ringe pressure or gravity into the bladder through a urethral catheter. Fluoroscopic films or overhead radiographs demonstrate bladder filling, then show excretion of the contrast as the patient voids. This test may be performed to investigate possible causes of chronic urinary tract infection. Other indications for voiding cystourethrography include a suspected congenital anomaly of the lower urinary tract, abnormal bladder emptying, and incontinence. In males, this test can assess hypertrophy of the lobes of prostate, urethral stricture, and the degree of compromise of a stenotic prostatic urethra.

Purpose
□ To detect abnormalities of the bladder and urethra, such as vesicoureteral reflux, neurogenic bladder, prostatic hyperplasia, urethral strictures, or diverticula.

Patient preparation
Explain to the patient that this test permits assessment of the bladder and the urethra. Inform him that he needn't restrict food or fluids before the test. Tell

him who will perform the test and where, and that it takes approximately 30 to 45 minutes.

Inform the patient that a catheter will be inserted into his bladder, and that a contrast medium will be instilled through the catheter. Tell him he may experience a feeling of fullness and an urge to void when the contrast is instilled. Explain that X-ray films will be taken of his bladder and urethra, and that he'll be asked to assume various positions.

Make sure the patient or responsible member of the family has signed a consent form. Check the patient's history for hypersensitivity to iodine-based contrast media or iodine-containing foods, such as shellfish; notify the doctor of any sensitivities.

Just before the procedure, administer a sedative, as ordered.

Equipment
X-ray equipment (fluoroscope and screen, and accessories for spot-film radiography)/Foley catheter/standard urographic contrast medium (up to 1,000 ml of 15% solution)/50-ml syringe (for infants) or gravity-feed apparatus.

Procedure
The patient is placed in supine position, and a Foley catheter is inserted into the bladder. The contrast medium is instilled through the catheter until the bladder is full. The catheter is clamped, and X-ray films are exposed, with the patient in supine, oblique, and lateral positions. Then, the catheter is removed, and the patient assumes right oblique position—right leg flexed to 90°, left leg extended, penis parallel to right leg—and begins to void. Four high-speed exposures of the bladder and urethra, coned down to reduce radiation exposure, are usually made on one film during voiding. (Male patients should wear a lead shield over their testes to prevent irradiation of the gonads; female patients can't be shielded without blocking the urinary bladder.) If the right oblique view does not delineate both ureters, the patient is asked to stop urinating and to begin

NORMAL AND ABNORMAL CYSTOURETHROGRAM

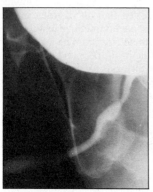 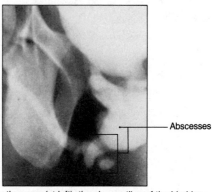

Abscesses

In the oblique view of a normal cystourethrogram (at left), the clear outline of the bladder and urethra shows normal structure. The oblique view of an abnormal cystourethrogram (at right) shows abscesses in the prostate and proximal urethra.

again in left oblique position.

The most reliable voiding cystourethrograms are obtained with the patient recumbent. Patients who can't void recumbent may do so standing (not sitting). Expression cystourethrography may have to be performed, under a general anesthetic, for young children who cannot void on command.

Precautions

Voiding cystourethrography is contraindicated in patients with an acute or exacerbated urethral or bladder infection, or an acute urethral injury. Hypersensitivity to contrast medium may also contraindicate this test.

Findings

Delineation of the bladder and urethra shows normal structure and function, with no regurgitation of contrast medium into the ureters.

Implications of results

Voiding cystourethrography may show urethral stricture or valves, vesical or urethral diverticula, ureteroceles, prostatic enlargement, vesicoureteral reflux, or neurogenic bladder. The severity and location of such abnormalities are then evaluated to determine whether surgical intervention is necessary.

Post-test care

□ Observe and record the time, color, and volume of the patient's voidings. If hematuria is present after the third voiding, notify the doctor.

□ Encourage the patient to drink large quantities of fluids to reduce burning on urination and to flush out any residual contrast medium.

□ Monitor for chills and fever related to extravasation of contrast material or urinary sepsis.

Interfering factors

□ Embarrassment may inhibit the patient's ability to void on command.

□ Pain on voiding resulting from urethral trauma during catheterization may cause an interrupted or less vigorous stream, muscle spasm, or incomplete sphincter relaxation.

□ Previous radiographic testing using contrast media or the presence of feces or gas in the bowel may obscure visualization of the urinary tract.

FRANK LOWELL BROWN, CUT

Whitaker Test

[Pressure/flow study]

This study of the upper urinary tract correlates radiographic findings with measurements of pressure and flow in the kidneys and ureters. It assesses the upper tract's efficiency in emptying. Radiographs are taken after urethral catheterization, I.V. administration of contrast medium, percutaneous cannulation of the kidney, and renal perfusion of contrast medium. Intrarenal and bladder pressures are then measured.

The Whitaker test may be performed as a primary study to detect intrarenal obstruction and to help determine if surgery is needed. It may also follow other procedures, such as percutaneous nephrostomy, for further evaluation of obstruction.

Purpose
☐ To identify and evaluate renal obstruction.

Patient preparation
Explain to the patient that the test evaluates kidney function. Instruct him to avoid food and fluids for at least 4 hours before the test. Tell him who will perform the test and where, and that it will take about 1 hour.

Describe the procedure to the patient. Inform him that he will be given a mild sedative before the test, that he may feel some discomfort during insertion of the urethral catheter and injection of the local anesthetic, and that he may sense transient burning and flushing after injection of the contrast medium. Warn him that the X-ray machine makes loud clacking sounds as films are exposed.

Make sure the patient or a responsible family member has signed a consent form. Check the patient's history and recent coagulation studies for bleeding disorders. Also check the patient's history for hypersensitivity reactions to iodine, iodine-containing foods such as shellfish, and contrast media. Inform the doctor of any sensitivities.

Just before the procedure, instruct the patient to void, if ordered, and administer a sedative, as ordered. Administer prophylactic antibiotics, as ordered, to prevent infection from instrumentation.

Equipment
X-ray equipment/perfusion pump with 50 ml Luer-Lok syringe/transducer and recorder/manometer/three-way and four-way stopcocks/I.V. extension set/manometer lines/one double-male connector to connect urethral catheter and stopcock/sterile water and normal saline solution/contrast medium/local anesthetic/percutaneous puncture tray with 4" to 6" 18G Longdwel cannula/gloves/preparatory tray/emergency resuscitation equipment.

Procedure
The patient is placed in a supine position on the X-ray table. The table is horizontal and must remain at the same height throughout the test. To prepare for measurement of bladder pressure, a urethral catheter is placed in the bladder, which may or may not be emptied. (If obstruction is suspected, the patient will be asked to void before the test. If a condition such as bladder hypertonia is the suspected cause of inefficient emptying, he should not void.) A plain film of the urinary tract is taken to obtain anatomic landmarks. The catheter is then connected to a three-way stopcock on a manometer line linked to the transducer and recorder. The line is filled with sterile water.

Contrast medium is injected intravenously, and the patient is placed prone and made comfortable with pillows. The side to be examined is closest to the doctor. When urography demonstrates contrast medium in the kidney, the skin is cleansed with antiseptic solution and draped. Pressure recording equipment is calibrated. The renal perfusion tubing is filled with sterile water or saline solution and held at the level of the kidney.

ASSESSING RENAL OBSTRUCTION WITH THE WHITAKER TEST

In the Whitaker test, serial X-rays of the upper urinary tract are correlated with measurements of intrarenal and bladder pressure.

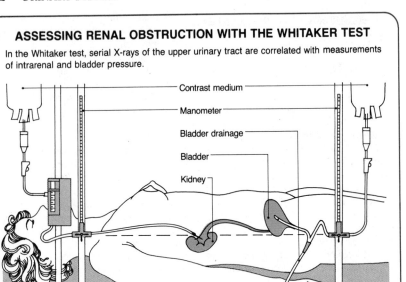

Local anesthetic is injected, and an incision is made through the flank for cannulation of the kidney. The patient is asked to hold his breath while the needle is inserted into the renal pelvis. Aspiration of urine confirms that the needle is in position. The cannula is then connected by a four-way stopcock to the perfusion tubing and the manometer line.

Perfusion of contrast medium is begun, serial X-rays are taken, and intrarenal pressure is measured. Bladder pressure is then measured. Perfusion continues at the steady rate of 10 ml/minute until bladder pressure is constant. When pressure holds steady for a few minutes and adequate films have been taken, perfusion is discontinued. Residual fluid is aspirated from the kidney, the cannula is removed, and the wound is dressed.

Precautions
Contraindications for the Whitaker test include bleeding disorders and severe infection.

Findings
Visualization of the kidney after gradual perfusion of contrast medium shows normal outlines of the renal pelvis and calyces. The ureter should fill uniformly and appear normal in size and course.

Normal intrarenal pressure is 15 cmH$_2$O; normal bladder pressure, 5 to 10 cmH$_2$O.

Implications of results
Enlargement of the renal pelvis, calyces, or ureteropelvic junction may indicate obstruction. Subtraction of bladder pressure from intrarenal pressure results in a differential that aids diagnosis. A differential of 12 to 15 cmH$_2$O indicates obstruction. A differential of less than 10 cmH$_2$O indicates a bladder abnormality, such as hypertonia or neurogenic bladder.

Post-test care
☐ Keep the patient in a supine position for 12 hours after the test.
☐ Check vital signs every 15 minutes for the first hour, every 30 minutes for the next hour, and then every 2 hours for 24 hours.
☐ Check the puncture site for bleeding, hematoma, or urine leakage each time

vital signs are checked. If bleeding occurs, apply pressure. If a hematoma develops, apply warm soaks. If urine leakage occurs, report this to the doctor.

☐ Monitor fluid intake and urine output for 24 hours. If hematuria persists after the third voiding, notify the doctor.

☐ Watch for signs of sepsis (chills, fever, tachycardia, tachypnea, hypotension) or similar signs of extravasation of the contrast medium.

☐ Inform the patient that colicky pains are transient. Administer analgesics, as ordered.

☐ Administer antibiotics for several days after the test, as ordered, to prevent infection.

Interfering factors

☐ Recent barium studies or the presence of feces or gas in the bowel hinder accurate needle placement and visualization of the upper urinary tract.

☐ Patient movement interferes with accurate needle placement.

ELLEN SHIPES, RN, ET, MN, MEd

External Sphincter Electromyography

This procedure measures electrical activity of the external urinary sphincter. The electrical activity can be measured in three ways: by needle electrodes inserted in perineal or periurethral tissues, by electrodes in an anal plug, or by skin electrodes. Skin electrodes are commonly used.

The primary indication for external sphincter electromyography is incontinence. Often, this test is done with cystometry and voiding urethrography as part of a full urodynamic study.

Purpose

☐ To assess neuromuscular function of the external urinary sphincter

☐ To assess the functional balance between bladder and sphincter muscle activity.

Patient preparation

Explain to the patient that this test will determine how well his bladder and sphincter muscles work together. Tell him who will perform the test and where, and that it takes 30 to 60 minutes.

If skin electrodes are to be used, tell the patient where they will be placed. Explain the preparatory prodecure, which may include shaving a small area.

If needle electrodes will be used, tell the patient where they will be placed and that the discomfort is equivalent to an intramuscular injection. Assure him that he'll feel discomfort only during insertion. Advise the patient that the needles are connected to wires leading to the recorder but that there is no danger of electrical shock. Explain to the female patient that she may notice slight bleeding at the first voiding.

If an anal plug will be used, inform the patient that only the tip of the plug will be inserted into the rectum, that he may feel fullness but no discomfort, and that a bowel movement is rare but easily managed.

Check the patient's medications. If he is taking cholinergic or anticholinergic drugs, notify the doctor. Discontinue medications, as ordered.

Equipment

Electromyograph and recorder/skin, needle, or anal plug electrodes/ground plate/electrode paste/tape/antiseptic solution, such as povidone-iodine/preparatory tray, if shaving is necessary.

Procedure

The patient is placed in lithotomy position for electrode placement, then may lie supine. Be sure to record patient position, type of electrode used, measuring equipment used, and any other tests done at the same time. (To obtain comparable results, subsequent studies must be done the same way.)

Electrode paste is applied to the ground plate, which is taped to the thigh and grounded. The electrodes are then placed, as described below, and connected to electrode adaptors.

Placing skin electrodes: The skin is cleansed with antiseptic solution and dried. A small area may be shaved for optimum electrode contact. Electrode paste is applied and the electrodes taped in place: for females, in the periurethral area; for males, in the perineal area beneath the scrotum.

Placing needle electrodes: With the male patient, a gloved finger is inserted into the rectum. The needles and wires are inserted 1.5″ through the perineal skin toward the apex of the prostate. Needle positions are 3:00 and 9:00. While the needles are withdrawn, the wires are held in place and then taped to the thigh.

With the female patient, the labia are spread, and the needles and wires inserted periurethrally at 2:00 and 10:00. The needles are withdrawn and the wires taped to the thigh.

Placing anal plug electrodes: The plug is lubricated, and the patient is informed again that only the tip will be inserted into the rectum. The patient is asked to relax by breathing slowly and deeply. He is asked to relax the anal sphincter to accommodate the plug by bearing down as if for a bowel movement.

After the appropriate electrodes are placed and connected to adapters, the adapters are then inserted into the preamplifier and recording is begun. The patient is asked to alternately relax and tighten the sphincter. When sufficient data have been recorded, he is asked to bear down and exhale while anal plug and needle electrodes are removed. Remove skin electrodes gently to avoid pulling hair and tender skin. Cleanse and dry the area before the patient dresses.

In some urodynamic laboratories, cystometrography is done with electromyography for thorough evaluation of detrusor and sphincter coordination.

Precautions
□ Insert needles quickly to minimize discomfort.

□ The ground plate should be properly applied and anchored; wires should be taped securely to prevent artifact.

Findings
The electromyogram shows increased muscle activity when the patient tightens the external urinary sphincter and decreased muscle activity when he relaxes it. (The International Continence Society doesn't specify normal findings for sphincter electromyography.) If electromyography and cystometrography are done together, a comparison of results shows that muscle activity of the normal sphincter increases as the bladder fills. During voiding and with bladder contraction, muscle activity decreases as the sphincter relaxes. This comparison is important in assessing external sphincter efficiency and functional balance between bladder and sphincter muscle activity.

Implications of results
Failure of the sphincter to relax or increased muscle activity during voiding demonstrates detrusor–external sphincter dyssynergia. Confirmation of such muscle activity by electromyography may indicate neurogenic bladder, spinal cord injury, multiple sclerosis, Parkinson's disease, or stress incontinence.

Post-test care
□ Watch for and report hematuria after the first voiding in the female patient tested with needle electrodes.
□ Watch for and report symptoms of mild urethral irritation, such as dysuria, hematuria, and urinary frequency.
□ Advise the patient to take a warm sitz bath, and encourage fluids (2 to 3 liters/day) unless contraindicated.

Interfering factors
□ Patient movement during electromyography may distort recordings.
□ Anticholinergic or cholinergic drugs affect detrusor and sphincter activity.
□ Improperly placed and anchored electrodes will cause inaccurate recordings.

ELLEN SHIPES, RN, ET, MN, MEd

Selected References

Berkow, Robert, ed. *The Merck Manual of Diagnosis and Therapy*, 14th ed. Rahway, N.J.: Merck, Sharp & Dohme, 1982.

Brunner, Lillian S., and Suddarth, Doris S. *Textbook of Medical-Surgical Nursing*, 5th ed. Philadelphia: J.B. Lippincott Co., 1984.

Diseases, 2nd ed. Nurse's Reference Library. Springhouse, Pa.: Springhouse Corp., 1986.

Engram, Barbara White. "Do's and Don'ts of Urologic Nursing: Ten Ways to Improve Your Urologic Nursing Care," *Nursing83* 13:49, October 1983.

Grossman, Zachary D., et al. *The Clinician's Guide to Diagnostic Imaging*. New York: Raven Press Pubs., 1983.

Guyton, Arthur C., *Textbook of Medical Physiology*, 6th ed. Philadelphia: W.B. Saunders Co., 1981.

Harrison, J., et al., eds. *Campbell's Urology*, 4th ed. Philadelphia: W.B. Saunders Co., 1978.

Harvey, A. McGehee, ed. *The Principles and Practice of Medicine*, 21st ed. East Norwalk, Conn.: Appleton-Century-Crofts, 1984.

Henry, John Bernard, ed. *Todd-Sanford-Davidsohn Clinical Diagnosis and Management by Laboratory Methods*, vol. 1, 17th ed. Philadelphia: W.B. Saunders Co., 1984.

Implementing Urologic Procedures. Nursing Photobook series. Springhouse, Pa.: Springhouse Corp., 1982.

Jacob, Stanley W., et al. *Structure and Function in Man*, 5th ed. Philadelphia: W.B. Saunders Co., 1982.

Lancaster, Larry E. *The Patient with End Stage Renal Disease*, 2nd ed. New York: John Wiley & Sons, 1984.

Luckmann, Joan, and Sorensen, Karen C. *Medical-Surgical Nursing: A Psychophysiologic Approach*, 2nd ed. Philadelphia: W.B. Saunders Co., 1980.

Petersdorf, Robert G., and Adams, Raymond D., eds. *Harrison's Principles of Internal Medicine*, 10th ed. New York: McGraw-Hill Book Co., 1983.

Price, Sylvia, and Wilson, Lorraine. *Pathophysiology: Clinical Concepts of Disease Processes*, 2nd ed. New York: McGraw-Hill Book Co., 1982.

Ravel, Richard. *Clinical Laboratory Medicine*, 4th ed. Chicago: Year Book Medical Pubs., 1984.

Renal and Urologic Disorders. Nurse's Clinical Library. Springhouse, Pa.: Springhouse Corp., 1984.

Smith, Donald R. *General Urology*, 10th ed. Los Altos, Calif.: Lange Medical Publications, 1981.

Thomas, Clayton L. *Taber's Cyclopedic Medical Dictionary*, 14th ed. Philadelphia: F.A. Davis Co., 1981.

Tilkian, Sarko M. *Clinical Implications of Laboratory Tests*, 3rd ed. St. Louis: C.V. Mosby Co., 1983.

Wyngaarden, James, and Smith, Lloyd. *Cecil Textbook of Medicine*, 16th ed. Philadelphia: W.B. Saunders Co., 1982.

30 Drugs and Toxicology

LEARNING OBJECTIVES

After completing this chapter, the reader will be able to:
- identify the major purposes of measuring drug levels.
- list the factors that influence drug effects.
- identify the clinical effects of alcohol.
- identify the street names of eighteen abused drugs.
- state the purpose of each test discussed in the chapter.
- prepare the patient physically and psychologically for each test.
- describe the procedure for performing each test.
- specify appropriate precautions for accurate administration of each test.
- recognize signs of adverse reaction and respond appropriately.
- implement appropriate post-test care.
- state the normal values for each test.
- discuss the implications of abnormal test results.
- list factors that may interfere with accurate test results.

Drugs and Toxicology

Introduction

Diagnostic tests that measure drug levels generally serve two major purposes: to monitor therapeutic levels and to identify or measure toxic substances.

Therapeutic monitoring

In therapeutic monitoring, analytic measurements of blood drug levels are taken serially to determine and maintain dosage at an effective level. Such monitoring is necessary periodically during treatment with certain drugs, because effects vary widely and can be influenced by many factors:

☐ patient compliance with the prescribed regimen

☐ specific disorder

☐ amount prescribed and route of administration

☐ extent and rate of absorption. For example, passive absorption of drugs administered P.O. is markedly influenced by gastric pH, gastrointestinal motility, intestinal blood flow, biliary function, and other substances in the gastrointestinal tract.

☐ distribution throughout the body, which is affected by cardiac output, tissue permeability, and the number of available receptor and binding sites

☐ metabolism

☐ drug excretion rate

☐ urine pH

☐ presence of other drugs that compete for protein binding sites.

Drug monitoring is especially useful when the margin of safety between therapeutic and toxic levels is narrow. Such monitoring is commonly restricted to drugs for which a known correlation exists between blood levels and therapeutic effects. These drugs include antiarrhythmics, bronchodilators, antibiotics, anticonvulsants, and cardiac glycosides. In patients who require these special groups of drugs, blood level monitoring can evaluate the patient's compliance, adequacy of dosage, and current clinical status.

Blood level monitoring is especially important during treatment with cardiac glycosides. These drugs have a narrow margin of safety between maximal therapeutic levels and toxic levels; when they reach toxic levels, they cause arrhythmias, the condition for which they are sometimes prescribed. Thus, in such patients, only blood level monitoring can clearly distinguish between toxicity and progression of the disease.

Results of steady state therapeutic monitoring tests are not reliable until an equilibrium (steady state) is attained (a balance between daily intake and excretion). To calculate the time required to achieve a steady state, multiply the half-life of the drug (time required to eliminate half its plasma concentration) by five. Before drawing a blood sample, check the time of the last dose, since the interval between administration and sample collection must be the same for each test in a series. Normally, blood samples for such tests are collected at the drug's peak level (highest therapeutic concentration) to monitor for toxicity or at the trough level (lowest therapeutic concentration) to check maintenance of

PERFORMING GASTRIC LAVAGE

Gastric lavage may be necessary to treat overdose in a patient who has CNS depression, an absent or diminished gag reflex, or who can't cooperate for emetic therapy. The following equipment is needed to perform this procedure: 3,000 ml of lavage fluid (normal saline solution, half-strength saline solution, or tap water, as ordered), irrigation and drainage collection sets, a large-bore double lumen (Moss) tube or a large-bore single lumen (Ewald) tube with Y connector, Kelly clamp, water-soluble lubricant or anesthetic

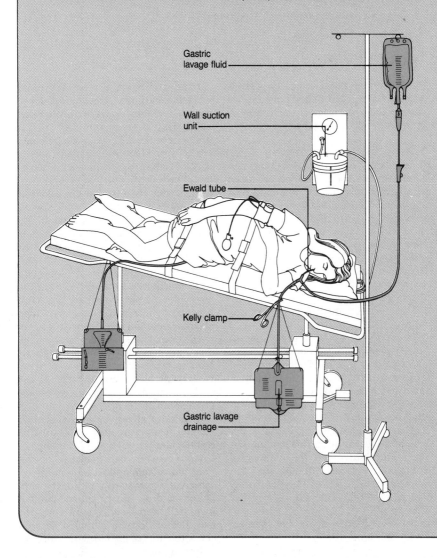

Gastric lavage fluid

Wall suction unit

Ewald tube

Kelly clamp

Gastric lavage drainage

therapeutic dosage). Identification of peak and trough levels may require collection of more than one sample, since the time required to reach a certain level depends on the drug, route of administration, and the patient's rate of drug metabolism.

Identifying toxic drugs

Toxicity determinations include emergency tests to evaluate the type and amount of legal or illegal drugs taken in accidental or intentional overdoses, as well as emergency and monitoring tests for industrial poisoning. Generally, blood or urine is the specimen of choice, but appropriate specimens may include gastric contents or lavage fluid, if the test is performed soon after ingestion. To test for certain toxic substances, special specimens may be required (for example, hair and nail clippings for detection of chronic arsenic poisoning).

After deliberate or accidental drug overdose, the patient's symptoms aid identification of the toxic drug or drugs. Early identification of the toxic drug—or at least exclusion of other drugs—can help the laboratory provide quick, accurate information. A complete drug history of the patient is essential, since it may identify the toxic substance and save valuable time and perhaps a life. If the toxic agent is not readily identified, a screening test for an entire class of drugs, such as narcotics, hallucinogens, or tranquilizers, may be ordered, as well as a general screening test for a class of drugs unidentifiable through symptoms. Urine is the specimen of choice for such screening tests. But, one or two blood samples should also be collected at the same time and refrigerated for later quantitative analysis.

Results of screening tests for drugs are presumptive and require careful correlation with symptoms. Results of screening tests for selected drugs such as phenobarbital, salicylates, and ethanol are usually available from the laboratory within 1 hour. Results of a general screening test are usually available within 3 to 5 hours.

For both quantitative analysis and screening tests, collect the samples in clean, properly labeled containers. Always include the following information on the laboratory slip: patient's name

---

jelly, bulb syringe, adhesive tape, I.V. pole, and suction unit.

Lubricate the distal end of the Ewald tube. Insert the tube slowly and gently into the patient's nasal passage. Rotate the tube inward to enter the pharynx. The patient may vomit, so be ready to suction. Once the tube has passed the posterior pharynx, position the patient on his left side in a three quarters prone position, with the stretcher in Trendelenburg position. Again rotate the tube inward, this time toward the esophagus, so the tube passes into the stomach.

To ensure proper tube placement, aspirate stomach contents with the bulb syringe. If the tube's positioned correctly, secure it to the patient's face with adhesive tape. Connect the Ewald tube to the Y connector. Then connect the irrigating fluid tubing and the drainage tubing to the Y connector. If a Moss tube is used, connect the dual tubing ends to irrigating fluid and drainage tubings.

Use the Kelly clamp to clamp the drainage tubing. Open the irrigating fluid tubing and allow 250 to 500 ml of lavage fluid to flow into the stomach. Larger amounts of lavage fluid may force the ingested substance into the duodenum. Clamp the irrigating fluid tube and open the drainage tube, for gravity flow of contents.

Watch for signs of intolerance, such as vomiting. If your patient starts to vomit, clamp the irrigating fluid tubing immediately and unclamp the drainage tubing.

Keep accurate inflow/outflow volume records. If outflow is significantly less than inflow, notify the doctor. Assess cardiac rhythm, vital signs, level of consciousness, and urinary output every 15 minutes. Also, obtain arterial blood gas measurements and serum electrolyte levels if the patient requires a large volume of lavage fluid.

Continue lavage (up to 10 liters) until the drainage fluid is clear. Then, clamp the irrigating fluid tubing and leave the drainage tubing open. If instillation of an adsorptive or purgative is ordered, administer it, then clamp the drainage tube for 20 to 30 minutes. Save all lavage fluid for possible analysis. Finally, document the procedure and your findings.

<hr>

ABNORMALITIES OF DRUG USE

Addiction: psychological and physical dependence, characterized by compulsion to obtain and use a drug

Drug abuse: repeated, inappropriate, and excessive use of therapeutic or illegal drugs

Drug tolerance: diminishing duration or level of effectiveness of a drug after repeated use. Tolerance of side effects usually occurs concurrently.

Psychological dependence: compulsive need to maintain a euphoric state or to fulfill an emotional need by using a drug

Physical dependence: biologic adaptation to the presence of a drug that produces symptoms on withdrawal

<hr>

and medical history (especially hepatic or renal conditions that affect metabolism and excretion), time of drug ingestion, suspected drug, current medications, time of sample collection, type of specimen, test requested, and clinical observations. Deliver specimen to the laboratory immediately. If transport of specimen is delayed, refrigerate the sample, but don't add a preservative.

Medicolegal considerations

If you are collecting a sample to be used for a medicolegal investigation, observe these additional precautions:

☐ Be sure a consent form has been signed before collecting the specimen, and that the collection is properly witnessed.

☐ Maintain continuity of possession. Keep the number of people handling the specimen to a minimum, and check that each person signs the laboratory slip and records the time and date he receives the sample.

☐ Seal the collection container with tape, and sign the label.

☐ Seal the specimen and laboratory slip in a package, and label it "Medicolegal case" on all sides.

☐ If transport of the specimen to the laboratory is delayed, lock the specimen in a container and refrigerate it.

Industrial toxicity

Toxicity determinations are also used to analyze poisoning in industrial workers who handle toxic substances, such as heavy metals, anions, and organic compounds. When an industrial accident causes acute poisoning, the laboratory performs emergency tests to measure the level of the toxic substance. Some laboratories monitor levels of absorption in workers who are exposed to toxicants.

HARVEY SPECTOR, MD

<hr>

THERAPEUTIC DRUG MONITORING

Serum Antiarrhythmics

Because of a low therapeutic index, a narrow margin of safety between therapeutic and toxic serum levels of antiarrhythmic drugs, this quantitative test is performed to monitor antiarrhythmic therapy. Depending on the drug being measured and the laboratory performing the assay, the analytic method used can be high-performance liquid chromatography, gas-liquid chromatography, spectrofluorometry, or enzyme-multiplied immunoassay technique.

Antiarrhythmic drugs reduce myocardial response to stimuli in patients with atrial fibrillation or flutter, supraventricular and ventricular tachycardia, or premature ventricular contractions.

They are used to treat atrial and ventricular arrhythmias of various causes; and to treat and prevent arrhythmias after myocardial infarction.

Lidocaine, procainamide, quinidine, disopyramide, and propranolol are readily absorbed and widely distributed throughout the body, and are primarily metabolized in the liver. Portions of the unmetabolized drugs and their active and inactive metabolites are excreted in the urine.

Purpose
□ To monitor therapeutic levels of anti-arrhythmic drugs
□ To check for toxicity suspected from history or after onset of symptoms.

Patient preparation
Explain to the patient that this test helps determine the most effective dosage of the drug he is receiving. Inform him that he needn't restrict food or fluids. Tell him the test requires a blood sample; who will perform the venipuncture and when; and that he may feel transient discomfort from the needle puncture and the pressure of the tourniquet. Reassure him that collecting the sample takes less than 3 minutes. Results are usually available in 2 or 3 days. Check the patient's history for recent use of other drugs.

Procedure
Perform a venipuncture, collecting ei-

ther a trough-level or peak-level sample, as appropriate, in the tube designated by the testing laboratory. Record the date and time of the last drug dose and the time of sample collection on the laboratory slip.

If the patient is receiving quinidine, also note the use of acetazolamide, antacids, or sodium bicarbonate on the laboratory slip; if the patient is receiving lidocaine, note the use of barbiturates or phenytoin.

Precautions
□ Handle the sample gently to prevent hemolysis, and send it to the laboratory immediately.
□ Observe the same time span between drug administration and sample collection for each test in the series.

Values
Peak time, steady state, and therapeutic

ANTIARRHYTHMIC BLOOD LEVELS

DRUG	PEAK TIME	STEADY STATE	THERAPEUTIC LEVEL	TOXIC LEVEL
Disopyramide	P.O.: 2 hours	25 to 30 hours	2 to 4.5 mcg/ml	> 9 mcg/ml
Lidocaine	I.V.: immediate	5 to 10 hours	2 to 6 mcg/ml	> 7 mcg/ml
Procainamide	P.O.: 60 minutes I.V.: 25 to 60 minutes	11 to 20 hours	4 to 8 mcg/ml	> 12 mcg/ml
N-acetyl-procainamide	—	—	2 to 8 mcg/ml	> 30 mcg/ml
Propranolol	P.O.: 60 to 90 minutes I.V.: 2 to 4 hours	10 to 30 hours	40 to 85 ng/ml (If patient's condition doesn't improve with serum level of 100 ng, treatment is unsuccessful.)	> 150 ng/ml (Toxic concentrations vary and require correlation with clinical status.)
Quinidine	P.O.: 1 to 3 hours I.V.: immediate I.M.: 30 to 90 minutes	20 to 35 hours	2.4 to 5 mcg/ml	> 6 mcg/ml
Verapamil	P.O.: 1 to 2 hours I.V.: 5 minutes	15 to 35 hours	0.08 to 0.3 mcg/ml	Unknown

and toxic serum levels depend on the specific antiarrhythmic drug and on the route of administration (see chart on page 1001).

Implications of results
Trough levels guide the adjustment of therapeutic dosage; peak levels can prevent or detect toxicity and monitor its treatment.

Post-test care
If a hematoma develops at the venipuncture site, ease discomfort by applying warm soaks.

Interfering factors
□ Hemolysis caused by rough handling of the sample can produce artifactual lowering of results for analysis by fluorometry or enzyme-multiplied immunoassay.
□ Serum quinidine levels are elevated by acetazolamide, antacids, and sodium bicarbonate.
□ Serum lidocaine and serum quinidine levels are suppressed by barbiturates and phenytoin.

HARVEY SPECTOR, MD

Serum Bronchodilators

Through high-performance liquid chromatography and immunoassay, this highly accurate test monitors serum levels of bronchodilators and detects toxicity. Since the margin of safety between therapeutic and toxic levels is narrow, this analysis is usually performed on patients beginning therapy with these drugs.

Bronchodilators—especially theophylline and aminophylline—relax smooth muscle, particularly that in the bronchi; consequently, these drugs are useful for treating asthma and bronchospasm. Theophylline can also effectively treat

neonatal and Cheyne-Stokes respiration apnea, probably because it directly stimulates the medullary respiratory center. Bronchodilators are absorbed in the gastrointestinal tract, metabolized in the liver, and excreted by the kidneys.

Purpose
□ To monitor therapeutic levels of bronchodilators
□ To check for toxicity suspected from the medication history or after onset of symptoms.

Patient preparation
Explain to the patient that this test helps determine the most effective dosage of bronchodilators. Inform him that he needn't restrict food or fluids. Tell him the test requires a blood sample; who will perform the venipuncture and when; and that he may experience transient discomfort from the needle puncture and the pressure of the tourniquet. Reassure him that collecting the sample takes only a few minutes. Test results are usually available within 24 hours.

Check the patient's history for recent ingestion of dietary xanthines, caffeine, and drugs that may affect test results.

Procedure
Perform a venipuncture, and obtain a trough-level sample by drawing blood just before a scheduled drug dose; obtain a peak-level sample by drawing blood 2 hours after the last dose. Collect the sample in a 7-ml *red-top* tube.

Record on the laboratory slip the specific bronchodilator administered, the time and amount of the last dose the patient's received, and the time of sample collection.

Precautions
□ Send the sample to the laboratory immediately.
□ Observe the same time span between drug administration and sample collection for serial testing.

Values
Serum concentrations of aminophylline

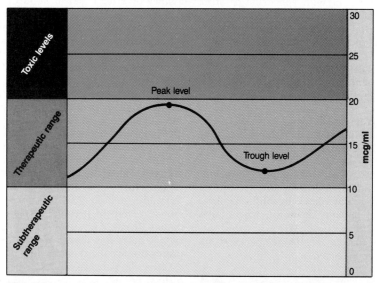

THERAPEUTIC RANGE OF SERUM BRONCHODILATORS

Toxic levels

Therapeutic range

Subtherapeutic range

Peak level

Trough level

mcg/ml

30
25
20
15
10
5
0

After attaining a steady state, serum bronchodilator levels are monitored to ensure that they remain in the therapeutic range. Graphs that plot therapeutic range, such as the graph above, show a normal cycle of peak and trough levels. In this graph, the cycle between peak and trough levels shows that the desired therapeutic range (peak level measurement) is being maintained.

or theophylline depend on the patient's age and metabolism. Generally, normal values range as follows:

□ *peak time:* 2 to 3 hours, if administered P.O.; 15 minutes, I.V.

□ *steady state:* 15 to 40 hours in adults; 5 to 40 hours in children

□ *therapeutic level:* 10 to 20 mcg/ml

□ *toxic level:* usually over 20 mcg/ml. However, smaller serum concentrations have been associated with toxicity and greater serum concentrations aren't toxic for all patients. In some patients, doses of 20 mcg/ml are required to relieve bronchospasm.

Implications of results

Peak and trough concentrations guide adjustment of therapeutic dosage, especially in children and patients with cardiac, hepatic, pulmonary, or renal dysfunction.

Simultaneous dietary intake of xan-

thine derivatives (coffee, tea, or chocolate) can account for 2 mcg/ml of serum concentration.

SYMPTOMS OF BRONCHODILATOR TOXICITY

Eye, ear, nose, and throat: tinnitus, flashing lights

Gastrointestinal system: anorexia, nausea, vomiting, diarrhea, epigastric pain and irritability, hematemesis

Central nervous system: headache, insomnia, restlessness, irritability, agitation, fainting, convulsions (especially in infants and young children), hyperreflexia, fasciculations, coma

Cardiovascular system: tachycardia, arrhythmias, marked hypotension, circulatory failure, cardiac arrest.

Genitourinary system: albuminuria, microhematuria

Other: cyanosis, dehydration, extreme thirst, tachypnea, respiratory arrest, fever

Simultaneous administration of more than one bronchodilator, by more than one route, or with ephedrine or other sympathomimetics increases the hazard of serious toxicity. Gastric symptoms result from irritation, not direct toxicity.

Post-test care
If a hematoma develops at the venipuncture site, apply warm soaks.

Interfering factors
□ Caffeine and other xanthines may falsely elevate serum bronchodilator concentrations.
□ Cimetidine, troleandomycin, erythromycin, and lincomycin raise serum bronchodilator levels by inhibiting these drugs' hepatic clearance; barbiturates lower them.

HARVEY SPECTOR, MD

Serum Antibiotics

This quantitative immunoassay directly measures serum levels of antibiotics to determine therapeutic concentrations and to detect toxic accumulations. Therapeutic levels are also measurable through assay of body fluids, but serum assay is more reliable.

The group of antibiotics that most often requires therapeutic monitoring is the aminoglycoside group: amikacin, gentamicin, kanamycin, netilmicin, and tobramycin. These drugs are used to treat infections from gram-negative bacilli and gram-positive cocci; resistant strains require high serum levels, with increased potential for ototoxicity, neurotoxicity, and nephrotoxicity. Although these antibiotics are normally excreted unmetabolized by the kidneys, toxic blood levels can damage the kidneys, allowing even higher blood levels to accumulate and produce ototoxicity.

Purpose
□ To monitor therapeutic levels of aminoglycoside antibiotics
□ To check for toxicity suspected from history or after onset of nephrotoxic symptoms—such as renal failure, proteinuria, oliguria or anuria, elevated serum creatinine and BUN, and low specific gravity and creatinine clearance—or ototoxic or neurotoxic symptoms.

Patient preparation
Explain to the patient that this test measures blood concentration of antibiotics to help determine the most effective dosage. Inform him that he needn't restrict food or fluids. Tell him the test requires a blood sample; who will perform the venipuncture and when; and that he may feel transient discomfort from the needle puncture and the pressure of the tourniquet. Reassure him that collecting the sample takes less than 3 minutes. Test results are usually available in 1 day.

Check the patient's recent medication history, noting drug, dosage, and route of administration.

Procedure
Perform a venipuncture, and collect a trough-level or peak-level sample in a 7 ml *red-top* tube. Record the date, time, and administration route of the last dose, and the sample collection time on the laboratory slip.

Precautions
□ Send the sample to the laboratory immediately.
□ When monitoring therapeutic levels, observe the same time span between drug administration and sample collection in serial testing.

Values
Peak time, steady state, and therapeutic and toxic serum levels vary, depending on the antibiotic being administered (see chart on page 1006).

Implications of results
Antibiotic blood levels allow adjustment of dosage to maintain effective therapeutic levels and prevent excessive accumulation and toxicity.

OTOTOXICITY: DAMAGE TO THE ORGAN OF CORTI BY AMINOGLYCOSIDES

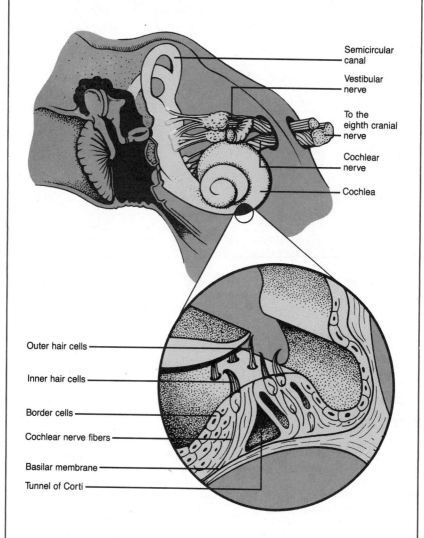

Semicircular canal

Vestibular nerve

To the eighth cranial nerve

Cochlear nerve

Cochlea

Outer hair cells

Inner hair cells

Border cells

Cochlear nerve fibers

Basilar membrane

Tunnel of Corti

High aminoglycoside levels damage the neuroepithelial sensory hair cells in the organ of Corti (shown in bottom illustration). These hair cells, the sensory receptors for hearing, synapse with cochlear nerve endings and eventually with branches of the eighth cranial nerve, which leads to the cortex. When the hair cells leading to the semicircular canals and receptors in the vestibule and connected to the vestibular branch are damaged, the patient develops dizziness and blurred vision; when damage to the hair cells connected to the cochlear branch occurs, the patient develops tinnitus and hearing changes or impairment.

ANTIBIOTIC BLOOD LEVELS

DRUG	PEAK TIME	STEADY STATE	THERAPEUTIC	TOXIC PEAK	TOXIC TROUGH*
Amikacin	I.M.: 30 minutes to 1 hour I.V.: 15 to 30 minutes	1 to 2 days	8 to 16 mcg/ml	> 35 mcg/ml	> 8 mcg/ml
Gentamicin	I.M.: 30 minutes to 1 hour I.V.: 15 to 30 minutes	1 to 2 days	4 to 10 mcg/ml	> 12 mcg/ml	> 2 mcg/ml
Kanamycin	I.M.: 30 minutes to 1 hour	1 to 2 days	8 to 16 mcg/ml	> 35 mcg/ml	> 8 mcg/ml
Netilmicin	I.M.: 30 minutes to 1 hour I.V.: 15 to 30 minutes	1 to 2 days	0.5 to 10 mcg/ml	> 16 mcg/ml	> 4 mcg/ml
Tobramycin	I.M.: 30 minutes to 1 hour I.V.: 15 to 30 minutes	1 to 2 days	4 to 8 mcg/ml	> 12 mcg/ml	> 2 mcg/ml

*Note: Trough toxic levels can be below therapeutic levels, due to nephrotoxic nature of antibiotics.

Post-test care
If a hematoma develops at the venipuncture site, apply warm soaks.

Interfering factors
None.

HARVEY SPECTOR, MD

Serum Anticonvulsants

This quantitative test uses an enzyme multiplied immunoassay technique to measure serum levels of anticonvulsants—notably carbamazepine, ethosuximide, phenobarbital, phenytoin, and primidone. It's useful in monitoring antiepileptic therapy in children and mentally retarded persons—in whom toxicity is difficult to detect.

Purpose
□ To monitor therapeutic levels of anti-convulsants

□ To confirm toxicity suspected from history or after onset of symptoms.

Patient preparation
Explain to the patient and to the family, if appropriate, that this test helps determine the most effective dosage of anticonvulsants. Inform him he that needn't restrict food or fluids. Tell him the test requires a blood sample; who will perform the venipuncture and when; and that he may experience transient discomfort from the needle puncture and the pressure of the tourniquet. Reassure him that collecting the sample takes less than 3 minutes. Test results are usually available in 1 day. Check the patient's recent medication history, noting dosage, interval, and route of administration.

Procedure
Perform a venipuncture, and collect a trough-level sample in a 7 ml *red-top* tube. Record the date, time, and route of administration of the last drug dose, and the time of sample collection on the laboratory slip.

THERAPEUTIC DRUG MONITORING **1007**

Precautions
☐ Send the sample to the laboratory immediately.
☐ Observe the same time span between drug administration and sample collection in serial testing.

Values
Steady state, peak time, and therapeutic and toxic serum levels of anticonvulsants vary (see chart on this page).

Implications of results
Anticonvulsant blood levels allow adjustment of dosage to maintain effective therapeutic levels and to prevent excessive accumulation and toxicity.

The slow rate of elimination of most anticonvulsants is an important consideration in treating drug toxicity.

Post-test care
If a hematoma develops at the venipuncture site, apply warm soaks.

Interfering factors
☐ Serum levels of carbamazepine are elevated by troleandomycin, erythromycin, and propoxyphene, and are lowered by phenytoin, phenobarbital, and primidone.
☐ Serum levels of phenobarbital are elevated by MAO inhibitors and primidone, and are lowered by rifampin.
☐ Serum levels of phenytoin may be

raised by oral anticoagulants, antihistamines, chloramphenicol, chlordiazepoxide, chlorpromazine hydrochloride, diazepam, diazoxide, disulfiram, ethosuximide, isoniazid, phenylbutazone, phenobarbital, propoxyphene, salicylates, sulfamethizole, and valproic acid; serum phenytoin levels may be sup-

---

SYMPTOMS OF ANTICONVULSANT TOXICITY

Carbamazepine: blood dyscrasias, drowsiness, nausea, vomiting, vertigo, ataxia, hallucinations, peripheral neuritis, congestive heart failure, hypo- or hypertension, hepatic abnormalities, urinary retention, convulsions
Ethosuximide: drowsiness, dizziness, blurred or double vision, myopia, hiccups, ataxia, anorexia, nausea, abdominal cramps or pain, blood dyscrasias, profound CNS depression
Phenobarbital: drowsiness, confusion, muscle weakness, headache, hypotension, respiratory depression, blood dyscrasias, profound CNS depression, shock syndrome
Phenytoin: gingival irritation and hyperplasia, nystagmus, ataxia, confusion, irritability, hallucinations, nausea, dry skin, rash, agranulocytosis, drowsiness, extreme lethargy, deep coma
Primidone: sedation, nystagmus, ataxia, vertigo, nausea, diplopia, hypertension, mental confusion, unusual excitement, mild tachycardia, crystalluria, leukopenia, eosinophilia, profound CNS depression, shock syndrome

---

ANTICONVULSANT BLOOD LEVELS

DRUG	PEAK TIME	STEADY STATE	THERAPEUTIC	TOXIC
Carbamazepine	2 to 6 hours	2 to 4 days	2 to 10 mcg/ml	> 12 mcg/ml*
Ethosuximide	1 to 2 hours	8 to 10 days	40 to 80 mcg/ml	> 100 mcg/ml
Phenobarbital	6 to 18 hours	14 to 21 days	20 to 40 mcg/ml	> 55 mcg/ml
Phenytoin	4 to 8 hours	5 to 11 days	10 to 20 mcg/ml	> 80 mcg/ml*
Primidone	2 to 4 hours	4 to 7 days	7 to 11 mcg/ml	> 12 mcg/ml*

*Toxic concentrations vary; serum levels should be correlated with clinical symptoms.

pressed by alcohol, phenobarbital, carbamazepine, folic acid, loxapine, and antacids.

☐ Serum levels of primidone are elevated by carbamazepine and phenytoin.

HARVEY SPECTOR, MD

Serum Cardiac Glycosides

This radioimmunoassay for monitoring cardiac glycoside therapy is especially useful for elderly patients or those with renal or hepatic disease. Cardiac glycosides (principally digoxin and digitoxin) improve myocardial contractility, increase cardiac output in congestive heart failure, and manage atrial arrhythmias. After P.O. administration of these drugs, the serum cardiac glycoside level rises rapidly but drops sharply as the drug enters the myocardium and other tissues. Toxicity usually results from hepatic or renal dysfunction, hypokalemia, hypothyroidism, severe hypoxic heart or respiratory disease, and variations in patient response rather than excessive dosage. Although digoxin and digitoxin assays are highly accurate (generally within 3% to 6% of true serum concentration), serum levels may not always correlate with the clinical state.

Purpose

☐ To monitor therapeutic levels of cardiac glycosides

☐ To check for toxicity suspected from history or after onset of symptoms, such as headache, drowsiness, anorexia, nausea, vomiting, diarrhea, yellow vision, generalized weakness, hypotension, delirium, slow and irregular pulse, or cardiac arrhythmias.

Patient preparation

Explain to the patient that this test helps determine the most effective drug dosage. Inform him that he needn't restrict food or fluids. Tell him the test requires a blood sample; who will perform the venipuncture and when; and that he may experience transient discomfort from the needle puncture and the pressure of the tourniquet. Reassure him that collecting the sample takes less than 3 minutes. The laboratory requires 2 days to complete the analysis.

Check the patient's recent medication history. Make sure the test is ordered for the appropriate cardiac glycoside.

Procedure

Perform a venipuncture, and collect a trough-level sample in a 7 ml *red-top* tube. Note on the laboratory slip the spe-

---

BLOOD LEVELS OF COMMON CARDIAC GLYCOSIDES

DRUG	PEAK TIME	STEADY STATE (without loading dose)	THERAPEUTIC	TOXIC
Digoxin	1½ to 5 hours	7 days	0.5 to 2 ng/ml	> 2.5 ng/ml
Digitoxin	4 to 12 hours	25 to 35 days	5 to 30 ng/ml	> 35 ng/ml

Digoxin and digitoxin, the two most commonly used cardiac glycosides, have similar clinical effects but are metabolized differently. These differences stem from the fact that digoxin is eliminated primarily through the kidneys, while digitoxin is primarily metabolized in the liver and excreted in feces. Consequently, renal dysfunction can cause digoxin toxicity; hepatic dysfunction can cause digitoxin toxicity. Moreover, toxicity may result from hypokalemia, hypothyroidism, and from heart and respiratory disease. With either drug, toxicity isn't necessarily dose related.

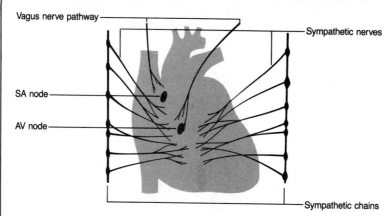

HOW VARYING BLOOD LEVELS OF DIGOXIN AFFECT THE HEART

Vagus nerve pathway

Sympathetic nerves

SA node

AV node

Sympathetic chains

At low therapeutic blood levels (0.5 to 1.5 ng/ml), digoxin enhances cardiac output and myocardial contractility by strengthening the force of ventricular contractions. Higher therapeutic blood levels (1 to 2 ng/ml) may be necessary to control supraventricular arrhythmias by slowing conduction through the atrioventricular node, and limiting the number of depolarization waves that reach the ventricle.

At therapeutic levels (0.5 to 2 ng/ml) in congestive heart failure, digoxin slows the action of the heart by permitting reduction in sympathetic drive as contractility increases, and somewhat by directly enhancing vagal tone.

cific cardiac glycoside being monitored; the date, time, amount, and route of administration of the last dose; and the time of sample collection.

Precautions
□ Send the sample to the lab promptly.
□ Observe the same time span between drug administration and sample collection in serial testing.

Values
Therapeutic and toxic serum levels of digoxin and digitoxin vary, depending on the patient and the disorder being treated; for example, some patients with supraventricular arrhythmias don't exhibit symptoms of toxicity even though they require high cardiac glycoside dosages to control ventricular rate.

Implications of results
Serum cardiac glycoside levels must be considered in relation to the patient's current clinical status, past levels and status, and renal function tests.

Post-test care
If a hematoma develops at the venipuncture site, apply warm soaks.

Interfering factors
□ Absorption of digitoxin and digoxin is decreased by aminosalicylic acid, antacids, cholestyramine, colestipol, kaolin-pectin, and neomycin.
□ Phenobarbital, phenytoin, cholestyramine, and phenylbutazone suppress digitoxin levels; quinidine and verapamil raise digoxin levels; spironolactone interferes with the test, producing false elevations.
□ Drugs that deplete body extracellular potassium levels predispose the patient to toxicity. Testing before steady state is achieved produces misleading findings.
□ Testing for the wrong cardiac glycoside—such as digitoxin rather than digoxin—results in erroneous findings.

HARVEY SPECTOR, MD

TOXICITY DETERMINATIONS

Serum Salicylates

This quantitative test uses a ferric chloride color reaction to measure serum salicylate levels. In unconscious or uncooperative patients, such testing may follow detection of salicylates in a qualitative urine screening.

Absorbed rapidly from the upper gastrointestinal tract, acetylsalicylic acid in therapeutic doses produces peak blood levels in 30 to 45 minutes, and is quickly hydrolyzed to salicylic acid and bound to albumin. However, with toxic doses, serum salicylate levels may rise for 6 to 10 hours after ingestion; thus, serial sampling is recommended for 24 hours following overdose to accurately determine toxicity. Salicylates are the most common cause of drug toxicity in young children; mortality for severe salicylism may be as high as 7% in children and 1% to 2% in adults.

Purpose

□ To confirm toxicity suspected from

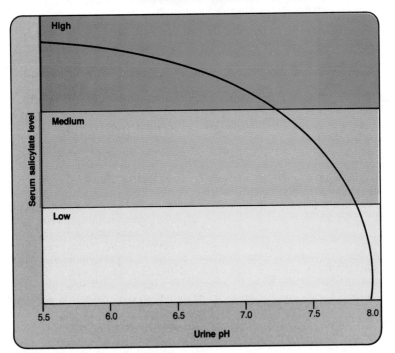

HOW ALKALINIZATION OF URINE DECREASES SERUM SALICYLATE LEVELS

When a patient has taken an overdose of aspirin, alkalinization of his urine by the administration of sodium bicarbonate increases his renal excretion, thus lowering his serum salicylate levels. In the chart above, notice that as the urine's pH approaches 7.5, the serum salicylate level decreases *rapidly.*

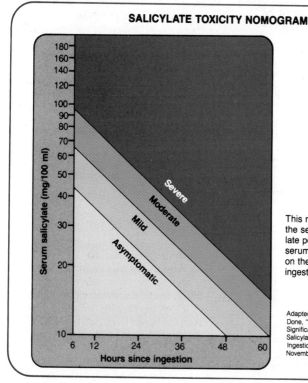

SALICYLATE TOXICITY NOMOGRAM

This nomogram estimates the severity of acute salicylate poisoning based on the serum salicylate level and on the time elapsed since ingestion.

Adapted with permission from A.K. Done, "Salicylate Intoxication: Significance of Measurement of Salicylate in Blood in Cases of Acute Ingestion," *Pediatrics*, Vol. 26, No. 5, November 1960.

history or onset of symptoms
☐ To monitor therapeutic levels of serum salicylate.

Patient preparation
Explain to the patient and to his family, if appropriate, that this test determines salicylate levels in the blood. Tell him the test requires a blood sample; who will perform the venipuncture and when; and that he may experience transient discomfort from the needle puncture and the pressure of the tourniquet. Reassure him that collecting the sample takes less than 3 minutes. Test results are usually available in 1 day.

If the test is being performed for medicolegal purposes, make sure the patient or responsible member of the family has signed a consent form. Check the patient's drug history for recent use of salicylates. Record the amount of salicylate ingested.

Procedure
Perform a venipuncture, and collect the sample in a 7 ml *red-top* tube.

Precautions
☐ Handle the sample gently to prevent hemolysis, and send it to the laboratory immediately or refrigerate it.
☐ For a medicolegal test, observe proper precautions.

Values
Therapeutic serum salicylate concentrations range from 2 to 30 mg/100 ml; toxicity is associated with concentrations greater than 40 mg/100 ml.

Implications of results
Therapeutic dosage is adjusted based on level reported. Treatment of toxicity is adjusted based on level of toxicity noted, clinical status, and time-dependent nomogram.

**CLINICAL EFFECTS OF
SALICYLATE TOXICITY**

Mild toxicity: moderate hyperpnea;
burning pain in throat, mouth, or abdomen;
vomiting; tinnitus; hearing loss; lethargy
Moderate toxicity: severe hyperpnea,
sweating, dehydration, fever, ecchymosis,
blurred vision, incoordination, restlessness,
excitability, delirium, marked lethargy,
respiratory alkalosis
Severe toxicity: severe hyperpnea;
cyanosis; pulmonary edema; oliguria;
convulsions; coma; hypothermia; sodium,
potassium, and bicarbonate urinary
loss; hypoglycemia; ketosis; and metabolic
acidosis (more severe in young children)

Post-test care

If a hematoma develops at the venipuncture site, apply warm soaks.

Interfering factors

□ Hemolysis due to rough handling of
the sample can falsely elevate serum salicylate levels.
□ Antacids and food lower serum salicylate levels; ammonium chloride and
other urine acidifiers elevate levels.

HARVEY SPECTOR, MD

Serum
Acetaminophen

*This test uses high-performance liquid
chromatography or an enzyme-multiplied immunoassay technique to measure serum acetaminophen levels. It's
essential for anticipating potential hepatotoxicity from an overdose; clinical effects (jaundice, coagulation defects,
encephalopathy, renal failure, coma)
don't appear until after liver damage
has occurred—generally 2 to 5 days after the ingestion of a toxic dose.*

*Absorbed rapidly from the GI tract,
acetaminophen is metabolized by the
liver and excreted in the urine. Acetaminophen overdose saturates the liver
conjugation pathway, causing metabo-*

*lism to hydroxamine-N-acetyl-P-ami-
nophenol, a reactive toxic intermediate
that injures liver cells and depletes hepatic glutathione, a substance that normally works to inactivate the toxic
intermediate.*

*Concomitant ingestion of alcohol or
barbiturates can significantly increase
the amount of acetaminophen metabolized to the toxic intermediate, exagger-
ating the risk of hepatotoxicity.*

Purpose

□ To confirm acetaminophen toxicity
suspected from history or onset of symptoms
□ To monitor detoxification treatment
with I.V. acetylcysteine (Mucomyst).

Patient preparation

Explain to the patient and to his family,
if appropriate, that this test determines
blood levels of acetaminophen to prevent
or check for toxicity. Inform the patient
that he needn't restrict foods or fluids.
Tell him that the test requires multiple
blood samples at timed intervals; who
will perform the venipunctures and
when; and that he may feel transient discomfort from the needle punctures and
the pressure of the tourniquet. Assure
him that collecting each sample takes
less than 3 minutes. And tell him that
test results are usually available within
1 day.

If the test is being performed for medicolegal purposes, make sure the patient
or a responsible member of his family
has signed a consent form. Check the
patient's drug history, noting the time of
acetaminophen ingestion and the dosage. Also check for use of alcohol and
barbiturates.

Procedure

Perform the venipuncture and collect the
sample in a 7-ml *red-top* tube. Repeat
the procedure 4, 8, and 12 hours after
drug ingestion.

If the time of drug ingestion is unknown, collect two samples at least 4
hours apart, so the elimination half-life
of the drug can be estimated.

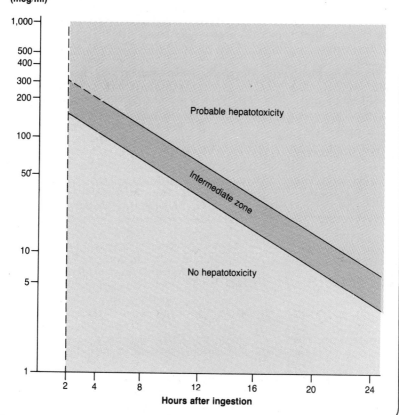

ACETAMINOPHEN HEPATOTOXICITY NOMOGRAM

This nomogram estimates the probability of hepatotoxicity from acetaminophen poisoning based on the serum acetaminophen level and the time elapsed since ingestion.

**Serum
Acetaminophen
(mcg/ml)**

Probable hepatotoxicity

Intermediate zone

No hepatotoxicity

Hours after ingestion

Precautions

□ Send the samples to the laboratory immediately.

□ Observe the correct time intervals between drug ingestion and sample collection in serial testing.

□ If test results are to be used for medicolegal purposes, carefully document all findings and maintain continuity of possession.

Values

Generally, serum acetaminophen levels

below 120 mcg/ml 4 hours after ingestion rule out hepatotoxicity.

When ingestion time isn't known, elimination half-life helps determine possible toxicity. Normal elimination half-life is 2 to 4 hours.

Implications of results

Serum acetaminophen levels above 150 mcg/ml 4 hours after ingestion indicate probable hepatotoxicity, as does an elimination half-life over 4 hours. An elimination half-life over 10 hours may indicate impending hepatic coma and death.

Liver function studies, such as serum bilirubin and alkaline phosphatase, may be necessary to further assess liver damage.

Post-test care

□ If acetaminophen levels indicate toxicity, begin treatment with I.V. acetylcysteine, as ordered. Draw additional blood samples, as needed, to monitor the effectiveness of detoxification measures.

□ If a hematoma develops at the venipuncture sites, ease discomfort by applying warm soaks.

Interfering factors

Failure to observe the correct time intervals in serial testing of serum acetaminophen can interfere with accurate determination of test results.

HARVEY SPECTOR, MD

Narcotic Analgesics

These tests, performed using thin-layer chromatography or enzyme-multiplied immunoassay technique, detect the presence of narcotic analgesics in patients with acute drug toxicities or adverse drug reactions, and help determine drug dependence and progress of detoxification. Testing for narcotic analgesics is usually qualitative, but quantitative testing for confirmation can also be performed on certain narcotic analgesics, such as morphine, codeine, meperidine, methadone, and propoxyphene. Although urine is the specimen of choice for detecting narcotic analgesics, gastric contents may also be analyzed.

Used primarily as CNS depressants for relieving pain, narcotic analgesics— a group of natural, semi-natural, and synthetic drugs with morphinelike action—can produce physical and psychological dependence. These drugs (which include morphine, heroin, hydromorphone, codeine, meperidine, methadone, propoxyphene, and oxycodone) are absorbed slowly from the gastrointestinal tract, with peak effects occurring approximately 1 hour after ingestion. When administered P.O., narcotic analgesics are less effective, but their duration is longer. Like most basic amines, free morphine leaves the blood quickly and concentrates in tissues, so it's undetectable in serum; heroin is metabolized and excreted as morphine. Narcotics are detoxified by the liver and eliminated in urine within 48 hours of administration, with 90% excreted in 24 hours.

Purpose

□ To determine the cause of acute drug toxicity or adverse drug reaction suspected from history

□ To help monitor drug dependence or the progress of narcotic detoxification

□ To detect the presence of narcotics for medicolegal purposes.

SYMPTOMS OF NARCOTIC ANALGESIC TOXICITY AND ABUSE

Central nervous system: respiratory depression, progressing to Cheyne-Stokes respiration; apnea; CNS depression, ranging from stupor to coma; muscle tremors and twitches; flaccid muscles; disorientation; delirium; hallucinations; grand mal seizures (meperidine derivatives)
Cardiovascular system: circulatory collapse, cyanosis, hypotension, bradycardia, tachycardia (meperidine derivatives)

Eye, ear, nose, and throat: miosis (morphine, derivatives and methadone), mydriasis (meperidine derivatives and terminal narcosis or severe hypoxia)
Gastrointestinal system: dry mouth (meperidine derivatives), nausea, vomiting, urinary retention, constipation
Other: hypothermia; cold, clammy skin; euphoria; unconsciousness; nephrogenic diabetes insipidus (propoxyphene)

Patient preparation

Explain to the patient that this test determines the presence of narcotic analgesics in the urine. For a monitoring test, inform him that he needn't restrict food or fluids. For methadone testing, tell him a 24-hour urine specimen is required, and teach him proper collection technique; for all other tests to detect the presence of narcotic analgesics, random urine specimens are used. Explain that test results are available the same day in emergencies.

For a medicolegal test, make sure the patient or responsible member of the family has signed a consent form. Record the patient's recent drug history, including dosage schedule and route of administration.

Procedure

Instruct the patient to collect a 24-hour urine specimen to measure methadone levels; a random urine specimen is required for other drugs in this group.

Precautions

□ Send the specimen to the laboratory immediately, or refrigerate the specimen during the collection period.
□ For a medicolegal test, observe proper precautions.

Values

Some narcotic analgesics can be measured quantitatively. Toxic concentrations of these drugs are as follows:

Morphine	>0.005 mg/dl
Codeine	>0.005 mg/dl
Hydromorphone	>0.1 mg/dl
Meperidine	>0.5 mg/dl
Methadone	>0.2 mg/dl
Propoxyphene	>0.5 mg/dl

Tests for heroin and oxycodone are qualitative.

Implications of results

Detoxification is based on urine levels. Identification of presence of narcotics may have medicolegal implications.

Post-test care

None.

DRUG TOLERANCE AND DEPENDENCE

Repeated use of a narcotic analgesic induces tolerance that first reduces the duration of effect and then the effectiveness of the prescribed dose. To detect such tolerance, observe the patient for relief of pain. If pain persists at the time of peak effect (about 1 hour after injection) or if relief doesn't last as long as expected, notify the doctor. He may increase the dose or shorten the interval between doses.

Narcotic analgesics can also induce physiologic dependence: a state in which absence of the drug causes withdrawal symptoms. Such symptoms are milder after withdrawal of drugs with long half-lives—such as methadone and codeine; consequently, methadone is often substituted for morphine to ease withdrawal, particularly after narcotic abuse. Such substitution prolongs withdrawal but mitigates symptoms. After use of narcotics for relief of acute pain, withdrawal symptoms are relatively uncommon—possibly because the dosage is gradually reduced as pain subsides.

Interfering factors

Delayed transport may produce false-negative test results in a urine specimen analyzed by thin-layer chromatography.

HARVEY SPECTOR, MD

Urine Amphetamines

This quantitative analysis measures the urine levels of amphetamine, dextroamphetamine, methamphetamine, and phenmetrazine—sympathomimetic drugs that stimulate the medullary respiratory center. Serum concentrations of these drugs are usually too small to measure toxic levels. Laboratory methods for quantitative testing of urine amphetamines consist of enzyme-multiplied immunoassay technique or gas chromatography; for screening, thin-layer chromatography.

Amphetamines are used to treat narcolepsy, hyperkinesia in children, and nocturnal enuresis. Amphetamines and similar drugs have also been used for

URINE AMPHETAMINE LEVELS		
DRUG	**THERA-PEUTIC**	**TOXIC**
Amphetamine	2 to 3 mcg/ml	> 30 mcg/ml
Dextroamphet-amine	1 to 1.5 mcg/ml	> 15 mcg/ml
Methamphet-amine	3 to 5 mcg/ml	> 40 mcg/ml
Phenmetrazine	5 to 30 mcg/ml	> 50 mcg/ml

treatment of obesity because of their appetite depressant effect. However, such use is controversial, and these drugs are commonly abused. Administered P.O., amphetamines are absorbed rapidly in the gastrointestinal tract. After distribution, highest concentrations appear in the brain and the cerebrospinal fluid. Normally, amphetamines are excreted in the urine in about 3 hours; in a shorter time in acid urine.

Purpose
□ To monitor therapeutic levels of am-

TOXIC EFFECTS OF AMPHETAMINES

Central nervous system
Restlessness, tremors, hyperactivity, talkativeness, insomnia, irritability, dizziness, headache, chills, overstimulation, dysphoria, psychosis

Cardiovascular system
Tachycardia, palpitations, hypertension, hypotension, arrhythmias, cerebrovascular accident

Gastrointestinal system
Nausea, vomiting, cramps, dry mouth, diarrhea, constipation, metallic taste, anorexia, weight loss

Other
Urticaria, impotence, changes in libido

---

phetamines
□ To determine amphetamine toxicity suspected from history or after onset of symptoms
□ To confirm the presence of amphetamines for medicolegal purposes.

Patient preparation
Explain to the patient and to his family, if appropriate, that this test detects the presence or measures the levels of amphetamines in the body. Tell him the test requires a urine specimen. Inform him that test results are usually available within 1 day.

If the test is being performed for medicolegal purposes, make sure the patient or responsible member of the family has signed a consent form. Check the patient's recent drug history.

Procedure
Collect a random urine specimen.

Precautions
□ Seal the container to prevent air contamination, and send the specimen to the laboratory immediately or refrigerate it.
□ For a medicolegal test, observe proper precautions.

Values
Therapeutic and toxic levels vary depending on the amphetamine being measured (see chart on this page).

Implications of results
Idiosyncratic toxic manifestations may follow administration of as little as 2 mg but are rare with doses under 15 mg. Severe reactions have followed 30-mg doses; yet 400- to 500-mg doses may not be fatal. Prolonged use promotes tolerance to larger doses.

Quantitative analysis of serum amphetamine levels provides a basis for regulation of therapeutic dosage and for detoxification.

Presence of nonprescribed amphetamines has medicolegal implications.

Post-test care
None.

Interfering factors

The rate at which amphetamines are excreted depends on urine pH; acid urine increases the rate of excretion; alkaline urine decreases it.

HARVEY SPECTOR, MD

Serum Barbiturates

This quantitative analysis measures serum barbiturate levels. The most common cause of drug-induced coma, barbiturates are classified by their length of action: long-acting (mephobarbital, phenobarbital); short- to intermediate-acting (amobarbital, pentobarbital, and secobarbital); and ultrashort-acting (thiamylal, hexobarbital, and thiopental). Barbiturates are used as sedatives, hypnotics, or anticonvulsant agents; however, only long-acting barbiturates are effective as anticonvulsants in doses that do not induce sleep. Short- to intermediate-acting barbiturates are used as sedatives and hypnotics; ultrashort-acting barbiturates, as anesthetics. Barbiturates do not produce analgesia at doses below anesthesia level.

The appropriate laboratory method for measuring serum barbiturate levels varies—for example, long-acting barbiturates require gas chromatography; short- to intermediate-acting barbiturates require the enzyme-multiplied immunoassay technique. Although the serum level usually correlates with the patient's clinical condition, many factors can influence it (including route of administration, the degree of CNS excitability, the patient's barbiturate tolerance, and the additive effect of such compounds as alcohol, opiates, and tranquilizers).

Purpose

☐ To check for barbiturate toxicity suspected from history or after the onset of toxic symptoms, such as headache, confusion, ataxia, respiratory and CNS depression, flaccid muscles, hypothermia to hyperthermia, hypotension, low uri-

BARBITURATE BLOOD LEVELS AND POSSIBLE EFFECTS

DRUG	MILD SEDATION	SLEEPINESS	COMATOSE, WITH REFLEXES	COMATOSE, WITHOUT REFLEXES	COMATOSE, WITH CIRCULATORY AND RESPIRATORY DIFFICULTY
Long-acting					
Phenobarbital	10	34	55	80	150
Short- to intermediate-acting					
Amobarbital	7	15	30	52	66
Pentobarbital	4	6	15	20	30
Secobarbital	3	5	10	15	20

All values are given in mcg/ml

KEY: Therapeutic ☐   Therapeutic/toxic ☐

Toxic ☐   Potentially lethal ☐   Probably lethal ☐

nary output, areflexia, or shock syndrome

☐ To monitor therapeutic barbiturate levels

☐ To confirm the presence of barbiturates for medicolegal purposes.

Patient preparation

Explain to the patient and to his family, if appropriate, that this test determines the concentration of barbiturates in the body. Tell him the test requires a blood sample; who will perform the venipuncture and when; and that he may experience transient discomfort from the needle puncture and the pressure of the tourniquet. Reassure him that collecting the sample takes less than 3 minutes. In an emergency, test results are usually available the same day; normally, however, the laboratory requires 1 day to complete the analysis.

If the test is being performed for medicolegal purposes, make sure the patient or responsible member of the family has signed a consent form. Obtain a recent drug history, including doses, times, and administration routes.

Procedure

Perform a venipuncture, and collect the sample in a 7 ml *red-top* tube.

Precautions

☐ Handle the sample gently to prevent hemolysis, and send the sample to the laboratory immediately or refrigerate it.

☐ For a medicolegal test, observe proper precautions.

Values

Generally, short-acting barbiturates produce both therapeutic and toxic effects at lower serum concentrations than long-acting barbiturates. (See chart on page 1017 for representative values.) These values are not absolute, but severe toxicity usually follows ingestion of 10 times the usual hypnotic dose.

Implications of results

Individual tolerance influences the clinical effects of barbiturates and should be considered in regulating therapeutic dosage. Prolonged use of barbiturates often induces tolerance and physical dependence, which are closely related. Abrupt withdrawal after chronic intoxication causes withdrawal syndromes that are consistently dose-related; the higher the intoxicating dose, the more severe the withdrawal syndrome. While tolerance to the sedative and intoxicating effects of barbiturates may be considerable, the lethal dose is not much greater in persons addicted to drugs than in other persons. Thus, acute toxicity may develop abruptly in barbiturate addicts. Physical dependence also occurs with long-term use and is a concern for withdrawal of the drug.

The anesthesia induced by ultrashort-acting barbiturates begins rapidly (onset at less than 1 minute) and disappears rapidly. Toxicity after intravenous use varies according to the patient's susceptibility to respiratory depression and apnea. I.V. use requires precautions to maintain pulmonary ventilation.

Paradoxically, children, the elderly, and patients with severe pain may respond to administration of barbiturates with excitement, restlessness, hyperactivity, or delirium.

Post-test care

If a hematoma develops at the venipuncture site, apply warm soaks.

Interfering factors

☐ Hemolysis caused by rough handling of the sample falsely elevates levels in a sample analyzed by the enzyme-multiplied immunoassay technique.

☐ Salicylates and sulfonamides interfere with the test.

☐ MAO inhibitors, disulfiram, and ingestion of alcohol can raise barbiturate blood levels; rifampin may lower them.

☐ Primidone may elevate phenobarbital blood levels.

☐ Concurrent use of barbiturates and other CNS depressants causes additive sedative effects that can exceed the safe level.

HARVEY SPECTOR, MD

Plasma or Serum Antidepressants

This quantitative toxicity test, which measures plasma antidepressant levels, confirms medication overdose and monitors therapy. Major laboratory methods used to perform this test include gas chromatography, high-performance liquid chromatography, and, for screening, thin-layer chromatography.

Drugs currently used in the treatment of depression include lithium salts, tricyclic antidepressants (TCAs)—doxepin, amitriptyline, desipramine, imipramine, nortriptyline, and protriptyline—and the monoamine oxidase (MAO) inhibitors—isocarboxazid, phenelzine, and tranylcypromine. TCAs are preferred for treating depression, since they are less toxic than MAO inhibitors or lithium salts. However, lithium salts are used extensively to treat manic-depressive psychosis, although the margin of safety between therapeutic and toxic levels is very narrow. After P.O. administration, all antidepressants are distributed through the body, metabolized in the liver, and excreted in urine; TCAs are also eliminated in feces.

Purpose
□ To check for antidepressant toxicity
□ To monitor therapeutic levels of antidepressants
□ To detect the presence of antidepressants for medicolegal purposes.

Patient preparation
Explain to the patient and to his family, if appropriate, that this test checks the level of antidepressants in the blood. Tell him the test requires a blood sample; who will perform the venipuncture and when; and that he may experience transient discomfort from the needle puncture and the pressure of the tourniquet. Reassure him that collecting the sample

---

SYMPTOMS OF ANTIDEPRESSANT TOXICITY

TCAs
Central nervous system: tremors, confusion, dizziness, headaches, ataxia, slurred speech, coma, convulsions
Cardiovascular system: hypotension, arrhythmias, EKG changes
Eyes, ears, nose, and throat: dry mouth, blurred vision, increased intraocular pressure, mydriasis
Genitourinary system: urinary retention
Other: diaphoresis, hyperpyrexia to hypothermia, paralytic ileus

MAO Inhibitors
Central nervous system: severe headaches, ataxia, weakness, fatigue, vertigo, confusion, insomnia, memory impairment, tremors
Cardiovascular system: rapid heartbeat, hypertensive crisis, orthostatic hypotension
Eyes, ears, nose, and throat: photosensitization, blurred vision
Gastrointestinal system: dry mouth, nausea and vomiting related to liver damage, diarrhea, incontinence, constipation
Genitourinary system: urinary retention, incontinence

Lithium salts
Central nervous system: tremors, seizures, fasciculations, ataxia, vertigo, headaches, stiff neck, restlessness, confusion, apathy, impaired consciousness progressing to stupor and coma
Cardiovascular system: arrhythmias, hypotension, pulse deficit, weak pulse
Eyes, ears, nose, and throat: transient vertical nystagmus, blurred vision, widely opened eyes, tinnitus
Respiratory system: irregular respirations
Gastrointestinal system: dry mouth, anorexia, nausea, vomiting
Genitourinary system: oliguria, glycosuria
Other: depressed thyroid function tests, hyperglycemia

---

takes less than 3 minutes. In an emergency, test results are usually available the same day; normally, however, the laboratory requires 1 day to complete the analysis.

If the test is being performed for medicolegal purposes, make sure the patient or responsible member of the family has signed a consent form. Check and record the patient's recent drug history, including dosage schedule and route of administration.

TRICYCLIC ANTIDEPRESSANT AND LITHIUM BLOOD LEVELS

DRUG	THERAPEUTIC	TOXIC
TCAs Amitriptyline (and metabolite, nortriptyline)	75 to 200 ng/ml	> 1000 ng/ml
Desipramine	20 to 160 ng/ml	> 1000 ng/ml
Doxepin (and metabolite, desmethyldoxepin)	90 to 250 ng/ml	> 1000 ng/ml
Imipramine (and metabolite, desipramine)	200 ng/ml	> 1000 ng/ml
Nortriptyline	75 to 150 ng/ml	> 300 ng/ml
Lithium	0.9 to 1.4 mEq	1.5 mEq

Procedure

Perform a venipuncture, and collect the sample in a 7 ml *red-top* tube. For a monitoring test, draw the sample 2 hours before the next drug dose; for lithium monitoring, 12 hours after the last dose.

Precautions

□ Send the sample to the laboratory immediately, or refrigerate it.
□ For a medicolegal test, observe proper precautions.

Values

Therapeutic and toxic antidepressant levels vary widely (see chart above). Currently, no data are available on lethal levels of protriptyline, isocarboxazid, phenelzine, and tranylcypromine.

Implications of results

Antidepressant blood levels allow regulation of therapeutic dosage and guide treatment of toxicity.

Post-test care

If a hematoma develops at the venipuncture site, apply warm soaks.

Interfering factors

□ Barbiturates lower blood TCA levels; methylphenidate raises them.
□ Diuretics increase blood lithium levels; aminophylline, sodium bicarbonate, and sodium chloride decrease lithium levels.

HARVEY SPECTOR, MD

Tranquilizers and Hypnotics

Depending on the drug being measured, this test determines the serum, plasma, or whole blood level of a tranquilizer or hypnotic by colorimetry, photometry, or spectrophotometry. These CNS depressants (including benzodiazepines, chloral derivatives, glutarimides, and quinazolones) are used to treat anxiety, alcohol withdrawal symptoms, and sleep disorders, and to prepare patients for anesthesia.

Tranquilizers and hypnotics, alone or in combination with other drugs or alcohol, are commonly used in suicide attempts. After prolonged or high-dose usage, they produce physical dependence; and as drugs of abuse, they may also cause psychologic dependence. Generally absorbed rapidly after P.O. administration, tranquilizers and hypnotics are metabolized in the liver and excreted in urine and feces.

Purpose

□ To check for toxicity suspected from history or after onset of symptoms of CNS depression, such as confusion, depression, diminished reflexes, hypotension, somnolence, or coma.

Patient preparation

Explain to the patient and to his family, if appropriate, that this test determines the level of tranquilizers or hypnotics in the blood. Tell him the test requires a blood sample; who will perform the venipuncture and when; and that he may experience transient discomfort from the needle puncture and the pressure of the tourniquet. Reassure him that collecting the sample takes less than 3 minutes. Test results are available in 1 day.

If the test is being performed for medicolegal purposes, make sure the patient or responsible member of the family has signed a consent form. Check the patient's recent drug history for names and dosage schedules of all drugs ingested.

Procedure

Perform a venipuncture, and collect the sample in a 7 ml *red-top* tube.

Precautions

□ Send the sample to the laboratory immediately, or refrigerate it.
□ For a medicolegal test, observe proper precautions.

Values

Toxic levels of tranquilizers and hypnotics depend on the specific drug.

Implications of results

Identification of a tranquilizer or hypnotic drug and its serum concentration confirms toxicity and guides its treatment.

Post-test care

If a hematoma develops at the venipuncture site, apply warm soaks.

Interfering factors

Ethanol elevates diazepam levels.

HARVEY SPECTOR, MD

Serum Phenothiazines

This screening test uses gas-liquid chromatography or fluorometry to measure serum phenothiazine levels in patients exhibiting symptoms of toxicity after treatment with phenothiazines. This group of drugs (including chlorpromazine, prochlorperazine, thioridazine, and trifluoperazine) is widely used to manage acute and chronic psychoses; to control nausea and vomiting; to augment the effects of anesthetics, analgesics, and sedatives; and to relieve acute symptoms during withdrawal from addicting drugs, including alcohol. Well absorbed from the gastrointestinal tract, these drugs are rapidly distributed to all body tissues. After conversion by the liver, the metabolites are excreted in urine, bile, and feces. Although phenothiazines can induce tolerance and some degree of physical dependence can develop, they are probably not addictive, since they don't produce the euphoric effects associated with drugs causing psychological dependence.

Purpose

□ To check for phenothiazine toxicity suspected from history or after onset of clinical symptoms
□ To monitor patient compliance with therapy
□ To determine the presence of phenothiazines for medicolegal purposes.

Patient preparation

Explain to the patient and to his family, if appropriate, that this test determines the phenothiazine level in the body. Tell him the test requires a blood sample; who will perform the venipuncture and when; and that he may experience transient discomfort from the needle puncture and the pressure of the tourniquet. Reassure him that collecting the sample takes less than 3 minutes. Test results are usually available in 1 day.

If the test is being performed for medicolegal purposes, make sure the patient or responsible member of the family has signed a consent form. Check and record the patient's drug history.

Procedure

Perform a venipuncture, and collect the sample in a 7 ml *red-top* tube.

Precautions

□ Send the sample to the laboratory immediately, or refrigerate it.
□ In serial testing, maintain a constant time span between drug administration and sample collection.
□ For a medicolegal test, observe proper precautions.

Values

Therapeutic levels of prochlorperazine, chlorpromazine, and trifluoperazine are less than 0.5 mcg/ml; toxic levels exceed 1.0 mcg/ml. Therapeutic levels of thioridazine are less than 1.25 mcg/ml; toxic levels exceed 10 mcg/ml.

Implications of results

Serial serum levels of phenothiazines

SYMPTOMS OF PHENOTHIAZINE TOXICITY

• **Central nervous system:** confusion, excitement, restlessness in early or mild intoxication; areflexia; difficulty in breathing and swallowing, accompanied by fever, pallor, and profuse sweating; akathisia; parkinsonism (abnormal posture, akinesia, excessive salivation, masklike facies, pill-rolling movements, rigidity, shuffling gait, tremors); dystonia in children, dyskinesia of the face and neck muscles in adults (drooping of head, mandibular tics, opisthotonos, protrusion of tongue, stiff neck, torsion spasms); acute psychotic reactions, convulsive seizures, coma with areflexia

• **Cardiovascular system:** hypotension, tachycardia, cardiac arrhythmias, EKG changes, vasomotor collapse

• **Other:** dry mouth, miosis, hypothermia, cyanosis and respiratory collapse, sometimes with sudden apnea

---

guide adjustment of therapeutic dosage. Identification of toxic levels guides treatment of toxicity.

Post-test care

If a hematoma develops at the venipuncture site, apply warm soaks.

Interfering factors

Antacids, anticholinergics, and barbiturates decrease serum phenothiazine levels.

HARVEY SPECTOR, MD

Urine Hallucinogens

This qualitative medicolegal screening test detects hallucinogens in a random urine specimen. The analytic laboratory method used depends on the particular hallucinogen and may include chromatography, thin-layer chromatography, or enzyme-multiplied immunoassay technique (EMIT). At present, no routine method is available to measure hallucinogen levels in blood or urine.

The hallucinogens—lysergic acid diethylamide (LSD), phenyclidine (PCP), mescaline, dipropyltryptamine (DPT), diethyltryptamine (DET), dimethyltryptamine (DMT), and marijuana (Cannabis sativa)—are a group of natural and synthetic drugs that distort perception, cause illusions, and may produce euphoria or panic, or induce psychotic behavior. They can also induce elevated blood pressure and pulse rate, reflex hyperactivity, and mydriasis. Their metabolic effects vary. For example, LSD, which has a half-life of 3 hours, is metabolized by the liver and excreted in feces. Marijuana, which is rapidly metabolized, may produce lingering symptoms, since some of its own metabolites are active hallucinogens.

Purpose

□ To detect presence of hallucinogens in the body for medicolegal purposes.

STREET NAMES OF ABUSED DRUGS

OFFICIAL NAMES	STREET NAMES
Amphetamines amphetamine (Benzedrine) methamphetamine (Desoxyn, Methedrine) dextroamphetamine (Dexedrine)	Beans, bennies, black beauties, black mollies, copilots, crank, crossroads, crystal, dexies, double cross, hearts, love drug, meth, minibennies, peaches, pep pills, speed, rosas, roses, thrusters, truck drivers, uppers, wake-ups, whites
Barbiturates amobarbital (Amytal) pentobarbital (Nembutal) phenobarbital (Luminal) secobarbital (Seconal)	Barbs, blockbusters, bluebirds, blue devils, blues, Christmas trees, downers, green dragons, Mexican reds, pink ladies, pinks, rainbows, red and blues, redbirds, red devils, reds, sleeping pills, yellow jackets, yellow
Camphorated tincture of opium (Paregoric)	"Blue velvet" when mixed with pyribenzamine and taken I.V.
Cannabis (marijuana)	Acapulco gold, Colombian, grass, hash, herb, J, jay, joint, Mary Jane, Panama red, pot, reefer, smoke, tea, weed
Cocaine	Blow, C, coca, coke, flake, girl, heaven, dust, lady, mujer, nose candy, paradise, perico, rock, snow, stardust, upper, white
Diacetylmorphine (heroin)	Big H, boy, brown, brown sugar, crap, estuffa, H, heroina, hombre, horse, junk, Mexican mud, scag, smack, stuff, thing
Dimethyltryptamine (DMT)	Businessman's special
Lysergic acid diethylamide (LSD)	Acid, big D, blotter acid, brown dot, California sunshine, cubes, haze, microdots, paper acid, purple haze, sugar, sunshine, trips
Meperidine (Demerol)	Dollies
Methadone (Dolophine)	Dollies
Methaqualone (Quaalude)	Ludes, quads, quas, soapers, sopes, sopor
Methylphenidate (Ritalin)	California sunshine
Morphine	Cube, first line, goma, morf, morfina, morpho
Pentazocine (Talwin)	Dollies
Phenycyclidine (PCP, Sernylan)	Angel dust, crystal, crystal joint, cyclone, elephant, hog, KJs, peace pill, rocket fuel
3, 4, 5-trimethoxyphenethylamine (Mescaline, Peyote)	Big chief, buttons, cactus, mesc, mescal, mescal buttons
3-(2-dimethylaminoethyl) indol-4-yl dihydrogen phosphate (Psilocybin)	Silly putty, the mushrooms, magic Mexican mushrooms
2, 5-dimethoxy-4, α-dimethylphenthylamine (STP, DOM)	Serenity-tranquility-peace pill

Patient preparation

Explain to the patient or his family, if appropriate, that this test detects hallucinogen parenteral administration, ingestion, or inhalation. Tell him the test requires a urine specimen, and explain the proper collection technique.

Make sure that the patient or responsible member of the family has signed a consent form. Check the patient's recent drug history, noting time and route of administration.

Procedure

Collect a random urine specimen.

Precautions

□ Send the specimen to the laboratory immediately, or refrigerate it.
□ For a medicolegal test, observe proper precautions.

Values

Normally, no hallucinogens are found in urine.

Implications of results

Since hallucinogens aren't used therapeutically, their presence in any amount confirms drug abuse.

Post-test care

Restrain the patient, if necessary, to protect him from self-imposed or sensory injury.

Interfering factors

Unknown interfering substances in some normal urine give false-positive LSD value.

HARVEY SPECTOR, MD

Blood Ethanol

This quantitative test uses gas chromatography or microdiffusion to measure the blood ethanol level. This assay determines the degree of ethanol intoxication, for use in medicolegal procedures, or rules out intoxication in a person who is comatose. Although the degree of intoxication can be measured using a breath or urine specimen, medicolegal tests in the United States require a blood sample, since the findings are more specific.

About 80% of ingested ethanol is absorbed in the jejunum, and 20% is absorbed in the stomach. When the stomach is empty, about 50% of ethanol is absorbed within 15 minutes, and peak levels are reached in 40 to 70 minutes (food in the stomach slows absorption). About 90% of ethanol reaches the liver, where alcohol dehydrogenase converts it to acetaldehyde, which then metabolizes to water and carbon dioxide. The remaining 10% is excreted unchanged in breath, sweat, and urine.

Purpose

□ To rule out alcohol intoxication in a person who is comatose
□ To evaluate the degree of ethanol intoxication, for medicolegal purposes.

Patient preparation

Explain to the patient and to his family, if appropriate, that this test determines the amount of ethanol in the blood. Tell him the test requires a blood sample; who will perform the venipuncture and when; and that he may experience transient discomfort from the needle puncture and the pressure of the tourniquet. Reassure him that collecting the sample takes less than 3 minutes. Test results are usually available the same day.

If the test is being performed for medicolegal purposes, make sure the patient or a responsible member of the family has signed a consent form. Check the patient's recent drug history for time and amount of ethanol ingestion as well as for the dosage schedule of other drugs being used.

Procedure

After cleansing the venipuncture site with benzalkonium chloride (aqueous 1:75 dilution) or povidone-iodine solution, perform a venipuncture, and collect the sample in a 7 ml *red-top* tube.

CLINICAL EFFECTS OF ALCOHOL (ETHANOL)

Alcohol's clinical effects vary widely, depending on such factors as the patient's body weight, nutritional status, and rate of ingestion. Also, the type of alcohol affects the clinical state, since the oil and sugar content raise the ethanol level. The following chart, using whiskey as an example, estimates alcohol's effects on a 160-pound person drinking at a rate of 3 ounces per hour.

QUANTITY OF WHISKEY CONSUMED	BLOOD ALCOHOL LEVEL % wt/vol	mg/dl	CLINICAL EFFECT
3 oz (90 ml)	0.05	50	Sedation and tranquility
6 oz (180 ml)	0.10	100	Lack of coordination, slurred speech, slow mental response
12 oz (360 ml)	0.20	200	Obvious intoxication, disturbed equilibrium, poor color perception
15 oz (450 ml)	0.30	300	Unconsciousness, tremors, sweating, and vomiting
24 oz (720 ml)	0.40	400	Deep coma, which may be irreversible
30 oz (900 ml)	0.50	500	Death

KEY:

= 1 oz (30 ml) of whiskey   = 30 oz (900 ml of whiskey)

Precautions

□ Don't cleanse the venipuncture site with alcohol or tincture of iodine, since these interfere with test results.

ETHANOL INTOXICATION

How does the law define ethanol intoxication? Laws pertaining to intoxication vary from state to state, but all are based on the following guidelines issued by the National Safety Council's Committee on Alcohol and Drugs:

• When the blood alcohol (ethanol) level is below 0.05% wt/vol (50 mg/dl), a person is considered *not* intoxicated.

• If the blood alcohol level is between 0.05% and 0.1% wt/vol (50 to 100 mg/dl), a person is, by law, considered intoxicated; however, the court is advised to consider other evidence, such as behavior and circumstances leading to arrest.

• A blood alcohol level of 0.1% wt/vol (100 mg/dl) or more conclusively confirms ethanol intoxication.

☐ Send the sample to the laboratory immediately, or refrigerate it.

☐ For a medicolegal test, observe proper precautions.

Values

For intoxicating and lethal alcohol levels, see chart on page 1025.

Implications of results

The overall effect of ethanol is CNS depression. Chart values apply primarily to acute toxicity, and treatment is based on confirmation of toxicity. Acute toxicity can also result from inhaling ethanol fumes in a distillery.

Chronic alcoholics tolerate much higher (even lethal) levels, metabolizing ethanol to acetaldehyde in half the normal time. The resultant high acetaldehyde levels may cause liver damage.

Ethanol levels have medicolegal implications.

Post-test care

If a hematoma develops at the venipuncture site, apply warm soaks.

Interfering factors

☐ Blood ethanol levels are elevated by chloral hydrate and glutethimide, and false elevations of the specimen's ethanol

level can occur with contamination by alcohol or tincture of iodine at the venipuncture site.

☐ Both ethanol and barbiturates are metabolized in the microsomal enzyme system, and when taken together high levels occur, with greatly increased CNS depression.

HARVEY SPECTOR, MD

Serum Isopropanol and Methanol

This toxicity determination, through gas chromatography, quantitatively measures serum isopropanol or methanol levels in patients suspected of ingesting these alcohols. Toxic symptoms produced by ingestion of isopropanol include gastritis, confusion, CNS depression, respiratory arrest, and coma; symptoms of methanol toxicity include nausea, vomiting, diarrhea, stupor, convulsions, respiratory arrest, blindness, metabolic acidosis, and coma, and may occur 8 to 36 hours after methanol ingestion. Ingestion of isopropanol or methanol can be fatal.

After ethanol, isopropanol and methanol are the most common volatile liquids. Isopropanol—used as a disinfectant, a liniment, and an industrial solvent—is more toxic than ethanol. Methanol—used in antifreeze, as an industrial solvent, and as an additive in bootleg liquor (moonshine)—is less inebriating but more toxic than ethanol, since it's partially oxidized to formaldehyde in the body.

Purpose

☐ To confirm the cause and extent of intoxication suspected from the history or after onset of symptoms.

Patient preparation

Explain to the patient and to his family, if appropriate, that this test determines whether the blood contains a toxic level of isopropanol or methanol. Tell him the test requires a blood sample; who will perform the venipuncture and when; and that he may experience transient discomfort from the needle puncture and the pressure of the tourniquet. Reassure him that collecting the sample takes less than 3 minutes. Test results are usually available in 1 hour.

If the test is being performed for medicolegal purposes, make sure the patient or a responsible member of his family has signed a consent form. Check the patient's recent drug history, including the amount and time of isopropanol or methanol ingestion and the names and dosage schedules of any other drugs the patient's used.

Procedure
Cleanse the venipuncture site with benzalkonium chloride (aqueous 1:75 dilution) or povidone-iodine solution. Perform a venipuncture, and collect the sample in a 7 ml *red-top* tube.

Precautions
□ Don't cleanse the venipuncture site with alcohol or tincture of iodine. This contaminates the specimen and interferes with test results.
□ Send the sample to the laboratory immediately or refrigerate it.
□ For a medicolegal test, observe proper precautions.

Values
The toxic serum level of isopropanol is 30 mg/dl; the lethal level, 150 mg/dl. The toxic serum level of methanol is 20 mg/dl; the lethal level, 80 mg/dl.

Implications of results
Confirmation of toxic serum levels of isopropanol or methanol guides treatment.

Isopropanol is twice as toxic as ethanol. Methanol toxicity is likely to cause blindness in the presence of metabolic acidosis.

Post-test care
If a hematoma develops at the veni-

puncture site, apply warm soaks.

Interfering factors
Alcohol and tincture of iodine at the venipuncture site falsely elevate levels.

HARVEY SPECTOR, MD

Hemoglobin Derivatives

This quantitative test measures the percentage of total hemoglobin containing abnormal derivatives—primarily, carboxyhemoglobin, sulfhemoglobin, and methemoglobin—after onset of signs of toxicity, such as cyanosis and anoxia. By changing the pH or adding a reducing substance, and then analyzing the blood with a spectrophotometer, the specific form of hemoglobin present can be determined, and thus the diagnosis can be confirmed.

When combined with certain chemicals or drugs, hemoglobins are converted into compounds that are incapable of transporting oxygen. One such compound is carboxyhemoglobin, which results from the union of hemoglobin and carbon monoxide. (This compound's affinity for hemoglobin is 210 times greater than that of oxygen.) The major effect of carbon monoxide toxicity is tissue hypoxia, because carboxyhemoglobin cannot carry oxygen and also because it prevents the release of oxygen from as yet unaffected hemoglobin. Treatment with 100% oxygen or with 95% oxygen and 5% carbon dioxide can help to reverse carbon monoxide toxicity. The principal sources of carbon monoxide include tobacco smoke and exhaust from incomplete combustion of petroleum and natural gas fuels, such as that from gasoline and diesel motors, unvented natural gas heaters, and defective gas stoves.

Another compound, sulfhemoglobin, results from combining hemoglobin with certain drugs, such as phenacetin or sulfonamides. Methemoglobin results from the oxidation of ferrous iron to the ferric form. Such oxidation usually results from chemicals and drugs—such as nitrates, nitrites, sulfonamides, aniline, chlorates, or phenacetin—or from primary methemoglobinemia. Sulfhemoglobin can't be removed by therapy, and disappears only with the destruction of the affected RBCs.

Purpose
□ To rule out abnormal hemoglobin derivatives as a cause of cyanosis or anoxia
□ To monitor persons in danger of overexposure to a substance causing cyanosis or anoxia, such as carbon monoxide.

Patient preparation
Explain to the patient and to his family, if appropriate, that this test helps determine if the hemoglobin in the blood has normal capacity to combine with oxygen. Tell him the test requires a blood sample; who will perform the venipuncture and when; and that he may experience transient discomfort from the needle puncture and the pressure of the tourniquet. Reassure him that collecting the sample takes less than 3 minutes. Test results are available in 1 day.

If the test is being performed for medicolegal purposes, make sure the patient or responsible member of the family has signed a consent form. Check the patient's history for recent exposure to drugs and other potentially toxic substances.

Procedure
Perform a venipuncture, and collect the sample in a 4.5 ml *blue-top* tube for carboxyhemoglobin, or in a 7 ml *green-top* (heparinized) tube for sulfhemoglobin or methemoglobin.

Precautions
□ Seal the container to prevent air contamination, and send the sample to the laboratory immediately, or refrigerate it.
□ For a medicolegal test, observe proper precautions.

Values
Normally, carboxyhemoglobin concentration is 3% of the total hemoglobin (up to 15% in tobacco smokers); methemoglobin concentration, less than 3%; and sulfhemoglobin concentration, undetectable.

In acute carbon monoxide poisoning, symptoms occur when carboxyhemoglobin levels reach 20%; severe poisoning exists at 30%; fatal poisoning, at 60% to 80%. Methemoglobin values of 10% to 25% produce cyanosis (but are tolerated); values of 35% to 40% produce exertional dyspnea and headache; values over 60% produce lethargy and stupor; values over 70%, death. Sulfhemoglobin values of 10 g/dl produce cyanosis but cause few or no toxic symptoms.

Implications of results
Levels depend on duration of exposure as well as concentration. Treatment of toxicity and exposure limitations depend on identification of various hemoglobins and levels noted.

Lower carboxyhemoglobin concentrations can produce serious symptoms in chronic carbon monoxide poisoning or in children.

A serum level of 50% carboxyhemoglobin may be fatal.

Post-test care
If a hematoma develops at the venipuncture site, apply warm soaks.

Interfering factors
Air contamination of the specimen may affect the accuracy of test results.

HARVEY SPECTOR, MD

Industrial Toxicology

These specific, quantitative tests detect acute poisoning or monitor chronic poisoning from topical absorption (or absorption through the skin), ingestion, or inhalation of industrial toxins, includ-

GUIDE TO TOXIC INDUSTRIAL SUBSTANCES

SUBSTANCE AND SPECIMEN	VALUES	INDUSTRIAL USES	SYMPTOMS
Antimony 100 ml urine	*Reference: < 50 mcg/liter Toxic: > 1 mg/liter	• Bronze finishing, alloy casting • Manufacturing of ceramics, plastic, pigment, paint, and rubber • Ore mining, smelting, and refining	*Acute:* abdominal pain; cardiovascular collapse; choking; coma; cyanosis; dysphagia; hypothermia; metallic taste; nausea; severe diarrhea; slow, shallow respirations; spasms; and vomiting *Chronic:* anemia, bleeding gums, conjunctivitis, dermatitis, and weight loss
Arsenic 50 ml urine	Reference: < 100 mcg/liter Toxic: > 850 mcg/liter	• Manufacturing of ceramics, dye, paint, and pigment • Horticultural and agricultural spraying	*Acute:* cardiovascular collapse, convulsions, garlic breath, metallic taste, profuse diarrhea, rapid onset of gastroenteritis, severe abdominal pains, thirst, and tremors *Chronic:* arsenic melanosis of neck, eyelids, or nipple; bleeding gums and nose; dermatitis; hair loss; hyperkeratosis of palms and soles; motor paralysis; nausea; peripheral neuritis, weakness; weight loss
20 ml blood	Reference: < 3 mcg/100 ml Reference: < 65 mcg/100 g		
0.5 g hair or nails (Proper selection of specimen can date exposure by relating to time of formation of hair or nails)			
0.5 g nails	Reference: 90 to 180 mcg/100 g		
Boron 5 ml urine	Reference: < 0.3 mg/100 ml	• Manufacturing of glass, enamel, soap, cement, pottery, antiseptics, water softeners, fireproofing, and preservatives	Acidosis, acute gastroenteritis, blue-green diarrhea, chills, coma, convulsions, dermatitis, headaches, nausea, restlessness, tremors, vomiting, and weak pulse

Adapted with permission from the *Bio-Science Handbook of Clinical and Industrial Toxicology* (Van Nuys, Calif.: Bio-Science Laboratories, 1979)

*Reference values are subject to revision based on current research. For update, contact: Dept. of Industrial Toxicology, Bio-Science Labs., Van Nuys, Calif.

GUIDE TO TOXIC INDUSTRIAL SUBSTANCES *(continued)*

SUBSTANCE AND SPECIMEN	VALUES	INDUSTRIAL USES	SYMPTOMS
Boron *(continued)* 4 ml serum	*Reference: < 1 mg/dl Toxic: 10 to 20 mg/dl	• Manufacturing of glass, enamel, soap, cement, pottery, antiseptics, water softeners, fireproofing, and preservatives	Acidosis, acute gastroenteritis, blue-green diarrhea, chills, coma, convulsions, dermatitis, headaches, nausea, restlessness, tremors, vomiting, and weak pulse
Cadmium 100 ml urine	Reference: 10 to 580 mcg/liter (after exposure); < 20 mcg/liter (without exposure)	• Manufacturing of alloys, batteries, and dental amalgams • Engraving, painting, welding • Textile printing • Pesticide spraying	*Ingestion:* Anemia, anorexia, back and leg pain, dizziness, gastroenteritis, liver and kidney damage, metallic taste, osteoporosis, salivation, and vomiting *Inhalation:* Cardiovascular collapse, dyspnea, pulmonary edema, and shock
1 ml blood (with heparin or oxalate)	Reference: < 41 ng/ml Toxic: > 41 ng/ml		
Cyanide 5 ml blood	Reference: < 15 mcg/100 ml Toxic: > 0.5 mg/ 100 ml	• Metallurgy • Manufacturing of metal polish • Pesticide spraying	Bitter almond odor, coma, convulsions, cyanosis, dizziness, headache, nausea, respiratory distress or failure, tachycardia
Fluoride 10 ml urine	Reference: 5 mg/liter Toxic: > 10 mg/liter	• Manufacturing of aluminum, insecticides, incandescent lamps, phosphate, and fertilizer • Cleaning metal, etching glass, processing yeast, welding, smelting	*Acute:* Abdominal pain; convulsions; low blood magnesium, potassium, and calcium; nausea; salivation; shallow respiration; tetany; tremors; and vomiting *Chronic:* Anemia; discolored, friable teeth; weakness; weight loss
5 ml serum or blood (in plastic container)	Reference: .05 mg/dl Toxic: 0.2-0.3 mg/ dl		
Lead 24-hour urine (acidified and in lead-free container)	Reference: < 80 mcg/liter Toxic: > 120 mcg/liter	• Manufacturing of ceramics, insecticides, and lubricants • Painting • Plumbing • Soldering	*Acute:* Anemia, basophilic stippling, "blue line" gum margin, colic, coma, constipation, convulsions, delirium, headache, metallic taste, lethargy *Chronic:* Abdominal pain, anemia, anorexia, basophilic stippling, "blue line" gum margin, headache, irritability, metallic taste, weight loss

*Reference values are subject to revision based on current research. For update, contact: Dept. of Industrial Toxicology, Bio-Science Labs., Van Nuys, Calif.

SUBSTANCE AND SPECIMEN	VALUES	INDUSTRIAL USES	SYMPTOMS
Lead *(continued)* 2 ml blood (with 1.5 mg/ ml heparin, ox- alate, or EDTA)	*Reference: < 30 mcg/dl; (chil- dren); < 40 mcg/dl (unexposed adults); < 40 mcg/dl (in- dustrial exposure) Toxic: > 40 mcg/dl (children and unex- posed adults); > 60 mcg/dl (industrial exposure)		
Manganese 15 ml clotted blood	Reference: 0.08 to 0.26 mcg/dl	• Manufacturing of drugs, pottery, glass, varnish, feed additives, and ceramics • Welding	Cirrhosis, cramps, elevated hemoglobin, headache, muscle twitches, nausea, parkinsonian syndrome, and sleepiness
Mercury 24-hour urine (acidified to pH 2.0 with ni- tric acid)	Reference: < 150 mcg/liter Toxic: > 150 mcg/ liter	• Manufacturing of scientific instru- ments, electric lamps, amalgams, disinfectants, ger- micides, herbi- cides, agricultural poisons, dyes, batteries, caustic soda, and paper	*Acute:* Ataxia, burning sensation in mouth and throat, circulatory collapse, fluid and electrolyte imbalance, nausea, rapid weak pulse, salivation, severe abdominal pain, shock, slow respiration, vomiting *Chronic:* Albuminuria; behavioral changes; black, loose teeth, black- blue gums; bloody stool; bronchitis; circulatory shock; corneal opacity; edema; foul breath; gingivitis; headache; hematuria; insomnia; metallic taste; pneumonitis; shock; whitish necrosis of oral or pharyngeal mucosa
5g of frozen tissue	Reference: 20 mcg/liter (non- exposed adult), 150 mcg/liter (exposed adult) Toxic: > 150 mcg/ liter		
Nickel 24-hour urine	Reference: < 25 mcg/liter Toxic: > 350 mcg/ liter	• Manufacturing of ceramics, stainless steel instruments, enamel, batteries, and glass • Electroplating	Chest pains, confusion, convulsions, coughing, cyanosis, dermatitis, fever, fruity breath, headache, itching, malignancy of lungs or nasal passage, nausea, pulmonary edema, and respiratory failure

*Reference values are subject to revision based on current research. For update, contact: Dept. of Industrial Toxicology, Bio-Science Labs., Van Nuys, Calif.

GUIDE TO TOXIC INDUSTRIAL SUBSTANCES *(continued)*

SUBSTANCE AND SPECIMEN	VALUES	INDUSTRIAL USES	SYMPTOMS
Organic Phosphate Carbamates measured by response of cholinesterase and pseudocholinesterase:			
Cholinesterase 2 ml blood (with heparin)	*Reference: 0.6 to 1 cholinesterase units	Organophosphorus insecticide spraying	Coma, confusion, convulsions, decreased cholinesterase level, headache, nausea, pulmonary edema, respiratory paralysis, visual disturbances, and vomiting
Pseudo-cholinesterase 2 ml serum or plasma (with heparin)	Reference: 3 to 8 pseudocholin-esterase units/ml Toxic: progres-sively decreasing cholinesterase ac-tivity in serum or plasma as the in-secticide is inacti-vated by the enzyme		
Phenol (benzene metabolite) 15 ml urine (collected at end of working day)	Reference: 2 to 12 mg/liter Toxic: > 75 mg/ liter	● Manufacturing of explosives, fertilizer, coke, paint, textiles, drugs, disinfectants, preservatives, and antiseptics	Abdominal pain, acidosis, alkalosis, anemia, blanching and necrosis of skin, burning sensation, coma, convulsions, cyanosis, dizziness, headache, hypotension, leukopenia nausea, pulmonary edema, respiratory failure, vomiting, and weakness
Selenium 24-hour urine	Reference: < 100 mcg/liter (with exposure); < 50 mcg/liter (without exposure) Toxic: > 400 mcg/ liter	● Manufacturing of glass, pesticides, rubber, semiconductors, and copper ● Developing film	Bronchial pneumonia, bronchospasm, circulatory collapse, conjunctivitis, garlic odor on breath and in urine, headache, metallic taste, nose and throat irritation, pulmonary edema, vomiting, and weakness
Silica 10 g lung tissue	Reference: < 0.2% of dry weight lung tissue	Clay, cement, and mining industries	Coughing, cyanosis, dyspnea, emphysema, respiratory infection, and weight loss
Thallium 24-hour urine	Reference: < 14 mcg/liter Toxic: > 50 mcg/ liter	● Manufacturing diamonds, chlorinated chemicals, dyes, optical glass, and photoelectric cells	Convulsions; coma; delirium; hair loss; insomnia; muscular pain; nose and throat irritation; severe gastroen-teritis, with diarrhea or constipation; abdominal pain; nausea; anorexia; and vomiting

*Reference values are subject to revision based on current research. For update, contact: Dept. of Industrial Toxicology, Bio-Science Labs., Van Nuys, Calif.

ing antimony, arsenic, boron, cadmium, organic phosphate carbonates, cyanide, fluoride, lead, manganese, mercury, nickel, phenol, selenium, silica, and thallium. Generally, concentrations are measured in a blood sample or urine specimen; less frequently, in hair, nail, or tissue specimens. However, hair or nail specimens, if appropriate, can date exposure by determining the time the ends of the hair or nails were formed.

Periodic monitoring tests (usually every 6 months) determine toxic concentrations in persons exposed to these toxins. After acute exposure, elevated levels are usually transient; after chronic exposure, elevated levels persist for a longer period of time.

Purpose
□ To monitor industrial workers for chronic toxicity
□ To detect acute toxicity following an industrial accident.

Patient preparation
Explain to the patient that this test detects harmful exposure to an industrial substance. For a blood test, tell the patient who will perform the venipuncture and when, and that he may experience transient discomfort from the needle puncture and the pressure of the tourniquet. Reassure him that collecting the sample takes less than 3 minutes. For a urine test, explain how to collect the appropriate specimen. Check the patient's history for recent exposure and use of drugs, including dosage schedule and administration route.

Procedure
Collect a random or 24-hour urine specimen, or perform a venipuncture and collect an appropriate sample (see chart, pages 1029 to 1032).

Precautions
□ Send the urine or blood specimen to the laboratory immediately, or refrigerate it.
□ For a 24-hour urine specimen, tell the patient not to contaminate the specimen with toilet tissue or stool. Refrigerate the specimen, or place it on ice during the collection period (with a preservative, if required).
□ If a blood sample requires an anticoagulant, completely fill the collection tube, and invert it gently at least 10 times to mix the sample and the anticoagulant. Handle the sample gently to prevent hemolysis.

Values
Reference values, toxic levels, and symptoms of toxicity depend on the specific toxin (see chart, pages 1029 to 1032).

Implications of results
Toxic levels dictate specific treatment or mandate exposure restrictions. Industrial toxins can be hazardous even after indirect contact (such as handling worker's contaminated clothing), and pose a serious hazard to fetal development.

Post-test care
If a hematoma develops at the venipuncture site, ease discomfort by applying warm soaks.

Interfering factors
□ Hemolysis due to rough handling of blood sample falsely elevates iron levels.
□ Failure to collect all urine during the test period invalidates results.

HARVEY SPECTOR, MD

Selected References

Butler, T. *Barbiturates*. Chicago: American Society of Clinical Pathologists, 1972.

Butler, T. *Blood Alcohol*. Chicago: American Society of Clinical Pathologists, 1973.

Kaye, Sidney. *Handbook of Emergency Toxicology: A Guide for the Identification, Diagnosis and Treatment of Poisoning*, 4th ed. Springfield, Ill.: Charles C. Thomas, 1980.

Nursing85 Drug Handbook. Springhouse, Pa.: Springhouse Corp., 1985.

31 Miscellaneous Tests

LEARNING OBJECTIVES

After completing this chapter, the reader will be able to:
- discuss the use of skin tests for evaluating cellular immune response.
- state the purpose of each test covered in the chapter.
- prepare the patient physically and psychologically for each test.
- describe the procedure for performing each test.
- specify appropriate precautions for safe administration of each test.
- recognize signs of adverse reaction and respond appropriately.
- implement appropriate post-test care.
- state the normal values or findings for each test.
- discuss the implications of abnormal test results.
- list factors that may interfere with accurate test results.

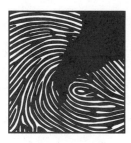

Miscellaneous Tests

Introduction

Some important diagnostic tests resist easy classification. For example, skin tests evaluate the immune response using different procedures from other immunologic tests. Nuclear medicine and contrast radiography tests, found elsewhere in this book, apply specifically to certain organs or body systems; but others, such as gallium scanning and lymphangiography, apply more widely. D-xylose absorption is the only diagnostic test that uses both serum and urine samples to detect the cause of malabsorption syndrome.

Skin tests

Skin tests evaluate cellular immunity by determining patient response to the intradermal injection or topical application of one or more antigens. In tuberculin skin tests, one antigen assesses the immune response to a specific infectious disease; in delayed hypersensitivity skin tests, a panel of antigens assesses general immunocompetency. In each test, in the presence of an intact secondary immune response (effective recall antigens), erythema and induration develop at the injection or application site within 24 hours, peak at 48 hours, and then begin to resolve thereafter.

Anergy—the inability to react to a battery of common antigens—suggests immunodeficiency. The anergic patient may require additional tests using greater concentrations of the same antigen(s), or using a test antigen that the patient hasn't encountered, such as dinitrochlorobenzene.

Radiology and nuclear medicine

Lymphangiography is the most important test for detecting obstruction, disease, and neoplasm in the lymphatic system. This system transports lymph—derived from tissue fluids—throughout the body and eventually empties it into the veins. The lymphatic system can spread inflammation and disease throughout the body.

In gallium scanning, a gamma camera or rectilinear scanner records distribution of radioactivity after I.V. injection of ^{67}gallium-citrate. Since gallium concentrates at sites of abscesses and carcinomas, it can help detect them or determine the extent of metastases and can also help evaluate their treatment.

The red blood cell (RBC) survival time test measures the life span of RBCs tagged with radioactive chromium-51 to help evaluate unexplained anemia. Serial blood tests and gamma camera scans help identify the type and site of RBC destruction.

Malabsorption test

The D-xylose absorption test distinguishes intestinal disease from other

GIVING INTRADERMAL INJECTIONS

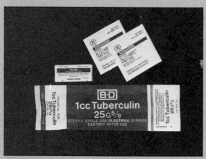

1 *Begin by assembling your equipment. You'll need the medication, a 1 cc tuberculin syringe, a 25G ⅝" needle, and several alcohol swabs. Attach the needle to the syringe. Check the medication to make sure it's not outdated or contaminated. If not, draw it up into the syringe, expelling any air in the needle. Then, cap the syringe and bring all the equipment to the patient's bedside. Explain the procedure to the patient. Position him, sitting or lying down, with his ventral forearm exposed and supported on a flat surface, and his elbow flexed.*

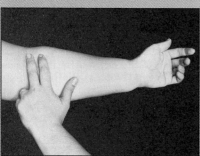

2 *Next, locate the patient's antecubital space. Then, measure several finger-widths away from it in the direction of the hand. Avoid any areas covered with hair or blemishes. These could make reading the test results difficult.*

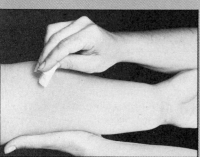

3 *Prepare the skin with an alcohol swab, beginning at the center of the site and moving outward in a circular motion. Never use a disinfectant like Betadine, which discolors the skin, and don't rub so hard that you cause irritation. This action could hinder the reading of the test.*
Allow the skin to dry thoroughly. If you inject the patient while the skin's wet, you may accidentally introduce antiseptic into the dermis.

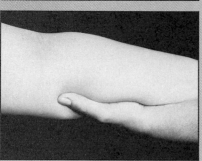

4 *Hold the patient's forearm in one hand, and stretch his skin with your thumb, as shown here.*

5 *Position the syringe so that the needle is almost flat against the patient's skin. Make sure that the bevel of the needle is up.*

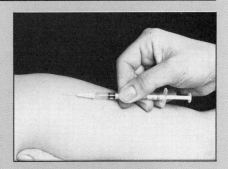

6 *Insert the needle by pressing it against the skin until you meet resistance. Then, advance the needle through the epidermis, so that the point of the needle is visible through the skin. Stop when it's resting ⅛" (3 mm) below the skin's surface, between the epidermis and the dermal layers.*

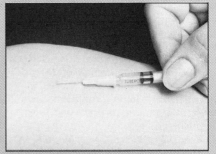

7 *Now, inject the medication as slowly and gently as possible. Expect to feel some resistance, which is your assurance that the needle's properly placed. If the needle moves freely, you've inserted it too deeply. Withdraw it slightly and try again. When you've finished injecting the medication, leave the needle in place momentarily. Watch for a small white blister or wheal to form, about 6 mm in diameter.*

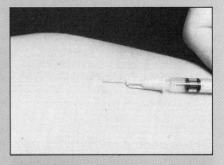

8 *When the wheal appears, withdraw the needle, and apply gentle pressure to the site. Don't massage it, because doing so may interfere with test results.*
   Document the name of the medication and the amount given. If the patient has an allergic reaction to the injection within 30 minutes, notify the doctor. Such reactions generally develop within 48 to 72 hours.

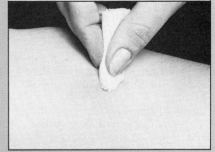

disorders that cause malabsorption. Blood and urine samples are analyzed after ingestion of a standard dose of D-xylose. In malabsorption caused by intestinal disease, D-xylose absorption decreases; in malabsorption caused by pancreatic insufficiency, cystic fibrosis, or liver disease, absorption remains normal.

KAREN DYER VANCE, RN, BSN

SKIN TESTS

Tuberculin Skin Tests

These skin tests are used to screen for previous infection by the tubercle bacillus. They are routinely performed in children, young adults, and persons with radiographic findings that suggest this infection. In both the old tuberculin (OT) and purified protein derivative (PPD) tests, intradermal injection of the tuberculin antigen causes a delayed hypersensitivity reaction in patients with active or dormant tuberculosis; sensitized lymphocytes gather at the injection site, causing erythema, vesiculation, or induration that peaks within 24 to 48 hours and persists for at least 72 hours.

The most accurate tuberculin test method, the Mantoux test, employs a single-needle intradermal injection of PPD, permitting precise measurement of dosage. Multipuncture tests—such as the Tine test, Mono-Vacc tests, and Aplitest—employ intradermal injections using tines impregnated with OT or PPD. Because multipuncture tests require less skill and are more rapidly administered than the Mantoux test, they're generally used for screening. However, a positive multipuncture test usually requires a Mantoux test for confirmation.

Purpose
□ To distinguish tuberculosis from blastomycosis, coccidioidomycosis, and histoplasmosis
□ To identify persons who need diagnostic investigation for tuberculosis.

Patient preparation
Explain to the patient that this test helps detect tuberculosis. Tell him the test requires an intradermal injection, which may cause him transient discomfort.

Check the patient's history for active tuberculosis, the results of previous skin tests, or hypersensitivities. If the patient has had tuberculosis, don't perform a skin test; if he's had a positive reaction to previous skin tests, consult the doctor or follow hospital policy; if he's had an allergic reaction to acacia, don't perform an OT test, since this product contains acacia.

If you're performing a tuberculin test on an outpatient, instruct him to return at the specified time so that test results can be read. Inform the patient that a positive reaction to a skin test appears as a red, hard, raised area at the injection site. Although the area may itch, instruct him not to scratch it. Stress that a positive reaction doesn't always indicate active tuberculosis.

Equipment
Alcohol swabs/vial of PPD (intermediate strength)—5 TU (tuberculin units) per 0.1 ml or vial of OT 1:2,000 dilution—5 TU per 0.1 ml, and 1-ml tuberculin syringe with ½" or ⅝" 25G or 26G needle for the Mantoux test/commercially available device (Tine, Mono-Vacc, or Aplitest) for multipuncture tests/epinephrine (1:1,000) and 3-ml syringe (for emergency use).

Procedure
The patient is placed in a sitting position, with his arm extended and supported on a flat surface. Cleanse the volar surface of the upper forearm with alcohol; allow the area to dry completely.

Mantoux test: Perform an intradermal injection.

Multipuncture tests: Remove the protective cap on the injection device to expose the four tines. Hold the patient's forearm in one hand, stretching the skin of the forearm tightly. Then, with your other hand, firmly depress the device into the patient's skin (without twisting it). Hold the device in place for at least 1 second before removing it. If you've applied sufficient pressure, you'll see four puncture sites and a circular depression made by the device on the patient's skin. Record where the test was given, the date and time, and when it's to be read. Tuberculin skin tests are generally read 48 to 72 hours after injection; however, the Mono-Vacc test can be read 48 to 96 hours after the test.

Precautions

□ Tuberculin skin tests are contraindicated in patients with current reactions to smallpox vaccinations, any rash, skin disorder or active tuberculosis.

□ Don't perform a skin test in areas with excess hair, acne, or insufficient subcutaneous tissue, such as over a tendon or bone. If the patient is known to be hypersensitive to skin tests, use a first-strength dose in the Mantoux test to avoid necrosis at the puncture site.

□ Have epinephrine available to treat a possible anaphylactoid or acute hypersensitivity reaction.

Findings

In tuberculin skin tests, normal findings show negative or minimal reactions.

Mantoux test: no induration, or induration less than 5 mm in diameter

Tine and Aplitest: no vesiculation; no induration or less than 2 mm diameter

Mono-Vacc tests: no induration.

Implications of results

A positive tuberculin reaction indicates previous infection by tubercle bacilli. It does not distinguish between an active and dormant infection, nor does it provide a definitive diagnosis. If a positive reaction occurs, sputum smear and culture, and chest radiography are necessary for further information.

In the Mantoux test, induration of 5 to 9 mm in diameter indicates a borderline reaction; larger induration, a positive reaction. Since patients infected with atypical myobacteria other than tubercle bacilli may have borderline reactions, repeat testing is necessary.

In the Tine or Aplitest, vesiculation indicates a positive reaction; induration of 2 mm in diameter without vesiculation requires confirmation by the Mantoux test. Any induration in the Mono-Vacc test indicates a positive reaction; however, it requires confirmation by the Mantoux test.

Post-test care

If ulceration or necrosis develops at the injection site, apply cold soaks or a topical steroid, as ordered.

Interfering factors

□ Subcutaneous injection, usually indicated by erythema greater than 10 mm in diameter without induration, invalidates the test.

□ Corticosteroids and other immunosuppressants, and live vaccine viruses (measles, mumps, rubella, or polio) given within the past 4 to 6 weeks may

---

READING TUBERCULIN TEST RESULTS

You should read the Mantoux, Tine, and Aplitest skin tests 48 to 72 hours after injection; the Mono-Vacc test, after 48 to 96 hours.

In a well-lighted room, flex the patient's forearm slightly. Observe the injection site for erythema and vesiculation, then gently rub your finger over the site to detect induration. If induration is present, measure the diameter in millimeters, preferably using a plastic ruler marked in concentric circles of specific diameter. In multipuncture tests, you may find separate areas of induration developed around individual punctures, or induration involving more than one puncture site. If so, measure the diameter of the largest single area of induration or coalesced induration.

SCHICK TEST

Although not performed routinely in the United States, the Schick test determines susceptibility or immunity to diphtheria—an acute, highly contagious bacterial infection. In this skin test, 0.1 ml of purified diphtheria toxin dissolved in buffered human serum albumin is injected intradermally into one forearm, and 0.1 ml of purified diphtheria toxoid is injected into the other forearm, as a control. Both sites are examined after 24 and 48 hours, and again 4 to 7 days after injection.

Patients susceptible to diphtheria—those who have slight amounts of or no circulating antitoxin—demonstrate inflammation and induration at the site of toxin injection within 24 hours and a peak reaction within 7 days. This reaction generally has a dark red center and may reach 3 cm in diameter. Conversely, the site of toxoid injection shows no reaction.

In patients immune to diphtheria (antitoxin levels between 1/30 and 1/100 unit), neither site shows a reaction.

suppress skin reactions.

□ Elderly persons and patients with viral infection, malnutrition, febrile illness, uremia, immunosuppressive disorders, or miliary tuberculosis may have suppressed skin reactions.

□ If less than 10 weeks has passed since infection with tuberculosis, the skin reaction may be suppressed.

□ Improper dilution, dose, or storage of the tuberculin interferes with accurate testing.

KAREN DYER VANCE, RN, BSN

Delayed Hypersensitivity Skin Tests

Skin testing is one of the most important methods for evaluating the cellular immune response of a patient with severe recurrent infection, infection caused by unusual organisms, or suspected dis-orders associated with delayed hypersensitivity. Since diminished delayed hypersensitivity may be associated with a poor prognosis in patients with certain malignancies, this test may also be useful in determining prognosis in such patients. A positive test reaction shows that the afferent, the central, and the efferent limbs of the immune response are intact, and that the patient can maintain a nonspecific inflammatory response to infection.

Skin tests employ new and recall antigens. New antigens—those not previously encountered by the patient, such as dinitrochlorobenzene (DNCB)—evaluate the patient's primary immune response when a sensitizing dose is given, followed by a challenge dose. Recall antigens—those to which a patient has had, or may have had, previous exposure or sensitization—evaluate the secondary immune response; these antigens include candidin, trichophytin, streptokinase-streptodornase (SK-SD), purified protein derivative (PPD), staphage lysate, mumps, and mixed respiratory vaccine, among others. The specific antigens chosen for this test are those to which exposure is common and which will usually provoke an immune response.

In skin tests, a small amount of antigen (or group of antigens) is injected intradermally or applied topically, and the test site is later examined for a visible reaction. Skin tests have only limited value in infants because their immune systems are immature and inadequately sensitized.

Purpose

□ To evaluate primary and secondary immune responses

□ To assess effectiveness of immunotherapy, when the patient's immune response is augmented by adjuvants (such as bacille Calmette-Guérin [BCG] vaccine) or other means (transfer factor, levamisole)

□ To diagnose fungal diseases (coccidioidomycosis, histoplasmosis), bacterial diseases (tuberculosis, brucellosis, leprosy), and viral diseases (infectious mononucleosis)

☐ To monitor the course of certain diseases, such as Hodgkin's disease and coccidioidomycosis.

Patient preparation

Explain to the patient that this test evaluates the immune system after application or injection of small doses of antigens. Inform him he needn't restrict food or fluids before the test. Tell him who will perform the test and where; that it takes about 10 minutes for each antigen to be administered; and that reactions should appear in 48 to 72 hours. Explain that some antigens (such as DNCB) are readministered after 2 weeks or, if the test is negative, that a stronger dose of antigen may be given.

Check the patient's history for hypersensitivity to any of the test antigens; if not listed in his history, ask the patient if he's had a skin test previously and, if so, what his reactions were. Check for previous BCG vaccination or tuberculosis. If the patient's history reveals no sensitivity or hypersensitivity, it's appropriate to test with intermediate-strength antigens.

If skin tests are to be performed, the standardized hospital procedure must be checked. Since many antigens are approved by the Food and Drug Administration (FDA) for use as vaccines but not for skin testing, check with the pharmacy about FDA approval for this purpose. If the tests require the patient's informed consent, such as for use of DNCB in research studies, check with the appropriate hospital committee for guidelines.

Equipment

DNCB test: DNCB/sterile gauze pad and tape/gloves/surgical mask/alcohol swabs/acetone/cotton swabs.

Recall antigen test: 1-ml tuberculin syringes/25G ⅝″ needles/alcohol swabs/antigens/syringe filled with diluted epinephrine (1:1,000)/extra needle and syringe containing allergy test diluent/pen.

Procedure

DNCB test: Wear gloves and a mask to avoid sensitizing yourself to DNCB. Dissolve DNCB in acetone, as ordered. Position the patient's forearm comfortably, ventral side up, with his elbow slightly flexed. Cleanse a small, hairless area midway between the wrist and elbow

ADMINISTERING TEST ANTIGENS

Ca —— CA ◯   ◯ PPD —— PPD

SL —— SL ◯   ◯ SK-SD —— SK-SD

MR —— MR ◯   ◯ Trich —— Trich

KEY:
  Ca = Candidin
  SL = Staphage lysate
  MR = Mixed respiratory
  PPD = Purified protein derivative
  SK-SD = Streptokinase-streptodornase
  Trich = *Trichophyton*

This patient is undergoing a test of his secondary immune response, his recall reaction to previously encountered antigens. A sample panel of six test antigens has been injected into his forearm, and the test site marked and labeled for each antigen.

Adapted with permission from Noel R. Rose and Herman Friedman, *Manual of Clinical Immunology* (Washington, D.C.: American Society for Microbiology, 1980), p. 203.

with an alcohol swab, allow it to dry, and apply the prescribed amount of DNCB (sensitizing dose) with a cotton swab. Allow this to dry, then cover the area with a sterile gauze pad for 24 to 48 hours.

Instruct the patient to watch for a spontaneous flare reaction 10 to 14 days

after application of DNCB. (If a reaction occurs, a lower dose of the test solution can be used for the challenge dose of DNCB.)

After 14 days, apply a challenge dose of DNCB to the same spot and in the same manner. Inspect the site 48 to 96 hours after application of DNCB for reactivity. The challenge dose can be repeated 2 weeks later (1 month after the sensitizing dose) when test results are negative.

Recall antigen test: Inject each antigen being tested intradermally, using a separate tuberculin syringe, on the patient's forearm. Circle each injection site with a pen and label each according to the antigen given. Instruct the patient to avoid washing off the circles until the test is completed. Then, inject the control allergy diluent on the other forearm.

Inspect injection sites for reactivity after 48 and 72 hours. Record induration and erythema in millimeters. A negative test at the first concentration of antigen should be confirmed using a higher concentration.

Precautions

☐ Store antigens in lyophilized (freeze-dried) form at 39.2° F. (4° C.), protected from light. Reconstitute them shortly before use, and check their expiration dates. If the patient is suspected of hypersensitivity to the antigens, apply them first in low concentrations.

☐ Since excess DNCB can burn the patient's skin, apply only the prescribed amount.

☐ If the forearms are not free from disease (for example, if the patient has atopic dermatitis), use other sites, such as the back.

 ☐ Observe the patient carefully for signs of anaphylactic shock—urticaria, respiratory distress, and hypotension. If such signs develop, administer epinephrine, as ordered, and notify the doctor immediately.

Findings

In the DNCB test, a positive reaction

(erythema, edema, induration) appears 48 to 96 hours after the second (challenge) dose; 95% of the population reacts positively to DNCB. In the recall antigen test, a positive response (5 mm or more of induration at the test site) appears 48 hours after injection.

Implications of results

In the DNCB test, failure to react to the challenge dose indicates diminished delayed hypersensitivity. In the recall antigen test, a positive response to less than two of the six test antigens, a persistent unresponsiveness to introdermal injection of higher-strength antigens, or a generalized diminished reaction (causing less than 10 mm combined induration) indicates diminished delayed hypersensitivity.

Diminished delayed hypersensitivity can result from conditions such as Hodgkin's disease (common); sarcoidosis; liver disease; congenital immunodeficiency disease, such as DiGeorge's syndrome, ataxia-telangiectasia, and Wiskott-Aldrich syndrome; uremia; acute leukemia; viral diseases, such as influenza, infectious mononucleosis, measles, mumps, and rubella; fungal diseases, such as coccidioidomycosis and cryptococcosis; bacterial diseases, such as lep-

---

HOW TO PERFORM A PATCH TEST

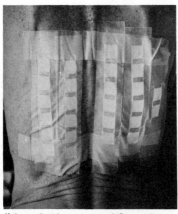 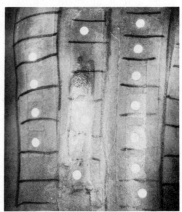

If the patient has an acute inflammation, postpone the patch test until the inflammation subsides, since patch testing may exacerbate the inflammation.

- *Use only potentially irritating substances for a patch test. Testing with primary irritants is not possible.*
- *To avoid skin irritation, dilute items that may be irritating to 1% to 2% in petrolatum, mineral oil, or as a last choice, water. When there are no clues to a likely allergen in a person with possible contact dermatitis, use a series of common allergens available in standard patch tests.*
- *Make applications to normal, hairless skin on the back or on the ventral surface of the forearm. First, apply potential allergens to a small disk of filter paper attached to aluminum and coated with plastic. Tape the paper to the skin (photograph at left above), or use a small square of soft cotton and cover with occlusive tape. Apply liquids and ointments to the disk or cotton. Apply volatile liquids to the skin and allow the areas to dry before covering. Before application, powder solids and moisten powders and fabrics.*
- *Patches should remain in place for 48 hours. However, remove the patch immediately if pain, pruritus, or irritation develops. Positive reactions may take time to develop, so check findings 20 to 30 minutes after removing the patch. Since a delayed reaction may occur, check findings again at 96 hours (4 days) after the application.*
- *To relieve the effects of a positive reaction, such as the reaction in the photograph at right above (at arrow), tell the patient to apply topical corticosteroids, as ordered.*

rosy and tuberculosis; and terminal cancer. Diminished delayed hypersensitivity can also result from immunosuppressive or steroid therapy or viral vaccination.

Post-test care
□ Watch the patient closely for severe local reactions that may occur at the test site, such as pain, blistering, swelling, induration, itching, and ulceration. Scarring or hyperpigmentation may result. Also observe for swelling and tenderness in the lymph nodes at the elbow or axillary region. Check for tachycardia and fever, although these rarely occur. Symptoms generally appear in 15 to 30 minutes.
□ Tell the patient experiencing hypersensitivity that steroids will control the reaction, but skin lesions may persist for 10 to 14 days. Instruct him to avoid scratching or otherwise disturbing the affected area.

Interfering factors
□ Use of antigens that have expired, or have been exposed to heat and light or to bacterial contamination interferes with accurate testing.
□ Poor injection technique—subcutaneous instead of intradermal injection—may produce negative results.
□ Inaccurate dilution of antigens, or error in reading or timing test results causes inaccurate test results.
□ A strong immediate reaction to the antigen at the site of injection may cause a false-negative delayed reaction.
□ Oral contraceptives may cause negative results by inhibiting lymphocyte mitosis.

BEVERLY A. ZENK WHEAT, RN, MA
SR. REBECCA FIDLER, MT(ASCP), PhD

RADIOLOGY AND NUCLEAR MEDICINE

Lymphangiography
[Lymphography]

Lymphangiography is the radiographic examination of the lymphatic system after the injection of an oil-based contrast medium into a lymphatic vessel in each foot or, less commonly, in each hand. Injection into the foot allows visualization of the lymphatics of the leg, inguinal and iliac regions, and the retroperitoneum up to the thoracic duct. Injection into the hand allows visualization of the axillary and supraclavicular nodes. This procedure may also be used to study the cervical region (retroauricular area), but this is less useful and less common. X-ray films are taken immediately after injection to demonstrate the filling of the lymphatic system, and then again 24 hours later to visualize the lymph nodes. Since the contrast remains in the nodes for up to 2 years, subsequent X-ray films can assess progression of disease and monitor effectiveness of treatment.

Lymphangiography is usually performed to stage disease in patients with an established diagnosis of lymphoma or cancer. It may also be performed for patients with enlarged lymph nodes, detected by computed tomography or ultrasonography.

Purpose
□ To detect and stage lymphomas, and to identify metastatic involvement of the lymph nodes
□ To distinguish primary from secondary lymphedema
□ To suggest surgical treatment or evaluate the effectiveness of chemotherapy and radiation therapy in controlling malignancy.

Patient preparation
Explain to the patient that this test permits examination of the lymphatic system through X-ray films taken after the injection of a contrast medium. Inform

him he needn't restrict food or fluids before the test. Tell him who will perform this procedure and where, and that it takes about 3 hours. Mention that additional X-ray films are also taken the following day, but these take less than 30 minutes.

Inform the patient that blue contrast will be injected into each foot to outline the lymphatic vessels; that the injection causes transient discomfort; and that the contrast discolors urine and stool for 48 hours, and may give his skin and vision a bluish tinge for 48 hours. Tell him a local anesthetic will be injected before a small incision is made in each foot. Inform him that the contrast medium is then injected for the next 1½ hours, using a cannula inserted into a lymphatic vessel. Advise the patient that he must remain as still as possible during injection of the contrast medium, and that he may experience some discomfort in the popliteal or inguinal areas at the beginning of the injection of the contrast medium. If this test is performed on an outpatient, advise him to be accompanied by a friend or relative. Warn him that the incision site may be sore for several days afterward.

Make sure the patient or responsible member of the family has signed a consent form. Check the history for hypersensitivity to iodine, seafood, or the contrast media used in other diagnostic tests, such as intravenous pyelography.

Just before the procedure, instruct the patient to void, and check his vital signs for a baseline. If ordered, administer a sedative and an oral antihistamine (if hypersensitivity to the contrast medium is suspected).

Procedure

A preliminary X-ray of the chest is taken with the patient in erect or supine position. Then, the skin over the dorsum of each foot is cleansed with antiseptics, and blue contrast is injected intradermally into the area between the toes, usually the first and fourth toe webs. The contrast infiltrates the lymphatic system and within 15 to 30 minutes the lym-

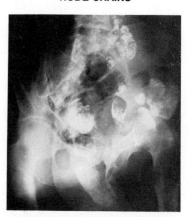

EVALUATING ABDOMINAL LYMPH NODE CHAINS

Lymphangiography is commonly used to detect and stage lymphoma. Normally, lymph node chains present a regular, uniform opacity and normal size and placement. In the photograph above of Stage IV lymphoma (24 hours after injection of contrast), lymph nodes are enlarged and displaced, and have the foamy appearance characteristic of lymphoma.

phatic vessels appear as small blue lines on the upper surface of the instep of each foot. A local anesthetic is then injected into the dorsum of each foot, and a 1″ (2.5 cm) transverse incision is made to expose the lymphatic vessel. Each vessel is cannulated with a 30G needle attached to polyethylene tubing and a syringe filled with ethiodized oil. Once the needles are positioned, the patient is instructed to remain still throughout the injection period to avoid dislodging the needles. The syringe is then placed within an infusion pump that injects the contrast medium at a rate of 0.1 to 0.2 ml/minute for about 1½ hours, to avoid injuring delicate lymphatic vessels.

Fluoroscopy may be used to monitor filling of the lymphatic system. If so, the infusion is stopped when the contrast reaches the level of the third and fourth lumbar vertebrae. At this point or when the injection is completed, the needles are removed, the incisions sutured, and

THE LYMPHATIC SYSTEM

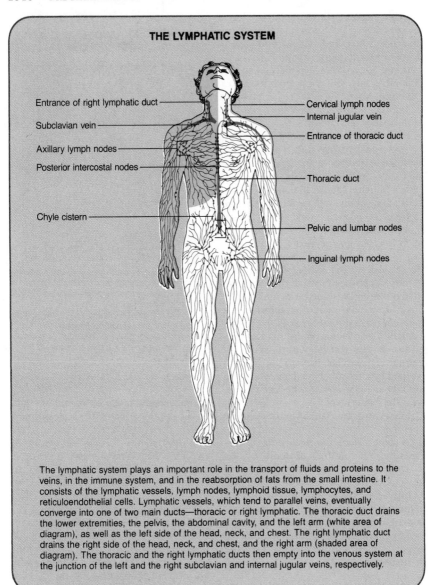

Entrance of right lymphatic duct

Subclavian vein

Axillary lymph nodes

Posterior intercostal nodes

Chyle cistern

Cervical lymph nodes

Internal jugular vein

Entrance of thoracic duct

Thoracic duct

Pelvic and lumbar nodes

Inguinal lymph nodes

The lymphatic system plays an important role in the transport of fluids and proteins to the veins, in the immune system, and in the reabsorption of fats from the small intestine. It consists of the lymphatic vessels, lymph nodes, lymphoid tissue, lymphocytes, and reticuloendothelial cells. Lymphatic vessels, which tend to parallel veins, eventually converge into one of two main ducts—thoracic or right lymphatic. The thoracic duct drains the lower extremities, the pelvis, the abdominal cavity, and the left arm (white area of diagram), as well as the left side of the head, neck, and chest. The right lymphatic duct drains the right side of the head, neck, and chest, and the right arm (shaded area of diagram). The thoracic and the right lymphatic ducts then empty into the venous system at the junction of the left and the right subclavian and internal jugular veins, respectively.

sterile dressings applied. X-ray films of the legs, pelvis, abdomen, and chest are taken. The patient is then taken to his room but must return 24 hours later for additional films.

Precautions
Lymphangiography is contraindicated in patients with hypersensitivities to iodine, pulmonary insufficiencies, cardiac diseases, severe renal or hepatic diseases.

Findings
The lymphatic system normally demonstrates homogeneous and complete

STAGING MALIGNANT LYMPHOMA

Stage I: Involvement of a single lymph node region or of a single extralymphatic organ or site
Stage II: Involvement of two or more lymph node regions on the same side of the diaphragm, or localized involvement of an extralymphatic organ or site of one or more lymph node regions on the same side of the diaphragm
Stage III: Involvement of lymph node regions on both sides of the diaphragm, which may also be accompanied by localized involvement of extralymphatic organ or site or by involvement of the spleen or both
Stage IV: Diffuse or disseminated involvement of one or more extralymphatic organs or tissues with or without associated lymph node enlargement

Reprinted with permission from *Manual for Staging of Cancer* (Chicago: American Joint Committee for Cancer Staging, 1983).

filling with contrast medium on the initial films. On the 24-hour films, the lymph nodes are fully opacified and well-circumscribed; the lymphatic channels are emptied a few hours after injection of the contrast agent.

Implications of results

Enlarged, foamy-looking nodes indicate lymphoma, classified as Hodgkin's or non-Hodgkin's. Filling defects or lack of opacification indicates metastatic involvement of the lymph nodes. The number of nodes affected, unilateral or bilateral involvement, and the extent of extranodal involvement help determine staging of lymphoma. However, definitive staging may require additional diagnostic tests such as computed tomography, ultrasonography, selective biopsy, and laparotomy.

In differential diagnosis of primary and secondary lymphedema, shortened lymphatic vessels and a deficient number of vessels indicate primary lymphedema. Abruptly terminating lymphatic vessels, caused by retroperitoneal tumors impinging on the vessels, inflammation, filariasis, and trauma resulting from surgery or irradiation, indicate secondary lymphedema.

Post-test care

□ Check the patient's vital signs every 4 hours for 48 hours.
□ Watch for pulmonary complications, such as shortness of breath, pleuritic pain, hypotension, low-grade fever, and cyanosis, due to embolization of contrast medium.
□ Enforce bed rest for 24 hours, with the patient's feet elevated to help reduce swelling, as ordered.
□ Apply ice packs to the incision sites to help reduce swelling and administer an analgesic, as ordered.
□ Check the incision sites for infection, and leave the dressings in place for 2 days, making sure the wounds remain dry. Tell the patient the sutures will be removed in 7 to 10 days.
□ Prepare the patient for follow-up X-rays, as ordered.

Interfering factors

Inability to cannulate the lymphatic vessels interferes with accurate determination of test results.

KAREN DYER VANCE, RN, BSN

Gallium Scanning

This test, a total body scan, is usually performed 24 to 48 hours after the I.V. injection of radioactive gallium (^{67}Ga) citrate; occasionally, it's performed 72 hours after the injection or, in acute inflammatory disease, after 4 to 6 hours. Although the liver, spleen, bones, and large bowel normally take up gallium, *certain neoplasms and inflammatory lesions also attract it. However, many neoplasms and a few inflammatory lesions may fail to demonstrate abnormal gallium activity. Because gallium has an affinity for both benign and malignant neoplasms and inflammatory lesions, exact diagnosis requires additional confirming tests, such as ultrasonography and computerized tomography.*

Gallium scanning is usually indicated when the site of the disease (usually malignancy) hasn't been clearly defined, and when the patient's condition won't be jeopardized by the time required for the procedure. It can also clarify focal hepatic defects when liver-spleen scanning and ultrasonography prove inconclusive and can evaluate suspected bronchogenic carcinoma when sputum culture proves positive for malignancy but other tests are normal, or when hydrothorax is present and bronchoscopy is contraindicated.

Purpose

□ To detect primary or metastatic neoplasms and inflammatory lesions
□ To evaluate malignant lymphoma and identify recurrent tumors following chemotherapy or irradiation therapy
□ To clarify focal defects in the liver and evaluate bronchogenic carcinoma.

Patient preparation

Explain to the patient that this test helps detect abnormal or inflammatory tissue. Inform him he needn't restrict food or fluids. Tell him the test requires a total body scan (usually performed 24 to 48 hours after the I.V. injection of radioactive gallium); who will perform the test and where; and that the scan takes 30 to 60 minutes. Warn him that he may experience transient discomfort from the needle puncture during injection of the radioactive gallium. Reassure him, however, that the dosage is only slightly radioactive and isn't harmful.

If a gamma scintillation camera is to be used, assure the patient that while the uptake probe and detector head may touch his skin, he will experience no discomfort. If a rectilinear scanner is to be used, mention that it makes a soft, irregular clicking noise as it registers the radiation emissions.

Make sure the patient or responsible member of the family has signed a consent form. Administer a laxative and/or cleansing enema, as ordered.

Procedure

The patient may be positioned erect or recumbent, or an appropriate combination of these positions, depending on his physical condition. Scans or scintigraphs of the patient are taken 24 to 48 hours after ^{67}Ga citrate injection (adult dose varies from 2 to 10 mc; the dose is scaled down for a child), from anterior and posterior views and, occasionally, lateral views.

Precautions

□ This test should precede barium studies, since barium retention may hinder visualization of gallium activity in the bowel.
□ Gallium scanning is relatively contraindicated in children and during pregnancy or lactation; however, it may be performed if the potential diagnostic benefit outweighs the risks of exposure to radiation.

Findings

Gallium activity is normally demonstrated in the liver, spleen, bones, and large bowel. Activity in the bowel results from mucosal uptake of gallium and the fecal excretion of gallium.

Implications of results

Gallium scanning may reveal inflammatory lesions—discrete abscesses or diffuse infiltration. In pancreatic or perinephric abscess, gallium activity is relatively localized; in bacterial peritonitis, gallium activity is spread diffusely within the abdomen.

Abnormally high gallium accumulation is characteristic in inflammatory bowel diseases, such as ulcerative colitis and regional ileitis (Crohn's disease), and in carcinoma of the colon. However,

USING GALLIUM SCANNING TO EVALUATE LYMPHOMA TREATMENT

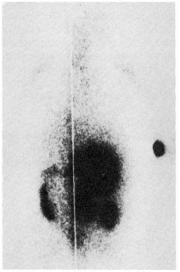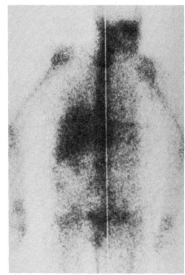

Gallium scanning can help evaluate the efficacy of treatment for lymphoma. In the pretreatment total body scanning of a patient with histiocytic lymphoma (photograph at left), radioactive gallium concentrates in tumors. After chemotherapy (photograph at right), the scan shows normal distribution of radiotracer through the body and supports the clinical impression of remission.

since gallium normally accumulates in the colon, the detection of inflammatory and neoplastic diseases is sometimes difficult.

Abnormal gallium activity may be present in various sarcomas, Wilms' tumor, and neuroblastomas; carcinoma of the kidney, uterus, vagina, and stomach; and testicular tumors, such as seminoma, embryonal carcinoma, choriocarcinoma, and teratocarcinoma, which often metastasize via the lymphatic system. In Hodgkin's and non-Hodgkin's lymphoma, gallium scanning can demonstrate abnormal activity in one or more lymph nodes or in extranodal locations. However, gallium scanning supported by results of lymphangiography can gauge the extent of metastases more accurately than either test alone, since neither test consistently identifies all neoplastic nodes.

After chemotherapy or radiation therapy, gallium scanning may be used to detect new or recurrent tumors. However, these forms of therapy tend to diminish tumor affinity for gallium without necessarily eliminating the tumor.

In the differential diagnosis of focal hepatic defects, abnormal gallium activity may help narrow the diagnostic possibilities. Gallium localizes in hepatomas, but not in pseudotumors; in abscesses, but not in pleural effusions; and in tumors, but not in cysts or hematomas. In examining patients with suspected bronchogenic carcinoma, abnormal activity confirms the presence of tumor. However, since gallium also localizes in inflammatory pulmonary diseases, such as pneumonia and sarcoidosis, chest radiography should be performed to distinguish a tumor from an inflammatory lesion.

Post-test care

If the initial gallium scan suggests bowel disease and additional scans are necessary, give the patient a cleansing enema, as ordered, before continuing the test.

Interfering factors
□ Hepatic and splenic uptake may obscure the detection of abnormal paraaortic nodes in Hodgkin's disease, causing false-negative scans.
□ Fecal accumulation can hinder visualization of the retroperitoneal space.
□ Barium studies within 1 week before this scan can interfere with visualization of gallium activity in the bowel.

MAE E. PAULFREY, RN, MN

Red Blood Cell Survival Time

Normally, red blood cells (RBCs) are only destroyed when they reach senility. However, in hemolytic diseases, RBCs of all ages are randomly destroyed, resulting in anemia. This test measures the survival time of circulating RBCs and detects sites of abnormal RBC sequestration and destruction, aiding evaluation of unexplained anemia.

Survival time is measured by labeling a random sample of RBCs with radioactive chromium-51 sodium chromate (^{51}Cr). The ^{51}Cr quickly crosses RBC membranes, reduces to chromium ion, and binds to hemoglobin. This labeled group of RBCs is then injected back into the patient. Serial blood samples measure the percent of labeled cells per unit volume over 3 to 4 weeks, until 50% of the cells disappears (disappearance rate corresponds to destruction of a random cell population). A normal RBC survives about 120 days (half-life of 60 days); the ^{51}Cr-labeled RBCs have a shorter half-life (25 to 30 days) because about 1% of senescent RBCs are removed from the circulation each day and about 1% of ^{51}Cr is spontaneously eluted from the labeled RBCs each day.

During the test period, a gamma cam-era scans the body for sites of abnormally high radioactivity, which indicate sites of excessive RBC sequestration and destruction. Other tests performed with the RBC survival time test may include spot-checks of the stool to detect gastrointestinal (GI) blood loss; hematocrit; blood volume studies; and radionuclide iron uptake and clearance tests to aid differential diagnosis of anemia.

Purpose
□ To help evaluate unexplained anemia, particularly hemolytic anemia
□ To identify sites of abnormal RBC sequestration and destruction.

Patient preparation
Explain to the patient that this test helps identify the cause of his anemia. Advise him that he needn't restrict food or fluids. Inform him that the test involves labeling a blood sample with a radioactive substance, and that it requires regular blood samples at 3-day intervals for 3 to 4 weeks. Tell him who will perform the procedures and when, and that he may experience slight discomfort from the needle punctures. Reassure him that collecting each sample takes less than 3 minutes, and that the small amount of radioactive substance used is harmless.

If the doctor orders a stool collection to test for GI bleeding, teach the patient the proper collection technique.

Procedure
A 30-ml blood sample is drawn and mixed with 100 microcuries (μCi) of ^{51}Cr for an adult; less for a child. After an incubation period, the mixture is injected intravenously into the patient. A blood sample is drawn 30 minutes after injection to determine blood and RBC volumes.

A 6-ml sample is collected in a *green-top* tube after 24 hours; follow-up samples are collected at 3-day intervals for 3 to 4 weeks. (Interval between samples may vary, depending on the laboratory.) To avoid error from physical decay of the ^{51}Cr, each sample is measured with a scintillation well counter on the day it's drawn. Radioactivity per ml of RBCs is calculated; these values are then plotted to determine mean RBC survival time. Simultaneous gamma camera scans of the precordium, sacrum, liver, and spleen detect radioactivity at sites of excess RBC sequestration. A hematocrit is done on a small portion of each blood sample to check for blood loss.

At the end of the study, a sample is drawn to compare ending blood and RBC volumes with beginning volumes.

Precautions

□ This test is contraindicated during pregnancy, because it exposes the fetus to radiation.

□ Because excess blood loss can invalidate test results, this test is usually contraindicated for a patient with active bleeding or poor clotting function. However, if the test is necessary for a patient with poor clotting function, observe the venipuncture sites carefully for signs of hemorrhage.

□ The patient should not receive blood transfusions during the test period and should not have blood samples drawn for other tests.

Findings

Normal half-life for RBCs labeled with ^{51}Cr is 25 to 35 days. Normal gamma camera scans reveal slight radioactivity in the spleen, liver, and sometimes the bone marrow.

Implications of results

Decreased RBC survival time indicates a hemolytic disease, such as chronic lymphocytic leukemia, congenital nonspherocytic hemolytic anemia, hemoglobin C disease, hereditary spherocytosis, idiopathic acquired hemolytic anemia, paroxysmal nocturnal hemoglobinuria, elliptocytosis, pernicious anemia, sickle cell anemia, sickle cell hemoglobin C disease, or hemolytic-uremic syndrome. If hemolytic anemia is diagnosed, additional tests using cross transfusion of labeled RBCs can determine if anemia results from an intrinsic RBC defect or an extrinsic factor.

A gamma camera scan that detects a site of excess RBC sequestration provides direction for treatment. For example, abnormally high RBC sequestration in the spleen may require a splenectomy.

Post-test care

If a hematoma develops at the venipuncture site, apply warm soaks.

Interfering factors

□ Dehydration, overhydration, or blood loss (from hemorrhage or blood samples drawn for other tests) can change the circulating RBC volume and invalidate test results.

□ Blood transfusions during the test period alter the proportion of labeled RBCs to total RBCs, thus altering results.

BONNIE L. ANDERSON, MD

MALABSORPTION TEST

D-Xylose Absorption

One of the most important tests for malabsorption, D-xylose absorption evaluates patients with symptoms of malabsorption, such as weight loss and generalized malnutrition, weakness, and diarrhea. In this test, the patient ingests a standard dose of D-xylose—a pentose sugar that's absorbed in the small intestine without the aid of pancreatic enzymes, passed through the liver without being metabolized, and excreted in the urine. Because of its absorption in the small intestine without digestion, measurement of D-xylose in the urine and blood indicates the absorptive capacity of the small intestine. Normally, blood levels of D-xylose peak 2 hours after ingestion, and 80% to 95% of the dose is excreted in 5 hours; the remaining dose, in 24 hours.

To ensure accurate results, the test requires the patient to fast, to remain in bed during the specimen collection period, and to have adequate renal function for the absorption and excretion of D-*xylose.*

Purpose
□ To aid differential diagnosis of malabsorption
□ To determine the cause of malabsorption syndrome.

Patient preparation
Explain to the patient that this test helps evaluate digestive function by analyzing blood and urine specimens after ingestion of a sugar solution. Advise him to fast overnight before the test. Instruct him to abstain from all food and fluids and remain in bed during the test, since activity affects test results. Tell him the test requires several blood samples; who will perform the venipunctures and when; and that he may experience some discomfort from the needle punctures and the pressure of the tourniquet. Reassure him that collecting each blood sample takes less than 3 minutes. Inform him that all his urine will be collected for 5 or 24 hours, as ordered.

As ordered, withhold aspirin and indomethacin, which alter test results, and record any medications the patient is taking on the laboratory slip.

Procedure
Perform a venipuncture to obtain a fasting blood sample, and collect the sample in a 10 ml *red-top* tube. Then, collect a first-voided morning urine specimen. Label these specimens, and send them to the laboratory immediately to serve as a baseline.

Give the patient 25 g D-xylose dissolved in 8 oz (240 ml) water, followed by an additional 8 oz (240 ml) of water. If the patient is a child, administer 0.5 g D-xylose/lb body weight, up to 25 g. Record the time of D-xylose ingestion.

In an adult, draw a blood sample 2 hours after D-xylose ingestion; in a child, 1 hour. Collect the sample in a 10 ml *red-top* tube (or a 10 ml *gray-top* tube if the sample won't be tested immediately). Occasionally, a 5-hour sample may be drawn to support the findings of the 1- or 2-hour sample. Collect and pool all urine during the 5 or 24 hours following D-xylose ingestion, as ordered.

Precautions
□ Handle the blood collection tubes gently to prevent hemolysis.
□ Tell the patient not to contaminate the urine specimens with toilet tissue or stool.
□ Be sure to collect all urine, and refrigerate the specimen during the collection period.
□ Check with the doctor to determine the length of the collection period, since patients aged 65 and older, or those with borderline or elevated creatinine levels tend to have low 5-hour urine levels but normal 24-hour levels. At the end of the collection period, send the urine specimen to the laboratory immediately.
□ Maintain bed rest and withhold food and fluids (other than administration of D-xylose) throughout the test period.

Values
The following are normal values for the D-xylose absorption test.
For *children:* blood concentration, greater than 30 mg/dl in 1 hour; urine, 16% to 33% of ingested D-xylose excreted in 5 hours
For *adults under age 65:* blood concentration, 25 to 40 mg/dl in 2 hours; urine, more than 4 g in 5 hours
For *adults aged 65 and older:* blood concentration, 25 to 40 mg/dl in 2 hours; urine, more than 3.5 g excreted in 5 hours and more than 5 g excreted in 24 hours.

Implications of results
Depressed blood and urine D-xylose levels most commonly result from malabsorptive disorders affecting the proximal small intestine, such as sprue and celiac disease. However, depressed levels may also result from regional enteritis involving the jejunum, Whipple's disease,

multiple jejunal diverticula, myxedema, diabetic neuropathic diarrhea, rheumatoid arthritis, alcoholism, severe congestive heart failure, and ascites.

Post-test care

□ If a hematoma develops at the venipuncture site, ease discomfort by applying warm soaks.

. □ Observe the patient for abdominal discomfort or mild diarrhea caused by D-xylose ingestion.

□ As ordered, resume administration of medications discontinued before the test.

□ Patient may resume usual diet.

Interfering factors

□ Failure to adhere to restrictions of diet and activity affects absorption of D-xylose.

□ Aspirin decreases D-xylose excretion by the kidneys; indomethacin depresses its intestinal absorption.

□ Failure to obtain a complete urine specimen or to collect blood samples at designated times interferes with accurate testing.

□ Intestinal overgrowth of bacteria or renal retention or insufficiency may cause depressed urine levels.

WILLIAM M. DOUGHERTY, BS

Selected References

Byrne, C. Judith, et al. *Laboratory Tests: Implications for Nurses and Allied Health Professionals*. Reading, Mass.: Addison-Wesley Publishing Co., 1981.

Diseases, 2nd ed. Nurse's Reference Library. Springhouse, Pa.: Springhouse Corp., 1986.

Griffiths, Harry J., and Sarno, Robert C. *Contemporary Radiology: An Introduction to Imaging*. Philadelphia: W.B. Saunders Co., 1979.

Hermann, Christy S. "Performing Intradermal Skin Tests—The Right Way," *Nursing83* 13:50-53, October 1983.

Immune Disorders. Nurse's Clinical Library.

Springhouse, Pa.: Springhouse Corp., 1985.

Luckmann, Joan, and Sorensen, Karen C. *Medical-Surgical Nursing: A Psychophysiologic Approach*, 2nd ed. Philadelphia: W.B. Saunders Co., 1980.

Ravel, Richard A. *Clinical Laboratory Medicine*, 4th ed. Chicago: Year Book Medical Pubs., 1984.

Rose, Noel, and Friedman, H., eds. *Manual of Clinical Immunology*, 2nd ed. Washington, D.C.: American Society for Microbiology, 1980.

Stites, Daniel P., et al., eds. *Basic and Clinical Immunology*, 4th ed. Los Altos, Calif.: Lange Medical Publications, 1982.

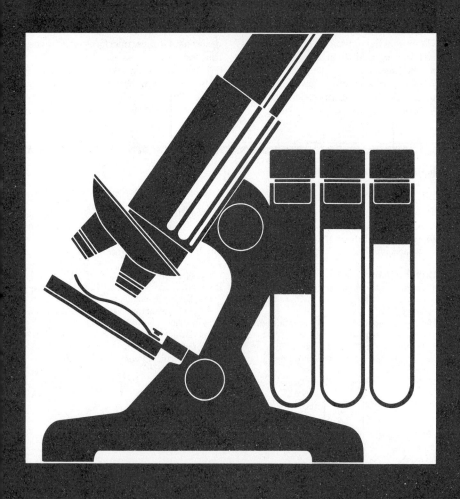

Appendices and Index

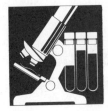

Abbreviations

Ab - antibody
ABLB - alternate binaural loudness balance
ABR - auditory brain stem response
ACG - apexcardiogram
ACTH - adrenocorticotropic hormone
ADH - antidiuretic hormone
AFP - alpha-fetoprotein
Ag - antigen
A/G ratio - albumin/globulin ratio
ANA - antinuclear antibodies
ARS-A - arylsulfatase-A
ASHA - American Speech, Language & Hearing Association
ASO - antistreptolysin O
ATP - adenosine triphosphate

BCG - bacille Calmette-Guerin
bpm - beats per minute
BUN - blood urea nitrogen

CAD - coronary artery disease
cAMP - cyclic adenosine monophosphate
CBC - complete blood count
CEA - carcinoembryonic antigen
CM - competing message
CNS - central nervous system
COPD - chronic obstructive pulmonary disease
CPK - creatine phosphokinase
CPK-BB - creatine phosphokinase, brain
CPK-MB - creatine phosphokinase, heart muscle
CPK-MM - creatine phosphokinase, skeletal muscle
cpm - counts per minute
CRP - C-reactive protein
CSF - cerebrospinal fluid
CT - computed tomography

dB - decibels
DET - diethyltryptamine
dl - deciliter
DNA - deoxyribonucleic acid
DNCB - dinitrochlorobenzene
DSA - digital subtraction angiography
DVT - deep vein thrombosis

EBV - Epstein-Barr virus
EDTA - ethylenediamine tetraacetic acid
EEG - electroencephalogram
EKG - electrocardiogram
EL - effective level
ELISA - enzyme-linked immunosorbent assay
EM - effective masking
EMIT - enzyme-multiplied immunoassay technique
ERPF - effective renal plasma flow
ESR - erythrocyte sedimentation rate

FHR - fetal heart rate
FSH - follicle-stimulating hormone
FT$_3$ - free triiodothyronine
FT$_4$ - free thyroxine
FTA - fluorescent treponemal antibody
FTA-ABS - fluorescent treponemal antibody absorption
FUO - fever of undetermined origin

G - gauge
GFR - glomerular filtration rate
GGT - gamma glutamyl transpeptidase
GI - gastrointestinal
G-6-PD - glucose-6-phosphate dehydrogenase
GVH - graft-versus-host

HBD - hydroxybutyric dehydrogenase
HB$_s$A$_g$ - hepatitis B surface antigen
hCG - human chorionic gonadotropin
hCS - human chorionic somatomammotropin
Hct - hematocrit
HDL - high-density lipoproteins
HDN - hemolytic disease of the newborn
Hgb - hemoglobin
hGH - growth hormone
HI - hemagglutination inhibition
5-HIAA - 5-hydroxyindoleacetic acid
HL - hearing level
hPL - human placental lactogen
HVA - homovanillic acid
Hz - hertz

131I - radioactive iodine
ICD - isocitrate dehydrogenase
Ig - immunoglobulin

I.V. - intravenous
IVGTT - intravenous glucose tolerance test

17-KGS - 17-ketogenic steroids
17-KS - 17-ketosteroids
KUB - kidney-ureter-bladder
KVO - keep vein open

LA - left atrium
LAP - leucine aminopeptidase
LDH - lactic dehydrogenase
LDL - low-density lipoproteins
LE - lupus erythematosus
LH - luteinizing hormone
LSD - lysergic acid diethylamide
LV - left ventricle
LVET - left ventricular ejection time

MAO - monoamine oxidase
mcg - microgram
MCH - mean corpuscular hemoglobin
MCHC - mean corpuscular hemoglobin
concentration
MCV - mean corpuscular volume
mg - milligram
MI - myocardial infarction
ml - milliliter
MLC - mixed lymphocyte culture
MLD - masking level differences
mm - millimeter
MRI - magnetic resonance imaging
MUGA - multiple-gated acquisition scanning

NADH - nicotinamide-adenine-dinucleotide
laced with hydrogen
NG - nasogastric
NPN - nonprotein nitrogen
5'NT - 5'-nucleotidase

OCT - ornithine carbamoyltransferase
OGTT - oral glucose tolerance test
17-OHCS - 17-hydroxycorticosteroids
OPG - oculoplethysmography
OPG-GEE - ocular pneumoplethysmography

PA - posteroanterior
PAP - pulmonary artery pressure

PAWP - pulmonary artery wedge pressure
PCG - phonocardiogram
PCP - phencyclidine
PEP - pre-ejection period
PET - positron emission tomography
pg - picogram
PHA - phytohemagglutinin
PID - pelvic inflammatory disease
PKU - phenylketonuria
PMI - point of maximum impulse
PPD - purified protein derivative
PSP - phenolsulfonphthalein excretion
PTH - parathyroid hormone
PTS - permanent threshold shift

RA - right atrium
RAST - radioallergosorbent test
RBC - red blood cell
RES - reticuloendothelial system
RL - right lateral
RNA - ribonucleic acid
RV - right ventricle

SBMPL - simultaneous binaural midplane
localization
SCAT - sheep cell agglutination test
SGOT - serum glutamic-oxaloacetic trans-
aminase
SGPT - serum glutamic-pyruvic transaminase
SHBG - sex hormone-binding globulin
SK-SD - streptokinase-streptodornase
SLE - systemic lupus erythematosus
STH - somatotropic hormone

T_3 - triiodothyronine
T_3UR - T_3 uptake ratio
T_4 - thyroxine
TBG - thyroxine-binding globulin
^{99m}Tc - technetium 99m pertechnetate
^{99m}Tc-DTPA - technetium and diethylene-
triamine pentaacetic acid
TSH - thyroid-stimulating hormone
TTS - temporary threshold shift

VCG - vectorcardiogram
VDRL - Venereal Disease Research Labo-
ratory test
VLDL - very low-density lipoproteins
VMA - vanillylmandelic acid

WBC - white blood cell

UNITS OF MEASURE

METRIC MEASURES: WEIGHT AND VOLUME

PREFIX SYMBOL	FACTOR	WEIGHT	VOLUME
k	1 x 1,000	kilogram (kg)	kiloliter (kl)
	1	gram (g)	liter (l)
d	1 ÷ 10	decigram (dg)	deciliter (dl)
c	1 ÷ 100	centigram (cg)	centiliter (cl)
m	1 ÷ 1,000	milligram (mg)	milliliter (ml)
μ (mc)	1 ÷ 1 million	microgram (μg, mcg)	microliter (μl, mcl)
n	1 ÷ 1 billion	nanogram (ng)	nanoliter (nl)
p	1 ÷ 1 trillion	picogram (pg)	picoliter (pl)
f	1 ÷ 1 quadrillion	femtogram (fg)	femtoliter (fl)

CONVERSION OF METRIC TO CUSTOMARY UNITS

WEIGHT	VOLUME
grams x 0.035 = ounces	milliliters x 0.03 = fluidounces
kilograms x 2.2 = pounds	liters x 2.1 = pints
	liters x 1.06 = quarts
	liters x 0.26 = gallons

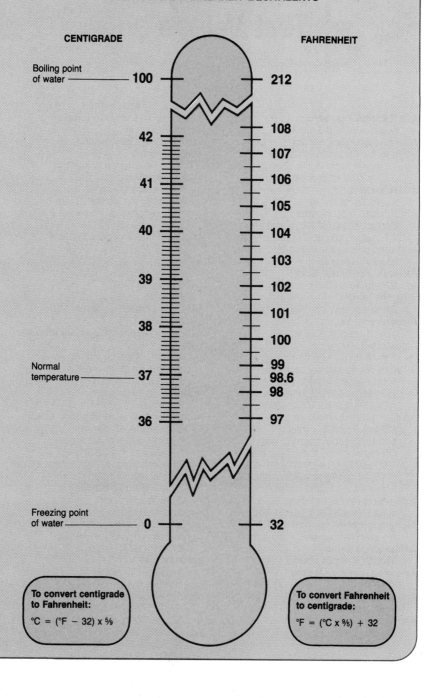

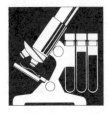

Laboratory Test Values

A

AChR antibodies, serum
negative or ≤ 0.5 nmol/liter

Acid phosphatase, serum
0 to 1.1 Bodansky units/ml
1 to 4 King-Armstrong units/ml
0.13 to 0.63 BLB units/ml

ACTH, plasma
< 120 pg/ml

ACTH, rapid test, plasma
Cortisol rises 7 to 18 mcg/dl above baseline, 60 minutes after injection

Activated partial thromboplastin time
25 to 36 seconds

Albumin, peritoneal fluid
50% to 70% of total protein

Albumin, serum
3.3 to 4.5 g/dl

Aldosterone, serum
1 to 21 ng/dl (standing)

Aldosterone, urine
2 to 16 mcg/24 hours

Alkaline phosphatase, peritoneal fluid
Men: > age 18, 90 to 239 units/liter
Women: < age 45, 76 to 196 units/liter; > age 45, 87 to 250 units/liter

Alkaline phosphatase, serum
1.5 to 4 Bodansky units/dl
4 to 13.5 King-Armstrong units/dl
Chemical inhibition method: Men, 90 to 239 units/dl; Women < age 45, 76 to 196 units/liter; Women > age 45, 87 to 250 units/liter

Alpha-fetoprotein, amniotic fluid
≤ 18.5 mcg/ml at 13 or 14 weeks

Alpha-fetoprotein, serum
Nonpregnant women: < 30 ng/ml

Amino acids, urine
50 to 200 mg/24 hours

Ammonia, peritoneal fluid
< 50 mcg/dl

Ammonia, plasma
< 50 mcg/dl

Amniotic fluid
Lecithin/sphingomyelin ratio: > 2
Meconium: Absent
Phosphatidiglycerol: Present

Amylase, peritoneal fluid
138 to 404 amylase units/liter

Amylase, serum
60 to 180 Somogyi units/dl

Amylase, urine
10 to 80 amylase units/hour

Androstenedione
Men: 0.9 to 1.7 ng/ml
Menstruating women: 0.6 to 3 ng/ml
Postmenopausal women: 0.3 to 8 ng/ml

Angiotensin converting enzyme
> age 20: 18 to 67 U/liter

Anion gap
8 to 14 mEq/liter

Antibodies to ENA
Negative

Antibody screening, serum
Negative

Anti–deoxyribonucleic acid antibodies, serum
< 1 mcg DNA bound/ml

Antidiuretic hormone, serum
1 to 5 pg/ml

Antiglobulin test, direct
Negative

Antimitochondrial antibodies, serum
Negative at 1:5 dilution

Antinuclear antibodies, serum
Negative at ≤ 1:32 titer

Anti–smooth-muscle antibodies, serum
Normal titer < 1:20

Antistreptolysin-O, serum
< 85 Todd units/ml

Antithrombin III
> 50% of normal control values

Antithyroid antibodies, serum
Normal titer < 1:100

Arginine test
Men: hgH increases to > 10 ng/ml
Women: hgH increases to > 15 ng/ml

Arterial blood gases
Pao_2: 75 to 100 mmHg
$Paco_2$: 35 to 45 mmHg
O_2CT: 15% to 23%
O_2 Sat: 94% to 100%
HCO_3^-: 22 to 26 mEq/liter

Arylsulfatase A, urine
    Men: 1.4 to 19.3 units/liter
    Women: 1.4 to 11 units/liter
Aspergillosis antibody, serum
    Normal titer < 1:8

B

B-lymphocyte count
    270 to 640/mm³
Bence Jones protein, urine
    Negative
Bilirubin, amniotic fluid
    Absent at term
Bilirubin, serum
    Adult: Direct, < 0.5 mg/dl; indirect,
        ≤ 1.1 mg/dl
    Neonate: Total, 1 to 12 mg/dl
Bilirubin, urine
    Negative
Blastomycosis antibody, serum
    Normal titer < 1:8
Bleeding time
    Modified template: 2 to 10 minutes
    Template: 2 to 8 minutes
    Ivy: 1 to 7 minutes
    Duke: 1 to 3 minutes
Blood urea nitrogen
    8 to 20 mg/dl

C

C-reactive protein, serum
    Negative
Calcitonin, plasma
    Baseline: Males, ≤ 0.155 ng/ml;
        females, ≤ 0.105 ng/ml
    Calcium infusion: Males, 0.265 ng/ml;
        females, 0.120 ng/ml
    Pentagastrin infusion: Males, 0.210 ng/
        ml; females, 0.105 ng/ml
Calcium, serum
    4.5 to 5.5 mEq/liter
    Atomic absorption: 8.9 to 10.1 mg/dl
Calcium, urine
    Men: < 275 mg/24 hours
    Women: < 250 mg/24 hours
Capillary fragility
Petechiae:	0 to 10	*Score:*	1 +
	10 to 20		2 +
	20 to 50		3 +
	50		4 +
Carbon dioxide, total, blood
    22 to 34 mEq/liter
Carcinoembryonic antigen, serum
    < 5 ng/ml
Carotene, serum
    48 to 200 mcg/dl

Catecholamines, plasma
    Supine: Epinephrine, 0 to 110 pg/ml;
        norepinephrine, 70 to 750 pg/ml;
        dopamine, 0 to 30 pg/ml
    Standing: Epinephrine, 0 to 140 pg/ml;
        norepinephrine, 200 to 1,700 pg/ml;
        dopamine, 0 to 30 pg/ml
Catecholamines, urine
    24-hour specimen: 0 to 135 mcg
    Random specimen: 0 to 18 mcg/dl
Catheterization, pulmonary artery
    Right atrial: 1 to 6 mmHg
    Systolic right ventricular: 20 to
        30 mmHg
    End diastolic right ventricular:
        < 5 mmHg
    Systolic PAP: 20 to 30 mmHg
    Diastolic PAP: approximately
        10 mmHg
    Mean PAP: < 20 mmHg
    PAWP: 6 to 12 mmHg
    Left atrial: approximately 10 mmHg
Cerebrospinal fluid
    Pressure: 50 to 180 mm water
    Appearance: Clear, colorless
    Gram stain: No organisms
Ceruloplasmin, serum
    22.9 to 43.1 mg/dl
Chloride, cerebrospinal fluid
    118 to 130 mEq/liter
Chloride, serum
    100 to 108 mEq/liter
Chloride, sweat
    10 to 35 mEq/liter
Chloride, urine
    110 to 250 mEq/24 hours
Cholesterol, total, serum
    120 to 330 mg/dl
Cholinesterase (pseudocholinesterase)
    8 to 18 units/ml
Chorionic gonadotropin, serum
    < 3 mIU/ml
Chorionic gonadotropin, urine
    Pregnant Women: First trimester,
        ≤ 500,000 IU/24 hours; second
        trimester, 10,000 to 25,000 IU/
        24 hours; third trimester, 5,000 to
        15,000 IU/24 hours
Clot retraction
    50%
Coccidioidomycosis antibody, serum
    Normal titer < 1:2
Cold agglutinins, serum
    Normal titer < 1:16
Complement, serum
    Total: 41 to 90 hemolytic units

Complement serum—continued
Cl esterase inhibitor: 16 to 33 mg/dl
C3: Men, 88 to 252 mg/dl; women, 88 to 206 mg/dl
C4: Men, 12 to 72 mg/dl; women, 13 to 75 mg/dl

Complement, synovial fluid
10 mg protein/dl: 3.7 to 33.7 units/ml
20 mg protein/dl: 7.7 to 37.7 units/ml

Copper, urine
15 to 60 mcg/24 hours

Copper reduction test, urine
Negative

Coproporphyrin, urine
Men: 0 to 96 mcg/24 hours
Women: 1 to 57 mcg/24 hours

Cortisol, plasma
Morning: 7 to 28 mcg/dl
Afternoon: 2 to 18 mcg/dl

Cortisol, free, urine
24 to 108 mcg/24 hours

Creatine phosphokinase
Total: Men, 23 to 99 units/liter; women, 15 to 57 units/liter
CPK-BB: None
CPK-MB: 0 to 7 IU/liter
CPK-MM: 5 to 70 IU/liter

Creatine, serum
Men: 0.2 to 0.6 mg/dl
Women: 0.6 to 1 mg/dl

Creatinine, amniotic fluid
> 2 mg/100 ml in mature fetus

Creatinine clearance
Men (age 20): 90 ml/minute/1.73 m^2
Women (age 20): 84 ml/minute/1.73 m^2

Creatinine, serum
Men: 0.8 to 1.2 mg/dl
Women: 0.6 to 0.9 mg/dl

Creatinine, urine
Men: 1 to 1.9 g/24 hours
Women: 0.8 to 1.7 g/24 hours

Cryoglobulins, serum
Negative

Cryptococcosis antigen, serum
Negative

Cyclic adenosine monophosphate, urine
Parathyroid hormone infusion: 3.6- to 4-μmol increase

D

Delta-aminolevulinic acid, urine
1.5 to 7.5 mg/dl/24 hours

D-xylose absorption
Blood: Children, 730 mg/dl in 1 hour; adults, 25 to 40 mg/dl in 2 hours

D-xylose absorption—continued
Urine: Children, 16% to 33% excreted in 5 hours; adults, > 3.5 g excreted in 5 hours

E

Erythrocyte sedimentation rate
Men: 0 to 10 mm/hour
Women: 0 to 20 mm/hour

Esophageal acidity
pH > 5.0

Estriol, amniotic fluid
16 to 20 weeks: 25.7 ng/ml
Term: < 1,000 ng/ml

Estrogens, serum
Menstruating women: day 1 to 10, 24 to 68 pg/ml; day 11 to 20, 50 to 186 pg/ml; day 21 to 30, 73 to 149 pg/ml
Men: 12 to 34 pg/ml

Estrogens, total urine
Menstruating women: follicular phase, 5 to 25 mcg/24 hours; ovulatory phase, 24 to 100 mcg/24 hours; luteal phase, 12 to 80 mcg/24 hours
Postmenopausal women: < 10 mcg/24 hours
Men: 4 to 25 mcg/24 hours

Euglobulin lysis time
≥ 2 hours

F

Factor II assay
225 to 290 units/ml

Factor V assay
50% to 150% of control

Factor VII assay
65% to 135% of control

Factor VIII assay
55% to 145% of control

Factor IX assay
60% to 140% of control

Factor X assay
45% to 155% of control

Factor XI assay
65% to 135% of control

Factor XII assay
50% to 150% of control

Febrile agglutination, serum
Salmonella antibody: < 1:80
Brucellosis antibody: < 1:80
Tularemia antibody: < 1:40
Rickettsial antibody: < 1:40

Ferritin, serum
Men: 20 to 300 ng/ml
Women: 20 to 120 ng/ml

Fibrin split products
 Screening assay: < 10 mcg/ml
 Quantitative assay: < 3 mcg/ml
Fibrinogen, plasma
 195 to 365 mg/dl
Fibrinogen, pleural fluid
 Transudate: Absent
 Exudate: Present
Fluorescent treponemal absorption, serum
 Negative
Folic acid, serum
 2 to 14 ng/ml
Follicle-stimulating hormone, serum
 Menstruating women: Follicular phase,
 5 to 20 mIU/ml; ovulatory phase, 15
 to 30 mIU/ml; luteal phase, 5 to 15
 mIU/ml
 Menopausal women: 5 to 100 mIU/ml
 Men: 5 to 20 mIU/ml
Free thyroxine, serum
 0.8 to 3.3 ng/dl
Free triiodothyronine
 0.2 to 0.6 ng/dl

G
Galactose-1-phosphate uridyl transferase
 Qualitative: negative
 Quantitative: 18.5 to 28.5 mU/g of
 hemoglobin
Gamma glutamyl transferase
 Men: 6 to 37 units/liter
 Women: < age 45, 5 to 27 units/liter;
 > age 45, 6 to 37 units/liter
Gastric acid stimulation
 Men: 18 to 28 mEq/hour
 Women: 11 to 21 mEq/hour
Gastric secretion, basal
 Men: 1 to 5 mEq/hour
 Women: 0.2 to 3.8 mEq/hour
Gastrin, serum
 < 300 pg/ml
Globulin, peritoneal fluid
 30% to 45% of total protein
Globulin, serum
 Alpha$_1$: 0.1 to 0.4 g/dl
 Alpha$_2$: 0.5 to 1 g/dl
 Beta: 0.7 to 1.2 g/dl
 Gamma: 0.5 to 1.6 g/dl
Glucagon, fasting, serum
 < 250 pg/ml
Glucose, amniotic fluid
 < 45 mg/100 ml
Glucose, cerebrospinal fluid
 50 to 80 mg/100 ml

Glucose, peritoneal fluid
 70 to 100 mg/dl
Glucose, plasma, fasting
 70 to 100 mg/dl
Glucose, plasma, oral tolerance
 Peak at 160 to 180 mg/dl, 30 to
 60 minutes after challenge dose
Glucose, plasma, 2-hour postprandial
 < 145 mg/dl
Glucose, synovial fluid
 70 to 100 mg/dl
Glucose, urine
 Negative
Glutathione reductase activity index
 0.9 to 1.3
Growth hormone, serum
 Men: 0 to 5 ng/ml
 Women: 0 to 10 ng/ml
Growth hormone suppression
 0 to 3 ng/ml after 30 minutes to
 2 hours

H
Haptoglobin, serum
 38 to 270 mg/dl
Heinz bodies
 Negative
Hematocrit
 Men: 42% to 54%
 Women: 38% to 46%
Hemoglobin electrophoresis
 Hgb A: 95%
 Hgb A$_2$: 2% to 3%
 Hgb F: > 1%
Hemoglobin, glycosylated
 Hgb A$_{1a}$: 1.6% of total RBC Hgb
 Hgb A$_{1b}$: 0.8% of total RBC Hgb
 Hgb A$_{1c}$: 4% of total RBC Hgb
 Total glycosylated Hgb: 5.5% to 9%
Hemoglobin, total
 Men: 14 to 18 g/dl
 Women: 12 to 16 g/dl
Hemoglobin, urine
 Negative
Hemoglobins, unstable
 Heat stability: Negative
 Isopropanol: Stable
Hemosiderin, urine
 Negative
Hepatitis-B surface antigen, serum
 Negative
Heterophil agglutination, serum
 Normal titer < 1:56
Hexosaminidase A and B, serum
 Total: 5 to 12.9 units/liter
 (Hex-A is 55% to 76% of total)

Histoplasmosis antibody, serum
Normal titer: < 1:8
Homovanillic acid, urine
< 8 mg/24 hours
Hydroxybutyric dehydrogenase
Serum HBD: 114 to 290 units/ml
LDH/HBD ratio: 1.2 to 1.6:1
17-Hydroxycorticosteroids, urine
Men: 4.5 to 12 mg/24 hours
Women: 2.5 to 10 mg/24 hours
5-Hydroxyindoleacetic acid, urine
< 6 mg/24 hours

I
Immune complex assays, serum
Negative
Immunoglobulins, serum
IgG: 6.4 to 14.3 mg/ml
IgA: 0.3 to 3 mg/ml
IgM: 0.2 to 1.4 mg/ml
Inulin clearance, urine
≥ *Age 21:* 90 to 130 ml/minute
Insulin, serum
0 to 25 μU/ml
Iron, serum
Men: 70 to 150 mcg/dl
Women: 80 to 150 mcg/dl
Iron, total binding capacity, serum
Men: 300 to 400 mcg/dl
Women: 300 to 450 mcg/dl
Isocitrate dehydrogenase
1.2 to 7 units/liter

K
17-Ketogenic steroids, urine
Men: 4 to 14 mg/24 hours
Women: 2 to 12 mg/24 hours
Ketones, urine
Negative
17-Ketosteroids, urine
Men: 6 to 21 mg/24 hours
Women: 4 to 17 mg/24 hours

L
Lactic acid, blood
0.93 to 1.65 mEq/liter
Lactic dehydrogenase
Total: 48 to 115 IU/liter
LDH$_1$: 18.1% to 29%
LDH$_2$: 29.4% to 37.5%
LDH$_3$: 18.8% to 26%
LDH$_4$: 9.2% to 16.5%
LDH$_5$: 5.3% to 13.4%
Leucine aminopeptidase
< 50 units/liter
Leukoagglutinins
Negative

Lipase
32 to 80 units/liter
Lipids, amniotic fluid
> 20% of lipid-coated cells stain
orange
Lipids, fecal
< 20% of excreted solids; < 7 g/
24 hours
Lipoproteins, serum
HDL-cholesterol: 29 to 77 mg/dl
LDL-cholesterol: 62 to 185 mg/dl
Long-acting thyroid stimulator, serum
Negative
Lupus erythematosus cell preparation
Negative
Luteinizing hormone, plasma
Menstruating women: Follicular phase,
5 to 15 mIU/ml; ovulatory phase, 30
to 60 mIU/ml; luteal phase, 5 to 15
mIU/ml
Postmenopausal women: 50 to
100 mIU/ml
Men: 5 to 20 mIU/ml
Lymphocyte transformation
60% to 90% lymphocytes respond
Lysozyme, urine
< 3 mg/24 hours

M
Magnesium, serum
1.5 to 2.5 mEq/liter
Atomic absorption: 1.7 to 2.1 mg/dl
Magnesium, urine
< 150 mg/24 hours
Manganese, serum
0.4 to 0.85 ng/ml
Melanin, urine
Negative
Myoglobin, serum
30 to 90 ng/ml
Myoglobin, urine
Negative

N
Neonatal thyroid-stimulating hormone
≤ Age 2 days: 25 to 30 gmIU/ml
> Age 2 days: 25 gmIU/ml
5′-Nucleotidase
2 to 17 units/liter

O
Occult blood, fecal
< 2.5 ml/24 hours
**Ornithine carbamoyltransferase,
serum**
0 to 500 Sigma units/ml

Oxalate, urine
≤ 40 mg/24 hours

P

Para-aminohippuric acid excretion, urine
Age 20: 400 to 700 ml/minute (17 ml/minute decrease each decade after age 20)

Parathyroid hormone, serum
20 to 70 μlEq/ml

Pericardial fluid
Amount: 10 to 50 ml
Appearance: Clear, straw-colored
White blood cell count: < 1,000/mm³
Glucose: approximately whole blood level

Peritoneal fluid
Amount: < 50 ml
Appearance: Clear, straw-colored

Phenylalanine, serum, screening
Negative: < 2 mg/dl

Phenolsulfonphthalein excretion, urine
15 minutes: 25% of dose excreted
30 minutes: 50% to 60% of dose excreted
1 hour: 60% to 79% of dose excreted
2 hours: 70% to 80% of dose excreted

Phosphate, tubular reabsorption, urine and plasma
80% reabsorption

Phosphates, serum
1.8 to 2.6 mEq/liter
Atomic absorption: 2.5 to 4.5 mg/dl

Phosphates, urine
< 1,000 mg/24 hours

Phospholipids, plasma
180 to 320 mg/dl

Placental lactogen, serum
Pregnant women: 5 to 27 weeks, < 4.6 mcg/ml; 28 to 31 weeks, 2.4 to 6.1 mcg/ml; 32 to 35 weeks, 3.7 to 7.7 mcg/ml; 36 weeks to term, 5 to 8.6 mcg/ml
Nonpregnant women: < 0.5 mcg/ml
Men: < 0.5 mcg/ml

Plasma plasminogen
2.7 to 4.5 μ/ml (activity units); ≥ 65% (normal control values)

Plasma renin activity
Sodium-depleted, peripheral vein (upright position): Ages 20 to 39, 2.9 to 24 ng/ml/hour; age 40 and over, 2.9 to 10.8 ng/ml/hour

Plasma renin activity—continued
Sodium-replete, peripheral vein (upright position): Ages 20 to 39, 0.1 to 4.3 ng/ml/hour; age 40 and over, 0.1 to 3 ng/ml/hour

Platelet aggregation
3 to 5 minutes

Platelet count
130,000 to 370,000/mm³

Platelet survival
50% tagged platelets disappear within 84 to 116 hours
100% disappear within 8 to 10 days

Pleural fluid
Appearance: Clear (transudate); cloudy, turbulent (exudate)
Specific gravity: < 1.016 (transudate); > 1.016 (exudate)

Porphobilinogen, urine
≤ 1.5 mg/24 hours

Porphyrins, total
16 to 60 mg/dl of packed RBCs

Potassium, serum
3.8 to 5.5 mEq/liter

Pregnanediol, urine
Men: 1.5 mg/24 hours
Women: 0.5 to 1.5 mg/24 hours
Postmenopausal women: 0.2 to 1 mg/24 hours

Pregnanetriol, urine
< 3.5 mg/24 hours

Progesterone, plasma
Menstrual cycle: Follicular phase, < 150 ng/dl; luteal phase, 300 ng/dl; midluteal phase, 2,000 ng/dl
Pregnancy: First trimester, 1,500 to 5,000 ng/dl; second and third trimesters, 8,000 to 20,000 ng/dl

Prolactin, serum
0 to 23 ng/dl

Protein, cerebrospinal fluid
15 to 45 mg/dl

Protein, pleural fluid
Transudate: < 3 g/dl
Exudate: > 3 g/dl

Protein, total, peritoneal fluid
0.3 to 4.1 g/dl

Protein, total, serum
6.6 to 7.9 g/dl
Albumin fraction: 3.3 to 4.5 g/dl
Globulin levels: Alpha₁–globulin, 0.1 to 0.4 g/dl; alpha₂–globulin, 0.5 to 1 g/dl; beta globulin, 0.7 to 1.2 g/dl; gamma globulin, 0.5 to 1.6 g/dl

Protein, total, synovial fluid
10.7 to 21.3 mg/dl

Protein, urine
≤ 150 mg/24 hours
Prothrombin consumption time
20 seconds
Prothrombin time
Men: 9.6 to 11.8 seconds
Women: 9.5 to 11.3 seconds
Protoporphyrins
16 to 60 mg/dl
Pyruvate kinase
Ultraviolet: 2 to 8.8 units/g hemoglobin
Low substrate assay: 0.9 to 3.9 units/g
hemoglobin
Pyruvic acid, blood
0.08 to 0.16 mEq/liter

R

Radioallergosorbent test
Negative: < 150% of control
Red blood cell count
Men: 4.5 to 6.2 million/μl venous blood
Women: 4.2 to 5.4 million/μl venous
blood
Red blood cell survival time
25 to 35 days
Red blood cells, pleural fluid
Transudate: Few
Exudate: Variable
Red blood cells, urine
0 to 3 per high-power field
Red cell indices
MCV: 84 to 99 μ³/red cell
MCH: 26 to 32 pg/red cell
MCHC: 30% to 36%
Reticulocyte count
0.5% to 2% of total RBC count
Rheumatoid factor, serum
Negative
Rubella antibodies, serum
Titer of 1:8 or less indicates little or no
immunity

S

Semen
Volume: 1.5 to 5 ml
pH: 7.3 to 7.7
Liquefaction: 30 minutes
Sperm: 60 million to 150 million/ml
Cervical mucus: ≥ 5 motile sperm per
high-power field
**Serum glutamic-oxaloacetic
transaminase**
8 to 20 units/liter
Serum glutamic-pyruvic transaminase
Men: 10 to 32 units/liter
Women: 9 to 24 units/liter

Sickle cell test
Negative
Sodium, serum
135 to 145 mEq/liter
Sodium, sweat
10 to 30 mEq/liter
Sodium, urine
30 to 280 mEq/24 hours
Sodium chloride, urine
5 to 20 g/24 hours
Sporotrichosis antibody, serum
Normal titers < 1:40
Synovial fluid
Color: Colorless to pale yellow
Clarity: Clear
Quantity (in knee): 0.3 to 3.5 ml
Viscosity: 5.7 to 1,160
pH: 7.2 to 7.4
Mucin clot: Good
Pao$_2$: 40 to 60 mmHg
Paco$_2$: 40 to 60 mmHg

T

T-lymphocyte count
1,400 to 2,700/mm³
T$_3$ resin uptake
25% to 35% of T$_3$* binds resin
**Terminal deoxynucleotidyl transferase,
serum**
0 to 10 IU/10¹³ cells
Testosterone, plasma or serum
Men: 30 to 1,200 ng/dl
Women: 30 to 95 ng/dl
Thrombin time, plasma
10 to 15 seconds
**Thyroid-stimulating hormone,
serum**
0 to 15 μIU/ml
Thyroxine, total, serum
5 to 13.5 mcg/dl
Thyroxine-binding globulin, serum
Electrophoresis: From 10 to 26 mcg T$_4$
(binding capacity)/dl to 16 to 24 mcg
T$_4$ (binding capacity)/dl
Radioimmunoassay: 1.3 to 2 ng/dl
Tolbutamide tolerance
Plasma glucose drops to one half
fasting level for 30 minutes, recovers
in 1½ to 3 hours
Transferrin, serum
250 to 390 mcg/dl
Triglycerides, serum
Ages 0 to 29: 10 to 140 mg/dl
Ages 30 to 39: 10 to 150 mg/dl
Ages 40 to 49: 10 to 160 mg/dl
Ages 50 to 59: 10 to 190 mg/dl

Triiodothyronine, serum
 90 to 230 ng/dl

U

Urea, urine
 Maximal clearance: 64 to 99 ml/minute

Uric acid, serum
 Men: 4.3 to 8 mg/dl
 Women: 2.3 to 6 mg/dl

Uric acid, synovial fluid
 Men: 2 to 8 mg/dl
 Women: 2 to 6 mg/dl

Uric acid, urine
 250 to 750 mg/24 hours

Urinalysis, routine
 Color: Straw
 Appearance: Clear
 Specific gravity: 1.005 to 1.020
 pH: 4.5 to 8
 Epithelial cells: Few
 Casts: Occasional hyaline casts
 Crystals: Present

Urine concentration
 Specific gravity: 1.025 to 1.032
 Osmolality: > 800 mOsm/kg water

Urine dilution
 Specific gravity: < 1.003
 Osmolality: < 100 mOsm/kg
 80% of water excreted in 4 hours

Urine hydroxyproline, total
 Adult: 14 to 45 mg/24 hours

Urine potassium
 Excretion: 25 to 125 mEq/24 hours
 Concentration: < 10 mEq/liter in
  patients with hypokalemia

Urobilinogen, fecal
 50 to 300 mg/24 hours

Urobilinogen, urine
 Men: 0.3 to 2.1 Ehrlich units/2 hours
 Women: 0.1 to 1.1 Ehrlich units/
  2 hours

Uroporphyrin, urine
 Men: 0 to 42 mcg/24 hours
 Women: 1 to 22 mcg/24 hours

Uroporphyrinogen I synthase
 Men: 7.9 to 14.7 nm/sec/liter
 Women: 8.1 to 16.8 nm/sec/liter

V

Vanillylmandelic acid, urine
 0.7 to 6.8 mg/24 hours

VDRL, cerebrospinal fluid
 Negative

VDRL, serum
 Negative

Vitamin A, serum
 125 to 150 IU/dl

Vitamin B$_1$, urine
 100 to 200 mcg/24 hours

Vitamin B$_6$ (tryptophan), urine
 < 50 mcg/24 hours

Vitamin B$_{12}$, serum
 200 to 1,100 pg/ml

Vitamin C, plasma
 0.2 to 2 mg/dl

Vitamin C, urine
 30 mg/24 hours

Vitamin D$_3$, serum
 10 to 55 ng/ml

W

White blood cell count, blood
 4,100 to 10,900/μl

White blood cell count, cerebrospinal fluid
 0 to 5/mm^3

White blood cell count, peritoneal fluid
 < 300/μl

White blood cell count, pleural fluid
 Transudate: Few
 Exudate: Many (may be purulent)

White blood cell count, synovial fluid
 0 to 200/μl

White blood cell count, urine
 0 to 4 per high-power field

White blood cell differential, blood
 Neutrophils: 47.6% to 76.8%
 Lymphocytes: 16.2% to 43%
 Monocytes: 0.6% to 9.6%
 Eosinophils: 0.3% to 7%
 Basophils: 0.3% to 2%

White blood cell differential, synovial fluid
 Lymphocytes: 0 to 78/μl
 Monocytes: 0 to 71/μl
 Clasmatocytes: 0 to 26/μl
 Polymorphonuclears: 0 to 25/μl
 Other phagocytes: 0 to 21/μl
 Synovial lining cells: 0 to 12/μl

Whole blood clotting time
 5 to 15 minutes

Z

Zinc, serum
 0.75 to 1.4 mcg/ml

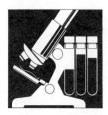

Guide to Color-top Collection Tubes

Red

Red-top *tubes contain no additives. Draw volume may be 2 to 20 ml. These tubes are used for tests performed on serum samples.*

ABO blood typing
Acetaminophen
Acetylcholine receptor antibodies
Acid phosphatase
Alkaline phosphatase
Alpha-fetoprotein
Amylase
Androstenedione
Angiotensin converting enzyme
Antibiotics
Antibody screening test
Anticonvulsants
Antidepressants
Antidiuretic hormone (vasopressin)
Anti-DNA antibodies
Antiglobulin
Antimitochondrial antibodies
Antinuclear antibodies
Anti–smooth-muscle antibodies
Antistreptolysin-0 test
Antithyroid antibodies
Arginine test (growth hormone stimulation test)
Barbiturates
Bilirubin
Blood ethanol
Blood urea nitrogen
Bronchodilators
Calcium
Carcinoembryonic antigen
Cardiac glycosides
Ceruloplasmin
Chloride
Cholinesterase
Cold agglutinins
Complement assays
C-reactive protein
Creatine
Creatine phosphokinase
Creatinine
Creatinine clearance
Crossmatching
Cryoglobulins
Direct antiglobulin
D-xylose absorption
Estrogens
Extractable nuclear antigen antibodies
Febrile agglutination tests
Ferritin
Fluorescent treponemal antibody absorption test
Folic acid
Follicle-stimulating hormone
FT_4 and FT_3
Fungal serology
Gamma glutamyl transferase
Gastrin
Growth hormone/somatotropic hormone
Growth hormone suppression test (glucose loading)
Haptoglobin
Hepatitis B surface antigen
Heterophil agglutination tests
Hexosaminidase A & B
Human chorionic gonadotropin
Human placental lactogen
Hydroxybutyric dehydrogenase
Hypnotics
Immunoglobulins G, A, and M
Immune complex assays
Insulin
Iron and total iron-binding capacity
Isocitrate dehydrogenase
Isopropanol
Lactic dehydrogenase
LE cell preparation
Leucine aminopeptidase
Leukoagglutinins
Lipase
Lipoprotein-cholesterol fractionation
Long-acting thyroid stimulator
Magnesium
Methanol
Myoglobin
Neonatal thyroid-stimulating hormone
5'-nucleotidase
Ornithine carbamoyltransferase
Parathyroid hormone (parathormone)
Phenothiazines
Phosphates
Phospholipids
Plasma LH
Plasma antidepressants
Potassium
Prolactin (lactogenic hormone, lactogen)
Protein electrophoresis
Prothrombin consumption time
Radioallergosorbent test
Rh typing
Rheumatoid factor
Rubella antibodies
Salicylates
SGOT
SGPT
Sodium
T_3 resin uptake

Testosterone
Thyroid-stimulating hormone (thyrotropin)
Thyroxine
Thyroxine-binding globulin
Total cholesterol
Tranquilizers
Transferrin
Triglycerides
Triiodothyronine
Tubular reabsorption of phosphate
Urea clearance
Uric acid
VDRL
Vitamin A and carotene
Vitamin B_2
Vitamin B_{12}
Vitamin D_3

Lavender

Lavender-top *tubes contain EDTA. Draw volume may be 2 to 10 ml. These tubes are used for tests performed on whole blood samples.*

ABO blood typing
Anti-DNA antibodies
Erythrocyte sedimentation rate
G-6-PD
Glucagon
Glycosylated hemoglobin
Heinz bodies
Hematocrit
Hemoglobin electrophoresis
Lipoprotein phenotyping
Plasma renin activity
Platelet count
Platelet survival
Pyruvate kinase
Red blood cell count
Red cell indices
Reticulocyte count
Rh typing
Sickle cell test (hemoglobin S)
Total hemoglobin
Unstable hemoglobins
White blood cell count
White blood cell differential

Green (heparinized)

Green-top *tubes contain heparin (sodium, lithium, or ammonium). Draw volume may be 2 to 15 ml. These tubes are used for tests performed on plasma samples.*

ACTH
Ammonia
Androstenedione
Angiotensin converting enzyme
Calcitonin (thyrocalcitonin)
Chromosomal analysis

Cortisol
Erythropoietic porphyrins
Galactose-1-phosphate uridyl transferase
Insulin tolerance test
Inulin clearance
Lymphocyte transformation tests
Osmotic fragility
Para-aminohippuric acid excretion
Progesterone
Rapid ACTH (cosyntropin test)
RBC survival time
T- and B-lymphocyte counts
Terminal deoxynucleotidyl transferase
Testosterone
Uroporphyrinogen I synthase

Blue

Blue-top *tubes contain sodium citrate and citric acid. Draw volume may be 2.7 or 4.5 ml. These tubes are used for coagulation studies requiring plasma samples.*

Activated partial thromboplastin time
Euglobulin lysis time
Fibrinogen
Hemoglobin derivatives
One-stage assay: Extrinsic coagulation system
One-stage assay: Intrinsic coagulation system
Plasminogen
Platelet aggregation
Prothrombin time
Thrombin time

Black

Black-top *tubes contain sodium oxalate. Draw volume may be 2.7 or 4.5 ml. These tubes are used for coagulation studies performed on plasma samples.*

Plasma vitamin C

Gray

Gray-top *tubes contain a glycolytic inhibitor (such as sodium fluoride, powdered oxalate, or glycolytic/microbial inhibitor). Draw volume may be 3 to 10 ml. These tubes are used most often for glucose determinations in serum or plasma samples.*

Anti-DNA antibodies
Fasting plasma glucose (fasting blood sugar)
Insulin tolerance test
Lactic acid and pyruvic acid
Oral glucose tolerance test
Tolbutamide tolerance test
Two-hour postprandial plasma glucose

A GUIDE TO REAGENT STRIP TESTS

REAGENT STRIPS	BILIRUBIN	BLOOD	GLUCOSE	KETONES	NITRITE	pH	PROTEIN	UROBILIN-OGEN
ALBUSTIX							X	
BILI-LABSTIX	X	X	X	X		X	X	
CHEMSTRIP GK			X	X				
CHEMSTRIP GP			X				X	
CHEMSTRIP 5		X	X	X		X	X	
CHEMSTRIP 6	X	X	X	X		X	X	
CHEMSTRIP 7	X	X	X	X		X	X	X
CHEMSTRIP 8	X	X	X	X	X	X	X	X
CLINISTIX			X					
COMBISTIX			X			X	X	
DEXTROSTIX Use fingerstick or venous blood			X					
DIASTIX			X					
HEMA-COMBISTIX		X	X			X	X	

SUBSTANCE DETECTED

REAGENT STRIPS	BILIRUBIN	BLOOD	GLUCOSE	KETONES	NITRITE	pH	PROTEIN	UROBILIN-OGEN
HEMASTIX May also test fecal matter		x						
HEMOCCULT		x						
KETO-DIASTIX			x	x				
KETOSTIX				x				
LABSTIX		x	x	x		x	x	
MICROSTIX-NITRITE					x			
MULTISTIX	x	x	x	x		x	x	x
NITRAZINE PAPER						x		
N-MULTISTIX	x	x	x	x	x	x	x	x
N-URISTIX			x		x		x	
TES-TAPE			x					
URISTIX			x				x	
UROBILISTIX								x

SUBSTANCE DETECTED

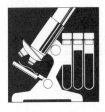

Photo acknowledgments

Collection Techniques

p. xxxvi to xli Paul A. Cohen

Chapter 1: Hematology

pp. 2, 3 Ann Bell, MS, SH(ASCP), CLS, University of Tennessee Center for Health Sciences, Memphis
p. 16 William Dougherty
p. 17 © Clifford Goldwaithe, 1981
p. 24 (bottom left) © Carroll H. Weiss, RBP, 1980
p. 24 (bottom right) © Carroll H. Weiss, RBP, 1973

Chapter 5: Hormones

p. 143 Arthur C. Guyton, *Textbook of Medical Physiology* (Philadelphia: W.B. Saunders, 1981).
p. 144 Sterling Publishing Co.
p. 177 Paul A. Cohen
p. 188 © Carroll H. Weiss, RBP, 1981

Chapter 11: Immune Response

pp. 316, 319, 321 Lynne Burek, PhD, Department of Immunology and Microbiology, Wayne State University, School of Medicine, Detroit

Chapter 18: Histology

pp. 475, 478 Maurice Barcos, MD, Roswell Park Memorial Institute, Buffalo
p. 480 © Carroll H. Weiss, RBP, 1981
p. 485 Emmanuel Rubin, MD, Hahnemann Medical College, Philadelphia
p. 489 Timothy King, MD, Cornell University Medical Center, N.Y.

Chapter 19: Microbes and Parasites

pp. 504, 515, 516 The Gram Stain Library, © Schering Corp., Kenilworth, N.J. 07033
pp. 505, 529 William G. Leibowitz (formerly Eliot Scientific), New York

p. 511 Centers for Disease Control, Atlanta
p. 514 Paul A. Cohen

Chapter 20: Thyroid

p. 542 Marc S. Lapayowker, MD, Department of Radiology, Abington (Pa.) Memorial Hospital

Chapter 21: Eye

pp. 557, 560, 565, 566, 568, 569 David Silva, Ophthalmic Photographer, Wills Eye Hospital, Philadelphia
p. 559 Joel I. Hamburger, MD, Northland Radioisotope Lab, Southfield, Mich.
p. 561 © Carroll H. Weiss, RBP, 1981
p. 572 © Joe Savoy, Ophthalmic Photographer, Detroit Institute of Ophthalmology, Grosse Point Park, Mich.

Chapter 22: Ear

pp. 592-93 Paul A. Cohen

Chapter 23: Respiratory System

pp. 649, 661, 663, 664, 666 Marc S. Lapayowker, MD, Department of Radiology, Abington (Pa.) Memorial Hospital

Chapter 24: Skeletal System

pp. 676, 677 Marc S. Lapayowker, MD, Department of Radiology, Abington (Pa.) Memorial Hospital
p. 680 John J. Joyce, III, MD, University of Pennsylvania, Philadelphia

Chapter 25: Reproductive System

p. 713 Peter H. Kohn, PhD, University of Florida College of Medicine, Gainesville.
pp. 731, 733 Marc S. Lapayowker, MD, Department of Radiology, Abington (Pa.) Memorial Hospital

Index

A

Abbreviations, list of, 1056-1058
Abdominal aorta, ultrasonography of, 870, **917-919**
Abetalipoproteinemia
  lipoprotein phenotyping and, 207
  small bowel biopsy and, 483
  triglyceride levels in, 201
ABG. *See* Arterial blood gases.
ABO blood group
  characteristics, 271
  frequency of types in U.S., 275i
  recipient-donor compatibility, 275i
  typing, **274-277**
Abortion
  hPL levels in, 194
  progesterone levels in, 187
  threatened, 393, 405
Abruptio placentae
  amniotic fluid color and, 715t, 718
  FSP test and, 65
  intrauterine pressure and, 729
  pelvic ultrasonography and, 736
Abscess, WBC count in, 32. *See also specific type.*
Acetaminophen, **1012-1014**
  hepatotoxicity nomogram, 1013i
Acetest, 439
Acetylcholine receptor antibodies, **330-331**
Acetylcholinesterase, 122
  role of, in nerve impulse transmission, 123i
Achalasia
  barium swallow and, 820
  esophageal manometry and, 796
  esophagogastroduodenoscopy and, 811
  upper GI series and, 822
Achlorhydria, 184
Achromatopia, 555
Acid-base balance, 70-71
  CO_2 levels and, 76
  disorders, 74t
  regulation of, 80
Acid-fast stain, 503, 504i
Acidified serum lysis test, **312**

Acidosis, 70t. *See also specific types.*
  pulmonary function tests and, 632t
  urine pH in, 359
Acid perfusion test, **796-798**
Acid phosphatase, 96, **116-117**
Acoustic immittance tests, **597-602,** 601i
  interpretation of findings in, 598-599t
Acoustic reflexes, **597-602**
Acquired immunodeficiency syndrome
  as complication of transfusion, 273t
  test for, in donated blood, 296
Acromegaly
  creatinine levels in, 226
  facial characteristics of, 143i
  fasting plasma glucose levels in, 239
  FSH levels in, 148
  hGH levels in, 144
  LH levels in, 150
  phosphate levels in, 83
  postprandial plasma glucose levels in, 241
  skull radiography and, 746
  TBG levels in, 163
ACTH. *See* Adrenocorticotropic hormone.
Activated partial thromboplastin time, 42t, **55-56**
Addison's disease
  ACTH levels in, 139
  ADH levels in, 156
  aldosterone levels in, 173, 385
  chloride levels in, 81, 457
  cortisol levels in, 175
  HLA testing and, 313
  17-KGS levels in, 400
  17-KS levels in, 399
  magnesium levels in, 82, 462
  OGTT and, 244
  17-OHCS levels in, 397
  potassium levels in, 83
  renin levels in, 120
Adenosine triphosphate, role of, in muscle contraction, 225i
ADH. *See* Antidiuretic hormone.
Admittance testing. *See* Acoustic immittance tests.

Adrenal carcinoma
  aldosterone levels in, 173
  androstenedione levels in, 179
  free cortisol levels in, 387
  17-KGS levels in, 400
  17-KS levels in, 399
  17-OHCS levels in, 397
  testosterone levels in, 190
Adrenal failure, sodium levels in, 457
Adrenal hormones, 137
  tests, **171-179**
Adrenal hyperplasia
  ACTH levels in, 139
  aldosterone levels in, 173, 385
  androstenedione levels in, 179
  estrogen levels in, 186, 390
  fasting plasma glucose levels in, 239
  free cortisol levels in, 387
  17-KGS levels in, 400
  17-KS levels in, 399
  postprandial plasma glucose levels in, 241
  pregnanediol levels in, 405
  progesterone levels in, 187
  testosterone levels in, 190
Adrenal insufficiency. *See also* Addison's disease.
  ACTH levels in, 139
  calcium levels in, 77
  fasting plasma glucose levels in, 239
  fetal, placental estriol levels in, 392
  insulin tolerance test and, 145
  magnesium levels in, 82, 462
  postprandial plasma glucose levels in, 241
  rapid ACTH test and, 140
  sodium levels in, 87
  sweat test and, 640
Adrenal tumors
  catecholamine levels in, 178
  estrogen levels in, 390
  nephrotomography and, 957
  renal CT scan and, 959
  testosterone levels in, 190
Adrenocorticotropic hormone, 135, **138-139**
Adrenogenital syndrome
  clinical aspects of, 396i
  pregnanetriol levels in, 396
Adrenoleukodystrophy, 757
Aeromonas hydrophila, in stool culture, 509, 510

Boldface page numbers indicate major entries; t refers to a table, i to an illustration.

Boldface page numbers indicate major entries; t refers to a table, i to an illustration.

Boldface page numbers indicate major entries; t refers to a table, i to an illustration.

N

O

Boldface page numbers indicate major entries; t refers to a table, i to an illustration.